Postgraduate

MEDICINE

Postgraduate
MEDICINE

Volume 1

Editor-in-Chief

Gurpreet S Wander MD DM FACC FAMS
Professor and Head of Cardiology
Hero DMC Heart Institute
Dayanand Medical College and Hospital
Ludhiana, Punjab, India

Section Editors

PK Deb	Cardiology
SK Sharma	Clinical Medicine
Surinder K Jindal	Pulmonary Medicine
Ajay Kumar	Gastroenterology
Vivekanand Jha	Nephrology
Rohini Handa	Rheumatology
Jyotirmoy Pal	General Medicine
Gagandeep Singh	Neurology
Dhruva Chaudhry	Critical Care
Sanjay K Bhadada	Endocrinology
Bibhuti Saha	Infectious Diseases

Associate Editors

Rajesh Mahajan
NK Singh

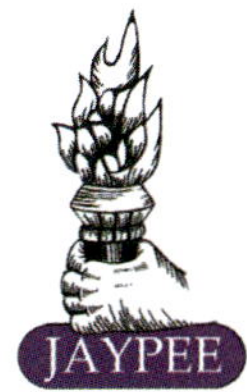

JAYPEE BROTHERS MEDICAL PUBLISHERS
The Health Sciences Publisher
New Delhi | London

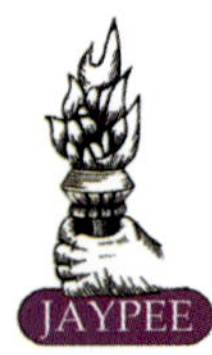

Jaypee Brothers Medical Publishers (P) Ltd

Headquarters
EMCA House
23/23-B, Ansari Road, Daryaganj
New Delhi 110 002, India
Landline: +91-11-23272143, +91-11-23272703
+91-11-23282021, +91-11-23245672
E-mail: jaypee@jaypeebrothers.com

Corporate Office
Jaypee Brothers Medical Publishers (P) Ltd.
4838/24, Ansari Road, Daryaganj
New Delhi 110 002, India
Phone: +91-11-43574357
Fax: +91-11-43574314
E-mail: jaypee@jaypeebrothers.com

Overseas Office
JP Medical Ltd.
83, Victoria Street, London
SW1H 0HW (UK)
Phone: +44-20 3170 8910
Fax: +44(0)20 3008 6180
E-mail: info@jpmedpub.com

Website: www.jaypeebrothers.com
Website: www.jaypeedigital.com

Inquiries for bulk sales may be solicited at: jaypee@jaypeebrothers.com

Postgraduate Medicine / *Gurpreet S Wander*

First Edition: **2022**

ISBN: 978-93-90595-46-4

Printed at: Sanat Printers

DEDICATED TO

Dr Harjit Singh

(1926–2018)

Professor and HOD Medicine
Government Medical College
Patiala, Punjab, India

"My father who taught me the value of hard work and integrity"

Dr BK Sharma

(1937–2021)

Professor and HOD Medicine
Postgraduate Institute of Medical Education and Research
Chandigarh, India

"My teacher in MD medicine from whom I learned bedside manners"

Dr SB Khurana

(1938–2011)

Professor and HOD Medicine
Dayanand Medical College Hospital
Ludhiana, Punjab, India

"Who taught me that practice of clinical medicine needs common sense and simple thinking"

Dr Siddharth N Shah

(1946–2021)

Past President API
Mumbai, Maharashtra, India

"From whom I learned how to work with others in a team with mutual respect"

Smt Raman Vij

(1957–2021)

W/o Sh Jitender Pal Vij and M/o Mr Ankit Vij
New Delhi, India

"Who was the driving force and inspiration for the Jaypee Brothers Medical Publishers (P) Ltd"

Editor-in-Chief

Gurpreet S Wander MD DM FACC FAMS
Professor and Head of Cardiology
Hero DMC Heart Institute
Dayanand Medical College and Hospital
Ludhiana, Punjab, India

Section Editors

Pradeep Kumar Deb MD DM
Ex. Chief Cardiologist
ESI PG Institute of Medical Sciences
Past President, Cardiological Society of India, Kolkata, West Bengal, India

SK Sharma MD PhD FNASc
Former Professor and Head
Department of Medicine
All India Institute of Medical Sciences, New Delhi, India

Surinder K Jindal MD
Medical Director, Jindal Clinics
Emeritus-Professor
Postgraduate Institute of Medical Education and Research
Chandigarh, India

Ajay Kumar MD DM
Chairman
BLK Liver and Digestive Diseases Institute
New Delhi, India

Vivekanand Jha MD DM
Executive Director
George Institute for Global Health India, New Delhi, India
Chair of Global Kidney Health
Imperial College, London, UK

Rohini Handa MD DNB FAMS FRCP
Professor and Senior Consultant
Department of Rheumatology
Apollo Indraprastha Hospitals
New Delhi, India

Jyotirmoy Pal MD FICP FRCP
WHO Fellow
Professor of Medicine
RG Kar Medical College
Kolkata, West Bengal, India

Gagandeep Singh MD DM
Professor and Head
Department of Neurology
Dayanand Medical College and Hospital
Ludhiana, Punjab, India

Dhruva Chaudhry MD DM
Senior Professor and Head
Department of Pulmonary and Critical Care Medicine, Post Graduate Institute of Medical Sciences
Rohtak, Haryana, India

Sanjay K Bhadada MD DM FAMS
Professor and Head
Department of Endocrinology
Postgraduate Institute of Medical Education and Research
Chandigarh, India

Bibhuti Saha DTM&H (Cal) MD
Head, Department of Tropical Medicine
Dean, Students' Affairs
School of Tropical Medicine
Kolkata, West Bengal, India

Associate Editors

Rajesh Mahajan MD
Professor of Medicine
Dayanand Medical College and Hospital
Ludhiana, Punjab, India

NK Singh MD FICP
Director, Diabetes and Heart Research Center
Jharkhand, Bihar, India

CONTRIBUTORS

VOLUME 1 (SECTION 1–4)

Section 1: Clinical Medicine (Section Editor: SK Sharma)

Alladi Mohan MD FRCP FAMS
Professor (Senior Grade) and Head of Medicine, Chief, Division of Pulmonary and Critical Care Medicine
Sri Venkateswara Institute of Medical Sciences
Tirupati, Andhra Pradesh, India

A Surekha MD
Assistant Professor
Department of Dermatology
Sri Venkateswara Institute of Medical Sciences, Sri Padmavathi Medical College for Women
Tirupati, Andhra Pradesh, India

B Soma Raju MD DM
Clinical Director and
Head of Cardiology
AIG Hospitals
Hyderabad, Telangana, India

B Vengamma DM FAMS FRCP
Director cum Vice-Chancellor
Professor (Senior Grade) and Head of Neurology, Sri Venkateswara Institute of Medical Sciences, Tirupati, AP, India

Chakravarthy DJK MD MACP
Assistant Professor of General Medicine, GSL Medical College
Rajahmundry, Andhra Pradesh, India

Chandan J Das MD DNB FICR
Additional Professor
Department of Radiology
All India Institute of Medical Sciences
New Delhi, India

Cynthia Amrutha MD
Assistant Professor
Department of Medicine
Kasturba Medical College, Manipal
Manipal, Karnataka, India

Devamsh GN MBBS MD
Senior Resident
Department of Medicine
Bangalore Medical College and Research Institute, Victoria Hospital
Bengaluru, Karnataka, India

Gaurav Gupta MBBS MD
Assistant Professor
Department of Medicine
All India Institute of Medical Sciences
New Delhi, India

G Eswar MD
Professor of Medicine
Dr Pinnamaneni Siddhartha Institute of Medical Science and Research Foundation, Chinna Avutapalli
Vijayawada, Andhra Pradesh, India

G Ramesh Kumar MD
Professor and Head
Department of Dermatology
Sri Venkateswara Medical College
Tirupati, Andhra Pradesh, India

K Ravi MBBS MD FICP
Professor and Head of Medicine
Bangalore Medical College and Research Institute
Victoria Hospital
Bengaluru, Karnataka, India

KSR Swamy MD
Professor of Medicine
Konaseema Institute of Medical Sciences & Research Foundation
Amalapuram, Andhra Pradesh, India

K SSS Surya Prakash MD
Senior Resident
Department of General Medicine
Govt Siddhartha Medical College
Vijayawada, Andhra Pradesh, India

KV Seshaiah MD
Former Professor of Medicine
Govt Siddhartha Medical College
Vijayawada, Andhra Pradesh, India

Neelkanth Patil MD DM
Consultant Cardiologist, AIG Hospitals
Hyderabad, Telangana, India

Ragul Ganesh MD
Senior Resident, Department of Psychiatry, All India Institute of Medical Sciences New Delhi, India

Rajeev Menon MD DNB
Consultant Cardiologist, AIG Hospitals
Hyderabad, Telangana, India

Rajesh Sagar MD
Professor, Department of Psychiatry
All India Institute of Medical Sciences
New Delhi, India

Sagnik Biswas MD DM
Senior Resident
Department of Gastroenterology and Human Nutrition, All India Institute of Medical Sciences, New Delhi, India

Sanchit Kumar MD
Senior Resident, Department of Medicine, All India Institute of Medical Sciences, New Delhi, India

Sanchit Sharma MD DM
Senior Resident
Department of Gastroenterology and Human Nutrition, All India Institute of Medical Sciences, New Delhi, India

Sanjeev Sinha MD
Professor of Medicine
All India Institute of Medical Sciences
New Delhi, India

SK Sharma MD PhD FNASc
Former Professor and Head
Department of Medicine
All India Institute of Medical Sciences
New Delhi, India

Sudhakar Rao MBBS MD DM
Associate Professor of Cardiology
Kasturba Medical College, Manipal
Manipal, Karnataka, India

Sudha Vidyasagar MD
Professor of Medicine
Kasturba Medical College, Manipal
Manipal, Karnataka, India

SV Ramanamurty MD FICP
Professor of General Medicine
Academic Director—PG Education
GSL Medical College
Rajahmundry, Andhra Pradesh, India

Vasili Pradeep MD
Assistant Professor
Department of Medicine
Sri Venkateswara Institute of
Medical Sciences
Tirupati, Andhra Pradesh, India

Veerappa Annasaheb Kothiwale
MD PhD (Card)
Registrar, KLE Academy of Higher
Education and Research
Professor, Department of General
Medicine, Jawaharlal Nehru
Medical College
Belgaum, Karnataka, India

Vivek Veereshkumar Shirol MD
Assistant Professor
Department of General Medicine
Jawaharlal Nehru Medical College
Belgaum, Karnataka, India

Y Rahul MBBS
Sri Ramachandra Institute of Higher
Education and Research
Chennai, Tamil Nadu, India

Y Sairam III year MBBS
Bhaskar Medical College
Moinabad Mandal, RR District
Hyderabad, Telangana, India

Y Sathyanarayana Raju MD FICP
Professor and Head
Department of General Medicine
Nizam's Institute of Medical Sciences
Hyderabad, Telangana, India

Zohra Ahmad MBBS MD DNB
Assistant Professor
Department of Radiology
Guwahati Medical College
Guwahati, Assam, India

Section 2: General Medicine (Section Editor: Jyotirmoy Pal)

Agnibha Maiti MD CCEBDM
Assistant Professor of Medicine
Institute of Postgraduate Medical
Education and Research and SSKM
Hospital, Kolkata, West Bengal, India

Ajay Kumar Baranwal MD
Professor
Department of Immunohematology
and Blood Transfusion
Armed Forces Medical College
Pune, Maharashtra, India

Akhil Krishna MBBS MD
Postdoctoral Trainee
Department of Endocrinology,
Institute of Postgraduate Medical
Education and Research
Kolkata, West Bengal, India

Aritra Kumar Ray MBBS
Junior Resident
Department of Internal Medicine
RG Kar Medical College and Hospital
Kolkata, West Bengal, India

Arkapravo Hati MBBS MD
Post Graduate Trainee
Department of General Medicine
RG Kar Medical College and Hospital
Kolkata, West Bengal, India

Ashish Sahani PhD
Assistant Professor
Department of Biomedical
Engineering
Indian Institute of Technology
Rupnagar, Punjab, India

Atanu Chandra MD DNB MRCP (UK)
Assistant Professor
Department of Internal Medicine
RG Kar Medical College and Hospital
Kolkata, West Bengal, India

Biman Kanti Ray MD DM
Professor
Bangur Institute of Neurosciences
Institute of Postgraduate Medical
Education and Research Annex 1
Kolkata, West Bengal, India

Deepika Bansal MD
MD Resident, Department of Psychiatry
Dayanand Medical College and Hospital
Ludhiana, Punjab, India

D Thangam MD
Senior Assistant Professor
Department of Geriatric Medicine
Rajiv Gandhi Government General
Hospital, Madras Medical College
Chennai, Tamil Nadu, India

Gaurav Sharma MD
Assistant Professor
Department of Translational and
Regenerative Medicine
Postgraduate Institute of Medical
Education and Research
Chandigarh, India

G Usha MD
Professor
Department of Geriatric Medicine
Madras Medical College
Chennai, Tamil Nadu, India

Jyotirmoy Pal MD FICP FRCP WHO Fellow
Professor of Medicine
RG Kar Medical College
Kolkata, West Bengal, India

Manali Chandra MD PGT
Junior Resident, Department of Internal Medicine, Medical College
Kolkata, West Bengal, India

Manicka Saravanan Subramanian MBBS MD
Senior Resident, Department of Geriatric Medicine, All India Institute of Medical Sciences, New Delhi, India

Monika Bansal MD DM
Associate Professor of Neurology
Dayanand Medical College and Hospital
Ludhiana, Punjab, India

Nandini Chatterjee MD FICP
Professor of Medicine
Institute of Postgraduate Medical Education and Research/SSKM Hospital, Kolkata, West Bengal, India

Narinder Kumar Mehra FNASc FIMSA FNA FHASc FTWAS FISOT FAMS
Hon Emeritus Scientist, ICMR
Former Dean (Res) AIIMS and National Chair, Founder Head, Department of Transplant Immunology and Immunogenetics, All India Institute of Medical Sciences, New Delhi, India

Navkiran Sooch Mahajan MD
Professor of Psychiatry
Dayanand Medical College and Hospital
Ludhiana, Punjab, India

Parveen Goel PhD
Neuropsychologist, Department of Neurology, Dayanand Medical College and Hospital, Ludhiana, Punjab, India

Prasun Chatterjee MD
Associate Professor
Department of Geriatric Medicine
All India Institute of Medical Sciences
New Delhi, India

Purbasha Biswas
2nd Year Junior Resident
RG Kar Medical College and Hospital
Kolkata, West Bengal, India

Rahul Shukla PhD
Research Scholar,
Department of Biomedical Engineering
Indian Institute of Technology
Rupnagar, Punjab, India

Ranjive Mahajan MD
Professor and Head
Department of Psychiatry
Dayanand Medical College and Hospital
Ludhiana, Punjab, India

Rina Das MD DMCW
Assistant Professor
Department of Forensic Medicine and Toxicology
RG Kar Medical College
Kolkata, West Bengal, India

Rudrajit Paul MD DNB MRCP (UK)
Consultant Physician
Ruby General Hospital
Kolkata, West Bengal, India

Somnath Das MD
In-Charge Poison Information and Research Centre
Professor Forensic Medicine and Toxicology, RG Kar Medical College
Kolkata, West Bengal, India

Souvik Dubey MD DM
Assistant Professor
Bangur Institute of Neurosciences
Institute of Postgraduate Medical Education and Research Annex 1
Kolkata, West Bengal, India

Subhadeep Gupta MD
Post-Doctoral Trainee
Bangur Institute of Neurosciences
Institute of Postgraduate Medical Education and Research
Kolkata, West Bengal, India

Subhra Sankar Sen MBBS
Postgraduate Trainee
Midnapore Medical College and Hospital
Kolkata, West Bengal, India

Sujoy Ghosh DM FRCP FACE
Professor
General Medicine Endocrinology
Institute of Postgraduate Medical Education and Research
Kolkata, West Bengal, India

Tanuka Mandal MD
Senior Resident Medicine
RG Kar Medical College and Hospital
Kolkata, West Bengal, India

Tarun Kumar Paria MBBS DA
Postgraduate Trainee
Department of General Medicine
RG Kar Medical College and Hospital
Kolkata, West Bengal, India

Udas Chandra Ghosh MD DNB (Med) DNB (Resp Dis) FRCP
Professor of Medicine
Medical College
Kolkata, West Bengal, India

Uddalak Chakraborty MBBS MD
Post-Doctoral Trainee
Bangur Institute of Neurosciences,
Institute of Postgraduate Medical Education and Research
Kolkata, West Bengal, India

Venugopalan Gunasekaran MD
Assistant Professor
Department of Geriatric Medicine
Jawaharlal Institute of Postgraduate Medical Education and Research
Puducherry, India

Vikas Gupta MD DM
Assistant Professor
Department of Rheumatology and Immunology
Dayanand Medical College and Hospital, Ludhiana, Punjab, India

Section 3: Infectious Diseases (Section Editor: Bibhuti Saha)

Aakash Rai MBBS
Junior Resident
Department of Medicine
Institute of Medical Sciences Banaras Hindu University
Varanasi, Uttar Pradesh, India

Abhipsa Mohapatra MD
Senior Resident
Department of Microbiology
VSS Institute of Medical Sciences and Research, Burla, Odisha, India

Abi Manesh MD
Assistant Professor
Department of Infectious Diseases
Christian Medical College
Vellore, Tamil Nadu, India

Agnibho Mondal MBBS
Postgraduate Trainee
Department of Tropical Medicine
School of Tropical Medicine
Kolkata, West Bengal, India

Akanksha MD
Senior Resident
Sri Guru Ram Das Institute of Health Sciences and Research
Amritsar, Punjab, India

Amit Kumar Adhikari MD
Assistant Professor
Department of Medicine
Raiganj Govt Medical College
Raiganj, West Bengal, India

Anupa Thampy MD
Consultant Infectious Diseases
Physician, Vellore, Tamil Nadu, India

Anup Kumar Das MD
Professor and Head of Medicine
Lakhimpur Medical College
Lakhimpur, Assam, India

Arti Kapil MD
Professor, Department of Microbiology
All India Institute of Medical Sciences
New Delhi, India

Ashish Bhalla MD
Professor
Department of Internal Medicine
Postgraduate Institute of Medical Education and Research
Chandigarh, India

Ashutosh Biswas MBBS MD
Professor
Department of Medicine
All India Institute of Medical Sciences
New Delhi, India

Atul K Patel MD FIDSA
Chief Consultant and Director
Infectious Diseases Clinic
3rd Floor "VEDANTA" Institute of Medical Sciences, Navrangpura, Ahmedabad,Gujarat, India

Ayan Basu MD DM (Infectious Diseases)
RMO cum Clinical Tutor
Department of Tropical Medicine
School of Tropical Medicine
Kolkata, West Bengal, India

BB Rewari MD FRCP(I) FICP FIACM
Former Professor of Medicine, PGIMER and RML Hospital, New Delhi, India
Former National Programme Officer (ART), National AIDS Control Organization, Govt of India

Bhaskar Thakuria MD
Associate Professor of Medicine
Guwahati Medical College and Hospital
Guwahati, Assam, India

Bibhuti Saha DTM&H (Cal) MD
Head of Tropical Medicine
Dean, Students' Affairs
School of Tropical Medicine
Kolkata, West Bengal, India

Bikram Das DTCD MD FNB
Fellow Infectious Diseases
Apollo Hospitals
Chennai, Tamil Nadu, India

Bipanchi Mahanta MD
Demonstrator of Microbiology
Jorhat Medical College
Jorhat, Assam, India

Dwijen Das MD FACP FRCP
Associate Professor of Medicine
Silchar Medical College and Hospital
Silchar, Assam, India

G Balajee MD DIH MBA (Hosp Admin)
Chief of Labs and Senior Consultant Microbiologist
Gleneagles Global Health City
Chennai, Tamil Nadu, India

Gagandeep Singh MD
Associate Professor
Department of Microbiology
All India Institute of Medical Sciences
New Delhi, India

Gaurav Gupta MBBS MD
Assistant Professor
Department of Medicine
All India Institute of Medical Sciences
New Delhi, India

George M Varghese MD DNB FRCP
Professor and Head
Department of Infectious Diseases
Christian Medical College
Vellore, Tamil Nadu, India

Gurinder Mohan MD
Professor and Head of Medicine
Sri Guru Ram Das Institute of Health Sciences and Research
Amritsar, Punjab, India

Haripriya Reddy Challa MD FNB
Fellow Infectious Diseases
Apollo Hospital
Chennai, Tamil Nadu, India

Hitakalpa Baishya MD
Registrar of Medicine
Guwahati Medical College and Hospital
Guwahati, Assam, India

Immaculata Xess MD
Professor, Department of Microbiology
All India Institute of Medical Sciences
New Delhi, India

Indrajit Debnath MD
Senior Resident
Department of General Medicine
Silchar Medical College and Hospital
Silchar, Assam, India

Indranil Sen MD
Assistant Professor
Department of Medicine
North Bengal Medical College
Siliguri, West Bengal, India

J Rajkumar DNB (Ped) Fell Ped Inf Dis,
Consultant—Infectious Diseases
Gleneagles Global Health City
Chennai, Tamil Nadu, India

Jacquiline D Shira MD
Senior Resident
Department of General Medicine
Silchar Medical College and Hospital
Silchar, Assam, India

Jagdish Chander MD
Consultant Microbiologist
Professor and Former Head
Department of Microbiology
Government Medical College
Chandigarh, India

Jaspreet Kaur MD
Senior Resident, Sri Guru Ram Das
Institute of Health Sciences and
Research, Amritsar, Punjab, India

Jaya Chakravarty MD FRCP
Head of the Department
Department of Medicine
Institute of Medical Sciences Banaras
Hindu University
Varanasi, Uttar Pradesh, India

Jyoti Sharma MD
Assistant Professor
Department of Pharmacology, PGIMS
Rohtak, Haryana, India

Ketan Patel MD
Associate Consultant
Infectious Diseases Clinic
Vedanta Institute of Medical Sciences
Ahmedabad, Gujarat, India

KVP Saikiran MD
Senior Resident
Department of Microbiology
All India Institute of Medical Sciences
New Delhi, India

Madhumitha R MBBS DNB FNB
Consultant Infectious Diseases- The
Capstone Clinic
Chennai, Tamil Nadu, India

Mahesh Moorthy MBBS MD
Professor
Department of Clinical Virology
Christian Medical College
Vellore, Tamil Nadu, India

Manasvini Bhatt MBBS MD
Senior Resident
Department of Medicine
All India Institute of Medical Sciences
New Delhi, India

Manoj Kumar Mohapatra MD FICP
FICD (WHO)
Professor of Medicine
VSS Institute of Medical Sciences and
Research, Burla, Odisha, India

Mehebubar Rahman MD
Associate Professor
Department of Tropical Medicine
School of Tropical Medicine
Kolkata, West Bengal, India

Mohuya Bhattacharya MD
Consultant, Critical Care
AMRI Hospitals
Kolkata, West Bengal, India

Murali Narasimhan MD DNB
Professor and Head of Dermatology
SRM Medical College Hospital and
Research Centre
Chengalpattu, Tamil Nadu, India

Navneet Arora MD
Senior Resident
Department of Internal Medicine
Postgraduate Institute of Medical
Education and Research
Chandigarh, India

OC Abraham MD MPH FRCP
Professor of Medicine
Christian Medical College
Vellore, Tamil Nadu, India

Priscilla Rupali MD DTMH FRCP
Professor of Infectious Diseases
Christian Medical College
Vellore, Tamil Nadu, India

Priyam Batra MD
Assistant Professor
Department of Microbiology
All India Institute of Medical Sciences
New Delhi, India

Priyanka Ojha MBBS MD
Consultant Physician
New Delhi, India

Rajeev Soman MD FIDSA
Consultant ID Physician
Jupiter Hospital
Pune, Maharashtra, India

Rama Chaudhry MD
Professor and Head
Department of Microbiology
All India Institute of Medical Sciences
New Delhi, India

Rama Prosad Goswami MD
Professor
Department of Tropical Medicine
School of Tropical Medicine
Kolkata, West Bengal, India

Ram Gopalakrishnan MD MRCP (UK)
Senior Consultant
Institute of Infectious Diseases
Apollo Hospitals
Adjunct Professor, The Tamil Nadu
Dr MGR Medical University, Chennai,
Tamil Nadu, India

Renu Yadav MD
Senior Demonstrator
Department of Microbiology
All India Institute of Medical Sciences,
New Delhi, India

Ritin Mohindra MD
Professor of Internal Medicine
Postgraduate Institute of Medical Education and Research
Chandigarh, India

Runal John Steve MBBS MD
Assistant Professor
Department of Clinical Virology
Christian Medical College
Vellore, Tamil Nadu, India

S Subramanian MD DNB MNAMS
Director
Infectious Diseases and Infection Control, Gleneagles Global Health City
Chennai, Tamil Nadu, India

Sajithkumar R MD PhD FICP
Professor and Head
Department of Infectious Diseases
Department of Medical Education
Govt Medical College, Kottayam
Kerala, India

Sanjay K Mahajan MD FICP
Department of Medicine
Indira Gandhi Medical College
Shimla, Himachal Pradesh, India

Sanyam K Mahajan MD
Department of Medicine
Indira Gandhi Medical College
Shimla, Himachal Pradesh, India

S Anuradha MD FACP FRCP Edin
Director-Professor of Medicine
Infectious Diseases Specialist
Maulana Azad Medical College
New Delhi, India

Savita Verma MD MS
Professor
Department of Pharmacology
PGIMS, Rohtak, Haryana, India

Shubham Gupta MBBS MD
Junior Resident
Department of Medicine
Institute of Medical Sciences Banaras Hindu University
Varanasi, Uttar Pradesh, India

SK Baruah MD
Professor of Medicine
Guwahati Medical College and Hospital
Guwahati, Assam, India

Smarajit Banik MD
Associate Professor
Department of Medicine
North Bengal Medical College
Siliguri, Darjeeling, India

Soumendra Nath Haldar MBBS MD
Senior Resident Infectious Diseases
Department of Medicine and Microbiology
All India Institute of Medical Sciences
New Delhi, India

Subhash Chandra Parija MD PhD DSc FRC Path
Vice Chancellor, Sri Balaji Vidyapeeth University, Puducherry, India

Subhash Todi MD MRCP
Director, Critical Care, AMRI Hospitals
Kolkata, West Bengal, India

Subhasish Kamal Guha MD FICP
Director, Professor
Department of Tropical Medicine
Medical Superintendent-cum-Vice-Principal, School of Tropical Medicine
Kolkata, West Bengal, India

Swati Khullar MD
Senior Resident
Department of Microbiology
All India Institute of Medical Sciences
New Delhi, India

Tuhina Banerjee MD PhD
Professor, Department of Microbiology
Institute of Medical Sciences
Banaras Hindu University
Varanasi, Uttar Pradesh, India

Umang Agrawal DNB FNB MRCP
Associate Consultant in ID
Hinduja Hospital
Mumbai, Maharashtra, India

Vikas Suri MD
Additional Professor, Department of Internal Medicine, Postgraduate Institute of Medical Education and Research, Chandigarh, India

V Ramasubramanian MD FRCP
Director - The Capstone Clinic
Consultant Infectious Diseases and Tropical Medicine, Apollo Hospitals
Adjunct Prof Infectious Diseases
Chennai, Tamil Nadu, India

Section 4: Critical Care (Section Editor: Dhruva Chaudhry)

Aakanksha Chawla Jain MD
Consultant
Department of Respiratory Critical Care and Sleep Medicine
Indraprastha Apollo Hospitals
New Delhi, India

Apurba Sankar Sastry MD DNB
Antimicrobial Stewardship Lead
Infection Control Officer
Associate Professor of Microbiology
JIPMER, Puducherry, India

Atul Prabhakar Kulkarni MD
Professor and Head, Division of Critical Care Medicine, Department of Anaesthesiology, Critical Care and Pain
Tata Memorial Hospital, Homi Bhabha National Institute, Dr Ernest Borges Road, Mumbai, Maharashtra, India

Binila Chacko MD DNB DM
Professor, Medical Intensive Care Unit
Christian Medical College
Vellore, Tamil Nadu, India

Camilla Rodrigues MD
Consultant Microbiologist and Chairperson Infection Control Committee, PD Hinduja National Hospital and Medical Research Centre
Mumbai, Maharashtra, India

Deepashree R MD DNB NMAMS
Infection Control Officer
Assistant Professor of Microbiology,
JSS Medical College
Mysuru, Karnataka, India

Dhruva Chaudhry MD DM
Senior Professor and Head
Department of Pulmonary and Critical Care Medicine
Post Graduate Institute of Medical Sciences
Rohtak, Haryana, India

Diksha Tyagi MD DM
Assistant Professor
Pulmonary and Critical Care Medicine
Postgraduate Institute of Medical Sciences, Rohtak, Haryana, India

GC Khilnani MD
Chairman
PSRI Institute of Pulmonary Critical Care and Sleep Medicine
PSRI Hospital, New Delhi, India

Haritha Madigubba MD
Fellow HIC (JIPMER)
Consultant Microbiologist
Yashoda Hospitals
Hyderabad, Telangana, India

Harpreet Singh MD
Senior Professor
Department of Medicine
Pt BDS PGIMS
Rohtak, Haryana, India

J Aarthi MD
Post Graduate
Department of Medicine, Maulana Azad Medical College
New Delhi, India

JV Peter MD DNB MAMS FRCP
Professor
Medical Intensive Care Unit
Christian Medical College
Vellore, Tamil Nadu, India

Ketan Priyadarshi MD DNB
Fellow HIC (First year)
Jawaharlal Institute of Postgraduate Medical Education and Research
Puducherry, India

Kunal Ahuja MD
Senior Resident
PSRI Institute of Pulmonary, Critical Care and Sleep Medicine, PSRI Hospital, New Delhi, India

Manjunath BG DM
Assistant Professor
Department of Pulmonary and Critical Care Medicine, Pt BDS PGIMS
Rohtak, Haryana, India

Mathew Joseph MCh
Head, Neurocritical Care and Trauma
Department of Neurological Science
Christian Medical College
Vellore, Tamil Nadu, India

Mohan Gurjar MD PDCC
Additional Professor
Department of Critical Care Medicine
Sanjay Gandhi Postgraduate Institute of Medical Sciences (SGPGIMS)
Lucknow, Uttar Pradesh, India

Mradul Kumar Daga MD
Director Professor
Department of Medicine
Maulana Azad Medical College
New Delhi, India

Nishanth Baliga MD DM
Fellow in Critical Care
Department of Anaesthesiology
Tata Memorial Hospital
Homi Bhabha National Institute
Mumbai, Maharashtra, India

Pawan Kumar Singh MD DM
Assistant Professor
Department of Pulmonary and Critical Care Medicine
Pt BDS Post Graduate Institute of Medical Sciences
Rohtak, Haryana, India

Prabhudev MBBS
Resident, Department of Medicine
Pt BDS PGIMS
Rohtak, Haryana, India

Raghu RV MBBS
Post Graduate, Department of Medicine, Maulana Azad Medical College, New Delhi, India

Rahul Pandit MD FCICM FCCP
Chairman ISCCM, Mumbai Branch
Treasurer ISCCM
Director Intensive Care Unit, Fortis Hospital, Mumbai, Maharashtra, India

Rajesh Chawla MD
Senior Consultant
Department of Respiratory Critical Care and Sleep Medicine
Indraprastha Apollo Hospitals
Delhi, India

Raj Kumar Mani MD FRCP FCCP
Director-Strategy and COVID-19 Management
Pulmonology and Critical Care
Yashoda Super Specialty Hospital
Kaushambi, Uttar Pradesh, India

Rakesh Kumar DA MD
Professor
Anesthesiology
Dr Baba Saheb Ambedkar Medical College and Hospital
New Delhi, India

Ritu Sangwan MBBS
Resident
Department of Medicine
Pt BDS PGIMS
Rohtak, Haryana, India

Roop Gursahani MD DM
Consultant Neurologist and Epileptologist
PD Hinduja National Hospital
Mumbai, Maharashtra, India

Roseleen Kaur Bali MD
Consultant
Department of Respiratory Critical Care and Sleep Medicine
Indraprastha Apollo Hospitals
New Delhi, India

Ruchira Wasudeo Khasne DA DNB
Senior Consultant and Head of Department, Critical Care Medicine
SMBT Institute of Medical Sciences and Research Centre
Igatpuri, Maharashtra, India

Rupali Patnaik MD DM
Senior Resident
Department of Critical Care Medicine
Sanjay Gandhi Postgraduate Institute of Medical Sciences
Lucknow, Uttar Pradesh, India

Saswati Sinha MD
Consultant Critical Care
AMRI Hospitals
Kolkata, West Bengal, India

Satya Ranjan Sahu MD
Consultant, PSRI Institute of Pulmonary Critical Care and Sleep Medicine
PSRI Hospital, New Delhi, India

Shaoli Basu MD DNB
Associate Consultant Microbiologist and Infection Control Officer
PD Hinduja National Hospital and Medical Research Centre
Mumbai, Maharashtra, India

Sheenam Walia MD
DM Fellow, Department of Cardiac Anaesthesia, Postgraduate Institute of Medical Education and Research
Chandigarh, India

Sheila Nainan Myatra MD FCCM
Professor
Department of Anaesthesiology
Critical Care and Pain
Tata Memorial Hospital
Homi Bhabha National Institute
Mumbai, Maharashtra, India

Shreyas H Gutte MD
Senior Resident
Department of Critical Care Medicine
Sanjay Gandhi Postgraduate Institute of Medical Sciences
Lucknow, Uttar Pradesh, India

Srinagesh Simha MS (Gen Surg) FRCP
Medical Director, Karunashraya
Bengaluru, Karnataka, India
Adjunct Faculty, Department of Palliative Medicine and Supportive Care, Kasturba Medical College
Manipal, Karnataka, India

Subhash Todi MD MRCP
Director, Critical Care
AMRI Hospitals
Kolkata, West Bengal, India

Sunil Kumar DA
CMO (HAG)
Lok Nayak Hospital
New Delhi, India

Sunil Shroff MS FRCS
Senior Consultant Urologist and Transplant Surgeon
Madras Medical Mission Hospital
Managing Trustee, MOHAN Foundation
Chennai, Tamil Nadu, India

Sushmita Jakka DM
Assistant Professor
Department of Pulmonary Medicine
GIMSR
Visakhapatnam, Andhra Pradesh, India

FOREWORD

"He who studies medicine without books sails an uncharted sea, but he who studies medicine without patients does not go to sea at all."

Sir William Osler emphasized the value of reading medicine from textbooks way back in the late 18th and early 19th century. However, he felt that clinical medicine can be learnt only by spending time with the patient. Knowledge, without its appropriate application for the patient welfare, is of no value.

Medicine is an ever-evolving field. Many earlier impressions, opinions dogmas, and axioms have been challenged and proven wrong. We today live in an era of "evidence-based medicine." Large registries, cohort studies, double-blind randomized trials, and at times sham-controlled trials are conducted every year. A modern-day textbook needs to incorporate the latest evidence in a comprehensive and simplified manner. The data from these trials needs to be interpreted by experts in the field so that meaningful clinical lessons can be derived. Dr Gurpreet Singh Wander, the editor of this book, has edited some nice books earlier also. The section editors are experts in their fields, and many have contributed to the API Textbook of Medicine, of which I was an editor-in-chief for two editions.

The disease pattern, presentation, and prevalence is different among South Asians as compared to the western world. This is due to our peculiar dietary, environmental, genetic, and social factors. We need to imbibe medicine with a regional flavor for a better understanding of the clinical presentation and response to management. While we think globally and understand the evidence and concepts from across the world, we need to act locally in a manner that is best for our population. This book fulfills the requirement very aptly and ably. In fact, most of the authors have done original work and collected data on the diseases they have written chapters on. I find the language is simple and comprehensible. The figures and tables are illustrative, and the layout is pleasant to the eyes.

Infectious diseases are posing new challenges to us and we need to update our knowledge. Multidrug-resistant bacterial infections in the ICUs, the Corona virus-related COVID-19 pandemic, and surprisingly high number of fungal infections with mucormycosis are all indicators of the need for continuing research in infectious diseases. Noncommunicable diseases have also become more common, as our population is aging with the improvement in longevity of life. We learn medicine in compartments and subspecialties, but patients will never present with single-system involvement. A good physician needs to have knowledge of all the subspecialties and the ability to assimilate and translate it into a comprehensive management plan for all the problems of a given patient. The science and art of medicine is to deliver evidence-based, state of art, and high-tech care with compassion and empathy. As Sir William Osler said, "*Medicine is a science of uncertainty and an art of probability.*" We have to use both at the same time, for the good of the patient.

We live in a rapidly evolving and changing world. The patients are more aware and better informed. They are getting more demanding and are little less tolerant. At the same time, we are much better equipped with access to high-end databases, simplified practice guidelines, and more informative but less invasive imaging and laboratory methodologies. Though these are challenging times, yet they are more exciting. Electronic medical records (EMRs) will ensure better continuity of care in the future. We need to incorporate information technology, artificial intelligence, and machine learning in our practice. We have to use them for the ultimate and only goal of medicine and that is, "better patient care." Do not feel threatened by these new modalities, learn to use them for better care. Textbooks, practice guidelines, medical journals, internet, and databases should all be used for better understanding. Take all this information that you gain from various sources to the bedside of the patient and use them for evidence-based care of the patient. There will still be many new lessons that you will learn by the side of the patient. Putting it in Giorgio Baglivi's words

"Let the young know, they will never find a more interesting, more instructive book than the patient himself."

I congratulate the editors, authors, and the publisher for this nice effort. For the readers I would say, enjoy reading the book and use the knowledge for better patient care. Learning medicine is a process that has to continue throughout the life of a physician.

YP Munjal MD MAMS FRCP (Edin)
Medical Director and Honorary Senior Consultant
Diabetes and Life Style Disease Center
Banarsidas Chandiwala Institute of Medical Sciences
New Delhi, India

PREFACE

Learning medicine is a process and not an event. Clinical medicine is of course learned in the wards and bedside of the patients. However, a good theoretical knowledge of the subject is a basic requirement. Knowledge is of value only if it is applied for the benefit of patients. The emphasis in this book is on providing evidence-based basic understanding of the subject. The pathophysiology of diseases has been simplified. Modes of presentation and approach to investigations are given in a clinically applicable manner. The therapeutic plan, as given in guidelines, is summarized and presented in a way it has to be used in practice.

We have tried to bring a book for postgraduate students and those practicing medicine after that. Each chapter has been written by an expert in the field. The abstract summarizes the contents. The main content will serve as an easy reading to understand the topic. The language is simple to comprehend. The graphs and tables will make it easier for you to have a comprehensive hold on the topic. You will get an Indian perspective of the diseases in each chapter. There are MCQs out of the contents of the chapter for revision. The selected readings can be used for more information on the topic.

The process involved was sharing of responsibilities. My job was only to request the best experts in each specialty to agree to be the "section editors." The choice of topics and authors of each respective section was left to the section editors. For all the good things in the section, they are responsible. They have chosen experienced teachers and clinicians who have done original work on the topic for years, for sharing the literature and their experience. The contents of the chapters were the domain of the authors. The authors are from some of the top medical colleges and teaching institutions from across the country. They have extensive experience of teaching postgraduate students. Each chapter was reviewed and approved by the section editor. We have no words to express our gratitude to the authors for sparing their valuable time.

We live in an era of evidence-based medicine, medical audit, heightened expectations, and information explosion. Electronic medical records, big data, artificial intelligence, and machine learning tools for diagnosis of diseases will be applied more and more in the future. 3D reconstruction will aid in developing prosthesis. Wearables, ingestible devices, and remote monitoring backups will provide greater information about the patients. During such challenging and exciting times, the physician must have a basic and a baseline knowledge of the subject on which one can build further. This book attempts to provide you with that correct information in a simple language and layout.

Since the COVID pandemic is ongoing, many chapters related to effects of COVID-19 on various systems have been included. COVID-19 has placed infectious diseases at the center stage. You will need to have a wide knowledge of infectious diseases, systemic inflammatory responses, components of the immune system, and the role of genetics and epigenetics in disease causation. In the last two decades emphasis was more or noncommunicable disease since these are age-related diseases. Now a student of medicine must lay equal emphasis on both communicable and noncommunicable diseases. You will get an overall perspective of both, in this book.

The book was a brainchild of Mr Jitender Pal Vij, since he felt that such a book does not exist in our country. He insisted upon us to work on this project. My personal thanks to my secretary Mr Raja Gupta, who has spent many hours with me working on this project. Muskan Sharma was a great help even after she migrated to USA after her marriage. Mr Gurinder Singh joined us halfway into the project and helped us after that. Prerna Bajaj, development editor from Jaypee Brothers, has been a very tolerant, and adjustable colleague. She solved a lot of problems with her patience and perseverance.

Special thanks to Dr Pankaj Malhotra from PGI Chandigarh and Dr Davinder from DMCH who helped us with the hematology and oncology sections, respectively. Some important topics must have been left and we do not claim that the book covers everything for you. Please read the "Yearbook of Medicine" which we bring every year for 20 important articles from each specialty. If you will combine it with this book, then possibly it becomes a comprehensive knowledge package for you.

We have enjoyed and learned a lot while preparing this book. We hope and expect that you also have the same experience reading it. The e-book is being released along with for your convenience of reading. We have included some videos of interesting cases in the e-book which will provide dynamic images. All MCQs are from the contents of the chapter and will provide you a chance to assess.

We realize there must be many flaws in the text. Any keen reader who gives us feedback will be helping the further readers since we will include that in the next edition. **Please write to us an email postgraduatemed@yahoo.com or message us on WhatsApp number 9915169600, any corrections, changes, or suggestions that you have.** It will be a two-way interaction and we will be happy to get back to you for any clarifications.

Gurpreet S Wander MD DM FACC FAMS
Professor and Head of Cardiology
Hero DMC Heart Institute
Dayanand Medical College and Hospital
Ludhiana, Punjab, India

CONTENTS

VOLUME 1

SECTION 1: CLINICAL MEDICINE

SECTION 2: GENERAL MEDICINE

GENERAL TOPICS

GERIATRICS

SECTION 3: INFECTIOUS DISEASES

BASIC CONSIDERATIONS

BACTERIAL INFECTIONS

VIRAL INFECTIONS

CORONAVIRUS INFECTION

OTHER INFECTIONS

VOLUME 2

SECTION 5: CARDIOLOGY

SECTION 6: ENDOCRINOLOGY AND METABOLIC DISORDERS

SECTION 7: GASTROENTEROLOGY

VOLUME 3

SECTION 9: NEPHROLOGY

SECTION 10: NEUROLOGY

SECTION 11: PULMONARY MEDICINE AND TUBERCULOSIS

SECTION 12: RHEUMATOLOGY

Free Online Resources

1. **E-version of the book chapters:** Kindly refer to the back side of the front cover to redeem the scratch code on http://www.emedicine360.com **and access the E-version.** All the chapters in the printed version can be accessed online.

2. **MCQs:** Each chapter in the printed book is followed by 5–10 MCQ's. These MCQ's have 4–5 options and one correct answer. They are from the contents of the chapter. You are advised to solve these after reading the whole chapter.

   In order to access MCQs in the E-version, kindly click the link given at the end of each chapter on www.emedicine360.com.

3. **E-Chapters:** Free elaborated E-version of the following 6 chapters is available on http://www.emedicine360.com
   - e-15 (CH-15): Chest X-ray Evaluation and Some Spotters
   - e-23 (CH-23): Electronic Health Records, Artificial Intelligence, and Big Data—Role in Medicine
   - e-38 (CH-38): Prevention and Management of Infection in Transplant Recipients
   - e-48 (CH-48): Other Virus Infections—Chikungunya, Hantavirus, Nipah Virus, and Zika Virus
   - e-88 (CH-88): Noninvasive Cardiac Imaging
   - e-118 (CH-118): Endocrine Tumors and Malignancies

4. **Videos:** Some of the chapters have videos. These videos can be accessed online in respective chapters.
   - ch-28: Falls in Elderly
   - ch-89: Cardiac Catheterization and Coronary Angiography
   - ch-185: Seizures and Epilepsy
   - ch-193: Movement Disorders: The Clinical Vignette

CHAPTER 1

Practice of Medicine in 21st Century: Opportunities and Challenges

G Eswar, KV Seshaiah, K SSS Surya Prakash

ABSTRACT

For thousands of years, practice of medicine has followed the long-standing tradition typical of a profession. A physician possessed a unique body of knowledge and skills and put them to use in the case of patients. As such the doctor–patient interaction was paramount and served as the foundation of a personal, caring relationship that has stood the test of time. New innovations in the field of medicine in relation to causative factors of diseases as well as technology starting from 19th and 20th century have completely changed practice of medicine in the 21st century.

"It is not the strongest of the species that survives, nor the most intelligent, but the one most responsive to change"

—Charles Darwin

INTRODUCTION

Recent advances in healthcare resulted in morbidity and mortality reduction through disease-specific interventions, with increased life expectancy of human beings. Despite increased opportunities in healthcare in 21st century, new challenges are being faced by physicians. These opportunities of healthcare in 21st century have both positive and negative impacts from physician's as well as patient's perspective.

It is very arduous to modify both the process and the content of medical education. There must be compelling reasons and clear path toward the goal, as it is needed to equip the clinicians to adopt successfully to the healthcare demands of 21st century. This must look deep into the cost vs. performance; science vs. art; research vs. clinical practice, and these ideals should consolidate the gains of 20th century without losing flexibility or constraining the promise of new information and new models of care for the future physician, who is immersed in demands of daily practice, i.e., where rubber meets the road.

With all reforms in medical education, with backup of technological advancement in healthcare, a new focus is needed to favor a paradigm shift from a case-oriented model of health to a preventive, predictive, personalized, and participatory medicine (P4 medicine).

ORIGIN OF MODERN MEDICINE

The history of medicine can be traced back to the early civilizations of Egypt, Babylon, and Greece. Though, the Hippocratic oath, that continues to remind the doctors of their roles and responsibilities toward the society, has its origin way back in the 5th century BC, the formal and systematic training started in 1220 in the universities of Italy. It was only after the industrial revolution of 18th century, the world saw the emergence of modern medicine. The 19th century was significant as Germ theory of disease was established, which was followed by introduction of public health measures.

MEDICINE IN 19TH CENTURY

The 19th century witnessed numerous scientific discoveries and inventions owing to the rapid growth in the economic and industrial sectors. Scientists developed a better understanding of microbes and their virulence mechanisms. However, they were way behind as far as treatment of infectious diseases was considered. During the 19th century, lifestyles changed dramatically. These changes affected the risk of infectious diseases and other conditions. Meanwhile scientific advances at that time started including germ theory, hygiene and sepsis, and electrocardiograph etc., which made possible for new treatments.

Some of the important milestones in 19th century were anesthetic nitrous oxide; stethoscope; first successful blood transfusion; discovery of X-rays; first aspirin etc.

MEDICINE IN 20TH CENTURY

Advanced research centers were opened in the early 20th century and they were connected to major hospitals. Mid-20th century was characterized by new biological treatments such as antibiotics. These developments along with those in chemistry, medical knowledge, and genetics have laid a path for modern medicine.

Medicine was heavily professionalized in the 20th century and new professional careers were opened up for women as nurses and as physicians. Disease specialization has developed, with aim of providing medical care with respect to its specific characteristics of its diseases, from specializes medical professionals.

Substantial advances in public health methods and practice have occurred in 20th century. Some of its most notable contributions are development and widespread use of Vaccines, Smallpox eradication, and large reduction in communicable disease epidemics. Many methodological advances have facilitated better understanding of disease process and opportunities for control. Occupational and Environmental health disciplines were created, leading to significant contribution to current and future public health. Healthcare system became more organized, technologically sophisticated, and at same time costly.

Paradigm changed in the 20th century. Successful treatment of infectious diseases has led to unprecedented increases in longevity during the first half of 20th century. A new set of challenges including heart diseases, stroke, cancer, diabetes mellitus, chronic respiratory diseases, and other non-communicable diseases (NCDs) became the major cause of morbidity and mortality. An increasingly fragmented public health infrastructure had to deal new changes, including increased ageing population, dramatic population growth, and changes in environmental health determinants.

Some of the important milestones in the inventions of 20th century were blood grouping and typing, practical electrocardiogram, vitamins, insulins, penicillins, electroencephalogram (EEG), paracetamol, first human transplantation, first pacemaker, first in vitro fertilization (IVF), cardiopulmonary resuscitation (CPR), magnetic resonance imaging (MRI), polymerase chain reaction (PCR) and its improvements, and stem cell lines.

The 20th century produced such plethora of discoveries and advances that the face of medicine changed out of all recognition. The 19th and 20th centuries experienced breakthrough occurring in infection control. At the end of 20th century, 30% deaths were due to infection. By the end of 20th century, this has reduced to 4%.

Rapid progress of medicine in this era was reinforced by extensive improvements in communication between scientists throughout the world, by associations and societies in many fields of medicine resulting in the origin of guidelines for patient care.

In the first half of the 20th century emphasis continued to be placed on combating infection and notable landmarks were also attained in endocrinology, nutrition, and other branches. Insights derived from cell biology altered basic concepts of its disease. New discoveries in cell physiology and biochemistry have led to more precise diagnostic tests and effective therapies. Advances in biomedical engineering enabled to assess the structure and function of the body by noninvasive methods of imaging such as ultrasonography, computed tomography (CT), and MRI. The advances in medicine during the 20th century have more than doubled the average person's lifespan. In the 20th century, the progress in medical technology outpaced the progress in medicine.

Healthcare scenario in India: India has a rich, centuries-old heritage of medical and health sciences. Ayurveda is a traditional Indian form of holistic medicine. The philosophy of ayurveda and contribution by Charaka (ancient physician) and Sushrutha (ancient surgeon), bear testimony to the ancient tradition of scientific healthcare among Indian people. Historically, the most outstanding hospitals in India were those built by King Ashoka in 273–232 BCE.

During the 17th and 18th centuries, there was a slow and steady growth of modern system of medicine in India. Organized medical training began with opening of first medical college in Kolkata in 1835.

India has made striking progress in the postindependence era. Yet public sanitation, preventive healthcare, and control of communicable diseases remained as incomplete in 20th century.

MEDICINE IN 21ST CENTURY

The 21st century is characterized by highly advanced research involving numerous fields of science. The advancement of medical care was moving hand in hand with technological advancement. It was the marriage of biology and engineering that brought above technological advances in medicine. Intercoupling of biological sciences with engineering had laid a road to improvement of medical care and consequently to personalize medicine.

Today, we do not simply treat a patient based on his symptoms. We evaluate not just the matrix of possible causes with the help of newer diagnostics and therapeutics, but also consider the complexity and chronicity of the disease. Understanding the pathophysiology is equally important, but there is need to look further beyond this.

It is said that the physicians need to learn to integrate science and art of medicine, along with data and intuition. However, this is hardly observed in this 21st century. The healthcare systems disorganized at many levels might be blamed for this, but we must work toward making doctors "integrative healers" who are able to provide comprehensive, patient-centric care, based on the Concepts of prospective healthcare, Personalized medicine, System Biology, Nutritional Genomics, Integrative medicine, Chronic care model, and others.

CHALLENGES AND OPPORTUNITIES

Challenges and opportunities in health sphere can be categorized into three groups for the sake of convenience of understanding:

1. Social level (geographic)
2. Professional level
3. Personal (physician) level

CHALLENGES AT SOCIAL LEVEL

As declared by World Health Organization (WHO) regional office for Europe in June 2018, the following are the today's health challenges:

- Aging population
- Unhealthy lifestyles
- Burden of behavioral determinants leading to increased mortality and morbidity from NCDs
- Rapid transfer of infectious pathogens and the potential for global pandemics
- Natural disasters, conflicts, and mass population movements
- Antimicrobial resistance
- Injuries
- Health impact of climate change and environmental pollution
- Bioterrorism

Global health challenges: Coronary artery disease alone kill 26,000 people worldwide per day close to the number of deaths caused by COVID-19 thus far. Top 10 global causes of death annually (in lacs) are shown in **Table 1**.

Health challenges in India: Swine flu continues to kill over 1,000 each year in India. Tuberculosis (including drug-resistant) continues to pose challenge, killing close to 4.5 lacs every year in India.

Top 10 causes of death annually in India (in lacs) are shown in **Table 2**.

Diseases are not the only big killers. Close to 500 Indians die in traffic accidents daily. Accidental deaths in India are increasing on par with population density and increasing vehicles (**Table 3**).

Opportunities at social level: Advancements in 21st century have led to important changes at social level. Locus of medical knowledge is steadily moving out of the minds of physicians into the public and digital sphere. Patients are having increased access to healthcare providers, through advanced network technology, for disease information, treatment, and for self management. Some of the new technologies include smartphones, tablet, personal computers (PCs), wearable sensors, patient portals, mobile home healthcare, social media, telemedicine, Internet of Things (IOT) etc. Patients can have health services and can have consultation from any time and place 24×7 hours.

CHALLENGES AT PROFESSIONAL LEVEL

WHO under title "Health Agenda for the 21st Century–Future Health Challenges", revealed certain health challenges.

For young and old alike, the world 2025 will be very different for that of previous figures. Death rate in the age group 20–64 years will increase by 21% in early 21st century. Small children will be outnumbered by people over 65 by 2025, because of increased life expectancy. Major health problems by the year 2025 will be diseases of circulatory

TABLE 1 Top 10 global causes of death annually.

Disease	Annual burden in lacs
Cancer	96
Heart disease	94
Stroke	58
COPD	31
LRTIs	30
Dementia	20
Diabetics mellitus	16
Road injuries	15
Diarrheal diseases	14
Tuberculosis	13

(COPD: chronic obstructive pulmonary disease; LRTIs: lower respiratory tract infections)

Source: Global burden of disease; www.who.int.

TABLE 2 Top 10 causes of death annually in India.

Disease	Annual burden in lacs
Ischemic heart disease	15.4
Chronic obstructive pulmonary disease	9.6
Cancer	7.8
Stroke	7.3
Diarrheal diseases	7.2
Lower respiratory tract infections	5.1
Tuberculosis	4.5
Neonatal disorders	4.3
Asthma	2.5
Diabetic mellitus	2.5

Source: Global burden of disease; www.who.int.

TABLE 3 Accidental deaths annually in India.

Disease	No. of cases
Electrocution	12,154
Accidental fire	12,748
Falls	20,201
Poisoning	21,646
Drowning	30,187
Railroad accidents	1,78,832

system, cancers, viral pandemics, e.g., severe acute respiratory syndrome (SARS) coronavirus-2 (SARS-CoV-2) disease-2019 (COVID-19), environmental diseases, and psychiatric disorders. Global situation with respect to cancers of lung, trachea, bronchus, colon, rectum and prostate, and lymphoma will worsen.

Emerging and re-emerging infectious diseases is a challenge. Changes in microbial populations can lead to evolution of new pathogens, development of new virulence factors, and development of antibiotic resistance outpacing the new antibiotics development. Vulnerable population like immunocompromised, elderly with multiple dysfunctional organs is very much increased. Physicians must become expert in variety of skills of advanced technology currently not emphasized in medical training. Mathematical skills are necessary to understand the meaning of diagnostic and therapeutic probabilities. Communicating skills are necessary to interpret disease probabilities to patients. They should know how to work with Artificial intelligence and high-end technological devices with a basic knowledge in computer systems, which is not a regular curricular subject in medical education.

Inadequate health resources and trained health personnel should be addressed to meet the demands and diversity of changes in healthcare needs of 21st century.

In Indian scenario poor doctor and healthcare professionals to population ratio, is to be addressed along with inadequate health budget in this second most populous country.

Opportunities at professional level: Healthcare is in the midst of a technologic convergence, compelling one historian to pronounce the 21st century as the age of dataism. A vast and growing list of health-related technologies will enable remote monitoring of patients and their access to healthcare, patient identification and data collection, treatment administration and guidance to patient in self-management etc. The following are some of the advanced health technologies in patient care:

- Rapid diagnostic methods
- Nanomedicine
- Genome based personalized medicine
- Virtual clinics
- Telemedicine
- Artificial intelligence
- New trends in medical imaging like dual energy CT (DECT), tomosynthesis, and hybrid imaging
- Robots in healthcare
- Silico drug designs for evolution in drug development

CHALLENGES AT PERSONAL LEVEL (PHYSICIAN)

The new trends of healthcare settings are creating new challenges at personal level.

- Patient-doctor relationship is being lost.
- Changing expectations and demands of patients
- Neglected human touch in treatment process
- Dependence on machines
- Maladjustment with new technologies
- Continuation of knowledge improvement in skills and new developments
- Deficient time for personal life (doctors)

Opportunities at personal level: Opportunities at personal level are vast in the healthcare scenario in 21st century.

- Care from anywhere
- Participation in teamwork
- Rapid diagnostic methods availability
- Telemedicine
- Easier data storage and analysis

GLOBAL SYNDEMICS IN 21ST CENTURY

Malnutrition in all its forms including obesity, undernutrition, and other dietary risks is the leading cause of poor health globally. Climate change can be considered as a pandemic because of its sweeping effects on human health. These pandemics—obesity, malnutrition, and climate change—represent global syndemic. Global syndemic is synergy of epidemics, because they co-occur in time and place, interact with each other. Upward trends in healthcare in 21st century are shown in **Figure 1**.

PARADIGM SHIFT

"If it were not for the great variability among individuals, medicine might as well be a science, not an art."

—William Osler 1892

Challenges of "standardization" and "individualization" have always been characteristic for medical services. In terms of individualization, the best possible individual care is the ethical imperative of medicine and it is a good right of all patients to receive it. In terms of standardization, all the available treatments are based on guideline recommendations derived from large multicentric trials. Optimal way is that standardization and individualization should go hand-in-hand, in order to identify the right patient, treating him/her with right medication and the right dose at the right point of time.

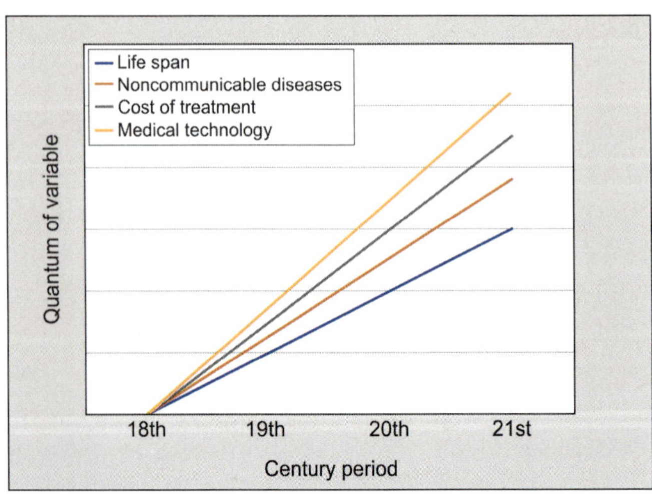

FIGURE 1: Upward trends in healthcare in 21st century.

Paradigm shift is needed to move from unpredictable, unpreventable, and impersonal medicine (unPPM) to predictive, preventive, personalized, and participatory medicine (P4 medicine), covering both healthcare and disease care, promoting an integrated approach combining advantages of individual biomedical fields and technologies and consolidating a multiprofessional collaboration.

EVIDENCE-BASED MEDICINE

Evidence-based medicine, originated in 18th century in France and formally conceptualized by the Evidence-based medicine working group in 1992, has been gaining importance in clinical practice and medical knowledge.

It is basically that integrates clinical expertise with the external clinical evidence obtained from best available literature based on systematic research.

MEDICAL EDUCATION IN 21ST CENTURY

As science progressed in medicine, the valuable doctor-patient relationship was lost, in the application of medical knowledge and technology. To solve this, medical universities should aim to revolutionize medical education through launching classes in medical humanities. Lancet's commission on medical education proposed a shared vision that all health professionals should be educated to mobilize knowledge and to engage in critical reasoning and ethical conduct. Emphasis should be with in the medical curricula that shapes the medical knowledge and skills are acquired and practiced. Downward trends in healthcare in 21st century are as shown in **Figure 2**.

Breadth and depth of medical knowledge combined with clinical acumen will always beat the heart of medical consultation. With all reforms in medical education, with backup of technological advancement in healthcare, a new focus is needed to favor a paradigm shift from a case-oriented model of health to a preventive, predictive, personalized, and participatory medicine.

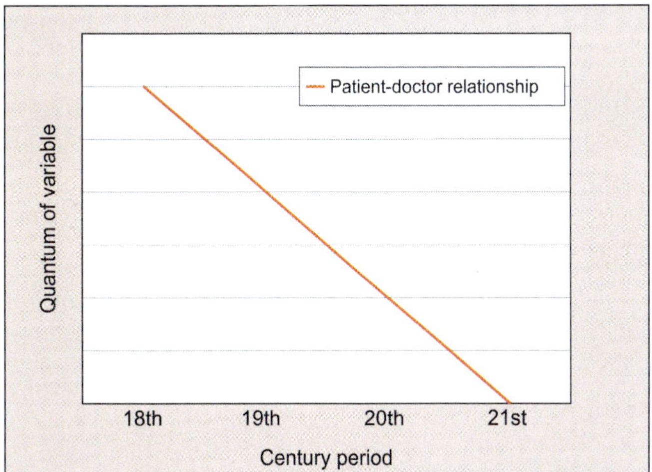

FIGURE 2: Downward trends in healthcare in 21st century.

RECOMMENDED READINGS

1. Koutsouris D. The evolution of medical care: from the beginnings to personalized medicine. Health Technol. 2017;7:3-4.
2. Bynum WF, Hardy A, Jacyna S, Lawrence C, Tansey EM. The Western Medical Tradition 1800-2000. United States of America: Cambridge University Press. 2006; 7-10,150-6.
3. Victoria and Albert Museum, online Museum (2011-07-04). Health and Medicine. [online] Available from www.vam.ac.uk.
4. Fielding JE. Public health in the twentieth century: Advances and challenges. Annu Rev Public Health. 1999;20:XIII-XXX.
5. Papyrus ES. Britannica online encyclopedia. [online] Available from www.britannica.com.
6. Jawahar SK. Healthcare scenario in India. published in ICU Management and practice, ICU. 2006;6(4):2007.
7. Mehic B. Trend of medicine of the 21st century. Bosn J Basic Med Sci. 2013;13(1):3-4.
8. Snyderman R, Williams RS. Prospective Medicine: The next healthcare transformation. Acad Med. 2003;78(11):1079-84.
9. Bajwa M. Emerging 21st century Medical technology. Pak J Med Sci. 2014;30(3):649-55.
10. Bunn TW, Sikarwar AS. Diagnostics: Conventional versus modern methods. J Adv Med Pharm Sci. 2016:1-7.
11. Tibbals HF. Medical nanotechnology and nanomedicine, 1st edition. CRC Press; 2011. p. 528.
12. Mishra SG, Takke AK, Auti ST, Suryavanshi SV, Oza MJ. Role of Artificial intelligence in healthcare. Biochem Ind J. 2017;11(5):120.
13. Swinburn BA, Kraak VI, Allender S, Atkins VJ, Baker PI, Bogard JR, et al. The Global syndemic of obesity, undernutrition, and climate change: The Lancet commission Report. Lancet. 2019;393(10173):791-846.
14. Golubnitschaja O, Baban B, Boniolo G, Wang W, Bubnov R, Kapalla M, et al. Medicine in the early twenty-first century: paradigm and anticipation-EPMA position paper 2016. EPMA J. 2016;7(1):23.
15. Andrews RJ, Quintana LM. Unpredictable, unpreventable, and impersonal medicine: global disaster response in thc 21st century. EPMA J. 2015;6(1):2.
16. Groopman J. How doctors think. Boston: Houghton Mifflin. 2007;117(10):2738.
17. Jones DS, Hofmann L, Quinn S. 21st Century Medicine: A new model for medical education and practice. Gig Harbor, Washington: The Institute for Functional Medicine (IFM). 2009.

CHAPTER

2

Good History Taking and General Physical Examination

SV Ramanamurty, KSR Swamy, Chakravarthy DJK

ABSTRACT

Clinical examination of a patient consists of history taking and physical examination. History taking is an art, which is to be mastered over years of repeated practice. In majority of cases, diagnosis can be made based on history alone. Over years, the doctor should develop the "clinical eye" by not only seeing but observing, not only touching but feeling and associating different observations and findings. Attentive conversation gains the confidence of the patient and establishes trust which makes physical and systemic examination easier by cooperation. Chronological order of the presenting complaints helps us to arrive at a probable diagnosis early and the differential diagnoses can be ruled out by negative history and general physical examination. Significant past illnesses, family, and social history and knowledge about workplace can include/rule out genetic and occupational etiologies. Head-to-toe examination can give clues about malnutrition, congenital abnormalities, endocrine disorders, and organ dysfunction, which along with proper history, can guide to the abnormal system which needs detailed systemic examination in majority of the cases. Thus, clinical examination plays a vital role in making a final diagnosis and should be learnt in detail.

"Certainly it is by their signs and symptoms, that internal diseases are revealed to the physician"

—Elisha Bartlett

INTRODUCTION

"Listen to the patient by taking a careful medical history. 90% of the time, you can arrive at an uncannily accurate diagnosis by paying close attention based on physical examination and sophisticated lab tests confirm your hunch."

—VS Ramachandran

From times immemorial, it has been the practice of taking history before proceeding for further examination. In the present day of "computer era" and "high tech" practice of medicine, the medical system is forced to become almost impersonal.

HISTORICAL BACKGROUND

From the classic Greek times, interrogation of the patient has been considered the most important, because disease was, and still is, viewed in terms of the discomfort it creates.

"Medicine is an art and science."

—Rogers (2006)

The art and science of medicine are not antagonistic but supplementary to each other. Unfortunately, the art has left slowly; and the science is threatened. Hence, it's time, to fill up the gap with "the art of good history taking coupled with the science of physical examination;" which will remain as invaluable tools for early diagnosis, besides creating a closer bond with the patient, which go a long way, in the onward march of clinical medicine.

HISTORY TAKING

"Listen to your patient, he is telling you the diagnosis."

—Sir William Osler

Father of the Modern medicine (1849–1919)

Speak clearly and audibly and appear unhurried. Understand your patient's context; that is nothing but empathy.

- Ask open questions to start with:
  - What has brought you along to see me today?
  - What problem you have? Tell me about yourself.
  - How can I help you today?

These questions give the impression that you have concern for the patient and you will get the confidence of the patient.

Structure of typical history taking:
- Patient data
- Chief complaints
- History of present illness
- Past history
- Personal history
- Family history (pedigree chart)

PATIENT DATA

Name, age, sex, marital status, occupation, phone number, address, photo identification, and identification marks (for further follow-up).

CHIEF COMPLAINTS

Complaints should be recorded in a chronological order.

1. *Example*:
   - Cough: 3 months
   - Cough with sputum: 2 months
   - Shortness of breath: 6 weeks
   - Blood spitting during cough: 5 days

   This indicates how the respiratory disease like pulmonary tuberculosis (TB) disease has progressed.
2. *Example*:
   - Chest pain/discomfort on walking for a distance (around 100 meters) relieving with rest: 6 months
   - Chest discomfort on walking for shorter distance (around 50 meters) relieving with rest: 2 months
   - Chest discomfort occurring even with minimal distance and not relieving with rest: 3 weeks
   - Of late chest pain developing even at rest: 1 week
   - Chest pain with profuse sweating at rest persisting for more than 15 minutes: 1 day

   This indicates how an angina has progressed to acute coronary syndrome (ACS).

An overview of other complaints to be documented in this situation.

- *General*: Body pains, fever, chills and rigors, lack of appetite, weight loss, weight gain, unexplained weakness, sleeplessness, fatigue, headache etc.
- *Respiratory system*: Shortness of breath, wheezing, cough, sputum or blood spitting, snoring while sleeping, fever, night sweats, and clearing cough early in the morning
- *Cardiovascular system*: Palpitations, swelling of feet, chest pain or discomfort, and shortness of breath at rest or on exertion or on lying down
- *Genitourinary system*: Dribbling of urine, difficulty, strain, or pain while passing urine, burning micturition, passing larger or smaller quantities of urine, blood in urine, or any color change in the urine, delay while starting urination (mainly in males)
- *Gastrointestinal system*: Abdominal pain, nausea, vomiting, indigestion, heart burn, acid belching, abdominal bloating or distension, change in bowel habits, diarrhea, constipation, blood in stools, jaundice, and yellowish urine
- *Hematological disorders*: History of bleeding from gums, rash, difficulty in healing, prolonged bleeding from cuts, blood clots or ulcers over legs, bony pain, and lumps in axilla or groin (enlarged lymph nodes)
- *Musculoskeletal*: Swelling of joints, pain in the neck or back, recent skin rash, red or dry eyes, mouth ulcers, history of rheumatoid arthritis, or painful red swelling of great toe (gout)
- *Endocrinal*: Easy fatigability, swelling in neck, hoarseness of voice, intolerance to cold or heat, excess sweating, trembling of fingers, palpitations, excess or decreased appetite, recent weight gain or loss, change in appearance, and coarse skin
- *Neurological system*:
  - Change in consciousness, altered speech, and memory loss
  - Change in vision, blackouts, deviation of angle of mouth or jaw, or difficulty in closure or opening of eyes, change in hearing, or ringing noise in ears, reeling sensation (vertigo), difficulty in swallowing, loss of voice, and difficult tongue movements
  - Loss of power in limbs, difficult coordinated movements, and involuntary movements if any
  - Decreased sensations, abnormal sensations, and difficulty to walk in darkness
  - Slurring of speech, swaying to one side, neck stiffness, vomiting, associated with fever
  - Dribbling of urine, urinary incontinence, and urgency
  - Fits, and falls, with loss of consciousness

HISTORY OF PRESENT ILLNESS

Note: We can ask closed questions.

- When he was free, i.e., when the presenting complaint started?
- What was the nature of onset?
  - Is it acute, subacute, or insidious?
  - Time of onset
  - Precipitating, relieving, or aggravating factors
- How each complaint progressed? (lateral profile)
  - Relentlessly progressing
  - Regressing
  - Static
  - Remissions and exacerbations present
  - Present state

  These points usually give clues regarding the nature of the disorder. Some examples are listed below:
- *Acute onset*: Stroke, acute myocardial infarction, and pulmonary embolism
- *Subacute onset*: Acute inflammatory demyelinating polyneuropathy (AIDP), pneumonia, meningitis, and intestinal obstruction
- *Insidious onset*: Peripheral neuropathy and chronic anemia
- Abdominal pain increasing with food (gastric ulcer), relieved with food (duodenal ulcer)
- Angina is precipitated with strain and relieved with rest or sublingual nitroglycerine.
- Headache due to intracranial space occupying lesion (ICSOL) and pneumothorax, (relentlessly progressing)
- Asthma, flushing episodes, convulsions, and migraine headache (episodic)
- Static (completed stroke)

Bowel and bladder habits: Whether regular or irregular or constipated.

History in the recent preceding past:
- This varies from system to system involved.
- For example, in a central nervous system (CNS) case visit to an endemic area, trauma to head or spine, snake bite, vaccination, excess drug intake, exposure to pesticide, or extremes of weather

HISTORY OF PAST ILLNESS

This usually varies from organ system involved:
- Whether the individual suffered in the past from
- Rheumatic fever, hypertension, epilepsy, stroke, diabetes mellitus, jaundice, and pulmonary TB
- Any previous surgeries, trauma, drug treatment, and drug allergies
- Bleeding episodes, easy bruises

Childhood:
- Injuries, birth trauma
- Diseases like measles, mumps, recurrent respiratory infections, cyanotic spells, congenital heart disease, and milestones of childhood

PERSONAL HISTORY

- Addiction to alcohol may indicate likely liver disease.
- Chronic smoking with history of morning cough may indicate likely chronic bronchitis or carcinoma lung.
- Sedentary lifestyle indicates likely atherosclerosis and coronary artery disease (CAD)
- Exposure to extramarital sex may suggest conditions like human immunodeficiency virus (HIV), syphilis, or so.

In case of females: Year of menarche, menstrual history, pregnancies, abortions, and year of menopause

FAMILY HISTORY

Whether any other family member suffered from:
- Pulmonary TB, epilepsy, CAD, stroke, diabetes mellitus, hypertension, psychiatric disorders, color blindness, and hemophilia
- *Autoimmune disorders*: Myasthenia, rheumatoid arthritis, and vitiligo
- Color blindness, muscular dystrophies, and periodic paralysis

SOCIAL AND OCCUPATIONAL HISTORY

Individual's economic status and occupation:
- Low socioeconomic status may indicate worm infestation, diarrhea, scabies, and certain communicable diseases
- High economic status may indicate likely atherosclerosis and CAD.
- Work in industries may give clues about pneumoconiosis.

GENERAL PHYSICAL EXAMINATION

"More mistakes are made for want of a proper examination than for any other reason."

—Russell John Howard (1875–1942)

History of clinical diagnosis starts with Hippocrates and his school. History taking and inspection are fundamental diagnostic tools.

Physical examination starts right from entry of the patient into the examination room.
- Facial appearance may give clues to the diagnosis:
- Agitated or fright and anxiety may suggest thyrotoxicosis.
- Mask-like face may point out to parkinsonism.
- Apathy may give a clue towards depression.
- Puffy face may direct towards myxedema or nephrotic syndrome.

ATTITUDE

Whether the patient is conscious, coherent, oriented, and cooperative?

GAIT

- Ataxic (cerebellar lesion, alcohol intoxication)
- Circumduction (hemiplegia)
- Scissoring (hydrocephalus and spastic paraplegia)
- High stepping (foot drop)
- Waddling (proximal muscular dystrophy)
- Festinant (parkinsonism)
- Hysterical (astasia-abasia)
- Stamping (posterior column defects)

NUTRITION

Nutrition is assessed by:
- Anthropometric measurements like height, weight, and body mass index (BMI)
- Mid upper arm circumference
- Subcutaneous fat (triceps skin fold thickness)
- Waist-to-hip ratio (**Table 1**)

SKELETAL HEIGHT

Skeletal height is measured from vertex to the sole of the foot.
- *Upper segment*: Distance between the top (vertex) and the upper border of pubic symphysis
- *Lower segment*: From upper border of pubic symphysis to the sole of the foot (floor)
- *Arm span*: Stretch the upper limbs horizontally outward and measure the distance between the tips of the middle fingers of the two outstretched hands
- Usually, arm span = height

Body mass index is calculated by dividing weight in kilograms by square of the height in meters (**Table 2**).

TABLE 1 Waist-to-hip ratio.

Waist-to-hip ratio	Type of obesity	Prognosis
0.8 or less	Pear-shaped obesity	Good
0.9 or greater	Apple-shaped obesity	Greater risk of developing complications of obesity

TABLE 2 Body mass index (BMI) kg/m².

Category	WHO criteria	Indian criteria
Normal	18–25	18–23
Over weight	<30 (26–29)	≤25
Obesity	>30 (30–39)	<25
Morbid obesity	>40	≥32.5

TABLE 3 Body mass index (BMI) and undernutrition.

Severity or grade	Percentage reduction	BMI level
Mild	From 90 to 81%	From 20 to 18 kg/m²
Moderate	80–71%	18–16 kg/m²
Severe	<70%	<16 kg/m²

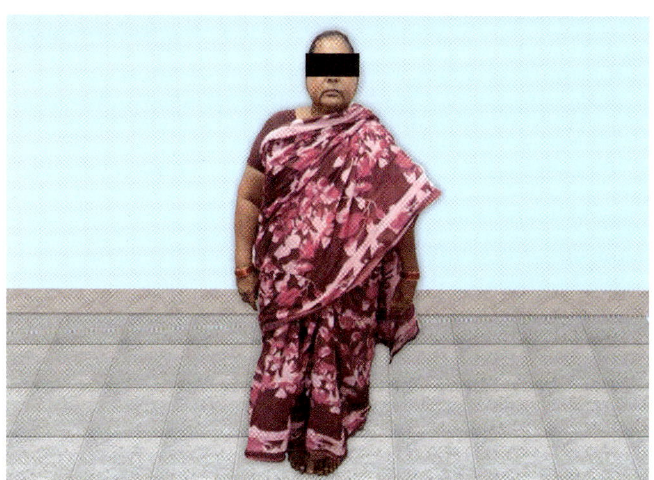

(BMI: body mass index; CAD: coronary artery disease; T2DM: type 2 diabetes mellitus; HTN: hypertension)

FIGURE 1: Morbid obesity—Female 58 years with T2DM, HTN, CAD, height 138 cm, weight 78 kg, BMI 40.96.

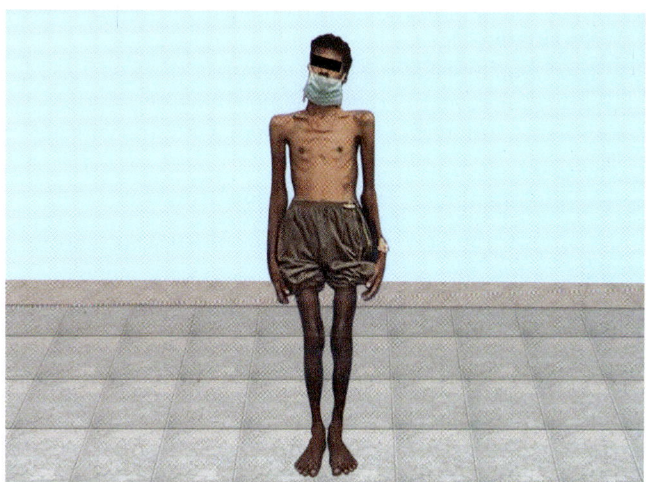

(BMI: body mass index; TB: tuberculosis)

FIGURE 2: Advanced pulmonary TB—Male 25 years, height: 171 cm, weight 40 kg, BMI 13.72 kg/m².

- Body mass index > 30 kg/m² indicates obesity and those individuals require weight reduction measures (**Fig. 1**).
- Body mass index < 18 kg/m² indicates undernutrition (TB and HIV) and requires nutritional supplementation (**Fig. 2**) (**Table 3**).

Tall stature (height >97th percentile of the normal population, >7 feet):

Causes of tall stature:
- Constitutional (just like other family members)
- Homocystinuria
- Marfan syndrome
- Klinefelter syndrome

Short stature (when an adult is <4 feet):

Causes of short stature:
- Turner syndrome [chromosomal disorder (45 XO)]
- Cretinism
- Achondroplasia (built stocky and short)
- Malabsorption syndrome (celiac disease)—actual height less than the expected figure as per age

Marfan syndrome is of clinical importance and characterized by:
- Arm span more than height
- *Metacarpal index*: More than 8.4 is suggestive of Marfan's
- Thumb sign, wrist sign, and arachnodactyly are positive, high arched palate
- Subluxation of lens (ectopia lentis)
- Aneurysm of aorta—dilatation of ascending aorta and mitral valve prolapse (MVP)

SPINE

- Kyphosis (tuberculous spine and ankylosing spondylitis)
- Scoliosis (long-standing cerebellar lesion)
- Kypho-Scoliosis (Friedreich's ataxia)

VITAL PARAMETERS

Pulse:

Rate:
- *Adults (age 18 and over)*: 60–100 beats/min.
- *Bradycardia*: Pulse rate is ≤60 beats/min.
- *Tachycardia*: Pulse rate is ≥100 beats/min.

Rhythm: Normally, it is regular. However, at times, it can be irregular, regularly irregular (second degree heart block), or irregularly irregular (atrial fibrillation, multiple premature ventricular contractions (PVCs), and supraventricular tachycardia (SVT) with varying block etc.).

Volume:
- The pulse volume roughly corresponds to pulse pressure (normal 40 mm Hg)
- High volume pulse [severe mitral regurgitation (MR) or aortic regurgitation (AR)]
- Low volume pulse [severe mitral stenosis and severe aortic stenosis (AS)]

Special character: Some important examples are:

- *Slow rise and slow fall with sustained summit*: Anacrotic pulse (AS)
- *Rapid rise and rapid fall and ill-sustained summit collapsing pulse*: AR and severe MR
- *Pulsus bisferiens (two peaks in systole)*: Hypertrophic obstructive cardiomyopathy (HOCM), severe AR, and moderate AS with severe AR
- *Pulsus paradoxus*: When the systolic pressure falls >10 mm Hg during inspiration, the pulse is referred to as pulsus paradoxus (bronchospasm and cardiac tamponade).
- Vessel wall thickening (due to aging)
- Radio radial and radiofemoral delay:
  - Radio radial delay (supravalvular AS and pulseless disease)
  - Radiofemoral delay (coarctation of aorta)

Different sites: Radial, brachial, left subclavian, carotid, femoral, popliteal, posterior tibial, and dorsalis pedis

Blood pressure:

- Normal 120/80 mm Hg
- It should be taken in all 4 limbs initially. Later, right or left upper limb, whichever shows a higher reading.
- Eighth Joint National Committee (JNC VIII) is referred to tell whether an individual is hypertensive (**Table 4**).

Hypertension:

- Hypertensive emergencies
- *Primary (essential) hypertension*: It runs in families.
- *Secondary*: Hyperthyroidism, hypothyroidism, chronic kidney disease, renal artery stenosis, pheochromocytoma, Cushing's syndrome, chronic use of corticosteroids, or nonsteroidal anti-inflammatory drugs (NSAIDs).

Hypotension:

- Anaphylaxis
- Cardiogenic shock
- Hypovolemia
- Cardiac tamponade
- Adrenal insufficiency (Addison's disease)
- Chronic under nutrition

Respiratory rate:

- Normal respiratory rate (RR) is 18 breaths/min (range 16–22 breaths/min), RR >22 breaths/min is called tachypnea, RR <14 breaths/min is bradypnea

TABLE 4 Eighth Joint National Committee (JNC VIII) classification of hypertension.

Category	Systolic (mm Hg)	Diastolic (mm Hg)
Normal	<120	<80
Prehypertension	120–139	80–89
Hypertension		
Stage 1	140–159	90–99
Stage 2	≥160	≥100

- *Types of respiration*:
  - Male (abdominothoracic)
  - Female (thoracoabdominal)

Temperature:

- Normal 36.6–37.2°C (98–99°F)
- Oral temperature is commonly used in clinical practice.

Types of fever:

- *Continuous fever*: Fluctuations of temperature <1°C, does not touch baseline, e.g., lobar pneumonia, first week of typhoid
- *Remittent fever*: Fluctuations of temperature >2°C, does not touch baseline, e.g., second week of enteric fever
- *Intermittent fever*: Temperature touches normal at least once in 24 hours, e.g., malaria
- *Prolonged fever*: Fever persisting for > 7 days (*febricula)*

Types of intermittent fever:

- *Temperature touches baseline*:
  - *Quotidian*—once in 24 hours
  - *Tertian*—once in 48 hours
  - *Quartan*—once in every 72 hours
- *Hyperpyrexia*: Common in cerebral malaria, lobar pneumonia, and sepsis syndrome
- *Hypothermia*: Seen in myxedema coma, exposure to severe cold

Relapsing fever: A fever occurring in bouts lasting for days with afebrile phases is called relapsing fever (Pel-Ebstein fever in Hodgkin's disease and saddleback fever in dengue fever).

Drug fever: A prolonged fever pertaining to any type, with relative bradycardia and hypotension, usually it starts 1–3 weeks after starting the offending drug (sulfonamides, penicillins, and anticonvulsants).

PALLOR

Waxy pale appearance of skin and mucosa suggests pallor.

Causes of pallor: Anemia of severe grade, cardiogenic shock, acute severe blood loss, and severe left heart failure

Sites to look for pallor: Palpebral conjunctiva, tip and dorsum of the tongue, palms and soles, and nail bed (**Figs. 3 A** and **B**)

JAUNDICE

Yellowish discoloration of skin, mucous membranes, and sclera due to circulating bilirubin excess >2 mg/dL (**Figs. 4 A** and **B**).

Causes of jaundice:

- *Unconjugated hyperbilirubinemia* (lemon yellow) (hemolytic jaundice)
- *Conjugated hyperbilirubinemia*:
  - Hepatocellular (orange yellow)(viral hepatitis)
  - Obstructive (greenish dark yellow) (biliary stasis)

Sites to look for jaundice: Sclera, underneath the tongue, oral cavity, palms and soles, and skin

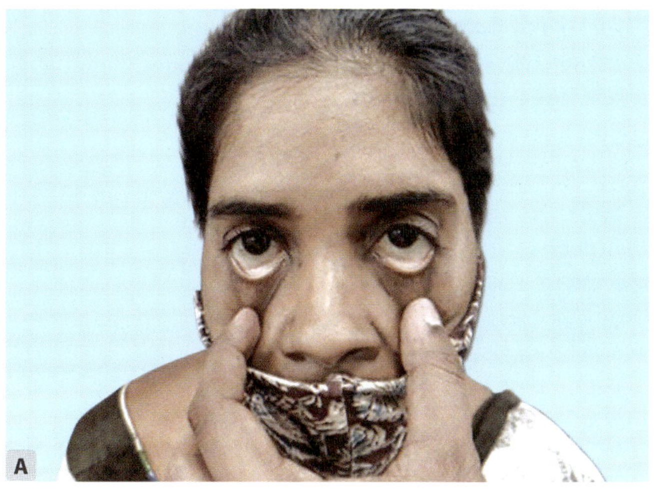

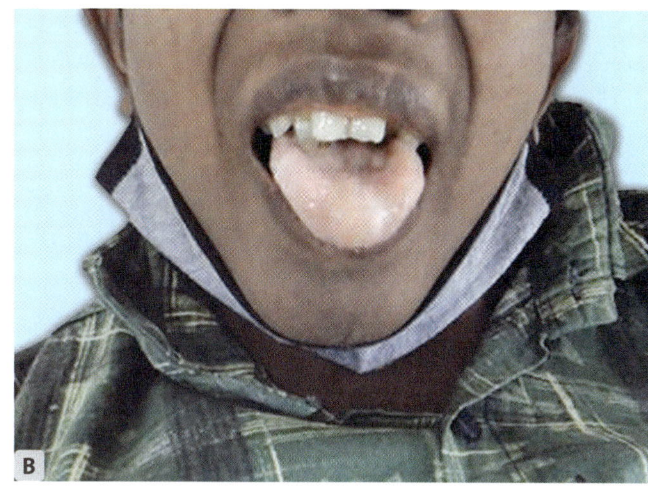

FIGURES 3 A & B: (A) Pallor due to severe anemia; (B) pallor.

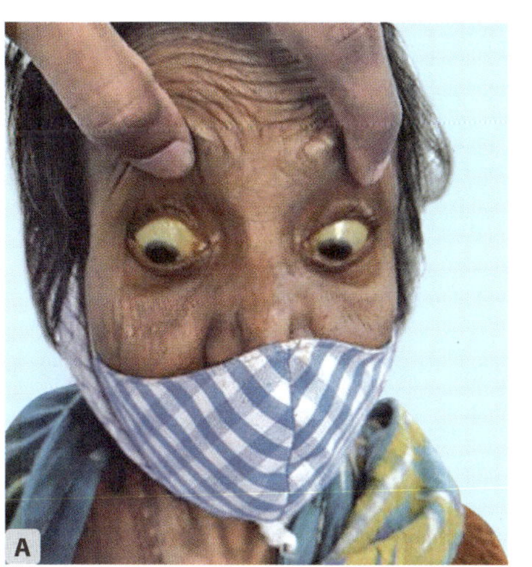

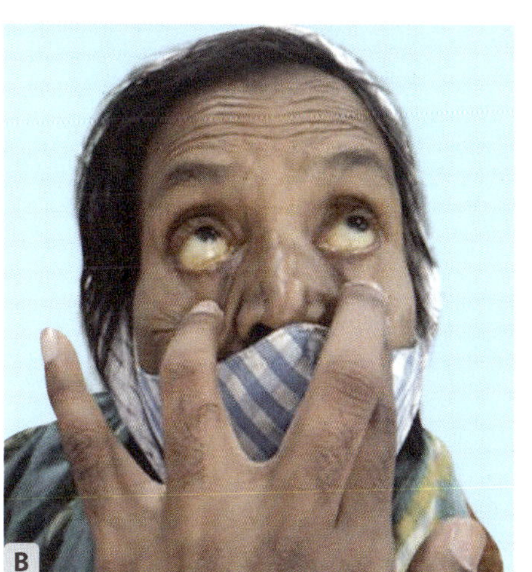

FIGURES 4 A & B: Jaundice.

CYANOSIS

Bluish discoloration of skin and mucosa, due to excess amount of reduced hemoglobin (Hb) >4 g/dL or presence of abnormal Hbs like methemoglobin and sulfhemoglobin (**Fig. 5**)

- *Central cyanosis*: Warm and cold areas, discoloration of tongue, and oral mucosa (congenital cyanotic heart disease)
- *Peripheral cyanosis*: Bluish discoloration of the cold areas of the body like fingertips, tip of the nose (exposure to severe cold)
- *Differential cyanosis*:
  - *Cyanosis seen in lower extremities* with patent ductus arteriosus (PDA) with reversal of shunt
  - *Cyanosis seen in upper extremities* with transposition of great arteries with PDA with reversal of shunt.

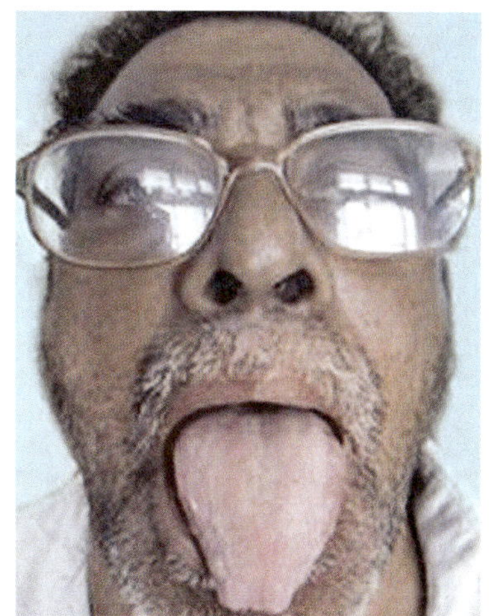

FIGURE 5: Cyanosis (methemoglobinemia).

EDEMA

Edema implies excessive collection of interstitial fluid.

- Pedal edema developing late in the evening after work indicates early stages of congestive cardiac failure (CCF).
- Early morning facial puffiness points to renal insufficiency (**Figs. 6** and **7 A** and **B**).

Types of edema:

- *Soft pitting edema*: Recent edema
- *Non pitting edema*: Myxedema and filarial edema
- *Unilateral pedal edema*: Filarial, deep vein thrombosis (DVT), inflammatory [immune mediated or presence of infection (cellulitis)] (**Figs. 7 C** and **D**). Drug-induced

bilateral pedal edema can be caused by calcium channel blockers.

Anasarca: Wet beriberi, nephritis, and nephrotic syndrome

LYMPH NODES

Lymphatic system consists of lymph nodes, lymphatic vessels, and lymphatic tissue.

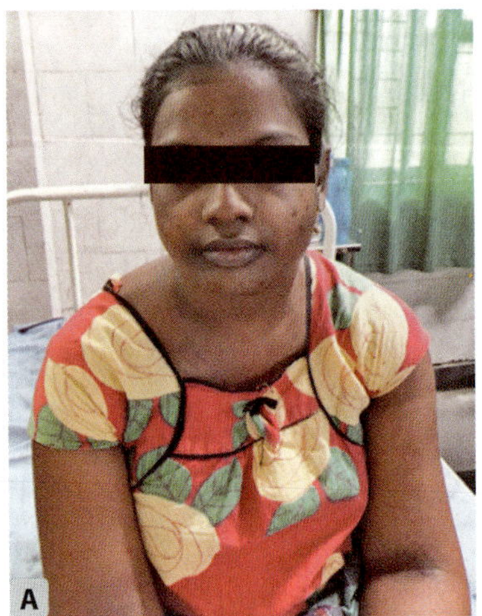

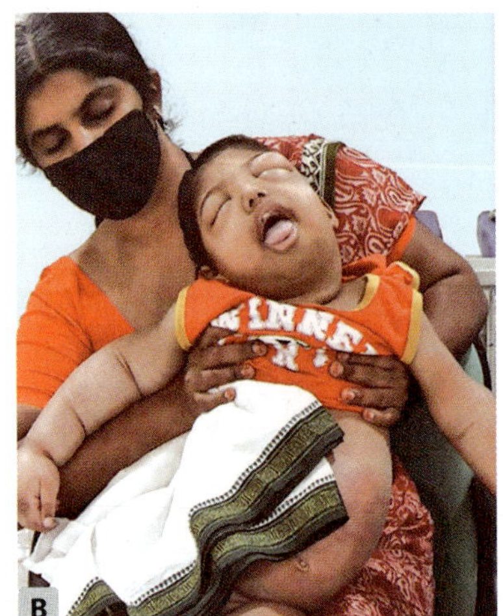

FIGURES 6 A & B: (A) Anasarca; (B) anasarca child with nephrotic syndrome.

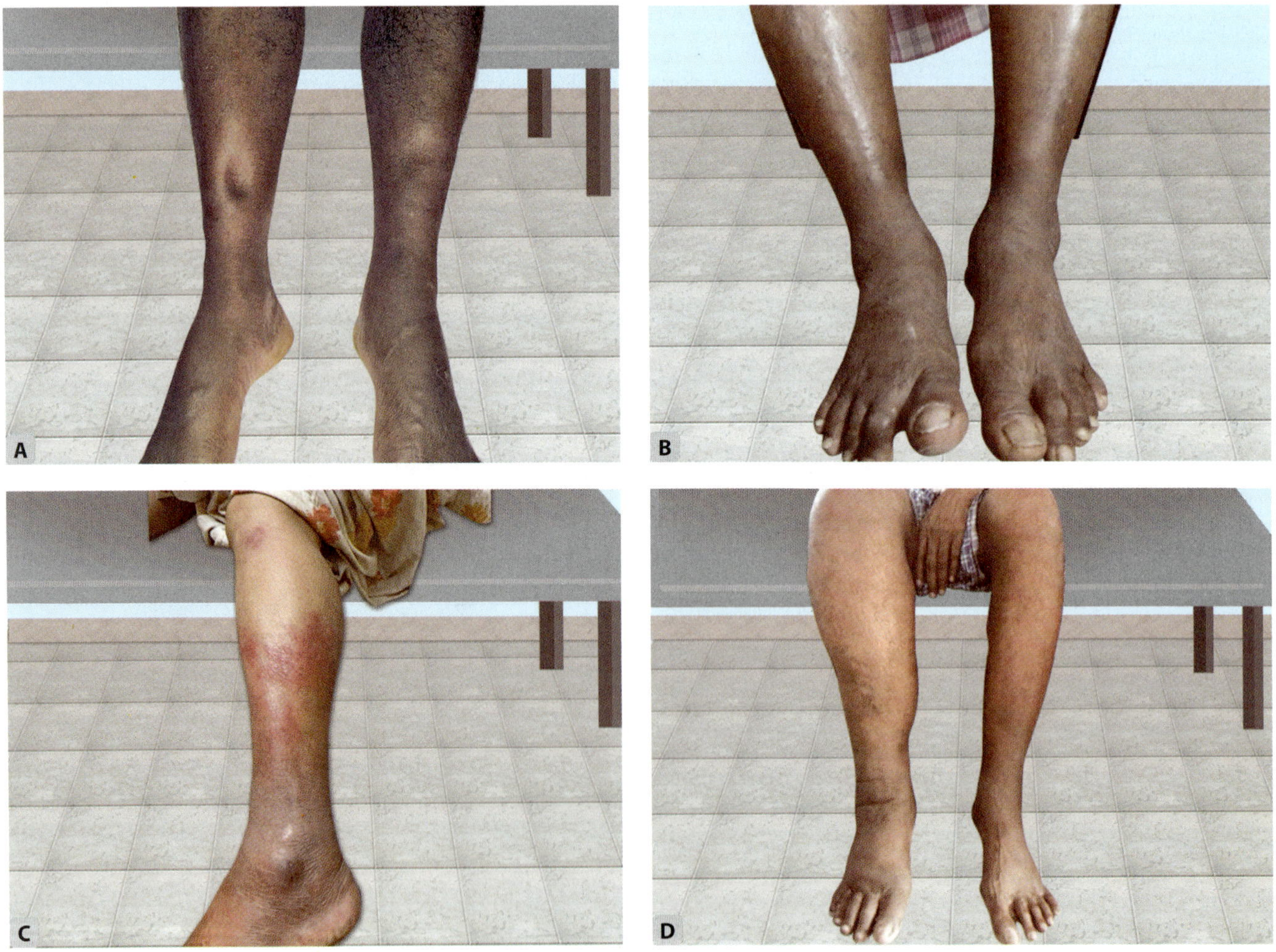

FIGURES 7 A to D: **(A)** Bilateral pedal edema; **(B)** inflammatory edema; **(C)** cellulitis left leg; and **(D)** filarial leg (right) unilateral edema.

Peripheral lymph nodes present at different regions: Cervical, axillary, mediastinal, abdominal, and inguinal. Diagnostic approach to lymphadenopathy is covered in the chapter "Lymphadenopathy: Causes and evaluation (Chapter 6)."

EXAMINATION OF FACE AND NECK

Hairline, eyes, eyebrows, nose, ears, parotid glands, and short neck.

Hypertelorism: [(The distance between the two mid-pupillary regions is increased (**Figs. 8 A** and **B**)].
- Supravalvular AS
- Noonan syndrome
- Turner syndrome
- Congenital—baby born to mother taking antiepileptics

Different types of facial appearances:
- Cushing's syndrome (Moon face)
- Acromegaly—frontal bossing with prognathism (**Fig. 9**)
- *Hippocratic facies*: In terminal stages of illness (shrunken eyes, dry skin, with flattening of cheeks)

Enophthalmos (inward movement of eyeball):
- Horner's syndrome (associated anhidrosis, miosis, and ptosis)
- Severe emaciation (entire body luster less, decreased weight)
- Extreme dehydration (associated dry tongue and loss of skin turgor)

Eyebrows: Lateral parts of the eye brows are lost in hypothyroidism.

Certain characteristic faces:
- *Mitral facies*: Malar flush with peripheral cyanosis
- *Saddle nose with rhagades*: Congenital syphilis
- *Frontal bossing* with thalassemia major

Plethoric facies with erythematous face:
- Alcoholism
- Cushing's syndrome

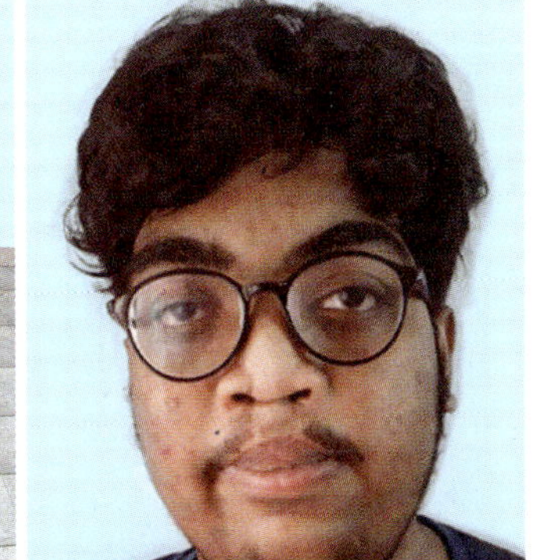

FIGURES 8 A & B: (A) Cleft lip, cleft palate, hypertelorism, congenital nystagmus in a child born to a mother taking antiepileptics during pregnancy; **(B)** Postoperative—same individual.

- Superior vena cava syndrome
- Polycythemia vera

Face with heliotrope rash (violet or bluish-purple rash):
- Juvenile dermatomyositis
- Photodermatosis
- Polycythemia rubra vera

Face with butter fly/malar rash (**Fig. 10**): Systemic lupus erythematosus (SLE), Lyme disease, pellagra, and sun exposure.

Bilateral parotid swellings: Mumps, Sjögren's syndrome, Sarcoidosis, and chronic alcoholism.

ORAL CAVITY EXAMINATION

- High arched palate (usually associated with congenital disorders)
- Leukoplakia (precancerous)
- Teeth and gums (dental caries, abscess, and gingivitis)
- Tonsils (infected and enlarged)

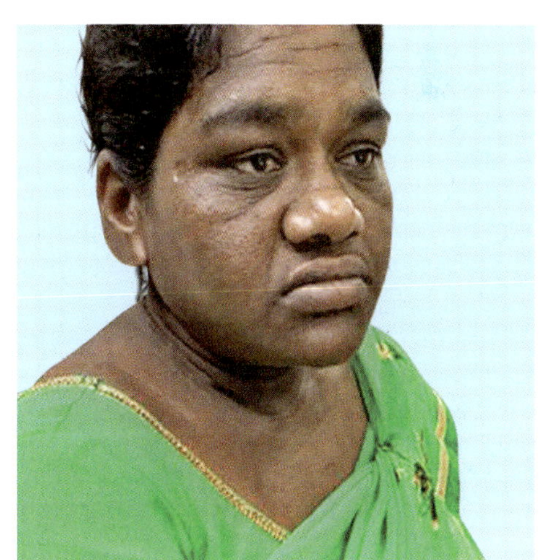

FIGURE 9: Acromegaly.

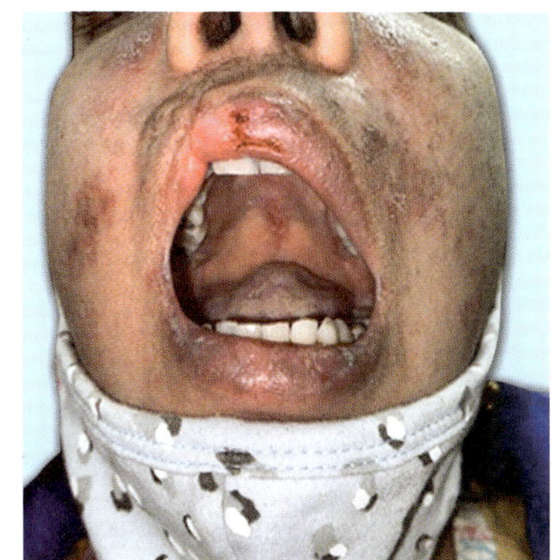

(SLE: systemic lupus erythematosus)

FIGURE 10: Malar rash, oral ulcer (SLE).

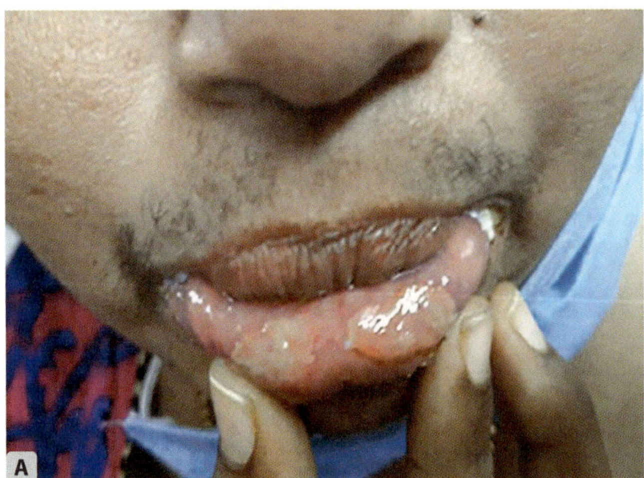

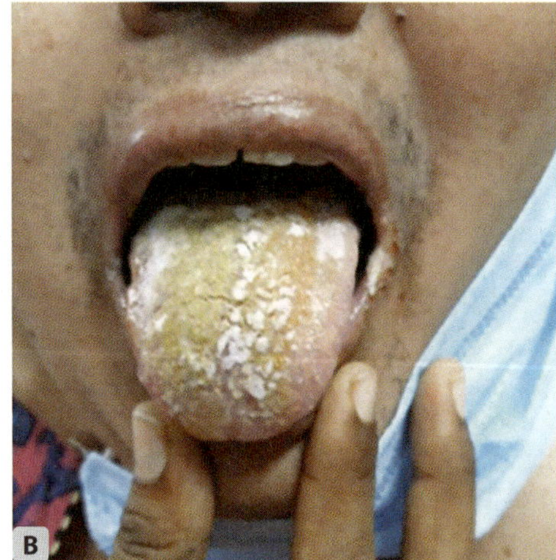

FIGURES 11 A & B: **(A)** Oral candidiasis; **(B)** COVID-19 with steroid therapy oral candidiasis and hirsutism.

- Tongue (ulcers, coating, oral candidiasis, and movements) (**Figs. 11 A** and **B**)
- Low-set ears with Down syndrome

NECK

- Thyroid selling (Goiter) (**Fig. 12**)
- Palpable lymph nodes (cervical group)
- *Short neck*: Klippel-Feil syndrome and Morquio syndrome
- The ratio of height to the distance between external occipital protuberance and C2 spinous process (Bird's index) ≤12.8 is normal, so if it is ≥13.6 indicates short neck.
- Webbed neck (Noonan syndrome, Turner syndrome and Trisomy 18, and Edward syndrome)
- Low-set hair line (Noonan syndrome, Turner syndrome, Klippel-Feil syndrome, and Cornelia de Lange syndrome)
- Low hairline is said to be present when the posterior hairline extends below the level of C5 spinous process or the ratio of distance from external occipital protuberance to the hair line and the distance from the hairline to C7 spinous process is >1/6 in males and >1/4 in females.

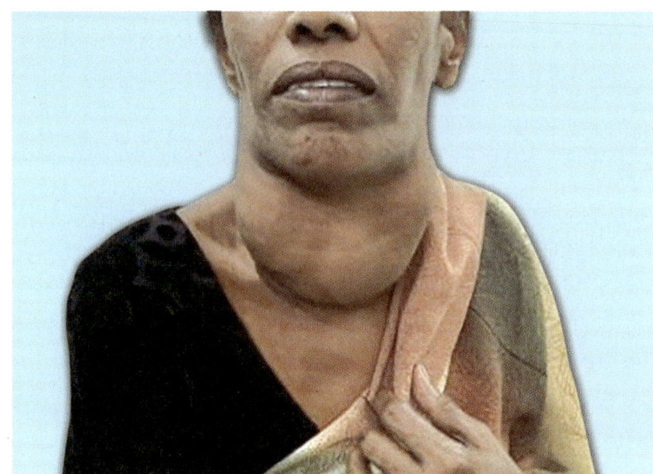

FIGURE 12: **Goiter.**

HAND

- Palmar erythema (cirrhosis of liver)
- Short trident hand, clinodactyly, polydactyly, syndactyly, arachnodactyly, and webbed fingers
- *Deformities*: Boutonniere defect, Z-deformity in rheumatoid arthritis, and Heberden's nodes (osteoarthritis) (**Fig. 13**)

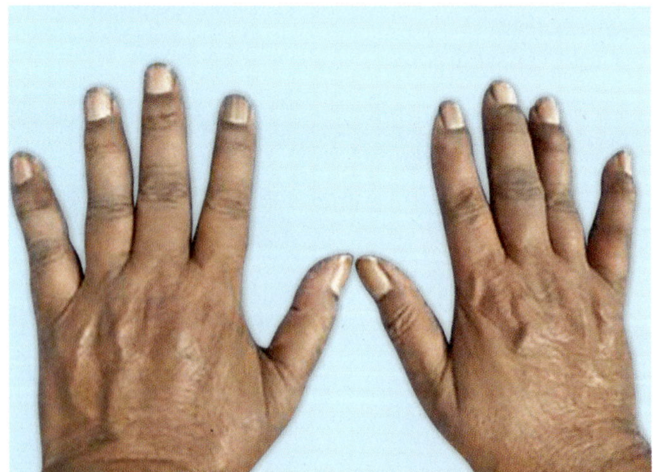

FIGURE 13: **Osteoarthritis—Heberden's nodes.**

NAILS

Clubbing, koilonychia, half-and-half nails, splinter hemorrhages, and pitting of nails.

Clubbing: Bulbous proliferation of subungual tissue is called clubbing.

Causes: Infective endocarditis, cirrhosis, lung abscess, cyanotic congenital heart disease, Empyema, bronchogenic carcinoma etc. (**Figs. 14** and **15**).

Grades:

- Grade 1—obliteration of the Lovibond's angle
- Grade 2—fluctuation
- Grade 3—parrot beak/drumstick appearance
- Grade 4—drum stick appearance

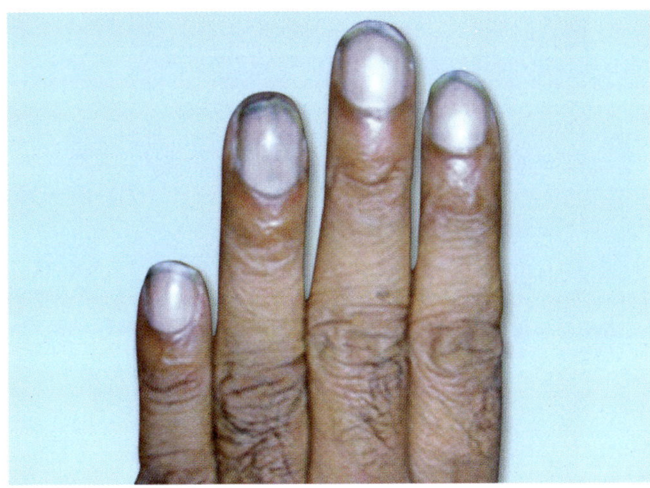

FIGURE. 14: Cyanosis and clubbing (methemoglobinemia).

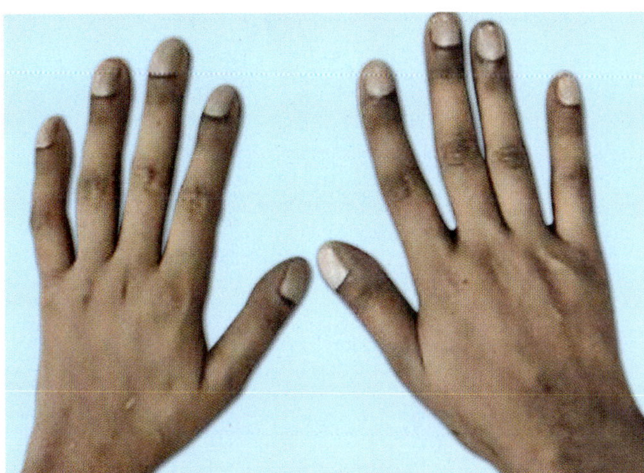

FIGURE 15: Digital clubbing.

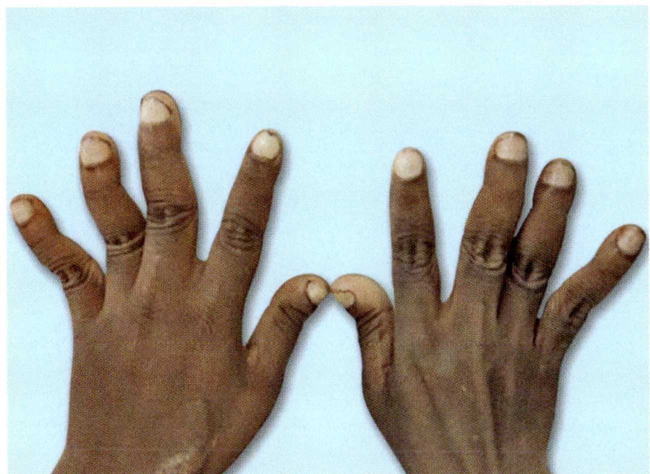

FIGURE 16: Leukonychia with deformity (connective tissue disorder).

Hypertrophic osteoarthropathy is now not considered to be a grade of clubbing.

Koilonychia: Spoon-shaped nails with iron deficiency anemia.

Splinter hemorrhages: Linear subungual hemorrhage on longitudinal direction of the nail (infective endocarditis) and transverse direction (trichinosis).

Half-and-half nails: Associated with chronic renal failure (distal—brown) and (proximal-dull tint) of the nail.

Leukonychia: White nails seen in cases with hypoalbuminemia (cirrhosis of liver), severe anemia (**Fig. 16**).

Pitting of nails: Small punctate depressions on the nail plate, seen in cases of psoriasis is given the name pitting of nails. Also seen in sarcoidosis, alopecia areata, eczema.

FEET

- Genu varum (achondroplasia, osteogenesis imperfecta)
- Genu valgum (rickets, Laurence-Moon-Biedl syndrome)
- Pes cavus, pes planus, and polydactyly
- Nail changes (clubbing and koilonychias)

SKIN

- Skin is considered as mirror of systemic disease.
- Examination of skin will reveal specific signs.

Primary skin lesions (Figs. 17 to 19):
- Macule (flat lesions <1 cm)
- *Papule*: Palpable elevated solid lesion (<1 cm)
- Maculopapular (presence of macules and papules)
- Vesicles (fluid filled lesions <1 cm)
- Bulla (>1 cm filled elevation) (**Fig. 16**)
- Plaque (papular lesion >1 cm)
- Patch (larger macule >2 cm)
- Nodule (solid lesion >1 cm)

Secondary lesions (Fig. 20):
- Scale, scar, crust, abrasion, eschar, fissure, and ulcer
- Eschar is a blackened scar with regional lymphadenopathy (scrub typhus).

Hyperpigmentation:
- *Megaloblastic anemia*, Addison's disease (**Fig. 21**), chronic liver disease, and hemochromatosis
- *Flushing of skin*: *Polycythemia vera, carcinoid, and alcoholism*

*Hypopigmented lesions (**Figs. 22 to 24**)*: Tinea versicolor, Ash leaf macules, Hansen's disease, and vitiligo.

Some skin markers:
- Café-au-lait spots (neurofibromatosis)
- Butterfly rash over face (SLE)
- Livedo reticularis (antiphospholipid syndrome)
- Dry skin and palmar erythema (cirrhosis)
- Striae and acne (Cushing's syndrome)
- Acanthosis nigricans (insulin resistance)
- Cutaneous bleeds (hematological—thrombocytopenia)
  - Petechiae <2 mm (**Fig. 25 A**)
  - Purpura 2–5 mm in size
  - Ecchymosis >5 mm in size (**Fig. 25 B**)

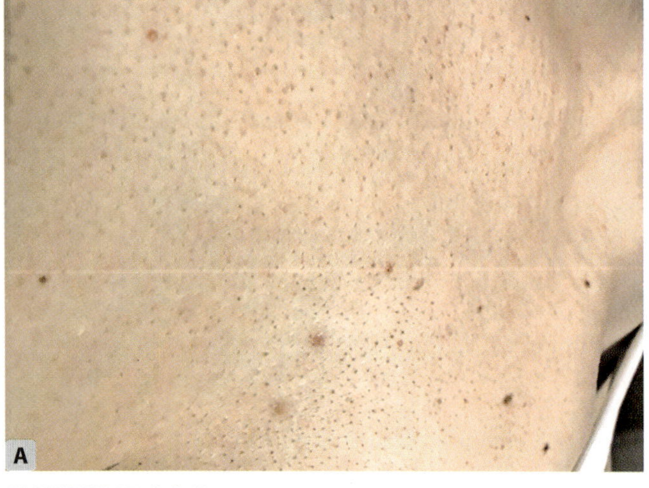

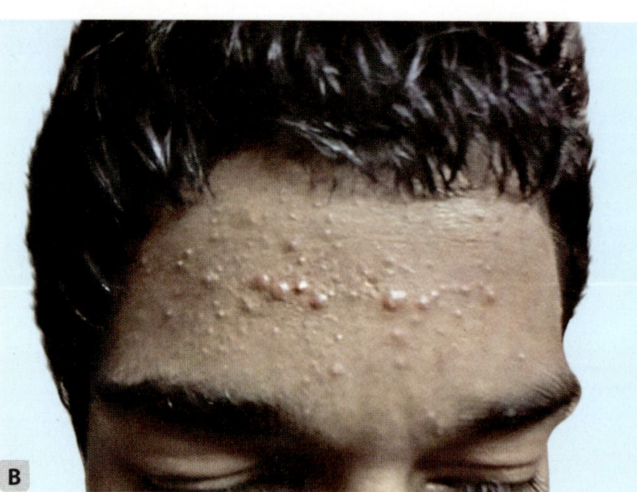

FIGURES 17 A & B: **(A) Papules; (B) nodules.**

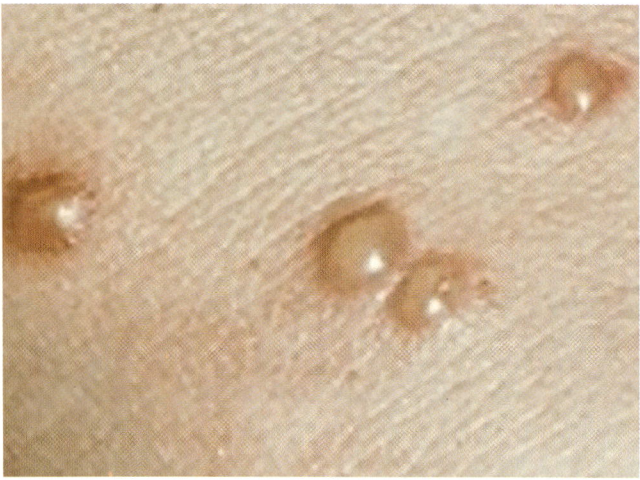

FIGURE 18: **Vesicles.**

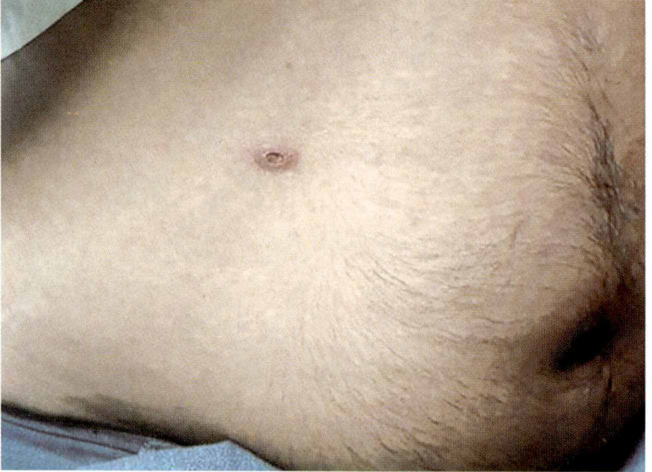

FIGURE 20: **Eschar (secondary skin lesion).**

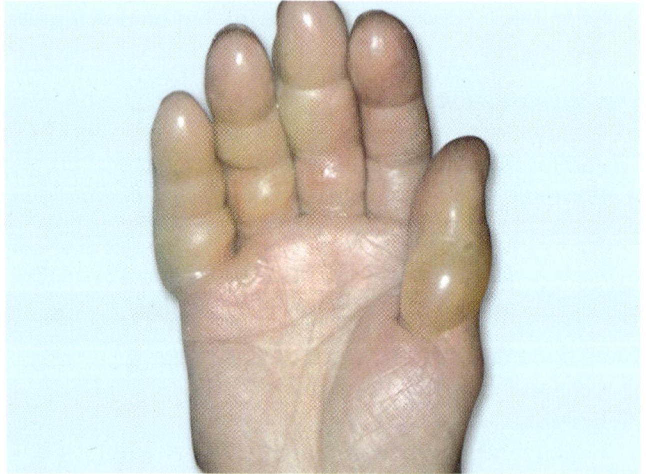

FIGURE 19: **Bullae (blisters).**

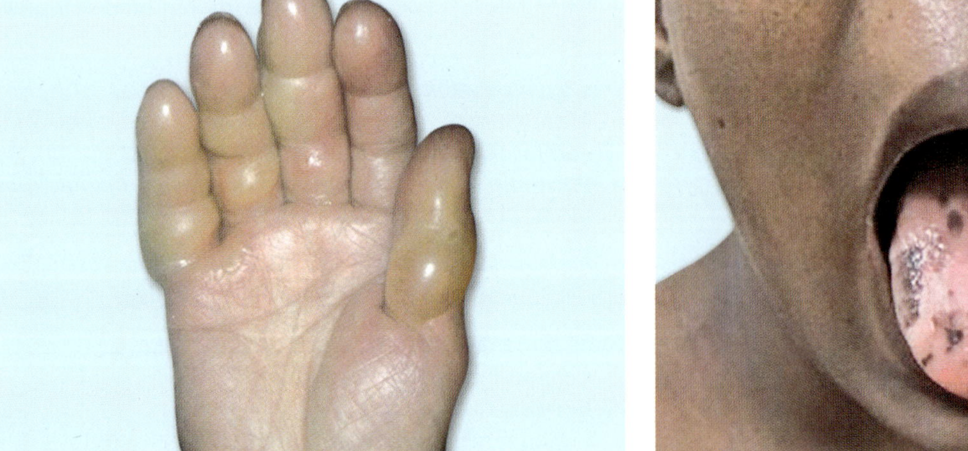

FIGURE 21: **Addison's disease.**

HAIR

Examination of hair consists of:

- Distribution (normal or abnormal)
- Alopecia (loss of hair from scalp)
- Hypertrichosis (excess hair)
- Color depends on age and race
- Hirsutism [growth of terminal hair in females similar to males (adrenal and ovarian tumors)]

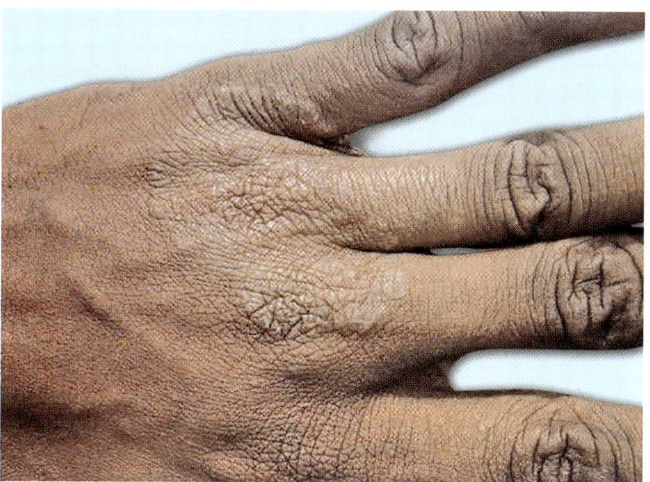

FIGURE 22: Hypopigmented patch.

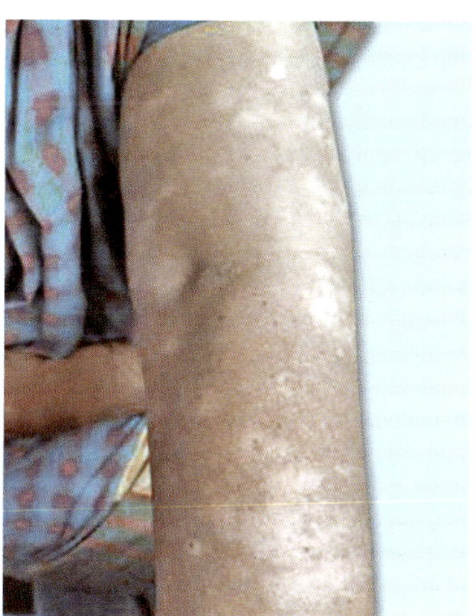

FIGURE 23: Vitiligo.

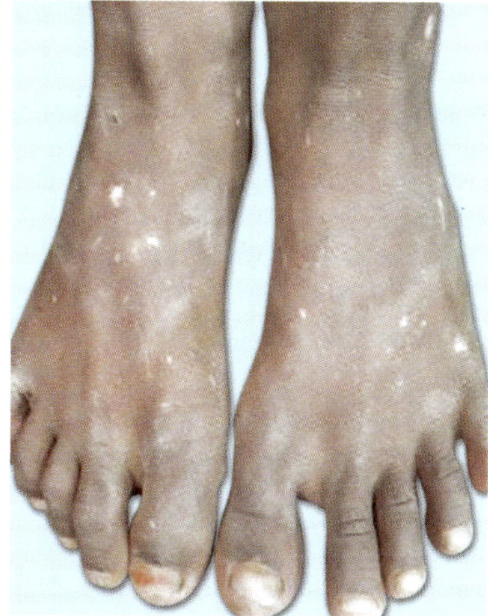

FIGURE 24: Acral vitiligo.

Head to toe examination can give clues about malnutrition, congenital abnormalities, endocrine disorders, and organ dysfunction, which along with proper history, can

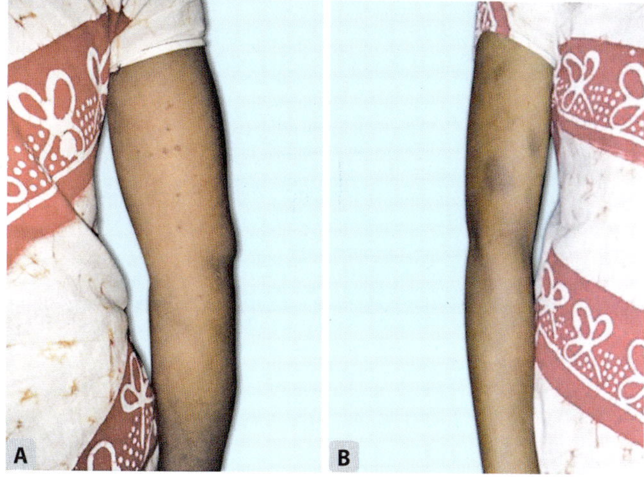

FIGURES 25 A & B: **(A)** Petechiae; **(B)** ecchymosis.

guide to identification of the abnormal system which needs detailed systemic examination in majority of the cases. Thus, clinical examination plays a vital role in making a final diagnosis and should be learnt in detail.

RECOMMENDED READINGS

1. Bellet PS, Maloney MJ. The importance of empathy as an interviewing skill in medicine. JAMA. 1991;266(13): 1831-2
2. Platt FW, Gaspar DL, Coulehan JL, Fox L, Adler AJ, Weston WW, et al. "Tell me about yourself": the patient-centered interview. Ann Intern Med. 2001;134:1079-85.
3. Roberts WC. Facts and ideas from anywhere. Proc (Bayl Univ Med Cent). 2009;22(4):377-84.
4. Kremling H. Zur entwicklung der klinischen diagnostik [Development of clinical diagnosis]. Wurzbg Medizinhist Mitt. 2004;23:233-61
5. Bailey KV, Ferro-Luzzi A. Use of body mass index of adults in assessing individual and community nutritional status. Bull World Health Organ. 1995;73(5):673-80.
6. Yallamraju SR, Mehrota R, Sinha A, Gattumeedhi SR, Gupta A, Khadse SV. Use of mid upper arm circumference for evaluation of nutritional status of OSMF patients. J Int Soc Prev Community Dent. 2014;4(Suppl 2):S122-5.
7. Kościński K. Assessment of waist-to-hip ratio attractiveness in women: an anthropometric analysis of digital silhouettes. Arch Sex Behav. 2014;43(5):989-97.
8. Sheth TN, Choudhry NK, Bowes M, Detsky AS. The relation of conjunctival pallor to the presence of anemia. J Gen Intern Med. 1997;12(2):102-6.
9. Dreizen S. The butterfly rash and the malar flush. What diseases do these signs reflect? Postgrad Med. 1991;89(1):225-34.
10. Senthilkumaran S, Balamurugan N, Karthikeyan V, Thirumalaikolndusubramanian P. Eschar–A forgotten focus of concern. J Glob Infect Dis. 2010;2(2):195-6.

CHAPTER 3

Weight Loss, Cachexia, and Fatigue: Clinical Approach and Evaluation

Y Sathyanarayana Raju, Y Rahul, Y Sairam

ABSTRACT

Clinically, important weight loss is conventionally defined as loss of >5% of usual body weight over a period of 6–12 months. Cachexia is weight loss that occurs due to loss of muscle mass (with or without fat loss). Sarcopenia, seen in the elderly, is characterized by loss of muscle mass, strength, and performance. Fatigue is a perception of generalized weakness, in the absence of objective demonstrable findings. The causes of weight loss, cachexia, and fatigue are protean. Weight loss can be unintentional or voluntary. Progressive unintentional involuntary weight loss often indicates a serious underlying medical disease or psychiatric illness and is associated with a higher mortality. The diagnostic evaluation of a patient with weight loss should be individualized, based on history and physical examination and relevant laboratory diagnostic testing. When these are inconclusive, carefully following up these patients in 1–6 months time is considered more appropriate than doing a battery of tests with a low diagnostic yield.

"The greatest discovery of all time is that a person can change his future by merely changing his attitude"

—Oprah Winfrey

INTRODUCTION

Weight loss, cachexia, and fatigue are common problems encountered by physicians in clinical practice. Weight loss may be voluntary or involuntary. Progressive involuntary weight loss points to an underlying medical illness and is associated with higher mortality. Voluntary weight loss in a normal weight person is an indicator of psychiatric disease. Cachexia derived from the Greek words *kakos* ("bad things"), and *hexus* ("state of being") is a severe form of wasting is an accelerated loss of skeletal muscle in the context of a chronic inflammatory response. Fatigue is a perception of generalized weakness, in the absence of objective demonstrable findings. In this chapter, clinical approach to and evaluation of weight loss, cachexia, and fatigue will be outlined.

ETIOLOGY

Weight loss occurs due to decreased food intake or increased energy expenditure. The causes of weight loss are protean (**Box 1**). Acute fatigue is most often seen in conjunction with an acute medical condition, or a recent life stressor. Some of the common causes of subacute and chronic fatigue are shown in **Box 2**.

DEFINITIONS

Clinically, important weight loss is conventionally defined as loss of >5% of usual body weight over 6–12 months. Cachexia is weight loss that occurs due to loss of muscle mass (with or without fat loss). Sarcopenia, seen in the elderly, is characterized by loss of muscle mass, strength, and performance. Fatigue is characterized by inability to initiate, impaired capacity to maintain activity along with reduced concentration, memory, and emotional stability.

CLINICAL APPROACH

UNINTENTIONAL OR INVOLUNTARY WEIGHT LOSS

Progressive unintentional/involuntary weight loss often points to an underlying serious medical or psychiatric illness.

Infections: In tropical countries, chronic infections are an important cause of unintentional involuntary weight loss. Unexplained weight loss is often a presenting constitutional symptom of active tuberculosis (TB), helminthic infections. Human immunodeficiency virus (HIV) infection and acquired immunodeficiency syndrome (AIDS) are associated with significant weight loss often associated with fatigue and malaise. In people living with HIV infection and AIDS (PLHA) weight loss may be episodic during the course of their illness and could be due to HIV/AIDS, secondary infections (e.g., TB) or gastrointestinal diseases, among others.

Endocrine diseases: Unintentional weight loss with increased appetite can be seen in some endocrine conditions like hyperthyroidism, poorly controlled type 1 diabetes mellitus (T1DM). In hyperthyroidism, increased catabolism, increased intestinal motility, and

BOX 1	Common causes of weight loss.
• Involuntary weight loss	
• Excessive physical activity*	
• **Medical disorders**	
○ Due to underlying malignancy	
○ Gastrointestinal tract diseases (e.g., malabsorption syndromes*, dysphagia, inflammatory bowel disease, hepatitis, Zenker's diverticulum, and paraesophageal hernia)	
○ Endocrine diseases (e.g., hyperthyroidism* uncontrolled diabetes mellitus*, and adrenal insufficiency)	
○ Infectious diseases (HIV, viral hepatitis, tuberculosis, chronic fungal or bacterial disease, chronic helminth infection, and lung abscess)	
• Severe cardiac, pulmonary or renal disease (e.g., cardiac cachexia from congestive cardiac failure; pulmonary cachexia from severe obstructive or restrictive lung disease)	
• Neurological diseases (e.g., dementia, Parkinson's disease, and amyotrophic lateral sclerosis)	
• Chronic inflammatory diseases (e.g., sarcoidosis and severe rheumatoid arthritis)	
• **Psychiatric disorders** [e.g., affective disorders (e.g., depression), anorexia nervosa, bulimia, and food-related delusional manifestations of other psychiatric diseases]	
• **Drugs, toxins,** drug-withdrawal syndromes (e.g., alcohol, cocaine, amphetamine, opiates, withdrawal after psychotropic medications; adverse effects drugs like metformin, topiramate, levodopa, digoxin, anticancer, and antiretroviral drugs)	
• Herbal and other preparations (e.g., caffeine, cascara, and herbal diuretics, nicotine)	
• **Social factors** (e.g., advertisement ramp models and professional dancers)	

*Weight loss is associated with increased appetite.

BOX 2	Common causes of subacute and chronic fatigue.
• **Cardiopulmonary disorders**	
○ Congestive heart failure	
○ Chronic obstructive pulmonary disease	
○ Sleep apnea	
• **Endocrinological disorders**	
○ Hypothyroidism	
○ Hyperthyroidism	
○ Adrenal insufficiency	
• **Metabolic diseases, electrolyte abnormalities**	
○ Chronic kidney disease	
○ Chronic liver disease	
○ Hyponatremia	
○ Hypercalcemia	
• **Hematological/oncological**	
○ Anemia	
○ Underlying malignancy	
• **Infections**	
○ Tuberculosis	
○ HIV/AIDS	
○ Viral hepatitis	
○ Subacute bacterial endocarditis	
• **Psychiatric diseases disorders**	
○ Depression	
○ Anxiety	
○ Somatization disorder	
• **Rheumatological disorders**	
○ Fibromyalgia rheumatica	
○ Polymyalgia	
○ Chronic fatigue syndrome	
• **Drug toxicity** (e.g., benzodiazepines, antidepressants, muscle relaxants, first-generation antihistamines, and beta-blockers)	
• **Substance abuse** (e.g., alcohol)	

malabsorption all contribute to weight loss. Unintentional weight loss up to 16% of usual body weight has been described in hyperthyroidism. However, weight is usually regained rapidly with appropriate treatment.

Weight loss is common with new onset T1DM; patients with type 2 diabetes mellitus (T2DM) rarely present with unintentional progressive weight loss. Anorexia, malabsorption, gastroparesis, enteropathy, diabetic neuropathic cachexia, among others are thought to be underlying mechanisms.

Primary adrenal insufficiency often presents with significant weight loss, anorexia, lassitude, fatigue, and weakness. Occasionally, a small proportion of patients with classical hyperparathyroidism, pheochromocytoma can also present with weight loss.

Gastrointestinal diseases: Gastrointestinal diseases are a common cause of progressive unintentional weight loss. Several gastrointestinal diseases can present with unintentional weight loss; the underlying mechanisms are multifactorial. Often, patients with malabsorption may present with weight loss with increased or normal appetite. However, weight loss is rare in coeliac disease. Weight loss may be evident in patients with inflammatory bowel disease as an early (Crohn's disease) or late (ulcerative colitis) manifestation. In vascular insufficiency (e.g., mesenteric artery syndrome), decreased food intake due to intestinal angina can cause weight loss.

Malignancy: Weight loss, often with anorexia, is a common presenting symptom in patients with underlying malignancy. For example, significant weight loss is common in lymphoma. Several mechanisms are important in the causation of weight loss and cachexia in patients with malignancy. These include molecular mechanisms due to tumor necrosis factor-alpha, interleukin (IL)-1, IL-6, among others that result in decreased muscle mass. Other factors, such as early satiety, dysphagia, abdominal pain, nausea, vomiting, malabsorption, adverse effects of chemotherapy, and radiotherapy would also contribute. However, other abnormalities are usually evident during the clinical and diagnostic evaluation; occult malignancy remains a rare cause of unintentional progressive weight loss.

Advanced systemic disease: Almost half the patients with congestive cardiac failure with New York Heart Association Class III or IV lose lean body mass and manifest weight loss and are associated with an increased mortality rate. The underlying mechanisms are anorexia, early satiety, hepatic congestion and increased levels of angiotensin II, among others. The loss of lean body mass may be masked by fluid retention. Pulmonary cachexia and chronic weight loss and malnutrition occur in 30–70% patients with chronic obstructive pulmonary disease. Increased respiratory muscle work, systemic inflammation corticosteroid treatment and immobility contribute to the loss of muscle mass. Weight loss also occurs in advanced kidney disease and this may be masked by fluid retention.

Neurological diseases like stroke, dementia, Parkinson's disease, among others can result in weight loss. Associated anorexia, alterations in cognitive function, motor dysfunction, and dysphagia are thought to contribute. Sometimes, chronic inflammatory disorders like rheumatoid arthritis and giant cell arthritis present with unintentional weight loss.

Psychiatric disease: Psychiatric illness is a common cause of unintentional weight loss. Depression, manic phase of bipolar disorder, delusions, or paranoia may develop peculiar ideations about food that lead to decreased food intake may all present with weight loss. In normal weight or underweight persons, eating disorders (anorexia nervosa, bulimia), self-induced vomiting, may result in weight loss.

Drugs and substance abuse: Several drugs, toxins, and drug-withdrawal syndromes can manifest weight loss. A careful history of over-the-counter drugs/medications (**Box 1**), remedies like and herbal medications, food additives that can contribute to weight loss must be obtained. Significant weight loss can occur after reduction or withdrawal of some antipsychotic drugs (**Box 1**). Weight loss is common with some drugs of abuse, like alcohol, cocaine, opiates, amphetamines, heavy tobacco use, among others. However, in alcoholic cirrhosis patients, ascites and fluid retention may mask weight loss.

VOLUNTARY WEIGHT LOSS

Voluntary weight loss is advised in overweight and obese patients who desire to lose weight. In normal weight or underweight subjects belonging to some vocations (e.g., advertisement ramp models, movie artistes, and professional dancers), drug/herbal medication use may be resorted to for losing weight. Gymnasts, athletes, and sports persons may engage in intense physical training to voluntarily lose weight.

EVALUATION

Given the wide range of causes for involuntary weight loss (**Box 1**), the evaluation should be individualized for the given patient based on history and physical examination. As subjective symptoms of weight loss are often unreliable, documenting objective weight loss is important. Review of earlier weight records, obtaining history from family members, friends can help. It is necessary to document the duration and pattern of weight loss including whether the weight loss has been progressive; history of diet patterns, physical activity, substance abuse, other medical, psychological, and functional factors is helpful.

In geriatric population with progressive unintentional weight loss, the *nine Ds* associated with weight loss namely, (1) *D*entition, (2) *D*ysgeusia, (3) *D*ysphagia, (4) *D*iarrhea, (5) *D*epression, (6) *D*ementia, (7) *D*isease, (8) *D*ysfunction, and (9) *D*rugs, should be sought for.

While evaluating a patient with fatigue, attention should be paid to the characteristics, severity, onset, course, duration and daily pattern, alleviating and aggravating factors, and impact on daily life should all be enquired into.

PHYSICAL EXAMINATION

A thorough clinical examination, including rectal examination may provide valuable clues to underlying systemic disease, malignancy, among others. Valuable physical examination clues, like eye signs of hyperthyroidism, Sister Mary Joseph nodule, generalized lymphadenopathy, and stigmata of nutritional deficiencies, when present, point to an underlying diagnosis.

LABORATORY TESTING

In patients with diagnostic clues on history, physical examination, further diagnostic testing should be aimed at ascertaining the suspected clinical diagnosis. Some of the useful laboratory investigations include complete hemogram, serum biochemistry including renal and liver function testing, thyroid profile, oral glucose tolerance test, hemoglobin A1c, urinalysis, stool for occult blood, tests for malabsorption syndrome, age-appropriate malignancy screening, among others. Diagnostic imaging initially includes chest radiograph, abdominal ultrasonography, and later on other modalities like computed tomography (CT), positron emission tomography (PET)-CT etc., as deemed appropriate. Upper gastrointestinal endoscopy and colonoscopy are done where indicated.

Further evaluation is based on results of these tests. Often, in spite of all these investigations, cause for weight loss is not evident. When these are inconclusive, carefully following up these patients in 1–6 months time is considered more appropriate than doing a battery of tests with a low diagnostic yield.

MANAGEMENT

The specific treatment of weight loss depends on the etiological cause specific underlying cause. Treatment strategies include pharmacological treatment (e.g., infections and endocrinopathies), surgery, radiation, chemotherapy (e.g., malignancy), behavioral therapy (e.g., depression and anorexia nervosa), taking off offending agents (e.g., laxatives), among others.

Goals of management of fatigue include accomplishing activities of daily living ensuring interpersonal relationships are maintained and return to work as soon as possible. Exercise therapy, treatment with antidepressants, cognitive behavior therapy should be instituted where appropriate.

RECOMMENDED READINGS

1. Wong CJ. Involuntary weight loss. Med Clin North Am. 2014;98:625-43.
2. Baracos VE, Martin L, Korc M, Guttridge DC, Fearon KCH. Cancer-associated cachexia. Nat Rev Dis Primers. 2018;4:17105.
3. Cruz-Jentoft AJ, Baeyens JP, Bauer JM, Boirie Y, Cederholm T, Landi F, et al. Sarcopenia: European consensus on definition and diagnosis: Report of the European Working Group on Sarcopenia in Older People. Age Ageing. 2010;39:412-23.
4. Nijrolder I, van der Windt D, de Vries H, van der Horst H. Diagnoses during follow-up of patients presenting with fatigue in primary care. CMAJ. 2009;181:683-7.
5. Cathébras PJ, Robbins JM, Kirmayer LJ, Hayton BC. Fatigue in primary care: prevalence, psychiatric comorbidity, illness behavior, and outcome. J Gen Intern Med. 1992;7:276-86.

CHAPTER 4 Abdominal Pain: Evaluation and Management

Sanchit Kumar, Gaurav Gupta, Sanjeev Sinha

ABSTRACT

Abdominal pain is a commonly encountered symptom in the emergency and outpatient departments. A knowledge of the underlying mechanisms and common causes with due diligence in ruling out sinister pathologies enables adequate patient care. Rapid diagnostic work-up to confirm the etiology of acute and chronic abdominal pain involves judicious use of laboratory investigations, including imaging modalities like radiography, ultrasonography, computed tomography (CT), and magnetic resonance imaging with interventional procedures being required in certain situations. Early diagnosis facilitates early institution of appropriate specific treatment and can be lifesaving.

"Treatment without prevention is simply unsustainable."

—Bill Gates

INTRODUCTION

Acute abdominal pain is defined as pain that has been occurring for no more than several days, subacute if occurring continuously/intermittently from several days to <6 months, and chronic abdominal pain if lasting >6 months continuously/episodically.

Acute abdominal pain accounts for 10–14% of visits to the emergency departments while chronic abdominal pain has an incidence of 22.3/1,000 person-years with a prevalence between 8% and 54%.

PATHOGENESIS

INNERVATION

Visceral afferents include vagal afferent nerves and spinal visceral sensory nerves. Spinal afferents may be splanchnic nerves (following sympathetic efferent pathways, containing Aδ and C type nerve fibers) or pelvic visceral afferents (running with parasympathetic efferents).

Somatic spinal nerves correspond to the T6–T12 spinal segments with small parts of the diaphragmatic peritoneum being innervated by branches from 6th to 8th intercostal nerves. Small area near the central diaphragm also receives innervation from the phrenic nerve (C3–C5). The parietal peritoneum of the true pelvis has large contributions from the obturator nerve (L2–L4).

MECHANISM OF PAIN

Distension, stretch, chemical irritation, and inflammation are stimuli for pain with factors such as inflammation, lowering threshold for pain where non-noxious stimuli may be perceived as painful.

TYPES OF PAIN

Visceral pain: Sensations carried by spinal visceral nerves (also known as splanchnic nerves) are poorly localized, referred to sites distant from their origin and often perceived in the midline. This is due to splanchnic nerve endings having wide overlapping areas of innervation, relaying onto a large range of dorsal root ganglia (causing poor localization) and entering the cord bilaterally (causing pain perception in the midline). Foregut pain is usually felt in the epigastric region, midgut pain in the periumbilical region, and hindgut in the hypogastrium.

Referred pain: As visceral and somatic afferents converge onto the same spinal segment with visceral pain being poorly localized, signals originating from visceral afferents are commonly referred to the areas innervated by the somatic nerve endings with which they share spinal segment relays.

Somatic-parietal pain: Somatic-parietal pain is subserved by Aδ fibers within somatic spinal nerves and in comparison to referred/visceral pain, is more intense and precisely localized. Signals travel with spinal sensory nerves and therefore it is localized (as well as lateralized) to more precise areas.

ACUTE ABDOMINAL PAIN

ETIOLOGY

Acute abdominal pain can have a multitude of underlying causes with pretest probability of particular diagnoses being dictated by age, sex, comorbidities, and clinical presentation. The important causes with areas of typical localization are summarized in **Table 1**.

Etiology of acute abdominal pain varies as per studies with the common ones being acute appendicitis (28–38.9%), acute pancreatitis (29%), gastritis (21%), renal/ureteric colic (14–43%), and gallbladder pathologies (13–21%). Knowledge of these common presentations and associated management decisions is essential for medical practitioners.

Commonly overlooked causes of abdominal pain include cardiac ischemia, lower lobe pneumonia, pulmonary embolism, lead poisoning, hypercalcemia, hypokalemia, hypophosphatemia, adrenal insufficiency, diabetic

TABLE 1 Common etiologies of abdominal pain.

Site		Etiology	Recommended investigation
Right upper quadrant			**Ultrasonography**
	Biliary	Cholecystitis, cholelithiasis, and cholangitis	
	Hepatic	Abscess, hepatitis, and mass	
	Renal	Nephrolithiasis, pyelonephritis	
	Pulmonary	Pneumonia, embolus	
	Colonic	Colitis, diverticulitis	
Epigastric			-
	Cardiac	Myocardial infarction/ischemia, pericarditis	
	Vascular	Aortic dissection, mesenteric ischemia	
	Gastric	PUD, GERD, and esophagitis	
	Pancreatic	Pancreatitis, mass	
	Biliary	Cholecystitis, cholelithiasis, and cholangitis	
Left upper quadrant			**CT scan**
	Cardiac	Myocardial infarction/ischemia, pericarditis	
	Vascular	Aortic dissection, mesenteric ischemia	
	Gastric	PUD, GERD, and esophagitis	
	Pancreatic	Pancreatitis, mass	
	Spleen	Infarction, abscess, and torsion	
	Renal	Nephrolithiasis, pyelonephritis	
Periumbilical			–
	Gastric	Esophagitis, PUD, GERD, small bowel obstruction/mass	
	Colonic	Early appendicitis	
	Vascular	Aortic dissection, mesenteric ischemia	
Right lower quadrant			**CT with contrast**
	Colonic	Appendicitis, colitis, diverticulitis, IBD, and IBS	
	Gynecological	Ectopic pregnancy, fibroids, ovarian mass, ovarian torsion, and pelvic inflammatory disease	
	Renal	Nephrolithiasis, pyelonephritis	

Continued...

Continued...

Site		Etiology	Recommended investigation
Suprapubic			**Ultrasonography**
	Colonic	Appendicitis, colitis, diverticulitis, IBD, and IBS	
	Gynecological	Ectopic pregnancy, fibroids, ovarian mass, ovarian torsion, and pelvic inflammatory disease	
	Renal	Nephrolithiasis, pyelonephritis	
Left lower quadrant			**CT with oral and IV contrast**
	Colonic	Colitis, diverticulitis, IBD, IBS	
	Gynecological	Ectopic pregnancy, fibroids, ovarian mass, ovarian torsion, and pelvic inflammatory disease	
	Renal	Nephrolithiasis, pyelonephritis	

(CT: computed tomography; GERD: gastroesophageal reflux disease; IBD: inflammatory bowel disease; IBS: inflammatory bowel syndrome; IV: intravenous; PUD: peptic ulcer disease)

ketoacidosis, acute intermittent porphyria, aortic aneurysms/dissections, and testicular torsion.

OVERVIEW

All cases with acute abdominal pain must be rapidly evaluated to identify compromised physiology suggestive of shock or hemodynamic instability. Attention must be paid to the presence of tachycardia, tachypnea, narrowed pulse pressure, postural symptoms, cold extremities, pallor, reduced urine output or an elevated lactate/high anion gap metabolic acidosis. Presence of these findings requires urgent intervention including fluid resuscitation, vasopressors, consideration for invasive mechanical ventilation apart from a focused workup to determine the cause.

HISTORY

As with most pain, it is useful to take a focused history using the mnemonic—SOCRATES: *S*ite, *O*nset, *C*haracter, *R*adiation/*R*eferral, *A*ssociated symptoms, *T*iming, *E*xacerbating/*R*elieving factors, and *S*everity of pain.

Onset of symptoms provides important clues to diagnoses. Acute onset of pain, especially when severe, should prompt consideration of serious diagnoses such as ruptured aortic aneurysms, perforated viscus, torsion, or mesenteric ischemia. The site and character of pain can point toward diagnoses. In general, gut pathologies have pain perceived in the midline (foregut in epigastrium, midgut in the periumbilical, and hindgut in the hypogastric region) while retroperitoneal structures may have prominent pain in the back (like aorta and kidneys). Colicky pain may be seen with intestinal obstruction and urolithiasis while sharp, boring pain is typical of acute pancreatitis.

It is extremely important to ask about flatus/feces passage, abdominal distension, and recurrent vomiting especially in cases with prior abdominal surgeries which may suggest possible intestinal obstruction. History must also be taken for urgency, frequency, dysuria, and hematuria which suggest a genitourinary source of pain. Past medical history including prior surgeries and episodes of abdominal pain may also provide help in diagnostics. Drug, menstrual, and sexual history are important (may suggest ectopic pregnancies/sexually transmitted infections as important differentials).

Based on these, several possible clues to diagnoses may be found:

- Nausea, recurrent vomiting with moderate-severe, boring pain radiating from epigastrium through to the back between interscapular region—*acute pancreatitis*
- Moderate to severe pain radiating from loin to groin—*urolithiasis*
- Dull, intense discomfort in the right upper quadrant which may radiate to the back and is exacerbated by meals—*cholelithiasis*
- Right upper quadrant pain (persisting for >6–12 h), fever, tenderness—*acute cholecystitis*
- Alcoholic with right upper quadrant pain and fever—*liver abscess (usually amebic)*
- Periumbilical pain associated with fever, nausea/vomiting, then localizing to right lower quadrant—*acute appendicitis*
- Missed menstrual period followed by lower abdominal pain/shock—*ruptured ectopic*
- Previous abdominal surgery, now with abdominal distension, and constipation/obstipation—*intestinal obstruction*

EXAMINATION

Vitals: Careful attention must be paid to the vitals in all cases of acute abdominal pain as subtle clues may be suggestive of potentially catastrophic diagnoses (like a narrowed pulse pressure in a case of a ruptured ectopic pregnancy):

Blood pressure:

- Careful evaluation for lowered mean arterial pressure, narrowed pulse pressure, or postural hypotension (fall in systolic blood pressure >20 mm Hg or diastolic blood pressure >10 mm Hg after 3 minutes of standing from a sitting/supine position)
- Patients with chronically elevated blood pressures may be in shock with apparently normal blood pressures. Therefore, it is pertinent to establish baseline blood

pressures as someone with a routine blood pressure of 170/96 mm Hg may be in shock if the presenting BP is 110/92 mm Hg without antihypertensive medications.

Heart rate: Hemorrhage, fever, sepsis, and pain may all act through the sympathetic nervous system to increase the heart rate. An elevated heart rate may be one of the first signs of hypovolemia and its presence must always be noted.

Respiratory rate: Tachypnea in a patient with acute abdominal pain may result from pain, metabolic derangements (e.g., lactic acidosis with hypovolemic shock, ketoacidosis with diabetic ketoacidosis), and impaired oxygenation [e.g., acute pancreatitis with associated acute respiratory distress syndrome (ARDS), lower lobe pneumonia, ruptured liver abscess]. Decreased respiratory rates may also be presented in cases such as opioid intoxication.

Temperature: While presence of fever may suggest systemic inflammation, its absence does not rule it out. Elderly patients especially may not mount fevers and present with decreased responsiveness and altered sensorium instead.

Oxygen saturation: It may be decreased with myocardial infarction, pneumonias, pulmonary emboli etc., which may present with abdominal pain.

Jugular venous pressure (JVP) must be assessed in all cases. If not elevated, using the hepatojugular reflex may enable recognition of occult heart failure—pressure over the upper abdomen firmly and look for increase in JVP for 10 seconds. Elevation by >4 cm through the complete 10 seconds suggests impaired cardiac function.

- General physical examination

Abdominal examination:

Inspection:

- Adequate exposure of the abdomen, ideally from the level of the nipples till the knees was traditionally advocated but is not considered acceptable in modern times. However, an abdominal examination is incomplete without evaluation of the groin and genitalia. Therefore, after proper explanation and consent (with inclusion of a female chaperone for examining female patients), these areas maybe exposed for the minimal time that they are being examined.
- Note the presence of symmetrical movements of all quadrants, scars, dilated vessels, and position of umbilicus.
- Distended abdomen with prior surgical scars suggests presence of intestinal obstruction.
- Cullen sign (periumbilical ecchymosis) and Grey Turner sign (flank ecchymosis) suggest retro-/intraperitoneal hemorrhage (e.g., from acute pancreatitis)
- Note any dermatomal vesicular rash that may suggest active Zoster infection.
- "Hipprocratic facies" may be seen in late stages of perforation peritonitis.

Palpation:

- This must proceed from areas without pain to the area with pain.
- Superficial palpation is followed by deep palpation
- All areas must be sequentially covered and a note made of any abdominal masses (hepatomegaly, splenomegaly, abdominal lymph nodes, aortic aneurysms etc.), any increase in local temperature or any tenderness.
- McBurney point tenderness (point lying one-third of the way from the anterior superior iliac spine to the navel) may be suggestive of acute appendicitis.
- Renal angle tenderness suggests pyelonephritis.
- Intercostal/thump tenderness (thumping over the right lower side of the chest) may be suggestive of a liver abscess.
- Palpation may reveal signs of an enlarged aorta which can be caused due to aneurysms and pain may suggest dissection/inflammation of the involved areas.
- Rigidity of the abdomen suggests muscle tension secondary to peritoneal irritation, likely from perforation and requires urgent intervention.

Percussion:

- Percussion allows a more sensitive method of assessing splenomegaly (using the Barkun, Nixon and Castell methods of percussion). As little as 500 mL fluid may be detected by shifting dullness on percussion.
- Rebound tenderness is elicited using percussion and suggests peritoneal irritation which may be localized (e.g., acute appendicitis) or generalized (e.g., perforation peritonitis).

Auscultation: This has a limited role in evaluation of an acute abdomen; however, presence of grossly increased bowel sounds (borborygmi) may suggest intestinal obstruction and bruits may be indicative of compromised arterial lumens.

- Symptoms disproportionate to the signs may suggest mesenteric ischemia and must never be ignored as "functional pain."

Pelvic examination:

- It may show presence of vaginal discharge and cervicitis.
- Cervical motion tenderness reflects adjoining peritoneal irritation which may be seen with pelvic inflammatory disease or inflammation involving surrounding areas such as with cystitis, appendicitis etc.
- Bimanual examination may show presence of mass suggesting fibroids or pregnancy in which complications may cause abdominal pain.
- Pain in unilateral adnexal mass may suggest ovarian torsion, ovarian cysts, tubo-ovarian abscess, or ectopic pregnancy.

Examination of the groin:

- Hernial orifices must be assessed to rule out hernia-related complications as cause for abdominal pain.
- The testes must be examined for masses (infectious or malignant), torsion and swelling (hydrocele, pyocele, and hematocele), all of which may present with abdominal pain.

Chest examination:

- The chest must always be examined after stabilization as a multitude of pathologies involving the thoracic organs can present with abdominal pain.

- Respiratory examination must evaluate position of the trachea, movements of the chest wall, any tenderness/rise of temperature, areas of impaired percussion notes, and/or altered air entry/breath sounds.
- Cardiac examination must include search for murmurs, pericardial rubs, and search for features of heart failure—low blood pressure, narrowed pulse pressure, tachycardia, pedal edema, cold extremities, crepitations on pulmonary examination from edema, raised JVP, tender hepatomegaly etc.

INVESTIGATIONS

- In general, these include a complete blood count, levels of bilirubin, alanine aminotransferase, aspartate aminotransferase, alkaline phosphatase, urea, creatinine, sodium, potassium, calcium, blood sugar, and lipase/amylase levels. Females of childbearing age should get a urine pregnancy test.
- Specific investigations including imaging and biomarkers are based on suspected pathologies. These may include electrocardiographs, troponin levels, chest radiographs/CT scans, CT angiography (including pulmonary, coronary and mesenteric vasculature), ultrasound of the kidneys/urinary bladder, ultrasound of the hepatobiliary system/pancreas etc.
- General approach to patient presenting with acute abdominal pain is given in **Flowchart 1**.

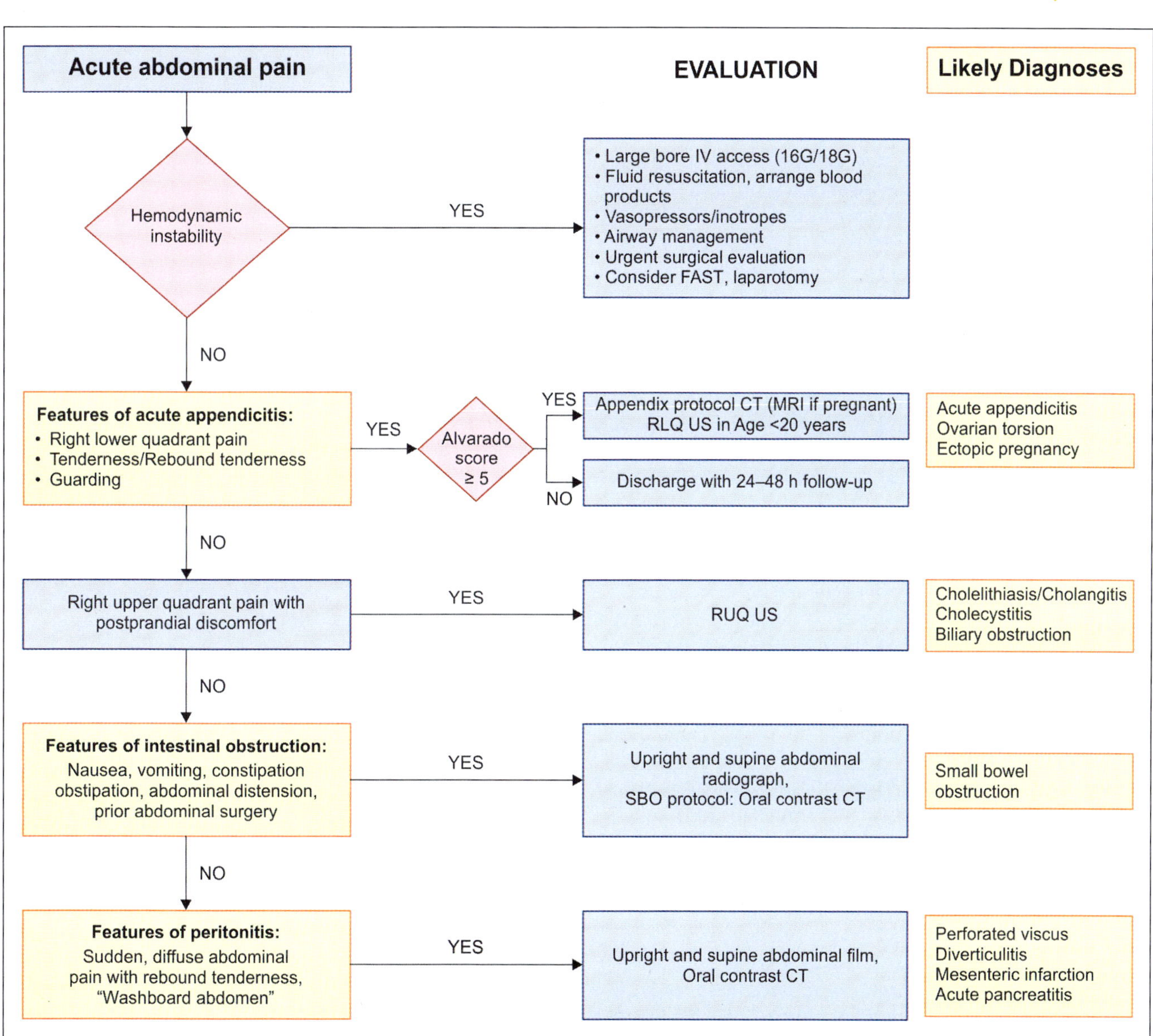

(CT: computed tomography; FAST: focused assessment with sonography in trauma; MRI: magnetic resonance imaging; RLQ: right lower quadrant; RUQ: right upper quadrant; SBO: small bowel obstruction; US: ultrasound)

FLOWCHART 1: Approach to acute abdominal pain.

Source: Adapted from Sleisenger and Fordtran's Gastrointestinal and Liver Disease, 11th edition.

MANAGEMENT

- Hemodynamic instability must be urgently addressed that includes correction of underlying metabolic derangements as definite steps are taken to address the underlying causes.
- Large bore intravenous (IV) access is crucial in those with features suggestive of hemodynamic instability. In cases with collapsed veins and difficult cannulation, urgent establishment of intraosseous or central venous access must be considered.
- Cases with shock must have blood products arranged for expected needs. It must be noted that acute bleeds do not cause a fall in hemoglobin concentration due to loss of equal amounts of plasma and red cell mass. It is only after adequate fluid resuscitation/sympathetic system and AVP mediated renal fluid retention that this deficit manifests as a fall in hemoglobin concentrations.
- Fluids and vasopressors/inotropes must be used as needed to manage shock with correction of electrolytes, acid-base disturbances, and hypoxia.
- Low Glasgow Coma Scale (<8), inability to protect airways or shock, may warrant consideration for intubation after optimizing hemodynamic parameters if the condition permits.
- Urgent consultation must be obtained from surgical teams for cases with expected requirement for surgical interventions.
- Definite management is ultimately dictated by the underlying pathology.

CHRONIC ABDOMINAL PAIN

This refers to pain lasting >6 months constantly or intermittently.

Different organ systems may cause chronic abdominal pain and a detailed history with focused examination can help guide physicians toward a diagnosis.

ETIOLOGY

Limited studies available from India show that the majority of cases of abdominal pain are due to gastrointestinal (GI) tract diseases (48%), followed by genitourinary tract (30%), functional GI disorders (11%), and hepatobiliary disease (8%). Within the GI system, the most common causes were found to be gastritis (13.5%), chronic recurrent appendicitis (11.8%), and worm infestations (8.5%). A list of important causes of chronic abdominal pain is summarized in **Table 2**.

TABLE 2 Causes of chronic abdominal pain.

Inflammatory	Vascular
• Appendicitis • Celiac disease • Diverticular disease • Eosinophilic gastroenteritis • Inflammatory bowel disease • Primary sclerosing cholangitis • Sclerosing mesenteritis • Pelvic inflammatory disease	• Celiac artery syndrome • Mesenteric Ischemia • Superior mesenteric artery syndrome **Metabolic** • Lead poisoning • Porphyria • Diabetic neuropathy
Urogenital	**Pelvic**
• Nephrolithiasis/ pyelonephritis • Pyelonephritis • Perinephric abscess	• Female reproductive tract: Pelvic inflammatory disease, ovarian cysts, malignancies • Male reproductive tract: Prostatitis, epididymitis, recurrent testicular torsion, and prostate cancer • Chronic pelvic pain: Interstitial cystitis, endometriosis, and pelvic muscle dysfunction
Neuromuscular	**Functional gastrointestinal disorders**
• Anterior cutaneous nerve entrapment • Myofascial pain syndrome • Splitting rib syndrome • Thoracic nerve radiculopathy	• Biliary pain • Irritable bowel syndrome • Levator ani syndrome • Gastroparesis
Others	
• Abdominal adhesions • Anaphylaxis • Chronic pancreatitis • Endometriosis • Gallstones • Intestinal obstruction	• Abdominal migraine • Angioedema • Cyclic vomiting syndrome • Familial Mediterranean Fever • Hernias • Lactose intolerance

Source: Adapted from Feldman M, Friedman L, Brandt L. (2020). Sleisenger and Fordtran's Gastrointestinal and Liver Disease, 11th edition, 2 Volume. [online] Available from https:// www.elsevier.com/books/sleisenger-and-fordtrans-gastrointestinal-and-liver-disease-2-volume-set/ feldman/978-0-323-60962-3.

Adapted from Ringel-Kulka T, Ringel Y. Evaluation of chronic abdominal pain. [online] Available from https:// bestpractice.bmj.com/topics/en-us/767/ pdf/767/ Evaluation%20of%20chronic%20abdominal%20pain. pdf.

HISTORY

- A detailed history is extremely important as thoughtless use of laboratory tests and imaging is unlikely to yield a proper diagnosis and has a high chance of showing incidental abnormalities that may not be the actual culprits. This can lead to excessive testing, overmedication, and loss of patient trust that hampers further evaluations.
- As with acute abdominal pain, the SOCRATES mnemonic provides the headings under which a detailed history may be elaborated.
- Knowledge of the innervation of viscera and the sites of perceived pain helps guide localization (as described in section on acute abdominal pain) of involved systems.
- Patients with chronic abdominal pain may have worsening of pain resulting from complications of underlying disorders (e.g., perforation in a case with inflammatory bowel disease) and therefore symptoms and signs of hemodynamic compromise must be sought and addressed in such cases as well.

- Bowel and bladder habits must be enquired about. Specific questioning regarding passage of worms in stool, blood/mucus in stool, blood in urine, and abnormal vaginal discharge
- History must account for sexual practices, menstrual history, pregnancy, prior abdominal surgeries, drug intake, exposure to toxins such as lead, and family history of similar disorders.
- Attention must be paid to red flags that are suggestive of major organic disorders which require more careful and detailed evaluation:
  - Fever, night sweats, loss of weight/loss of appetite
  - Nocturnal awakening
  - Blood in stool/melena, coffee ground emesis
  - Jaundice
  - Edema
  - Dysphagia/odynophagia
- Clues to diagnosis:
  - Increase in pain after meals: Gastric ulcers, gallstones, chronic mesenteric ischemia, irritable bowel syndrome, and chronic pancreatitis
  - Decrease in pain after eating: Duodenal peptic ulcer
  - Pain without red flags, associated with exaggerated gastrocolic reflex, relieved by defecation: irritable bowel syndrome

EXAMINATION

Vitals:

- These must be recorded first as with patients having acute abdominal pain and derangements can suggest worsening/complication of the underlying cause.
- Patients with hemodynamic instability often require urgent, lifesaving interventions and therefore recording of the vitals is essential to avoid missing potentially serious cases.

General physical examination:

- Temporal muscle wasting, pallor, prominent bones, and sunken eyes may suggest significant weight loss as may be seen with malignancy and etiologies causing malabsorption.
- Presence of icterus, weight loss, and right upper quadrant pain suggest a biliary source of pain.
- Presence of lead line over the gums may suggest lead toxicity.
- Hyperpigmentation over knuckles, skin creases of the hand, axillae, and oral mucosa may suggest adrenal insufficiency.
- Cold extremities with diminished pulses may be suggestive of arterial disease where involvement of abdominal vasculature may cause abdominal pain ("intestinal angina").

Abdominal examination:

Inspection:

- Exposure of the patient must follow principles highlighted previously.
- Patients must be examined for distension (5 F's: feces, flatus, fluid, fat, fetus)
- Note presence of any scars, rashes, dilated vessels, fistulas, hernial site fullness or abnormalities of the genitalia which might suggest an etiology.

Palpation:

- Must always proceed from normal to painful areas with care taken to avoid patient discomfort.
- Note must be made of tenderness or local increase in temperature.
- All quadrants must be sequentially palpated to avoid missing important findings.
- Note presence of any hepatomegaly, splenomegaly, enlarged lymph nodes, enlarged gallbladder, and pelvic masses (cannot get below the swellings).
- Presence of guarding/tenderness to palpation/rebound tenderness suggests peritoneal irritation and requires urgent investigation.

Percussion: May enable detection of small amounts of ascitic fluid, early spleen enlargement, and elicitation of rebound tenderness.

Auscultation: Limited utility in chronic abdominal pain cases. Presence of bruits may enable consideration of mesenteric arterial insufficiency.

- *Carnett's sign* is elicited by making the patients tense their abdomen and lifting their heads off the table. An intra-abdominal/visceral source of pain is suspected by a decrease in pain.

Rectal examination: It may be needed in cases such as suspected prostatitis, diverticulitis, hemorrhoids etc.

- The hernial orifices must be examined for any masses/lumps.
- Pelvic and genitalia examination may be required in cases where the genitourinary system is the likely source of the pain.

INVESTIGATIONS

Routine investigations: These may include a blood count, kidney and liver function tests, electrolytes, thyroid-stimulating hormone level, and lipase and glucose levels. Further testing may be guided by clinical suspicion and presence of red flags.

Specific investigations:

Urine analysis with/without urine cultures, stool for ova/cysts/parasites based on clinical suspicion

Disease markers: Anti-immunoglobulin A (IgA) tissue transglutaminase for celiac disease, p-antineutrophil cytoplasmic antibody (p-ANCA) for primary sclerosing cholangitis, IgG4 levels for IgG4 -related disease, fecal calprotectin for inflammatory bowel disease, and urea breath test for *Helicobacter pylori* infection maybe obtained based on clinical suspicion.

Endoscopy: This may be used judiciously in cases with chronic abdominal pain at >50 years of age. Colonoscopy may be used if predominantly lower abdominal pain/association with a microcytic-hypochromic iron deficiency anemia and upper GI endoscopy if symptoms of dysphagia/odynophagia, unintentional weight loss, overt GI bleeding, palpable mass/lymphadenopathy, persistent vomiting are present or there is family history of upper GI cancer.

Ultrasonography: For cases with right upper quadrant (RUQ)/epigastric pain where hepatobiliary/pancreatic pathologies are suspected, ultrasound examination may provide adequate assessment. Nephrolithiasis, pyelonephritis, perinephric abscesses, cystitis, and gynecological disorders may also be diagnosed using ultrasonography which is especially useful in patients with lower abdominal pain.

- Computed tomography (CT) of the abdomen/pelvis with or without contrast may help to investigate inflammatory processes (e.g., inflammatory bowel disease), retroperitoneal organs (e.g., aortic aneurysms), bowel obstruction/perforation etc.
- *Magnetic resonance cholangiopancreatography:* Useful in cases of suspected biliary pathology.

MANAGEMENT

- Definitive management is as per etiology after diagnostic workup. Patients with red flags require more frequent follow-up and more urgent investigations to rule out sinister pathologies.
- Irritable bowel syndrome is an important functional cause of chronic abdominal pain. It must be included in the differential for such presentations and has an important component of mood disturbances that must also be adequately addressed.
- Usual measures for nonspecific chronic pain include prescriptions for proton pump inhibitors, stool softeners, promoters of GI motility (e.g., metoclopramide and domperidone), antihelminth medications, and analgesics.

RECOMMENDED READINGS

1. Charles G, Chery M, Do MKC. Chronic abdominal pain: Tips for the primary care provider. Osteopathic Family Physician. 2019;11(1):7.
2. Kamin RA, Nowicki TA, Courtney DS, Powers RD. Pearls and pitfalls in the emergency department evaluation of abdominal pain. Emerg Med Clin North Am. 2003;21(1):61-72, vi.
3. Thakur JK, Kumar R. Epidemiology of acute abdominal pain: a cross-sectional study in a tertiary care hospital of Eastern India. Int Surg J. 2019;6(2):345-8.
4. Heading RC. Prevalence of upper gastrointestinal symptoms in the general population: a systematic review. Scand J Gastroenterol Suppl. 1999;231:3-8.
5. Wallander MA, Johansson S, Ruigómez A, García Rodríguez LA. Unspecified abdominal pain in primary care: the role of gastrointestinal morbidity. Int J Clin Pract. 2007;61(10):1663-70.
6. Standring S. (2015). Gray's Anatomy, 41st edition [online] Available from https://www.elsevier.com/books/grays-anatomy/standring/978-0-7020-5230-9.
7. Feldman M, Friedman L, Brandt L. (2020). Sleisenger and Fordtran's Gastrointestinal and Liver Disease, 11th edition, 2 Volume. [online] Available from https://www.elsevier.com/books/sleisenger-and-fordtrans-gastrointestinal-and-liver-disease-2-volume-set/feldman/978-0-323-60962-3.
8. Struller F, Weinreich FJ, Horvath P, Kokkalis MK, Beckert S, Königsrainer A, et al. Peritoneal innervation: embryology and functional anatomy. Pleura Peritoneum. 2017;2(4):153-61.
9. Chanana L, Jegaraj MA, Kalyaniwala K, Yadav B, Abilash K. Clinical profile of non-traumatic acute abdominal pain presenting to an adult emergency department. J Family Med Prim Care. 2015;4(3):422-5.
10. Kumar NR, Krishna BS, Satyanarayana V, Reddy VV, Madhusudhan M, Subramanyam P. Study of clinical features and outcomes in patients presenting to the emergency department with acute abdomen. J Clin Sci Res. 2019;8(4):173.
11. Sapmaz F, Başyiğit S, Başaran M, Demirci S. Non-Surgical Causes of Acute Abdominal Pain. Actual Problems of Emergency Abdominal Surgery. [online]. Available from https://www.intechopen.com/books/actual-problems-of-emergency-abdominal-surgery/non-surgical-causes-of-acute-abdominal-pain.
12. Cartwright SL, Knudson MP. Evaluation of acute abdominal pain in adults. Am Fam Physician. 2008;77(7): 971-8.
13. Macaluso CR, McNamara RM. Evaluation and management of acute abdominal pain in the emergency department. Int J Gen Med. 2012;5:789-97.
14. Schofield M, Shetty A, Spencer M, Munglani R. (2014). Pain Management: Questions and Answers [online] Available from https://www.bjfm.co.uk/pain-managment-part-1.
15. Ringel-Kulka T, Ringel Y. Evaluation of chronic abdominal pain. [online] Available from https://bestpractice.bmj.com/topics/en-us/767/pdf/767/Evaluation%20of%20chronic%20abdominal%20pain.pdf.
16. Gotfried J. (2020). Chronic Abdominal Pain and Recurrent Abdominal Pain - Gastrointestinal Disorders Merck Manuals Professional Edition. [online]. Available from https://www.merckmanuals.com/professional/gastrointestinal-disorders/symptoms-of-gastrointestinal-disorders/chronic-abdominal-pain-and-recurrent-abdominal-pain.
17. Clinical Gate. (2015). Abdominal distension. [online] Available from https://clinicalgate.com/abdominal-distension.
18. Kamboj AK, Hoversten P, Oxentenko AS. Chronic Abdominal Wall Pain: A Common Yet Overlooked Etiology of Chronic Abdominal Pain. Mayo Clinic Proceedings. 2019;94(1):139-44.

CHAPTER 5

Diarrhea and Constipation: Clinical Approach and Management

Veerappa Annasaheb Kothiwale, Vivek Veereshkumar Shirol

ABSTRACT

Diarrhea and constipation are common entities in clinical practice and are faced by clinicians all over the world. They are issues of public health importance. Thus their proper evaluation and treatment is very vital in the maintenance of proper nutrition and health in all people.

Diarrhea is defined as having three or more bowel movements in a day with abnormally liquid stools and unformed consistency. Fecal incontinence and pseudo-obstruction must be differentiated from it. Diarrhea can be classified as acute and chronic diarrhea, large volume and small volume diarrhea, osmotic and secretory diarrhea, and fatty acid diarrhea. In the evaluation of acute diarrhea, it is important to assess for red flag signs such as oliguria, dark urine, giddiness, disorientation, and blood and mucus in stools. Appropriate laboratory investigations are to be done to rule out complications like hemolytic uremic syndrome (HUS), acute kidney injury (AKI) etc. The mainstay of management is by fluid replenishment by oral or intravenous (IV) route. Antibiotics are indicated only in cases of invasive diarrhea. The evaluation of chronic diarrhea depends on the identification of organic cause. Treatment is specific for all conditions along with supplementation of essential vitamins and minerals.

Constipation is described as an unsatisfactory defecation with infrequent and difficult stool passage. It is important to rule out the secondary causes of constipation like, hypothyroidism, Parkinson disease, multiple sclerosis etc. Primary constipation is of three types: normal transit, slow transit, and rectal evacuation disorder for which colon transit tests (CTT) like radio-opaque marker study, wireless motility capsule study, and defecography are performed. Treatment is by high fiber diet, bulk-forming laxative, lactulose, and sorbitol. Pharmacotherapy of chronic constipation includes drugs like linaclotide, plecanatide, lubiprostone etc. Subtotal colectomy is considered only as a last resort in severe symptomatic constipation when all medications have failed.

"All disease begins in the gut"

—Hippocrates

INTRODUCTION

The complaints of diarrhea and constipation are very commonly encountered in the day-to-day clinical practice. They are faced by clinicians all over the world. While infective diarrhea is commonly seen in the tropical countries like India and becomes an issue of public health importance, the noninfective and malabsorptive diarrhea is more commonly encountered in the Western world. Proper evaluation and treatment of diarrhea and constipation is very vital in the maintenance of adequate nutrition and health in all people. This chapter deepens our understanding of various types of diarrhea and constipation and their management.

DIARRHEA

Diarrhea is defined as having three or more bowel movements in a day with abnormally liquid stools and unformed consistency. Diarrhea can also be assessed by the stool weight. In a developing country like India where there is increased consumption of dietary fiber, stool weight of more than 300 g/day can be considered as abnormal.

There are two important clinical entities, fecal incontinence and pseudo-diarrhea, which should be differentiated from diarrhea. The importance of doing so is in the fact that the treatment is different for these conditions.

1. Fecal incontinence
2. Pseudodiarrhea

Fecal incontinence is a complaint that is usually reported by the elderly. Here the major defect is not in the intestinal handling of the water and electrolytes, but is in the structural and neuromuscular dysfunction involving the rectum. In other words, fecal incontinence is increased frequency of stool passage, but without tenesmus or urgency.

Pseudodiarrhea, on the other hand, is the passage of frequent but small quantity of stools with or without the alteration in the consistency of the stools but accompanied by a feeling of incomplete evacuation. This pattern is most attributable to irritable bowel syndrome.

Normal physiology: In a day average of 10 L of fluid enters the jejunum. It comprises the ingested food and liquid along with saliva, pancreatic juice, and bile. Approximately 6 L is absorbed by the jejunum, 2.5 L by ileum, and the remaining 1.5 L goes into the colon where 90% is reabsorbed and only 100–150 mL is excreted with the stools (**Fig. 1**).

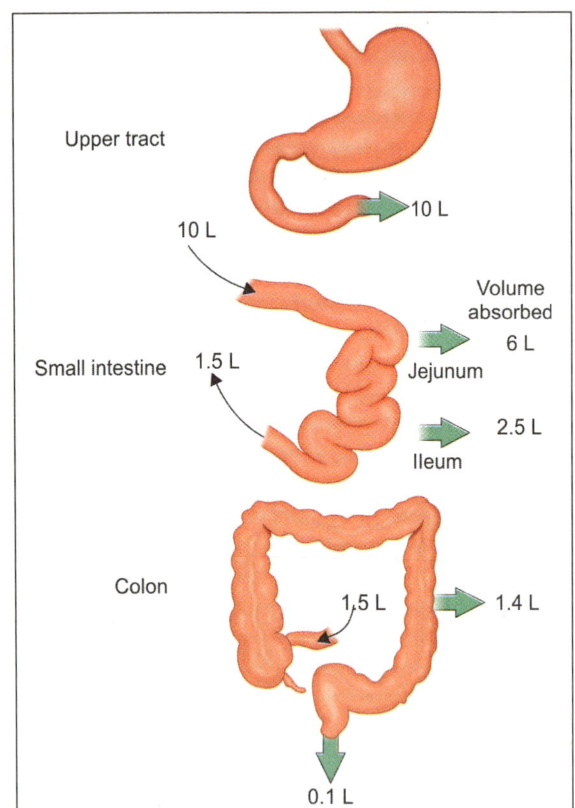

FIGURE 1: Normal physiology.

PATHOPHYSIOLOGY

There is either reduced absorption or increased secretion by the intestinal epithelial cells.

- *Secretory diarrhea*: The main mechanism of this type of diarrhea is increased secretion of chloride or nonabsorption of sodium and water. The most common cause of secretory diarrhea is infection, e.g., cholera. The other noninfectious cause is carcinoid syndrome.
- *Osmotic diarrhea*: The consumption of large quantities of poorly absorbed sugars and ions like magnesium, phosphate, mannitol, and sorbitol leads to the development of osmotic diarrhea. Even lactase deficiency causes osmotic diarrhea.

CLASSIFICATION OF DIARRHEA

Diarrhea can be classified into: (1) acute and chronic diarrhea; (2) large volume and small volume diarrhea; (3) osmotic and secretory diarrhea; (4) fatty acid diarrhea; (5) drug-induced diarrhea

Acute and chronic diarrhea: The duration of acute diarrhea is <4 weeks and that of chronic diarrhea is >4 weeks. The main causes of acute infectious diarrhea are viruses like norovirus, rotavirus, adenoviruses, and astrovirus; bacteria like *Salmonella, Campylobacter, Shigella,* Enterotoxigenic *Escherichia coli, Clostridium difficile* and protozoa like *Cryptosporidium, Giardia, Cyclospora, Entamoeba,* and others (**Box 1**; **Tables 1** and **2**).

Large volume and small volume diarrhea: The passage of small, frequent, and painful stools with blood and mucus points toward large bowel/colon as the source of diarrhea. The passage of painless large volume stools accompanied by malabsorption and dehydration suggests the presence of small bowel as the source of diarrhea.

BOX 1	Acute diarrhea: Differential diagnosis.
• Campylobacter species	
• Clostridium difficile	
• Escherichia coli	
• Salmonella species	
• Shigella species	
• Food allergies	
• Food poisoning	
• Medications	
• Norovirus	
• Rotavirus	
• Cryptosporidium	
• Cyclospora	
• Entamoeba histolytica	
• Giardia lamblia	

Osmotic and secretory diarrhea: The stool osmolar gap of >50 mOsm/L suggests osmotic diarrhea. Osmotic diarrhea reduces with fasting, but secretory diarrhea does not respond to fasting.

Fatty acid diarrhea: It typically results due to malabsorption of fat in the small intestine, most commonly due to pancreatic exocrine insufficiency.

Drug-induced diarrhea: In this type of diarrhea the initiation of the offending drug and the occurrence of diarrhea usually coincide. Metformin, a commonly prescribed agent for treating type 2 diabetes mellitus, can cause diarrhea. The exact mechanism is not well understood. Some drugs increase cyclic adenosine monophosphate (cAMP) activity in the small intestinal epithelial cells and cause diarrhea, e.g., caffeine and theophylline.

EVALUATION OF ACUTE DIARRHEA

- *History*: Information about the frequency, duration of symptoms, and characteristics of the stool is obtained.
  - *Red flag signs* in history include:
    - Oliguria
    - Dark-colored urine
    - Giddiness and disorientation
    - Blood and mucus in diarrhea
    - Fever and abdominal pain

  The above symptoms suggest the presence of invasive diarrhea by organisms like *Salmonella, Shigella,* enterotoxigenic *E. coli.*
  - *Food history*: Consumption of raw or undercooked meat and unpasteurized milk is important. Diarrhea occurring within 6 hours of food ingestion indicates the presence of a preformed toxin due to *Bacillus cereus.* At 8–16 hours, it points out to *Clostridium*

TABLE 1 Chronic diarrhea: Differential diagnosis.

Fatty diarrhea	Inflammatory bowel diseases	Osmotic diarrhea	Secretory diarrhea
• Malabsorption syndromes • Mesenteric ischemia • Mucosal diseases (e.g., celiac disease, Whipple's disease) • Short bowel syndrome • SIBO	• Crohn's disease • UC • Ulcerative jejunoileitis • Ischemic colitis	• Carbohydrate malabsorption • Osmotic laxatives (e.g., magnesium, PO_4, SO_4)	• Bacterial toxins • Diabetic autonomic neuropathy • IBS • Diverticulitis • Addison's disease • Carcinoid syndrome • Gastrinoma • Hyperthyroidism

(IBS: inflammatory bowel syndrome; SIBO: small intestinal bacterial overgrowth; UC: ulcerative colitis)

TABLE 2 Causes of diarrhea in specific patients.

Traveler's diarrhea	Epidemics and outbreaks	Patients with diabetes mellitus	Patients with acquired immunodeficiency syndrome
• Bacterial infection (mostly acute infection with *E. coli*) • Protozoal infections (e.g., amebiasis, giardiasis) • Tropical sprue	• Bacterial infection • Epidemic idiopathic secretory diarrhea (e.g., Brainerd diarrhea) • Protozoal infection (e.g., cryptosporidiosis) • Viral infection (e.g., rotavirus)	• Altered motility (increased or decreased) • Associated diseases • Celiac disease • Pancreatic exocrine insufficiency • SIBO	• Drug side effects • Lymphoma • Opportunistic infections (e.g., cryptosporidiosis, cytomegalovirus

(SIBO: small intestinal bacterial overgrowth)

perfringens. At intervals of >16 hours indicates enterotoxigenic *E. coli*. Medical history about the immunocompromised state is very important which points out to opportunistic infections.

- *Physical examination*: It is important to assess the volume status of the patient.
  The *red flag signs* are:
  - Fever 101°F
  - Hypotension
  - Dry mucous membranes
  - Altered sensorium
  - Abdominal tenderness
- *Laboratory investigations*:
  - Metabolic panel is useful to rule out hypokalemia and acute renal failure.
  - A low platelet count may suggest a development of HUS.
  - Stool routine and microscopy is done to assess for the presence of fecal white blood cell (WBC), ova, cyst etc.
  - Stool cultures for the detection of specific organism. A routine stool culture will identify organisms like *Salmonella*, *Shigella*, and *Campylobacter*.
  - For patients who have a concern for possible cytomegalovirus (CMV) infection in HIV patients, endoscopy with biopsy is the best approach.
- *Indications for imaging*: Patients who have significant peritoneal signs or paralytic ileus, abdominal imaging including contrast-enhanced computed tomography of the abdomen can be helpful.

MANAGEMENT OF ACUTE DIARRHEA

The mainstay of treatment is fluid repletion and nutrition maintenance. Antibiotic therapy is not indicated in most cases since the illness is usually self-limiting. Specific antibiotic therapy is appropriate in the presence of invasive bacterial infection.

Fluid replacement: Oral Rehydration Solution (ORS) is useful in majority of the cases. The mechanism of action is that water is absorbed in the small intestine via sodium-glucose cotransporter. Patients with severe hypovolemia should initially receive IV fluid therapy. IV bolus of Ringer lactate or 0.9% normal saline is the fluid of choice. Initially fluid at the rate of 20 mL/kg/h IV bolus is given. Continuous monitoring of every 10 minutes for a total of 1 hour is done. Goal is to maintain the urine output at 0.5 mL/kg/h.

Once hemodynamic stability is achieved, the patient can be switched over to ORS 10 mL/kg/h. Correction of all the electrolyte imbalances is of utmost importance.

Antibiotic therapy: The choice of antibiotic is either azithromycin or a fluoroquinolone and metronidazole. Azithromycin can be given in the dose of 500 mg once daily for 3 days. Ciprofloxacin 500 mg bid for 3–5 days or levofloxacin 500 mg od for 3–5 days, and metronidazole 500 mg tid for 7 days should usually be sufficient to treat invasive diarrhea.

Antimotility drugs: When an infective cause of diarrhea is ruled out, loperamide 4 mg initially, then 2 mg after each unformed stools is given for 3–4 days.

Probiotics: Lactobacillus GG and *Saccharomyces boulardii* have shown some efficacy in decreasing the duration of *C. difficile* infection.

It has been observed that inulin and fructans are a type of fibers which are known as the prebiotics. These when used along with the probiotics, together are called the synbiotics. They positively impact the colonic microbiota and reduce inflammation. They have been known to induce remissions in Inflammatory Bowel Disease (IBD) and also have a role in the prevention of traveler's diarrhea. Probiotics may also increase the digestion of lactose and may play a prominent role in persistent diarrhea.

Another study done by Bhatnagar S et al. shows that probiotics may increase the digestion of lactose and may play a prominent role in persistent diarrhea.

EVALUATION OF CHRONIC DIARRHEA

The following red flag signs must be carefully looked for in a patient of chronic diarrhea to find out an organic cause.

- Age > 50 years
- Rectal bleeding
- Nocturnal diarrhea
- Fever and weight loss
- Family history of carcinoma colon

History:

- Osmotic diarrhea usually stops on fasting for 12–24 hours. The stool osmotic gap is usually >50 mOsm/L.
- Fatty diarrhea usually presents with long-standing bulky, greasy, and foul-smelling stools.
- Inflammatory diarrhea usually presents with fever, diarrhea with pain abdomen and blood in stools.
- If the patient has depression, stress, and alternating diarrhea and constipation, it suggests inflammatory bowel syndrome (IBS) as the likely cause.
- Presence of upper gastrointestinal (GI) symptoms in a patient with IBS indicates consumption of food with high amount of irritant (chili), especially in the Indian subcontinent, which is also a factor in the frequent exacerbations of IBS-D symptoms.

Physical examination: Table 3 shows physical examination findings in patients with chronic diarrhea.

Laboratory investigations:

- Complete blood count may show anemia of chronic disease.
- Thyroid profile for screening of hyperthyroidism
- Celiac serology, anti-endomysial antibody, anti-tissue transglutaminase (TTG) antibody, and anti-gliadin antibody for the evaluation of celiac disease
- Stool for occult blood
- Fecal calprotectin and fecal lactoferrin to support the diagnosis of IBD.
- Stool microscopy for evidence of giardia, cyclospora, and cryptosporidium.
- Serum iron, total iron-binding capacity (TIBC), serum vitamin B12 levels, serum albumin, and serum 25-hydroxyvitamin D.

TABLE 3 Physical findings in patients with chronic diarrhea.

Findings	Inference
• Orthostasis, hypotension	• Dehydration, neuropathy
• Muscle wasting, edema	• Malnutrition
• Flushing, right-sided heart murmur, wheezing	• Carcinoid syndrome
• Dermatitis herpetiformis	• Celiac disease
• Tremor, lid lag	• Hyperthyroidism
• Arthritis	• Inflammatory bowel disease, Whipple's disease
• Hyperpigmentation	• Addison's disease

Imaging and endoscopy:

- The above-mentioned red flag signs are the indication to perform a sigmoidoscopy or a colonoscopy and obtain a biopsy for the diagnosis of organic disorders.
- Contrast-enhanced CT abdomen is indicated if a diagnosis of chronic pancreatitis is suspected.
- Magnetic resonance enterography is done for the evaluation of Crohn's disease.

MANAGEMENT OF CHRONIC DIARRHEA

- Empiric antibiotic treatment with rifaximin is indicated for the treatment of small intestinal bacterial overgrowth.
- Lactose-free diet is recommended for the patients suffering from lactose intolerance.
- Gluten-free diet is recommended for the management of celiac disease.
- Glucocorticoids and anti-inflammatory agents are used in the management of IBD.
- Replacement of pancreatic enzymes is advocated for chronic pancreatitis.
- 5-HT_3 antagonist alosetron is helpful in controlling of IBS-D symptoms.
- Symptomatic management with diphenoxylate and loperamide is helpful in reducing the frequency of stools.
- Along with the above treatments, the replacement of fat-soluble vitamins, A, D, E, and K is also essential.

CONSTIPATION

Constipation refers to altered bowel movements with persistent difficulty in defecation and a sense of incomplete evacuation. The American College of Gastroenterology's definition of constipation describes it as unsatisfactory defecation with infrequent and difficult stool passage.

Constipation is significantly more frequent in females than in males (20% vs. 13%) and more in nonworking population than in the working population (20% vs. 12%). Poor dietary habits, lesser fluid intake per day, and lesser physical activity were found to be significant factors leading to the constipation.

Constipation tends to become chronic when it persists for >3 months.

TYPES

- *Primary*:
  - Normal transit constipation
  - Slow transit constipation
  - Rectal evacuation disorder
- *Secondary*:
  - Hypothyroidism
  - Parkinson disease
  - Hypercalcemia
  - Multiple sclerosis
  - Spinal cord injury
  - Rectocele
  - Rectal prolapse
  - Drugs like calcium channel blockers and antidepressants

Chronic constipation is not an uncommon issue in India. In a study conducted in North India, 555 people out of 4,767 (11%) reported symptoms of constipation. When compared between males and females in India, the females were shown to be suffering more from chronic constipation. The factor responsible was found to be that the intestinal transit time is slower in females. The pelvic floor is also weaker in females due to obstetric trauma as shown by the study.

According to the Bristol stool chart, the passage of type 1 or 2 stool should be considered as constipation (**Fig. 2**).

Normally colon absorbs most of the water content amounting up to 1–1.5 L/day and leaves only 100–200 mL of water in feces.

PATHOPHYSIOLOGY

- *Normal-transit constipation*: There is incomplete evacuation and accompanied by abdominal pain. Physiologic test results are normal. The patients tend to have abnormal rectal compliance. Usually the diet of such patients is deficient in adequate water and fiber content.

Whole-gut transit time	Type of stool	Description	Pictorial representation
Long transit (e.g., 100 hours)			
	Type 1	Separate hard lumps, like nuts, hard to pass	
	Type 2	Sausage-shaped but lumpy	
	Type 3	Like sausage but with cracks on its surface	
	Type 4	Like sausage or snake, smooth and soft	
	Type 5	Soft blobs with clear-cut edges (passed easily)	
	Type 6	Fluffy pieces with ragged edges, a mushy stool	
	Type 7	Watery, no solid pieces	Entirely liquid
Short transit (e.g., 10 hours)			

FIGURE 2: The Bristol stool chart.

- *Slow-transit constipation*: The stool frequency is usually less than once per week. There is poor response to dietary fiber supplementation. The radio-opaque marker is retained in the colon >20% after 5 days of intake.
- *Rectal evacuation disorder*: There is a need for frequent straining and manual maneuvers to initiate the process of defecation. There is presence of abnormal balloon expulsion test and/or anorectal manometry test. The patient usually has high tone of anal sphincter or the perineal descent is inadequate. The patient may also have pelvic floor dysfunction due to the paradoxical contraction and anterior motion of the puborectalis muscle.

EVALUATION

- *Drug history*: The drugs causing constipation are:
  - Antispasmodics
  - Antidepressants
  - Antipsychotics
  - Opioids
  - Iron supplements
- *Ruling out systemic causes* of constipation with appropriate investigations:
  - Type 2 diabetes mellitus
  - Multiple sclerosis
  - Parkinson disease
  - Hypothyroidism
  - Hypoparathyroidism
  - Hypokalemia
  - IBS
  - Systemic sclerosis
- *Exclude local causes* like:
  - Carcinoma rectum
  - Anal fissures
  - Hemorrhoids
- *Indications for flexible sigmoidoscopy* are:
  - Age > 60 years
  - Family history of colon cancer
  - Rectal bleeding
  - Significant weight loss
  - Iron deficiency anemia
- *Colon transit study*: Indicated in patients with constipation refractory to laxatives and other drugs. The different CTT are:
  - *Radio-opaque marker study*: Retention of >20% of radio-opaque marker on day 6 is considered abnormal.
  - *Wireless motility capsule study*: It is well tolerated and has a good compliance and avoids the risk of radiation exposure.
  - *Defecography*: It is useful in knowing the anatomical and functional aspects of the anorectum. The measurement of anorectal angle is done before and during the procedure. There should be at least an increase of 15° or more in the anorectal angle to label it as adequate. The diagnosis of enterocele and rectocele is also done by this investigation.
  - *Anorectal manometry*: The vital information regarding anal sphincter junction is obtained by this test. This test helps in diagnosing rectal sensory

defects and dyssynergic defecation. Information about the sphincter response is also obtained. If a high sphincter tone of >80 mm Hg is present, it indicates anal sphincter spasm.

- *Balloon expulsion test*: It is a simple bedside test to assess the patient's ability to expel simulated stool. Normally a person is able to expel a 50-mL fluid-filled balloon from the rectum in <2 minutes. And the weight required for assistance is usually <200 g.

MANAGEMENT OF CHRONIC CONSTIPATION

- *General measures*: Initially when the patient presents, the following general measures are tried. These are effective in majority of the cases.
  - High fiber diet
  - Use of bulk-forming laxative, e.g., methylcellulose, psyllium
  - Increased fluid intake
  - Foods containing high fiber content like apple, banana, oranges, cabbage, cucumber, and spinach.
  - The citrus fruits also help in increasing normal flora of colon and thus increase fecal mass.
  - Daily approximately 30 g of fiber intake is recommended.
  - The bulk-forming laxatives act by absorbing water and increase the fecal mass.
  - PEG (polyethylene glycol) acts as osmotic agent. The recommended daily dosage is about 50 g/day.
  - Lactulose and sorbitol are the stool softeners used for the treatment of chronic constipation.
  - Stimulant laxatives like bisacodyl and sodium picosulfate increase the motor activity of the colon. A randomized controlled trial (RCT) successfully evaluated the efficacy of 10 mg of bisacodyl daily in inducing complete and spontaneous stool passage.
  - Patients failing to respond to the above treatment require the usage of suppositories or enema to effectively evacuate their bowel.
- *Pharmacological therapy*:
  - *Linaclotide*: It is a guanylate cyclase-C receptor agonist. Dosage is 72–145 μg/day. It increases the stool volume by binding to the surface of the intestinal epithelial cells and increases the level of cyclic guanosine monophosphate (cGMP) and this increases the water content of the stools.
  - *Plecanatide*: It is also a guanylate cyclase-C receptor agonist. Dosage is 3 mg/day.
  - *Lubiprostone*: It is a chloride channel opener which acts locally in the colon. It thus increases the fluid secretion into the lumen. The recommended dose is 24 mg daily. The most common side effect is nausea.
  - *Prucalopride*: It is a class of medication belonging to the prokinetic group. It is a 5HT-4 receptor agonist. The dosage is 1–4 mg daily. It improved the quality of life at 18 months in a trial.
  - *Biofeedback training*: It is a form of behavioral therapy. It helps in training the patients in proper bowel habits. It is helpful in the treatment of anorectal dysfunction, anismus, and pelvic floor dysfunction.

Indications for surgical intervention:

- Chronic severe and disabling constipation refractory to medical therapy
- Slow colonic transit time
- Presence of megacolon or megarectum
- No pseudo-obstruction and no pelvic floor dysfunction

The surgical procedure of choice is subtotal colectomy with ileorectal anastomosis.

The common postoperative complications are small bowel obstruction, prolonged ileus, and fecal staining. Surgical option should be kept as the last option when all the other treatment modalities have failed to yield results.

RECOMMENDED READINGS

1. Kasper DL, Fauci AS, Hauser SL, Longo DL, Jameson JL, Loscalzo J (Eds). Harrison's Principles of Internal Medicine, 19th edition, Volume 2. New York: McGraw-Hill Education; 2015. pp. 2399, 2400, 2422.
2. Feldman M, Friedman LS, Brandt LJ (Eds). Sleisenger and Fordtran's Gastrointestinal and Liver Disease, 11th edition, Volume 1. Philadelphia: Elsevier; 2020. Pp. 204-23, 250-70.
3. Schiller LR. Secretory diarrhea. Curr Gastroenterol Rep. 1999;1:389-97.
4. Schiller LR, Pardi DS, Spiller R, Semrad CE, Surawicz CM, Giannella RA, et al. Gastro 2013 APDW/WCOG Shanghai Working Party Report: Chronic diarrhea: Definition, classification, diagnosis. J Gastroenterol Hepatol. 2014;29(1):6-25.
5. Theilman NM, Guerrant RL. Clinical practice. Acute infectious diarrhea. N Engl J Med. 2004;350:38-47.
6. Shane AL, Mody RK, Crump JA, Tarr PI, Steiner TS, Kotloff K, et al. 2017 Infectious Diseases Society of America Clinical Practice Guidelines for the Diagnosis and Management of Infectious Diarrhea. Clin Infect Dis. 2017;65(12):e45-e80.
7. Allen SJ, Martinez EG, Gregorio GV, Dans LF. Probiotics for treating acute infectious diarrhoea. Cochrane Database Syst Rev. 2010;CD003048.
8. Pandey KR, Naik SR, Vakil BV. Probiotics, prebiotics and synbiotics – a review. J Food Sci Technol. 2015;52(12):7577-87.
9. Rahman MM, Mahadeva S, Ghoshal UC. Epidemiological and clinical perspectives on irritable bowel syndrome in India, Bangladesh and Malaysia: A review. World J Gastroenterol. 2017;23(37):6788-6801.
10. American College of Gastroenterology Chronic Constipation Task Force. An evidence-based approach to the management of chronic constipation in North America. Am J Gastroenterol. 2005;100(Suppl 1):S1-4.
11. Ghoshal UC, Sachdeva S, Pratap N, Verma A, Karyampudi A, Misra A, et al. Indian consensus on chronic constipation in adults: A joint position statement of the Indian Motility and Functional Diseases Association and the Indian Society of Gastroenterology. Indian J Gastroenterol. 2018;37(6):526-44.
12. Wald A. Approach to the patient with constipation. In: Yamada T (Ed). Textbook of Gastroenterology, 2nd edition. Philadelphia, PA: JB Lippincott; 1995. p. 864.

CHAPTER

6

Lymphadenopathy: Causes and Evaluation

Alladi Mohan, Vasili Pradeep

ABSTRACT

Clinical detection of lymphadenopathy is a cause for concern. In a majority of the patients, the etiological cause of lymphadenopathy is evident on eliciting a careful history and conducting a thorough physical examination. Lymphadenopathy is considered significant when the lymph nodes are >1 cm. When lymphadenopathy involves only one region such as the neck or axilla, it is considered to be local. In generalized lymphadenopathy, there is involvement of two or more noncontiguous regions. The causes of lymphadenopathy are protean. In patients presenting with localized lymphadenopathy, prompt search in the drainage area for the etiological cause is warranted. In generalized lymphadenopathy, further clinical, laboratory, and imaging investigations are indicated. Imaging methods like ^{18}F-labeled 2-deoxy-D-glucose positron emission tomography (^{18}FDG-PET)-computed tomography (CT) and PET-magnetic resonance imaging (MRI) are helpful in defining the disease extent. While fine needle aspiration cytology (FNAC) is often helpful, definitive diagnosis is established by excisional biopsy of the most abnormal lymph node and examination by histopathological, immunohistochemical, microbiological, and molecular methods.

"Reasons are the pillars of the mind"

—Edward Counsel

INTRODUCTION

Lymphadenopathy is a commonly encountered clinical problem by physicians. Presence of palpable peripheral lymphadenopathy on general physical examination and intrathoracic, intra-abdominal lymphadenopathy on imaging offers valuable clue to the underlying etiological cause. The causes of lymphadenopathy are numerous ranging from reactive, benign, and malignant etiologies. The etiological cause of lymphadenopathy is often evident on FNAC, but lymph node biopsy may be required in some cases. In this chapter, the etiological causes and the general approach to evaluating a patient with lymphadenopathy are presented.

Anatomical basis: The peripheral lymph node groups are located in the cervical (including the supraclavicular region), deltopectoral, axillary, epitrochlear, inguinal, and popliteal regions. Normally lymph nodes are <1 cm in diameter and are not palpable. Sometimes, cervical lymph nodes are palpable as a consequence of head and neck infections (e.g., chronic tonsillitis and pediculosis of the head).

ETIOLOGY

A wide range of causes including drugs are known to cause lymphadenopathy. These are listed in **Box 1**.

Significant lymphadenopathy: Lymphadenopathy is considered significant when the lymph nodes are >1 cm, although this varies by lymphatic region. Palpable lymph nodes of any size in the supraclavicular region, epitrochlear nodes >5 mm are considered significant. Clinically, it is important to distinguish between local and generalized lymphadenopathy to formulate a set of differential diagnosis. When lymphadenopathy involves only one region such as the neck or axilla, it is considered to be local. In generalized lymphadenopathy, there is involvement of two or more noncontiguous regions.

LOCALIZED LYMPHADENOPATHY

Anterior cervical lymphadenopathy is often caused by local infections of the head and neck; or to some systemic infections, such as, infectious mononucleosis (IMN), cytomegalovirus (CMV) infection, or toxoplasmosis. Tuberculosis (TB), lymphoma, Kikuchi–Fujimoto disease, and head and neck malignancy (lymphomas or metastatic malignancy) involve posterior cervical lymph nodes.

Cervical lymphadenopathy characterized by multiple enlarged lymph nodes that develop over weeks to months, lymph nodes that are matted (periadenitis), fluctuant without evident signs of inflammation or tenderness (cold abscess) are seen in TB or nontuberculous mycobacterial (NTM); fever and constitutional symptoms are rare. Cervical nodes are firm/rubbery in consistency in lymphomas. Hard, fixed especially in elderly patients and in smokers, suggests metastatic malignancy; primary being in head and neck.

Right supraclavicular lymphadenopathy is associated with cancer in lungs, esophagus, or mediastinum. Left supraclavicular lymphadenopathy ("Virchow's node") may be a harbinger of abdominal malignancy primary being in

BOX 1 Some of the common causes of lymphadenopathy in adults.

- **Infections:**
    - Mycobacterial: Tuberculosis, nontuberculous mycobacteria
    - Spirochaetal: Primary and secondary syphilis
    - Chlamydial: Lymphogranuloma venereum
    - Fungal histoplasmosis, coccidioidomycosis, and cryptococcosis
    - Protozoan: Toxoplasmosis
    - Helminthic: Filariasis
    - Other bacterial: Scrub typhus, cat-scratch fever, chancroid, and melioidosis
    - Viral: Human immunodeficiency virus/acquired immunodeficiency syndrome, infectious mononucleosis, cytomegalovirus, and hepatitis B virus
- **Malignancies:**
    - Hodgkin disease, non-Hodgkin's lymphoma, acute and chronic leukemia, and metastatic "solid" tumors
- **Connective tissue diseases:**
    - Rheumatoid arthritis
    - Systemic lupus erythematosus
    - Dermatomyositis
    - Sjögren's syndrome
- **Other granulomatous disorders:**
    - Sarcoidosis
    - Granulomatosis with polyangiitis (Wegener's granulomatosis)
    - Silicosis
    - Berylliosis
- **Rare causes:**
    - Angiofollicular lymph node hyperplasia (Castleman disease)
    - Progressive transformation of germinal center
    - Angioimmunoblastic lymphadenopathy
    - Inflammatory pseudotumor of lymph nodes
    - Histiocytic necrotizing lymphadenitis (Kikuchi–Fujimoto disease)
    - Sinus histiocytosis with massive lymphadenopathy (Rosai–Dorfman disease)
    - Kawasaki disease
    - Immunoglobulin G4 disease-related lymphadenopathy:
        - Multicentric Castleman disease-like (type I)
        - Follicular hyperplasia (type II)
        - Interfollicular expansion (type III)
        - Progressive transformation of germinal center-like (type IV)
        - Nodal inflammatory pseudotumor-like (type V)
- **Drugs:**
    - Allopurinol
    - Atenolol
    - Carbamazepine
    - Cephalosporins

Continued...

Continued...

    - Gold
    - Hydralazine
    - Phenytoin
- **Others:**
    - Hypersensitivity syndromes
    - Serum sickness
    - Silicone reaction
    - Vaccination related
    - Graft-versus-host disease

stomach, gallbladder, pancreas, kidneys, and testes. Axillary nodes drain the arm, thoracic wall, and breast. Infections (e.g., cat scratch disease) and breast malignancy are common causes of axillary lymphadenopathy. Normally, the epitrochlear nodes are not palpable. The differential diagnosis of epitrochlear lymphadenopathy includes local infections of the hand, forearm, secondary syphilis, sarcoidosis among others.

In some otherwise healthy people, inguinal lymph nodes are often palpable, especially in barefoot walkers, because chronic trauma and infection are common in their draining area, i.e., lower limbs. Inguinal lymphadenopathy is otherwise a consequence of regional infection, sexually transmitted diseases, or cancer in the draining area.

GENERALIZED LYMPHADENOPATHY

Generalized lymphadenopathy is the manifestation of a number of systemic diseases. Evaluation of some common causes of generalized lymphadenopathy are described below.

LYMPHORETICULAR MALIGNANCIES

Generalized lymphadenopathy is seen in patients with Hodgkin's and non-Hodgkin's lymphomas, leukemias, and other lymphoreticular malignancies. The lymph nodes are firm, fixed, circumscribed, nontender, and rubbery in consistency. Generalized lymphadenopathy may also be seen with advanced disseminated metastatic solid tumors.

INFECTIONS

Mycobacterial disease: In India, disseminated and miliary TB are common causes of generalized lymphadenopathy. These forms of TB are more common in immunosuppressed individual. The enlarged lymph nodes are firm, matted. Cold abscess, collar-stud abscess formation can be evident. Generalized lymphadenopathy can be seen due to NTM infection.

Acquired immunodeficiency syndrome: Generalized lymphadenopathy is common in human immunodeficiency virus (HIV) infection, acquired immunodeficiency syndrome. In people living with HIV infection (PLHIV), during the second week of the illness generalized nontender lymphadenopathy involving cervical, occipital, and axillary lymph nodes develops in the majority of individuals. Though the lymph node size may later on decrease, generalized lymphadenopathy tends to persist. Other causes of generalized lymphadenopathy in PLHIV include TB, cryptococcosis, CMV, and toxoplasmosis. In Kaposi's sarcoma, generalized lymphadenopathy may be evident before visible skin lesions appear.

Infectious mononucleosis: In classic IMN, the triad of fever, pharyngitis, and lymphadenopathy are seen. Lymph node involvement is typically symmetrical. Lymph nodes in the cervical, axillary, and inguinal regions are enlarged. Occurrence of generalized lymphadenopathy helps to clinically distinguish IMN from other causes.

Others: Generalized lymphadenopathy may be a feature of CMV, human herpesvirus 6, adenovirus, herpes simplex virus (HSV), *Streptococcus pyogenes*, and *Toxoplasma gondii* infections also.

CONNECTIVE TISSUE DISEASES

Enlargement of lymph nodes occurs in about 50% of patients with systemic lupus erythematosus (SLE), rheumatoid arthritis among others. The lymph nodes are soft, nontender, and discrete of varying sizes and are evident in cervical, axillary, and inguinal regions.

DRUGS

A number of drugs are implicated in the causation of generalized lymphadenopathy. Drugs can cause serum sickness and generalized lymphadenopathy can be a component of that; other features being fever, arthralgias, and rash. Several drugs are known to cause generalized lymphadenopathy per se, without serum sickness (**Box 1**).

RARE CAUSES

Generalized lymphadenopathy is a characteristic feature of several rare systemic diseases. Some of these conditions, seen in adults, are described below.

Angiofollicular lymph node hyperplasia (Castleman disease) is a lymphoproliferative disorder characterized by lymphadenopathy and systemic features such as fever, hepatosplenomegaly, and polyclonal hypergammaglobulinemia. Angioimmunoblastic lymphadenopathy is characterized by fever, generalized lymphadenopathy, hepatosplenomegaly, hemolytic anemia, and polyclonal hypergammaglobulinemia. Another systemic disease that presents with generalized lymphadenopathy, Kawasaki disease (mucocutaneous lymph node syndrome) is rare in adults.

Kikuchi–Fujimoto's disease is a rare, benign condition of unknown etiology that occurs most commonly in young women and is usually characterized by cervical lymphadenopathy; generalized lymphadenopathy is also common and fever. Progressive transformation of germinal centers (PTGC) is more commonly seen in men, presents with asymptomatic, persistent, or recurrent lymphadenopathy, often in the head and neck area. These two conditions are confused with lymphomas.

Kimura disease is an inflammatory condition that involves subcutaneous tissue, cervical lymphadenopathy, peripheral blood eosinophilia, and elevated serum immunoglobulin (Ig) E levels.

Inflammatory pseudotumor of lymph nodes and amyloidosis are also rare causes of generalized lymphadenopathy. Sinus histiocytosis with massive lymphadenopathy (SHML, Rosai–Dorfman syndrome) is also a rare cause of generalized lymphadenopathy.

In patients with IgG4-related disease (IgG4-RD), lymphadenopathy may be the initial or only manifestation (**Box 1**); other systemic manifestations are also present. Patients with IgG4-RD often manifest elevated serum IgG4, IgG and IgE, polyclonal hypergammaglobulinemia, and elevated erythrocyte sedimentation rate (ESR). Histopathologically, lymph node biopsy seldom reveals the storiform fibrosis that is evident in IgG4-RD and, therefore, may be difficult to interpret.

Kawasaki disease (earlier called mucocutaneous lymph node syndrome) is rare in adults. About 25% of adult Kawasaki disease cases have been documented in PLHIV.

EVALUATION

Ascertaining the etiology of lymphadenopathy entails eliciting a detailed history and carrying out a thorough physical examination, laboratory investigations, imaging and lymph node FNAC, and biopsy. While evaluating a patient with lymphadenopathy, the following constitute key considerations (acronym *ALL AGES*): *A*ge, *L*ocation, *L*ength of time present, *A*ssociated symptoms and signs, *G*eneralized lymphadenopathy, *E*xtranodal associations, and *S*plenomegaly and fever. Older age is associated with a higher likelihood of malignant etiology. Documenting the length of time lymphadenopathy is present (time-course) of the adenopathy also facilitates narrowing down the differential diagnosis. But, patients seldom notice the presence of lymphadenopathy, even in obviously accessible places like the neck.

In a patient presenting with lymphadenopathy, history should focus on localizing symptoms suggestive of an infectious etiology or an underlying malignancy. Fever is commonly present in lymphadenopathy due to infectious causes. Constitutional symptoms such as fever, night sweats, anorexia, or weight loss suggest the possibility of TB, lymphoma, or other malignancies. Other history tick bite (Lyme disease), cat scratches (cat scratch disease), high-risk behavior for HIV (e.g., multiple sexual partners, intravenous drug use sharing), and use of medication (e.g., phenytoin) may give a clue to etiology.

A thorough physical examination should be carried out to look for signs suggestive of a systemic disease. When localized lymphadenopathy is present, the catchment area should be carefully examined. Generalized lymphadenopathy is indicative of systemic disease. However, some systemic diseases (lymphomas) can present initially with localized lymphadenopathy. Lymphadenopathy due to malignancy is hard in consistency; rubbery consistency is noted in lymphoma, chronic leukemias. Fixity to adjacent tissues suggests cancer or inflammation. Tender lymphadenopathy is suggestive of recent rapid enlargement causing stretching of the lymph node capsule and stimulating the pain receptors, but also may indicate hemorrhage into the node, immunological stimulation, or malignancy also.

Associated skin lesions, peripheral and hilar lymphadenopathy, are seen in sarcoidosis. Common causes of hepatomegaly/splenomegaly associated with lymphadenopathy include disseminated/miliary TB, lymphoma, chronic lymphocytic leukemia, acute leukemia, and sarcoidosis.

DIAGNOSTIC TESTING

Laboratory testing: Work-up of a patient with lymphadenopathy depends upon whether the lymphadenopathy is localized or generalized (**Fig. 1**). A detailed description of these laboratory tests is beyond the scope of this chapter.

Imaging and endoscopic procedures: Imaging modalities such as chest radiograph, ultrasonography, CT, MRI, ^{18}FDG-PET–CT, and PET-MRI are helpful in detecting intrathoracic and intra-abdominal lymphadenopathy, defining the disease extent (**Fig. 2**). Further, associated disease processes in other organs systems can also be detected. Common causes of hilar and mediastinal lymphadenopathy are shown in **Box 2**.

Further, when peripheral lymph nodes are not accessible for sampling, image-guided FNAC and biopsy are done. Endoscopic examination of the oropharynx nasopharynx, larynx, upper gastrointestinal endoscopy, and bronchoscopy including endobronchial ultrasonography (EBUS) has facilitated more precise mediastinal lymph node sampling.

LYMPH NODE ASPIRATION

If the enlarged lymph nodes are fluctuant, aspiration and pyogenic, mycobacterial culture of the aspirated pus along with application of molecular diagnostic methods like cartridge-based nucleic acid amplification test (CBNAAT) can help in diagnosis.

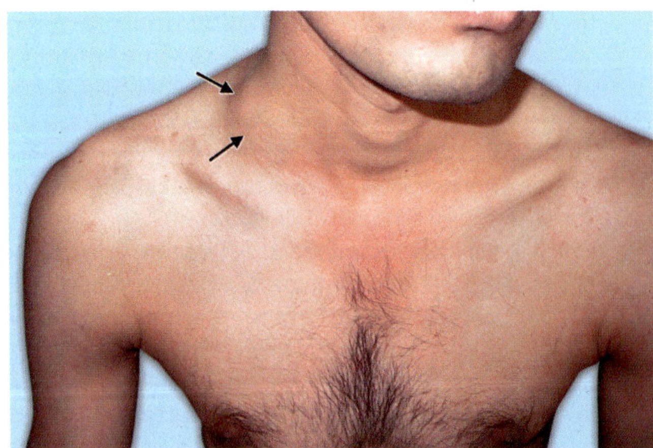

FIGURE 1: Clinical photograph showing right supraclavicular lymphadenopathy (arrows).

FINE NEEDLE ASPIRATION CYTOLOGY

Fine needle aspiration cytology is widely available and is useful in detecting malignant etiology. With availability of CBNAAT like Xpert MTB/RIF, rapid diagnosis of TB lymphadenitis is possible. However, false-negative results occur with FNAC because of sampling error and subsequently biopsy and histopathological examination will be required.

LYMPH NODE BIOPSY

The options for lymph node biopsy include core needle biopsy and excision biopsy. Some clinicians-pathologists combine FNAC and core needle biopsy with ancillary studies in preference to ewxcision biopsy, which is an invasive procedure. However, excision biopsy remains the gold standard for the etiological diagnosis of lymphadenopathy.

In addition to conventional staining, special stains, immunohistochemistry, among others are applied to the excised lymph node biopsy specimens.

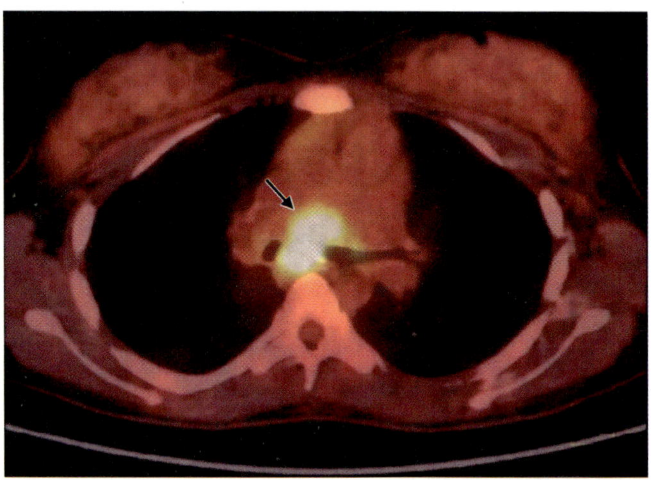

(CT: computed tomography; PET: positron emission tomography)

FIGURE 2: Transaxial fused PET-CT image showing mediastinal lymphadenopathy with abnormal ^{18}F-labeled 2-deoxy-D-glucose uptake (arrow).

Courtesy: Dr TC Kalawat, Dept. of Nuclear Medicine, Sri Venkateswara Institute of Medical Sciences, Tirupati.

BOX 2	Common causes of hilar and mediastinal lymphadenopathy.
• **Infections**	
◦ Tuberculosis*	
◦ Nontuberculous mycobacterial infections	
◦ Fungal infections (e.g., histoplasmosis)	
◦ Tularemia	
◦ Psittacosis	
◦ Sarcoidosis* and other granulomatous diseases*	
• **Malignancy**	
◦ Bronchogenic carcinoma	
◦ Metastatic cancers	
◦ Lymphoma	
• **Silicosis***	

*Bilateral hilar lymphadenopathy common.

RECOMMENDED READINGS

1. Mohan A, Reddy MK, Phaneendra BV, Chandra A. Aetiology of peripheral lymphadenopathy in adults: analysis of 1724 cases seen at a tertiary care teaching hospital in southern India. Natl Med J India. 2007;20:78-80.
2. Habermann TM, Steensma DP. Lymphadenopathy. Mayo Clin Proc. 2000;75:723-32.
3. Gaddey HL, Riegel AM. Unexplained lymphadenopathy: Evaluation and differential diagnosis. Am Fam Physician. 2016;94:896-903.
4. Bledsoe JR, Della-Torre E, Rovati L, Deshpande V. IgG4-related disease: review of the histopathologic features, differential diagnosis, and therapeutic approach. APMIS. 2018;126:459-76.

CHAPTER 7

Patient with Hepatosplenomegaly: Possibilities and Evaluation

Sagnik Biswas, Sanchit Sharma

ABSTRACT

Hepatosplenomegaly is a commonly encountered entity in clinical practice. Various disorders can cause enlargement of spleen and liver. Careful history and clinical examination complemented by relevant laboratory and imaging investigations lead to correct diagnosis in most conditions. While any degree of hepatic enlargement is usually appreciable clinically, spleen needs to be enlarged significantly before it can be detected on clinical examination. Degree of splenic enlargement points toward a group of disorders which can be separated out from a wide list of differential etiologies for the same. Common disorders associated with hepatosplenomegaly are hemolytic anemia, lymphoreticular malignancies, tropical infections, and portal hypertension (more commonly with isolated splenomegaly).

"What happens to a person is less significant than what happens within him."

—Louis L Mann

INTRODUCTION

Hepatosplenomegaly is a commonly encountered clinical entity in the medicine ward and outpatient department. The differentials for the condition are diverse primarily because both involved organs occupy central roles in various systems—gastrointestinal, reticuloendothelial, hematology etc. Thus when confronted with a patient presenting with hepatosplenomegaly, the approach should focus on good history-taking and clinical assessment to assess the organ system involved—for example a patient with temporal hollowing, muddy discoloration of facies along with mild hepatosplenomegaly and ascites is likely to have alcohol-related chronic liver disease (CLD), while a patient who presents with hepatosplenomegaly with multiple lymph nodes, ascites, and pleural effusion is more likely to have a lymphoma or disseminated tuberculosis. In the latter example, it is not possible to distinguish between the two causes clinically and laboratory tests will be required to differentiate between them. However, in most cases the above approach gives a clear idea of the organ system involved and therefore streamlines further investigations for confirmation of diagnosis and initiation of therapy.

For the purpose of this chapter we will describe the various etiologies which should be considered when evaluating a case of hepatosplenomegaly. While an exhaustive list of causes, where this condition is encountered, is not feasible, the commonly encountered causes and approach have been dealt with in detail.

HEPATOMEGALY

The liver is housed in right hypochondrium and carries out several important bodily functions which include drug detoxification, bile secretion, protein, and fat synthesis. The location, vascularity, and multifaceted functions of liver make it susceptible to various pathological insults that result in hepatomegaly. This may be detected either on physical examination or on imaging.

Size and location: The liver is a wedge-shaped organ weighing approximately 1.5–2.0 kg located in the right upper quadrant. Typically found to extend from right fifth intercostal space to right costal margin, it is usually 12–15 cm in span. Thus, a liver span of >16 cm in the midclavicular line is used to define hepatomegaly on abdominal ultrasonography.

Consistency: Normal liver consistency is soft with a smooth contour. Firm or hard consistency, nodularity or tenderness are all signs of pathology.

Anatomy: Traditionally divided into right and left lobes—the right lobe is larger and occupies right hypochondrium. The left lobe is smaller, flatter, and situated in epigastrium and left hypochondrium.

Segments: The liver is divided into eight segments based on its vascular supply—each segment containing a branch of portal vein, hepatic vein, hepatic artery, and bile duct. There are no distinct anatomical landmarks that demarcate segments.

Anatomic variations: May be palpable and mistaken for hepatomegaly—Riedel's lobe, caudate lobe papillary process.

SPLENOMEGALY

The spleen is a highly vascular organ which takes part in hematologic and immune homeostasis. Just like liver, its vascularity, anatomical location, and function make it the target for various pathologic conditions. Unlike liver, however, there is no consensus for splenic size. In clinical practice a size of 11–12 cm is considered as normal for spleen and any enlargement beyond this measure noted on ultrasound is considered as splenomegaly. It is to be noted that the spleen needs to undergo significant enlargement to be palpable and lesser degrees of enlargement are not appreciable on clinical examination.

Size and location: It lies within the peritoneal cavity in left upper quadrant, below diaphragm. It is adjacent to 9th to 11th ribs, stomach, splenic flexure of colon, and left kidney. The tail of the pancreas terminates close to the splenic hilum.

Anatomy: The spleen has the following parts which help explain the involvement of spleen in multiple disease processes:

- *White pulp*: It is a major secondary lymphoid compartment containing 25% of lymphocytes in circulation. It is organized in the form of lymphoid sheaths with T- and B-cell areas surrounding the arterioles.
- *Red pulp*: It is the site for blood filtration and accounts for 75% of splenic volume. Phagocytosis of bacteria and red blood cells occurs here. Red pulp enlarges in autoimmune hemolytic anemia (AIHA) and cirrhosis causing splenomegaly.

Terminology: Certain terminology is associated with disease processes involving the spleen:

- Accessory spleen: Separate deposits of splenic tissue in abdomen, also called splenunculi
- Asplenia: May be structural or functional. This could be surgical or pathological such as in sickle cell disease
- Hyposplenia: Reduced splenic function which typically affects antibody production without affecting other functions, e.g., celiac disease
- Hypersplenism: Splenic sequestration of cellular components of blood which may be extensive enough to cause cytopenia of one or more cell lines.

CAUSES

The various causes of hepatosplenomegaly in adults are listed in **Table 1**.

RELEVANT CLINICAL HISTORY

As can be seen from the **Table 1**, the differentials of hepatosplenomegaly cover a vast spectrum of diseases. The approach in taking clinical history in such cases is to therefore identify or narrow down the etiology. This

TABLE 1 Causes of hepatosplenomegaly in adults.

Infections	Hematological disorders	Congestive states	Storage disorders	Connective tissue disorders

• Malaria
• Kala azar
• Infective endocarditis
• Disseminated tuberculosis
• Infectious mononucleosis
• Histoplasmosis
• Human immunodeficiency virus
• Acute viral hepatitis
• Cytomegalovirus
	• Chronic hemolytic anemia:
	  ◦ Glucose-6-phosphate dehydrogenase deficiency
	  ◦ Pyruvate kinase deficiency
	• Myeloproliferative disorders:
	  ◦ Essential thrombocythemia
	  ◦ Chronic myeloid leukemia
	  ◦ Primary myelofibrosis
	  ◦ Polycythemia
	• Non-Hodgkin's lymphoma
	• Hodgkin's lymphoma
	• Pernicious anemia
	• Sickle cell disease
	• Beta thalassemia major
	• Defects of red cell structure:
	  ◦ Spherocytosis
	  ◦ Elliptocytosis
		• Congestive cardiac failure
		• Constrictive pericarditis
		• Cirrhosis of liver with portal hypertension
		• Budd–Chiari syndrome
			• Gaucher's disease
			• Amyloidosis
			• Glycogen storage disorders
				• SLE
				• Sarcoidosis

is primarily achieved by taking appropriate positive and negative history followed by verification of the same along with elicitation of signs on physical examination. The following points should be focused on while taking the history:

- *Presenting complaint*:
  - Abdominal swelling or lump
  - Generalized lymphadenopathy
  - Fatigue
  - Shortness of breath
- *History of present illness*:
  - Infective: Fever, abdominal heaviness, loss of weight, and loss of appetite
  - Hematological: Fatigue, easy bruising, and jaundice
  - Congestive: Abdominal distension, pedal edema, abdominal pain, shortness of breath, and paroxysmal nocturnal dyspnea (PND)
  - Storage: Symptom complex since childhood, fatigue on exertion, neurological dysfunction
  - Connective tissue: Joint pain, redness of eye, cough, and cola-colored urine
- *Past history*:
  - Infective: History of tuberculosis in family/friends, past history of malaria
  - Hematological: Recurrent need for blood transfusion, episodes of sickle crisis
  - Congestive: History of PND, arrhythmias, and recurrent episodes of jaundice
  - Storage: Symptom complex since childhood, seizures, and feed intolerance
  - Connective tissue: Joint pains, redness of eye, cough, and cola-colored urine
- *Social history*:
  - Residence: Endemic areas for malaria, kala azar
  - Recreational drug use: Alcohol-related liver disease, infective endocarditis
  - High-risk sexual behavior: HIV, hepatitis B and C
  - Housing: Overcrowding is a risk factor for respiratory illness
  - Consanguinity: Risk factor for thalassemia
  - Water source: Hepatitis A and E

PHYSICAL EXAMINATION

Physical examination of liver and spleen is done as a part of examination of abdomen as a whole and comprises of the following:

- *General physical examination*:
  - Pallor, cyanosis, icterus, clubbing, edema, and prominent neck veins may all be seen.
  - Lymph node groups: All groups should be examined carefully.
  - Vitals
  - Skeletal system: Knuckles, gibbus, and swelling
  - Skin, hair, and nails: Apple jelly nodules, lupus pernio, terry nails, paper money skin, spider naevi, palmar erythema, and pigmentation of kala azar/hemochromatosis
  - Oral cavity: Candidiasis, oral hairy leukoplakia
  - Tremors: In hepatic encephalopathy and in Wilson's disease
  - Facies: Alcoholism, thalassemia
  - Eyes: K-F rings (although difficult to identify without a slit lamp)
  - Sternal tenderness: Acute lymphoblastic leukemia (ALL)
  - Fundus: Infective endocarditis
- *Inspection*: Inspection of the abdomen comprises of noting the following:
  - *Distension*: Ascites/lump/obesity
  - *Flanks*: Presence of fluid/pelvic masses causing dullness in females
  - *Location and position of umbilicus*: Usually in midline. May be pushed upward by a pelvic tumor or downward by an abdominal mass/ascites.
  - *Nature of umbilicus:* Usually inverted but may be flushed with the surface or everted in cases of raised abdominal pressure such as ascites. An everted umbilicus carries a risk of perforation and should always be examined for contents (hernia).
  - *Skin and venous prominences*: There may be discharging sinuses or other lesions on the skin suggestive of inflammatory involvement. Venous prominences are common in cirrhosis of liver and inferior vena cava (IVC) obstruction and may be seen in Budd–Chiari syndrome.
  - *Genitalia*: One of the most commonly overlooked sites in abdominal examination; genitalia in males may show atrophy and lack of pubic hair in cases of liver cirrhosis. Testicular volume loss is also a noted feature in hemochromatosis and may rarely be seen in patients of thalassemia major with iron overload.

The rest of the clinical examination is described as relevant to liver and spleen.

LIVER

- *Palpation*: Palpation is to assess liver size, tenderness, borders, surface nodularity, and space-occupying lesions (SOL). It is seen in supine position. The liver may be tender in acute hepatitis, congestive hepatitis, and liver abscess. The edge may be firm and nodular in cirrhosis and/or malignancy.
- *Percussion*: Assessed in the supine position. Upper border of liver dullness is usually seen in right fifth intercostal space. It may be displaced lower by a lung with enlarged air spaces such as in chronic obstructive pulmonary disease (COPD) or may be displaced upward by collapse of right lower lung lobes, or a subdiaphragmatic collection such as an abscess. Percussion is also used to assess liver span to confirm hepatomegaly.

SPLEEN

A spleen becomes palpable when it enlarges and/or its texture changes. For example, a spleen which is infiltrated with lymphomatous cells or a site for extramedullary hematopoiesis would be more engorged with cells and

TABLE 2 Causes of splenomegaly.

Mild (<2 fingers)	Moderate (2–5 fingers)	Massive (>5 fingers)
• Malaria • Kala azar • Enteric fever • SABE • Disseminated tuberculosis • Hemolytic anemia • Infective endocarditis	• Chronic malaria • Chronic kala azar • Portal hypertension • Lymphoma • CLL • Connective tissue disorders	• Chronic kala azar • Thalassemia major • CML • Tropical splenomegaly • Polycythemia vera • Amyloidosis • Gaucher's disease

(CLL: chronic lymphocytic leukemia; CML: chronic myelogenous leukemia; SABE: subacute bacterial endocarditis)

thus firmer to palpation. It would therefore be more easily palpable than a normal spleen which is soft in texture (**Table 2**).

- *Palpation*: A mildly enlarged spleen may not extend beyond left costal margin and thus may not be palpable. Several sources in literature suggests that spleen needs to be enlarged above 40% of its baseline size to be palpable. A massively enlarged spleen may extend into pelvis and extent of swelling may be difficult to assess.
- *Percussion*: Percussion of Traube's space (tympanitic area overlying the gastric bubble in left lateral hemithorax) may reveal dullness when spleen is enlarged.
- *Alternative methods for confirmation of splenomegaly*: The following are alternative methods for assessment of splenomegaly:
  - Castell's method: Percussion in 8th or 9th (lowest) intercostal space in the anterior axillary line demonstrates dullness in splenomegaly.
  - Nixon's method: Percussion of abdomen from lower level of pulmonary resonance starting in the posterior axillary wall proceeding diagonally along an anterior line toward lower mid anterior costal margin reveals dullness >8 cm in splenomegaly.
  - *Middleton's method*: Examiner stands on left side of patient and tries to "hook" the spleen under costal margin and feel the spleen.

LABORATORY INVESTIGATIONS

Once the history, general and systemic examination have been reviewed, laboratory and radiological investigations are carried out for confirmation of clinical findings as well as to screen for other organ system involvement which may be asymptomatic. Radiological investigations also provide us a means for obtaining tissue samples for biopsy which provide us definitive proof of the diagnosis. In some cases, radiological and laboratory investigations are used in composite scores which provide disease prognosis and guide therapy.

Laboratory investigations include primarily the following:

- Hemogram
- Liver function tests
- Renal function tests
- *Peripheral smear*: Nature of anemia, reticulocyte count, blasts, and parasites
- Blood culture
- *Special tests*:
  - GeneXpert: Tuberculosis
  - Rk 39: Kala azar
  - Epstein-Barr virus (EBV) and cytomegalovirus (CMV) serology
  - Glucose-6-phosphate dehydrogenase (G6PD) levels
  - JAK2 mutation
  - HIV-1 and -2 levels, venereal disease research laboratory (VDRL)
  - CLD etiology: Iron profile, copper studies, and viral markers
  - High-performance liquid chromatography (HPLC) for thalassemia
  - Lactate dehydrogenase (LDH) for hemolysis/lymphoma
- *Radiology*: X-ray—
  - Chest: Tuberculosis (TB), lymphoma, and sarcoidosis
  - Skull: "Hair-on-end" appearance in beta thalassemia major
  - Bones: "Erlenmeyer flask deformity" in Gaucher's disease
- Ultrasonography of abdomen—
  - Confirmation of hepatosplenomegaly
  - Ascites: CLD, TB, lymphoma, and systemic lupus erythematosus (SLE)
  - Enlarged lymph nodes: Lymphoma and TB
- CT, lymphangioscintigraphy
- *Others*:
  - Bone marrow biopsy
  - Liver biopsy
  - Lymph node biopsy

DIFFERENTIAL DIAGNOSIS

The various clinical scenario of hepatosplenomegaly are given in **Table 3**.

- *Tropical splenomegaly syndrome*:
  - Patient is a resident of a hyperendemic zone.
  - High-grade fever with chills and rigor along with periodicity as in malaria
  - Splenomegaly is the prominent finding—firm to hard and is nontender
  - Hypersplenism may be seen.
  - Renamed "hyper-reactive malarial splenomegaly"
- *Kala azar*:
  - Patient is a resident of an endemic area.
  - Fever and loss of weight are prominent features.
  - Massively enlarged, nontender spleen is characteristic.
  - Moderately enlarged liver
  - Pigmentation of skin as indicated in the name
- *Beta thalassemia major*:
  - Typically a young child

TABLE 3 Commonly encountered scenarios of hepatosplenomegaly.

Hepatosplenomegaly with lymphadenopathy	Hepatosplenomegaly with fever	Hepatosplenomegaly with ascites	Hepatosplenomegaly with anemia
• Lymphoma • HIV • Disseminated tuberculosis • Histoplasmosis • Sarcoidosis • Syphilis • Felty syndrome	• Malaria • Kala azar • Enteric fever • Tuberculosis • Lymphoma • HIV • Infective endocarditis	• Cirrhosis with portal hypertension • Lymphoma • Disseminated tuberculosis • SLE	• Chronic malaria • Chronic kala azar • Hematologic malignancies • SLE • Thalassemia

(SLE: systemic lupus erythematosus)

- If seen in adulthood, history of multiple transfusions
- Consanguinity may be present.
- Stunted growth, chipmunk facies, hepatosplenomegaly, ascites, pallor, and jaundice

- *Cirrhosis of liver*:
  - Hepatomegaly in alcohol and nonalcoholic steatohepatitis (NASH)-related CLD
  - Anemia, jaundice, coagulopathy, and altered sensorium
  - History of hematemesis, melena, and venous prominences
  - Important signs on physical examination in alcohol-related liver disease
- *Chronic myelogenous leukemia (CML)*:
  - Middle-aged individual
  - Dragging sensation or heaviness in left hypochondrium
  - May report early satiety as a symptom
  - Hepatosplenomegaly present
  - Cytopenia may be seen.
- *Lymphoma*:
  - Multiple generalized lymph node swellings
  - Fever, ascites, pleural effusion, superior vena cava (SVC) syndrome
  - B symptoms may be present.
- *Acute viral hepatitis*:
  - Fever, nausea, and anorexia vomiting followed by jaundice in afebrile phase
  - Arthralgia and rashes may also be seen.
- *Enteric fever*:
  - Headache, fever, constipation, and rose spots on abdomen
  - Soft and tender splenomegaly
- *Polycythemia vera*:
  - Headache, tinnitus, pruritus, and peripheral thrombosis
  - Epistaxis, hematemesis, melena, and conjunctival suffusion
  - Splenomegaly is more common than hepatomegaly.
- *Connective tissue disorders*:
  - Fever, joints pains, redness of eyes, and cola-colored urine
  - Renal, pulmonary, and cardiac involvement may be seen as disease progresses.
  - Felty syndrome in rheumatoid arthritis (RA) is associated with splenomegaly and neutropenia.
- *Myelofibrosis*:
  - Primary or secondary to toxins, malignancy, lymphoma, or irradiation
  - Leukoerythroblastic blood picture with thrombocytosis
- *Tuberculosis*:
  - High-grade fever, insidious onset, loss of appetite, and weight
  - Classic evening rise of temperature
  - Extrapulmonary TB strongly associated with HIV
  - Multisystem involvement is possible.
- *Amyloidosis*:
  - Usually develops in the background of chronic inflammation—leprosy, RA, bronchiectasis etc.
  - Primary amyloidosis is rare.
  - Visceromegaly, nephrotic range albuminuria, and anasarca
  - Peripheral neuropathy, cardiomyopathy, and lymphadenopathy may be seen.

RECOMMENDED READINGS

1. Levy L, Nasereddin A, Rav-Acha M, Kedmi M, Rund D, Gatt ME. Prolonged fever, hepatosplenomegaly, and pancytopenia in a 46-year-old woman. PLoS Med. 2009;6(4):e1000053.
2. Karakus V, Dere Y, Dere O, Sahin F, Ozsan N. Gaucher disease in an adult: A rare cause of hepatosplenomegaly in adults. North Clin Istanb. 2018;5(1):58-9.
3. Naylor CD. The rational clinical examination. Physical examination of the liver. JAMA. 1994;271:1859-65.
4. Wolf DC. Evaluation of the size, shape, and consistency of the liver. In: Walker HK, Hall WD, Hurst JW (Eds). Clinical Methods: The History, Physical, and Laboratory Examinations, 3rd edition. Boston: Butterworths; 1990.
5. Cesta MF. Normal structure, function, and histology of the spleen. Toxicol Pathol. 2006;34:34:455-65.
6. Vancauwenberghe T, Snoeckx A, Vanbeckevoort D, Dymarkowski S, Vanhoenacker FM. Imaging of the spleen: what the clinician needs to know. Singapore Med J. 2015;56:133-44.
7. Barkun AN, Camus M, Green L, Meagher T, Coupal L, De Stempel J, et al. The bedside assessment of splenic enlargement. Am J Med. 1991;91:512-8.
8. Yang JC, Rickman LS, Bosser SK. The clinical diagnosis of splenomegaly. West J Med. 1991;155:47-52.

CHAPTER 8

Ascites: Clinical Approach

K Ravi, Devamsh GN

ABSTRACT

Ascites refers to abnormal accumulation of fluid in the peritoneal cavity. Cirrhosis of liver is the most common cause for ascites. However, there are several other conditions that can lead to ascites apart from cirrhosis. The evaluation of a patient with ascites starts with clinical history and thorough physical examination. The foremost step while investigating a case of ascites is to calculate serum ascites albumin gradient (SAAG). Based on the value of SAAG, patients are classified into either high SAAG or low SAAG ascites and further investigations are planned to identify the cause of ascites. Not all patients with ascites require hospital admission. Uncomplicated ascites patients can be managed on outpatient basis.

The management of ascites is primarily aimed at creating a negative sodium balance by dietary sodium restriction and diuretic therapy. Spironolactone is the diuretic of choice for single-agent therapy in ascites. Combination therapy with spironolactone and furosemide is recommended for recurrent ascites. Treatment options for refractory ascites include large volume paracentesis, stent surgeries, and liver transplantation. Development of ascites in a patient with cirrhosis should alert the physician of other impending complications of cirrhosis and portal hypertension.

"The question is not how to get cured, but how to live"

—Joseph Conrad

INTRODUCTION

Ascites refers to abnormal accumulation of fluid in the peritoneal cavity. Ascites is one of the most common decompensating events in cirrhosis. However, there are several other conditions that can lead to ascites apart from cirrhosis. It results from conditions directly affecting the peritoneum or diseases affecting other organ systems (liver disease, heart failure, malignancies etc.). This chapter will deal with clinical approach to a patient with ascites with special focus on the causes, clinical presentation, evaluation, and management of ascites.

The most common cause of ascites in the Western world and in India is cirrhosis of liver. The development of ascites in cirrhotic patients indicates decompensation. Such patients are more prone to other complications like spontaneous bacterial peritonitis (SBP), hyponatremia, hepatorenal syndrome (HRS), and overall reduction in the quality of life.

MECHANISM OF ASCITES IN CIRRHOSIS

There are several theories postulated for the formation of ascites in portal hypertension. They are:

- *Underfill theory*: This theory refers to the arterial vasodilation leading to decreased effective arterial blood volume. This leads to activation of renin-angiotensin-aldosterone system (RAAS) causing sodium and water retention, renal vasoconstriction, plasma volume expansion, and ascites (**Flowchart 1**).
- *Overfill theory*: This refers to primary renal change in response to hepatic insufficiency and portal hypertension that leads to sodium retention causing ascites (**Flowchart 2**).
- *Backward theory*: Portal hypertension and low serum albumin result in disruption of equilibrium of Starling's forces causing increase in intestinal lymph formation.
- *Forward theory*: Splanchnic vasodilation and pooling of blood lead to increase in capillary pressure and filtration coefficient. This causes increased lymph formation.

The key mechanism leading to ascites is renal sodium retention due to activation of RAAS and sympathetic nervous system (**Flowchart 3**).

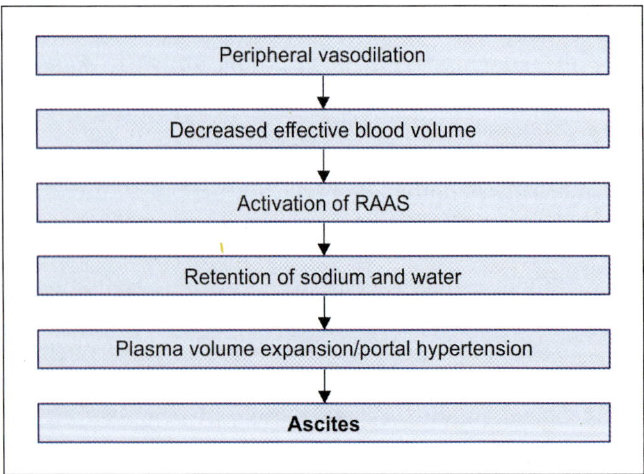

(RAAS: renin–angiotensin–aldosterone system)

FLOWCHART 1: Underfill theory.

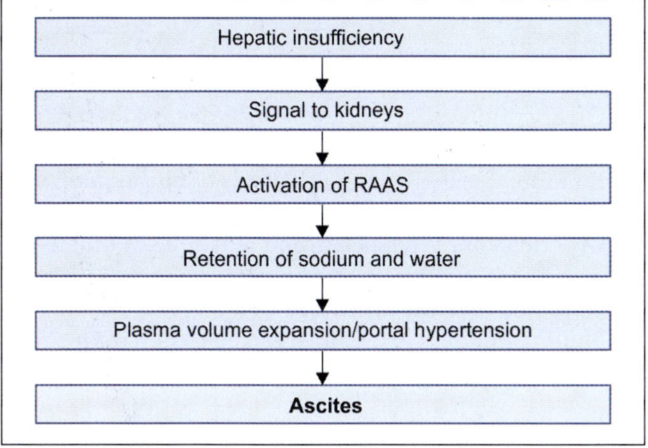

(RAAS: renin–angiotensin–aldosterone system)

FLOWCHART 2: Overfill theory.

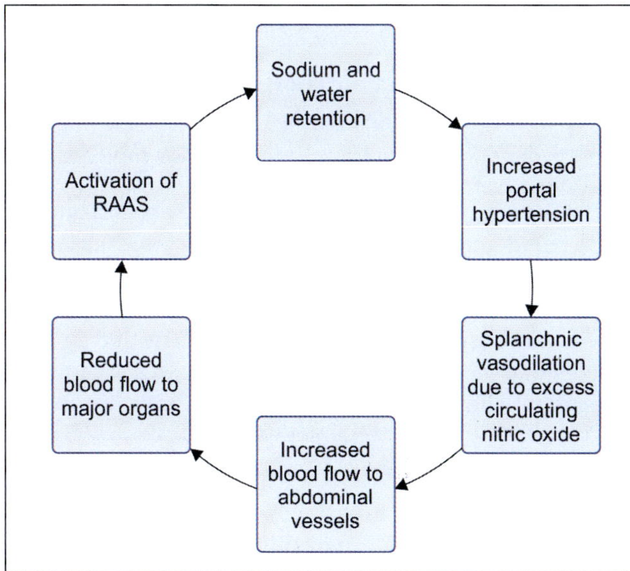

FLOWCHART 3: Summary of pathophysiology of ascites.

CAUSES OF ASCITES

Common causes of ascites are shown in **Table 1**.

- The most common cause of ascites is cirrhosis (~75%). Other causes include peritoneal malignancy (12%), cardiac failure (5%), peritoneal tuberculosis (TB) (2%) etc.
- Approximately 50% of patients with cirrhosis develop ascites within 10 years.
- Onset of ascites in patients with cirrhosis indicates decompensation and 5-year survival rate of such patients is around 30%.
- In a 1-year hospital-based cross-section observational study conducted in a tertiary care center of Himachal Pradesh, cirrhosis of liver was the leading cause of ascites (60.7%). TB was the second most common cause of ascites (13%), followed by malignancy and cardiac disorders (7.7%).
- Tuberculosis peritonitis should be considered in Indian population when patients present with ascites and constitutional symptoms like fever, weight loss, loss of appetite etc.

TABLE 1 Causes of ascites.

Peritoneal causes	Nonperitoneal causes

• Malignany (primary peritoneal mesothelioma, secondaries)
• Granulomatous peritonitis:
  ◦ Tuberculosis peritoneum
  ◦ Fungal/parasitic infections
  ◦ Sarcoidosis
  ◦ Foreign body
• Vasculitis/CTD
• Eosinophilic peritonitis
• Familial mediterranean fever
• Whipple disease
	• Hepatic
	  ◦ Cirrhosis of any cause
	  ◦ Alcoholic hepatitis
	  ◦ Budd–Chiari syndrome
	  ◦ Sinusoidal obstruction syndrome
	• Extrahepatic:
	  ◦ Heart failure
	  ◦ Hypoalbuminemia (nephrotic syndrome, malnutrition etc.)
	  ◦ Pancreatitis
	  ◦ Myxedema
	  ◦ Cancer related
	  ◦ Postoperative lymphatic leak

(CTD: connective tissue disease)

- Onset of ascites:
  - *Sudden*:
    - Acute Budd-Chiari syndrome
    - Acute right heart failure
  - *Insidious*: Cirrhosis of liver and other causes.

CLINICAL PRESENTATION

HISTORY

- *Abdominal distension*:
  - Progressive increase in the belt/clothing size/ abdominal girth
  - Development of umbilical/inguinal hernias
- *Swelling of lower limbs*:
  - Pedal edema precedes ascites in congestive cardiac failure (CCF), nephrotic syndrome etc.
  - Ascites precedes pedal edema in cirrhosis, constrictive pericarditis (ascites precox).
  - Edema is out of proportion to ascites in severe anemia with hypoproteinemia.
- *Jaundice*:
  - It indicates hepatic/biliary causes for ascites.
  - Jaundice can also be seen less often in extrahepatic causes of ascites like CCF, malignancies etc.
- *Hematemesis, melena*:
  - Presence of variceal upper gastrointestinal (UGI) bleed with splenomegaly indicates ascites might be secondary to portal hypertension.
- *Pain abdomen*:
  - Ascites + Diffuse pain—peritonitis of any cause and pancreatitis
  - Ascites + Right upper abdomen pain +/- hepatomegaly—in cases of acute Budd-Chiari, heart failure etc. It may also be a clue toward biliary causes.
- Ascites + Fever, weight loss, anorexia, chronic cough—consider TB in the differential diagnosis.

- Ascites + early morning periorbital puffiness—consider nephrotic syndrome.
- Facial puffiness, cold intolerance, and other symptoms of hypothyroidism must be recorded.
- Easy fatigability and other symptoms of anemia and hypoproteinemia must be recorded.
- Past history of pulmonary/abdominal TB, cardiac illness, hepatitis B, hepatitis C, autoimmune conditions, weight loss, and recurrent pain abdomen (pancreatitis) should be recorded. History of alcohol intake and drug abuse must be enquired. History often reveals clues to alcoholic liver disease or chronic viral hepatitis which helps in avoiding unnecessary investigations and planning appropriate treatment.

GENERAL PHYSICAL EXAMINATION

Ascites with the following findings in general physical examination (GPE) may suggest certain diagnosis as mentioned in **Table 2**.

TABLE 2 General physical examination in ascites.

Clinical finding	Differential diagnosis
Icterus	Cirrhosis (any cause), alcoholic hepatitis, Budd–Chiari syndrome, and congestive heart failure
Raised JVP	Congestive heart failure
Absent hepatojugular reflux	Budd–Chiari syndrome
Clubbing	Biliary cirrhosis, protein-losing enteropathy, malignancy
Pedal edema	Cirrhosis, heart failure, hypoproteinemia, and other causes of anasarca
Lymphadenopathy	Tuberculosis, supraclavicular lymph node (Virchow's node)—GI malignancy
Stigmata of chronic liver disease	Chronic liver disease of any cause
Periorbital puffiness	Nephrotic syndrome
Sister Joseph nodules, tylosis, sign of Leser–Trélat	External markers of internal malignancy

(GI: gastrointestinal; JVP: jugular venous pressure)

SYSTEMIC EXAMINATION

- Per abdomen examination should record findings as mentioned in **Table 3**.
- Divarication of recti, umbilical hernia, and striae albicantes suggest long-standing ascites.
- Prominent veins around umbilicus or epigastrium with blood flowing away from the umbilicus suggest portal hypertension. Whereas, prominent veins in the flanks with blood flow from below upward suggest inferior vena cava (IVC) obstruction.
- Shifting dullness is the most sensitive sign of free fluid in the peritoneal cavity on physical examination. It is present when ascitic fluid volume is >1,500 mL. False-positive shifting dullness may be seen in paralytic ileus (rare finding).
- Fluid thrill suggests tense ascites (ascitic fluid volume >2,000 mL). See **Box 1** for grades of ascites.
- Venous hum may be heard over distended veins around the umbilicus. This sign is called as *Cruveilhier-Baumgarten sign***.**
- Per rectal examination should be done to identify palpable mass, pelvic deposits (*Blumer's shelf*).
- Cardiovascular and respiratory system examination should be done to identify relevant clinical signs which include signs of heart failure, constrictive pericarditis, tricuspid regurgitation, hydrothorax, and basal lung collapse.
- Pleural effusion develops in about 5–10% of patients with cirrhosis. Pleural effusion is right sided in 85%, left sided in 13%, and bilateral in 2% cases. Grading of ascites is shown in **Box 1**.

INVESTIGATIONS

The evaluation of a patient with ascites starts with clinical history and thorough physical examination. The foremost step while investigating a case of ascites is to

BOX 1 Grades of ascites.

Grade 1:	Detectable on ultrasound and careful physical examination
Grade 2:	Easily detectable on physical examination but relatively small amount of free fluid
Grade 3:	Grossly or markedly distended abdomen

Source: Adapted from European Association for the Study of the Liver 2010.

TABLE 3 Per abdomen examination.

Inspection	Palpation	Percussion
• Abdominal distenison • Bulging flanks • Everted umbilicus • Tight-stretched skin (paper money skin) • Umbilical hernia, divarication of recti • Dilated veins • Near umbilicus (Caput medusa)—portal hypertension	• Fluid thrill • Hepatomegaly • Splenomegaly • Palpable primary gastrointestinal/pelvic tumors • Measurements include abdominal girth, spinoumbilical distance etc.	• Shifting dullness • Horse-shoe dullness • Puddle's sign

calculate SAAG. SAAG is calculated by subtracting ascitic fluid albumin from serum albumin (SAAG = serum albumin – ascitic fluid albumin). If SAAG is >1.1 g/dL, it is considered as high SAAG ascites which indicates presence of portal hypertension as the cause of ascites. If SAAG is <1.1 g/dL, it is considered as low SAAG ascites which indicates ascites due to other causes (**Table 4**). Based on the value of SAAG, appropriate investigations have to be planned to identify the cause of ascites.

ASCITIC FLUID ANALYSIS

Diagnostic paracentesis using 1.5 inch 22G steel needle should be performed in all patients with first episode of ascites. About 30 mL is obtained using Z-tract technique and analyzed. Diagnostic paracentesis can be performed in patients despite coagulopathy that is usually seen in patients with cirrhosis. However, it should be avoided in patients with clinically evident primary hyperfibrinolysis or disseminated intravascular coagulation (DIC). The following tests are performed on ascitic fluid (**Box 2**):

- *Appearance*:
  - Clear: Low protein, transudate
  - Cloudy: Infection
  - Milky: Chylous ascites
  - Brown: Biliary ascites
  - Straw color: Tuberculosis
  - Red: Hemorrhagic ascites or traumatic tap
- *Ascitic fluid albumin and protein*: SAAG is calculated as mentioned above. Ascitic fluid protein helps in further classification as shown in **Flowchart 4**.
- *Glucose*: Ascitic fluid glucose is usually similar to serum glucose levels. Low ascitic glucose indicates infection.
- *Cell count and typing*: In sterile ascites, white blood cell (WBC) count is usually <100 cells/mm^3 with predominant mononuclear cells. If WBC count is >500 cells/mm^3 and neutrophil count is >250 cells/mm^3, then diagnosis of SBP can be made. Ascites neutrophil count increases with peritoneal infection or other inflammatory conditions like diverticulitis and cholecystitis. Elevated WBC count with lymphocyte predominance suggests possibility of TB.
- *Gram staining and culture*: Gram staining is helpful in the diagnosis of gut perforation with high bacterial load. Ascitic fluid culture is performed by inoculating around 10 mL of ascitic fluid in culture media. Bedside inoculation into blood culture bottles is far superior

TABLE 4 Causes of ascites based on SAAG.

High gradient (>1.1 g/dL)	Low gradient (<1.1 g/dL)
• Cirrhosis	• Peritoneal carcinomatosis
• Alcoholic hepatitis	• Tuberculous peritonitis
• Cardiac ascites	• Pancreatic ascites
• Massive liver metastases	• Biliary ascites
• Fulminant hepatic failure	• Nephrotic syndrome
• Budd–Chiari syndrome	• Serositis in connective tissue disorder
• Portal vein thrombosis	
• Veno-occlusive disease	
• Fatty liver pregnancy	
• Myxedema	
• Mixed ascites	

BOX 2 Tests performed on ascitic fluid.

- Appearance
- Albumin and total protein
- Glucose
- Cell count and typing
- Gram stain and culture
- Lactate dehydrogenase
- Amylase
- Bilirubin
- Triglyceride
- Malignant cells
- Adenosine deaminase

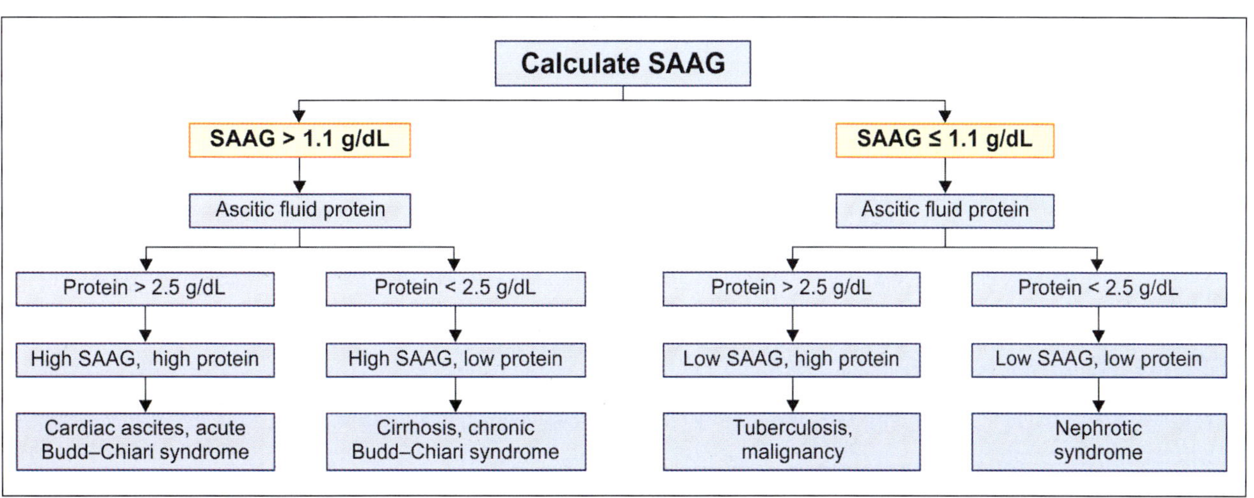

(SAAG: serum ascites albumin gradient)

FLOWCHART 4: Algorithm for diagnosis of ascites using SAAG.

to detect bacterial growth as compared to delayed inoculation in laboratory. In patients with SBP, culture is monobacterial. If culture is polybacterial, secondary bacterial peritonitis should be suspected.

- *Lactate dehydrogenase (LDH)*: Significantly elevated LDH levels suggest secondary peritonitis or SBP. Usually ascitic fluid LDH is less than half the serum LDH.
- *Amylase*: Ascitic fluid amylase level >2,000 U/L indicates pancreatic ascites or gut perforation.
- *Bilirubin*: Ascitic fluid bilirubin greater than serum bilirubin suggests biliary ascites.
- *Triglyceride*: Ascitic fluid triglyceride level >200 mg/dL is seen in chylous ascites.
- *Adenosine deaminase (ADA)*: It is used to diagnose TB. Although insensitive, ADA level >36 U/L in ascitic fluid is considered to be significant.

LABORATORY TESTS

- Liver biochemical and coagulation tests should be performed.
- Renal function tests including serum creatinine, serum and urine electrolytes, and 24-hour urine sodium and protein quantifications are helpful.
- Measurement of baseline sodium excretion helps to predict response to diuretic therapy as well as prognosis in cirrhotic patients with ascites. Urine sodium ≥10 mEq/day is more likely to respond better to lower doses of diuretics. Patients with baseline sodium excretion ≤10 mEq/day have poorer prognosis with median survival of only 1.5 years, as compared with 4.5 years in patients with urine sodium ≥ 10 mEq/day.

ULTRASOUND

- Ultrasonography (USG) detects as little as 100 mL of ascitic fluid.
- It helps in identifying cirrhosis, primary or secondary hepatic neoplasms, congestive hepatomegaly etc. Hepatic venous Doppler is useful in diagnosis of Budd-Chiari syndrome.
- USG abdomen should be performed in all patients with a first episode of ascites.

ENDOSCOPY

- Upper gastrointestinal endoscopy helps in identifying signs of portal hypertension. It also helps in diagnosis of gastric malignancies.
- Colonoscopy helps in identifying lower GI malignancies with peritoneal metastasis. It also helps in diagnosis of abdominal TB.

DIFFERENTIAL DIAGNOSIS

Heart failure patients with ascites may mimic cirrhotic patients. We should look for presence of cardiac symptoms like dyspnea, PND, orthopnea, and chest pain. Clinical examination may reveal signs of heart failure like raised jugular venous pressure (JVP), pedal edema, and pathological S3 or S4. In cardiac ascites, SAAG will be >1.1 g/dL and ascites protein will be >2.5 g/dL. Patients with cirrhosis have low ascitic protein, hematocrit, and platelet count which are usually absent in cardiac ascites. 2D echo, cardiac catheterization, and measurement of hepatic vein pressures may be required to differentiate between cardiac and cirrhotic ascites. It is noteworthy that patients with ascites of unknown etiology may have constrictive pericarditis. Paradoxical pulse, raised JVP, and a calcified pericardium on radiological studies are the clues to diagnose constrictive pericarditis.

Malignant ascites contributes to <10% of all cases of ascites. Patients may have symptoms and localizing signs of the primary tumor but many patients present with ascites alone (Example: Elderly postmenopausal woman presenting with ascites alone may have an underlying ovarian neoplasm). Cytology of the ascitic fluid is not very sensitive and normal endothelial cells can resemble malignant cells. Imaging studies like CT and FDG-PET (fluorodeoxyglucose-positron emission tomography) should be considered.

Tuberculous ascites is more commonly observed in India. It should be suspected in patients with fever, weight loss, loss of appetite, and severe malnutrition. Doughy feel on palpation of the abdomen suggests lumps of matted omentum. Ascitic fluid has predominantly lymphocytes and ADA level >36 U/L may be significant. Ascites should be stained for tubercle bacilli and appropriate cultures obtained. If diagnosis cannot be confirmed, abdominal laparoscopy and peritoneal biopsy should be considered.

Pancreatic ascites is uncommon and rarely gross. It is seen in patients with pseudocyst rupture or pancreatic duct disruption. Ascitic fluid amylase levels are usually >2,000 U/L.

Chylous ascites refers to milky appearance of ascitic fluid. It results from rupture of intra-abdominal lymphatics. Most common nonsurgical cause of chylous ascites is cirrhosis. Surgical causes include retroperitoneal surgery, radical surgery in patients with malignancy. Ascitic fluid is milky and triglyceride levels are >200 mg/dL.

COMPLICATIONS

The common complications of ascites include SBP, refractory ascites, and HRS. Other complications include hepatic hydrothorax, abdominal wall hernias etc. Development of ascites in a patient with cirrhosis should alert the physician of other impending complications of cirrhosis and portal hypertension. We should actively look for and treat these complications in a patient with ascites.

TREATMENT

Patients with uncomplicated ascites can be managed on outpatient basis (**Table 5**). Not all patients with ascites require hospital admission. Inpatient care should be considered in patients who develop complications of ascites or for in-hospital investigation in a patient who presents with ascites for the first time.

TABLE 5 Medical management of uncomplicated ascites.

Grade 1 ascites	Grade 2 ascites	Grade 3 ascites
• Dietary sodium restriction • No specific guidelines	• Dietary sodium restriction • Diuretic therapy • Close monitoring of body weight	• Dietary sodium restriction • Large volume paracentesis • Albumin and diuretic therapy

SODIUM RESTRICTION

It is clear from pathogenesis that sodium retention plays a key role in the development of ascites. Hence, management of ascites is primarily aimed at creating a negative sodium balance. The best way to achieve negative sodium balance is to reduce sodium intake and supplement it with diuretics to increase renal sodium excretion. Dietary sodium restriction alone might satisfactorily treat patients with ascites. Ideally, a patient with cirrhosis and ascites should not consume >1 g of sodium per day. But such food is unpalatable. Hence current recommendations suggest dietary sodium intake should be restricted to 70–90 mEq/day or 1.5–2 g/day. In common parlance, this would mean "*no added salt*". Salt should neither be used while cooking nor while serving food. Canned food should be avoided.

Dietary sodium restriction alone might be enough in a subset of patients who have normal creatinine clearance, urine sodium excretion >10 mEq/day, acute onset ascites secondary to a treatable complication like infection, ascites following excess sodium intake in a stable patient etc. In patients who do not respond to diet restriction alone will need diuretic therapy.

DIURETICS

Antimineralocorticoid and loop diuretics are the two classes of diuretics used in the treatment of ascites (**Flowchart 5**). There are two approaches that can be used while starting diuretic therapy: Spironolactone alone or a combination of spironolactone and furosemide. The choice of therapy has been a matter of controversy. Two studies were conducted to identify which is the better initial therapy—spironolactone alone followed by addition of furosemide or a combination of both drugs from day one of treatment. Both studies had contrasting outcomes. Current guidelines suggest use of spironolactone alone for patients with a first episode of ascites and combination therapy for recurrent ascites.

Spironolactone alone:

- It is a potassium-sparing, antimineralocorticoid diuretic acting on distal tubule and collecting duct.
- It is the diuretic of choice for single-agent therapy in ascites.
- It is less potent natriuretic than furosemide. Since it is potassium-sparing, hypokalemia is unlikely.
- The starting dose is 50–100 mg/day depending on degree of ascites. If the patient does not respond in 3–4 days, the dose can be increased by 100 mg/day every 4 days up to a maximum of 400 mg/day. At high doses, hyperkalemia may develop and drug may have to be stopped temporarily.

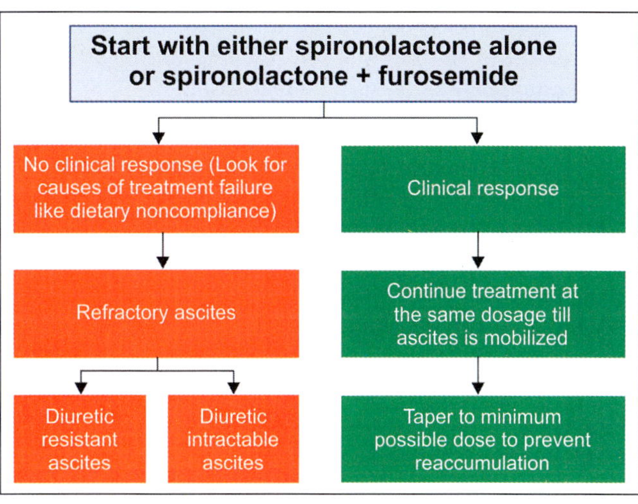

FLOWCHART 5: Algorithm for diuretic therapy.

- Spironolactone has delayed clinical response, hyperkalemia and poor natriuresis as disadvantages. On the other hand, it has a long half-life and allows once daily dosing.
- When patients do not respond to spironolactone or develop hyperkalemia, furosemide at a dose of 20–40 mg/day can be started.
- If patients develop painful gynecomastia, spironolactone can be replaced with amiloride at a dose of 10–15 mg/day.

Combination therapy:

Spironolactone + Furosemide:

- Starting dose of spironolactone 100 mg/furosemide 40 mg once daily is recommended. This ratio leads to fewer potassium abnormalities.
- In case of lack of response, spironolactone dose should be increased by 100 mg/day and furosemide dose by 40 mg/day once in 4 days.
- Maximum dosage of spironolactone and furosemide is 400 mg/day and 160 mg/day, respectively.

Weight monitoring and follow-up: Diuretic dose should be titrated to achieve:

- 0.5 kg/day weight loss in patients without peripheral edema
- 1 kg/day weight loss in patients with ascites and edema
- It should be noted that only up to 700 mL of ascitic fluid can be mobilized in a day with intensive diuretic therapy. Hence clinicians should not aim for a negative fluid balance of >1 L/day.
- Once ascites is mobilized, the diuretic dose should be down-titrated to minimum necessary dose required to keep the patient free of ascites and also avoid adverse effects.
- Serum electrolytes, urea, creatinine, and liver function tests are done every 4 weeks for stable outpatients on diuretics.

- As liver function improves and ascites resolves, plan to stop furosemide first and then spironolactone and maintain patient on sodium restriction.

Causes for failure of diuretic therapy:

- Dietary noncompliance (check by measuring 24 hour urinary sodium excretion)
- Concomitant use of nonsteroidal anti-inflammatory drugs (NSAIDs), angiotensin-converting enzyme (ACE) inhibitors, or angiotensin receptor blockers
- Very poor hepatocellular function.

REFRACTORY ASCITES

Refractory ascites refers to ascites that cannot be mobilized, or recurrence of which cannot be prevented because of a lack of response to maximum diuretic therapy (diuretic resistant) or development of diuretic-related complication that prevents the use of an effective diuretic dose (diuretic intractable). Patients should be labeled diuretic resistant when there is no clinical response in patients who are on spironolactone 400 mg/day and furosemide 160 mg/day for at least 1 week and on salt restricted diet of <80 mEq/day. Treatment options for refractory ascites include:

- Large volume paracentesis (LVP)
- TIPS (transjugular intrahepatic portosystemic shunt)
- Peritoneovenous shunts. Example: LeVeen shunt, Denver shunt, and Minnesota shunt
- Liver transplantation

NOTEWORTHY POINTS

- *Recidivant ascites/refractory ascites*: Ascites that recurs on three or more occasions within 12 months period despite dietary sodium restriction and adequate diuretic dosage.
- *Early recurrence of ascites*: Reappearance of grade 2 or 3 ascites within 4 weeks of initial mobilization.
- *Other pharmacotherapies in ascites*: Drugs like midodrine, long-term IV albumin therapy, and vaptans (Satavaptan) have been studied as treatment options for ascites. But the evidence is limited and controversial.
- *Alfapump system*: It is an automated low-flow ascites pump that moves ascites from peritoneal cavity to urinary bladder. Studies show that using alfapump system results in a significant reduction in the number and volume of LVP needed in patients with cirrhosis and recurrent or refractory ascites compared with standard care. Since alfapump is associated with side effects like device-related adverse events, AKI, and other complications of cirrhosis, it is currently only recommended in patients in whom TIPS is not indicated.

RECOMMENDED READINGS

1. Runyon BA. Ascites. In: Schiff L, Schiff ER (Eds). Diseases of the Liver. Philadelphia: Lippincott Company; 1993. pp. 990-1015.
2. European Association for the Study of the Liver. EASL Clinical Practice Guidelines for the management of patients with decompensated cirrhosis. J Hepatol. 2018;69:406-60.
3. D'Amico G, Garcia-Tsao G, Pagliaro L. Natural history and prognostic indicators of survival in cirrhosis: a systematic review of 118 studies. J Hepatol. 2006;44:217-31.
4. Kumar B, Sharma B, Raina S, Sharma N, Gupta D, Mardi K. Etiology of ascites in adults living in the Hills of Himachal Pradesh, India: A hospital-based study. CHRISMED J Health Res. 2016;3:41-4.
5. Lieberman FL, Hidemura R, Peters RL, Reynolds TB. Pathogenesis and treatment if hydrothorax complicating cirrhosis with ascites. Ann Intern Med. 1966;64:341-51.
6. Strauss RM, Boyer TD. Hepatic hydrothorax. Semin Liver Dis. 1997;17:227-32.
7. Arroyo V, Bosch J, Gaya-Beltrán J, Kravetz D, Estrada L, Rivera F, et al. Plasma renin activity and urinary sodium excretion as prognostic indicators in nonazotemic cirrhosis with ascites. Ann Intern Med. 1981;94(2):198-201.
8. Llach J, Ginès P, Arroyo V, Rimola A, Tító L, Badalamenti S, et al. Prognostic value of arterial pressure, endogenous vasoactive systems, and renal function in cirrhotic patients admitted to the hospital for the treatment of ascites. Gastroenterology. 1988;94(2):482-7.
9. Bhargava DK, Gupta M, Nijhawan S, Dasarathy S, Kushwaha AK. Adenosine deaminase (ADA) in peritoneal tuberculosis: diagnostic value in ascitic fluid and serum. Tubercle. 1990;71(2):121-6.
10. Angeli P, Fasolato S, Mazza E, Okolicsanyi L, Maresio G, Velo E, et al. Combined versus sequential diuretic treatment of ascites in non-azotaemic patients with cirrhosis: results of an open randomised clinical trial. Gut. 2010;59:98-104.
11. Santos J, Planas R, Pardo A, Durández R, Cabré E, Morillas RM, et al. Spironolactone alone or in combination with furosemide in the treatment of moderate ascites in nonazotemic cirrhosis. A randomized comparative study of efficacy and safety. J Hepatol. 2003;39:187-92.
12. Sola E, Gines P. Ascites and spontaneous bacterial peritonitis. In: Feldman M, Friedman L, Brandt L (Eds). Sleisenger and Fordtran's Gastrointestinal and Liver Disease, 11th edition. Philadelphia, Pa: Elsevier Health Sciences; 2020. pp. 1795-805.

CHAPTER
9

Dyspnea, Syncope and Palpitations: Evaluation

Sudha Vidyasagar, Sudhakar Rao, Cynthia Amrutha

ABSTRACT

Dyspnea, palpitations, and syncope are common complaints in any medicine outpatient department and reasons for admission in medicine and cardiology wards. Palpitations are more often due to cardiac causes, but syncope can occur due to cardiac, neurological, and autonomic dysfunction. Dyspnea has an even more wider etiology encompassing cardiac, respiratory, neuromuscular, and metabolic causes.

All of them can be due to simple or dangerous causes, and a keen clinical approach is needed to sort out the benign from the life-threatening ones. Diligent history taking, bedside examination, and sensible algorithm of investigations can help to arrive at a diagnosis and appropriate therapy. In this chapter, we will go through the causes, clinical manifestations, and differential diagnosis of each of these symptoms, and also summarize the relevant investigations needed to make a possible diagnosis.

"There is only one cardinal rule: One must always listen to the patient"

—Oliver Sacks

DYSPNEA

INTRODUCTION

Dyspnea is a clinical manifestation that occurs in up to 25% of ambulatory patients. It is seen in various clinical settings and has the potential to be life-threatening as well. Focused evaluation and diagnosis are important to reduce the clinical morbidity and mortality. However, despite identifying an underlying cardiac or pulmonary cause, overlapping clinical conditions and comorbidities have proven to be a challenge. Hence, it is important to evaluate this common clinical symptom sequentially with targeted diagnostics to reach a timely diagnosis.

DEFINITION

The American Thoracic Society defines dyspnea as "a subjective experience of breathing discomfort that consists of qualitatively distinct sensations that vary in intensity."

CAUSES

Common causes of dyspnea are shown in **Table 1**.

TABLE 1 Causes of dyspnea.

System	Causes
Pulmonary	Chronic obstructive pulmonary disease (COPD), asthma, pulmonary embolism, pneumonia, acute respiratory distress syndrome (ARDS), interstitial lung disease, pleural effusion, pneumothorax, and stridor
Cardiac	Acute coronary syndrome, heart failure, cardiomyopathy, arrhythmias, valvular heart disease, and cardiac tamponade
Neuromuscular	Stroke, central hyperventilation syndromes, amyotrophic lateral sclerosis, Guillain–Barré syndrome, and myasthenia gravis
Metabolic	Metabolic acidosis such as diabetic ketoacidosis, uremia, lactic acidosis, salicylate poisoning, sepsis, and renal tubular acidosis
Chest wall	Rib fracture, flail chest, and kyphoscoliosis
Psychiatric	Anxiety and panic attacks
Physiological	Exercise, ageing, deconditioning, obesity, and pregnancy
Anaphylaxis	Due to allergy or bites

MECHANISM

Mechanoreceptors: J receptors in chest wall receptors and upper airway receptors contribute to decreased compliance. Mechanoreceptors (in skeletal muscles) respond to local changes in the tissue environment.

Chemoreceptors (in carotid bodies at the bifurcation of common carotid artery): Changes in arterial blood pH, arterial carbon dioxide tension ($PaCO_2$,) and arterial oxygen tension (PaO_2) can be sensed by the central and peripheral chemoreceptors and the stimulation of these causes an increase in respiratory motor activity (**Flowchart 1**).

APPROACH TO HISTORY TAKING

A detailed and precise history should focus on classifying the dyspnea in order to reach a plausible diagnosis. This can be done by dividing the questions into:

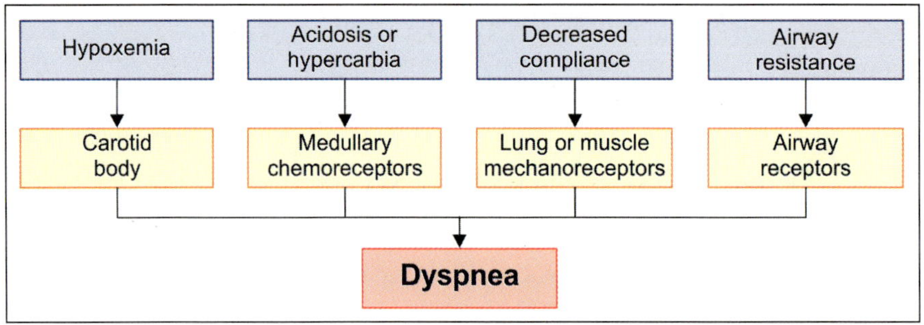

FLOWCHART 1: Receptors involved in dyspnea.

Onset and course:

- Acute onset—left heart failure, acute coronary syndrome, pneumothorax, acute severe asthma, pulmonary embolism, and acute exacerbation of chronic obstructive pulmonary disease (COPD)
- Chronic (present for >4 weeks)—pleural effusion, interstitial lung disease (ILD), and COPD
- Acute on chronic—asthma and COPD
- Acute intermittent episodes—myocardial ischemia, bronchospasm, and recurrent pulmonary embolism
- Chronic persistent episodes—COPD, ILD, and chronic thromboembolism

Symptomatology according to cause of dyspnea:

- Pulmonary—cough with/without expectoration, wheeze, and pleuritic chest pain
- Cardiac—orthopnea, paroxysmal nocturnal dyspnea (PND), and severe chest pain
- Nocturnal dyspnea—congestive heart failure and asthma
- Fever—pneumonia, acute bronchitis, and acute respiratory distress syndrome (ARDS)
- Hemoptysis—mitral stenosis, pulmonary thromboembolism, and malignancy
- Drugs and substance abuse—salicylate poisoning and nonselective beta-blockers
- Psychiatric illness—this should be a diagnosis of exclusion. It becomes important with a history of previous underlying panic and/or anxiety disorder.
- Trauma—injury to airway/mediastinal structures

Severity of dyspnea: Depending on the cause of dyspnea being cardiac or respiratory, the following grades can be used. The Modified Medical Research Council (MMRC) scale is useful for assessing severity of dyspnea due to noncardiac causes. Assessment of dyspnea is one of the components of the New York Heart Association (NYHA) functional status classification.

Orthopnea:

- Dyspnea that is relieved in sitting position or to feel comfortable patient assumes sitting or upright posture (it is not breathlessness in supine as patient is uncomfortable in prone or lateral decubitus as well).
- It occurs rapidly, within 1-2 minutes of lying down and is somewhat relieved on sitting.
- Cause of orthopnea—left heart failure causing pulmonary congestion
- Differential diagnosis—ascites and bilateral diaphragmatic paralysis

Paroxysmal nocturnal dyspnea: Paroxysmal nocturnal dyspnea is the occurrence of dyspnea during sleep, commonly 2-3 hours after going to bed, associated with cough, and usually relieved by assuming upright posture for 15-30 minutes. PND mimickers can be seen in bronchial asthma, postnasal drip, gastroesophageal reflux disease, nocturnal arrhythmias, obstructive sleep apnea, nocturnal angina, anxiety with hyperventilation, and Cheyne-Stokes respiration.

Mechanisms of orthopnea and paroxysmal nocturnal dyspnea: Increased distribution of blood into the pulmonary circulation:

- Increased venous return (in supine position)
- Shift of fluid from interstitium to venous circulation at night in PND
- Depression of respiratory center during sleep
- Nocturnal dreams and related increase in sympathetic activity with increased blood pressure (BP)
- Elevation of diaphragm in supine position

↓

- Pooling of blood in pulmonary vasculature
- Increase in intrapulmonary intravascular pressure
- Ventilation perfusion mismatch

↓

Leads to dyspnea and makes patient sit up (diaphragm moves down, venous return decreases due to sitting posture, and being awake stimulates the respiratory center) to maintain better ventilation—perfusion ratio.

Trepopnea:

- Trepopnea is a term used to define breathlessness in either lateral decubitus position.
- *Causes*: Congestive cardiac failure and severe unilateral pleural effusion
- *Mechanism*: Trepopnea may occur with asymmetric lung disease when the patient lies with the more affected lung down. In cardiac failure, the patient is dyspneic in the left lateral position, it is probably caused by distortion of the great vessels in one lateral decubitus position versus the other.

Platypnea:

- *Platypnea/platypnea-orthodeoxia syndrome (POS)*: Dyspnea that is accentuated by standing or sitting from the recumbent position and relieved on lying down.

- *Causes*: Left atrial myxoma, intracardiac shunts like patent foramen ovale, atrial septal defect or atrial septal aneurysm with fenestration, and hepatopulmonary syndrome
- *Mechanism*: Increase in the positional right-to-left shunting through intrapulmonary or intracardiac shunts

GENERAL PHYSICAL EXAMINATION

Identification and integration of clinical signs aid in diagnosis of cause of dyspnea.

Vital signs:

- Low volume pulse—cardiogenic shock
- Bounding pulse—type 2 respiratory failure
- Pulsus alternans—left heart failure
- Pulsus paradoxus—right heart failure, tension pneumothorax, and cardiac tamponade
- Blood pressure—low (cardiogenic/septic shock)/ tension pneumothorax and acute severe asthma
- Respiratory rate is high—all dyspneic patients
- Accessory muscles acting—all dyspnea
- *Hyperventilation*: Metabolic acidosis, sepsis, and anxiety

General examination:

- Pallor—anemia
- Clubbing—interstitial pulmonary fibrosis
- Cyanosis—hypoxia due to any cause
- Joint swelling or deformity—collagen vascular disease and Raynaud's disease
- Signs of liver cell failure—spider angiomata and gynecomastia
- Stridor—foreign body and epiglottitis

Respiratory examination:

- Asymmetrical chest expansion—unilateral disease
- *Bilateral decreased expansion*: Emphysema and ILD
- Paradoxical movement of abdomen—diaphragmatic weakness
- *Trachea and mediastinum*:
  - *To opposite side*: Pleural effusion and pneumothorax
  - *To same side*: Fibrosis/collapse
- *Percussion dull*: Collapse/effusion/consolidation
- *Resonant*: Pneumothorax and emphysema
- *Breath sounds*:
  - Decreased—COPD emphysema
  - Absent—pneumothorax (unilateral) and severe asthma (bilateral)
- *Adventitious sounds*:
  - Crepitations—left heart failure, ARDS, and pneumonia
  - Rhonchi—asthma and COPD

The dangerous signs of respiratory distress on clinical examination are listed below.

Dangerous signs:

- Altered mental status
- Increased respiratory effort
- Cyanosis
- Inability to complete sentences
- Use of accessory muscles of respiration
- Supraclavicular retractions
- Assuming tripod position (sitting with hands braced on knees)
- Orthopnea
- Diaphoresis
- Stridor

Cardiovascular examination:

- Raised jugular venous pressure (JVP)/hepatojugular reflux—right heart failure
- Cardiac murmur—valvular heart disease
- S_3—left ventricular systolic dysfunction (heart failure and mitral/aortic regurgitation)
- S_4—left ventricular diastolic dysfunction [severe hypertension and aortic stenosis (AS)]
- Muffled heart sounds—cardiac tamponade

DIAGNOSTIC APPROACH

The diagnostic approach consists of first ruling out hypoxia by a pulse oximetry. This will decide the urgency needed to treat the patient and the need for supplemental oxygen as immediate therapy. The other investigations are done, as required, to assess the cause of dyspnea (cardiac/ respiratory/others). The severity may be assessed bedside with an arterial blood gas (ABG) and 6-minute walk test. This is done to assess functional capacity of the patient, by making the patient walk for 6 minutes. The distance covered can be noted, as a baseline, to be used in future for comparison. In addition, a pulse oximetry done at the end of 6 minutes will help to assess desaturation during daily activities, and need for oxygen, in conditions such as ILD.

Table 2 below gives a list of investigations that may be needed.

Diagnostic approach to dyspnea is shown in **Flowchart 2**.

SYNCOPE

DEFINITION

Transient loss of consciousness due to acute global impairment of cerebral blood flow with loss of postural tone and spontaneous and complete recovery (self-limited).

CAUSES

The causes of syncope can be divided into three general categories:

1. Cardiac syncope—arrhythmias or structural cardiac diseases that cause a decrease in cardiac output. This is most dangerous and life-threatening, and needs urgent diagnosis.
2. Neurally-mediated syncope (also called reflex or vasovagal syncope)—a transient change in the reflexes responsible for maintaining cardiovascular homeostasis
3. Orthostatic hypotension—autonomic failure, cardiovascular homeostatic reflexes are chronically impaired.

TABLE 2 List of investigations.

Diagnostic tool	Clinical significance
Pulse oximetry	Bedside test to confirm hypoxia
6-minute walk test	• To detect hypoxia on exertion and exercise capacity • Usually, patients with ILD may have hypoxia on exertion
Complete blood count	To detect anemia, increased total counts in infection, and platelets decreased in systemic illness/sepsis
Arterial blood gas analysis	• Hypoxia—respiratory failure • CO_2 retention—hypoventilation-type 2 respiratory failure • Acidosis (metabolic/respiratory)
Chest X-ray	Cardiomegaly, pulmonary congestion in left heart failure, pneumonia, ARDS, pneumothorax, and pleural effusion
Ultrasound of chest	Pericardial tamponade, heart failure, pneumothorax, and pleural effusion
Electrocardiogram	Cardiac ischemia, MI, ventricular hypertrophy, arrhythmias, and electrical alternans in pericardial effusion
Cardiac biomarkers raised	Troponin T—cardiac ischemia
NT-proBNP raised	Cardiac failure
D-dimer increased	Pulmonary embolism
CT chest	Pulmonary thromboembolism, malignancy, and interstitial lung disease

(CT: computed tomography; ARDS: acute respiratory distress syndrome; ILD: interstitial lung disease)

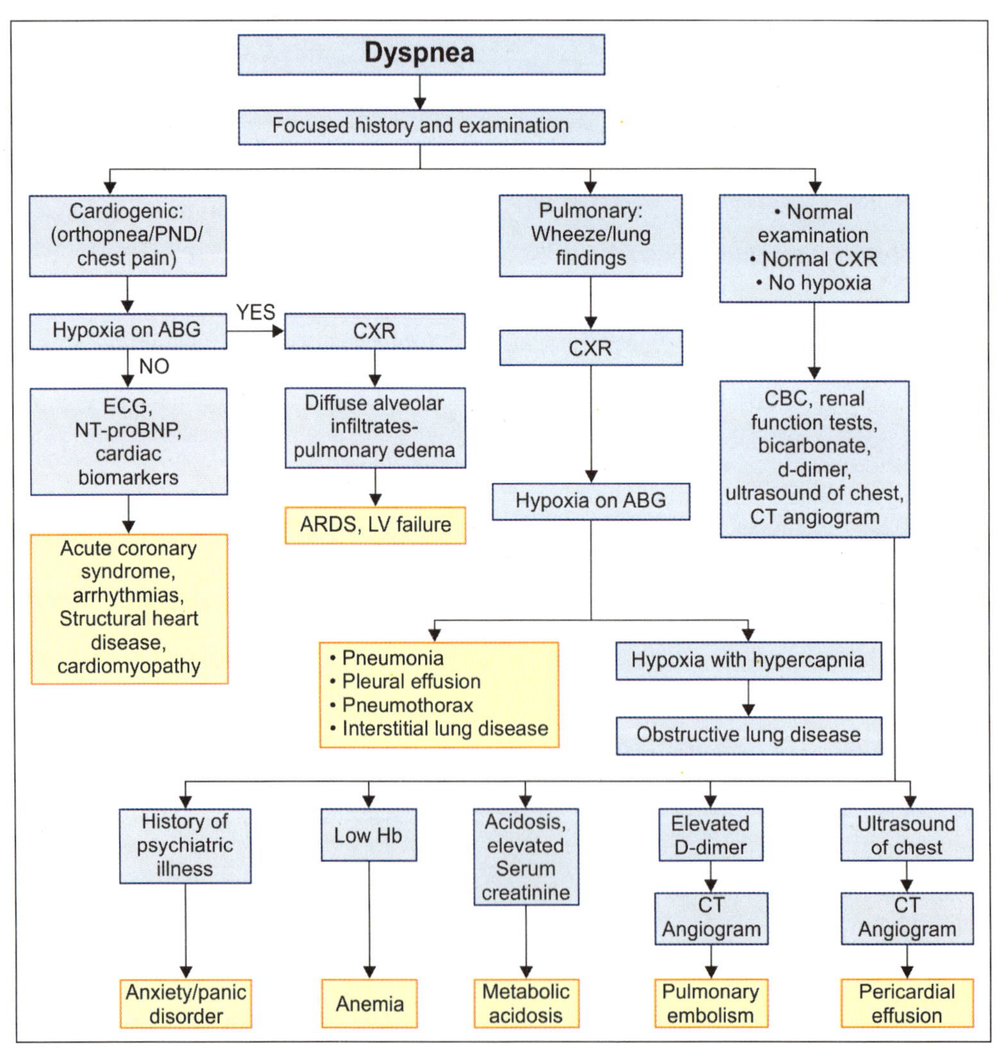

(ABG: arterial blood gas; ARDS: acute respiratory distress syndrome; CT: computed tomography; CXR: chest X-ray; Hb: hemoglobin; LV: left ventricular; PND: paroxysmal nocturnal dyspnea)

FLOWCHART 2: Diagnostic approach to dyspnea.

CARDIOVASCULAR CAUSES OF SYNCOPE

The cardiovascular causes of syncope can be divided into structural causes and arrhythmias.

Structural and obstructive causes:

- Severe AS
- Hypertrophic cardiomyopathy (HCM)
- Massive myocardial infarction (MI)/shock due to any cause
- Mitral stenosis—severe
- Acute pulmonary embolism
- Severe pulmonary arterial hypertension (PAH)
- Cardiac tamponade
- Severe pulmonary stenosis
- Eisenmenger syndrome
- Atrial myxoma
- Rarely restrictive and constrictive pericardial diseases

Mechanism of syncope in valvular heart diseases:
Mitral stenosis:

- Severe PAH—low cardiac output
- Severe PAH—dilated pulmonary artery obstructing the left main coronary artery
- Atrial arrhythmias
- Cerebral embolism

Aortic stenosis:

- Fixed cardiac output state
- Low cardiac output causes activation of baroreceptor causing fall in systemic vascular resistance
- Arrhythmias
- Associated conduction disease (due to calcific AS)

Other structural lesions interfere with the cardiac output and hence the cerebral blood flow, causing syncope. Any form of shock, hypovolemic, septic, or anaphylactic can cause syncope.

Cardiac arrhythmias: They cause syncope when they decrease cardiac output, as in atrial tachyarrhythmias with fast ventricular response, or ventricular arrhythmias. This happens especially, if ventricular rate is above 200 bpm, as this seriously interferes with diastolic filling of ventricle, and also coronary blood flow. Long QT syndromes can lead to polymorphic VT called torsade de pointes and degenerate into ventricular fibrillation. Brugada's syndrome is an inherited cause of sudden death, presenting with ST elevation in right ventricular leads, which may present episodic syncope. In sick sinus syndrome, there are exit blocks, during which there is no cardiac contraction, causing syncope.

In complete heart block, there can be Stokes-Adams syndrome, which is when second degree heart block, transitions into third degree heart block, and the ventricular pacemaker has not taken over. The following list shows the arrhythmias that can cause syncope.

Bradyarrhythmias:

- Sinus bradycardia, sinus arrest, sinoatrial block, and sick sinus syndrome
- Atrioventricular block and complete heart block

Tachyarrhythmias:

- Supraventricular tachycardia (SVT) with 1:1 conduction
- Atrial fibrillation (AF) with Wolff-Parkinson-White (WPW) syndrome
- Atrial flutter with 1:1 conduction
- Ventricular tachycardia (VT)

NEURALLY-MEDIATED SYNCOPE (REFLEX OR VASOVAGAL)

This occurs in conditions where there is pooling of blood in the lower limbs such as in prolonged standing, or where autonomic reflexes are *transiently* dysfunctional causing drop in BP in upright posture. This is the most common cause of syncope in all groups, especially in the young, and refers to fainting episodes. These attacks occur in situations of prolonged standing, fear, anxiety, and unpleasant sensations.

Typical features are light headedness, sweating, nausea, and vomiting. The up rolling of eyes that can occur at the beginning of syncope may be confused with seizure, along with a few jerky movements that may transiently occur. Vagally-mediated syncope can cause cough syncope, and micturition syncope, associated with these acts. Carotid sinus hypersensitivity can also cause syncope when the neck is touched in sensitive individuals.

ORTHOSTATIC HYPOTENSION

Orthostatic hypotension is defined as a fall in BP of 20 mm Hg systolic, and 10 mm Hg diastolic, within 3 minutes of standing, and is a manifestation of sympathetic failure. There is also an early orthostatic hypotension that can occur within 15 seconds, and may reflect transient mismatch between vascular capacity and cardiac output.

This occurs when autonomic failure is *permanent,* and leads to lack of compensation of BP fall, which normally will occur in upright posture. It is also characterized by light headedness, and black outs, occurring with change to upright posture, and can cause falls in the elderly. Nonspecific symptoms, such as cognitive clouding, or headache, or weakness when standing, can be equivalents of syncope.

The causes include conditions causing degeneration of autonomic system, such as multisystem atrophy or hereditary sensory motor neuropathies. Diabetes is one of the most common causes of secondary autonomic failure leading to orthostatic hypotension. Drugs causing autonomic failure, amyloidosis, human immunodeficiency virus (HIV) disease, paraneoplastic conditions, and Guillain-Barré syndrome variants are some other causes. Postprandial syncope can occur after large meals and alcohol, due to an unexplained mechanism. Subclavian steal can occur, if there is stenosis of subclavian artery before the origin of the vertebral artery. When the person exerts his arm, blood can flow from vertebral artery to the arm, causing syncope.

APPROACH TO HISTORY TAKING

Important clues in history in patient with syncope are shown in **Table 3**.

TABLE 3 Important clues in history in patient with syncope.

Condition	Clues
Cardiac conditions	History of structural cardiac disease, palpitations, syncope even in lying position
Diabetes mellitus	Hypoglycemia, CVA, CAD, TIA, postural hypotension due to autonomic neuropathy
Hypertension	Postural hypotension, encephalopathy, ICH, TIA, CAD
Postoperative/prolonged rest	Pulmonary embolism, postural hypotension
Drugs	Diuretics, methyldopa, vasodilators, nitrates, prazosin, ACE inhibitors, CCBs
Situational syncope	Episodes after coughing, urinating, defecating, or swallowing
Vasovagal syncope	Painful/unpleasant event/site
Subdural hematoma	History of fall/head injury
Hypertrophic cardiomyopathy, arrhythmias, long QT syndrome, Brugada syndrome	Family history of syncope/sudden cardiac death
Epilepsy	Aura, abrupt LOC, sensory hallucinations, Déjà vu, automatisms, prolonged amnesia, incontinence of urine/stool, family history
GI bleeding causing hypovolemic shock	History of peptic ulcer, hematemesis, melena, vomiting, abdominal pain, trauma to abdomen
Long QT syndrome	Deaf patient
Aortic stenosis, HCM, B/L carotid stenosis, pulmonary hypertension, severe CAD	Exertional syncope
Subclavian steal syndrome	Syncope with upper limb exercise

(ACE: angiotensin-converting enzyme; CAD: coronary artery disease; CCB: calcium channel blocker; CVA: cerebrovascular accident; GI: Gastrointestinal; HCM: hypertrophic cardiomyopathy; ICH: intracerebral hemorrhage; TIA: transient ischemic attack)

A detailed history regarding the patients' premorbid conditions would help to classify the cause of syncope. It is worthwhile eliciting a good history from a bystander who has witnessed the event as patients may not be able to recollect an accurate picture. Young patients with no premorbidity under circumstances of mental stress, fear or extreme emotion, would probably have vasovagal syncope. Older patients with cardiac diseases will present with cardiac symptoms. In the elderly, orthostatic hypotension is known to occur due to degeneration of the autonomic nervous system (ANS) or usage of drugs such as antihypertensives (prazosin, beta-blockers, clonidine etc.).

Syncope can be triggered by various circumstances such as coughing and micturition. The history may give the context in which the syncope occurred and the diagnosis can be made. Patients with cataplexy may have abrupt loss of muscle tone following strong emotions such as anger or laughter; however, these patients are fully conscious during these episodes though they have repeated falls. Patients with subclavian steal have syncope when they use their arm on the side of the stenosis.

Patients with neurological disorders like multisystem atrophy or parkinsonism or sensory neuropathies can be diagnosed by detailed neurological assessment. Several psychiatric disorders such as anxiety, depression, panic attacks, and somatization present with syncope for which history regarding the patient's social and emotional circumstances would be crucial.

EXAMINATION

- Syncope is accompanied by *hypotension* with *inappropriate bradycardia* in patients with neural origin.
- In cardiac patients the pulse rate must be recorded to document bradycardia or tachycardia. Irregularities in the pulse such as ectopics and AF must be looked for. The carotids must be palpated and auscultated for the presence of stenosis. All patients in whom orthostatic hypotension is suspected must have a supine and standing BP (<3 min of standing) recorded.
- A detailed cardiac examination should be done to diagnose the presence of underlying heart disease such as ischemic heart disease or valvular heart disease. Neurological evaluation for the presence of extrapyramidal and cerebellar diseases must be done to rule out degenerative conditions.
- *Psychiatric evaluation*: For patients with anxiety or somatization where an underlying psychiatric problem is suspected, consultation with a psychiatrist is advised.

DIFFERENTIAL DIAGNOSIS

The first step in the evaluation of syncope begins with differentiating it from a seizure. A detailed history regarding the onset, accompanying features and recovery would help to make the diagnosis (**Table 4**).

Patients with posterior circulation transient ischemic attack (TIA) can present with transient loss of consciousness along with other neurological symptoms such as diplopia, dysarthria, and ataxia. This should be suspected in patients with atherosclerotic risk factors and cardiac conditions causing embolization.

Patients with diabetes can present with loss of consciousness because of hypoglycemia. This is especially common in type 1 diabetic patients due to repeated hypoglycemia causing unawareness. The same problem can be encountered in elderly diabetics who have autonomic failure. However, in both these circumstances, recovery of consciousness is dependent on replacement of glucose and is not spontaneous.

The clinical features that may help to differentiate cardiac syncope from noncardiac causes are shown in **Table 5**.

TABLE 4 Features differentiating syncope from seizure.

Feature	Syncope	Seizure
Age group	• Neural—young • Cardiac—old	• Epilepsy—young • Secondary causes—old
Precipitating factors	Prolonged upright posture, anxiety, extreme pain, fear	Lack of sleep, photic stimulation
Onset	Presyncope—feeling of dizziness and blackouts	Aura
Accompanying symptoms	Sweating, palpitations, hyperventilation	Convulsions, urinary and fecal incontinence, tongue bite
Duration	Transient, few seconds to 5 min	3–5 min for convulsions followed by loss of consciousness >5 min
Recovery	Immediate clarity following episode	Postictal confusion, headache and sleep, muscle aches, and pains

TABLE 5 Differentiation of cardiac syncope from noncardiac causes.

Cardiac causes	Noncardiac causes
Older age (>60 years)	Younger age
Male sex	Psychogenic—female sex
Presence of ischemic heart disease, structural heart disease, previous arrhythmias, or reduced ventricular function	No underlying heart disease
Brief prodrome such as palpitations, or sudden loss of consciousness without prodrome	*Presence of prodrome*: Nausea, vomiting, or feeling warmth
Syncope in supine position	Positional change from supine or sitting to standing (orthostatic)
Lesser number of syncope episodes (1 or 2)	• Frequent recurrence or prolonged history of syncope with similar characteristics • *Situational triggers*: Cough, micturition, defecation, and deglutition
Cardiac symptoms such as chest, pain, palpitations common	• None in neurally mediated • In orthostatic hypotension—other autonomic symptoms common

EVALUATION

The evaluation begins with routine blood sugar to rule out diabetes, and other biochemical evaluations, for renal function. Cardiac conditions such as MI/arrhythmias must be looked for, by electrocardiogram, biomarkers, and echocardiography. ANS testing for evaluation of the integrity of the ANS must be done. These include assessment of the parasympathetic system (heart rate variability with respiration and Valsalva and sympathetic system with "tilt-table test" and "beat-to-beat" BP measurement.

An electroencephalogram (EEG) may be needed to differentiate a seizure from a syncope, if doubt exists regarding the diagnosis.

The other investigations (**Box 1**) are listed below.

With a good history, focused clinical examination, and appropriate evaluation, the cause of syncope can be diagnosed, following which treatment can be initiated.

BOX 1 Causes of palpitations.

Palpitations due to arrhythmic causes:
- Supraventricular extrasystoles
- Ventricular extrasystoles
- Sick sinus syndrome
- Supraventricular tachycardia (SVT) [atrioventricular nodal reentrant tachycardia (AVNRT), atrioventricular reentrant tachycardia (AVRT)]
- Ventricular tachycardia (VT)
- Bradyarrhythmia like complete heart block
- Anomalies in functioning/programming of implantable cardioverter defibrillator (ICD)

Palpitations due to structural heart disease:
- Severe mitral regurgitation (as a result of volume overload)
- Severe aortic regurgitation (as a result of volume overload)
- Mitral valve prolapse (due to volume overload and arrhythmias)
- Congenital heart diseases with significant shunt
- Atrial myxoma
- Mechanical prosthetic valves
- Cardiomegaly/heart failure of various causes

Palpitations due to systemic causes:
- *Metabolic disorders:* Hyperthyroidism, pheochromocytoma, and hypoglycemia
- *High output states:* Fever, anemia, pregnancy, Paget's disease, and AV fistula
- *Orthostatic syndromes:* Orthostatic hypotension, postural orthostatic tachycardia syndrome (POTS)

Palpitations induced by drugs/illicit substances:
- Beta agonists, anticholinergics, and hydralazine
- Recent withdrawal of beta-blockers
- Alcohol intoxication/withdrawal, cocaine, heroin, amphetamines, caffeine, nicotine, and cannabis

Palpitations of psychiatric origin:
- Anxiety and panic attacks

PALPITATIONS

DEFINITION

Palpitations are defined as an unpleasant perception of the heartbeat and are described by patients as a disagreeable sensation of throbbing or movement in the chest and/or adjacent areas.

TABLE 6 Investigations for syncope.

Laboratory investigations	Comments
Laboratory investigations	Complete hemogram, arterial blood gas analysis, cardiac enzymes, blood glucose, serum electrolytes
Electrocardiogram (5% yield)	QT prolongation/short QT, short PR with delta wave, RBBB with ST elevation (Brugada pattern), LVH (s/o AS, HCM), evidence of myocardial ischemia, High grade AV block, T inversion in right precordial leads (arrhythmogenic right ventricular dysplasia)
Echocardiogram (low yield with normal ECG and physical examination, 1–2% yield)	To rule structural heart disease
Cardiac CT/MRI	In patients with syncope of suspected cardiac etiology
Cardiac monitoring (2% yield)	24-hour holter monitoring, event loop recorders, implantable loop recorders
Tilt-table testing	Neurally-mediated syncope, rule out psychogenic syncope
Electro-physiological testing (low yield if done in all patients)	Sick sinus syndrome, carotid sinus hypersensitivity, heart block, SVT, VT, AF
EEG, CT, MRI	Rule out neurological causes
Signal averaged ECG, stress test, cardiac catheterization	ARVD, high suspicion of CAD

(AF: atrial fibrillation; ARVD: rrhythmogenic right ventricular dysplasia; CT: computed tomography; CAD: coronary artery disease; ECG: electrocardiography; LVH: left ventricular hypertrophy; MRI: magnetic resonance imaging; RBBB: right bundle branch block; SVT: Supraventricular tachycardia; VT: ventricular tachycardia)

MECHANISM

The mechanisms implicated in causation of palpitations include—alterations in heart rate and rhythm; and augmentation of myocardial contraction.

CAUSES

Causes for palpitations include cardiac 43%, psychiatric 31%, miscellaneous 10%, and unknown 16% (**Table 6**).

APPROACH TO HISTORY TAKING

Age of onset: Inappropriate sinus tachycardia can occur at any age though more prevalent in young adults. Palpitations due to psychiatric causes are usually encountered in young adults. Palpitations due to accessory pathways [atrioventricular reentrant tachycardia (AVRT)] predominate in childhood and adolescence and have a structurally normal heart.

Atrioventricular nodal reentrant tachycardia (AVNRT) increases with age. Patients with palpitations due to VT tend to be older and usually with structural heart disease.

Description: The description of palpitations can give a clue to their origin (**Table 7**).

TABLE 7 Description of palpitations and the causes.

Description	Causes
Rapid and regular	Sinus tachycardia, SVT, and VT
Rapid and irregular	Atrial fibrillation (AF), multifocal atrial tachycardia (MAT), atrial flutter with varying block
Flip-flopping	Atrial/ventricular premature ventricular complexes (PVCs)
Rapid fluttering	SVT/VT
Rapid and regular neck pulsations—Frog sign	AVNRT (systolic cannon waves which occur with AV dissociation result from simultaneous contractions of atria and ventricle against closed mitral and tricuspid valves causing reflux of blood into neck veins)
Irregular neck pulsations	AV dissociation in PVCs, complete heart block and VT (causes irregular systolic cannon waves due to varying relation between P and QRS due to atrioventricular dissociation)

(AVNRT: atrioventricular nodal reentrant tachycardia; SVT: supraventricular tachycardia; VT: ventricular tachycardia)

Onset and offset: This too helps to analyze the type of arrhythmia causing palpitations.

- Randomly and episodically and lasting for an instant—mostly premature beats
- Abrupt onset and offset—SVT or VT
- Gradual onset and offset—sinus tachycardia
- *Mode of termination*: Vagal stimulation—SVT

Positional palpitations:

- Palpitations upon standing up straight after bending over and ends by lying down—mostly AVNRT
- Intermittent pounding sensations on lying in bed—atrial or ventricular premature ventricular complexes (PVCs)

Associated symptoms: The accompanying symptoms of palpitations depend upon the underlying cause and the effect of palpitations on the coronary and cerebral blood flow.

- Chest pain—arrhythmogenic MI
- Dyspnea—heart failure due to arrhythmias

- Syncope—low cardiac output during arrhythmias, acute coronary syndrome, hypoglycemia, and pheochromocytoma
- Polyuria—SVT (due to release of atrial natriuretic peptide)
- Sweating—anxiety and hypoglycemia
- Diarrhea, weight loss, increased appetite—thyrotoxicosis

Palpitations at rest or exertional:

- Arrhythmic palpitations usually are gradual or sudden in onset and offset and usually occur at rest and rarely during exercise.
- Palpitations due to volume overload are related to exertion and disappear at rest.

History of psychiatric diseases:

- Anxiety
- Panic attacks
- Depression
- Somatization disorders

History of underlying disease: The main cause of palpitations is cardiac, and hence history pertaining to presence of underlying ischemic heart disease, rheumatic heart diseases, congenital heart diseases, or cardiomyopathies must be elicited. A history of stressors or anxiety will help to diagnose psychiatric causes. Hypoglycemia must be ruled out by context and thyrotoxicosis and pheochromocytoma can be diagnosed by typical clinical features. A drug history of intake of beta agonists, amphetamines, and theophylline may sometimes avoid unnecessary investigation. A history of alcohol intake must be recorded to rule out alcoholic cardiomyopathy or withdrawal from alcohol.

CLINICAL EXAMINATION

The aim of clinical examination is to find out if the arrhythmia is life-threatening, causing hemodynamic compromise, or due to serious underlying heart disease.

The examination should begin with recording of pulse rate, and its regularity. **Table 8** gives a summary of the clinical findings and their significance in the diagnosis of the cause of palpitations.

Blood pressure is important in deciding the seriousness of any arrhythmia, as hypotension signifies reduced cerebral blood flow, due to compromise of cardiac output. In conditions with irregular heartbeat, BP may have to be recorded multiple times, and averaged, as in AF. Patients with heart disease can be diagnosed by abnormal cardiac findings like cardiomegaly, murmurs, left and right heart failure and must be documented, as this will help us to decide further management. Clinical features of thyrotoxicosis and pheochromocytoma must be looked for in patients with normal hearts. Presence of cold extremities, and tremors, with anxious affect, may suggest a psychiatric basis for palpitation.

EVALUATION

Standard 12-lead electrocardiography: Standard 12-lead electrocardiography (ECG) is essential part of evaluation in all patients with palpitations. Suggestion of previous

TABLE 8 Clinical findings and their significance in the diagnosis of the cause of palpitations.

Arrhythmia	Pulse rate regularity	JVP	BP	Other clinical features
Atrial fibrillation	• 150–200 bpm • Rate depends upon the conduction through AV node • Irregular	• Absent "a" waves • Absent "x" descent	Hypotension in extreme rates with fast ventricular response	• Varying volume of pulse • Varying intensity of first heart sound • Apex pulse deficit >10
Atrial flutter	• 200–250 bpm • Regular • Irregular if variable conduction	Normal most of the times as regular	Hypotension in extreme rates	May resemble atrial fibrillation if variable conduction occurs
Atrioventricular block (CHB)	• Significant bradycardia • <40 bpm • Regular	Irregular slow systolic cannon a waves	High pulse pressure due to high systolic, due to increased stroke volume	Variable intensity of first heart sound
AVNRT	• 250–300 bpm • Regular	Frog sign with rapid regular systolic cannon a waves (1:1 VA conduction)	Mostly normal	–
VT	• 250–300 bpm • Regular	Irregular rapid systolic cannon a waves	• With structural heart disease may present with hypotension • In structurally normal hearts, no hemodynamic compromise	• Varying intensity of first heart sound • Systolic blood pressure unrelated to respiration
Ventricular premature complexes	• Variable • Irregular	normal	normal	• Apex pulse deficit <10 • Usually disappears with exercise • Post systolic accentuation of mitral regurgitation murmur

(AVNRT: atrioventricular nodal reentrant tachycardia; BP: blood pressure; CHB: complete heart block; JVP: jugular venous pressure; VT: ventricular tachycardia)

MI may be a clue for significant arrhythmias particularly VT. Presence of left or right ventricular hypertrophy with atrial enlargement may point toward underlying chamber enlargement leading to volume overload. Nonspecific ST changes and T wave abnormalities are important clues to presence of myocardial diseases. A prolonged QT may suggest polymorphic VT whereas a short PR with delta waves may suggest underlying accessory pathway. Frequent PVCs in a patient presenting with palpitations should always be localized and evaluated properly. Complete heart block will show low ventricular rate and AV dissociation. Sick sinus syndrome shows bradycardia, and episodes of tachycardia, with periods of sinus exit block.

Laboratory investigations: Baseline laboratory testing should include a complete blood count, blood sugar, blood urea nitrogen, serum creatinine, electrolyte levels, and thyroid profile to exclude anemia, renal disease, electrolyte, and thyroid disorders particularly thyrotoxicosis. Drug screen should be ordered in suspected cases presenting with palpitations.

Stress exercise testing: Patients with exertional symptoms should be evaluated with exercise testing because they are at higher risk of morbidity and mortality. Stress testing also provides prognostic value in some cases with palpitations. Patients with benign ventricular premature complexes can have disappearance of PVCs with exercise. Disappearance of pre-excitation on exercise testing (present on baseline ECG) may suggest a good prognosis in patients with WPW syndrome.

Two-dimensional echocardiography: Echocardiography should be considered a routine investigation in all patients with palpitations particularly when they are exertional. A high suspicion of abnormal test should be considered when patient has abnormal signs like elevated JVP and pedal edema. One should look for evidence of structural heart disease particularly regurgitant valvular lesions, underlying wall motion abnormalities, ventricular dysfunction, and congenital heart diseases.

Ambulatory holter monitoring: A 24-hour holter monitoring should be considered when the patient experiences specific triggers or if symptoms tend to occur daily. If symptoms are less frequent, event loop recorders can be worn for longer period up to 30 days. Implantable loop recorders are subcutaneous devices in patients with infrequent palpitations accompanied by syncope concerning arrhythmic etiology.

Cardiac imaging: Though not frequently used modality, cardiac magnetic resonance imaging (MRI) may be useful modality to know underlying etiology in patients presenting with palpitations/syncope and PVCs on baseline ECG. Diseases like arrhythmogenic right ventricular dysplasia should be considered in patients with right ventricular outflow tract (RVOT) type of PVCs [left bundle branch block (LBBB) morphology and positive ventricular premature contraction (VPC) morphology in inferior leads] on baseline ECG. Other diseases like sarcoidosis, myocarditis, and infiltrative diseases can also be diagnosed by cardiac MRI.

TABLE 9	Summary of investigations for palpitations.
Electrocardiogram	• Previous myocardial infarction • Left or right ventricular hypertrophy • Atrial enlargement • Atrioventricular blocks • Short PR and delta waves (WPW syndrome) • Prolonged QT interval • Isolated premature atrial/ventricular complexes
Laboratory investigations	• Complete blood count • BUN, creatinine • Blood sugar • Thyroid profile • Serum electrolytes • Drug screen
Exercise stress testing	Patients with palpitations on physical exertion or suspected coronary artery disease or myocardial ischemia
Two-dimensional echocardiography	Rule out structural abnormalities/look for ventricular function
Holter monitoring/ event loop recorders	• For patients with palpitations and structural heart disease • In patients with family history of syncope, arrhythmia or sudden cardiac death

(BUN: blood urea nitrogen; WPW: Wolff–Parkinson–White)

Table 9 summarizes these investigations and their relevance.

To summarise, all these symptoms are very common in clinical practice, and a sound understanding in the approach to these, would translate into good patient care.

RECOMMENDED READINGS

1. Kasper D, Fauci A, Hauser S, Longo D, Jameson J, Loscalzo J. Harrison's principles of internal medicine, 20 edition. United States: Mcgraw-hill; 2015.
2. Anil OM. Syncope: Approach to diagnosis. J Clin Prev Cardiol. 2016;5:84-93.
3. Guttikonda SNR, Vadapalli K. Approach to undifferentiated dyspnea in emergency department: aids in rapid clinical decision-making. Int J Emerg Med. 2018;11(1):21.
4. DeVos E, Jacobson L. Approach to adult patients with acute dyspnea. Emerg Med Clin North Am. 2016;34(1):129-49.
5. Mukerji V. Dyspnea, orthopnea, and paroxysmal nocturnal dyspnea. In: Walker HK, Hall WD, Hurst JW (Eds). Clinical Methods: The History, Physical, and Laboratory Examinations, 3rd edition. Boston: Butterworths; 1990.
6. Ewert R, Glaser S. Dyspnea from the concept up to diagnostics. Der Internist. 2015;56:865-71.
7. Manning HL, Schwartzstein RM. Pathophysiology of dyspnea. N Engl J Med. 1995;333(23):1547-53.

8. Raviele A, Giada F, Bergfeldt L, Blanc JJ, Blomstrom-Lundqvist C, Mont L, et al. Management of patients with palpitations: a position paper from the European Heart Rhythm Association. Europace. 2011;13(7):920-34.
9. Zipes DP, Libby P, Bonow RO, Mann DL, Tomaselli GF. Braunwald's Heart Disease E-Book: A Textbook of Cardiovascular Medicine. Edinburgh: Elsevier Health Sciences; 2018.
10. McLellan AJ, Kalman JM. Approach to palpitations. Aust J Gen Pract. 2019;48(4):204-9.
11. Giada F, Raviele A. Clinical approach to patients with palpitations. Card Electrophysiol Clin. 2018;10(2):387-96.

CHAPTER

10

Cough and Hemoptysis: Evaluation

SK Sharma

ABSTRACT

Cough is a vexing and bothersome symptom for the patients and constitutes one of the most common indications for which outpatient consultation is sought. Cough can be acute (<3 weeks), or chronic (>8 weeks); cough of >3 weeks and <8 weeks duration has been termed subacute cough. Both upper and lower respiratory tract infections are common causes of acute cough. Subacute, chronic cough can be caused by a wide range of etiological causes. Diagnostic work-up includes a detailed history, physical examination, coagulation profile, complete hemogram including platelet count, platelet function studies, use of imaging modalities, endoscopic evaluation of upper and lower respiratory tracts, pulmonary function testing including of reversibility of airflow obstruction, echocardiography, among others. Hemoptysis can be mild/moderate or massive/life-threatening. A wide range of etiological causes has been implicated in the causation of hemoptysis. A coordinated effort by a team consisting of a physician, interventional radiologist, and cardiothoracic and vascular surgeon is essential for successful management of life-threatening hemoptysis. Hemodynamic stabilization and monitoring, early localization of the cause and site of bleeding, judicious use of bronchial artery embolization, and timely surgery can be lifesaving in these patients.

"Love and a cough cannot be hid"

—George Herbert

INTRODUCTION

Coughing is a natural process that protects the airway by moving mucus out of the large airways. Coughing is helpful for maintaining patency of the airway and protecting the lungs from potentially harmful agents. Cough offers a valuable clue to the presence of underlying disease. Upper and lower respiratory tract disease, pleural disease, cardiac disease, among others can present with cough. Dry cough may be the initial manifestation of bronchial asthma in children. Gastroesophageal reflux disease (especially in obese individuals) can result in chronic pharyngitis and present with chronic cough. Tropical pulmonary eosinophilia, pulmonary eosinophilia due to migratory larvae, is also a common cause of cough in India.

However, sometimes, inflammatory pathologies can result in sensitization and activation of the neural pathways that regulate cough resulting in excessive and nonproductive coughing which has little protective utility. Cough can be refractory to disease-specific treatments currently available and may often not be responsive to antitussive treatment as well. Thus, cough is one the most vexing and bothersome symptom for the patients and constitutes one of the most common indications for which outpatient consultation is sought.

PATHOPHYSIOLOGY

Cough reflex is triggered when chemical (e.g., acid, cold, heat, and capsaicin-like molecules) or mechanical stimuli (particulate matter) irritate sensory nerve endings (primarily rapidly adapting cough receptors) and C fibers that exist in the larynx, trachea, carina, or main bronchi. This is thought to occur via activation of cationic ion channel, the transient receptor potential vanilloid 1 (TRPV1) and transient receptor potential ankyrin type 1 (TRPA1). Mechanical cough receptors can be stimulated by trigger factors like touch or displacement. Laryngeal and tracheobronchial receptors respond to both chemical and mechanical stimuli. Impulses from cough receptors traverse an afferent pathway via the vagus nerve to a "cough center" in the medulla. This cough center is thought to be under control

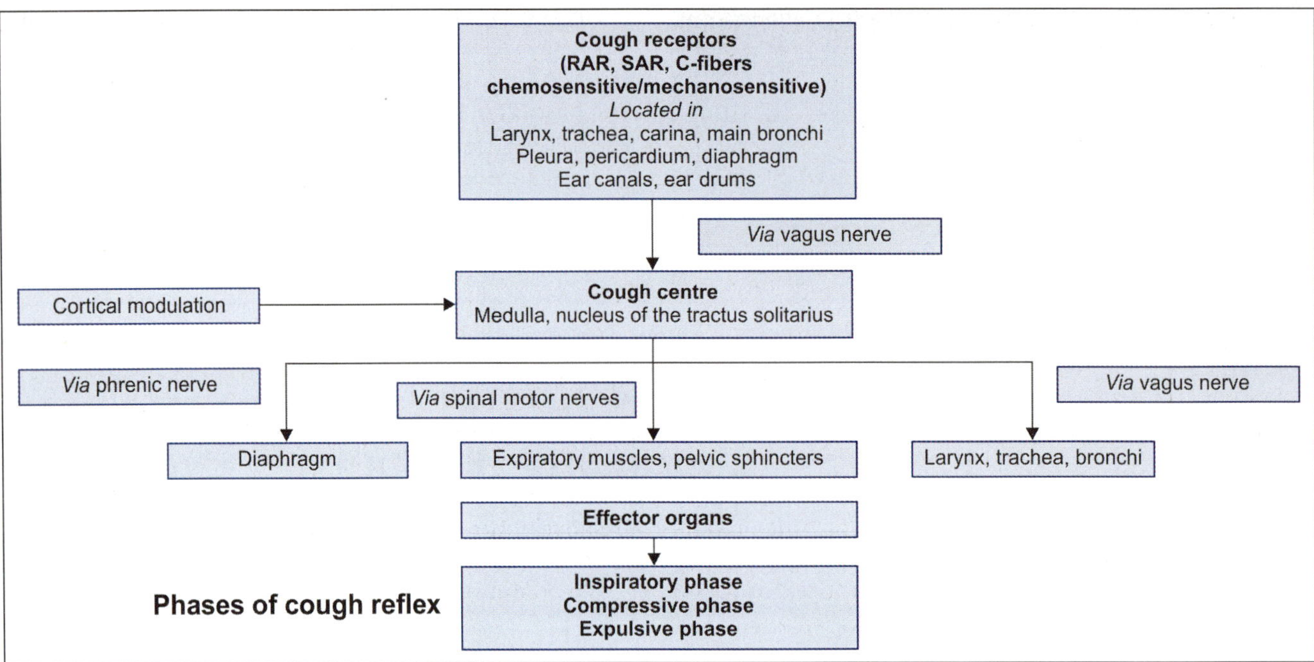

(RAR: rapidly adapting receptors; SAR: slow adapting receptors)

FLOWCHART 1: Cough reflex.

by higher cortical centers and coughing can be voluntarily initiated or partially inhibited. The efferent signals from the cough center travel via the vagus, phrenic, and spinal motor nerves to expiratory musculature generating cough (**Flowchart 1**).

Based on the duration, cough is classified as acute, subacute, and chronic.

ACUTE COUGH

Cough of <3 weeks duration is acute cough. Common causes of acute cough are listed in **Box 1**. In clinical practice, upper respiratory tract infections (URTI), including common cold constitute a common cause of acute cough. The URTI together with acute bronchitis accounts for almost two-thirds of the cases of acute cough seen by physicians. Though foreign body aspiration is an important cause of acute cough in the pediatric age group, it is an important cause for acute cough in geriatric population also.

BOX 1	Some common causes of acute cough in adults.

- Infections of the upper respiratory tract
- Acute bronchitis
- Pneumonia, lower respiratory tract infection
- Acute sinusitis
- Acute left ventricular failure, cardiogenic pulmonary edema
- Acute respiratory distress syndrome
- Pulmonary thromboembolism
- Tension pneumothorax
- Pleurisy
- Acute exacerbation of bronchial asthma, chronic obstructive pulmonary disease
- Inhaled toxic fumes, gases

CLINICAL PRESENTATION

The clinical approach to acute cough starts with eliciting history and conducting physical examination focusing on differentiating harmless etiological causes like common cold from serious life-threatening causes of acute cough. In patients with URTI, acute cough is often accompanied by sore throat, running nose, headache, myalgias, fatigue, and fever. While this presentation is typical of common cold, presently it would raise the clinical suspicion of severe acute respiratory syndrome Coronavirus 2 (SARS-CoV-2) Coronavirus disease (COVID-19).

History of dyspnea, orthopnea, tachypnea, pleuritic chest pain, hemoptysis, and changes in vital signs such as high-grade fever, tachycardia, and hypotension in the setting of underlying comorbid conditions constitute major warning signs ("red flags") of a life-threatening cause of acute cough and warrant immediate hospitalization, diagnostic evaluation, stabilization, and management.

SUBACUTE AND CHRONIC COUGH

Cough lasting for >3 weeks and up to 8 weeks is subacute cough. Chronic cough refers to cough lasting >8 weeks duration. Common causes of subacute and chronic cough are listed in **Box 2**.

CLINICAL PRESENTATION

The upper airway cough syndrome occurs due to postnasal drip and is a common cause of subacute and chronic cough. Frequent etiological causes of postnasal drip

BOX 2	Some common causes of subacute/chronic cough in adults.
• Upper airway cough syndrome	
• Bronchial asthma	
• Bronchial hyperreactivity	
• Chronic obstructive pulmonary disease	
• Gastroesophageal reflux and laryngopharyngeal reflux	
• Respiratory tract infections (e.g., pulmonary tuberculosis)	
• Suppurative lung disease (lung abscess and bronchiectasis)	
• Lung cancer	
• Drugs (e.g., angiotensin-converting enzyme inhibitors, beta-blockers, and nitrofurantoin)	

include allergy, vasomotor rhinitis and sinusitis, among others. Patients with upper airway cough syndrome present with a history of nasal discharge, a sensation of liquid dripping into the back of the throat, and need for frequent throat clearing; however, in some patients these symptoms may be absent.

In patients with bronchial asthma, cough is accompanied by episodic wheezing and dyspnea. In the "cough variant" of bronchial asthma, it can be the sole manifestation. Chronic bronchitis is diagnosed clinically in patients presenting with cough and sputum production for most days over at least a 3-month period for >2 consecutive years for which no other cause has been found.

Subacute/chronic cough associated with gastroesophageal reflux could be due to stimulation of cough receptors in the upper respiratory tract; aspiration of gastric contents resulting in stimulation of cough receptors in the lower respiratory tract, and reflux of gastric acid into the distal esophagus. The typical symptoms of gastroesophageal reflux like heartburn or sour eructations may be absent in >40% of patients in whom chronic cough is due to reflux. Further, esophageal dysmotility (with or without evidence of reflux) is also common in patients with subacute/chronic cough. Retrograde movement of gastric contents into the laryngopharynx is termed laryngopharyngeal reflux (LPR). Symptoms of LPR include chronic cough, throat clearing, hoarseness of voice, dysphonia, and mild dysphagia. LPR is considered primarily to be an upper esophageal sphincter problem and is manifest in the erect/upright position during periods of physical exertion. In contrast, gastroesophageal reflux disease, a problem of the lower esophageal sphincter manifests when the patient assumes a recumbent position. Patients with interstitial lung disease (ILD), especially idiopathic pulmonary fibrosis (IPF) often presents with subacute/chronic cough.

In patients with subacute/chronic cough, presence of associated symptoms of hemoptysis, constitutional symptoms such as fever, toxemia, anorexia, and weight loss may point to respiratory tract infections like pulmonary tuberculosis. Expectoration of copious quantities of foul smelling sputum suggests suppurative lung disease which is rarely being seen these days.

Dry (nonproductive cough) is a common adverse event in patients receiving treatment with angiotensin-converting enzyme (ACE) inhibitors, seen in up to 15% of patients. While the underlying mechanism is unclear, as per the "kinin hypothesis", accumulation of bradykinin (that is normally degraded partly by ACE) is thought to stimulate afferent C-fibers in the airway resulting in cough. This view is supported by the fact that cough is relatively rare in patients receiving angiotensin II receptor antagonists which do not increase kinin levels.

Cough is an infrequent symptom in patients with lung cancer. It is seen in lung cancer arising in the central airways (where cough receptors are present) present with cough. Lung cancer should be suspected in patients presenting with a new cough or a recent change in chronic "smoker's cough." In patients with bronchoalveolar cell carcinoma, a relatively rare type of lung cancer, cough with copious expectoration (bronchorrhea) is a cardinal symptom.

Uncommon causes of subacute chronic cough include lesions compressing the upper airway (arteriovenous malformations and retrotracheal masses), tracheobronchomalacia, tracheal diverticula, and laryngeal sensory neuropathy. Another intriguing cause of chronic cough is irritation of the external auditory canal by impacted cerumen ("ear-cough", oto-respiratory reflex) and is thought to be due to the stimulation of the auricular branch of the vagus nerve (Arnold's nerve). Rarely, patients with premature ventricular contractions (PVCs) can present with chronic cough.

DIAGNOSIS

Diagnosis of cough is based on eliciting a detailed clinical history including history of drug use, a thorough clinical examination, judicious use of imaging modalities, pulmonary function testing including testing for reversibility of airflow obstruction, work-up for respiratory infections where indicated, among others. Other useful tests include absolute eosinophil count, serum immunoglobulin E (IgE) (total), serum Aspergillus-related IgE, IgG, IgA and IgM, and stool examination for ova and cysts.

MANAGEMENT

Symptomatic treatment of cough includes administration of nasal drops, sprays, mucolytic agents, cough expectorants, antihistamines, among others. Specific treatment is administered as per the etiological diagnosis (for e.g., bronchodilator therapy for bronchial asthma, antibiotics, antiviral drugs as appropriate for respiratory infections, antihistamine drugs, montelukast with bronchodilators for bronchial hyperreactivity, deworming for worm infestations, diethylcarbamazine for tropical pulmonary eosinophilia, among others). A detailed description of these aspects is beyond the scope of this chapter.

HEMOPTYSIS

Hemoptysis is a commonly encountered symptom in patients with respiratory and some nonrespiratory diseases.

In usual clinical practice, "frightening" hemoptysis is more frequently seen than "life-threatening" hemoptysis. However, the unpredictable course of massive life-threatening hemoptysis necessitates prompt evaluation and aggressive management.

ETIOLOGY

Hemoptysis usually originates from the bronchial (90%) and pulmonary circulation (10%), respectively. When the bleeding is from the bronchial circulation, hemoptysis can be massive as it is a circulation at systemic pressure. Some common etiological causes of hemoptysis are listed in **Box 3**.

CLINICAL ASSESSMENT

History: A detailed history and thorough physical examination are essential for early diagnosis and effective management of hemoptysis. History helps in clarifying whether, it is really hemoptysis or other mimics such as epistaxis or hematemesis. History of fever and the presence of parenchymal infiltrates on the chest radiograph indicate the possibility of chronic inflammatory conditions like pulmonary tuberculosis, bronchiectasis, necrotizing pneumonia, or lung abscess. In a patient with a past history of cavitating lung disease, if there is a history of *melanoptysis*, the possibility of a pulmonary mycetoma should be considered.

In chronic tobacco smokers over 40 years of age, lung cancer is an important cause of hemoptysis. In patients presenting with associated eye, kidney involvement, and cavitating lung disease, granulomatosis with polyangiitis (GPA) (previously called Wegener's granulomatosis) is likely. Occurrence of hemoptysis in conjunction with hematuria suggests Goodpasture syndrome. Hemoptysis, spontaneous pneumothorax in a woman of child bearing age who also manifests diffuse interstitial pattern on the chest radiograph suggests lymphangioleiomyomatosis (LAM).

BOX 3 | Some common causes of hemoptysis.

- **Infections:**
  - Pulmonary tuberculosis
  - Pulmonary mycetoma (e.g., aspergilloma)
  - Lung abscess
  - Necrotizing pneumonias (*Klebsiella*, *Staphylococcus*, and *Legionella*)
  - Parasitic
    - Hydatid lung disease
    - Paragonimiasis
- **Neoplasm:**
  - Bronchogenic carcinoma
  - Bronchial adenoma
  - Pulmonary metastases
  - Sarcoma
- **Vascular:**
  - Pulmonary infarction
  - Pulmonary embolism
  - Arteriobronchial fistula
  - Arteriovenous malformations
  - Bronchial telangiectasia
- **Cardiological:**
  - Mitral stenosis
  - Left ventricular failure
- **Pulmonary:**
  - Bronchiectasis (including cystic fibrosis), bronchiectasis sicca (dry bronchiectasis)
  - Chronic bronchitis
  - Bullous lung disease
- **Bleeding/clotting disorders:**
  - von Willebrand disease

Continued...

Continued...

  - Hemophilia
  - Thrombocytopenia
  - Platelet dysfunction
  - Anticoagulant therapy
  - Disseminated intravascular coagulation (DIC)
- **Vasculitis:**
  - Granulomatosis with polyangiitis (previously called Wegener's granulomatosis)
  - Behçet's disease
- **Iatrogenic:**
  - Swan–Ganz catheterization
  - Bronchoscopy
  - Transbronchial lung biopsy
  - Transtracheal aspiration
- **Trauma:**
  - Blunt/penetrating injury
  - Suction ulcers
  - Tracheoarterial fistula
- **Miscellaneous:**
  - Lymphangioleiomyomatosis (LAM)
  - Catamenial (pulmonary endometriosis)
  - Pneumoconiosis (e.g., silicosis, silicotuberculosis, coal-worker's pneumoconiosis etc.)
  - Broncholith
  - Tracheobronchial amyloidosis
  - Idiopathic pulmonary hemosiderosis
  - Cocaine-induced, bevacizumab
  - Catamenial
  - Spurious (malingering)
  - Cryptogenic

If there is a history of travel to endemic areas, parasitic infections such as pulmonary paragonimiasis or hydatid disease of the lung are likely causes. Concurrent occurrence of massive hemoptysis during menstruation points to the possibility of catamenial hemoptysis (pulmonary endometriosis). Hemoptysis especially in conjunction with bleed from other sites suggests bleeding diathesis or clotting disorders (including drug induced, e.g., anticoagulant use).

Physical examination: Presence of a saddle nose, rhinitis, or perforated nasal septum (GPA), oral or genital ulceration, uveitis, cutaneous nodules (Behçet's syndrome) offer valuable diagnostic clues. Digital clubbing may indicate bronchogenic carcinoma or suppurative lung disorders. Stigmata such as ecchymosis, petechiae, or purpura point to of a bleeding diathesis and clotting disorders. Presence of respiratory signs (e.g., leathery crepitations) or a cardiac murmur (mid-diastolic rumble in the mitral area) may point out to bronchiectasis, mitral stenosis as causes respectively.

MANAGEMENT

Diagnosis: Diagnosis of hemoptysis involves localization of the site of bleeding. Imaging modalities (chest radiograph, computed tomography, and computed tomography pulmonary angiography) indicate the site of disease. Venous Doppler ultrasonography study of lower limbs is helpful for evaluation of deep vein thrombosis. D-dimer estimation has negative predictive value in ruling-out venous thromboembolism. Clinical examination and endoscopic examination of nose, paranasal sinuses, nasopharynx, larynx, and bronchoscopy are useful in precisely localizing the bleeding site and also facilitate therapeutic intervention. Both rigid bronchoscopy and flexible fiberoptic bronchoscopy (FOB) have been employed in evaluating patients with massive hemoptysis. In a young patient presenting with recurrent hemoptysis and a normal chest radiograph, bronchial adenoma may be identified as the etiological cause on bronchoscopy.

Echocardiography is helpful in the diagnosis of mitral stenosis. Esophageal manometry, pH monitoring (for gastroesophageal reflux disease) are helpful in the diagnostic work-up for gastroesophageal reflux disease. Laboratory investigations are required to ascertain the etiological cause. Work-up for bleeding/coagulation abnormalities, connective tissue disorders, lung cancer (cytopathology and histopathology), and other pulmonary infections can facilitate identification of etiological cause.

Treatment: In patients with mild-moderate hemoptysis, identifying the etiological cause and institution of specific treatment would control the hemoptysis. In patients presenting with life-threatening hemoptysis, simultaneous stabilization, identifying and controlling the bleeding by specific therapeutic interventions are of paramount importance.

Massive hemoptysis: Massive hemoptysis has been variously defined as expectoration of 200–1,000 mL of blood over a period of 24 hours, or, blood loss significant enough to decrease the hematocrit to <30%. A practical definition of massive hemoptysis is "bleeding that is life threatening by virtue of airway obstruction or blood loss."

Patients with life-threatening massive hemoptysis should be admitted into an intensive care unit (ICU). The vital parameters such as pulse, blood pressure, respirations, and oxygen saturation by pulse oximetry (SpO_2), hourly urinary output must be monitored. Intravenous access should be secured using a wide bore cannula. Blood sample should be drawn for blood grouping and crossmatching and various laboratory investigations. Crystalloid fluid replacement must be initiated awaiting the crossmatched packed red blood cell transfusion. In case coagulation disorders, appropriate blood cell component therapy must be instituted.

Protection of the airway: If the side of bleeding is identified, the patient must be positioned in the lateral decubitus position with the bleeding side down to prevent aspiration into the unaffected lung. Oxygen should be administered by a face mask. Worsening arterial hypoxemia (as indicated by a drop in SpO_2) in spite of supplemental oxygen administration, hypovolemic shock, and carbon dioxide retention usually warrants tracheal intubation.

Specific treatment for the underlying cause: Early institution the specific treatment for the underlying cause, e.g., antituberculosis treatment, antifungal treatment would be lifesaving.

Bronchial artery embolization: Bronchial artery embolization is an effective nonsurgical treatment in massive hemoptysis. Selective angiography should be performed initially to locate the bleeding bronchial artery before the injection of particles such as polyvinyl alcohol foam, isobutyl-2-cyanoacrylate, absorbable gelatin pledgets, or steel coils, among others. Angiographic findings implicating the bronchial arteries as the cause of bleeding includes identification of extravasated dye, the visualization of tortuous vessels of increased caliber, or aneurysmal dilatation. Bronchial artery embolization is associated with the risk of accidental embolization of the spinal artery resulting in ischemic injury to the spinal cord and recurrence of bleeding. Immediate results with bronchial artery embolization are encouraging; however, the patient should be watched for recurrence of bleeding.

Surgery: Surgical management is considered when bronchial artery embolization fails, especially for localized lesions in persons with adequate respiratory reserve. Surgery is the treatment of choice, if the massive hemoptysis is due to leaking aortic aneurysm, hydatid cyst, iatrogenic pulmonary rupture, chest trauma, bronchial adenoma, or hemoptysis related to aspergilloma.

Medical management: Appropriate medical management is indicated in the control of life-threatening hemoptysis caused by conditions such as bleeding or clotting disorders, anticoagulant therapy, or Goodpasture syndrome.

PROGNOSIS

When bronchiectasis, lung abscess, or necrotizing pulmonary infections have been the cause of massive hemoptysis, the mortality rate is low (<3%). Factors such as the volume of blood expectorated, the rate of bleeding, the amount of blood retained within the lungs, and the premorbid respiratory reserve have been identified to be predictors of mortality in patients with massive hemoptysis irrespective of the etiology. If malignant lung disease is the etiology, or if the hemoptysis is >1,000 mL in 24 hours, the mortality rates have been observed to be considerably higher (>50%).

RECOMMENDED READINGS

1. Holzinger F, Beck S, Dini L, Stöter C, Heintze C. The diagnosis and treatment of acute cough in adults. Dtsch Arztebl Int. 2014;111(20):356-63.
2. Michaudet C, Malaty J. Chronic cough: Evaluation and management. Am Fam Physician. 2017;96:575-80.
3. Jean-Baptiste E. Clinical assessment and management of massive hemoptysis. Crit Care Med. 2000;28: 1642-7.

CHAPTER 11

Clinical Approach to a Cardiac Murmur

Rajeev Menon, Neelkanth Patil, B Soma Raju

ABSTRACT

Murmurs are caused by prolonged vibrations secondary to turbulence in blood. A complete description of murmur is necessary to differentiate pathological from innocent murmurs, identify the underlying etiology, and assess the severity of the underlying lesion. Identification of a murmur can aid in diagnosis of an unsuspected underlying structural heart disease which can have enormous clinical implications.

"Even the invisible leave foot prints"

—WG Trotman

INTRODUCTION

As discussions about "is stethoscope dead" gain traction, cases like above demonstrate the importance of identifying a murmur in aiding the diagnosis and management of patients.

The presence of a heart murmur raises questions regarding prophylaxis for endocarditis, restriction from athletics, eligibility for life insurance or employment, risk of pregnancy to the mother or fetus, and the safety of noncardiac surgery. If the practitioner has acquired fundamental skills in cardiac auscultation, capable physician should not need to refer all suspicious murmurs to a specialist for evaluation.

CASE VIGNETTE

A 48-year-old man presented at 3 am to the emergency room with retrosternal pain radiating to back. He was evaluated by a physician and a cardiologist outside and treated as acute coronary syndrome (ACS) unstable angina. Electrocardiogram (ECG) was normal (**Fig. 1**). Cardiologist on call saw the patient and recognized an early diastolic murmur (EDM) in the aortic area. This prompted a suspicion of aortic dissection as cause of chest pain and prompted an urgent bedside echo which showed a dissection flap in the ascending aorta (**Fig. 2**). Patient was rapidly deteriorating and was taken up for emergency surgery. Aortic valve and root replacement along with arch replacement was done. Patient had an uneventful postoperative recovery and was discharged on the 10th postoperative day.

DEFINITIONS

Murmur is defined as prolonged vibrations caused by turbulence in the blood flow. Turbulence is thought to be the primary factor in the genesis of heart murmurs, although there are many other theories about the production of cardiovascular sound, including vortex shedding, collision and cavitation phenomena, and eddy production.

EVALUATION

Describing a murmur in its entirety is necessary to draw the following conclusions which in turn guide management decisions. It is required to know whether the murmur is

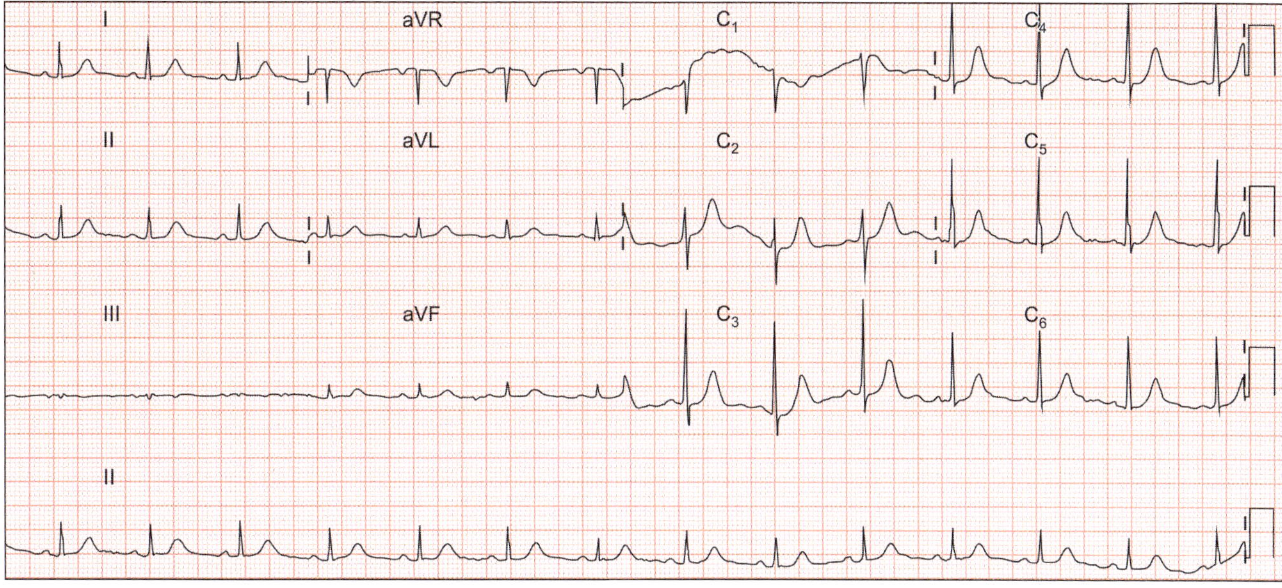

FIGURE 1: Electrocardiogram at presentation.

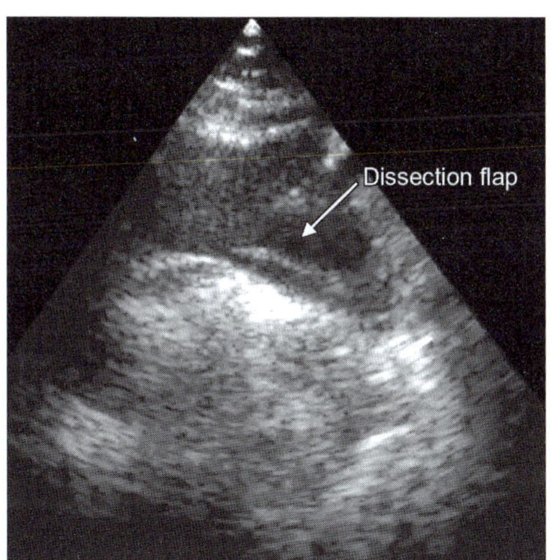

FIGURE 2: Echocardiography showing dissection flap (arrow).

BOX 1	Components of the murmur that need to be evaluated.
• Timing	
• Site	
• Intensity	
• Frequency	
• Quality	
• Length/duration	
• Peaking	
• Radiation/conduction	
• Changes with physiological/pharmacological maneuvers	
• Accompanying features	

physiological or pathological? It is required to ascertain the underlying lesion producing the murmur; and also assess the severity of the underlying lesion. The following components of the murmur need to be evaluated (**Box 1**) and are discussed below.

TIMING

The evaluation of murmurs starts with identifying the timing of the murmur in cardiac cycle. Conventionally, they are divided into systolic, diastolic, and continuous murmurs.

Systolic murmurs: Systolic murmurs are further classified into the following: Pansystolic murmur (PSM) starts with first heart sound and ends with second heart sound of that side (A2 or P2). Ejection systolic murmur (ESM) starts after first heart sound and ends with or before second heart sound of that side. Late systolic murmur (LSM) starts well after first heart sound and ends with second heart sound of that side. Short systolic murmur (SSM) may start with or after first heart sound and ends well before second heart sound. Early systolic murmur starts with the first heart sound and ends well before second heart sound.

The clue to identify if it is early, mid, or late is to compare the intensity of the corresponding sound. For example, in early systolic murmur, the first heart sound is not clear while the second heart sound is heard clearly, while in PSM both first and second heart sounds (of the corresponding side) are muffled.

The causes of systolic murmurs are shown in **Tables 1** to **3**. As described previously PSM by definition is associated with muffling of the first heart sound. However if the patient has a PSM of mitral regurgitation (MR) but the first heart sound is heard normally or is loud the following conditions should be considered: (1) mitral stenosis (MS) with MR (where MS is the dominant lesion); (2) mitral valve prolapse (MVP) with MR; and (3) ischemic MR. LSMs are noted with MVP with MR and tricuspid valve (TV) prolapse with tricuspid regurgitation (TR).

TABLE 1 Ejection systolic murmurs.

Site	Mechanism
Flow murmur across pulmonary valve	Hyperdynamic circulation: Anemia, thyrotoxicosis, pregnancy, atrial septal defect etc.
Still's murmur	Vibratory murmur in aortic area
Left ventricular outflow and right ventricular outflow	• Obstruction: Valvular, supravalvular, subvalvular (dynamic or static) • Increased pressure • Dilatation of vessel beyond

TABLE 2 Pansystolic murmurs.

Site	Mechanism
Ventricular septal defect	Persistent high pressure difference between LV and RV
Mitral regurgitation	Persistent high pressure difference between LV and LA
Tricuspid regurgitation	Persistent high pressure difference between RV and RA as in severe PAH or PS
Pansystolic-like murmurs	
○ **PDA (large)**	High PA pressures obliterate the diastolic component of CM
○ **Long ESMs of severe AS or PS**	Very high gradients, with prolonged gradient and murmur

(AS: aortic stenosis; CM: cardiomyopathy; ESM: ejection systolic murmur; LA: left atrium; LV: left ventricle; PAH: pulmonary arterial hypertension; PDA: patent ductus arteriosus; PS: pulmonic stenosis; RA: right atrium; RV: right ventricle)

Diastolic murmurs: Diastolic murmurs are further classified into the following: EDM starts with second heart sound of that side and ends at a variable interval. Mid-diastolic murmur (MDM) starts after second heart sound and ends with or before first heart sound. Presystolic murmur (Pre-SM) occurs just before systole ending in first heart sound and is usually due to atrial contraction. However, there is now evidence that pre-SM may occur even in atrial fibrillation and is attributed to a rapidly closing mitral valve in very early systole.

Early diastolic murmurs: The EDMs begin flush with semilunar valve closure of that side (aortic sound or pulmonic sound). They are related to backward flow of blood across the semilunar valves under high pressure. Only two sites in the circulation are capable of murmurs of this timing, *i.e.*, aortic and pulmonary regurgitations. Pulmonary regurgitation secondary to pulmonary arterial hypertension (PAH) is referred to as *Graham-Steell murmur*.

Mid-diastolic murmurs: Causes of MDMs are listed in **Table 4**. MDM can be because of pathological lesions or just flow murmurs. **Table 5** illustrates how to differentiate them.

Continuous murmurs: The term continuous murmurs by definition indicates that the murmur begins anywhere in systole and continues into diastole encompassing second heart sound without change in its frequency or quality.

TABLE 3 Early systolic murmurs.

Site	Mechanism
Very small muscular VSD	Early systolic murmur as valve-like mechanism closes the defect in late systole
Large VSD	Equalization of pressures after initial gradient
Acute MR/TR (early systolic)	Small atrium causes rapid rise in pressures causing equalization of pressure in later systole

(MR: mitral regurgitation; TR: tricuspid regurgitation; VSD: ventricular septal defect)

TABLE 4 Causes of mid-diastolic murmur.

Site	Mechanism
Mitral/tricuspid valve (mitral stenosis, tricuspid stenosis)	Forward flow of blood occurs at these valves only after the closure of aortic and pulmonary valves (A2, P2) and opening of mitral and tricuspid valves
Flow murmurs **Mitral valve MDM**	• Mitral regurgitation (indicates MR of at least moderate severity) • Ventricular septal defect, PDA, other post-tricuspid shunt (indicates shunt >2:1) • Presence of MDM in a shunt in spite of PAH indicates that it is more of a hyperkinetic (reversible) • PAH rather than fixed (irreversible) PAH
Tricuspid valve MDM	Indicates pre-tricuspid shunt (e.g., ASD) of >2:1
Carey Coombs murmur	Due to mitral valve inflammation in acute rheumatic fever
Austin Flint Murmur	MDM in severe AR due to fluttering of anterior mitral leaflet between the AR jet and diastolic flow from left atrium to ventricle
Mid-diastolic like murmur	
○ **Pulmonary regurgitation with normal PA pressure**	With low pressure, pulmonary regurgitation produces turbulence later in the diastole across the RV outflow

(AR: aortic regurgitation; ASD: atrial septal defect; MR: mitral regurgitation; MDM: mid-diastolic murmur; PDA: patent ductus arteriosus; PAH: pulmonary arterial hypertension; PA: pulmonary artery; RV: right ventricle)

The characteristics of a continuous murmur are represented in **Figure 3**. Continuous murmur from aorto-pulmonary communications is loudest around the S_2. Arterial continuous murmur is characterized by a more pronounced systolic component. Venous continuous murmur is characterized by a more pronounced diastolic component.

Classification of continuous murmurs is based on physiology. Continuous murmurs can be caused by rapid blood flow. Causes include venous hum, mammary soufflé, hemangioma, hyperthyroidism, acute alcoholic

TABLE 5 Differentiating mid-diastolic murmurs.

Murmur	S_1	OS	S_3	Character of MDM	Presystolic accentuation
Mitral stenosis	Loud	+	Never present	Rough	+
Flow murmurs	Soft	–	+	Soft	–
Carey Coombs	Normal/soft	–	+/–	Soft	–
Austin Flint	Normal/soft	–	+/–	Soft	–

(MDM: mid-diastolic murmur; OS: opening snap; S_1: first heart sound; S_3: third heart sound)

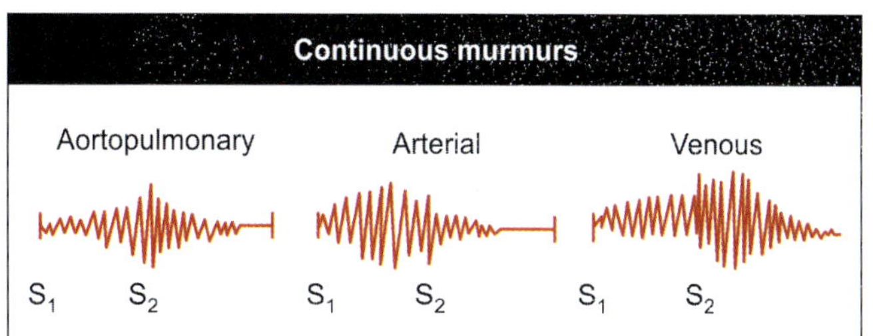

FIGURE 3: Continuous murmurs peaking based on underlying etiology.

Source: Adapted from Ginghină C, Năstase OA, Ghiorghiu I, Egher L. Continuous murmur - the auscultatory expression of a variety of pathological conditions. J Med Life. 2012;5:39-46.

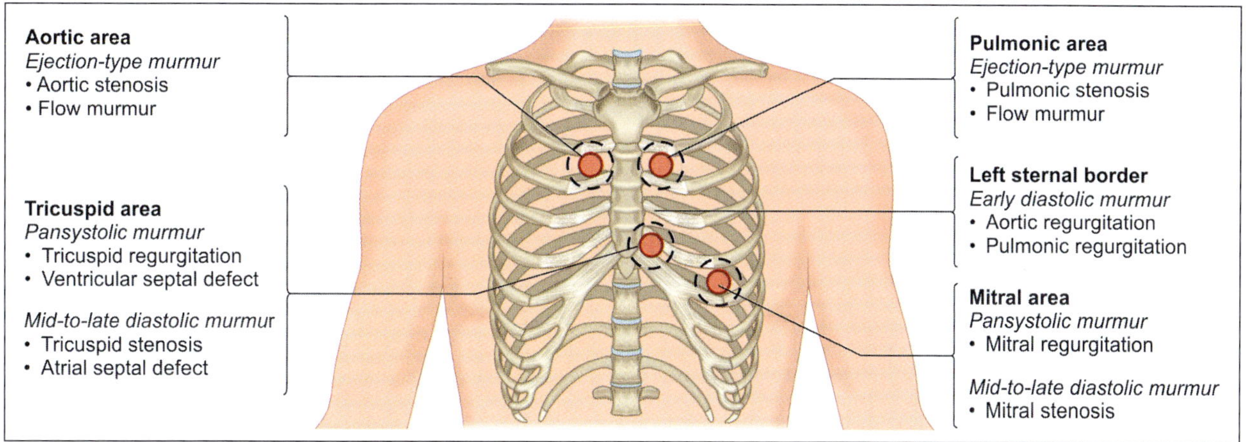

FIGURE 4: Site of best audibility of common murmurs.

hepatitis, and hyperemia of neoplasm (e.g., hepatoma, renal cell carcinoma, Paget's disease). These can also be produced by high-to-low pressure shunts, like systemic to pulmonary artery shunts [patent ductus arteriosus (PDA), aortopulmonary window, truncus arteriosus, pulmonary atresia, anomalous left coronary, bronchiectasis, sequestration of the lung)]; systemic artery to right heart shunts (e.g., ruptured sinus of Valsalva, coronary artery fistula); left to right atrial shunting (e.g., anomalous pulmonary veins, portosystemic shunts); and pulmonary or systemic arteriovenous fistulas. Further, continuous murmurs can also be heard secondary to localized arterial stenosis (e.g., renal stenosis, mesenteric artery stenosis etc.).

Continuous murmur needs to be differentiated from systolic-diastolic murmurs which are a combination of ejection or PSM with EDM and can be mistaken as continuous murmur. The change in character between the systolic and diastolic component helps in differentiating it from continuous murmurs.

The other close differential for a continuous murmur is a pericardial rub which is differentiated by its superficial, scratchy nature, and variation with respiration and posture.

SITE OF BEST AUDIBILITY

As seen in **Figure 4** each murmur is generally best heard at a particular site. The site of best audibility helps in differentiating the cause of that particular murmur. For example, a PSM can occur due to MR, TR, or ventricular septal defect (VSD). Presence of PSM at apex indicates that it is MR while presence of PSM in left lower sternal border indicates that it could be TR or VSD.

Aortic regurgitation (AR) murmurs can be heard in the right second intercostal space or left third intercostal space, the so called neoaortic area or Erb's area. The presence of EDM in right second intercostal space localizes the etiology

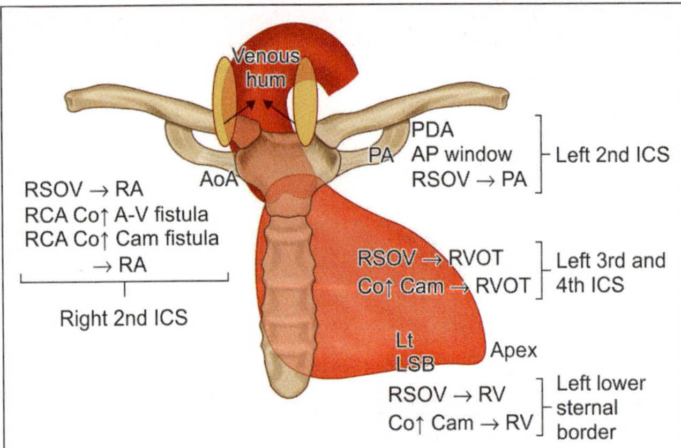

(AoA: aortic arch; AP: aortopulmonary; ICS: intercostal space; PDA: patent ductus arteriosus; PA: pulmonary artery; RA: right atrium; RCA: right coronary artery; RSOV: ruptured sinus of Valsalva; RVOT: right ventricular outflow tract)

FIGURE 5: Etiology of continuous murmurs based on site of best audibility.

of the AR to aorta/aortic root while the presence of EDM in neoaortic area indicates a primary valvular pathology (like rheumatic fever, and infective endocarditis). Hence, it is extremely important to look for an EDM in neoaortic area in all cases where AR is suspected.

The site of best audibility is particularly useful in identifying the cause of continuous murmurs as shown in **Figure 5**.

INTENSITY

Intensity or the loudness of the murmur is directly proportional to the amplitude of the murmur. The Levine and Freeman classification of murmurs was initially proposed in 1933 for systolic murmurs (Grade 1: Soft murmur heard in quiet surroundings; Grade 2: Soft murmur heard in noisy surroundings; Grade 3: Prominently heard murmurs; Grade 4: Loud murmur with a thrill; Grade 5: Loud murmur heard with edge of the stethoscope tilted against the chest wall + thrill; and Grade 6: Loud murmur heard 5–10 mm from the chest + thrill) on the premise that greater than Grade 3 systolic murmurs are pathological, while diastolic murmurs need not be graded as all diastolic murmurs are pathological. This has since been refuted and all murmurs are now graded similarly. It is pertinent to know here that contrary to conventional thinking, the intensity of the murmur does not correlate with the severity of the lesion.

FREQUENCY

Murmurs can be of high, low, or mixed frequencies. Frequency correlates with the pressure gradient across the lesion producing the murmur. Frequency is sometimes referred to as pitch. Frequency is an objective expression of the number of vibrations per second, and pitch is the subjective version of the same (**Fig. 6**).

High frequency (about 400 CPS) or high-pitched sounds or murmurs: The descriptions often used are: Soft, blowing, musical, and cooing.

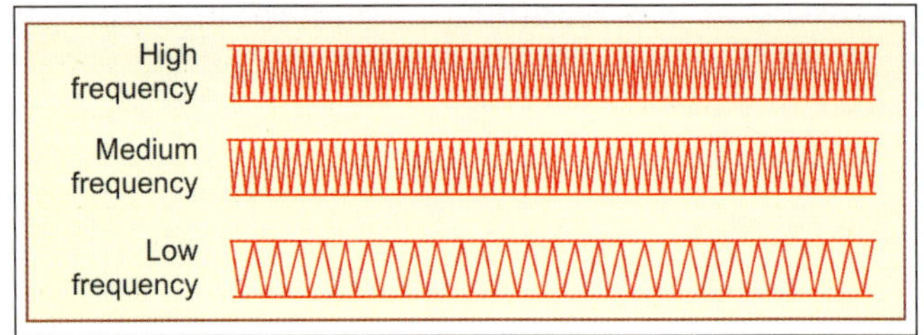

FIGURE 6: Diagrammatic representation of frequencies.

TABLE 6 Different frequencies of the murmurs and their corresponding pressure differences.

Feature	Mechanism
High frequency (high pitch):	High pressure difference between two sites
Soft	MR (LV 120 to LA 12 mm Hg)
Blowing	AR (aorta 80 to LV 12 mm Hg)
Musical	
Low frequency (low pitch):	Low pressure difference between two sites
Rough	MS (LA 20 to LV 5 mm Hg)
Rumbling	TS (RA 15 to RV 5 mm Hg)
Mixed frequency:	High pressure difference between two sites
Rough	AS (LV 200 to aorta 120 mm Hg)
Harsh	• PS (RV 120 to PA 25 mm Hg) • VSD (LV 120 to RV 25 mm Hg)

(AR: aortic regurgitation; AS: aortic stenosis; LA: left atrium; LV: left ventricle; MR: mitral regurgitation; MS: mitral stenosis; PA: pulmonary artery; PS: pulmonic stenosis; RV: right ventricle; TS: tricuspid stenosis; VSD: ventricular septal defect)

Low frequency (60–200 CPS) or low-pitched sounds or murmurs: The descriptions used are: Rough, rumbling, dull, and thud. Low-frequency murmurs are best heard with the bell while high-frequency murmurs are best heard with the diaphragm of stethoscope. **Table 6** illustrates the different frequencies of the murmurs and their corresponding pressure differences.

Low-frequency murmurs are generally localized while high-frequency murmurs are widely audible. Hence, in order to make sure that a low-frequency murmur like that of a MS is not missed, it is necessary to localize the apex and then look for the murmur exactly at that point with the bell of the stethoscope.

Mixed frequency murmurs have both components, and this is best demonstrated by the Gallavardin's dissociation. Here the aortic stenosis (AS) murmur of degenerative aortic valve has mixed frequencies. While the low frequency component is localized to aortic area, the high frequency component is widely audible and may sound as a PSM at apex and readily mistaken for MR.

CHARACTER

Character or quality of the murmur is different from the intensity or frequency.

It is akin to differentiating two musical instruments (e.g., flute and violin) which are playing the same song at the same intensity and frequency but with different sound because of their timbre or quality.

This is often under-recognized and often ignored part of auscultation, but significantly useful especially in significant tachycardia where differentiating systole and diastole itself becomes difficult. Training the ears from initial days of auscultation to appreciate the quality of the murmur goes a long way in identifying correctly in tough situations.

Some of the commonly used descriptions of murmurs are given below.

- *Rough and rumbling*: MDM of MS
- *Cooing/musical quality*:
  - In the presence of regurgitant lesions, indicates prolapse or aortic valve or flail mitral leaflet.
  - Stenotic lesions indicate sclerosis/calcification.
- *Machinery murmur, train in a tunnel*: Gibson's murmur of PDA
- *Honking murmur*: MVP/MR

LENGTH/DURATION AND PEAKING

Contrary to loudness, length, duration, and time of peaking of murmur correlate with severity of underlying disorder.

- *Length proportional to severity*:
  - Mid-diastolic murmurs (e.g., MS):
    - Mild lesions: When only presystolic accentuation is present.
    - Moderate: Short MDM with a gap between MDM and PSA
    - Severe lesion: Prolonged MDM continuous with presystolic accentuation
  - Early diastolic murmurs (e.g., aortic regurgitation):
    - <30% of diastole: Mild
    - 30–60% of diastole: Moderate
    - >60% of diastole: Severe
- *Time of peaking proportional to severity*:
  - Stenotic murmurs (e.g., AS):
    - Early peaking: Initial 50% of systole: Mild
    - Mid peaking: Around 50% of systole: Moderate
    - Late peaking: Beyond 50% of systole: Severe
- *No relation to severity*:
  - Pansystolic murmurs

Hence, in deciding the severity in MR, TR, and VSD, other factors need to be taken into consideration.

Severity of mitral regurgitation: Severity assessment of MR is shown in **Table 7**.

Severity of tricuspid regurgitation: The signs helpful in determining the severity of TR are shown in **Table 8**. However, since many of these signs are influenced by the size of right atrium, right ventricle, and the annulus, the sensitivity and specificity of these signs are restricted. TR with normal RV systolic pressure is often missed as these are early systolic and not pansystolic. They are important to identify as they may be the first clue to TV endocarditis. Septic abortions, indwelling central and peripheral lines are common causes of TV endocarditis in our population. They can produce recurrent septic emboli into lungs producing recurrent pneumonia and lung abscesses.

TABLE 7 Severity assessment of mitral regurgitation.

Severity of MR	PSM	S_3	MDM	Cardiac enlargement
Mild	+	–	–	–
Moderate	+	+	+	–
Severe	+	+	+	+

(MDM: mid-diastolic murmur; MR: mitral regurgitation; PSM: pansystolic murmur; S_3: third heart sound)

TABLE 8 Severity assessment of tricuspid regurgitation.

Severity of TR	PSM	S_3	MDM	CV wave on JVP	Hepatic pulsations
Mild	+	–	–	–	–
Moderate	+	+/–	+/–	+	–
Severe	+	+	+	+	+

(JVP: jugular venous pulse; MDM: mid-diastolic murmur; PSM: pansystolic murmur; S_3: third heart sound; TR: tricuspid regurgitation)

TABLE 9 Determining size of ventricular septal defect.

Shunt in VSD	PSM	S_3/MDM across mitral valve
<2:1	+	–
>2:1	+	+

(MDM: mid-diastolic murmur; PSM: pansystolic murmur; S_3: third heart sound; VSD: ventricular septal defect)

Size of ventricular septal defect: Size of VSD is determined based on whether shunt is more or less than 2:1 (**Table 9**).

RADIATION/CONDUCTION

Radiation by definition means that a murmur is heard at a remote site of origin with the same intensity as at the site of origin while conduction is when the murmur is heard widely because of the loudness rather than because of selective radiation.

Some murmurs which radiate are as follows:

- *PSM of MR*:
  - Axilla, back [anterior mitral leaflet (AML) involvement]
  - Anterior chest [posterior mitral leaflet (PML) involvement]
- *ESM of AS*: Radiates to carotids:
  - Generally radiation is slightly more toward right carotid
  - If the murmur is heard better in left rather than right carotid, associated carotid stenosis should be ruled out.
  - Radiation to carotids helps in differentiating from:
    - Supravalvular AS: Where murmur is better heard in right subclavian than left and blood pressure

is higher in right arm than left, so called Coandă effect (**Fig. 7**), due to hugging of jet toward the right subclavian.

- Hypertrophic cardiomyopathy (HCM): Where murmur does not radiate to the carotids.

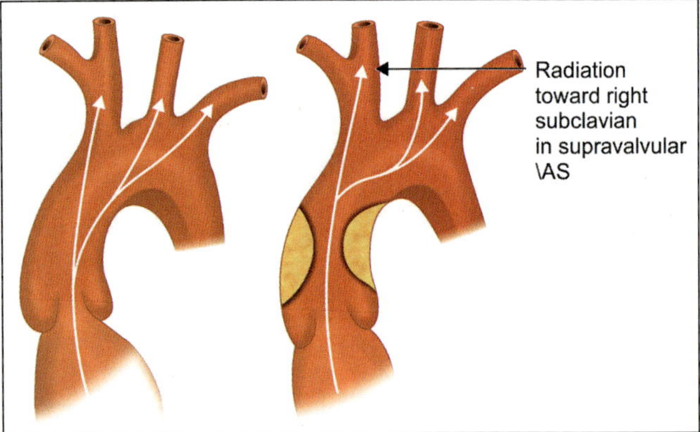

FIGURE 7: Coandă effect in supravalvular aortic stenosis (AS) (radiation toward right subclavian in supravalvular aortic stenosis (arrow).

CHANGES WITH PHYSIOLOGICAL/ PHARMACOLOGICAL MANEUVERS

Also referred to as "dynamic auscultation", this is used to differentiate the origin of murmurs based on how they change by changing the hemodynamics.

This is done by altering the following on the right and left sides of the heart:

- *Preload*: Venous return
- *Afterload*: Peripheral vascular resistance
- *Contractility*: Cardiac output
- Heart rate

The most common maneuvers employed and the most predominant change that occurs are as shown in **Table 10**.

It is important to recognize that all maneuvers which decrease the size of the heart (by decreasing preload or afterload or both) decrease all murmurs except those of HCM and MVP MR. By decreasing the ventricular size, the obstruction in HCM increases, causing an increase in intensity of murmur; while in MVR, MR the smaller ventricular size causes the nonejection click to occur earlier and prolongs the duration of the LSM, not necessarily increasing its intensity.

TABLE 10 Changes with physiological/pharmacological maneuvers.

Maneuver	Hemodynamic effect	Used where
Inspiration	Increase venous return to right side of heart	• All right-sided sounds and murmurs increase except pulmonary valvular ejection click • Used to differentiate right from left-sided murmurs • TR and PR murmurs secondary to PAH (i.e., functional or secondary) increase with inspiration while primary (or organic) murmurs do not increase • Increase in TR intensity with inspiration is referred to as Rivero–Carvallo's sign
Passive leg raising	Increased venous return to right side of heart	Similar to inspiration
Position: Lateral decubitus	Causes heart to come closer to chest wall	Used to listen to MDM in mitral stenosis when not heard in supine position
Position: Bending forwards	Causes the heart to come closer to chest	• Used to listen to murmur of AR or PR when not heard in supine position • Pericardial rubs better heard in this position
Hand grip	Significant increase in afterload on left side	• All stenotic murmurs (except MS) decrease in intensity • All regurgitant murmurs increase in intensity • Useful in differentiating PSM of MR (which increases) from PSM due to Gallavardin's dissociation (which decreases)
Squatting → Standing	• Sudden increase in afterload and preload (Squatting) → sudden decrease in both (Standing) • Squatting to standing causes a sudden decrease in LV size	• Helps in identifying the nonejection click/late systolic murmur of MVP/MR • Click occurs earlier and murmur is more prolonged with standing while the opposite occurs with squatting • The dynamic movement of click and murmur confirms the diagnosis of MVP/MR
Valsalva	During strain phase, there is a significant decrease in venous return to both right and left side of heart	• All murmurs decrease in intensity except • MVP/MR (click occurs earlier and murmur duration increases because of smaller LV cavity) • HCM (obstruction increases because of smaller LV cavity)
Amyl nitrite	Decrease in afterload	• No longer used after advent of echocardiogram • Effect opposite to that of handgrip
Phenylephrine	Increase in afterload by producing systemic vasoconstriction	• No longer used • Similar to handgrip

Continued...

Continued...

Maneuver	Hemodynamic effect	Used where
Ventricular premature complexes (VPCs)	The compensatory pause following a VPC produces increased ventricular filling and augmentation of ventricular contractility in the next beat	Murmurs of outflow tract obstruction (like AS and PS) increases in intensity while that of regurgitant murmurs like MR do not change. Helps in differentiating AS from MR
Atrial fibrillation	• The long cycle length produces increased ventricular filling and augmentation of ventricular contractility in the next beat • While short cycle length increases the LA to LV gradient	• Post long cycle length murmurs of outflow tract obstruction (like AS and PS) increases in intensity while that of regurgitant murmurs like MR do not change. Helps in differentiating AS from MR • In mitral stenosis, presence of MDM even in long cycle lengths (where the LA/LV gradients are expected to be less) indicates severe mitral stenosis

(AR: aortic regurgitation; AS: aortic stenosis; HCM: hypertrophic cardiomyopathy; LA: left atrium; LV: left ventricle; MDM: mid-diastolic murmur; MR: mitral regurgitation; MS: mitral stenosis; MVP: mitral valve prolapse; PAH: pulmonary arterial hypertension; PR: pulmonary regurgitation; PS: pulmonic stenosis; PSM: pansystolic murmur; TR: tricuspid regurgitation)

ACCOMPANYING FEATURES

The accompanying features in each murmur help in interpreting the murmur appropriately as shown in **Table 11**.

INNOCENT (FUNCTIONAL) AND PATHOLOGICAL MURMURS

There are only a few criteria that absolutely identify the organic or pathologic cardiac murmur. These are listed below.

- *All diastolic murmurs are pathological except flow murmurs*: Mid-diastolic flow murmurs across the mitral (VSD, PDA, and MR) or tricuspid (ASD, TR) valves do not imply organic disease of the A-V valves, but reflect the marked diastolic volume overload traversing the A-V valve during rapid ventricular filling.
- *All PSMs and LSMs are pathologic.* Murmurs that extend to S_2 are organic and indicate continuing turbulent blood flow at a time in the cardiac cycle when silence is expected.
- *Continuous murmurs usually indicate organic heart disease.* With few exceptions such as venous hum and mammary soufflé, murmur that continues up to S_2 and spills over into diastole must reflect a continuous pressure differential between two cardiovascular structures and is, therefore, abnormal.
- *Very loud murmurs are usually pathologic.* All murmurs associated with a thrill (Grade 4 or greater) have a pathologic basis. In rare cases of pure AR without AS, the huge stroke volume traversing the diseased aortic valve will result in a very loud ejection murmur and a thrill. In such situations the presence of the systolic ejection murmur may not indicate actual AS.
- *Associated cardiac abnormalities.* Evidence of underlying cardiac disease raises the likelihood that a given heart murmur is organic. For instance, the presence of left ventricular hypertrophy on precordial palpation, an ejection or midsystolic click, or an opening snap would suggest that the heart murmur represents a cardiac structural abnormality. However, these phenomena may be unrelated to the production of the murmur itself.
- *Frequency, shape* or *contour,* and *radiation* characteristics of heart murmurs are too nonspecific to definitively establish the organic etiology of a murmur. They are generally low to medium frequency. Still's murmur is a term that denotes a particularly vibratory murmur of a dominant harmonic, usually low to medium frequency.

The only difference between an innocent and a flow murmur is that the latter disappears when the underlying cause of the increased flow (e.g., anemia, fever, and thyrotoxicosis) disappears.

SOME COMMON MURMURS

Summarizing the above discussion, following paragraphs illustrate how commonly encountered murmurs are described.

Mid-diastolic murmur of mitral stenosis: A MDM is heard at the apex, Grade 4/6, low frequency, rough and rumbling, better heard with the bell of the stethoscope in the left lateral position. It is prolonged with a presystolic accentuation.

Pansystolic murmur of mitral regurgitation: A pansystolic (or holosystolic) murmur is heard at the apex. It is Grade 3/6, high frequency, soft and blowing, radiating to the axilla and the back. It does not vary with respiration but increases on handgrip.

Pansystolic murmur of tricuspid regurgitation: A PSM is heard at the left lower sternal border. It is Grade 2/6, high frequency, soft, increasing with inspiration and passive leg raising.

Pansystolic murmur of ventricular septal defect: A PSM is heard at the lower left sternal border. It is Grade 4/6, rough, not increasing with inspiration.

TABLE 11 Accompanying features of murmurs and their significance.

Auscultatory event	Accompanying feature	Significance
ESM of LV outflow	Slow rising pulse	Fixed LV outflow obstruction
	Bisferiens pulse	AS + AR or HOCM
	Normal pulse	Aortic valve sclerosis or mild AS
EDM along LSB	Collapsing pulse	AR
	Normal pulse	PR or mild AR
Long systolic murmur at 2nd or 3rd space	Prominent "a" wave in JVP	Severe RV outflow obstruction
	Sustained parasternal impulse	As above
	Ejection click	Valvular PS
	Absence of any of the above signs	VSD small
MDM at apex	Loud S_1, OS	MS
	Diastolic thrill	MS
	S_3	Flow murmur due to MR or post-tricuspid shunts
	Severe AR	Possible Austin Flint
	Atrial fibrillation	MS
Pansystolic murmur at LLSB	Pure RV impulse	TR
	Biventricular impulse	VSD
	Large "v" wave in JVP	TR
Long systolic murmur at apex	Forcible LV impulse	MR
	Sustained LV impulse	AS
	S_3	MR
	S_4	AS

(AR: aortic regurgitation; AS: aortic stenosis; HOCM: hypertrophic obstructive cardiomyopathy; JVP: jugular venous pulse; LV: left ventricle; MR: mitral regurgitation; MS: mitral stenosis; OS: opening snap; PR: pulmonary regurgitation; PS: pulmonic stenosis; S_3: third heart sound; S_4: fourth heart sound; TR: tricuspid regurgitation)

Ejection systolic murmur of aortic stenosis: There is an ESM, best heard in the right second intercostal space. It is Grade 3/6, harsh, mixed frequency crescendo decrescendo murmur peaking in late systole. The murmur radiates to both the carotids. It decreases in intensity with handgrip, Valsalva, and on standing from a squatting position.

Ejection systolic murmur of pulmonic stenosis: There is an ESM, best heard in the left second intercostal space, Grade 3/6, harsh, mixed frequency, crescendo-decrescendo, peaking late in systole, and increasing with inspiration.

Ejection systolic murmur of hypertrophic cardiomyopathy: There is an ESM, best heard in the left fourth intercostal space. It is Grade 3/6, harsh mixed frequency murmur with late peaking. There is no radiation to carotids. It does not vary with respiration, increases with Valsalva, and on standing from squatting position.

Late systolic murmur of mitral valve prolapse/mitral regurgitation: There is a LSM, best heard at the apex. It is Grade 3/6, high frequency, cooing type of murmur. It radiates to the axilla and the back. It does not change with respiration. It becomes long with Valsalva and on standing from squatting position.

Early diastolic murmur of aortic regurgitation: There is an EDM best heard in the left third intercoastal space. It is Grade 3/6, high frequency, soft murmur best heard in expiration in bending forward position. It extends to the latter one-third of diastole and increases with handgrip.

RECOMMENDED READINGS

1. Raju BS. Clinical methods in cardiology. Bangalore: Universities Press (India) Private Limited; 2009.
2. Abrams J. Essentials of cardiac physical diagnosis. Washington: Lea and Febiger; 1987.
3. Ginghină C, Năstase OA, Ghiorghiu I, Egher L. Continuous murmur - the auscultatory expression of a variety of pathological conditions. J Med Life. 2012;5:39-46.
4. Zipes DP, Libby P, Bonow RO, Mann DL, Tomaselli GF (Eds). Braunwald's Heart Disease: A Textbook of Cardiovascular Medicine, 11th edition. Elsevier Health Sciences; 2019.

CHAPTER 12

Patient with Altered Sensorium: Evaluation and Management

B Vengamma

ABSTRACT

Altered sensorium is a common, often misdiagnosed clinical entity characterized by an acute change in attention and consciousness. Altered sensorium can develop both as an acute and subacute condition and carries significant morbidity and mortality. Good clinical history, meticulous physical examination, and judicious use of laboratory investigations help in ascertaining the etiological cause of delirium early. Recognizing the etiological cause and institution of specific treatment can be lifesaving in patients presenting with altered sensorium.

"Only the inquiring mind solves problems"

—Edward Hodnett

INTRODUCTION

Prompt diagnosis and effective management of the patient presenting with altered sensorium is one of the challenging tasks faced by a physician. Arousal emerges from the action of the reticular activating system (RAS), which receives stimulations from the environment via the somatosensory, the autonomic pathways and inputs from the limbic system. The RAS stimulates the brain, activating the cerebral cortex. In clinical practice, arousal is induced in comatose patients by stimulating the RAS.

While consciousness is the state of awareness of the self and the environment, coma is its exact opposite. Between the states of consciousness (state of awareness of the self and the environment) and coma (unarousable state), a variety of altered states of consciousness exist (**Box 1**). Delirium is a disturbance of consciousness characterized by reduced ability to focus, sustain, or shift attention that is not accounted for by a preexisting, established, or evolving dementia. Delirium usually develops over hours to days and tends to fluctuate as the day progresses.

DIAGNOSTIC APPROACH

Several causes of altered sensorium (e.g., hypoglycemia) can be fatal if not recognized early and treated. Therefore, an early diagnosis of the etiological cause of altered sensorium is essential to ensure early initiation of specific treatment. The diagnostic approach to a patient with altered sensorium begins with obtaining a good detailed clinical history. Accurately eliciting and interpreting of physical signs that reflect the integrity or impairment of various levels of the brain; and the determining the pathophysiological basis of the lesion facilitates neurological localization and will direct the work-up. It is necessary to ascertain whether the cause of altered consciousness is supratentorial (starts rostrally and evolves caudally), subtentorial (starts focally in the brainstem), metabolic (produces form the onset signs of diffuse or multifocal dysfunction), or psychiatric (lacks signs of physiologic brain dysfunction).

Initial evaluation and stabilization: At the time of initial evaluation, it is required to concurrently assess whether the patient is clinically stable by assessing whether the circulation, airway, and breathing (CAB) is adequate.

In the setting of altered sensorium, carrying out the initial stabilization and laboratory testing and institution of immediate treatment for treatable conditions are done concurrently as this can be lifesaving. Examples include reversing metabolic coma due to hypoglycemia with intravenous glucose, naloxone for opiate overdosage, among others. These details are listed in **Box 2**.

HISTORY

As patients in altered sensorium cannot provide the history themselves, history may have to be elicited from an eyewitness account. The recent events (e.g., trauma) or preceding illnesses (e.g., psychiatric illnesses) that lead to altered state of sensorium should be enquired into. If available, the medication list of, or the medicines kept by the patient should be scrutinized.

Bedside examination should being with checking the blood pressure (BP). If the BP is high, evaluation for signs of raised intracranial tension, acute ischemic, or hemorrhagic stroke is warranted. Certain breathing patterns facilitate anatomical localization in a comatose patient. *Kussmaul breathing* (deep, rapid breathing) may be evident in metabolic acidosis. *Cheyne-Stokes breathing* (cyclical rapid shallow breathing to the point where there is a cessation of breathing and apnea followed by an abrupt spontaneous return of respirations with deep sighs) is seen in head injuries and metabolic conditions. *Biot's breathing*

BOX 1 Various states of altered sensorium.

- **Confusion:** Confusion refers to impaired attention and implies adequate arousal to perform mental status tests of this ability
- **Delirium:** Delirium is a condition characterized by a disturbance of consciousness with inattention, accompanied by acute change in cognition not accounted for by pre-existing, established, or evolving dementia that develops over a short period of time (hours to days) with fluctuation over time; and evidence that the disturbance is caused by the direct physiologic consequences of a general medical condition
    - Hypoactive delirium: Symptoms of lethargy and minimal psychomotor activity
    - Hyperactive delirium: Symptoms of significant agitation
    - Mixed delirium: Expressions fluctuate between the hypoactive and hyperactive delirium
- **Akinetic mutism:** Patients with akinetic mutism are silent, alert appearing immobility with retainment of sleep, wake cycles, and absent mental and spontaneous motor activity
- **Apallic syndrome:** In apallic syndrome, there is absent neocortical function with relatively intact brainstem function
- **Locked-in syndrome:** Locked in syndrome refers to a state in which weakness all four limbs with lower cranial paralysis; but, the patient manifests signs of being appropriately aware of himself and environment and communicates with vertical eye movements
- **Inattention:** Inattention is a state where a person can actually look like they are entirely alert or even hyperalert
- **Abulia:** Abulia (seen with frontal lesions) is a state where the patient is essentially quiet and has complete lack of spontaneity
- **Stupor:** Stupor is a state of severely impaired arousal with some responsiveness to vigorous stimuli
- **Obtundation:** Obtundation is a lesser state of decreased arousal with some responsiveness to touch or voice
- **Lethargy (somnolence):** In lethargy, patient arousal, though diminished, is maintained spontaneously or with repeated light stimulation
- **Coma:** Coma is a state of total or near total unresponsiveness characterized by total absence of awareness of self and environment even when the subject is externally stimulated
- **Vegetative state:** In vegetative state, there is wakefulness accompanied by an apparent total lack of cognitive function. The patient opens eyes spontaneously in response to verbal stimuli

(rapid, shallow breaths followed by periods of apnea) and *apneustic breathing* (irregular breathing intermixed with irregular periods of apnea) are seen in lesions of medulla oblongata (e.g., head injury and stroke).

Physical examination should also look for signs of traumatic injury, an infectious disease, or drug ingestion. Odor of the breath (e.g., alcohol ingestion; hepatic encephalopathy) can provide valuable clues.

NEUROLOGIC EXAMINATION

The neurologic examination in patients with altered sensorium should encompass all components of the conventional neurologic examination to the extent possible except perhaps the gait. More emphasis is placed on the level of arousal, the cranial nerve examination, and the motor system. Sensory system examination and evaluation of the pattern of reflexes are also meticulously to be done. The initial step involves assessing the level of consciousness (**Box 1**). This is done traditionally using the Glasgow Coma Scale (GCS). Funduscopic examination provides information about intracranial pressure and pathology. Blink test or menace reflex facilitates assessment of visual fields. Other aspects of cranial nerve examination include pupils, eye movements, sensory component of V, motor component of VII, and the gag response (cranial nerves IX and X).

Small and reactive pupils and absent corneal oxycephalic reflex indicate metabolic injury. Symmetry of the pupils helps in differentiating nonstructural from structural injuries. In midbrain injury, pupils tend to be fixed in midposition, may be irregular with intact reaction to light response. In opiate intoxication and pontine injury, pupils are constricted, pin-point and do not react to light response. Unilateral dilated pupil in a comatose patient indicates III cranial nerve palsy due uncal herniation and these patients may need urgent neurosurgical intervention.

Gaze deviation, away from the side that is weak, suggests a hemispheric lesion. If gaze deviation is toward the side

BOX 2 Initial management of acute onset altered sensorium.

- **Stabilization:**
    - "CAB"
        - Adequate circulation
        - Airway control
        - Breathing (oxygenation and ventilation)
    - Cervical spine stabilization
- **Immediate therapies:**
    - Thiamine 100 mg IV
    - Dextrose 50%, 50 mL IV (may be held if immediate finger-stick glucose check establishes adequate serum glucose)
    - Naloxone 0.4–2.0 mg IV (may be repeated)
    - Procuring blood sample for laboratory testing

(CAB: circulation, airway, and breathing; IV: intravenous)

of the hemiparesis, a brainstem lesion, involving pons or cerebellum is likely. In midbrain lesions, primary gaze is downward. Spontaneous eye rolling movements is evident in metabolic encephalopathies and is due to bilateral hemispheric dysfunction. *Ocular bobbing* (eyes at rest, dip down, and return to the resting position) and *ocular dipping* (eyes bounce up and have a slow downward phase) are suggestive of pontine injury. When spontaneous and saccadic and rolling eye movements on opening the eyelids are noted, true coma is unlikely.

Normally, when head is moved, eyes move contralateral to the side of head movement (oculocephalic reflex). Absence of oculocephalic reflex suggests bilateral hemispheric injury. Cold caloric test (oculovestibular reflex) assesses the integrity of brainstem especially pontine and cerebellar function. The patient's head is kept elevated at 30° and 60 cc of ice water is instilled in each ear using a syringe. Normally, a tonic movement of the eyes toward and fast saccades away from the side of stimulation is observed. Absence of fast movement component on both sides is suggestive of bihemispheric injury. An asymmetrical response and negative response indicate brainstem dysfunction and loss of brainstem integrity, respectively.

If there are no spontaneous motor movements, verbal commands are issued asking the patient to move a limb. If no perceptible movement is noticed, then progressively more noxious stimuli are applied to try and induce a response. A decorticate posturing indicates hemispheric injury. When the pathology is around the level of the red nucleus, decerebrate posturing is noticed.

LABORATORY INVESTIGATIONS

Laboratory testing (e.g., plasma glucose, serum electrolytes, drug, and toxin levels) and neuroimaging (computed tomography and magnetic resonance imaging) can provide diagnostic and localization clues. In patients with history of epilepsy who present with altered consciousness, electroencephalogram (EEG) can be helpful in detecting nonconvulsive status epilepticus.

DIFFERENTIAL DIAGNOSIS

Differential diagnosis of altered sensorium is shown in **Box 3**. In patients presenting with altered consciousness, a structural reason may be evident only in about one-third. The differential diagnosis includes traumatic or vascular in origin; neuroinfections including, meningitis, encephalitis; tumors, or hydrocephalus among others. Toxic or metabolic causes include exposure to toxin such as carbon monoxide, drugs, hypoglycemia, and electrolyte disorders. Psychiatric disorders can present with altered sensorium and are difficult to differentiate from the metabolic causes. However, certain features can be useful in detecting these conditions.

In altered sensorium due to metabolic causes, confusion and stupor commonly precede motor signs. Motor signs are usually symmetrical; pupillary reactions

BOX 3 Some common causes of altered sensorium.

- **Toxic:**
  - Sedatives, hypnotics
  - Opiates
  - Benzodiazepines, barbiturates, and other sedatives
  - Tricyclic antidepressant agents
  - Phenothiazines and butyrophenones
  - Stupefying poisons (e.g., *Datura*), acute alcohol intoxication
- **Stimulating exogenous toxins:**
  - Amphetamines, cocaine
  - Phencyclidine
  - Methylphenidate
- **Withdrawal syndromes:**
  - Alcohol withdrawal
  - Benzodiazepine, barbiturates, and other sedative withdrawal
- **Metabolic disorders:**
  - Diabetes mellitus: Hyperglycemia (diabetic ketoacidosis and hyperosmolar coma) and hypoglycemia
  - Thyroid disease (myxedema and thyroid storm)
  - Renal failure (uremia and disequilibrium syndrome)
  - Electrolyte abnormalities (dehydration and volume contraction, hyponatremia, and hypercalcemia
  - Acid-base disorders
  - Hepatic failure: Hyperammonemia
  - Hypoadrenalism
  - Hypoxia and hypercarbia
  - Hereditary metabolic disorders (i.e., porphyria, carbamoyltransferase deficiency carrier state)
  - Seizure (postictal state, non-convulsive status epilepticus)
- **Infections:**
  - Acute meningitis, encephalitis caused by neurotropic viruses, dengue fever etc.
  - Sever complicated falciparum malaria
  - Enteric encephalopathy
  - Leptospirosis
  - Scrub typhus
- **Focal disease:**
  - Trauma (contusion, ICH)
  - Nontraumatic ICH
  - Ischemic stroke
  - Infection (abscess, subdural empyema, and focal encephalitis)
  - Tumor
  - Demyelination (multiple sclerosis, acute demyelinating encephalomyelitis)
- **Nonfocal disease:**
  - Trauma (elevated ICP, diffuse axonal injury)
  - Vascular syndrome
    - Subarachnoid hemorrhage
    - Aneurysm in posterior fossa with mass effect

Continued...

Continued...

- Hypoxic-ischemic encephalopathy
- Stroke (focal strokes with nonfocal presentations, posterior fossa infarct with mass effect, and hydrocephalus)
- Hypertensive encephalopathy (including eclampsia)

◦ Infection (meningitis and diffuse encephalitis)

◦ Tumor-related
- Tumor (brain-stem invasion, posterior fossa mass effect, elevated ICP, and hydrocephalus)
- Paraneoplastic syndromes (brainstem and limbic encephalitis and vasculitis)

- **Others:**
  - Basilar migraine
  - TGA
  - TTP and other syndromes of medical illness
  - Sleep deprivation
  - Situational (i.e., ICU psychosis)
  - Psychiatric (conversion, depression, mania, and catatonia)
  - Neuroleptic malignant syndrome
  - Serotonin syndrome
  - Malignant hyperthermia
  - Pheochromocytoma
  - Psychiatric disorders: Acute psychosis, mania, and anxiety state
  - Porphyria
  - Nutritional deficiencies (Wernicke's encephalopathy, pellagra etc.)
  - Disordered temperature regulation

(ICH: intracranial hemorrhage; ICP: intracranial pressure; ICU: intensive care unit; TGA: transient global amnesia; TTP: thrombotic thrombocytopenic purpura)

are usually preserved. Asterixis, myoclonus, tremor, and seizures are commonly seen. Acid-base imbalance with hyper- or hypoventilation is frequent. In psychiatric unresponsiveness, lids close actively, pupils are reactive, and motor tone is inconsistent or normal. Eupnea or hyperventilation is usual, no pathologic reflexes are present and EEG is normal.

CHANGING TRENDS

Common causes of altered sensorium, like enteric encephalopathy and severe complicated falciparum malaria are less frequently being encountered in the present era. Altered sensorium caused by infections with neurotropic viruses is being increasingly recognized, probably because of increased awareness and access to virology diagnostic facilities. Dengue fever outbreaks, scrub typhus, and leptospirosis are commonly seen. Altered sensorium in these patients could not only be because of the encephalopathy caused by the disease process per se, but also due to intracranial bleeding related to thrombocytopenia. Myxedema coma and stupefying poisons (e.g., *Datura* poisoning) are some of the conditions that physicians may encounter in acute care setting. Altered sensorium has also been the presenting symptom in patients presenting with severe acute respiratory syndrome (SARS) coronavirus-2 (SARS-CoV-2) disease-2019 (COVID-19) pandemic.

PROGNOSIS

Altered sensorium is not a final diagnosis, it is a transitional state. Patients, who are postictal after a seizure, can be in an encephalopathic state for some time afterward. Infectious processes, especially meningitis or encephalitis, can lead to encephalopathy.

Sleep-wake cycles are absent in coma. In vegetative state, arousal mechanisms are preserved with a complete lack of self or environmental awareness. This is usually due to diffuse bilateral cerebral involvement that spares the brainstem. The toxic and metabolic causes of altered sensorium tend to have a better prognosis than structural causes. However, traumatic injury fares better than anoxic injury. Clinically, important prognostic signs include the motor component of the GCS, the duration of coma, and other signs of brainstem damage.

Certain EEG patterns that are helpful in assessing prognosis in patients with coma. Alpha coma in an essentially unarousable patient is associated with a higher mortality. Somatosensory evoked potentials (SSEP) testing can used for testing the brainstem and bilaterally absent cortical SSEP is strongly associated with the instance of vegetative state or death. Neuroimaging though useful in differentiating structural lesions has limited overall predictive value is less when compared to electrophysiologic tests or even the clinical examination itself in assessing the prognosis in a patient with altered consciousness.

In coma due to hypoxic ischemic injury, patients with a preserved light reflex, those with a motor response that is either flexor or extensor; and those who have spontaneous eye movements have better survival. In traumatic injury or head injuries, patients with loss of consciousness for <6 hours and a normal CT tend to have a good outcome.

RECOMMENDED READINGS

1. Oh ES, Fong TG, Hshieh TT, Inouye SK. Delirium in older persons: Advances in diagnosis and treatment. JAMA. 2017;318:1161-74.
2. Maldonado JR. Acute brain failure: Pathophysiology, diagnosis, management, and sequelae of delirium. Crit Care Clin. 2017;33:461-519.
3. Wijdicks EF, Cranford RE. Clinical diagnosis of prolonged states of impaired consciousness in adults. Mayo Clin Proc. 2005;80:1037-46.
4. Morandi A, Jackson JC. Delirium in the intensive care unit: a review. Neurol Clin. 2011;29:749-63.
5. Vengamma B. Clinical approach to coma. In: Munjal Y (Ed). API Textbook of Medicine, 10th ed. Mumbai: Association of Physicians of India: Jaypee Brothers, Medical Publishers; 2015.

CHAPTER
13

Cutaneous Manifestations and Diseases

A Surekha, G Ramesh Kumar

ABSTRACT

Cutaneous lesions are a common reason for presentation to a physician and skin manifestations may be a manifestation of a more serious underlying systemic disease. Disorders of the every organ system may result in cutaneous manifestations. Several drugs are also known to cause skin lesions. In this chapter, an overview of some of the common cutaneous manifestations of systemic diseases as seen by physicians in their daily clinical practice, common systemic diseases that have prominent cutaneous findings, common cutaneous diseases that have important systemic associations, and skin manifestations that alert the clinicians to the possibility of an internal malignancy are summarized.

"The physician should not treat the disease but the patient who is suffering from it"

—Moses Maimonides

INTRODUCTION

Many systemic diseases have cutaneous manifestations and the skin is considered to be a mirror, reflecting these. The cutaneous manifestations of systemic disease are often vague and nonspecific (e.g., toxic erythema that might follow a viral infection) (**Fig. 1**). Sometimes, while the cutaneous manifestations are highly specific and define the illness (**Fig. 2**), systemic manifestations are vague and nonspecific (e.g., chicken pox and measles). Further, many drugs that are used to treat systemic disease are known to produce a wide range of cutaneous manifestations (**Fig. 3**). In this chapter, an attempt has been made to provide an overview of some of the common cutaneous manifestations of systemic diseases (**Fig. 4**) as seen by physicians in their daily clinical practice, common systemic diseases that have prominent cutaneous findings, common cutaneous diseases that have important systemic associations, and skin manifestations that alert the clinicians to the possibility of an internal malignancy.

COMMON CUTANEOUS MANIFESTATIONS OF SYSTEMIC DISEASE

GENERALIZED PRURITUS

Generalized "itch" or pruritus is a common clinical problem for which physicians are consulted. Generalized pruritus can present with or without an accompanying rash. Generalized pruritus in the absence of an accompanying rash warrants a thorough workup for exclusion of an underlying systemic disease (**Box 1**).

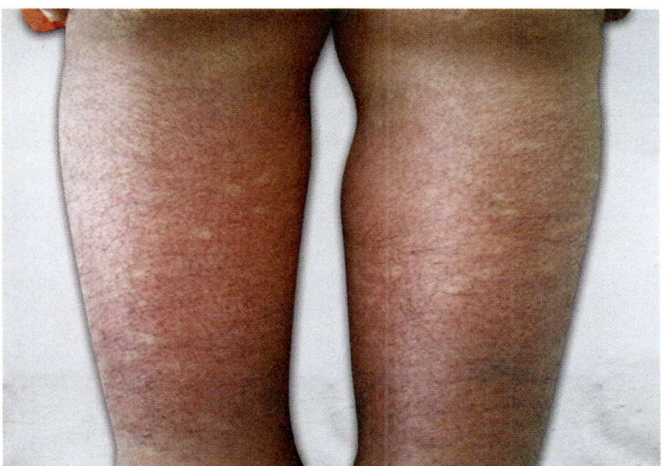

FIGURE 1: Clinical photograph showing erythematous rash with islands of sparing in a patient with dengue fever.

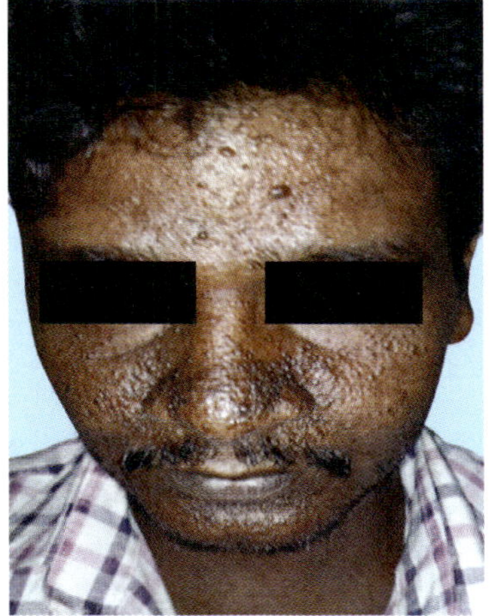

FIGURE 2: Clinical photograph in a patient with tuberous sclerosis showing facial angiofibromas.

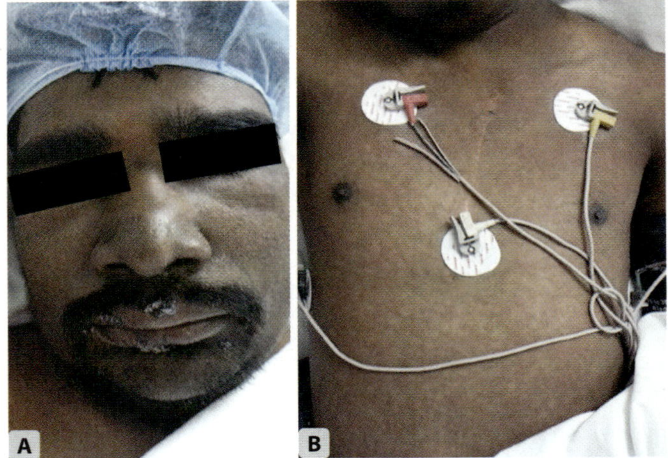

FIGURES 3 A & B: Clinical photographs showing **(A)** facial edema and **(B)** morbilliform rash over the trunk in a patient with drug rash with eosinophilia and systemic symptoms (DRESS) syndrome due to furosemide usage.

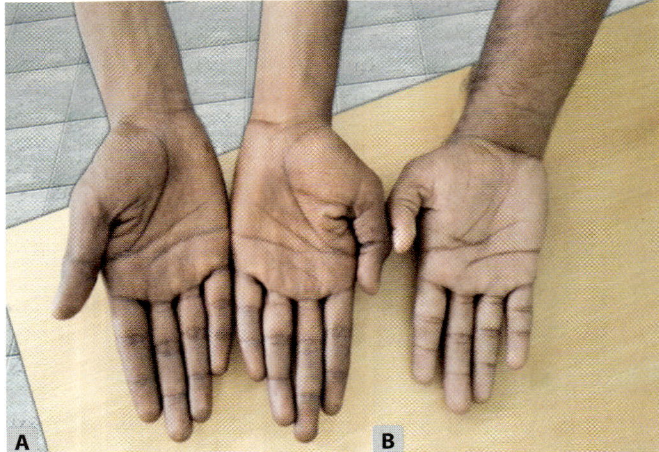

FIGURES 4 A & B: **(A)** Clinical photograph showing pigmentation in both palms in a patient with Addison's disease; **(B)** Normal hand of the patient's father is shown for comparison.

ERYTHEMA NODOSUM

Erythema nodosum (EN) is a commonly encountered form of septal panniculitis. EN most commonly affects young women. It presents as symmetric warm, tender, and erythematous nodules over the extensor surface of legs (**Fig. 5**). Lesions of EN do not ulcerate or undergo scarring or atrophy. Associated fever, arthralgias, and malaise may be evident. EN may be primary. However, a detailed history, physical examination, and laboratory diagnostic workup are required to establish whether EN is secondary to other systemic causes (**Box 2**).

CUTANEOUS VASCULITIS

Vasculitis can affect small, medium, or large vessels. Cutaneous manifestations are often evident in patients with small and medium vessel vasculitis. Patients presenting with a cutaneous vasculitis, warrant a search for evidence of systemic vasculitis, as this has prognostic significance.

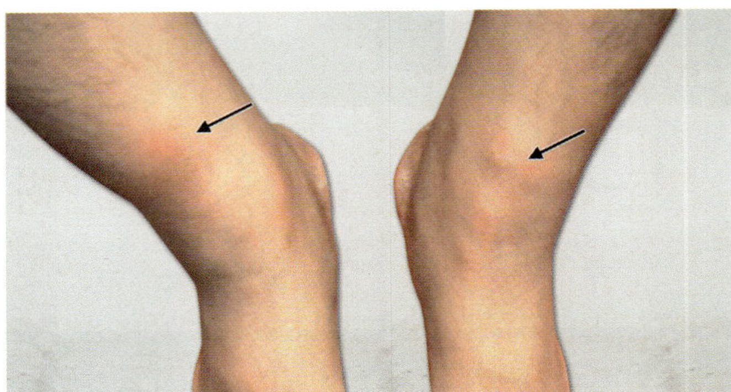

FIGURE 5: **Erythema nodosum (arrows).**

BOX 1	Common causes of generalized pruritus.
Liver diseases:	
• Cholestasis due to any cause	
Renal diseases:	
• Uremia due to any cause	
Endocrine diseases:	
• Hyperthyroidism and hypothyroidism	
Hematological diseases and lymphoreticular malignancies:	
• Iron deficiency anemia	
• Polycythemia rubra vera	
• Leukemia	
• Lymphoma	
• Multiple myeloma and monoclonal gammopathies	

BOX 2	Common causes of generalized pruritus.
• **Infections:**	
◦ Bacterial (e.g., *Streptococcus, Yersinia, Salmonella*, and *Campylobacter*)	
◦ Viral (e.g., Epstein–Barr virus)	
◦ Mycobacterial (e.g., tuberculosis)	
• **Sarcoidosis**	
• **Inflammatory bowel disease**	
• **Malignancy:**	
◦ Leukemia and lymphoma	
◦ Postradiotherapy	
• **Behçet's syndrome**	
• **Drugs:**	
◦ Oral contraceptive pill	
◦ Phenytoin	
◦ Tetracyclines	
◦ Sulphonamides	
◦ Salicylates	

Small vessel vasculitis affects the arterioles, capillaries, and venules. Most common cutaneous manifestations of small vessel vasculitis include palpable purpura and

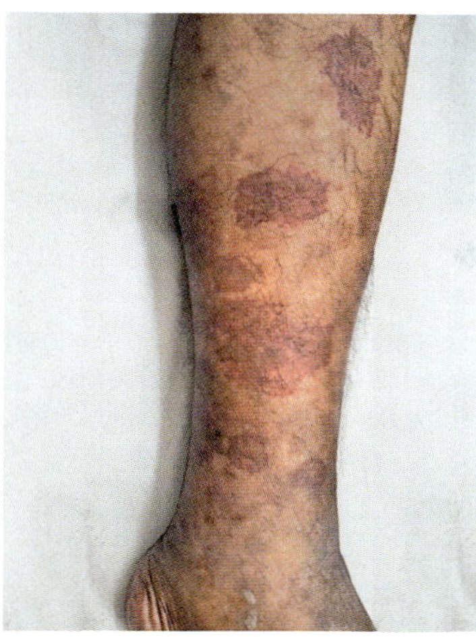

FIGURE 6: Clinical photograph showing palpable purpuric plaques on lower limb in a patient with small vessel vasculitis.

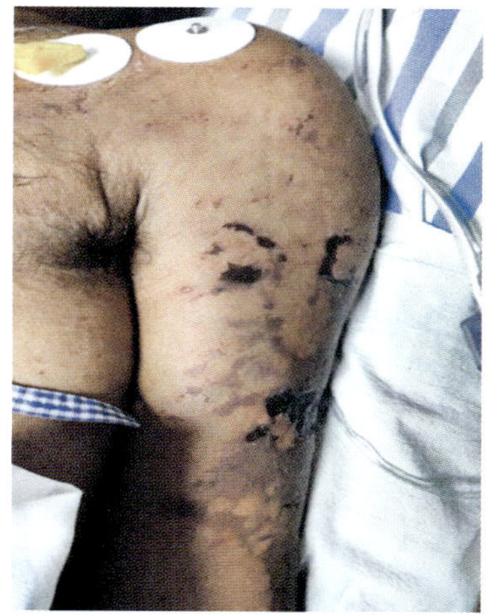

FIGURE 7: Clinical photograph showing purpura fulminans in a patient with meningococcemia.

plaques (**Fig. 6**), typically affecting the lower legs and dependent areas. In patients presenting with purpura, palpation by lightly running the index finger over the rash with eyes closed is helpful to clinically detect palpable purpura which is a physical sign indicating small vessel vasculitis. Leukocytoclastic vasculitis (LCV) (hypersensitivity vasculitis) is a small vessel vasculitis characterized by leukocytoclasis (vascular damage caused by nuclear debris from infiltrating neutrophils). LCV classically presents as palpable purpura; rare findings include urticarial plaques, vesicles, bullae, and pustules. LCV can be acute or chronic; it is idiopathic in up to half the cases; it may be secondary to drugs, underlying infection, connective tissue disorders, or malignancy. LCV may be localized to the skin or may be associated with systemic involvement. Henoch-Schönlein purpura (HSP) is a specific subtype of LCV.

Cutaneous manifestations of a medium vessel vasculitis include subcutaneous nodules, livedo reticularis, and ulcers. Systemic diseases such as systemic lupus erythematosus (SLE), granulomatosis with polyangiitis (GPA; earlier called Wegener's granulomatosis), polyarteritis nodosa and Churg-Strauss syndrome often manifest small and medium vessel vasculitis. Septic vasculitis is a frequently seen manifestation with meningococcemia (**Fig. 7**) and gonococcemia.

ERYTHEMA MULTIFORME, STEVENS–JOHNSON SYNDROME, AND TOXIC EPIDERMAL NECROLYSIS

Erythema multiforme represents an acute, self-limited mucocutaneous syndrome with distinctive skin lesions and histopathology. Patients present with erythematous macules on the extensor extremities, which may spread to involve flexural surfaces and the trunk. These macules evolve into target lesions (**Fig. 8**) characterized by a dusky center surrounded by a zone of pallor, which is surrounded by an erythematous ring. When mucosal involvement is evident, it is usually limited to the oral cavity (**Fig. 9**).

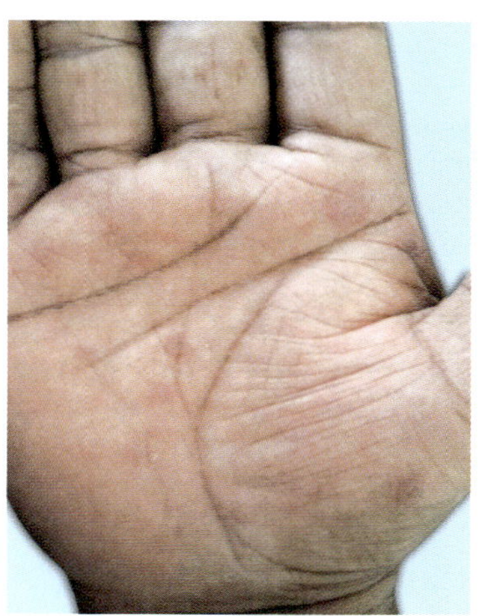

FIGURE 8: Clinical photograph showing target lesions in a patient with erythema multiforme.

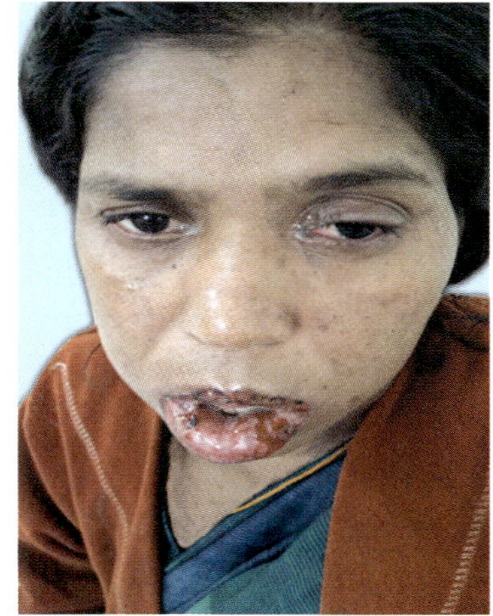

FIGURE 9: Clinical photograph of a patient with erythema multiforme major showing conjunctival and oral mucosal involvement.

Stevens-Johnson syndrome (SJS) is a potentially lethal acute mucocutaneous syndrome characterized by severe purulent conjunctivitis, stomatitis with extensive mucosal necrosis, and purpuric macules. *Toxic epidermal necrolysis (TEN)* is a drug-induced syndrome and most often caused by drugs such as sulfonamides, pyrazolones, barbiturates, and antiepileptic drugs. Presently, SJS and TEN are considered to be two ends of a spectrum of severe epidermolytic adverse cutaneous drug reactions, differing only by their extent of skin detachment (Nikolsky's sign). When the extent of cutaneous skin involvement is <10% of body surface area, it is termed as SJS; when >30% of body surface area is involved, it is termed TEN; when skin involvement is 10–30%, it is designated SJS/TEN.

XANTHOMAS

Xanthomas are localized accumulations of lipid-laden histiocytes that are located found in the dermis or tendons. Their presence offers a clue to an underlying dyslipoproteinemia. These are categorized as tendinous, planar, eruptive, and tuberous xanthomas. Tendinous xanthomas are found on the extensor tendons. These are smooth and firm nodules with normal overlying skin and are usually associated with increased serum cholesterol. Planar xanthomas are soft and yellow maculopapular lesions. These consist of xanthelasma, xanthoma striatum palmare, and diffuse plane xanthoma; and are associated with either elevated cholesterol or triglycerides. Diffuse plane xanthomas may or may not be associated with abnormal lipid levels and may be associated with a paraproteinemia. Eruptive xanthomas are associated with significantly elevated triglycerides. Tuberous xanthomas are associated with elevated cholesterol/triglyceride levels.

VITILIGO

Vitiligo, characterized by hypopigmented lesions, been associated with autoimmune disorders such as rheumatoid arthritis, insulin-dependent diabetes mellitus, pernicious anemia, autoimmune thyroiditis, alopecia areata, and Addison's disease.

SYSTEMIC DISEASES WITH CUTANEOUS MANIFESTATIONS

Some of the commonly encountered systemic diseases with cutaneous manifestations are listed in **Box 3**. Connective tissue disorders often have classic skin manifestations, some of which are disease specific such as SLE (**Figs. 10** and **11**), scleroderma (**Fig. 12**), and dermatomyositis (Gottron papules over knuckles and heliotrope rash) among others.

SKIN MANIFESTATIONS OF INTERNAL MALIGNANCIES

Cutaneous paraneoplastic syndromes (**Fig. 13**) are associated with several internal malignancies. The presence of these paraneoplastic cutaneous manifestations (**Table 1**) warrants a thorough search for the malignancy.

BOX 3 Commonly encountered systemic diseases with cutaneous manifestations.

Diabetes mellitus:
- Necrobiosis lipoidica diabeticorum, diabetic dermopathy, bullous diabeticorum, scleredema, and increased susceptibility to skin infections

Thyroid diseases:
- Hyperthyroidism: Warm, moist, soft, and smooth skin, pruritus, generalized or localized hyperhidrosis of the palms and soles, nonscarring alopecia, nail changes, and hyperpigmentation
- Graves' disease: Thyroid acropachy and pretibial myxedema
- Hypothyroidism cold, dry, pale, xerotic, pruritic skin, and generalized myxedema

Rheumatological diseases:
- Rheumatoid arthritis: Rheumatoid nodule, linear subcutaneous bands, and rheumatoid neutrophilic dermatitis
- Systemic lupus erythematosus, subacute cutaneous lupus erythematosus, and discoid lupus erythematosus; malar erythema, annular/psoriasiform rash affecting arms and "V" area of chest; and well demarcated plaques with adherent scales and scarring alopecia
- Dermatomyositis: Heliotrope rash, Gottron papules and sign (violaceous macules and papules over interphalangeal and metacarpophalangeal joints), macular violaceous or poikilodermatous rash over shoulders and hips, and hyperkeratosis on ulnar border of fingers (mechanics hands)
- Systemic sclerosis: Calcinosis cutis, Raynaud's phenomenon, esophageal dysmotility, sclerodactyly, and telangiectasia (CREST) syndrome

Renal disease:
- Pruritus, abnormal pigmentation, xerosis, metastatic calcification, blistering eruptions resembling porphyria cutanea tarda, and nail changes

Hepatic disease:
- Jaundice, pruritus, spider telangiectasias, palmar erythema, xanthelasmas, gynecomastia, hair pattern changes, and nail lesions. Mixed essential cryoglobulinemia, porphyria cutanea tarda, and lichen planus common with hepatitis C

Porphyrias:
- Increased skin fragility, vesicles and bullae, facial hypertrichosis, and hyperpigmentation of the periorbital and malar regions

Sarcoidosis:
- Papules, plaques, and nodules scar infiltration

SKIN DISEASES THAT MIMIC SYSTEMIC DISEASES

Careful evaluation is required to differentiate skin manifestations of common skin diseases that mimic systemic diseases. Malar rash, a manifestation of SLE should be differentiated from facial redness secondary to acne rosacea. In patients suspected to have vitiligo, tinea versicolor should be excluded as a cause of hypopigmentation. Patients with dermatomyositis may not present with the classic heliotrope rash but may present with a seborrheic dermatitis pattern of facial and scalp disease. Stasis dermatitis should be differentiated from cellulitis.

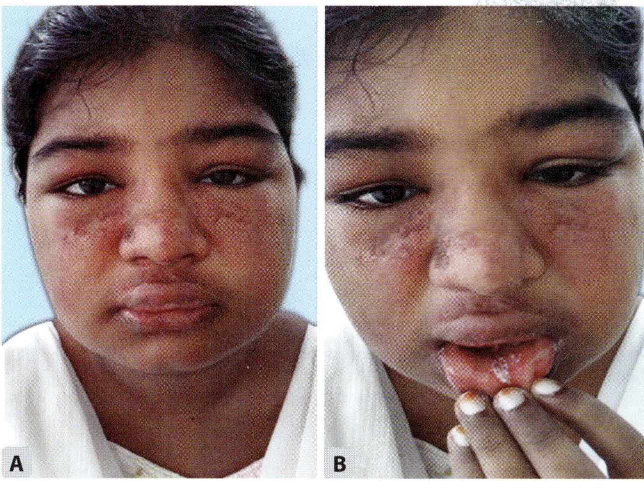

FIGURES 10 A & B: Clinical photographs of a patient with systemic lupus erythematosus showing malar rash with **(A)** facial puffiness and **(B)** oral ulcers.

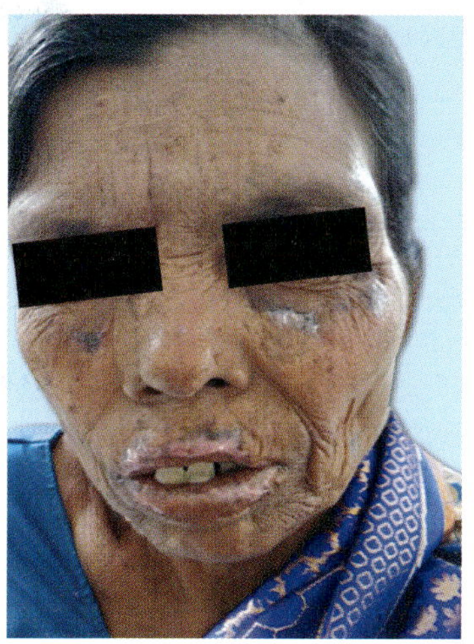

FIGURE 11: Clinical photograph showing discoid lupus erythematosus.

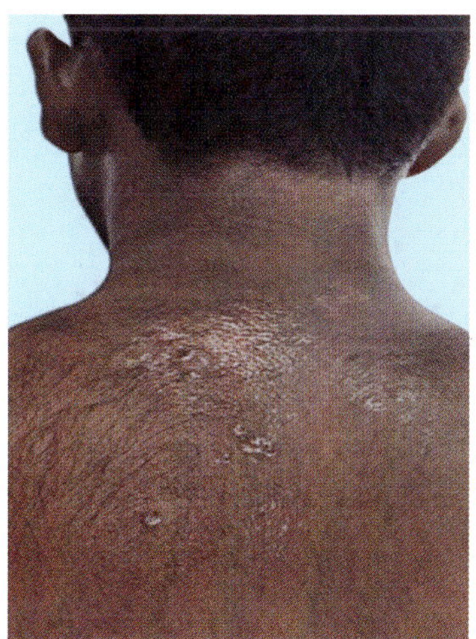

FIGURE 12: Clinical photograph showing salt and pepper appearance in a patient with scleroderma.

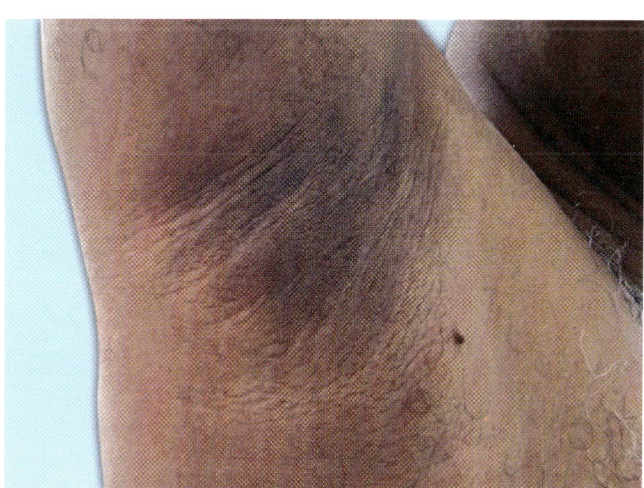

FIGURE 13: Clinical photograph showing acanthosis nigricans in the right axilla in a patient with lung cancer.

TABLE 1 Commonly encountered paraneoplastic cutaneous manifestations.

Most common associated malignancies	Paraneoplastic cutaneous manifestations
Intra-abdominal adenocarcinoma, lung carcinoma, and lymphoreticular malignancies	Acanthosis nigricans
Lung cancer	• Hypertrichosis lanuginose (sudden development of fine, downy, unpigmented hair on face, axillae, limbs, and trunk) • Erythema gyratum repens
Hodgkin's lymphoma	Acquired ichthyosis
Squamous cell carcinoma of upper aerodigestive tract	Acrokeratosis paraneoplastica (Bazex syndrome)
Glucagonoma	Necrolytic migratory erythema
Leukemia, lymphoma, and multiple myeloma	Sweet's syndrome and pyoderma gangrenosum, especially bullous variant
Gastrointestinal carcinomas	Muir–Torre syndrome (sebaceous tumors including adenomas, adenocarcinomas, and epitheliomas)
Intra-abdominal adenocarcinoma	Sign of Leser–Trélat (sudden appearance of multiple seborrheic keratoses or a sudden increase in size of previous seborrheic keratosis

RECOMMENDED READINGS

1. Stollery N. Skin signs associated with systemic disease. Practitioner. 2011;255:32-3.
2. Cahill J, Sinclair R. Cutaneous manifestations of systemic disease. Aust Fam Physician. 2005;34:335-40.
3. Lee A. Skin manifestations of systemic disease. Aust Fam Physician. 2009;38:498-505.
4. Sontheimer RD. Skin manifestations of systemic autoimmune connective tissue disease: diagnostics and therapeutics. Best Pract Res Clin Rheumatol. 2004;18:429-62.
5. Robson KJ, Piette WW. Cutaneous manifestations of systemic diseases. Med Clin North Am. 1998;82:1359-79, vi-vii.
6. Ostezan LB, Callen JP. Cutaneous manifestations of selected rheumatologic diseases. Am Fam Physician. 1996;53:1625-36.
7. Hansen RC. Dermatologic manifestations of rheumatic diseases. Adolesc Med. 1998;9:85-100, vi.
8. Van Hecke E. Cutaneous manifestations of internal diseases. Acta Clin Belg. 2003;58:302-7.
9. Abu-Hilal M, Krotva J, Chichierchio L, Obeidat N, Madanat M. Dermatologic aspects and cutaneous manifestations of sarcoidosis. G Ital Dermatol Venereol. 2010;145:733-45.
10. Daneshgaran G, Dubin DP, Gould DJ. Cutaneous manifestations of COVID-19: An evidence-based review. Am J Clin Dermatol. 2020;21:627-39.

CHAPTER 14

Psychiatric Disorders in Clinical Medicine

Rajesh Sagar, Ragul Ganesh

ABSTRACT

Psychiatry is the branch of medicine dealing with diagnosis and management of disorders with abnormal mental function. Mental, neurological, and substance misuse disorders are the leading cause of "years lost to disability" (YLDs). Assessment of patients with psychiatry disorders is distinct from medical disorders, with more emphasis on history taking and mental state examination. Biochemical and structural alterations in brain are found in various psychiatric disorders. Various treatment modalities are available for the management of psychiatric disorders including psychotropic medications, psychotherapy, and electroconvulsive therapy. Medical and psychiatric illnesses can influence each other. Psychiatric disorders can precipitate medical illness and medical conditions can lead to development of psychiatric illness. Physicians should be trained in the diagnosis and management of common psychiatric disorders at different settings.

"There is hope, even when your brain tells you there isn't"

— John Green

INTRODUCTION

Psychiatric disorders manifest with abnormal functioning in the areas of emotion, perception, thinking, and memory. Psychosomatic medicine or consultation liaison psychiatry deals with psychiatric disorders in patients with medical conditions. Psychiatrists worldwide use the diagnoses listed in the chapter "Mental and behavioral disorders" of International Classification of Diseases (ICD) published by World Health Organization (WHO). Mental, neurological, and substance misuse disorders are the leading cause of YLDs contributing to 28.5% of global YLDs. The prevalence of psychiatric disorders varies with the setting. In the clinical setting such as medical wards, delirium, and other organic disorders are common. In general population, depressive and anxiety disorders are most common.

CLINICAL EVALUATION

Psychiatric interview is the most essential part of assessment and management of patients with mental illness. It comprises clinical history, examination, and investigations, with more emphasis on taking history followed by detailed mental state examination.

PSYCHIATRIC INTERVIEW

Presenting complaints: The main problems for which help is requested. The patient's complaints should be in his or her own words.

History of present illness: This is a chronological description of the illness course from the onset of symptoms including nature, severity, and duration of the symptoms.

Past psychiatric history: The course of all psychiatric illnesses over the patient's lifetime, including the symptoms, severity, and frequency of the episodes should be assessed.

Treatment history: The details about the type of treatment including medications, psychological therapies, and other modalities should be reviewed.

Past medical history: The account of major medical conditions and past surgeries should be noted.

Family history: Many psychiatric illnesses have genetic predisposition. Family history should include psychiatric diagnoses, substance use disorders, and lethality history in family members. Medical illnesses in family history are important in management (e.g., choice of antipsychotic medication in patients with family history of diabetes mellitus).

Personal history: This includes childhood and developmental history, social history, sexual history, and occupational history. History of substance use and abuse should be carefully reviewed during psychiatric interview.

Mental status examination: The mental state examination involves systemic examination of thinking, emotion, and behavior of the patient with the aim to identify objective clinical signs.

Various components of mental status examination (MSE) include:

- *General appearance and behavior*: The appearance of the patient, state of the clothes and grooming, eye contact, and posture should be noted. Any abnormalities in psychomotor activity such as agitation or retardation should be assessed.
- *Speech*: Speech fluency, rate, tone, and volume should be observed. Abnormalities such as pressure of speech, dysarthria, and dysphasia should be assessed.
- *Mood*: Patients should be asked about how they feel (e.g., happy/sad/anxious). Patient's affect can be assessed by facial expression, posture, and movements.
- *Thoughts*: The content of thoughts should be assessed for ideas of self-harm, hopelessness, grandiose ideas etc. Abnormalities in the form of thinking such as loosening of association should be noted. Thought possession abnormalities including broadcasting of patient's thoughts to other people should be assessed.
- *Perception*: Hallucinations are sensory perceptions in the absence of external stimuli. Auditory hallucinations such as running commentary of the patient's own acts, thought echo are common in schizophrenia.
- *Cognitive function*: Patient's orientation can be briefly assessed by asking name, what building they are currently in, present date, month, and year. Attention can be assessed by asking the patient to subtract 7 from 100 and 7 from the answer and continue till they can do (serial 7s). Instruments such as Montreal Cognitive Assessment (MoCA) and Mini Mental State Examination (MMSE) are widely used for assessing cognitive functions.
- *Insight*: Patient's understanding about their symptoms and the need for treatment should be assessed.

ETIOLOGY

Psychiatric disorders result from interface between genetic, environmental, social, and psychological factors.

BIOLOGICAL FACTORS

Genetic factors: Genetic factors contribute to the etiology of many psychiatric disorders. Relative risk for first-degree relative to develop schizophrenia is higher than risk in general population. If both the parents have schizophrenia, the risk is 46% in children. Lifetime risk of unipolar disorder in first-degree relative of bipolar proband is 10–20%. Recurrence rate is 2–8% in siblings of autistic children. Various genes such as *NRG1, DTNBP1, COMT, DISC1,* and *G72* are implicated in the pathogenesis of psychiatric disorders. Mutations in presenilin 1 (chromosome 14) and amyloid precursor protein (chromosome 21) are responsible for Alzheimer's disorder.

Brain structure and function:

- Generalized atrophy of the cerebral cortex seen in Alzheimer's disease
- Ventricles are enlarged in schizophrenia.
- Increased anterior cingulate activity predicts good response to antidepressants and cognitive behavior therapy in depression.
- Hypoplasia of cerebellar vermis is seen in autism.
- Degenerative changes and small hemorrhages in structures surrounding the third ventricle and aqueduct are seen in Wernicke's encephalopathy.

Biochemical factors: Alternations in the level of neurotransmitters such as serotonin [5-hydroxytryptamine (5-HT)], dopamine, and norepinephrine are commonly found in psychiatric disorders. Studies have demonstrated increased dopamine level in striatum in schizophrenia and reduction in 5-HT receptor binding in amygdala in depression.

Neuropathology: Decrease in the volume of cerebral hemispheres with enlargement of lateral ventricles is noted in schizophrenia. White matter hyperintensities are seen in both unipolar and bipolar mood disorders. Hypoplasia of cerebellar vermis is noted in autism. Diffuse cortical atrophy is seen in Alzheimer's disorder. Disruptions in neuronal system have been observed in psychiatric disorders. Diffusion tensor imaging (DTI) has shown reduction in white matter density in psychiatric disorders. Resting state functional magnetic resonance imaging (fMRI) studies showed involvement of default mode, salience, and executive control networks in many psychiatric disorders.

PSYCHOSOCIAL FACTORS

Environmental factors: Most of the psychiatric disorders show association with emotional deprivation, childhood abuse, and other early childhood adversities.

Social factors: Lack of close relationship may act as a predisposing factor for psychiatric disorders, resulting in reduction in social support which precipitates further mental health issues.

RELATIONSHIP WITH MEDICAL ILLNESS

Medical illness and psychiatric disorder can influence each other. Psychiatric disorders can precipitate medical illness. Patients with anorexia nervosa can develop hypokalemia, which in turn can lead to arrhythmias. Medical illnesses such as recently diagnosed cancer can precipitate psychiatric disorder (e.g., depression). Certain medical conditions like hyperthyroidism can mimic psychiatric disorder (e.g., anxiety disorder). Medical disorders can limit the use of psychotropic medication (use of lithium in renal disorder). Medical conditions can develop as result of psychotropic medications (patients on antipsychotic medications can develop metabolic syndrome). Medical side effects can impact the compliance to psychiatric medications. Patients on antidepressants might stop the medication due to sexual side effects.

Studies have shown that 80% of schizophrenia patients have comorbid medical illnesses, however, 50% remain undiagnosed. Increased mortality rate in patients with schizophrenia might be related to diagnosis and treatment of medical condition. Most of the treatable psychiatric disorders such as depression remain underdetected in the primary care settings. Due to significant deficit in percentage of psychiatrists in India, primary care physicians should be sensitized regarding the management of psychiatric conditions like mild-to-moderate depression, somatoform disorder, and anxiety disorder in primary care settings.

PRINCIPLES OF MANAGEMENT

PHARMACOLOGICAL AGENTS

Pharmacological agents used in management of psychiatric disorders are listed in **Box 1**.

PSYCHOLOGICAL THERAPY

- Cognitive therapy
- Behavior therapy
- Psychodynamic psychotherapy
- Interpersonal psychotherapy
- Electroconvulsive therapy

BOX 1 Pharmacological agents used in management of psychiatric disorders.

Antipsychotics:
- Phenothiazines (aliphatic side chain): Chlorpromazine
- Phenothiazines (piperidine side chain): Thioridazine and pipothiazine
- Phenothiazines (piperazine side chain): Trifluoperazine and fluphenazine
- Butyrophenones: Haloperidol
- Thioxanthenes: Flupenthixol and zuclopenthixol
- Diphenylbutylpiperidines: Pimozide
- Dibenzodiazepines: Clozapine
- Benzoxasoles: Risperidone
- Thienobenzodiazepines: Olanzapine
- Dibenzothiazepines: Quetiapine
- Substituted benzamides: Sulpiride and amisulpride
- Arylpyperidylindole: Aripiprazole

Antidepressants:
- Tricyclic antidepressants: Amitriptyline, nortriptyline, imipramine, and clomipramine
- Selective serotonin reuptake inhibitors (SSRI): Sertraline, citalopram, escitalopram, fluoxetine, fluvoxamine, and paroxetine
- Serotonin and noradrenaline reuptake inhibitor (SNRI): Venlafaxine and duloxetine
- Noradrenaline and serotonin-specific antidepressant (NaSSa): Mirtazapine
- Noradrenaline reuptake inhibitor (NaRI): Reboxetine
- Serotonin antagonist and reuptake inhibitor (SARI): Trazodone
- Reversible inhibitor of monoamine oxidase type A: Moclobemide
- Melatonergic agonist: Agomelatine
- Norepinephrine-dopamine reuptake inhibitor (NDRI): Bupropion

Mood-stabilizing agents:
- Lithium
- Valproate
- Lamotrigine
- Carbamazepine
- Oxcarbazepine
- Topiramate

Others:
- Benzodiazepines
- Propranolol
- Trihexyphenidyl

COMMON PSYCHIATRIC DISORDERS

The ICD-10 listing of psychiatric disorders is shown in **Box 2**.

DEMENTIA

Clinical syndrome defined as progressive, nonreversible, global impairment of cognitive function. It is characterized by impairment in previously acquired intellectual function, affecting 5% of population above 65 years. Based on the clinical features, it can be divided into "cortical" and "subcortical" types. It is essential to obtain history from both the patient and a family member living along with the patient. Clinical features include impairment in memory, apraxia, visuospatial impairment, and anosognosia. Usual psychiatric presentations are disturbance of personality, depression, and aggression.

Alzheimer's disease is the most common subtype of dementia. The prevalence of disease increases with age and uncommon before 45 years. It comprises of two main groups—(1) early onset and (2) later-onset groups. Apolipoprotein E4 inheritance is associated with

BOX 2	ICD-10—Chapter V (F00–F99) Mental and behavioral disorders.

- F00–F09: Organic mental disorders
- F10–F19: Disorders due to psychoactive substances: Alcohol, opioids, cannabinoids etc.
- F20–F29: Schizophrenia and delusional disorders
- F30–F39: Mood (affective) disorders
- F40–F48: Neurotic, stress-related and somatoform disorders
- F50–F59: Behavioral syndromes associated with physiological disturbances
- F60–F69: Disorders of adult personality and behavior
- F70–F79: Mental retardation
- F80–F89: Disorders of psychological development
- F90–F98: Behavioral and emotional disorders of childhood

an increased risk of Alzheimer's disease. The disease is characterized by atrophic changes, senile plagues, and neurofibrillary tangles in cerebral cortex. Impairment in cholinergic transmission and abnormalities of noradrenaline, serotonin, and glutamate has been demonstrated. Anticholinesterases such as donepezil, rivastigmine, and galantamine are used for slowing the progression of cognitive impairment. N-methyl-D-aspartate (NMDA) receptor antagonist memantine is used to enhance memory.

Frontotemporal dementia characterized by abnormalities in behavior and language usually occurs before 60 years of age. It comprises of three clinical subtypes—(1) Behavioral variant frontotemporal dementia, (2) primary progressive aphasia, and (3) sematic dementia. Mutation in *MAPT* gene encoding microtubule-associated protein tau plays an important role in pathogenesis. It is characterized by abnormal accumulation of tau proteins (cytoplasmic inclusion bodies) in the brain.

Lewy body dementia is characterized by dementia with signs of Parkinson's disease. Mutation in *α-synuclein* gene results in neuronal accumulation of abnormal protein.

SUBSTANCE USE DISORDER

Alcohol: Various factors associated with alcohol use include social factors, genetic factors, and psychiatric disorders such as depression or anxiety. Harmful use of alcohol is associated with complications such as depression, alcoholic hallucinosis, alcoholic blackouts, delirium tremens, Wernicke's encephalopathy, and Korsakoff's syndrome. Alcohol misuse leads to social problems such as unemployment, financial difficulties, violence, and legal issues.

Alcohol withdrawal symptoms consist of restlessness, sweating, anxiety, agitation, hallucinations, seizures, and delirium tremens. Long-acting benzodiazepines are commonly used for management of alcohol withdrawal syndromes. High doses of thiamin are used for prevention of Wernicke-Korsakoff syndrome. Acamprosate and disulfiram are used to maintain abstinence in patient with alcohol use disorder.

Important medical consequences of alcohol use are listed in **Box 3**.

BOX 3	Medical consequences of alcohol use.

- **Hepatic:** Fatty liver, cirrhosis
- **Neurological:** Peripheral neuropathy, cerebellar degeneration
- **Gastrointestinal:** Mallory–Weiss syndrome, gastritis, pancreatitis, and malabsorption
- **Dermatological:** Palmar erythema and Dupuytren's contractures
- **Cardiovascular:** Hypertension, cardiomyopathy
- **Reproductive:** Fetal alcohol syndrome, infertility

Other substance use disorders: Sedatives such as benzodiazepines, opioids such as heroin, morphine and dihydrocodeine, stimulants such as amphetamines and cocaine, cannabis, solvents and hallucinogens such as lysergic acid diethylamide (LSD), psilocybin (magic mushrooms) are other commonly abused substances.

Diagnosis of dependence is usually made if three or more of strong desire to take substance; difficulties in controlling substance taking behavior, presence of physiological withdrawal state, tolerance, progressive neglect of alternative interests, and persisting with substance use despite harmful consequences are present during the previous year.

SCHIZOPHRENIA

Schizophrenia is characterized by distortions of thinking and perception, with insidious social withdrawal and inappropriate or blunted affect. Bleuler introduced the term schizophrenia. He considered associational disturbances of thought, affective disturbances, autism, and ambivalence as fundamental symptoms of schizophrenia. Schneider described first rank symptoms of schizophrenia: Auditory hallucinations, thought broadcast, thought insertion, controlled feelings, impulses or acts and delusional perception. Lifetime prevalence is about 1% in general population. It is equally prevalent in men and women; however, onset is earlier in men than in women. Genetic contribution is strong, with 50% concordance rate in monozygotic twins. Excessive dopaminergic activity is seen in schizophrenia. Other neurotransmitters implicated are serotonin, norepinephrine, and glutamate. Chronic schizophrenia presents with symptoms of flatted affect, apathy, avolition, social isolation, poverty of speech, and poor self-care. Other functional psychoses, depression, mania, and organic psychoses are the main differential diagnoses of schizophrenia. Antipsychotic agents are used effectively for the management of positive symptoms.

MOOD DISORDERS

Depression: Depressive disorder is a major cause of disability, with a prevalence of 5% in the general population. Variants in a large number of genes, emotional deprivation early in life, stressful life events, and medical illnesses are associated with onset of depression. Hypofunction of 5-HT and noradrenaline, elevated cortisol levels are demonstrated in depression. Low mood, loss of interest, and reduced energy leading to increased fatigability are common symptoms of depression. Other common symptoms are reduced attention, reduced self-esteem, unworthiness, pessimistic views of the future, ideas of self-harm, disturbed sleep, and diminished appetite. Investigations to rule out underlying medical disorder such hypothyroidism, vitamin deficiency, or Cushing's syndrome is required. Antidepressant drugs are effective in management of depression. The choice of antidepressant depends on the patient's preference, previous response, side effects, and potential drug interactions. Psychological treatments such as cognitive behavioral therapy and interpersonal therapy are also effective for mild to moderate depression.

Bipolar disorder: It is an episodic illness characterized by periods of depression and elevated mood. Manic episode is associated with expansive, elated or irritable mood, inflated self-esteem, decreased need for sleep, and increased activity, when mild or short lived, and it is referred to as hypomania. Bipolar disorder has strong heritability. Relatives of patients with bipolar disorder have increased risk of developing both unipolar and bipolar disorder. Diagnosis of bipolar disorder is made when there is at least one depressive episode present with at least one other hypomanic, manic, or mixed episode. Mood stabilizing agents such as lithium, sodium valproate, carbamazepine, and lamotrigine are used for the management of acute episode and prevention of recurrent episodes. Antipsychotics such as olanzapine, quetiapine, and risperidone are also used for management of bipolar disorder.

NEUROTIC, STRESS-RELATED, AND SOMATOFORM DISORDERS

- *Anxiety disorders*: Anxiety disorders include panic disorder, agoraphobia, specific phobia, social anxiety and generalized anxiety disorder.
- *Panic disorder*: Patients have recurrent episodes of severe anxiety characterized by sudden onset of palpitations, sweating, chest pain, choking sensations, and dizziness. The attacks are unpredictable and not restricted to any particular situation. It must be differentiated from numerous medical conditions (**Box 4**).
- *Agoraphobia*: Anxiety about the places from which it might be difficult to escape. Anxiety occurs mainly in situations such as crowds, public places, travelling away from home, and travelling alone.
- *Specific phobia*: Phobias restricted to highly specific situations, e.g., acrophobia, examination phobia, and animal phobias
- *Generalized anxiety disorder*: Anxiety is generalized, persistent, free floating, in any particular environmental circumstances. Somatic symptoms such as muscular tension, trembling, palpitations, and epigastric discomfort are commonly present.

BOX 4 Differential diagnosis for panic disorder.

- **Cardiovascular:**
  - Anemia, angina, hypertension, mitral valve prolapse, and myocardial infarction
- **Respiratory:**
  - Asthma, hyperventilation, and pulmonary embolus
- **Neurological:**
  - Epilepsy, Huntington's disease, migraine, multiple sclerosis, and transient ischemic attack
- **Endocrine:**
  - Addison's disease, carcinoid syndrome, Cushing's syndrome, diabetes, hyperthyroidism, hypoglycemia, hypoparathyroidism, menopausal disorders, and pheochromocytoma
- **Drug induced:**
  - *Intoxication*: Amphetamine, cocaine, hallucinogens, and nicotine
  - *Withdrawal*: Alcohol, antihypertensives, opiates and opioids sedative-hypnotics
- **Other conditions:**
  - Anaphylaxis, B12 deficiency, systemic lupus erythematosus, temporal arteritis, and uremia

- *Obsessive-compulsive disorder*: It is characterized by "obsessions"—recurrent, unpleasant thoughts, images, or impulses that are resisted unsuccessfully, but recognized as one's own. They are usually anxiety provoking leading to "compulsions"—the acts performed to relieve anxiety. Thoughts of contamination and ritualistic hand-washing, obsession of doubts, and repeated checking are common examples.
- *Stress-related disorders*: A disorder which develops in response to stressful event such as major accident or serious medical illness.
- *Somatoform disorders*: Present with somatic symptoms, not explained by a medical condition.
  - Somatoform autonomic dysfunction
  - Persistent somatoform pain disorder
  - Chronic fatigue syndrome
  - Somatization disorder
  - Hypochondriacal disorder

EATING DISORDERS

- *Anorexia nervosa*: Disorder characterized by reduced body weight, body image distortion, deliberate measures of weight loss such as self-induced vomiting, excessive exercise, use of diuretics, and appetite suppressants. Clinical findings include amenorrhea, elevated growth hormone and cortisol levels, and Russell's sign—calloused skin over interphalangeal joints, lanugo hair and electrolyte disturbances: Hypokalemia, hypophosphatemia, and hypomagnesemia.
- *Bulimia nervosa*: Disorder characterized by episodes of overeating, preoccupation with control of body weight, and extreme measures to prevent increase in weight—self-induced vomiting, periods of starvation, and use of drugs to reduce weight.

BOX 5 Management of patient with depressive symptoms.

Diagnosis:
- Patient with diagnosis of depression

Assessment:
- Severity
- Risk of harm to self, suicidal ideations, and suicidal attempts
- Comorbid mental and substance use disorder
- Personality factors
- Current level of functioning

Physical examination:
- To examine for medical illness that can contribute to depression (thyroid swelling, nutritional deficiency, and Cushing's syndrome)
- Mental state examination

Investigation:
- Hemogram, liver function test, renal function test, and thyroid function test

Inpatient:
- Suicidality, catatonia, and comorbid general medical condition

Pharmacological management:
- Antidepressant based on treatment response, side effects, cost, comorbidity, and patient preference

Nonpharmacological management:
- Psychoeducation, cognitive behavioral therapy

Electroconvulsive therapy:
- Catatonia, suicidality, and past response to ECT

BOX 6 Management of patient with psychotic symptoms.

Diagnosis:
- Patient with diagnosis of schizophrenia

Assessment:
- Severity
- Risk of harm to self and others
- Comorbid mental and substance use disorder
- Level of functioning

Physical examination:
- Diabetes mellitus, hypertension, obesity, and metabolic syndrome (to decide regarding the choice of medication)
- Mental state examination

Investigation:
- Hemogram, liver function test, renal function test, lipid profile, and electrocardiogram (QTc)

Inpatient:
- Severe agitation, risk of violence, catatonia, and comorbid general medical condition

Pharmacological management:
- Antipsychotic based on treatment response, side effects, cost, and metabolic profile

Nonpharmacological management:
- Psychoeducation

Electroconvulsive therapy:
- Catatonia, past response to ECT, and augmentation

PSYCHIATRY AND LAW

Protection of children from sexual offences act 2012: The act was formed to protect children from the offences of sexual assault, sexual harassment, and pornography. The gender-neutral law takes cognizance of sexual crimes committed against both girls and boys under the age of 18 years.

Rights of persons with disability act (2016): The act was formed to ensure that the persons with disabilities enjoy their rights equally with others. It includes mental illness, intellectual disability, autism spectrum disorder, and specific learning disability.

Mental healthcare act (2017): Mental illness is defined as substantial disorder of thinking, mood, perception, orientation, or memory that grossly impairs judgment, behavior, capacity to recognize reality, or ability to meet the ordinary demands of life. Substance use included in definition of mental illness. The act allows patient with mental illness to decide, "how they wish to be cared and treated" and "the way they do not wish to be cared and treated" defined as advanced directives. The act decriminalized suicide attempts.

MANAGEMENT

Management plan in patients with psychiatric illness includes treatment setting, medications, and psychological treatments. Patients and caregivers must be included in treatment decisions (**Boxes 5** and **6**).

RECOMMENDED READINGS

1. American Psychiatric Association. (2013). Diagnostic and statistical manual of mental disorders (DSM-5®). [online] Available from https://www.appi.org/diagnostic_and_statistical_manual_of_mental_disorders_dsm-5_fifth_edition.
2. Ambekar A, Agrawal A, Rao R, Mishra AK, Khandelwal SK, Chadda RK. Magnitude of substance use in India. New Delhi: Ministry of Social Justice and Empowerment, Government of India; 2019.
3. Gautam S, Jain A, Gautam M, Vahia VN, Grover S. Clinical practice guidelines for the management of depression. Indian J Psychiatry. 2017;59(Suppl 1): S34-S50.
4. Gururaj G, Varghese M, Benegal V, Rao GN, Pathak K, Singh LK, et al. National mental health survey of India, 2015-16: Summary. Bengaluru: National Institute of Mental Health and Neurosciences; 2016.
5. Grover S, Chakrabarti S, Kulhara P, Avasthi A. Clinical practice guidelines for management of schizophrenia. Indian J Psychiatry. 2017;59(Suppl 1):S19-S33.
6. Pattanayak RD, Sagar R. Depressive disorders in Indian context: A review and clinical update for physicians. J Assoc Physicians India. 2014;62:827-32.
7. Janardhan Reddy YC, Sundar AS, Narayanaswamy JC, Math SB. Clinical practice guidelines for obsessive-compulsive disorder. Indian J Psychiatry. 2017;59 (Suppl 1):S74-S90.

8. Sadock BJ, Sadock VA, Ruiz P. Kaplan and Sadock's comprehensive textbook of psychiatry. US: Wolters Kluwer Health; 2017.
9. Sagar R, Dandona R, Gururaj G, Dhaliwal RS, Singh A, Ferrari A, et al. The burden of mental disorders across the states of India: the Global Burden of Disease Study 1990-2017. Lancet Psychiatry. 2020;7(2):148-61.
10. Stahl SM, Stahl SM. Stahl's essential psychopharmacology: Neuroscientific basis and practical applications. England: Cambridge University Press; 2013.
11. Taylor DM, Barnes TR, Young AH. The Maudsley prescribing guidelines in psychiatry. United States: John Wiley and Sons; 2018.
12. World Health Organization. (1992). International statistical classification of diseases and related health problems: 10th revision (ICD-10). [online] Available from http://www. who. int/classifications/apps/icd/ icd.

CHAPTER

15

Chest X-ray Evaluation and Some Spotters

Chandan J Das, Zohra Ahmad

ABSTRACT

Chest radiograph or commonly called chest X-ray (CXR) is often the first radiological investigation performed in many clinical as well as preoperative situations. A fair knowledge of reading the CXR is very important in making a clinical diagnosis. This is a simple radiological investigation which can be interpreted at the level of clinician. With the introduction of digital technique, quality of the CXR is excellent most of the time. The CXR should be interpreted in a sequential manner so that most of the findings can be picked up without missing major points.

A CXR is an important tool in the armamentarium of the clinician. It provides a variety of information on both local as well as systemic disease process. Interpretation of a chest radiograph is a skill developed by systematic evaluation and interpreting the findings in light of the clinical findings. A radiologist and a clinician may adopt a different approach to interpret the chest radiograph but with methodical analysis with evaluation of core as well as hidden areas is mandatory.

"Great discoveries are made accidentally less often, than the populace likes to think"

—William Cecil Dampier

INTRODUCTION

A systematic approach to evaluation should start with patient identification and labeling, projection, and quality checking. Every physician has their own method of evaluating films. Although there is no such hard and fast rule to read a CXR, some people use the mnemonic "A, B, C, D, E, F, G, H, I" (where A = airway, B = bone, C = cardiac silhouette, D = diaphragm, E = edge of the heart, F = field of lung, G = gastric bubble, H = hilum of lung to do that).

SYSTEMATIC EVALUATION: RULE OF 10

We would like to present here a simple rule of 10 (**Fig. 1**) which can be an easy and effective way to evaluate the CXR in a sequential manner. The "rule of 10" should begin with evaluation of soft tissue shadows. All points mentioned in the rule of 10 need to be compared with the opposite side. These points are presented in such a manner that the structures evaluated are contiguous with each other for the sake of remembrance. These points are:

- Soft tissues including breast shadows

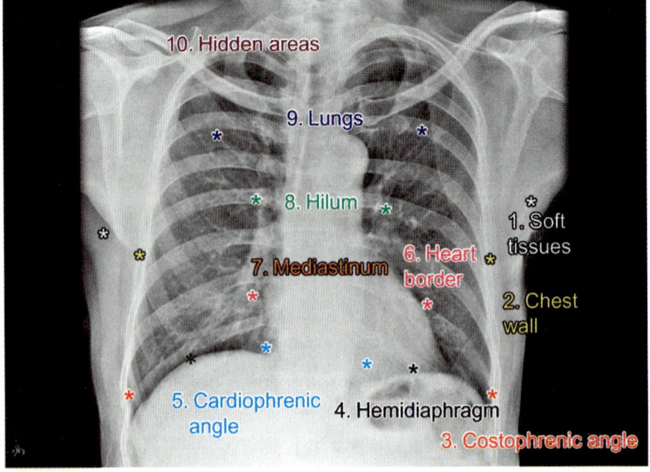

FIGURE 1: 10-point rule.

- Chest wall
- Costophrenic angle
- Hemidiaphragm
- Cardiophrenic angle

- Heart border
- Mediastinal shadow
- Hilum
- Lung fields
- *Four quadrants*: Hidden areas

STEP BY STEP EVALUATION

PATIENT IDENTIFICATION

The first step in evaluating the radiograph is to make sure that it belongs to the patient being examined. Radiograph carries the patient's name and date of the examination in a corner/below and needs to be checked. Side marker (L or R) is important information on the film. In the event of it not corresponding with the heart shadow, the label should be double checked before calling it dextrocardia (**Fig. 2**). The importance of date on a chest radiograph cannot be over emphasized. This investigation is often repeated and serial or comparative evaluation of the radiographs is a very useful tool in the radiologist's/clinician's tool kit.

PROJECTION

Posteroanterior (PA) is the projection commonly used, as this does not produce as much radiographic magnification of the heart and mediastinum as an anteroposterior (AP) projection. A PA film is taken with the film cassette placed in front of the patient while the beam is delivered from behind with the patient in an upright position. In a PA view of the scapulae are away from the lung fields with angulated clavicle. However, films taken in intensive care units or when the patient is unable to stand upright are AP projection. An AP film is also sometimes used to evaluate the ribs for fractures. There is apparent cardiac enlargement in an AP view.

A lateral CXR is sometimes utilized to localize lesions and lung lobes and to locate lesions hidden behind the heart or in the posterior recesses of the lungs. A left lateral (with the left side of the chest against the film and the beam projected from the right) is the standard projection. However, to localize a lesion specifically in the right lung, a right lateral projection may be used. Expiratory films are used to assess air trapping in bronchial obstruction such as a foreign body or to visualize a small pneumothorax. It may be noted that expiratory films would cause spurious enlargement of the heart and this should always be accounted for while interpreting the radiograph.

QUALITY OF FILM

Penetration and rotation: The thoracic vertebral bodies should just be visible through the cardiac silhouette. The medial aspect of the clavicles should be symmetrically positioned on either side of the vertebral spinous processes.

Inspiration: Ideally, the CXR is taken toward the end of inspiration (by asking the patient to take a deep breath in and hold). A good inspiratory film should have the anterior end of the fifth or sixth rib meeting the middle of the diaphragm. More than six anterior ribs show hyperinflation, and fewer than five indicate an expiratory film (underinflated). The diaphragm should lie at the level of the sixth rib anteriorly. A poor inspiratory effort results in magnification of the mediastinal structures. A good inspiration and optimal positioning may be difficult in small children and elderly patients, but all effort should be obtained to obtain a good quality film.

After checking these technical details of the radiograph, the next step is to look for pathology in the CXR as discussed here.

SOFT TISSUES AND BONES OF CHEST WALL

A chest radiograph is not only about the lungs and heart. There is a lot of information available in the bones and soft tissues. This is an area which is frequently overlooked! The soft tissues of the neck and chest wall are examined, particularly for surgical emphysema, abnormal density/calcification. Cervicothoracic lesions like thyroid mass with mediastinal extension may be appreciated on radiograph as mediastinal mass with its margins becoming indistinct above level of clavicles and merging with cervical neck tissues (**Fig. 3**). The breast shadows should always be

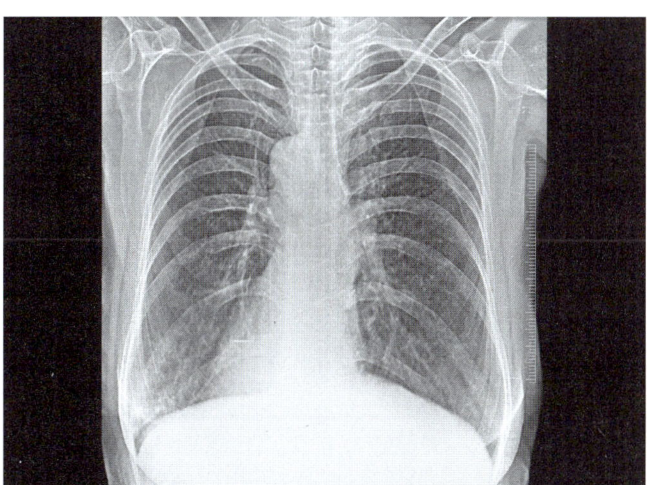

FIGURE 2: Dextrocardia. Cardiac apex and aortic knuckle are on the right side. Always double check side marker.

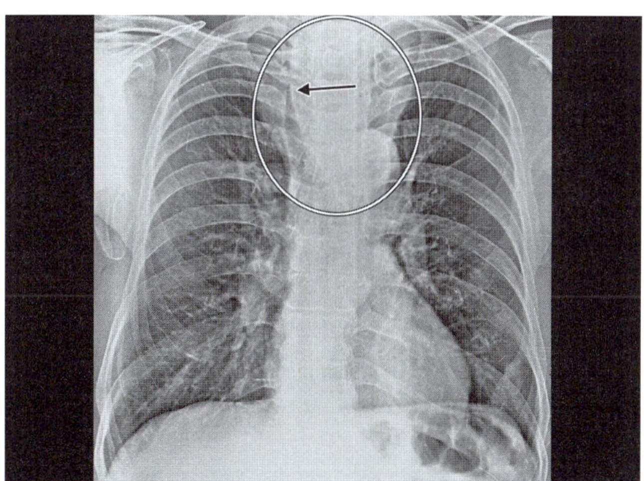

FIGURE 3: Thyroid mass with mediastinal extension. Superior mediastinal widening with mediastinal soft tissue opacity (encircled) extending above level of clavicles and merging with soft tissues of neck. There is also right side deviation of trachea (arrow).

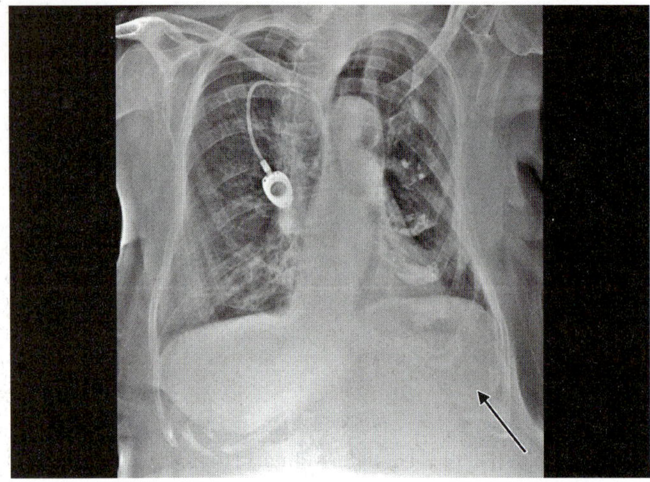

FIGURE 4: *Mastectomy*: Chest X-ray of an 80-year-old female reveals absent breast shadow on left side (arrow). Left lung appears darker or hyperlucent. Pacemaker also visualized in situ. Otherwise unremarkable radiograph.

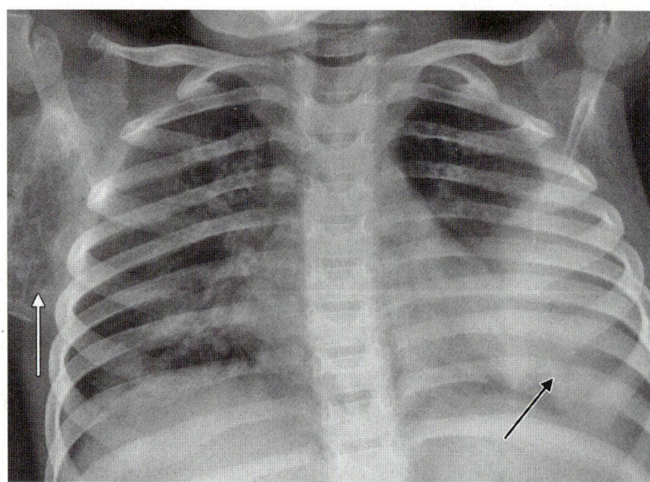

(CXR: chest X-ray; PNET: primitive neuroectodermal tumor)

FIGURE 6: *Scapula mass*: CXR of a 5-year-old child reveals moderate left pleural effusion (black arrow) with an aggressive neoplasm of right scapula (white arrow). This was a scapular PNET.

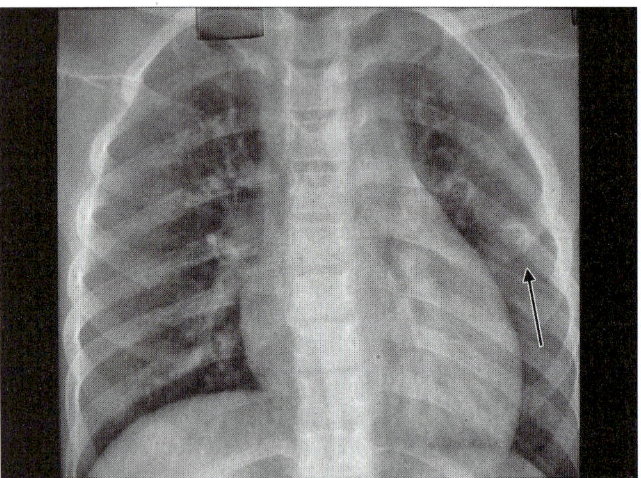

(CT: computed tomography; CXR: chest X-ray)

FIGURE 5: Rib osteochondroma. CXR of a 10-year-old child reveals well-defined focal lesion in left 3rd anterior rib (arrow) which was confirmed on CT (not shown) to be an exostosis.

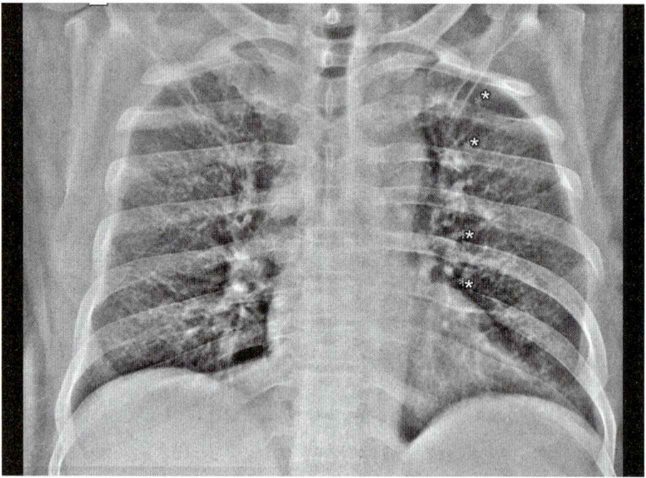

FIGURE 7: Rib fractures. Anteroposterior (AP) radiograph done in a trauma patient to evaluate ribs reveals fractures (*) in left posterior third, fourth, sixth, and seventh ribs.

examined for asymmetry of size, shape, and position. Many students have walked into a trap laid down by the examiner by failing to spot the missing breast shadow in a previously mastectomized patient. In addition to missing outline of the breast shadow, the lung field on the side of absent breast will appear a little darker than the other side (**Fig. 4**).

The ribs (**Fig. 5**), thoracic spine, clavicles, scapulae (**Fig. 6**), and humeri should be examined for fractures, focal lesions, metastatic deposits, and degenerative changes. The thoracic spine should be examined for alignment and abnormal curvature. The acromioclavicular and glenohumeral joint should also be checked for alignment and evidence of arthritis.

In trauma cases, ribs of each side should be traced individually in a systematic manner to rule out subtle factures. AP radiograph is better than PA at demonstrating rib fractures (**Fig. 7**).

COSTOPHRENIC ANGLES

The costophrenic angles are the meeting places of diaphragms and ribs. Each costophrenic angle can normally be seen on CXR as a sharply pointed, downward indentation between each hemidiaphragm and the adjacent chest wall. A small portion of each lung normally dips into the costophrenic angle. With pleural effusion (**Fig. 6**), fluid often builds up in the costophrenic angle (due to gravity). This can push the lung upward, resulting in blunting of costophrenic angle. The posterior angle is the deepest. The normal angle usually measures 30° and obtuse angulation is a sign of disease.

HEMIDIAPHRAGM

The diaphragmatic outline is clearly visible on a chest radiograph. It should be evaluated for shape, position, and sharpness of outline. Both costophrenic angles should be clear and sharp. The right hemidiaphragm is usually slightly higher than the left-up to 1.5 cm (**Fig. 1**). On the lateral film, the right hemidiaphragm is seen in its entirety but the anterior aspect of left hemidiaphragm merges with the heart and therefore not visualized. The diaphragmatic outline is obscured by pleural effusion, consolidation, or by lower lobe or cardiac lesion (**Fig. 8**).

CARDIOPHRENIC ANGLE

It is viewed on the radiographs as the angle formed by shadows of the diaphragm and the heart. Any altered appearance of cardiophrenic angle may be used to assess changes in the size and position of the heart. Mass in the lower lobe of lung or a giant esophageal diverticulum can obscure this angle. It may appear lucent due to overlying large bullae of lung. The common differentials for cardiophrenic angle masses include pleura, ventricular aneurysm (**Fig. 8**), pericardial cysts, foramina of Morgagni hernia, epicardial fat pad, and lymph node enlargement.

HEART AND MEDIASTINUM

The mediastinum contains structures between the lungs on either side and is divided into anterior, middle, and posterior compartments. The heart and mediastinal outline on radiograph are made up of a series of "bumps." The left atrium and right ventricle do not form heart borders. On the right side, from above downward is these are right brachiocephalic vessels, the ascending aorta and superior vena cava, the right atrium, and the inferior vena cava. Similarly, on the left side, these are the left brachiocephalic vessels, the aortic arch, the pulmonary trunk, the left atrial appendage, and left ventricle. The cardiac outline is examined identifying all the heart borders and the outline of the great vessels. A very important component of evaluation is to look at the outline of the aorta and the pulmonary artery. The size and shape of each of these structures may to be assessed with a view for enlargement of reduction in size. In case of unilateral lung collapse, the mediastinum is shifted to the collapsed side. Pleural effusion and pneumothorax push the mediastinum to the opposite side. Any mass in the mediastinum causes widening of the mediastinal outline (**Fig. 8**).

HILUM

The hila should be evaluated with respect to position, size, and density. In a normal individual, the left hilum is placed superior to the right hilum because the left main pulmonary artery passes over the left main bronchus while the right main pulmonary artery passes in front of the right main bronchus. The hila may be at the same level in about 5% individuals but an important rule to remember is that the left hilum should never be below the level of right hilum. About 99% of the hilar shadows are contributed by the pulmonary vessels, mainly the pulmonary artery and there is very minor contribution from fat, lymph vessels, and bronchial walls. The contour of a normal hilum is always smooth. Sometimes, an otherwise normal hilum may appear unduly prominent due to technical factors like rotation or scoliosis (**Fig. 9**). Tumors and enlarged lymph nodes can occur making the hila appear bulky (**Figs. 10** and **11**). It must be remembered that increased hilar density may be the only sign of a mass lying in front of, or behind the hilum.

LUNG FIELDS

The "lung shadows" are composed of the pulmonary arteries and veins. Apart from the pulmonary vessels, the lungs should appear black because they contain air. To assess the density variation, compare the rib interspaces on the right with those on the left and compare lung vascularity on either side. Compare the two sides—Is there any difference? Is the normal lung too lucent or too opaque? Unilateral hyperlucent lung or hyperinflation may be a finding noted in foreign body impacted in bronchus especially in pediatric setting. Hyperinflation is due to ball

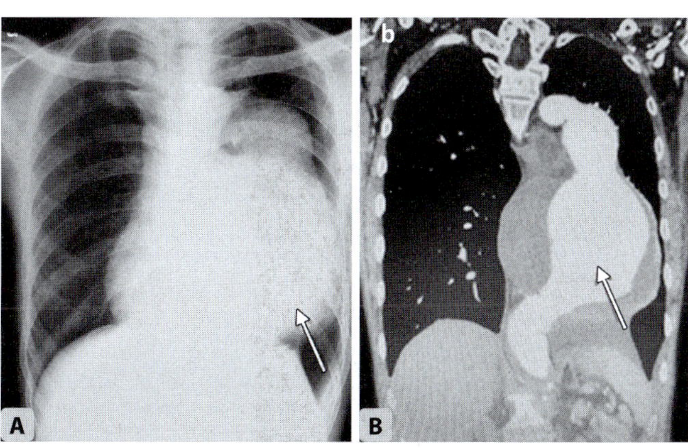

(CT: computed tomography; CXR: chest X-ray)

FIGURES 8 A & B: **(A)** CXR reveals widening of mediastinum with obscuration of left heart border and aortic outline. **(B)** CT angiography revealed a large partially thrombosed aneurysm of descending aorta.

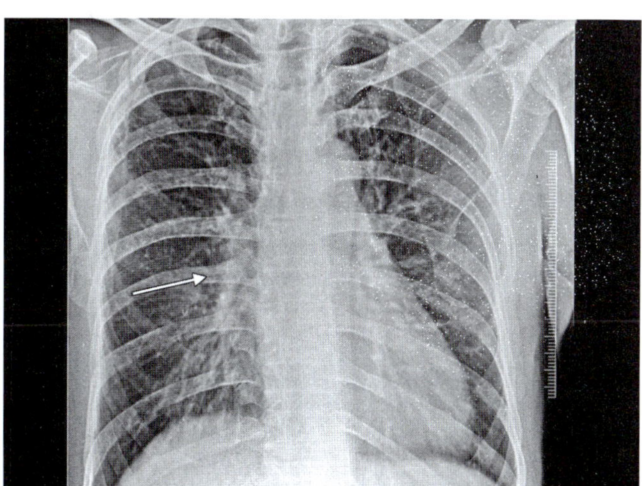

FIGURE 9: Prominent hilum due to rotation. Chest X-ray reveals unduly prominent right hilum due to leftward rotation (distance of medial left clavicle to spinous process is greater than distance of medial right clavicle to spinous process).

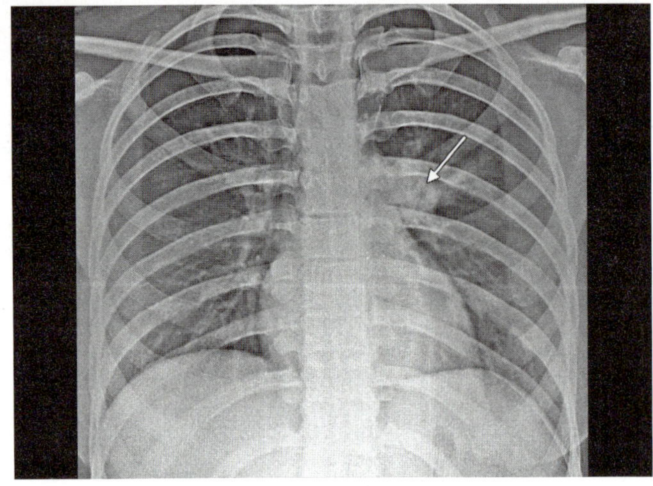

FIGURE 10: Left hilum is enlarged (arrow) with a rounded and convex contour. This is contrasted to right hilum which is concave.

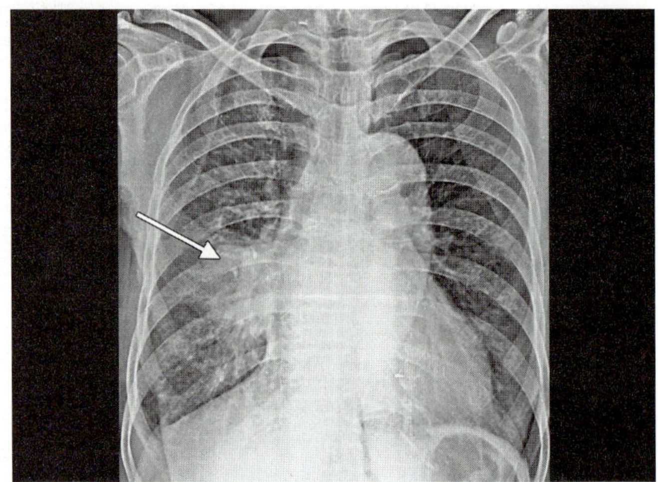

FIGURE 11: Right hilum is markedly enlarged with irregular outline. This was a hilar malignancy.

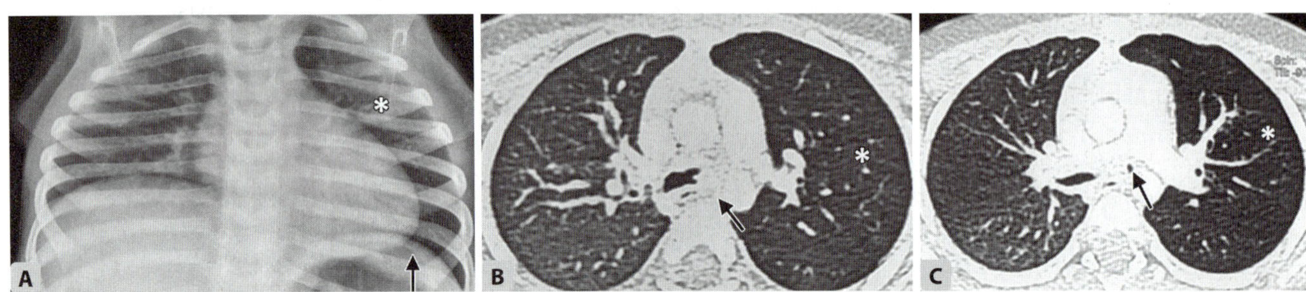

FIGURES 12 A to C: **(A)** Radiograph of a 2-year-old child with history of sudden onset breathlessness reveals left lung hyperinflation (*) and depressed left hemidiaphragm (arrow). **(B and C)** computed tomography (CT) scan showed narrowing of the left main bronchus (arrow) and hyperlucency of left lung (*) suggesting hyperinflation. On bronchoscopy, a peanut was extracted from the left bronchus.

valve phenomenon whereby air can enter the lung via the obstructed bronchus, however, cannot escape (**Fig. 12**).

It is helpful to divide the lungs into zones when describing abnormalities. The upper zone extends from the apex to the inferior border of the second rib anteriorly, the mid zone from the inferior border of the second rib to the inferior border of the fourth rib anteriorly, and the lower zone from the fourth anterior rib to the diaphragm.

Opacity is usually in the lung (e.g., collapse or consolidation; nodular shadows or linear shadows) or pleural space. Consolidation is visualized as fluffy air space opacity which may obscure or silhouette heart or diaphragmatic border. Air bronchograms may also be seen on radiograph in consolidated lung. Collapse is visualized as opacification of a particular lobe, with associated volume loss in form of rib crowding, mediastinal, or diaphragmatic shift to the same side. Predominantly reticular opacities are seen in interstitial lung disease (ILD) (**Fig. 13**). The abnormality is sometimes located in the chest wall (e.g., body wall edema).

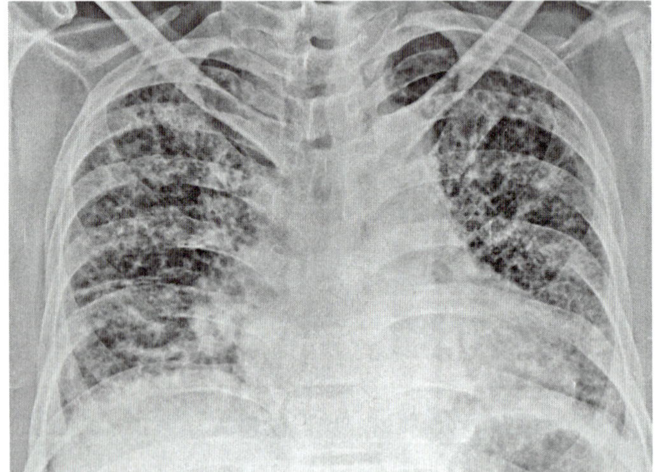

FIGURE 13: Interstitial lung disease. In an elderly patient, who presented with cough and breathing difficulty over a longtime frame, chest X-ray reveals underinflated lungs showing diffuse bilateral reticular opacities without any apicobasal or mediolateral gradient. These findings are in keeping with interstitial lung disease.

FOUR QUADRANTS—HIDDEN AREAS

These areas are sites where pathology is commonly missed and warranted a second look before any CXRs are reported as normal (**Fig. 14**):

- Below the diaphragm—particularly gas under diaphragm which is a sign of pneumoperitoneum, and upper abdomen for surgical clips/calcification/pneumoperitoneum (**Fig. 15**)

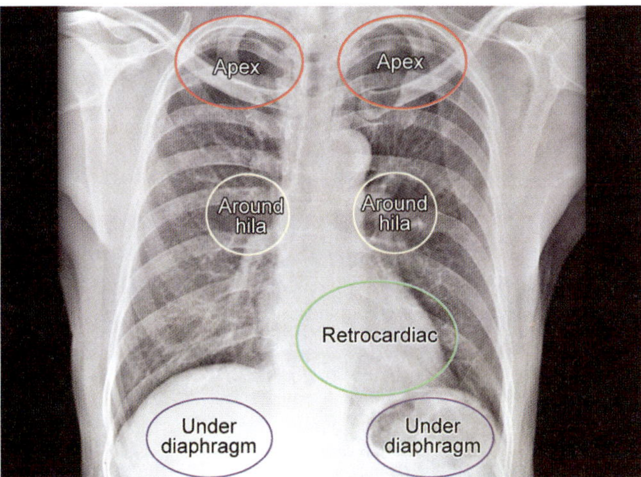

FIGURE 14: Hidden areas of radiograph must be given a second look.

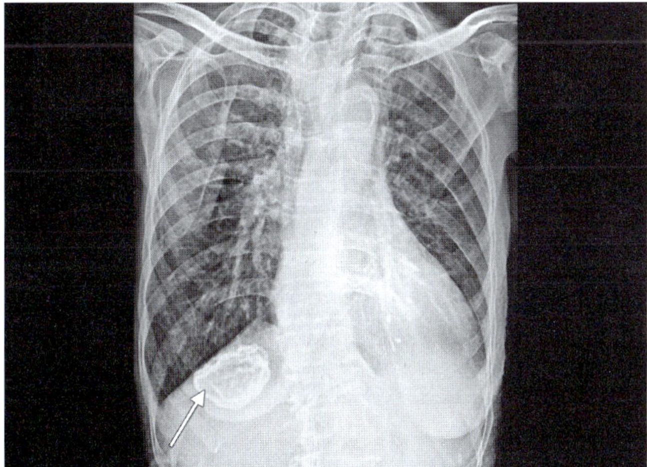

FIGURE 15: Chest X-ray (CXR) in an adult patient reveals hyperinflated lungs. The only abnormality is in right upper abdomen showing a well-defined calcified lesion which was confirmed to be a calcified hydatid.

- Behind the heart (hiatus hernia/lung nodule/left lower lobe collapse)
- Apices (pancoast tumor)
- Hila (assess position, size, and density)
  It is also important to assess thoracic spine and paraspinal lines (trauma), shoulder (dislocation), and clavicle (fracture, lung nodules behind medial end, and eroded lateral end in all radiographs).

PATHOLOGY

Having looked at the CXR, it remains to classify the signs into a radiographic pattern. Particular radiographic pattern has a list of diagnostic possibilities. At its simplest, a CXR abnormality can be classified into increased or decreased density. Patterns of increased density include nodules or masses, airspace opacification of consolidation, interstitial opacification, and pleural disease such as pleural effusion.

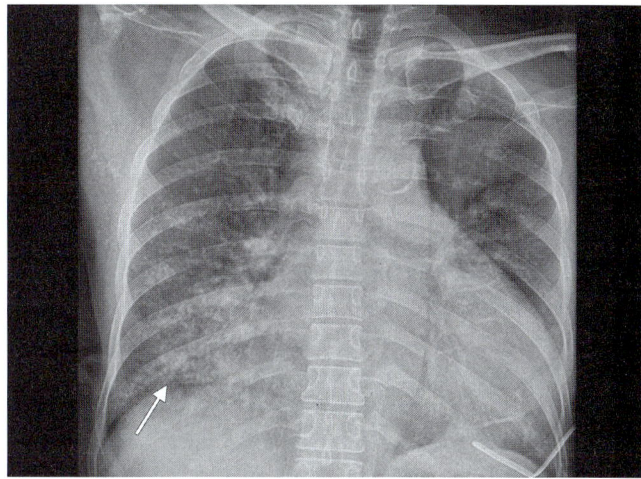

FIGURE 16: Right middle lobe pneumonia. Chest X-ray in an adult patient with fever and cough reveals air space opacification in right lower zone with obscuration of right heart border suggestive of right middle lobe pneumonia.

CONSOLIDATION

The consolidation represents a piece of sponge soaked in water or other fluid where the sponge represents the lung. When the fluid fills the airspaces, the spongy lung becomes dense (consolidated). The fluid could be water, blood, or pus (e.g., pneumonia). The volume of an affected segment is normally preserved. An important radiological sign that can help to detect and localize pulmonary abnormality is as a silhouette sign. The mediastinal silhouette is visible on a CXR because it is bordered by aerated lung. When consolidation (which is soft tissue density) abuts the mediastinal border that border may become obscured. For example, the right middle lobe is an anterior structure and lies adjacent to the right atrium. The only clue to pathology causing increased density in the right middle lobe (such as collapse or consolidation) may be obscuration of the right heart border. The right middle lobe has little contact with the diaphragm, so right middle lobe opacification does not result in obscuration of the right hemidiaphragm (**Fig. 16**). Right upper lobe consolidation may obscure right paratracheal stripe and is inferiorly outlined by minor fissure (**Fig. 17**). Similarly, obscuration of the left heart border usually indicates pathology in the lingular segment of the left upper lobe, which lies adjacent to the left ventricle. By contrast, pathologies causing increased density in a lower lobe results in loss of clarity of part or all of the relevant hemidiaphragm. Appearance of lung infections on radiographs is summarized in **Table 1**.

DIFFUSE LUNG OPACIFICATION

Diffuse opacification of lungs is commonly encountered finding in ICU patients. The differentials of this finding are generally acute respiratory distress syndrome, cardiogenic pulmonary edema, or widespread pneumonia. There may also be a combination of findings including pneumonia, collapse, and effusion.

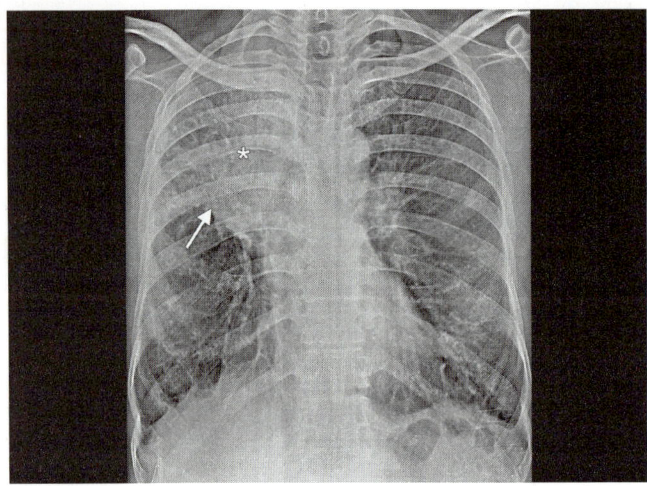

FIGURE 17: Right upper lobe consolidation. There is air space opacification (*) with air bronchograms of right upper zone with obscuration of right paratracheal stripe. The consolidation is outlined inferiorly by minor fissure (white arrow).

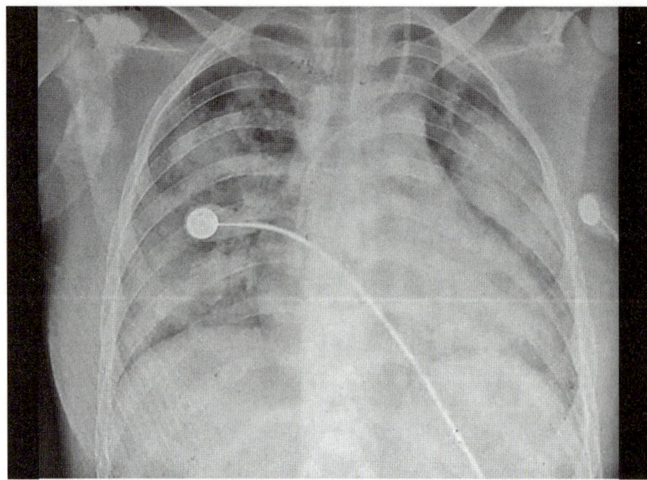

(ARDS: respiratory distress syndrome; CXR: chest X-ray; PA: posteroanterior)

FIGURE 18: ARDS. CXR reveals bilateral air space opacification involving all segments of lung. There is absence of pleural effusion. There is apparent cardiomegaly due to AP projection.

TABLE 1 Appearance of lung infections on radiographs.

Lobar pneumonia	Homogeneous opacification of part or whole of a single lobe
Bronchopneumonia	Widespread nodular opacities which may become coalescent
Aspiration pneumonia	Patchy consolidation in dependent lobes
Viral pneumonia	Multifocal GGO or consolidation, bronchial thickening
COVID-19	Bilateral multifocal, peripheral haziness, or consolidation
Pulmonary tuberculosis	
Primary	Focal consolidation in mid or upper zone with ipsilateral lymph node enlargement and pleural effusion
Postprimary	Consolidation ± cavitation in upper lobes or apical segments of lower lobes
Miliary TB	Bilateral tiny nodules scattered throughout lung

(GGO: ground-glass opacity; TB: tuberculosis)

Acute respiratory distress syndrome presents on radiographs as widespread bilateral air space opacification involving almost all areas of lung without any mediolateral gradient. Heart is normal sized and there is absence of pleural effusion (**Fig. 18**).

In contrast, cardiogenic pulmonary bilateral air space opacification (**Fig. 19**) which may initially have a perihilar or basal predominance. Cardiomegaly and bilateral pleural effusion are associated findings. Pneumonia reveals patchy consolidation with sparing of some areas with pleural effusion commonly associated with it.

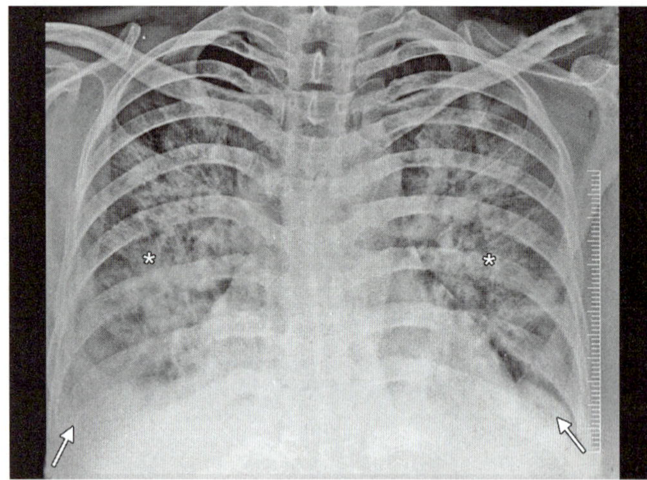

FIGURE 19: Congestive heart failure (CHF). chest X-ray reveals bilateral pleural effusion (arrow), cardiomegaly and bilateral perihilar consolidation (*) suggestive of cardiogenic pulmonary edema.

COLLAPSE

Collapse implies loss of volume and occurs for many reasons. The lung is dense but for a different reason—this time because all the air has been removed. Radiographically, collapse can be identified by opacification with signs of volume loss like fissural displacement (**Fig. 20**). In children, the cause is usually in the airway (intraluminal foreign body or mucous plug) (**Fig. 21**). Complete airway obstruction results in resorption of air in the affected lobe or segment. Collapse can also be due to extrinsic compression (e.g., a mediastinal mass) or pneumothorax.

NODULES AND MASSES

Solitary pulmonary nodules (SPN) are spherical radiographic opacities that measure up to 30 mm in diameter.

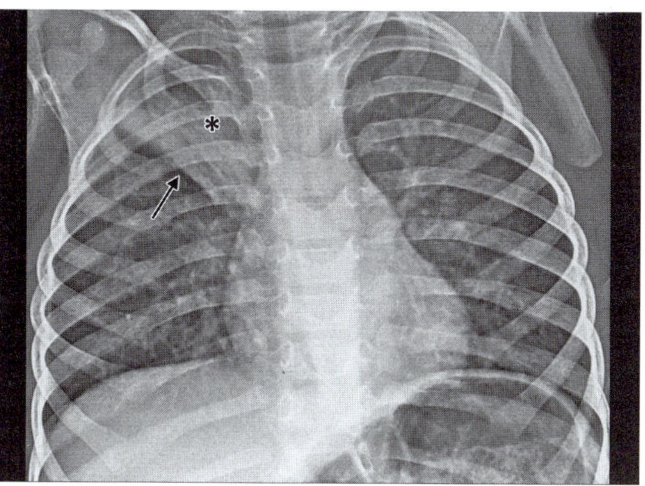

FIGURE 20: Right upper lobe collapse. Homogeneous opacification (*) of right upper zone with superior displacement of horizontal or minor fissure (arrow).

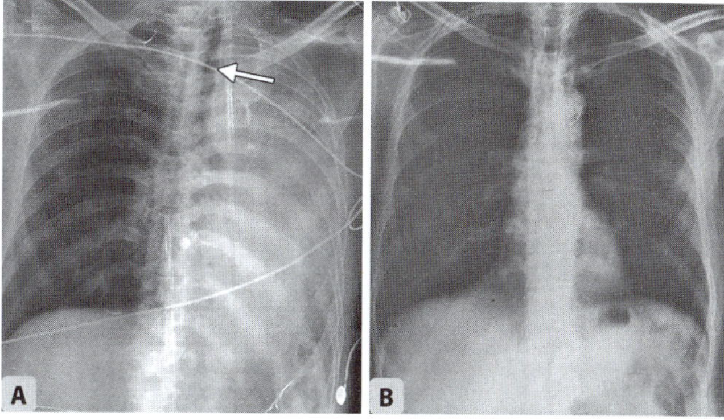

FIGURES 21 A & B: Postoperative collapse. **(A)** Chest X-ray reveals homogeneous opacification of left lung field with volume loss evidenced by ipsilateral tracheomediastinal shift. Left heart border is silhouetted. **(B)** Follow-up radiograph reveals complete resolution of collapse. The cause of collapse was a mucus plug which was removed bronchoscopically.

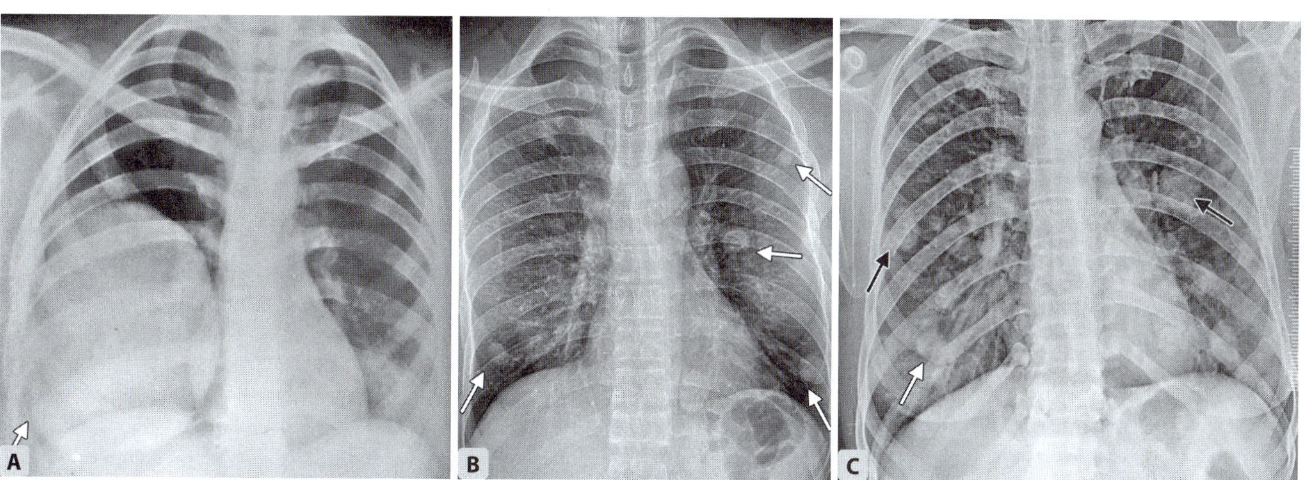

(CT: computed tomography; CXR: chest X-ray)

FIGURES 22 A to C: **(A)** Hydatid cyst. CXR reveals a large rounded mass in right mid and lower zone (arrow), which was confirmed on CT to be a pulmonary hydatid cyst. **(B)** Metastasis. CXR in an elderly patient reveals multiple well-defined nodules of varying sizes with middle and lower zone predominance suggestive of metastases. Primary malignancy was undiagnosed at the time of presentation. **(C)** Metastasis. CXR in a middle aged adult with a history of orchiectomy for germ cell tumor. CXR reveals multiple well-defined nodules of varying size in both lungs suggestive of pulmonary metastases.

Focal pulmonary lesions that are >30 mm in diameter are called lung masses and are presumed to represent bronchogenic carcinoma until proven otherwise. Most common causes of benign SPN are healed or nonspecific granulomas, tubercular, fungal, and hamartomas. Round pneumonia, round atelectasis, focal hemorrhage, hemangiomas, and arteriovenous malformations are less common causes. Most common causes of malignant SPN are primary malignancy (adenocarcinoma more than squamous), metastasis, and carcinoid. Most common cause of lung mass is lung carcinoma. Hydatid, metastasis, and carcinoid are other common causes of lung mass (**Fig. 22**). The mass can show cavitation or areas of calcification. The silhouette sign can also be apply to localize the mass in different lobes.

CAVITY

A cavity is defined as an air containing space within the lung surrounded by a complete wall of at least 1-mm thickness (**Fig. 23**). The wall can be smooth and regular (benign) and thick and irregular (malignancy). The common causes of cavity include abscess, tuberculosis (TB), malignancy, pneumatoceles, metastasis, and ruptured hydatid cyst. Some nodules like rheumatoid, Wegener's, and fungal can cavitate. Cavity can show a fluid level or intracavitary nodule. The spectrum of changes in tuberculosis are shown in **Figure 24 A** to **D**.

PLEURAL EFFUSION AND PNEUMOTHORAX

At least 300 mL of fluid must be present before upright chest films can pick up signs of pleural effusion (e.g., blunted

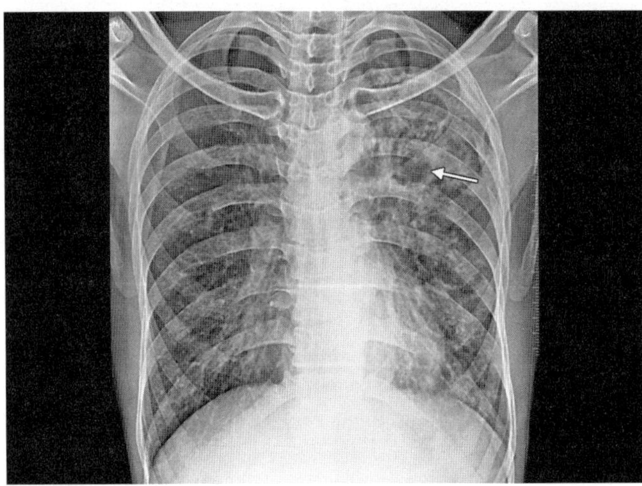

FIGURE 23: Chest X-ray (CXR) reveals a cavity (arrow) with surrounding patchy air space opacification in left upper zone.

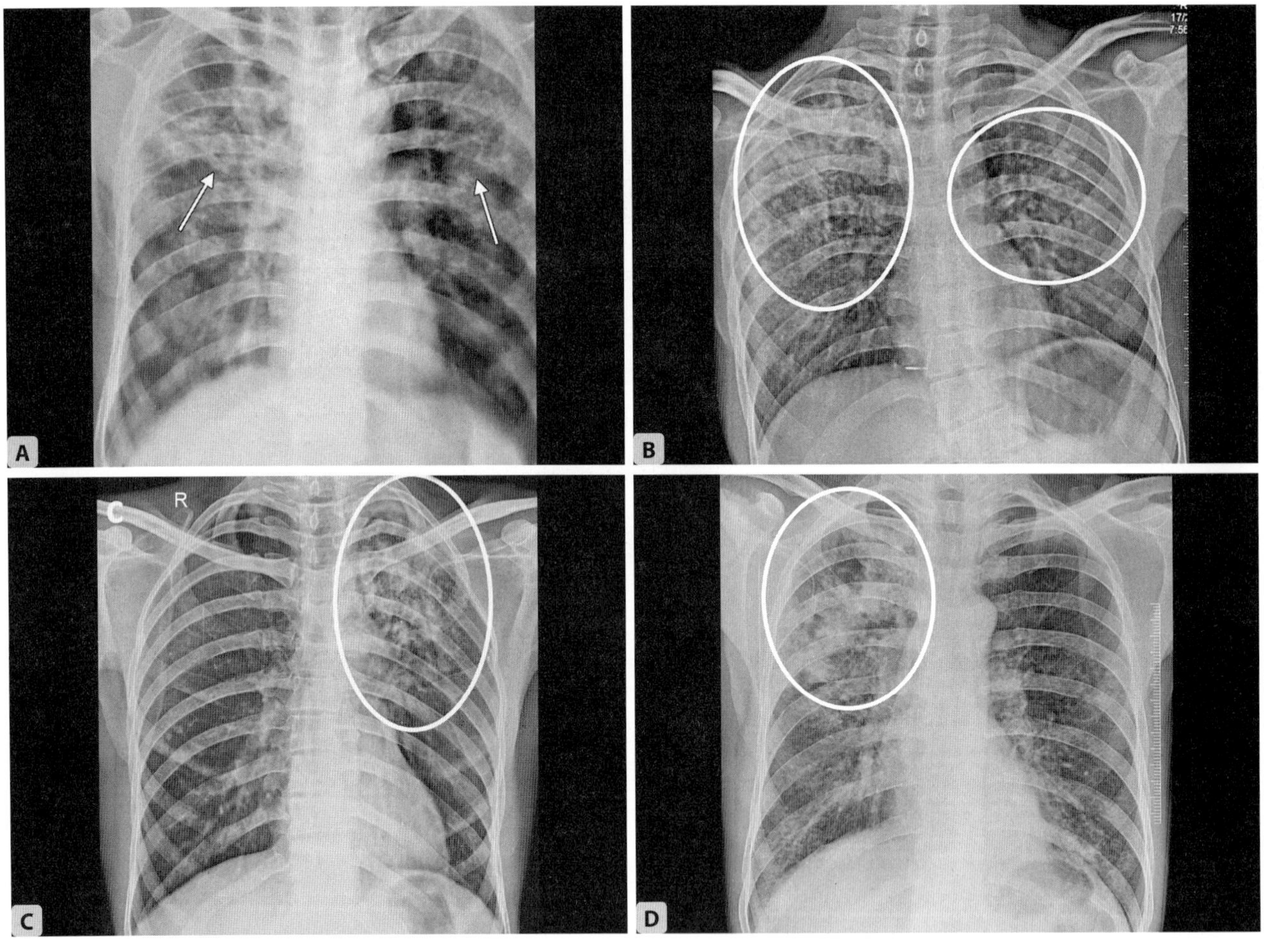

FIGURE 24 A to D: Tuberculosis. **(A)** Bilateral lungs reveal cavitation (arrow), interspersed with patchy consolidation and ill-defined nodules with upper lobe predominance. **(B)** Patchy nodular opacifiation noted in bilateral upper and mid zones (right > left). **(C)** Patchy nodules and consolidation in left upper zone with left hilar enlargement/adenopathy. **(D)** Patchy consolidation in right upper and mid zone.

costophrenic angles). Lateral decubitus position (with the patient lying on his side) is more sensitive, and can pick up as little as 50 mL of fluid. The fluid collection can be free or loculated (empyema) (**Fig. 25**). At times, fissural effusion may appear as a rounded opacity on radiograph and mimic a tumor (**Fig. 26**). Pneumothorax is visualized as absence of lung markings with a thin visceral pleural line visible at the medial edge of pneumothorax. It is sometimes difficult to detect and effort must be made to look for small amount of air and thin visceral pleural line in lung apices and along periphery of lung field (**Fig. 27**).

Hydropneumothorax is identified by the presence of air in pleural cavity along with an air-fluid level (**Fig. 28**). Tension pneumothorax is a medical emergency and is

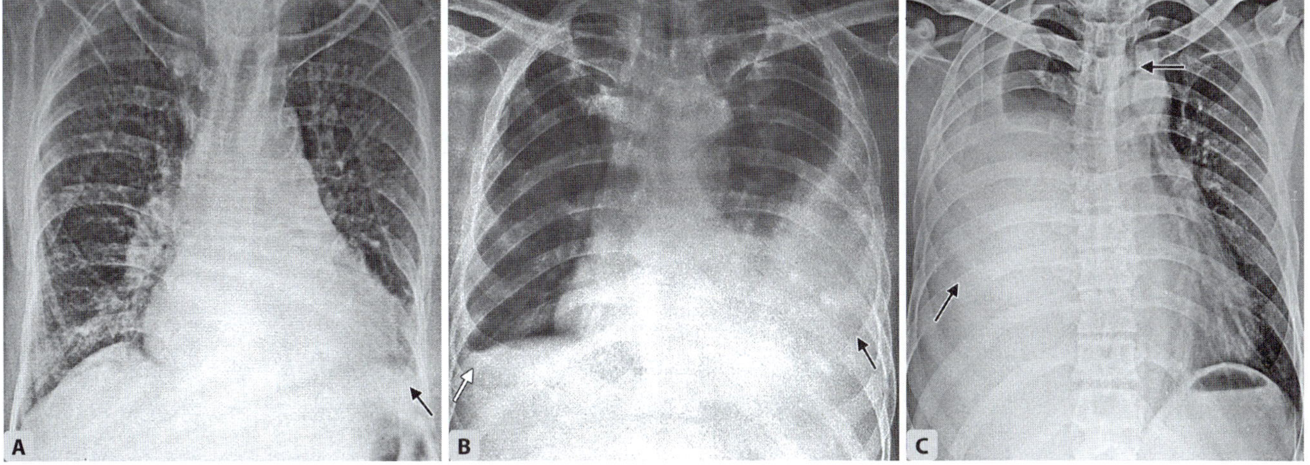

FIGURES 25 A to C: (A) Small left effusion; **(B)** moderate left effusion with fluid tracking along left lateral chest wall. There is blunting of right CP angle also with suggestion of small effusion. **(C)** Large right effusion with tracheomediastinal shift to left side.

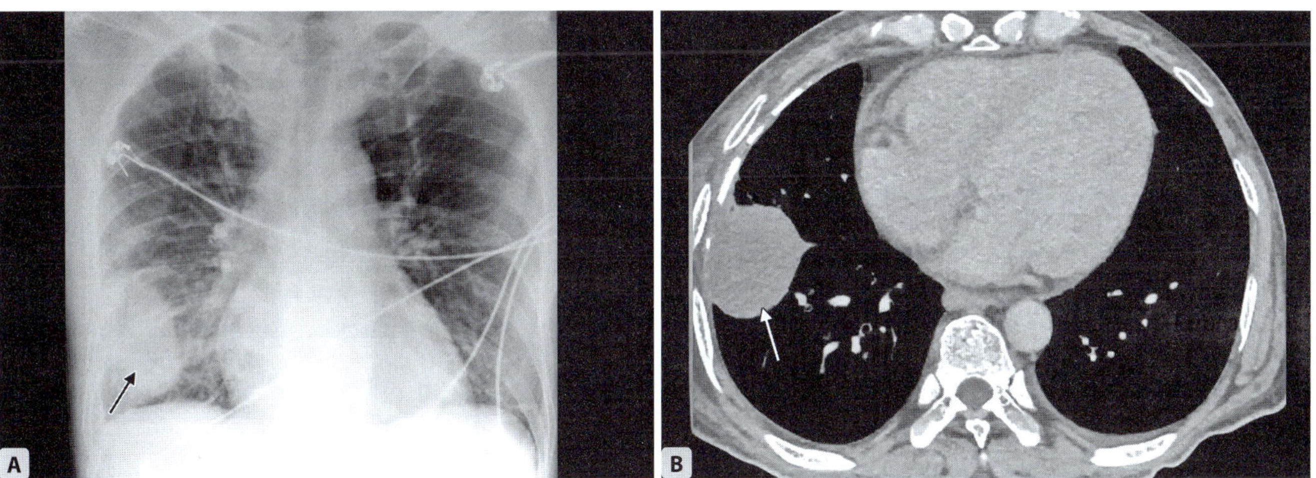

(CT: computed tomography)

FIGURES 26 A & B: (A) Rounded opacity in right lower zone (arrow), suspicious for mass. There is small right effusion. **(B)** CT confirms the opacity to be a loculated effusion in the fissure (arrow).

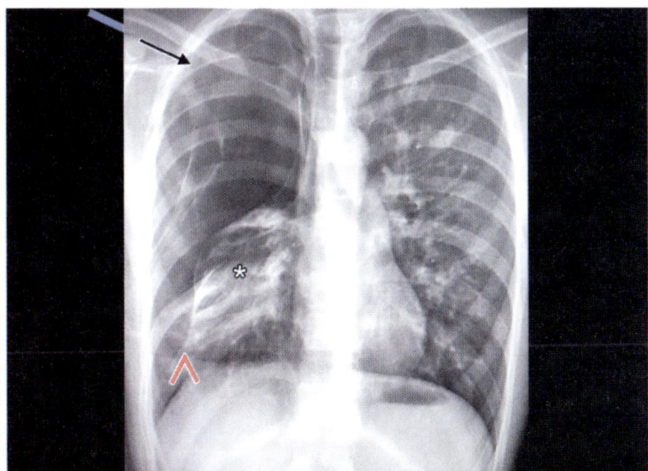

FIGURE 27: Pneumothorax. Chest X-ray reveals moderate pneumothorax in right pleural cavity (arrow) with collapsed lung (*) and visible visceral pleural line (arrowhead).

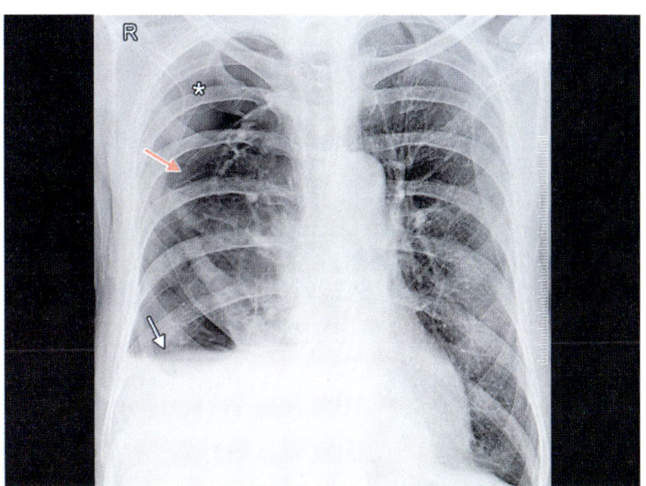

FIGURE 28: Hydropneumothorax. chest X-ray reveals free air in right pleural cavity (*). Visceral pleural line is seen at the lateral margin of the partially collapsed lung (red arrow). Air-fluid level noted (white arrow).

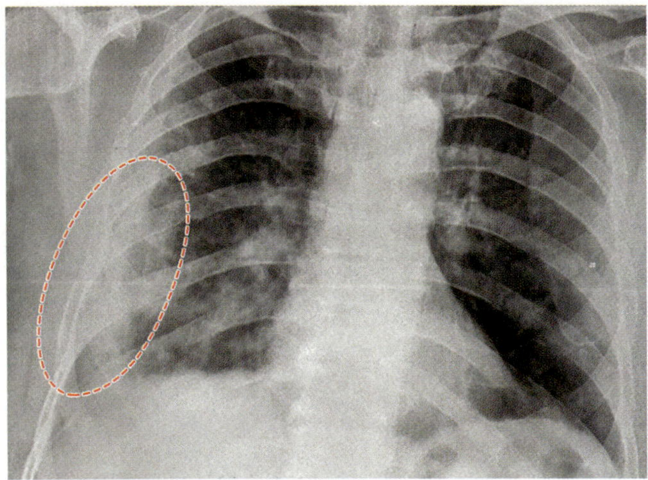

FIGURE 29: COVID-19 pneumonia. Portable Chest X-ray showing right mid and lower zone ground glass opacities (dotted red circle).

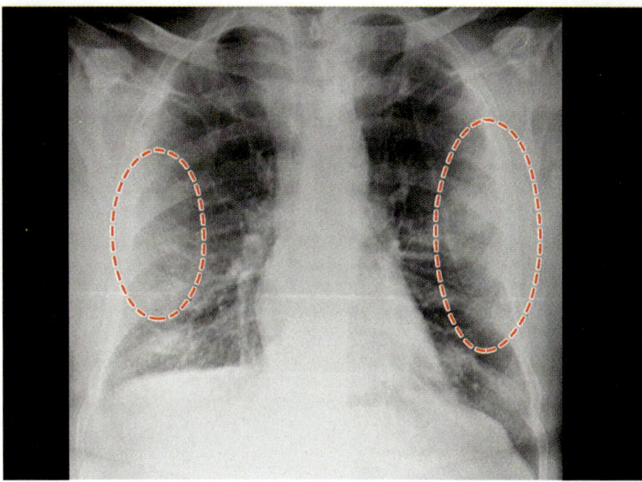

FIGURE 30: COVID-19 pneumonia. Portable chest X-ray showing bilateral mid and lower zone, peripheral, patchy consolidations, and ground glass opacities (red dotted circle).

identified on radiograph as pneumothorax with depression of ipsilateral hemidiaphragm and contralateral shift of mediastinum. Pneumothorax can be classified into small or large depending on whether its diameter (distance from visceral pleural line to chest wall) is less or more than 2 cm, respectively.

CARDIOMEGALY

Cardiomegaly is a medical condition where the heart is enlarged (Spotter 8) with dilatation of cardiac chambers, hypertrophy of cardiac walls, or due to pericardial effusion. The size of the heart can be estimated using the cardiothoracic ratio. Watch for rotation and adequate inspiration. The diaphragm should be lowered to at least the posterior position of the ninth rib. Calculate the ratio by first measuring the transverse cardiac diameter horizontally through the widest part of the cardiac silhouette. Divide this by the chest diameter measured at the widest part between the inner surfaces of the ribs. A ratio of 0.5–0.55 or less can be considered within the limits of normal for an adult. Ratios of up to 0.6 are normal in children and infants. Fluid accumulation in the pericardium causes distension, enlarging the cardiac silhouette, and overlapping and obscuring the hilar vessels. In congestive heart failure (CHF), the vessels become congested and appear more prominent than normal.

RADIOGRAPHY IN COVID-19 PNEUMONIA

Chest X-ray is often the initial investigation in suspected respiratory infection. In severe acute respiratory syndrome (SARS) coronavirus-2 (SARS-CoV-2) disease-2019 (COVID-19) pandemic, CXR has been very useful for follow-up and risk stratification of diagnosed patients. Positive radiography findings have included unifocal peripheral pneumonitis (**Fig. 29**) to bilateral patchy, peripheral and multifocal areas of haziness, or consolidation (**Fig. 30**). In late stages, the opacities may become more confluent with a "white out lung" when acute respiratory distress syndrome occurs. Pleural effusion, cavitation, and nodules are less commonly seen in this disease.

CONCLUSION

Chest X-ray is the primary basic investigation to for the evaluation of chest disorders. It is simple and cost-effective and can be safely repeated. The radiation dose in a CXR is very low (0.2 mSv). However, it should still be ordered judiciously to avoid unnecessary radiation to thyroid and breast. The findings need to be analyzed in the light of clinical information. To say the least, one needs a keen eye for its evaluation.

X-RAY SPOTTERS

The legends are not given here but are in the e-chapter. The reader can refer to the e-chapter for the actual diagnosis of these spotters. (Spotters are given in the next page)

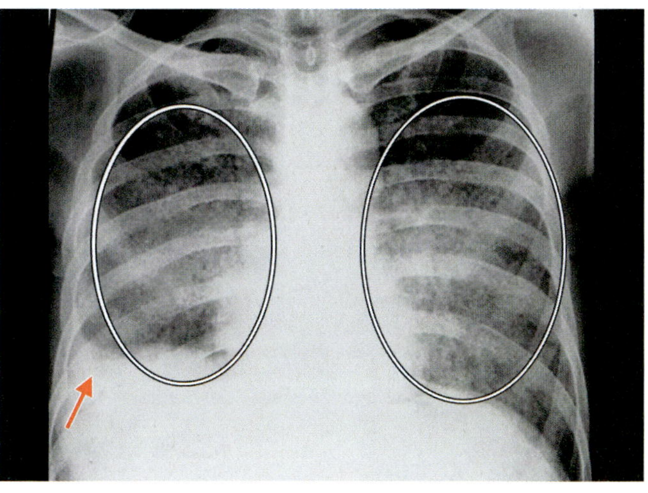

SPOTTER 1:

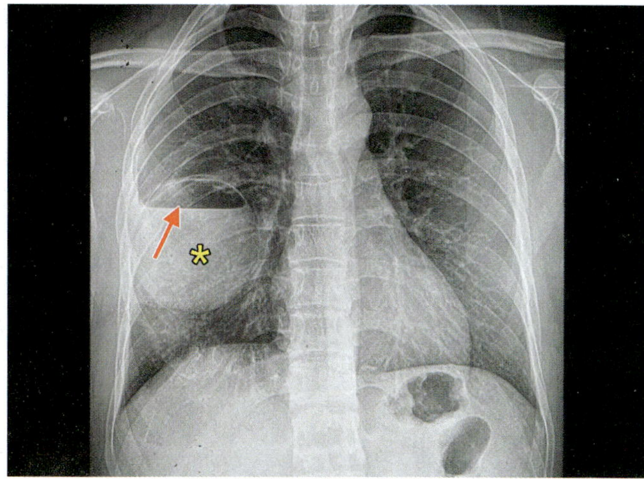

SPOTTER 2:

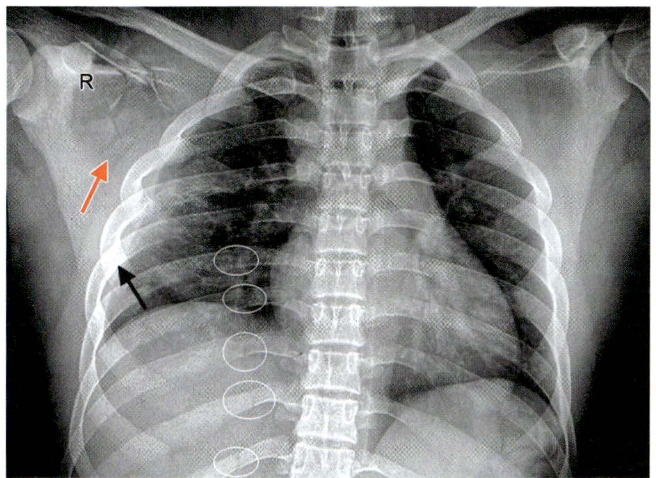

SPOTTER 3:

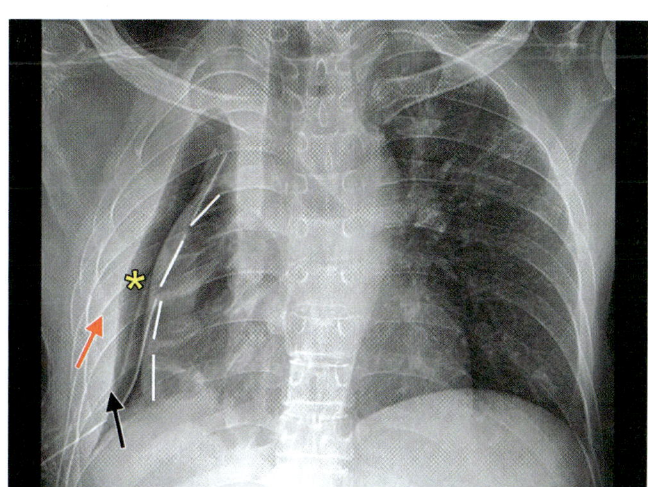

SPOTTER 4:

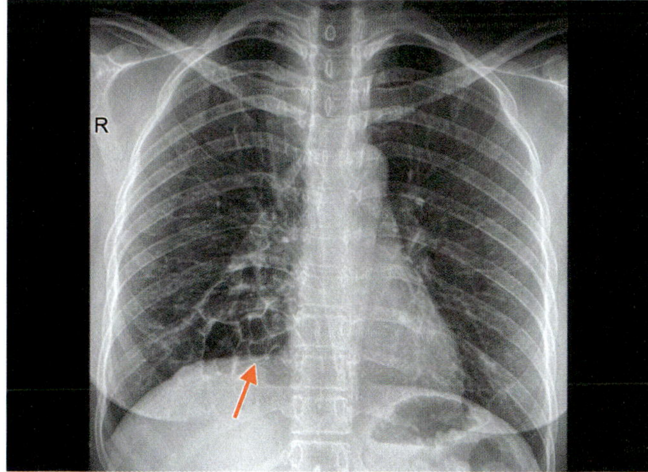

SPOTTER 5:

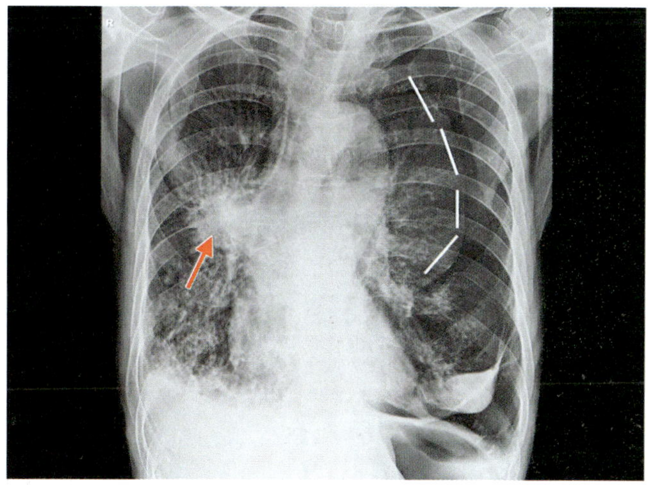

SPOTTER 6:

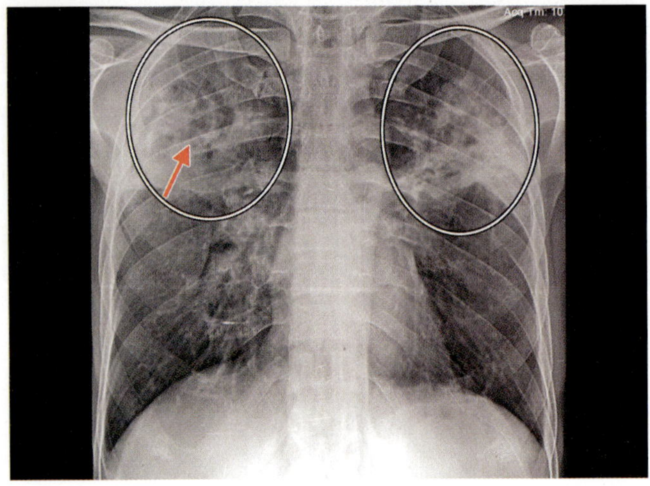

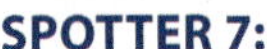

SPOTTER 7:

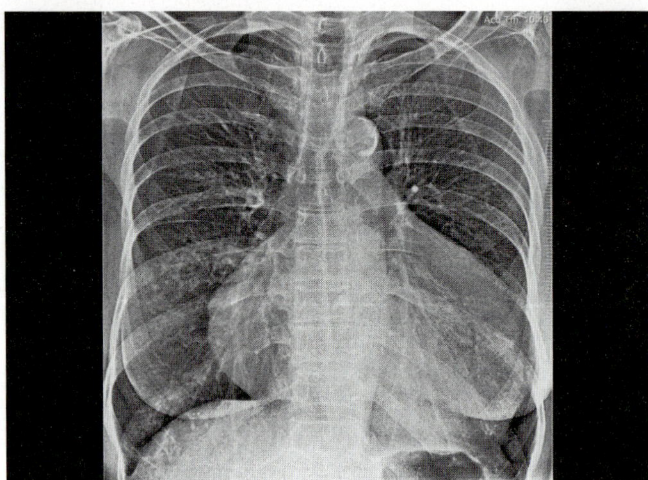

SPOTTER 8:

RECOMMENDED READINGS

1. deLacey G, Morley S, Berman L. The Chest X-Ray. A survival guide. United States: Saunders Elsevier; 2008.
2. DifuWu, Krystle, Eric, Davjohn. How to Read a Chest X Ray. [online] Available from https://www.wikihow.com/wikiHowTo?search=How+to+Read+a+Chest+X+Ray.
3. Lennon FA, Simon G. The height of the diaphragm in the chest radiographs of normal adults. Br J Radiol. 1965;38:937-43.
4. Flower CD, Verschakelan JA. The diaphragm. In: Grainger RG, Allison D (Eds). Diagnostic Radiology, 3rd edition. New York: Churchill Livingstone; 1997. pp. 270.
5. Felson B, Felson H. Localization of intrathoracic lesions by means of the postero-anterior roentgenogram; the silhouette sign. Radiology. 1950;55:363-74.
6. Felson B. Chest roentgenology. Philadelphia: WB Saunders Company; 1973.
7. Fraser RS, Muller NL, Colman N, Pare PD. The normal lung. In: Fraser RS, Muller NL, Colman N, Pare PD (Eds). Fraser and Pare's Diagnosis of Diagnosis of Diseases of Chest, 4th edition. Philadelphia: WB Saunders Company; 1999. pp. 299.
8. Edwards DK, Higgins CB, Gilpin EA. The cardiothoracic ratio in newborn infants. AJR Am J Roentgenol. 1981;136:907-13.
9. Farr PF, Allisy-Roberts PJ. Radiation hazards protection. In: Farr PF, Allisy-Roberts PJ (Eds). Physics for Medical Imaging. London: Saunders; 1998. pp.148-82

MULTIPLE CHOICE QUESTIONS

To access the multiple choice questions of this Section online, kindly scan the QR code.

CHAPTER

16

Nutritional Deficiency Disorders

Atanu Chandra, Aritra Kumar Ray

ABSTRACT

Normal cellular function of the human body is largely dependent on the adequate intake of macro- and micronutrients. Nutritional deficiency disorders are very prevalent in developing countries such as India mainly due to inadequate dietary intake, poor maternal health, and poor hygiene leading to protozoal and helminthic infestations. Other causes include medical conditions associated with malabsorption, alcoholism, and chronic illnesses such as chronic liver disease and chronic kidney disease. There is no definite laboratory indicator of comprehensive nutritional status. Therefore, careful history taking along with meticulous clinical examination and focused laboratory investigations are of paramount importance to plan for proper nutritional supplementation with treatment of the precipitating causes.

"Our bodies are our gardens, to which our wills are our gardeners"

—William Shakespeare

INTRODUCTION

Nutritional deficiency disorders are seen very commonly in Indian subcontinent owing to poor socioeconomic conditions leading to inadequate dietary intake and lack of appropriate awareness and education. Nutritional deficiency can also be seen in diseases causing poor absorption and utilization of nutrients in the body. Poor environmental and maternal health, premature termination of breastfeeding, large family size, adverse cultural practices related to weaning and child-rearing, delayed supplementary feeding, and discarding cooking water from cereals are the contributory factors leading to nutritional deficient conditions.

The major classes of nutrients comprise of carbohydrates, proteins, fats, minerals, vitamins, and minerals. Nutritional deficiency disorders can be classified into macronutrient and micronutrient deficiency. Macronutrients, namely carbohydrates, proteins, and fats, are required in large quantities and they are the primary building blocks of the body. The micronutrients, namely vitamins and minerals, are needed in small quantities and they play a key role in metabolic pathways.

FOR ASSESSING NUTRITIONAL STATUS

History: Weight loss (quantification); dietary intake; socioeconomic assessment; mental health, lifestyle, medications, and substance abuse; careful search for any medical, surgical, or chronic disorders, which may be responsible for malnutrition; constitutional signs/symptoms; and presence of gastrointestinal symptoms.

Physical examination: *Body mass index* (BMI) = Weight in kg/(height in m)^2 (BMI < 18.5 kg/m^2 needs assessment for malnutrition); *anthropometric measurements* such as skinfold thickness and circumference of limbs; weakness or loss of strength assessed by grip strength and leg extensor strength; *peripheral edema* associated with hypoproteinemia or thiamine deficiency; *abnormalities in hairs*; *dermatological abnormalities* such as petechiae (vitamin A and C deficiency), ecchymosis (vitamin C and K deficiency), acro-orificial dermatitis (zinc deficiency), acneiform lesions (vitamin A deficiency), and poor wound healing; abnormalities in *oral cavity and perioral region* such as angular stomatitis (B complex and iron deficiency), glossitis (vitamin B12, folate, or niacin deficiency), magenta tongue (riboflavin deficiency), and bleeding gums (vitamin C deficiency); *ocular findings* such as dry eyes and Bitot's spots (vitamin A) and angular palpebritis (riboflavin); *neurological dysfunction* such as cognitive disorder (vitamin B12 deficiency), peripheral neuropathy (thiamine and vitamin B12), ophthalmoplegia (thiamine), and impairment of posterior column sensation (vitamin B12); and lastly, careful systemic examination to find out the etiological and associated abnormalities.

Laboratory tests: Complete blood count, blood urea nitrogen, creatinine, glucose, C-reactive protein, albumin and prealbumin, retinol-binding protein, prothrombin time, 24-hour urinary urea nitrogen to assess nitrogen balance, 72-hour quantitative fecal fat estimation, Schilling test for impaired vitamin B12 absorption, dual-energy X-ray absorptiometry, assessment of specific micronutrients, and functional assessment of gastrointestinal tract.

VITAMIN DEFICIENCY DISORDERS

VITAMIN A

Sources:

- *Plant sources*: Green leafy vegetables (such as amaranth and spinach) and fruits (mango, papaya, and pumpkin)
- *Animal sources*: Eggs, liver, cheese, butter, meat, fish, and whole milk
- *Fortified foods*: Vitamin A fortified foods include milk, margarine, and vanaspati

Deficiency symptoms:

*Ocular manifestations (**Table 1**)*:

- *Night blindness*: Defect in dark adaptation is the most striking early clinical feature of vitamin A deficiency where a person finds difficulty to see in dim light. The condition even gets worsened with diarrhea and other infections.
- *Conjunctival xerosis*: It is the first clinical sign of vitamin A deficiency where the conjunctiva looks dry, wrinkled, muddy, and nonwettable. It has been classically described as "emerging-like sand banks at receding tide" when a child stops to cry.
- *Bitot's spots*: They are triangular, pearly-white spots on the bulbar conjunctiva and it generally indicate vitamin A deficiency.
- *Corneal xerosis*: This is a serious condition in which the cornea loses its moist appearance and appears dry, nonwettable, dull, and opaque. Corneal ulceration and scarring may eventually develop, which may lead to impaired vision.
- *Keratomalacia*: It is a medical emergency condition in which a part or the whole of cornea may become soft and may even burst open. It is a rapidly progressive condition, which may lead to loss of vision.

Extraocular manifestations:

- Follicular hyperkeratosis
- Growth retardation
- Infertility
- Keratinization of epithelial tissue (in skin, lung, and genitourinary system)
- Metaplastic bones
- Increased incidence of respiratory and intestinal infection

Requirement: The requirement is given in **Table 2**.

Prevention:

- By reducing the severity and frequency of contributing factors, e.g., diarrhea, respiratory tract infection, protein-energy malnutrition (PEM), and measles
- Adequate and regular intake of vitamin A-rich foods

Treatment: In adults, oral vitamin A at the dose of 10,000 IU per day for 3 months.

VITAMIN D

Sources: Vitamin D is primarily derived from both foods and sunlight. Foods rich in vitamin D include human milk, fish liver oils, egg yolk, cheese, butter, and some species of fish. Foods artificially fortified vitamin D include margarine, vanaspati, milk, and infant foods.

Deficiency symptoms:

- *Rickets*: It occurs due to reduced calcification of growing bones and usually affects young children between 6 months and 2 years of age. It is characterized by growth failure, muscular hypotonia, bone deformity, tetany, and convulsion. The bony deformities include rickety rosary, deformed pelvis, pigeon chest, Harrison's sulcus, double malleoli due to metaphyseal hyperplasia, genu valgum, genu varum, craniotabes, kyphoscoliosis, and delayed developmental milestones.
- *Osteomalacia*: This condition affects the adults in which the trabecular bones become soft and weak leading to deformity.

Prevention:

- Parents should be educated to expose their children to sunlight
- Prophylaxis of children with vitamin D should be done at periodic intervals
- Fortification of foods (especially milk) with vitamin D

TABLE 1 World Health Organization (WHO) classification of xerophthalmia.

Primary signs	Secondary signs
• X1A—conjunctival xerosis • X1B—Bitot's spots • X2—corneal xerosis • X3A—corneal ulceration (<one-third of cornea) • X3B—corneal ulceration(>one-third of cornea)	• XN—night blindness • XF—fundal changes • XS—corneal scarring

TABLE 2 Daily recommendation of vitamin A.

Groups	Retinol (µg)
0–12 months	350
1–6 years	400
7–9 years	600
10–17 years	600
Man	600
Woman	600
Pregnancy	800
Lactation	950

VITAMIN E

Sources: Sources of vitamin E are sunflower seed, cotton seed, vegetable oils, green leafy vegetables, butter, and egg yolk. Breast milk, especially colostrum, is particularly rich in vitamin E.

Often fat malabsorption may lead to vitamin E deficiency and it may manifest as:

- Hemolytic anemia in premature infants
- Spinocerebellar ataxia manifesting as truncal and limb ataxia, ophthalmoplegia, loss of vibration and position sense, loss of deep tendon reflexes, muscle weakness, dysarthria, and ptosis

Requirement: About 8–10 mg/day of tocopherol (depends on the edible oil which is used).

VITAMIN K

Sources: Fresh green vegetables and some fruits are particularly rich in vitamin K1. Cow's milk is richer in vitamin K (60 μg/L) than human milk. The main source of vitamin K2 in human is intestinal bacteria.

Vitamin K plays a key role in the synthesis of various coagulation factors and its deficiency leads to bleeding manifestations. The hemorrhagic disease of newborn is a condition seen predominantly in breastfed infants due to low vitamin K content of human milk. Low dietary intake, maternal use of antagonist drugs, cholestasis, antibiotic therapy, and fat malabsorption may act as contributory factors.

Requirement: About 0.03 mg/kg for adults. Newborn infants generally tend to be suffering from vitamin K deficiency due to lack of prothrombin stores and lack of adequate intestinal flora.

WATER-SOLUBLE VITAMINS

THIAMINE (VITAMIN B1)

Sources: Sources of vitamin B1 are wheat, whole-grain cereals, pulses, yeast, gram, groundnuts, and oilseeds. Cereals (wheat and rice) form the main source of thiamine for the Indian population.

The two deficiency disorders associated with thiamine deficiency include: (1) Wernicke's encephalopathy and (2) beriberi.

1. *Wernicke's encephalopathy*, seen primarily in chronic alcoholic patients, is characterized by ataxia, ophthalmoplegia, and confusion.
2. Three forms of *beriberi* may be seen which include:
   i. The dry form of beriberi is characterized by involvement of nerves (peripheral neuritis)
   ii. The wet form is characterized by involvement of heart (cardiac beriberi)
   iii. Infantile beriberi is seen in breastfed infants of thiamine-deficient mothers

Requirement: Around 1.2 mg/day for adults.

Diagnosis:

- Measurement of 24-hour urinary excretion of thiamine
- Response of red cell transketolase to the in vitro addition of thiamine. An increase of transketolase activity of 15–25% is considered as mild deficiency and over 25% is considered as severe deficiency

Prevention:

- A well-balanced and mixed diet rich in thiamine (e.g., undermilled and parboiled rice) should be advocated
- Thiamine supplementation of high-risk population (e.g., lactating mothers)

RIBOFLAVIN (VITAMIN B2)

Riboflavin is a water-soluble flavoprotein and it is found to be widely distributed in plants.

Sources: Sources of vitamin B2 are eggs, kidney, liver, milk, meat, fish, and green leafy vegetables. Cow's milk contains 250 μg/100 kcal of riboflavin and human milk contains around 40–70 μg/100 kcal of riboflavin.

Deficiency symptoms:

- Angular stomatitis and cheilosis
- Nasolabial dyssebacia
- Mouth ulcers and glossitis
- Impaired neuromotor function
- Dry skin
- Impaired wound healing

Requirement: About 0.6 mg/1,000 kcal of energy intake.

Diagnosis: History of dietary deficiency and clinical symptoms are the keys to the diagnosis of riboflavin deficiency. A 24-hour excretion of the vitamin in the urine is a reliable and practical indicator of riboflavin status in the body. Excretion of <10% of intake over 24 hours is a reliable indicator of riboflavin deficiency.

NIACIN (VITAMIN B3)

Sources: Sources of vitamin B3 are cereals, milk, poultry, meat, fish, groundnut, and legumes. Milk is a poor source of niacin. Cow's milk contains 0.12 mg/100 kcal of niacin and human milk contains around 30 mg/100 kcal of niacin.

Deficiency symptoms: Niacin deficiency leads to pellagra, which is characterized by three Ds: dementia, diarrhea, and dermatitis. The cutaneous lesions are bilaterally symmetrical and occur in sun-exposed parts of the body. Neurologic symptoms include headache, loss of memory, apathy, irritability, depression, and delirium. In chronic forms, peripheral nerve lesions and posterolateral cord degeneration may be seen.

Requirement: About 6 mg/1,000 kcal of energy intake.

Diagnosis: A 24-hour excretion of N^1-methylnicotinamide below 3 mg is indicative of niacin deficiency.

PANTOTHENIC ACID (VITAMIN B5)

Source: Pantothenic acid is present almost in all naturally occurring foods and it is also synthesized by microorganisms from β-alanine and pantoic acid.

Deficiency symptoms:
- Fatigue
- Irritability
- Apathy
- Neurological symptoms including paresthesia, sensation of numbness, and muscle cramps
- Malaise and restlessness
- Nausea and vomiting
- Abdominal cramps

Requirement: 10 mg daily.

Pantothenate deficiency, as an isolated entity, occurs very rarely, though it may be associated with other vitamin deficiencies.

PYRIDOXINE (VITAMIN B6)

It may exist in three forms: (1) Pyridoxal, (2) Pyridoxine, and (3) Pyridoxamine.

Sources: Sources of vitamin B6 are liver, meat, milk, egg yolk, sunflower seeds, soya beans, and walnuts.

Deficiency symptoms:
- Anemia
- Peripheral neuritis
- Seizures
- Skin rashes
- Glosssy tongue
- High homocysteine
- Weakened immune function

Requirement:
- Adults—2 mg/day
- Pregnancy and lactation—2.5 mg/day

Pyridoxine deficiency, as an isolated entity, occurs very rarely as balanced diet contains adequate amount of pyridoxine. Tuberculosis patients on isoniazid are given a supplementation of pyridoxine (10 mg/day).

FOLATE

Sources: Sources of folate are meat, liver, eggs, milk, cereals, fruits, and vegetables.

Deficiency symptoms:
- Megaloblastic anemia
- Cheilosis and glossitis
- Gastrointestinal symptoms such as distension, diarrhea, and flatulence
- Infertility
- Abortions
- Congenital malformations in newborn

Requirement:
- Healthy adults—200 µg/day
- Lactation—300 µg/day
- Pregnancy—500 µg/day
- Children—80-120 µg/day

Folate deficiency is diagnosed based on the red cell and serum folate assay.

COBALAMIN (VITAMIN B12)

Sources: Sources of vitamin B12 are kidney, liver, fish, meat, milk, eggs, and cheese. It is also synthesized by colonic bacteria.

Deficiency symptoms:
- Megaloblastic anemia
- Diffuse and progressive demyelinating neurological lesions
- Subacute combined degeneration of spinal cord
- Gastrointestinal symptoms
- Growth retardation, irritability, hypotonia, involuntary movements, and delayed developmental milestones in children

Requirement:
- Normal adults—1 µg/day
- Lactation—1.5 µg/day
- Pregnancy—1.3 µg/day
- Infants and children—0.2 µg/day

Diagnosis of deficiency: Vitamin B12 status is determined by measurement of serum cobalamin levels. Increased level of homocysteine and methylmalonic acid along with methylmalonic aciduria may be found in vitamin B12 deficiency.

BIOTIN

Sources: Sources of biotin are egg yolk, milk, meat, liver, and yeast extracts. Person who consume large amount of raw eggs (which is rich in avidin) are found to be suffering from biotin deficiency.

Deficiency symptoms:
- Anorexia and vomiting
- Glossitis
- Hypercholesterolemia
- Dry scale dermatitis

Requirement: About 0.15 mg in the multivitamin supplements for children and infants.

VITAMIN C

Vitamin C is a water-soluble heat-sensitive vitamin, which plays a key role in tissue oxidation.

Sources: Sources of vitamin C are green leafy vegetables, fresh fruits, germinating pulses, and amla (one of the richest sources).

Deficiency symptoms: Vitamin C deficiency for prolonged period leads to scurvy, the signs of which include bleeding into the skin or joints, subcutaneous bruising, swollen and bleeding gums, and delayed wound healing. Additionally, pallor, anorexia, diarrhea, irritability, and increased susceptibility to infection may be seen in infants. It is predominantly seen in individuals who are deprived of green leafy vegetables and citrus fruits.

Requirement: About 40 mg/day for adults.

Diagnosis of scurvy: Scurvy is diagnosed based on history of inadequate dietary intake, characteristic physical findings, and radiological imaging of long bones.

MINERAL DEFICIENCY DISORDERS

CALCIUM

Calcium is the most abundant mineral in our body and is involved in nerve conduction, muscle stimulation, and coagulation cascade.

Sources: Sources of calcium are milk and milk products (e.g., curd, butter milk, skimmed milk, cheese), fish, and eggs and cheaper dietary sources include cereals, millets, and green leafy vegetables.

Deficiency symptoms:
- Muscle aches, spasms, and cramps
- Tingling and numbness in the feet, legs, hands, arms, and around the mouth
- Extreme fatigue and lethargy
- Dizziness, lightheadedness, forgetfulness, and confusion
- Osteopenia and osteoporosis
- Eczema and psoriasis
- Painful premenstrual syndrome (PMS)
- Dental problems in the form of tooth decay, weak roots, and delay in tooth formation

Requirement: About 600 mg/day is recommended for adults.

MAGNESIUM

Magnesium plays a key role in signal transmission, membrane transport, and fuel oxidation.

Sources: Sources of magnesium are bananas, nuts, legumes, and whole grains. Majority of total body magnesium is found in skeletal muscles and bones.

Deficiency symptoms:
- Muscle weakness and fatigue
- Muscle cramps and twitches
- Irregular heartbeat
- Tetany
- Irritability
- Hyperreflexia and occasionally hyporeflexia

Requirement: About 340 mg/day is recommended for adults.

PHOSPHORUS

Sources: Sources of phosphorus are fruits, vegetables, nuts, milk and milk products, meats, fish, and some seafoods. Majority of the total body phosphate content is found in bones and teeth.

Deficiency symptoms:
- Fragile bones and bone pain
- Numbness
- Weakness
- Fatigue
- Joint pain and stiffness

Requirement: About 700 mg/day is recommended for adults.

SODIUM

Sodium is found in different foods and it is also added to foods while cooking in the form of sodium chloride.

Deficiency symptoms:
- Muscle weakness, cramps, or spasms
- Irritability and restlessness
- Headache and confusion
- Nausea and vomiting
- Fatigue and drowsiness
- Seizures
- Coma

Requirement: Around 5 g/day in adults.

POTASSIUM

Potassium is found widely in different foodstuffs and hence there is little likelihood of its dietary deficiency.

Deficiency symptoms:
- Nausea and vomiting
- Fatigue, weakness, and cramps in muscles
- Muscle paralysis
- Constipation, bloating, and abdominal cramps
- Tingling and numbness
- Heart palpitations

Requirement: At least 90 mmol/day for adults.

IODINE

Iodine is an important micronutrient and is essential for the synthesis of thyroid hormones, triiodothyronine, and thyroxine.

Sources: Seafoods (e.g., sea salt, sea fish) and cod liver oil are the best sources of iodine and smaller amounts are found in meat, milk, cereals, vegetables etc.

Requirement:
- Adults—150 µg/day
- Pregnancy—250 µg/day

Deficiency: Features of deficiency are shown in **Table 3**.

TABLE 3 Spectrum of manifestations seen in iodine deficiency disorders (IDDs).

Fetus	• Stillbirths • Spontaneous abortions • Endemic cretinism • Increased perinatal mortality • Congenital anomalies
Neonate	• Neonatal hypothyroidism • Neonatal goiter • Mental retardation
Child and adolescent	• Goiter • Impaired mental function • Subclinical hypothyroidism • Retarded physical development

IRON

Sources: Iron is found in two forms—(1) non heme iron and (2) heme iron. Meat, liver, fish, and poultry are rich source of heme iron. Foods of vegetable origin, e.g., green leafy vegetables, cereals, jaggery, nuts, legumes, oilseeds, and dried fruits, are rich source of non heme iron.

Common causes of iron deficiency:

- Increased requirements of iron as during pregnancy
- Blood loss (such as during childbirth, menstruation, bleeding hemorrhoids, and peptic ulcer)
- Inadequate intake of iron in the diet
- Excretion through bile, sweat, urine, and desquamated surface cells

Symptoms of iron deficiency:

- Headache and dizziness
- Tiredness and fatigue
- Shortness of breath
- Palpitations
- Restless legs
- Spoon-shaped finger nails called koilonychia

FLUORINE

It is the most abundant and highly reactive element in nature. It is found only in combined form but never in its elemental gaseous form. Fluorine is very essential for the formation of dental enamel and normal mineralization of bones.

Sources: The major source of fluorine is drinking water (about 0.5 mg/L). Though it is found in traces in different foodstuffs, cheese, tea, and sea fish are found to be rich in fluorides.

Deficiency symptoms:

- Dental caries
- Weak and brittle bones

Requirement: The recommended level of fluorides in drinking water is 0.5–0.8 mg/L.

Trace elements: The signs and symptoms of deficiency of trace elements is shown in **Table 4**.

TABLE 4	Deficiency of trace elements.
Zinc	• Poor physical growth is seen in school-age children • Delayed sexual maturation • Anemia • Hypogonadism • Hair loss • Diarrhea • Anorexia • Impaired perception of taste and/or smell • Pica is noted in some cases • Blepharitis, photophobia, and corneal opacities • Acrodermatitis enteropathica
Copper	• Microcytic hypochromic anemia • Skeletal lesions include submetaphyseal fractures, spontaneous fracture of ribs, flaring of the anterior ribs, periosteal elevation, cupping and flaring of long bone metaphyses, and spur formation • Depigmentation of hair and skin • Anorexia • Diarrhea • Failure to thrive • Central nervous system manifestations include psychomotor retardation, apneic episodes, and hypotonia
Cobalt	• Fatigue, dizziness, and weakness • Anorexia and weight loss • Shortness of breath • Loss of sensation and tingling in the hands and feet • Muscle weakness and cramps • Dementia • Altered thyroid function
Chromium	• Impaired glucose tolerance • Peripheral neuropathy • Impaired lipid metabolism leading to increased chance of atherosclerosis
Selenium	• Keshan disease which presents as cardiomyopathy in young children • Skeletal myopathies • Loss of hair and macrocytosis have been reported in mild selenium deficiency
Molybdenum	Deficiency of molybdenum is associated with oral and esophageal carcinoma

MACRONUTRIENT DEFICIENCY

PROTEINS

The main constituents of dietary protein are essential and nonessential amino acids, which are absolutely necessary for protein synthesis. The recommended dietary allowance for protein is 0.8–1 g/kg body weight. When the total energy intake is insufficient, the intake of protein of high biological values should be enhanced as they are diverted into cellular oxidation and gluconeogenesis. 10–15% of the total calories should be derived from dietary protein. Animal proteins are usually of high biological values. Protein intake should be increased during the phases of increased need such as puberty, pregnancy, lactation, and hypercatabolic states. Protein intake should be modified in disease conditions such as chronic liver disease or chronic kidney disease.

CARBOHYDRATES AND FAT

Fat intake should be not >30% of total calories for maintaining optimum health. Saturated and trans-fat intake should be <10% of calories and the same amount of <10% is also applicable for polyunsaturated fatty acids. Deficiencies of alpha-linolenic acid and linoleic acid lead to hair loss, dry skin, and impaired wound healing.

Carbohydrates are found abundantly in vegetables, fruits, whole-grain cereals, and legumes. Insufficient dietary carbohydrate leads to breakdown of glycerol (derived from fat) and amino acids (derived from dietary protein and body protein). Long-term deficiency of carbohydrates leads to a condition called ketosis. They should make 45–55% of the total calories. The glucose requirement of brain is 100 g/day and for other tissues, it is 50 g/day. Some tissues such as brain and red blood cells are solely dependent on glucose as the source of energy.

CONCLUSION

Good nutritional habits are not developed in a single day nor they get destroyed in one unbalanced meal. Food is a part of civilization and security. Malnutrition and hunger have always posed a great threat to mankind and civilization throughout history. It should be of prime international concern to address these issues as nations are linked to each other not only through ideas but also through breads.

RECOMMENDED READINGS

1. Shenkin A. Micronutrients in health and disease. Postgrad Med J. 2006;82(971):559-67.
2. Jen M, Yan AC. Syndromes associated with nutritional deficiency and excess. Clin Dermatol. 2010;28(6):669-85.
3. Dwyer J. Nutrient requirements and dietary assessment. In: Jameson JL, Fauci AS, Kasper DL, Hauser SL, Longo DL, Loscalzo J (Eds). Harrison's Principles of Internal Medicine, 20th edition. New York: McGraw Hill Education; 2018. pp. 2303-6.
4. Indian Council of Medical Research (ICMR). (2009). Nutrient Requirements and Recommended Dietary Allowances for Indians: A Report of the Expert Group of the ICMR. [online] Available from https://vetconcerns.org/wp-content/uploads/2015/06/Recommended-Dietary-Allowance-ICMR.pdf. .
5. Raman JK, Chaudhery DN. Need to revisit vitamin A supplementation programme in India. Indian J Med Res. 2014;139(2):323-4.
6. Vijayaraghavan K. National control programme against nutritional blindness due to vitamin A deficiency: current status and future strategy. Indian J Med Res. 2018;148:496-502.
7. Narayan J, John D, Ramadas N. Malnutrition in India: status and government initiatives. J Public Health Policy. 2019;40(1):126-41.
8. Gonmei Z, Toteja GS. Micronutrient status of Indian population. Indian J Med Res. 2018;148(5):511-21.
9. Benoist S, Brouquet A. Nutritional assessment and screening for malnutrition. J Visc Surg. 2015;152 Suppl 1:S3-7.

CHAPTER 17

Metabolic Disorders: Carbohydrate, Protein, and Others

Akhil Krishna, Sujoy Ghosh

ABSTRACT

Inherited metabolic disorders (IMDs) are rare disorders due to genetic defects in the enzymes mediating the metabolic pathways leading to a myriad of clinical manifestations. Hundreds of IMDs are described. Glycogen storage disorders (GSDs), which come under disorders of carbohydrate metabolism, can be mainly divided into those affecting the liver or muscle. Those affecting the liver mainly present with hepatomegaly and fasting hypoglycemia, whereas those affecting the muscle present with exercise intolerance, muscle pain, and progressive muscle weakness. Genetic testing is the preferred method to diagnose GSDs. Mainstay of treatment of GSDs is dietary, focusing on prevention of hypoglycemia. Inherited disorders of protein metabolism can be either amino acid disorders, organic acid disorders, or urea cycle disorders. The clinical manifestations differ widely between the conditions. Diagnosis relies on analysis of plasma or urine amino acids and can be confirmed by genetic testing. Lysosomal storage disorders (LSDs) occur when one or more of the lysosomal hydrolytic enzymes are defective. They can be divided onto sphingolipidoses, mucopolysaccharidoses (MPS), glycoproteinoses, mucolipidoses, lysosomal membrane transport disorder, and lysosomal GSDs. LSDs can present from infancy to adulthood. Enzyme assays or genetic testing can be used to make a definitive diagnosis. Treatment strategies include enzyme replacement therapy and substrate reduction.

"Diet is the essential key to all successful healing"

—JR Raymond

INTRODUCTION

Inherited metabolic disorders, previously known as inborn errors of metabolism, are a heterogenous group of monogenic disorders which occur due to enzyme defects in various stages of the metabolic pathways. The field of IMDs is vast, with hundreds of disorders described. Individually, they are rare, but collectively the prevalence ranges from 1 in 800 to 1 in 2,500 live births. The exact prevalence of IMDs in India is not yet known, but more and more cases are being diagnosed nowadays, because of increased awareness among the treating physicians and increased access to the diagnostic tests.

In this chapter, we will be discussing:

- Disorders of carbohydrate metabolism
- Disorders of protein metabolism
- Lysosomal storage disorders

DISORDERS OF CARBOHYDRATE METABOLISM

Disorders of carbohydrate metabolism can be divided as shown in **Flowchart 1**. The salient features of various disorders are shown in **Tables 1** to **5**.

GLYCOGEN STORAGE DISEASES

- Glycogen is the major storage form of glucose in mammals.
- It is stored mainly in the liver and muscle.

TABLE 1 Liver glycogen storage diseases.

Type	Common name	Defective enzyme	Onset	Clinical presentation	Treatment
0	**Glycogen synthase deficiency**	Hepatic glycogen synthase	Neonatal	• Severe fasting hypoglycemia and ketosis, but postprandial hyperglycemia and lactic acidosis • No hepatomegaly	• Uncooked cornstarch, especially at bedtime • High protein diet
Ia	**Von Gierke's disease**	Glucose-6-phosphatase	Neonatal	• Growth retardation • Hepatomegaly and enlarged kidney • Severe fasting hypoglycemia • Elevated blood lactate, triglycerides, and uric acid	• Uncooked cornstarch during the day and night or continuous overnight intragastric feeding
Ib		Glucose-6-phosphatase translocase		Same as type Ia, with additional findings of: • Neutropenia and recurrent bacterial infections • Inflammatory bowel disease	• Uncooked cornstarch as for Ia • Granulocyte colony stimulating factor • Mesalamine for inflammatory bowel disease (IBD)
IIIa	**Cori–Forbes disease (limit dextrinosis)**	Liver and muscle debranching enzyme	Infancy	• Hepatomegaly • Mild fasting hypoglycemia • Myopathy • Hypertrophic cardiomyopathy • Elevated liver aminotransferases	High protein diet with low dose uncooked cornstarch supplementation
IIIb		Liver debranching enzyme (normal muscle debrancher activity)		Liver symptoms same as IIIa; no muscle symptoms	
IV	**Andersen's disease (amylopectinosis)**	Branching enzyme	Infancy	Classical form: • Failure to thrive • Progressive cirrhosis (death usually before 5th year) • Adult form (presents between 40 years and 60 years) • Neurogenic bladder • Spastic paraparesis • Peripheral neuropathy	• High protein diet with restriction of carbohydrates • Liver transplantation decreases glycogen storage in heart and skeletal muscle
VI	**Hers' disease**	Liver phosphorylase	Early childhood	• Hepatomegaly • Mild fasting hypoglycemia • Hyperlipidemia • Ketosis	Uncooked cornstarch
IX	**Phosphorylase kinase deficiency**	Phosphorylase kinase			• Uncooked cornstarch • High protein diet

TABLE 2 Muscle glycogen storage diseases.

Type	Common name	Basic defect	Clinical presentation	Treatment
V	**McArdle disease**	Muscle phosphorylase	• Exercise intolerance • Muscle cramps • Myoglobinuria on strenuous exercise • "Second-wind" phenomenon (if they take a short break at the first appearance of muscle pain, they can resume the activity without pain)	• High protein diet • Oral sucrose before sustained aerobic exercise may be useful
VII	**Tarui disease**	Phosphofructokinase	As in type V, with additional features of: Hemolytic anemia	No specific treatment; avoid strenuous exercise

TABLE 3 Lysosomal glycogen storage disorder.

Type	Common name	Basic defect	Clinical presentation	Treatment
II	**Pompe disease**	Lysosomal acid maltase (α glucosidase)	Infantile: • Hypotonia • Hepatomegaly • Cardiomegaly • Cardiorespiratory failure leading to death by age 1–2 years Late onset (juvenile and adult): • Myopathy • Variable cardiomyopathy and respiratory insufficiency Serum creatine kinase is markedly increased	Intravenous enzyme replacement with recombinant human α glucosidase

TABLE 4 Galactose disorders.

Common name	Basic defect	Clinical presentation	Treatment
Galactosemia	Most commonly galactose 1-phosphate uridyltransferase	Neonatal presentation on ingestion of galactose (milk/formula) with: • Vomiting • Failure to thrive • Hepatomegaly • Cataracts • Aminoaciduria	Immediate removal of galactose from diet
		Treated adults can have: • Developmental delay • Neurological deficits • Premature ovarian failure Adult presentation is rare, but exclude diagnosis in patients with premature ovarian failure ± cataracts ± neurological deficits	Supportive therapy including options to cryopreservation of eggs before premature ovarian failure

TABLE 5 Fructose disorders.

Common name	Basic defect	Clinical presentation	Comments
Hereditary fructose intolerance	Aldolase B	• Ingestion of fructose/sucrose/sorbitol causes acute illness within minutes of abdominal pain, vomiting, and diarrhea • Persistent exposure leads to liver steatosis/fibrosis/failure and renal tubular disease	Withdraw all sources of fructose

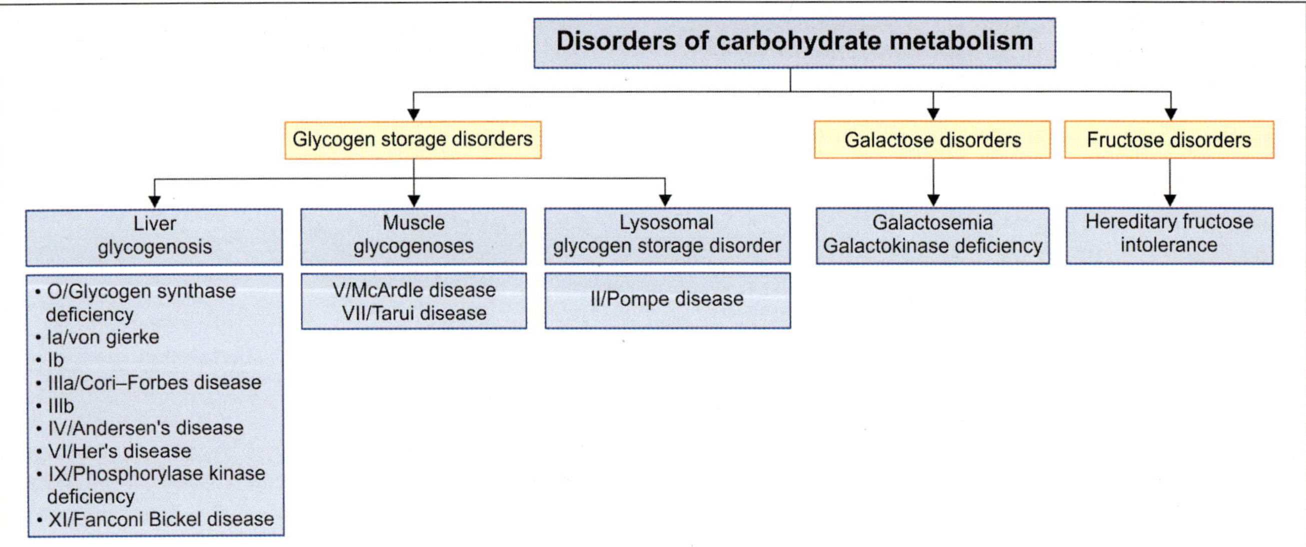

FLOWCHART 1: Disorders of carbohydrate metabolism.

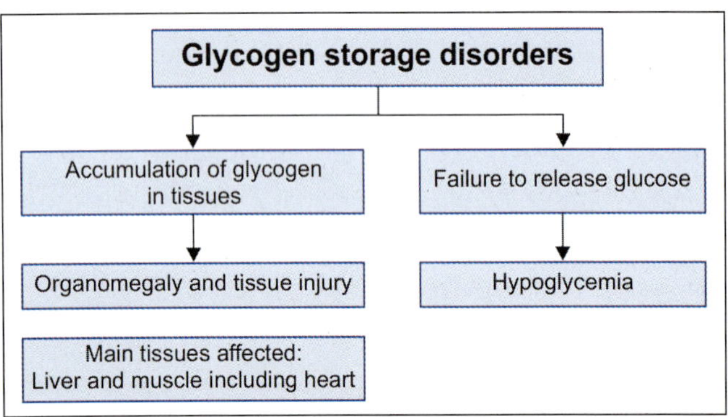

FLOWCHART 2: Pathophysiology of clinical features in glycogen storage diseases (GSDs).

Glycogen storage disorders

Those involving liver

- Fasting hypoglycemia and ketosis
- Hepatomegaly

Those involving muscle

- Exercise intolerance with muscle pain, cramps, rhabdomyolysis and myoglobinuria
- Progressive muscle weakness
- Cardiomyopathy if cardiac muscle involved

FLOWCHART 3: Clinical features of glycogen storage diseases (GSDs) in general.

- The glycogen stored in the liver is important to maintain euglycemia during fasting whereas muscle glycogen serves as the immediate source of glucose for the production of energy during exercise.
- Genetic disorders which affect various enzymes involved in the regulation of glycogen synthesis and breakdown cause marked accumulation of glycogen in various tissues.

Clinical features:

- Clinical features of GSDs are due to the abnormal accumulation of glycogen in various tissues, mainly liver and muscle including the cardiac muscle. In severe cases, other organs may also be involved (**Flowchart 2**).
- Those GSDs which predominantly involve the liver presents with fasting hypoglycemia due to the inability to breakdown hepatic glycogen.
- Those which involve the muscle presents with exercise intolerance, muscle pain, cramps, rhabdomyolysis, and progressive muscle weakness (**Flowchart 3**).

Glycogen storage diseases types:

- Sixteen types of GSDs have been identified so far. They are identified by a numbering system in the historical sequence of their identification, of which GSD I, III, VI, IX (all of which involve the liver) and GSD II (which involve skeletal muscle) account for about 95% of the cases.
- Recently described inherited multisystem disorders with neurodegeneration such as polyglucosan body disease and Lafora body disease are characterized by accumulation of abnormal glycogen structure in various cell types including neurons.
- Details of selected GSDs are given in **Tables 1** to **3**.

Investigations:

- Previously, GSDs were diagnosed by demonstrating excess glycogen storage in the tissue of interest and reduced activity of particular glycogen metabolizing enzyme.
- Currently, molecular genetic testing is the preferred method to diagnose GSDs.

Treatment:

General principles of treatment of liver glycogenoses:

- The goals of treatment of liver glycogenoses are to prevent hypoglycemia and glucose counter-regulation
- The mainstay of treatment is dietary.
- Infants and children may require continuous supply of carbohydrates by nasogastric route to maintain euglycemia.

- Adults can be managed by a combination of frequent sugary snacks and uncooked cornstarch (UCS), which is slowly digested and absorbed into the circulation as glucose.

Treatment of glycogen storage disease I differs from other liver glycogen storage diseases:

- In GSD I, abnormal glucose-6-phosphatase activity impairs both glycogenolysis and gluconeogenesis. But in other forms of hepatic GSDs, gluconeogenesis is intact. So, protein can be used as a substrate for endogenous glucose production. Fatty acid oxidation is also impaired in GSD I, whereas it is intact in others. Hence, ketosis accompanies hypoglycemia in GSDs other than GSD I.
- Treatment of GSD I includes providing a continuous dietary source of glucose to maintain euglycemia (blood glucose at 75–90 mg/dL) before meals and overnight. Glucose concentrations should be kept above 70 mg/dL to prevent counter-regulation, which causes diversion of glucose-6-phospahte into alternative pathways, leading to increased lactate, uric acid, and triglycerides.
- Patients with other forms of GSDs can be advised to take high protein diet (2 or 3 g/kg) with complex carbohydrates and UCS to maintain euglycemia.

INHERITED DISORDERS OF PROTEIN METABOLISM

- Disorders of protein metabolism are individually rare. The incidences range from 1 in 10,000 for phenylketonuria or cystinuria to 1 in 200,000 for alkaptonuria or homocystinuria. Collectively, they affect 1 in 1,000 newborns.
- Inherited disorders of protein metabolism can be of following types (**Flowchart 4**)
- Amino acid disorders are called amino acidemias when there is abnormal accumulation of amino acids in blood and amino acidurias when there is abnormal excretion of amino acids in urine (**Table 6**).

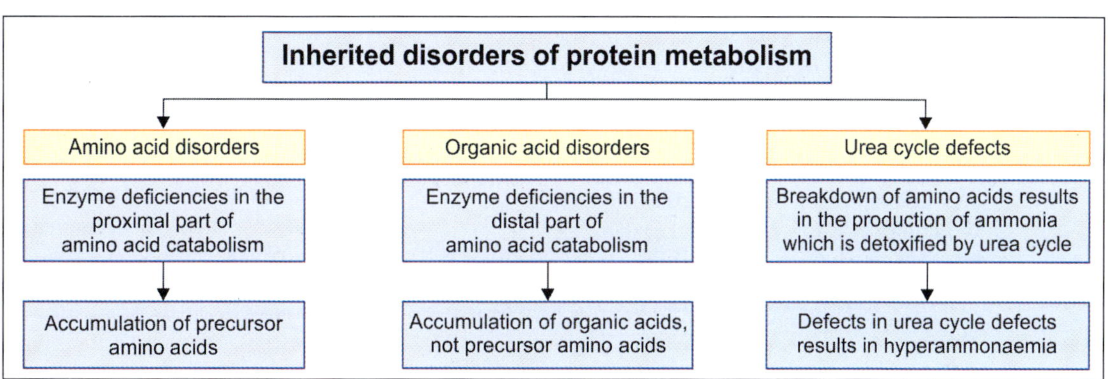

FLOWCHART 4: Types of inherited disorders of protein metabolism.

TABLE 6 Selected inherited disorders of amino acid metabolism.

Disease	Defective enzyme	Clinical presentation	Biochemical features	Treatment
Phenylketonuria (PKU)	Phenylalanine hydroxylase	• Intellectual disability • Microcephaly • Hypopigmented skin and hairs • Eczema • "Mousy" odor	Raised phenylalanine in serum	• Dietary restriction of phenylalanine • Pegvaliase—enzyme therapy approved for adult patients with PKU
Tyrosinemia type 1 (hepatorenal)	Fumarylacetoacetate hydroxylase	• Cirrhosis • Liver failure • Rickets • Failure to thrive • Peripheral neuropathy • "Boiled cabbage" odor	Raised tyrosine in serum and raised succinylacetone in urine	• Nitisinone • Tyrosine restriction • Tyrosine free amino acid supplementation • Liver transplantation may be considered
Alkaptonuria	Homogentisic acid oxidase	• Ochronosis • Arthritis • Cardiac valve involvement • Urine becomes black on standing	Raised urine homogentisic acid	Nitisinone

Continued...

Continued...

Disease	Defective enzyme	Clinical presentation	Biochemical features	Treatment
Classical homocystinuria	Cystathionine b synthase	• Lens dislocation • Thromboembolic events • Intellectual disability • Osteoporosis • Marfanoid habitus	• Raised plasma homocysteine • Raised plasma methionine • Raised plasma cysteine	• Pyridoxine • Betaine • Vitamin B12 • Folate
Cystinosis	Cystinosin	• Renal Fanconi's syndrome • Rickets • Photophobia • Hypotonia • Renal failure	• Elevated intraleukocyte cystine • Demonstration of cystine corneal crystals by slit lamp examination	• Cysteamine • Renal transplantation in end-stage renal disease (ESRD)
Defects in metabolism of branched-chain amino acid (BCAA)		• Acute decompensation ◦ Encephalopathy ◦ Acidosis ◦ Hyperammonemia • Developmental delay • Cardiomyopathy in PA • Pancreatitis in MMA/PA • Renal failure	• High anion gap metabolic acidosis • Hyperammonemia during acute decompensation • Characteristic abnormalities on amino acid/organic acid and acylcarnitine profile	• Natural protein restriction • Liver transplantation (MSUD and PA) • Renal/combined liver and renal transplantation (MMA) • Carnitine supplementation (PA/MMA) • BCAA free supplements (MSUD)
Maple syrup urine disease (MSUD)	Branched-chain α-ketoacid dehydrogenase			
Propionic aciduria (PA)	Propionyl-CoA carboxylase			
Methylmalonic aciduria (MMA)	Methylmalonyl-CoA mutase/racemase			
Urea cycle defects	Mutations in one of six urea cycle enzymes, most commonly ornithine transcarbamylase deficiency (OTC) deficiency	• Progressive encephalopathy • Cyclical vomiting • Nonspecific neuropsychiatric symptoms	• When unwell, hyperammonemia and characteristic abnormalities in amino acids/organic acids • May also have: ◦ Alkalosis ◦ Consistently very low urea	• Lifelong protein restriction • Ammonia scavengers • Arginine • Citrulline

CLINICAL FEATURES

- Clinical features result from accumulation of the substance which cannot be metabolized.
- Manifestations differ widely between various conditions.
- Central nervous system dysfunction in the form of developmental retardation, seizures, altered sensorium, or behavioral disturbances is seen in over half of these disorders.
- Protein-induced vomiting, neurological dysfunction, and hyperammonemia are seen in many urea cycle disorders.
- Metabolic ketoacidosis with hyperammonemia is common in organic acidemias.

INVESTIGATIONS

- Diagnostic tests include analysis of:
  - Plasma amino acids
  - Urine amino acids
  - Plasma acylcarnitine profile
- The diagnosis can be confirmed by:
  - Enzyme assay on cells or tissues
  - Deoxyribonucleic acid (DNA) testing

SPECIAL DIETARY PRODUCTS OR FOODS

- Many of the disorders of inborn errors of metabolism like those related to protein metabolism require specialty foods, which are not readily available in India.
- Previously, the patients had to procure these through acquaintances in the West or wait till their doctor got them directly from nutrition companies.
- Recently, by the efforts of organizations such as the Indian Society for Inborn Errors of Metabolism (ISIEM) and Indian Academy of Pediatrics, special dietary products or foods for special medical purposes (FSMP), have been made available for various metabolic disorders, after permission was granted by Food Safety and Standards Authority of India (FSSAI).

Two case vignettes on disorders of protein metabolism are presented next.

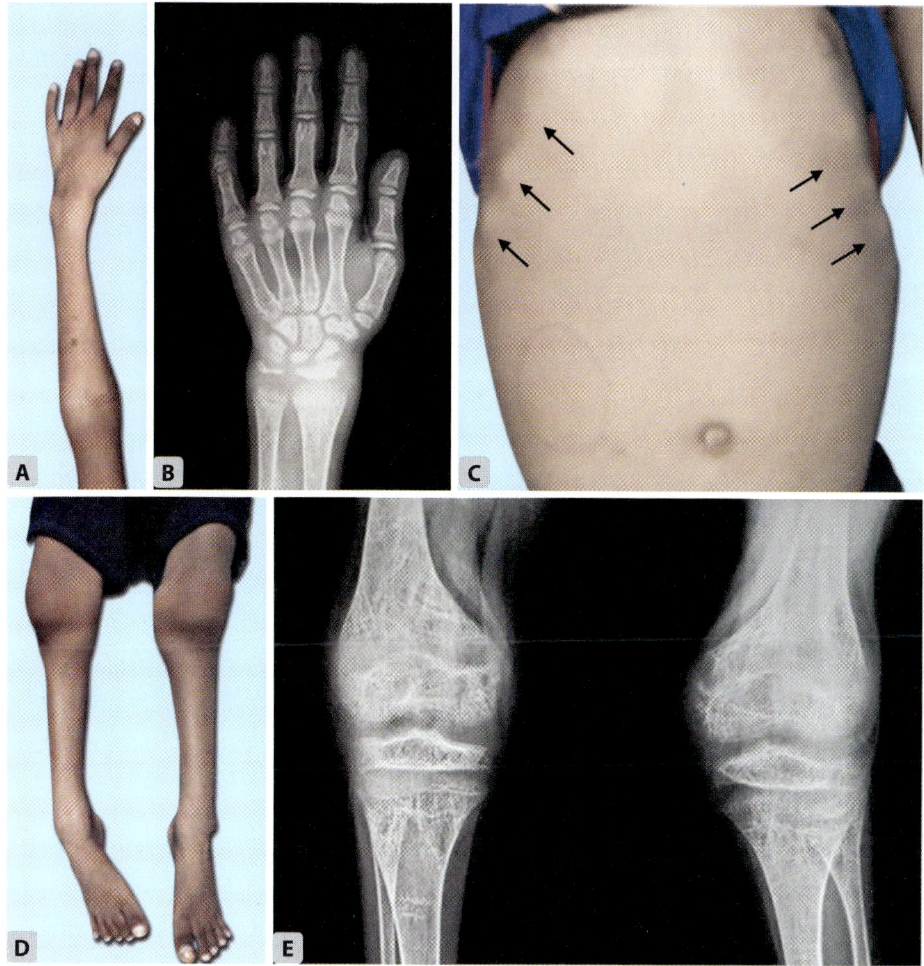

FIGURES 1 A to E: A case of tyrosinemia type 1. **(A)** Broadening of the wrist due to rickets; **(B)** X-ray of left wrist showing rachitic changes; **(C)** Rickety rosary (arrows); **(D)** Lower limb deformities due to rickets; **(E)** X-ray of knee showing rachitic changes.

CASE VIGNETTE 1

A 9-year-old boy from Bangladesh, product of second degree consanguineous marriage, with history of cirrhosis of liver was referred to us for evaluation of rickets. The boy had rachitic changes in both upper and lower extremities with rachitic rosary (**Fig. 1**). On evaluation, the boy had raised urinary succinylacetone, suggesting a diagnosis of tyrosinemia type 1, which was confirmed by genetic analysis.

CASE VIGNETTE 2

A 7-year-old girl from West Bengal, born out of second-degree consanguineous marriage, presented with history of failure to thrive since birth and knock knees since 2½ years of age. She also had photophobia. On evaluation, the child was found to have proximal renal tubular acidosis with Fanconi syndrome, hypophosphatemic rickets, and chronic kidney disease—end-stage renal disease (ESRD). Cystine corneal crystals were evident on slit lamb examination and the child was diagnosed to have cystinosis, which was confirmed on genetic testing (**Fig. 2**).

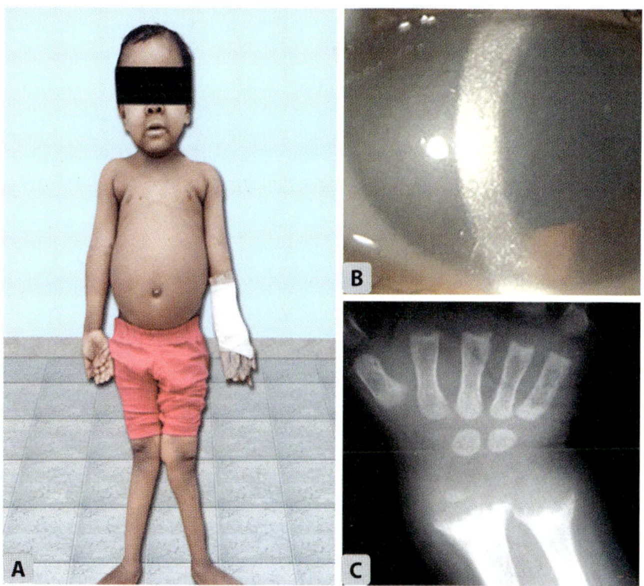

FIGURES 2 A to C: A case of cystinosis. **(A)** Child with cystinosis. Genu valgum and pot belly can be noted; **(B)** Slit lamp examination showing cystine corneal crystals; **(C)** X-ray of wrist showing rachitic changes.

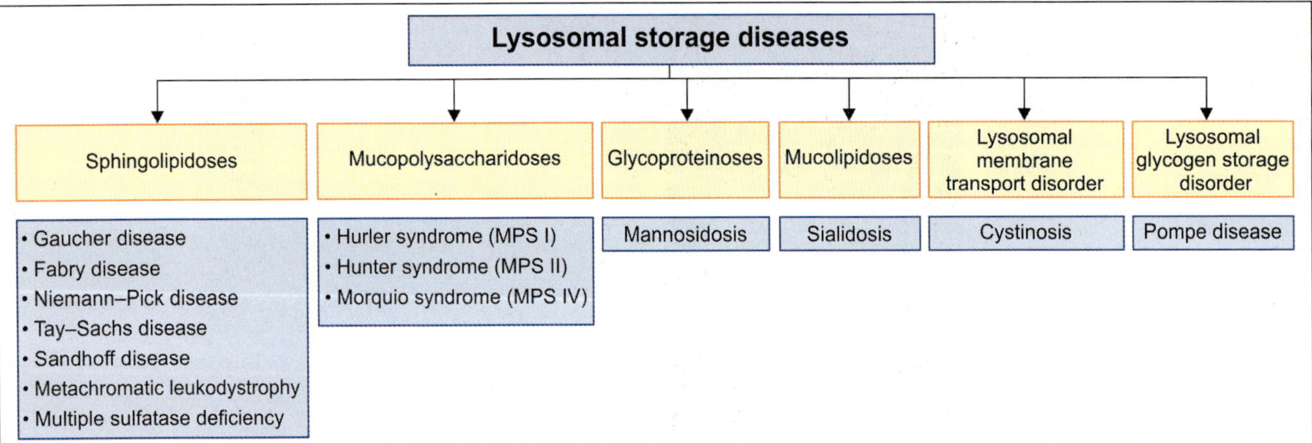

(MPS: mucopolysaccharidoses)

FLOWCHART 5: Classification of lysosomal storage disorders with selected examples.

LYSOSOMAL STORAGE DISORDERS

- Lysosomes are membrane bound organelles in the cytoplasm which contain enzymes that degrade macromolecules.
- The complex macromolecules such as mucopolysaccharides, glycolipids, and glycoproteins are delivered to the lysosome, where they undergo sequential modification by a series of hydrolases.
- LSDs occur when one or more of the hydrolytic enzymes are deficient or when the essential lysosomal transporters, receptors, cofactors, or protective proteins are lacking or defective.
- More than 50 different LSDs are identified. Classification of LSDs with selected examples is shown in the **Flowchart 5**.
- LSDs may present at different ages, from infancy to adulthood.
- They should be suspected in patients presenting with neurologic, renal, or muscular degeneration and/or unexplained organomegaly, cardiomyopathy, or skeletal dysplasias.
- The clinical features are disease specific (**Table 7**).
- Inheritance pattern of most of LSDs is autosomal recessive except Fabry, Hunter, and Danon diseases which show X-linked inheritance.
- Enzyme assays or genetic testing can be used to make a definitive diagnosis.
- Treatment strategies include enzyme replacement therapy and substrate reduction. Selected enzyme replacement therapies for various LSDs are shown in **Table 8**.

INDIAN SCENARIO

- About 2,000 cases of LSDs were reported from different studies in India. The burden of these disorders is predicted to be high in India because of the large population, coupled with the practice of consanguineous marriages. Gaucher disease is the most common LSD seen in Indian population, followed by mucopolysaccharidosis.

TABLE 8: Enzyme replacement therapy for selected lysosomal storage disorders approved by FDA.

	Enzyme replacement therapy
Gaucher disease	Recombinant glucocerebrosidase • Imiglucerase • Velaglucerase alpha • Taliglucerase alpha
MPS I	Recombinant human alpha-L-iduronidase • Laronidase
MPS II	Recombinant human iduronate sulfatase • Idursulfase
MPS IV	Recombinant human N-acetylgalactosamine-6-sulfatase • Elosulfase alpha
MPS VI	Recombinant human N-acetylgalactosamine-4-sulfatase • Galsulfase
MPS VII	Recombinant human beta-glucuronidase • Vestronidase alpha
Pompe disease	Recombinant human acid alpha-glucosidase • Alglucosidase alpha
Fabry disease	Recombinant human alpha-galactosidase A • Agalsidase alpha • Agalsidase beta

(FDA: Food and Drug Administration; MPS: mucopolysaccharidoses)

Let us wrap up this chapter with a case vignette on mucopolysaccharidoses (MPS).

CASE VIGNETTE 3

A 2-year-old girl child, born out of consanguineous marriage, was referred for evaluation of short stature and was diagnosed to have MPS type 1 (**Fig. 3**).

TABLE 7 Selected lysosomal storage disorders.

Disorder	Enzyme deficiency	Stored material	Clinical types (onset)	Clinical presentation			
				Neurologic	Visceromegaly (liver and spleen enlargement)	Skeletal dysplasia	Ophthalmologic
Mucopolysaccharidoses (MPS)							
Hurler syndrome (MPS I)	α-L-iduronidase	• Dermatan sulfate • Heparan sulfate	• Infantile • Intermediate	Cognitive degeneration	+++	++++	Corneal clouding
Hunter syndrome (MPS II)	Iduronate sulfatase	• Dermatan sulfate • Heparan sulfate	• Severe infantile • Mild juvenile	Cognitive degeneration	+++	++++	Retinal degeneration No corneal clouding
Sphingolipidoses							
Gaucher disease	Acid β-glucosidase	Glucosylceramide	Type 1	None	++++	++++	None
			Type 2	++++	+++	+	Eye movements
			Type 3	++	++++	++++	Eye movements
Fabry disease	α-galactosidase A	Globotriaosylceramide	Childhood	Painful acroparesthesias	None	None	Corneal dystrophy, vascular lesions
Niemann–Pick disease A and B	Sphingomyelinase	Sphingomyelin	• Neuronopathic, type A • Non-neuronopathic, type B	• Cognitive degeneration • Seizures	++++	None	Macular degeneration
Tay–Sachs disease	β-hexosaminidase A	GM_2 gangliosides	• Infantile • Juvenile	• Cognitive degeneration • Seizures	None	None	Cherry red spot in infantile form
Sandhoff disease	β-hexosaminidase A and B	GM_2 gangliosides	Infantile	• Cognitive degeneration • Seizures	++	±	Cherry red spot
Metachromatic leukodystrophy	Arylsulfatase A	Cerebroside sulfate	• Infantile • Juvenile • Adult	• Cognitive degeneration • Dementia • Psychosis in adults	None	None	Optic atrophy

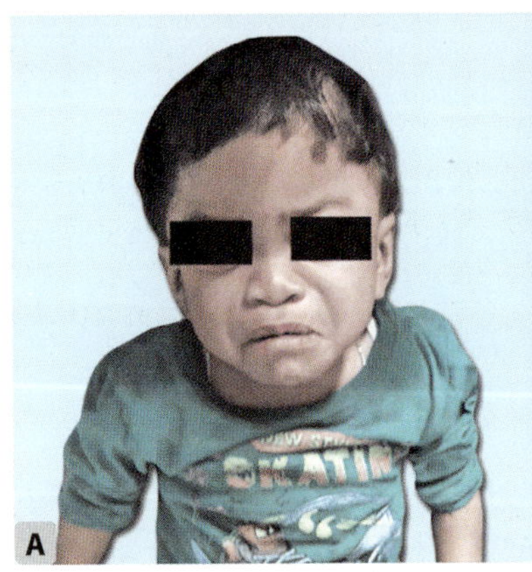

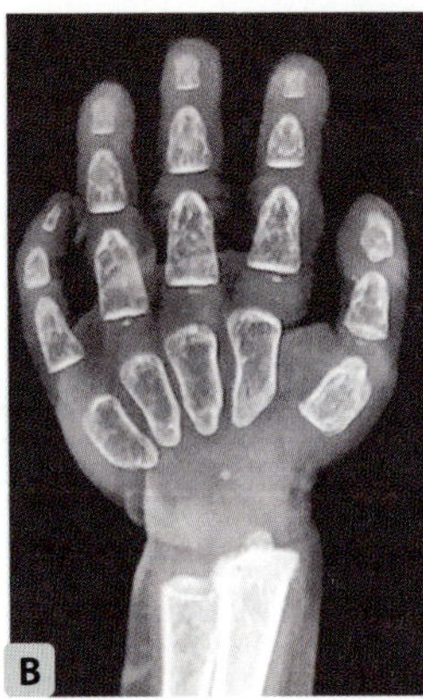

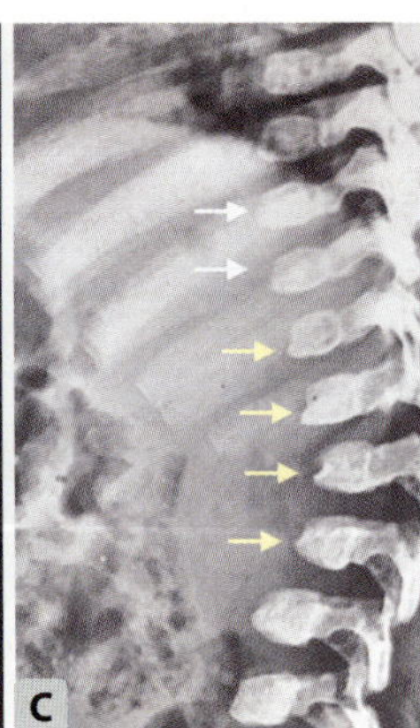

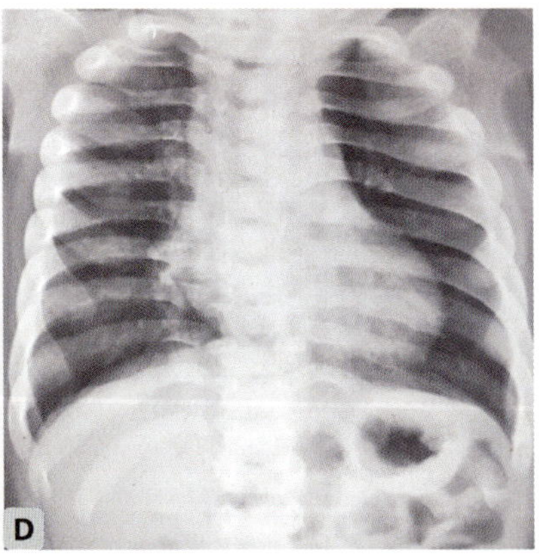

FIGURES 3 A to D: A case of mucopolysaccharidoses (MPS) type 1. **(A)** Coarse facies; **(B)** X-ray of hand showing bullet-shaped phalanges; **(C)** X-ray of spine showing anterior beaking of the vertebra (yellow arrows) and flat and rounded vertebral bodies (white arrows); **(D)** X-ray of chest showing paddle-shaped (oar-shaped) ribs.

RECOMMENDED READINGS

1. Jameson JL, Fauci AS, Kasper DL, Hauser SL, Longo DL, Loscalzo J. Harrison's Principles of Internal Medicine, 20th edition. New York: The McGraw-Hill Companies, Inc.; 2018.
2. Goldman L, Schafer A. Goldman-Cecil Medicine, 26th edition. Philadelphia, PA: Elsevier Health Sciences; 2019.
3. Feather A, Randall D, Waterhouse M. Kumar and Clark's Clinical Medicine, 10th edition. Edinburgh: Elsevier Health Sciences; 2020.
4. Firth J, Conlon C, Cox T. Oxford Textbook of Medicine, 6th edition. Oxford: Oxford University Press; 2020.
5. Bijarnia-Mahay S, Verma IC. Inborn Errors of Metabolism in India-Where We are At! Indian J Pediatr. 2019;86(10):875-6.
6. Shah I, Tolani D, Shetty NS, Karkare V. Prevalence and clinical profile of glycogen storage diseases in children from Western India. Clin Exp Hepatol. 2020;6(1): 9-12.
7. Koshy A, Ramaswamy K, Correa M, Rekha S. Glycogen storage disease: report of 17 cases from southern India. Indian J Gastroenterol. 2006;25(4):182-4.
8. ICMR Task Force on Inherited Metabolic Disorders. High Risk Stratified Neonatal Screening. Indian J Pediatr. 2018;85(12):1050-4.
9. Gupta N, Aggarwal B, Kabra M. Lysosomal Storage Disorders in India: A Mini Review. J Mucopolysaccharidosis and Rare Dis. 2018;4(1):1-6.
10. Sheth J, Mistri M, Sheth F, Shah R, Bavdekar A, Godbole K, et al. Burden of Lysosomal Storage Disorders in India: Experience of 387 Affected Children from a Single Diagnostic Facility. JIMD Rep. 2013;12:51-63.

CHAPTER
18

Common Metabolic Disorders: Amyloidosis, Porphyria, and Wilson's Disease

Uddalak Chakraborty, Tarun Kumar Paria

ABSTRACT

Amyloidosis, porphyria, and Wilson's disease (WD) are common metabolic disorders which are relatively neglected by the students. The authors have tried to provide a comprehensive outlook on these three conditions in this chapter. This chapter methodically makes an overview of the key aspects of all three conditions with reference to incidence, pathogenesis, clinical features, diagnosis, and treatment. These conditions have both local and systemic manifestations and with emergence of multiple specialties still need investigations on the diverse causes, as well as exploration of new therapeutic targets and available therapies.

"A correct diagnosis is three-fourths the remedy"

—Mahatma Gandhi

AMYLOIDOSIS

INTRODUCTION

Amyloidosis is a rare disorder in which there is deposition of insoluble fibrils composed of low molecular weight subunits of a variety of proteins in the extracellular tissues, eventually leading to organ dysfunction and death. These deposits may lead to a wide range of clinical manifestations depending upon the type, site, and amount of deposition. Determination of the underlying protein is essential to prognosticate and treat amyloidosis.

Chemical composition: The amyloid is 85–95% composed of the fibrillar protein. The amyloid P component is a glycoprotein that comprises 5–15% of the amyloid deposit, and contributes to its stability. The fibrillogenesis is enhanced by various glycosaminoglycans (GAGs), and the amyloid enhancing factor.

Epidemiology: About 0.5–1% autopsies and 2–3% of renal biopsies globally are suggestive of amyloidosis.

GENETICS

About 30 human and 10 animal protein precursors of amyloid fibrils are now known. Several types of familial amyloidosis have been linked to missense mutations of the precursor proteins. Genetic variants resulting in fibrillogenesis:

- Polymorphism of cofactors (e.g., apolipoprotein E) or subunit proteins [e.g., serum amyloid A (AA)]
- Heritable disorders that lead to accumulation of precursor proteins (e.g., presenilin mutations in familial Alzheimer disease).
- Familial disorders/autoinflammation leading to deposition of wild-type precursor protein as AA amyloidosis [e.g., pyrin and cryopyrin mutations in familial Mediterranean fever (FMF) and cryopyrin-associated periodic syndrome (CAPS), and tumor necrosis factor (TNF) receptor mutations in the TNF receptor-associated periodic syndrome (TRAPS), respectively].

PATHOGENESIS

- The primary pathogenesis of amyloid protein is the misfolding of protein that leads to its accumulation. The misfolding can be attributed to genetic mutation that codes a different amino acid altering protein conformation.
- Several factors determine the tissue deposition of amyloid:
  - Molecular configuration
  - Acidosis
  - Excess accumulation of protein
  - Specific proteolytic activity and the interaction of fibrils with GAGs and advanced glycation end products

Amyloid proteins have a high tendency to aggregate without a barrier to unfolding. Some fragmentation may expose the surface of growing fibrils and accelerate aggregation leading to cell-to-cell transmission, and disruption of the tissue architecture with subsequent organ failure.

CLASSIFICATION

Amyloidosis may be localized or systemic. Localized amyloid deposits may be seen in:

- Medullary carcinoma thyroid
- Alzheimer's disease
- Diabetes mellitus
- Prion diseases

Generalized/systemic amyloidosis may be again classified into primary amyloidosis and secondary amyloidosis. A comprehensive classification of amyloidosis is given in **Table 1**.

Primary amyloidosis/AL amyloidosis:

- The fibrils are derived from various fragments of monoclonal light chains. Most common light chains in AL amyloidosis is λ.
- Seen in plasma cell disorders (e.g., multiple myeloma) in which monoclonal immunoglobulin is detected in serum or urine.

Secondary/reactive/amyloid a amyloidosis:

- Associated with chronic inflammation (bronchiectasis, rheumatoid arthritis, tuberculosis etc.) malignancies (Hodgkin's lymphoma, renal cell carcinoma etc.)
- Most common cause of secondary amyloidosis is rheumatoid arthritis; however, in India, tuberculosis is considered to be the most common cause.
- Usually, the latent period between onset of inflammation and secondary amyloidosis is around 15–20 years. Increased production of interleukins (IL-1, IL-6) leads to increased production of serum amyloid associated (SAA) protein in secondary amyloidosis.

Dialysis-related amyloidosis: Accumulation of β2-microglobulin in patients on long-term hemodialysis leads to musculoskeletal symptoms.

Senile amyloidosis: It is deposition of normal transthyretin in tissues. Involvement of myocardium is more compared to renal involvement. Carpal tunnel syndrome is common.

Familial amyloidosis: Heredofamilial disorders with localized or systemic deposition of amyloid which may be neuropathic or nonneuropathic.

- *Familial amyloid polyneuropathy (FAP)*: Autosomal dominant inheritance due to mutated transthyretin (TTR)
- *Familial Mediterranean fever:* Autosomal recessive due to MEFV mutation leading to AA amyloidosis due to TTR accumulation

TABLE 1 Classification of amyloidosis.

Category	Associated disease	Biochemical type	Organs commonly involved
Systemic (Generalized) amyloidosis			
Primary	Plasma cell dyscrasias	AL type	Heart, bowel, skin, nerves, kidney
Secondary (Reactive)	Chronic inflammation, cancers	AA type	Liver, spleen, kidneys, adrenals
Hemodialysis-associated	Chronic renal failure	Aβ_2M	Synovium, joints, tendon sheaths
Heredofamilial			
• Hereditary polyneuropathies	–	ATTR	Peripheral and autonomic nerves, heart
• Familial Mediterranean fever	–	AA type	Liver, spleen, kidneys, adrenals
• Rare hereditary forms	–	AApoAI, AGel, ALys, AFib, ACys	Systemic amyloidosis
Localized amyloidosis			
Senile cardiac	Senility	ATTR	Heart
Senile cerebral	Alzheimer's, transmissible encephalopathy	Aβ, APrP	Cerebral vessels, plaques, neurofibrillary tangles
Endocrine	Medullary carcinoma Type 2 diabetes mellitus	Procalcitonin Proinsulin	Thyroid Islets of Langerhans
Tumor-forming	Lungs, larynx, skin, urinary bladder, tongue, eye	AL	Respective anatomic location

(AL: amyloid light chain; AA: amyloid-associated protein; Aβ_2M: amyloid β_2-microglobulin; ATTR: amyloid transthyretin; APrP: amyloid of prion proteins; Aβ: β-amyloid protein)

CLINICAL FEATURES

The organ involvement and clinical features of amyloidosis have been elaborated in **Table 2** and shown in **Figures 1** and **2**.

DIAGNOSIS

- Complete blood count may reveal reduced hemoglobin, plasma cells in AL amyloidosis; high ESR, increased globulin fraction, and high serum calcium with normal alkaline phosphatase may be seen.
- Bence Jones protein may be seen in a sample of urine in absence of a positive dipstick test for albumin.
- Echocardiography may show speckled appearance of myocardium (**Fig. 3**).
- Computed tomography/magnetic resonance imaging (CT/MRI) to detect musculoskeletal lesions; supraspinatus with or without subscapularis tendon thickening may be seen in dialysis-related amyloidosis (DRA).
- *Tissue biopsy*: Abdominal fat pad aspirate is now considered the most preferable investigation for a confirmatory diagnosis. Rectal biopsy and tongue biopsy are much less preferred techniques. Renal biopsy is the procedure of choice in case of renal involvement.
- *Stains for amyloid*:
  - Hematoxylin and eosin (H&E): Hyaline pink color
  - Periodic acid Schiff: Magenta (amyloid is diastase resistant)
  - Congo red: Salmon pink in light microscopy, apple green birefringence in polarized light
  - Methyl violet: Metachromatic
  - Thioflavin S and T: Immunofluorescent
  - Gross staining: Surface of tissue (mahogany brown color) painted with Lugol's iodine and sulfuric acid added will give blue color in amyloidosis.
- *Light microscopy*: Diffuse extracellular deposits of amorphous hyaline pink material in H&E (**Fig. 4 A**). Congo red stain gives a salmon pink color (**Fig. 4 B**).
- Polarized microscopy reveals apple green birefringence with Congo red stain (**Fig. 4 C**).
- Immunofluorescence is negative for immunoglobulins and complements in secondary amyloidosis. However, lambda and kappa chains are visible in AL amyloidosis (**Figs. 4 D** and **E**).
- Electron microscopy reveals nonbranching fibrils of indefinite length of 7.5–10 nm in diameter (**Fig. 4 F**).

TREATMENT

AL amyloidosis: Cytotoxic therapy or bone marrow transplant. Cytotoxic therapies include:

- Melphalan with dexamethasone
- Bortezomib and bendamustine may be combined with cyclophosphamide or melphalan along with dexamethasone.
- Thalidomide/pomalidomide/lenalidomide along with dexamethasone
- New drugs like daratumumab (anti-CD38), ixazomib, and carfilzomib are still being used on experimental basis.

Intensive chemotherapy with autologous stem cell transplant is more effective.

- *AA amyloidosis*: Aim is to suppress production of SAA.
  - Alkylating agents like chlorambucil, cyclophosphamide for rheumatological diseases

TABLE 2 Clinical features and organ involvement in amyloidosis.

Organ	Clinical features
Renal	Nephrotic syndrome, symptomatic/asymptomatic proteinuria, hematuria (microscopic/frank), chronic renal failure, tubular dysfunction, and renomegaly
Endocrine	Adrenal gland dysfunction, hypothyroidism, and panhypopituitarism
Cardiovascular	• Arrhythmias, restrictive cardiomyopathy, systolic/diastolic dysfunction, heart failure, infarction, and angina/infarction • Subendocardium affected most commonly
Nervous system	• Sensory motor polyneuropathy with or without autonomic neuropathy. Peripheral nerve compression, e.g., carpal tunnel syndrome. • Central nervous system involvement such as dementia, encephalopathy, and stroke more common in hereditary amyloidosis
Musculoskeletal	• Pseudohypertrophy of muscles, macroglossia (**Fig. 1**) (common in AL amyloid), and arthropathy • Shoulder pad sign—enlarged anterior shoulder, characteristic finding of AL amyloidosis, spondyloarthropathy, cauda equina syndrome, and simple bone cysts
Gastrointestinal	Hepatosplenomegaly, bleeding (vascular fragility), gastroparesis, dysmotility, malabsorption, and cirrhosis of liver Characteristic involvement: • Sago spleen (follicles affected) • Lardaceous spleen (sinusoidal infiltration with large geographic map like areas) • Space of Disse affected in liver, leading to pressure atrophy of hepatocytes
Respiratory	Pleural effusion, pulmonary hypertension
Hematological	Bleeding diathesis (factor X deficit due to binding of amyloid fibrils in liver and spleen), dysfunctional coagulation, thrombocytopenia, anemia, and acquired von Willebrand disease
Dermatological	Waxy thickening, easy bruising, subcutaneous nodules, and periorbital purpura (raccoon eyes) (**Fig. 2**)

- Podophyllotoxin with azathioprine, chlorambucil, and cyclophosphamide may be used.
- Tumor necrosis factor-alpha antagonists may be helpful.
- Odo-deoxydoxorubicin to bind and disrupt fibrils
- Tafamidis, diflunisal to stabilize TTR in hereditary amyloidosis
- Colchicine 1–2 mg/day in FMF

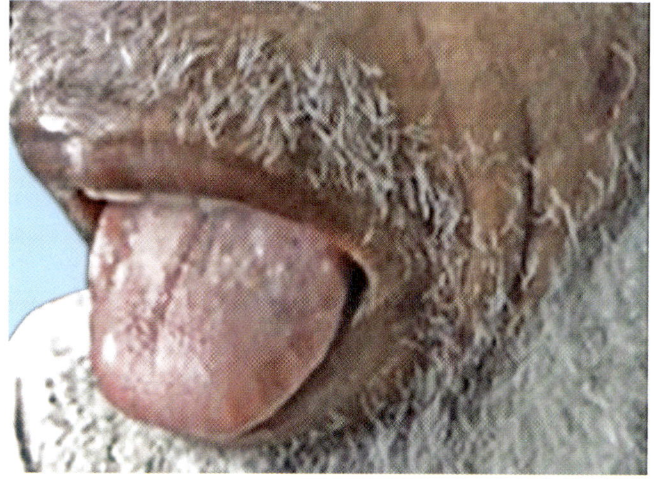

FIGURE 1: Macroglossia in AL amyloidosis (light chain amyloidosis).

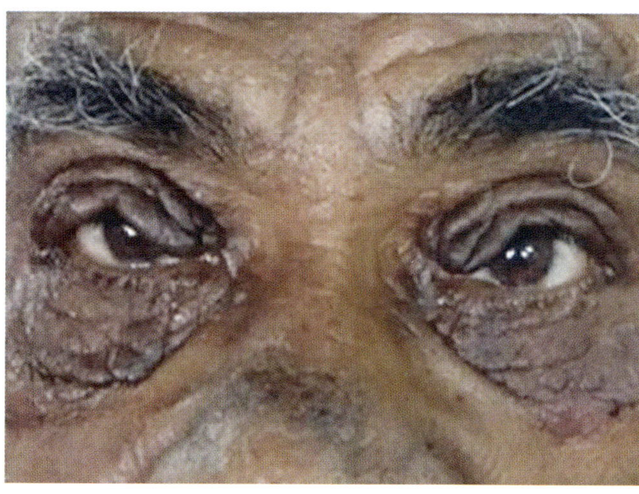

FIGURE 2: Raccoon eyes in AL amyloidosis (light chain amyloidosis).

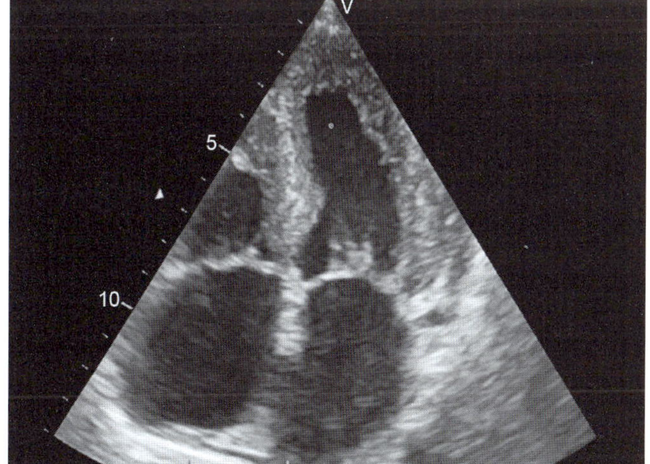

FIGURE 3: Echocardiography showing speckled appearance of interventricular septum in amyloidosis.

Source: Nandakumar S, Chandrasekharan R, Vijayakumar M, Thachathodiyl R. Speckle tracking as an adjunctive echocardiographic technique for differentiating cardiac amyloidosis from hypertrophic cardiomyopathy: A case study. J Indian Acad Echocardiogr Cardiovasc Imaging. 2017;1:163-6.

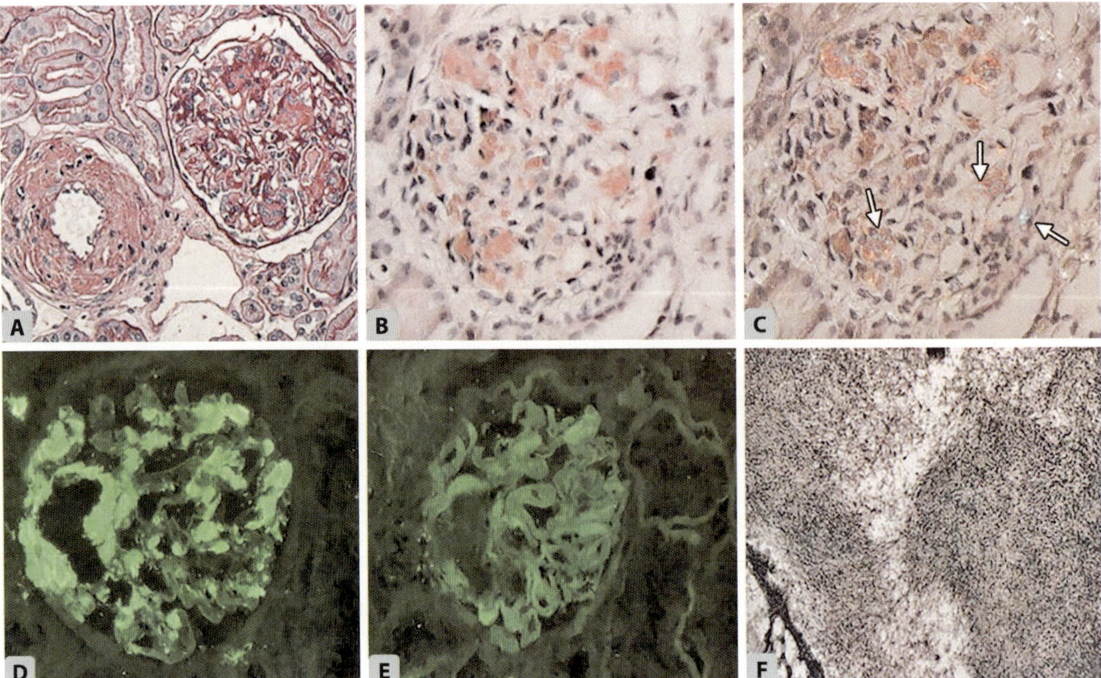

FIGURES 4 A to F: (A) Renal biopsy showing light microscopy findings in AL amyloidosis with H&E stain, **(B)** Congo red stain; **(C)** polarized microscopy showing apple green birefringence with congo red stain; **(D)** immunofluorescence microscopy showing deposition of lambda chains; **(E)**, weak reactivity of kappa chains; and **(F)** electron microscopy demonstrating amyloid fibrils.

Source: Dember LM. Amyloidosis-associated kidney disease. J Am Soc Nephrol. 2006;17(12):3458-71.

PROGNOSIS

The median survival of untreated primary amyloidosis is 6 months, and 5-year survival of secondary amyloidosis is 43%. The most common cause of death in primary amyloidosis is due to cardiac complications, while in secondary amyloidosis renal involvement leads to mortality.

PORPHYRIA

INTRODUCTION

The porphyrias encompass a broad-spectrum disorder of heme biosynthesis which involves an inherited or acquired defect (**Flowchart 1**). The biosynthesis of heme takes place in the mitochondria as well as cytosol. Although heme synthesis occurs in almost every human cell except mature erythrocytes, it is most abundantly produced in the red blood cells for hemoglobin synthesis and the hepatic parenchymal cells for synthesis of cytochromes and hemoproteins. Major heme-containing proteins include hemoglobin, myoglobin, cytochrome P450, cytochrome C, catalase, tryptophan pyrrolase, and nitric oxide synthase. Porphyria is often classified depending on site of accumulation of heme precursors such as hepatic or erythropoietic porphyria. Accumulation of the heme precursors is associated with characteristic clinical features such as neurovisceral involvement, cutaneous lesions, or both. The hepatic porphyrias occur due to hepatic overproduction of the precursors and the symptoms are due to involvement of the nervous system. Cutaneous porphyrias occur due to overproduction of photosensitizing precursors by the liver or bone marrow. However, a classification as acute porphyria, cutaneous porphyria, and rare recessive porphyria is more practical and easier than are other classifications.

Indian perspective: The prevalence of porphyria in India is around 1 in 4.4 million with predominance in some districts and communities of Rajasthan. Female predilection of 2:1 is usually observed in porphyria.

CLASSIFICATION

The porphyrias may be broadly classified into hepatic porphyrias and erythropoietic porphyrias (**Table 3**).

The characteristic features of the different porphyrias have been compared in **Table 4**.

GENETICS

About 20% porphyrias are sporadic in nature. All porphyrias are autosomal dominant, except:

- X-linked protoporphyria (XLP)—X-linked recessive
- Congenital erythropoietic porphyria (CEP) —autosomal recessive
- Aminolevulinic acid (ALA) dehydratase deficient porphyria (ADP) —autosomal recessive
- Erythropoietic protoporphyria (EP)—autosomal recessive

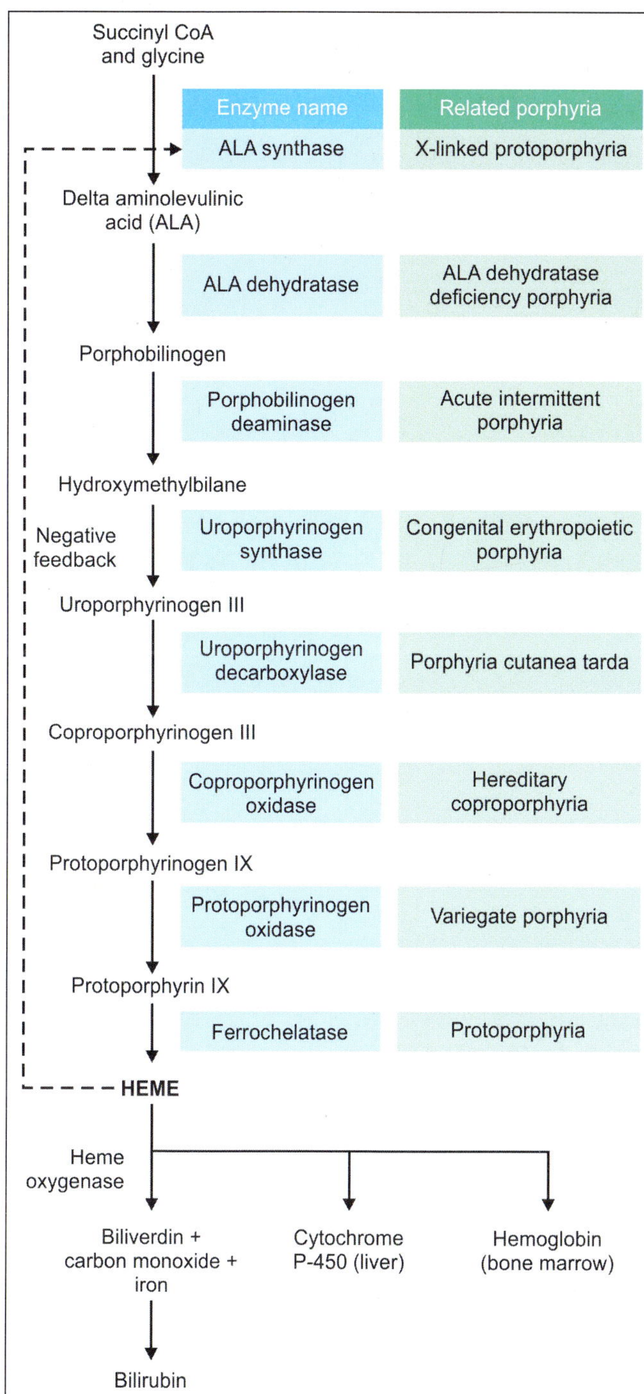

FLOWCHART 1: Biosynthesis of heme.

Source: Bissell DM, Anderson KE, Bonkovsky HL. Porphyria. N Eng J Med., 2017;377(9):86272.

Pearls:

- Enzyme defect early in the pathway of heme biosynthesis leading to accumulation of ALA and porphobilinogen (PBG) leads to predominant neurovisceral symptoms.
- Enzyme defect late in the pathway of heme biosynthesis leading to accumulation of porphyrins leads to predominant cutaneous symptoms.
- Acute porphyrias—acute intermittent porphyria (AIP), variegate porphyria (VP), hereditary coproporphyria (HCP)

TABLE 3 Classification of porphyrias.

Hepatic	Erythropietic
• ALA dehydratase deficient porphyria (ADP) • Acute intermittent porphyria • Porphyria cutanea tarda (PCT) • Hereditary coproporphyria (HCP) • Variegate porphyria (VP)	• Congenital erythropoietic porphyria • Erythropoietic porphyria • X-linked protoporphyria

(ALA: aminolevulinic acid)

- *Most common acute porphyria*: AIP
- *Most common porphyria*: Porphyria cutanea tarda (PCT)
- *Most common sporadic porphyria*: PCT
- *Most common porphyria in children*: EP

INDIVIDUAL SUBTYPES

Acute intermittent porphyria:

- Autosomal dominant porphyria due to defect in PBG deaminase/hydroxymethylbilane (HMB) synthase
- Disease manifestation is more common after puberty, with majority presenting in the age group of 20–40 years. Most of the patients experience few intermittent acute attacks while some may have a severe chronic illness.
- Acute attacks of porphyria may be triggered by multiple factors (**Box 1**).
- Pathogenesis includes accumulation of precursor of porphyrins in the tissues and circulation. ALA excess leads to neurotoxicity via multiple mechanisms.
- Clinical features include neurovisceral symptoms.
  - Most common symptom is recurrent attacks of poorly localized acute abdominal pain often associated with passage of port-wine-colored urine and may or may not be accompanied with neuropsychiatric and autonomic manifestations. Symptoms may mimic acute to subacute intestinal obstruction.
  - Alteration of urine color to dark red on exposure to light is a characteristic finding.
  - Neuropsychiatric symptoms include irritability, agitation, anxiety, depression, disorientation, and hallucination.
  - Predominantly symmetrical pure motor axonal neuropathy commonly affecting proximal portion of the limbs with or without encephalopathy may be seen. Seventh, tenth, and eleventh cranial nerves may be rarely involved. Symptoms may mimic acute inflammatory demyelinating polyradiculoneuropathy and may be associated with sphincter dysfunction, deglutition difficulties, and respiratory failure. Seizures secondary to hypertension, electrolyte dysfunction, or due to the disease per se may be seen. Rarely, sensory manifestations such as paresthesia, numbness, or neuropathic pain may be complained of. Autonomic dysfunction in the form of postural hypotension, resting tachycardia, and hypertension may be observed in some cases. Occasionally, acute

TABLE 4 Characteristic features and presentations of porphyria.

Disease (abbreviation)	Enzyme (abbreviation)	Mutations of this enzyme	Presentation	Classifications			
				Hepatic	Erythropoietic	Acute/ Neurologic	Cutaneous
δ-aminolevulinic acid dehydratase porphyria (ADP)	δ-aminolevulinic acid dehydratase (ALAD)	Homozygous	Mostly postpuberty	X	X*	X	
Acute intermittent porphyria (AIP)	Porphobilinogen deaminase (PBGD)	Heterozygous	Postpuberty	X		X	
Homozygous AIP		Homozygous	Childhood	X	X	X	
Congenital erythropoietic porphyria (CEP)	Uroporphyrinogen III synthase (UROS)	Homozygous	In utero or infancy		X		X
Porphyria cutanea tarda (PCT)L type 1	Uroporphyrinogen decarboxylase (UROD)	None	Adults	X			X
PCT type 2[†]		Heterozygous	Adults	X			
PCT type 3		None	Adults	X			
Hereditary copro-porphyria (HCP)	Coproporphyrino-gen oxidase (CPO)	Heterozygous	Postpuberty	X		X	X
Homozygous HCP		Homozygous	Childhood	X	X	X	X
Variegate porphyria (VP)	Protoporphyrino-gen oxidase (PPO)	Heterozygous	Postpuberty	X		X	X
Homozygous VP		Homozygous	Childhood	X	X	X	X
Erythropoietic protoporphyria (EPP)	Ferrochelatase (FECH)	Heterozygous (heteroallelic with low expression normal allele) or homozygous	Childhood		X		X
X-linked protoporphyria (XLP)	δ-Aminolevulinate synthase 2 (ALAS2)	X-linked	Childhood		X		X

*ADP and HEP are considered primarily hepatic porphyrias, but substantial increase in erythrocyte zinc protoporphyrin suggests an erythropoietic component.

† PCT is due to inhibition of hepatic UROD. Autosomal dominant inheritance of a partial deficiency of UROD is a predisposing factor in cases defined as familial (type 2) PCT.

Source: Anderson KE, Lee C, Balwani M, Desnick RJ. (2016). The Porphyrias [online].

BOX 1 Factors precipitating acute attack of porphyria.

- Drugs-barbiturates and estrogens (may be safe in replacement doses), progesterones, sulfonamides, methyldopa, danazol, diazepam, phenytoin, carbamazepine, sulfonylureas, chloramphenicol, tetracyclines, and some antihistamines
- Fasting
- Smoking
- Alcohol
- Substance misuse—particularly marijuana, ecstasy, amphetamines, and cocaine
- Infection
- Emotional and physical stress
- Cyclic factors—premenstrual attacks are common

Source: Thadani H, Deacon A, Peter T. Diagnosis and management of porphyria. BMJ. 2000;320(7250):1647-51.

life-threatening crises may arise. Rare complications include cardiac arrhythmias and rhabdomyolysis.

- Prognosis is good with therapy. Long-term sequelae such as hypertension, chronic kidney disease, hepatocellular carcinoma, and chronic pain syndrome may be seen.

Porphyria cutanea tarda:

- Autosomal recessive porphyria due to defect in uroporphyrinogen decarboxylase. Type 1 is sporadic while familial PCT includes type 2 and 3.
- Clinical features include blistering photosensitive skin rash, commonly on dorsum of hands which heals with crusting, scar, and atrophy (**Fig. 5**). Forearms, face, and legs may also be involved. Friable skin with papules and hypertrichosis of face is fairly common.

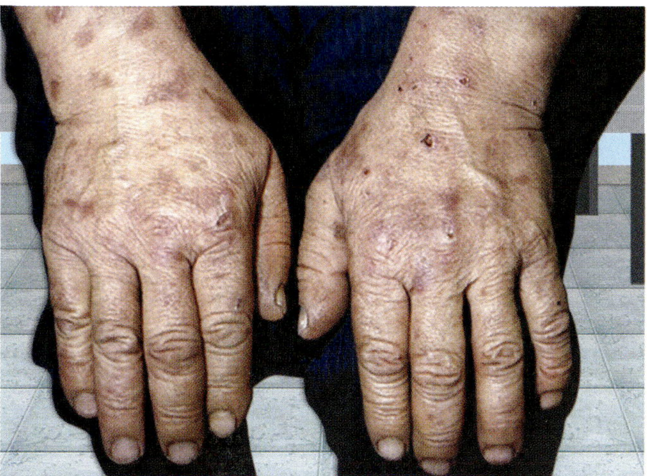

FIGURE 5: Photosensitive lesions of porphyria cutanea tarda (PCT) on dorsum of hand.

Source: Healthline (2020). Everything You Should Know About Porphyria Cutanea Tarda [online].

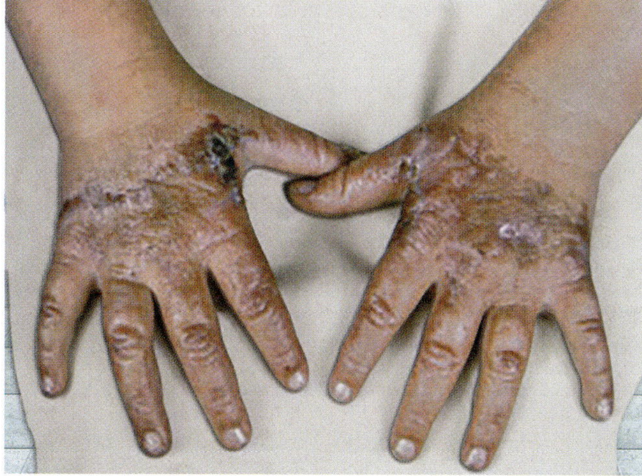

FIGURE 6: Nonblistering rash with erythema in erythropoietic protoporphyria (EPT).

Source: DermNet NZ [online].

- Precipitated by hepatitis C, HIV, alcohol, hemochromatosis, and drugs (digoxin, iron, and hexachlorobenzene)

Congenital erythropoietic porphyria/Gunther disease:
- Autosomal recessive porphyria due to deficient uroporphyrinogen III synthase
- Cutaneous photosensitivity early in infancy, bullous eruptions, lichenification, focal hypo-/hyperpigmentation, and hypertrichosis of face may occur.
- Hemolysis may be seen. Nonimmune hydrops and still birth may occur sometimes.

Erythropoietic protoporphyria:
- Autosomal recessive inheritance due to partial deficit of ferrochelatase
- Nonblistering photosensitivity with eczema, lichenification, and eczema is common feature (**Fig. 6**).
- Characteristic increase in erythrocyte protoporphyrin not complexed with zinc is seen.

X-linked protoporphyria:
- Gain of function mutation of ALA synthase leading to increased protoporphyrin synthesis
- Loss of function mutation of ALA synthase associated with X-linked sideroblastic anemia

Hereditary coproporphyria:
- Autosomal dominant porphyria due to defective activity of coproporphyrinogen oxidase
- Acute attacks of neurovisceral symptoms with or without cutaneous photosensitivity may be seen.

Variegate porphyria:
- Autosomal dominant porphyria due to deficiency of protoporphyrinogen oxidase
- Both acute neurovisceral crises and photosensitivity may coexist.

ALA dehydratase deficient porphyria/plumboporphyria:
- Severe deficit of ALA dehydratase
- Neuropathy and abdominal pain are common manifestations.
- Symptoms may mimic lead toxicity.

DIAGNOSIS

Acute attacks of porphyria are usually associated with raised urinary excretion of ALA and PBG, which may be detected from a fresh urine sample, protected from light. Darkening of urine on standing occurs due to polymerization of PBG to porphyrins and other pigments. Concentrations of urinary PBG and ALA may be normal in between attacks. The diagnosis may be based on heme precursors (**Table 5**).
- Acute intermittent porphyria, VP, and HCP can be differentiated by analysis of fecal porphyrins. The diagnosis of AIP can be confirmed by reduced RBC HMB synthase activity provided routine hematological indices are normal. Ehrlich test may be positive in AIP and qualitative estimation of PBG can be done by Watson-Schwartz test. Genetic analysis for mutation has limited role.
- Red fluorescence on illumination of tissue and blood with long ultraviolet rays is suggestive of porphyria. Absorption band at 400 nm (Soret band) is characteristic of porphyrin. Plasma fluorescence peak at neutral pH is characteristic of VP.
- Erythropoietic protoporphyria is diagnosed by erythrocyte free protoporphyrin. Analysis of urine and feces may help.

The first-line investigations are given in **Figure 7**.

TABLE 5 Heme precursors in urine and stool, found in different porphyrias.

Type of porphyria	Urine concentration		Porphyrins in feces	Porphyrin in erythrocytes
	Prophobilinogen and aminolevulinic acid	Porphyrins		
Plumboporphyria*	Aminolevulinic acid	Coproporphyrinogen III	Not increased	Zinc protoporphyrin
Acute intermittent porphyria	Porphobilinogen > aminolevulinic acid	Porphyrin mainly from porphobilinogen	Normal, occasionally slight increase (coproporphyrinogen, protoporphyrin)	Not increased
Congenital erythropoietic porphyria	Not increased	Uroporphyrinogen I > coproporphyrinogen I	Coproporphyrinogen I	Zinc protoporphyrin, coproporphyrinogen, uroporphyrinogen
Porphyria cutanea tarda	Not increased	Uroporphyrinogen > heptacarboxylate	Isocoproporphyrinogen, heptacarboxylate	Not increased
Hereditary coproporphyria	Porphobilinogen > aminolevulinic acid	Coproporphyrinogen III (porphyrin mainly from porphobilinogen)	Coproporphyrinogen III	Not increased
Variegate porphyria	Porphobilinogen > aminolevulinic acid	Coproporphyrinogen III (porphyrin mainly from porphobilinogen)	Protoporphyrin IX > coproporphyrinogen III and porphyrin X	Not increased
Erythropoietic protoporphyria	Not increased	Not increased	Protoporphyrin increased or decreased	Protoporphyrin

* Lead poisoning produces an identical overproduction pattern.

Source: Thadani H, Deacon A, Peter T. Diagnosis and management of porphyria. BMJ. 2000;320(7250):1647-51.

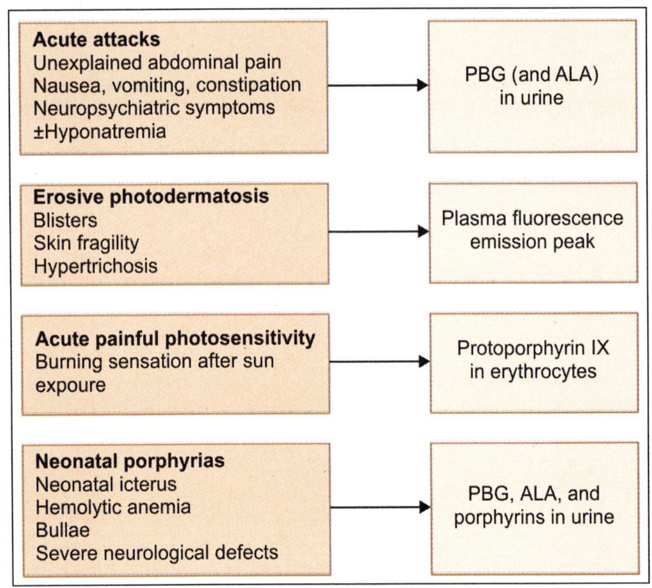

(ALA: aminolevulinic acid; PBG: porphobilinogen)

FIGURE 7: First-line investigations in porphyria.

Source: Puy H, Gouya L, Deybach JC. Porphyrias. Lancet, 2010;375(9718): 924-37.

MANAGEMENT

The comprehensive management of porphyrias has been outlined in **Table 6**.

- *Acute attacks*: About 1% of porphyria may be lethal. Nonporphyrogenic drugs should be prescribed. For severe pain, opiates (pethidine and morphine) are the drug of choice. Chlorpromazine may be added to promote sleep. Sympathetic overactivity may be alleviated with propranolol.
- Convulsions may be precipitated by hyponatremia, which should be duly corrected by fluid restriction. Convulsions are notoriously difficult to manage in porphyria as all commonly used anticonvulsant agents are porphyrogenic. Gabapentin and vigabatrin are now the treatment of choice for these patients.
- Oral and intravenous glucose along with heme arginate are the mainstay of treatment. Dextrose (10%) may be given for mild attacks with pending administration of heme arginate. Heme arginate should be given over 15 minutes preferably through a central venous line at an early stage, as it cannot reverse an established neuropathy.
- Tin protoporphyrin, an inhibitor of heme oxygenase may prolong remission when coadministered with heme arginate. Prophylactic heme arginate may prevent recurrent attacks.
- Induction of a chemical menopause with luteinizing hormone-releasing hormone agonists has been used with some success.
- Attacks may occur during pregnancy, with high estrogen concentrations. The patient should avoid pregnancy until she has been in remission for at least 2 years. ALA can cross the placenta and is possibly toxic to the fetal brain. Acute attacks during pregnancy have been successfully treated with heme arginase.
- The cutaneous porphyrias are best treated by photoprotection of skin. In PCT, phlebotomy to deplete

TABLE 6 Outline of management of porphyria.

	Treatment measures
Preventive	Prescribe drugs from safe drug list; avoid alcohol, smoking and soft drugs (cannabis), dieting, and fasting; carry medical alert cards or jewelry
Specific	
• Repress heme synthesis	• Hemin* (4 mg/kg/day for 3–4 consecutive days)
• Hyponatremia and fasting	• Maintain fluid and calorie intake • *Mild case*: 2 L normal saline containing 5–10% dextrose or glucose (>200 g/day) • *Severe hyponatremia*: Infusion of 3% saline (500 mmol/L) • Correction <12 mmol/L/day
Treatment of symptoms:	
• *Autonomic neuropathy:*	
◦ Abdominal pain	• Opiates (pethidine, morphine, and diamorphine); aspirin, paracetamol, and dihydrocodeine
◦ Vomiting and sedation	• Promazine, chlorpromazine, cyclizine, and ondansetron
◦ Constipation	• Bulk laxatives, senna, and lactulose
◦ Hypertension and tachycardia	• β-blockers (propranolol, atenolol, and labetalol)
◦ Abnormal sphincter function	• Urethral catheter
◦ Arrhythmia	• β-blockers, follow-up patient in intensive care unit
• *Peripheral sensory or motor neuropathy:*	• Opiates
◦ Limb pain, back pain, or both	• Early activating physiotherapy
◦ Muscle weakness	• Follow-up patient in intensive care unit; mechanical ventilator
◦ Respiratory muscle paresis	• Sign of poor prognosis, nasogastric tube, and speech therapy
◦ Bulbar paresis (dysarthria, dysphagia, and dysphonia)	
CNS involvement:	
• Insomnia and anxiety	• Lorazepam
• Hallucinations	• Chlorpromazine
• Conscious impairment • Convulsions	• Follow-up patient in an intensive care unit; monitor and correct hyponatremia; diazepam (IV 10 mg once only), clonazepam, magnesium sulfate, gabapentin, or clonazepam if prolonged treatment is needed
Extremely severe recurrent cases	Poor quality of life; consider liver transplantation

*Human hemin stabilized with arginine (Normosang) is available worldwide, apart from in USA where lyophilized hemin is available.

(CNS: central nervous system; IV: intravenous)

Source: Puy H, Gouya L, and Deybach JC. Porphyrias. Lancet. 2010;375(9718):924-37.

excess iron stores, oral chloroquine (125 mg twice a week), and avoidance of alcohol and estrogen are all particularly helpful. In EP, administration of carotene is seldom helpful along with above measures.

WILSON'S DISEASE

INTRODUCTION

Wilson's disease or hepatolenticular degeneration is an autosomal recessive condition of copper overload, resulting from mutations in the chromosome 13q14 in the region coding for *ATP7B*. In WD, copper overload in hepatocytes is associated with excess copper being released into the circulation with accumulation in other tissues like brain, which can lead to neuropsychiatric disturbances.

EPIDEMIOLOGY

The World Health Organization (WHO) estimates that the worldwide prevalence of WD is 1/10,000–1/30,000. The disease is most frequent in Germany, Japan, and Austria; however, Costa Rica has the highest incidence. In India, no community-based prevalence studies of WD are available yet. However, WD accounts for 7.6–19.7% pediatric liver diseases. Annually 15–20 new cases are registered in tertiary neurology centers.

PATHOPHYSIOLOGY

- Compound heterozygous or less commonly homozygous mutations lead to defective binding of copper with apoceruloplasmin thus hampering formation of holoceruloplasmin, impairing secretion of copper into the bile leading to defective copper metabolism and consequent copper intoxication.

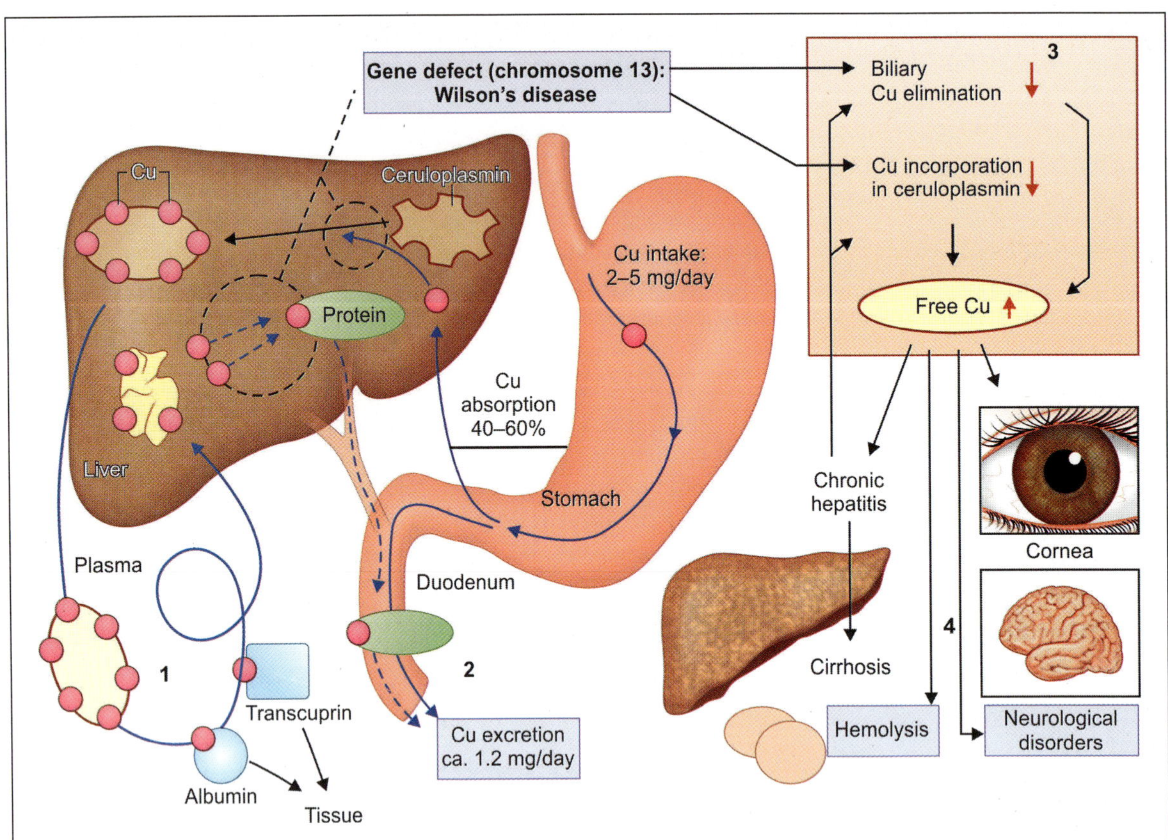

FIGURE 8: Defective copper metabolism and pathogenesis of Wilson's disease.

Source: Semela D (2013). Wilson Disease [online].

- Labile nonceruloplasmin-bound copper is taken up by all tissues via divalent metal transporter 1 (DMT1). Free copper in the bloodstream determines copper intoxication, as opposed to deposited copper in the tissues (**Fig. 8**). Free copper exerts its toxicity through:
  - Oxidative stress and lipid peroxidation of membranes, mitochondria, and DNA
  - Unregulated apoptosis leading to cell death
- Mitochondria are the most sensitive targets for copper toxicity.
- The liver is the central organ regulating copper homeostasis with the highest tissue expression of the ATP7B copper transporter. Impaired biliary excretion of copper leads to hepatic copper accumulation. Liver injury is one of the earliest and most common manifestations of WD.
- The copper concentration in brain may reach values 10-15 times higher in patients of WD compared to normal population. Long-term exposure to high copper concentrations results in damaged astrocytes, dysfunctional blood-brain barrier, and further damage of neurons and oligodendrocytes.

CLINICAL FEATURES

Clinical features of WD depend on the predominant organ involved and the disease has been diagnosed reportedly from 3 to 85 years of age. However, the disease is more commonly seen in between 12 and 20 years of age. Though copper starts to accumulate soon after birth, it usually takes at least 3 years to manifest symptoms. Hepatic presentation is common in younger age groups while neuropsychiatric presentation increases with advanced age, however, the latter may precede in some cases. Isolated hepatic involvement has been reported in 20-54% cases, isolated neurological presentation in 8-22%, although about 15-35% may be asymptomatic.

Asymptomatic WD has been found in about 3-40% patients. These patients have incidental hepatomegaly, transaminitis, or are siblings of WD patients. These cases are usually identified in their first decade of life or in adolescence.

The clinical manifestations in WD have been enlisted in **Table 7**.

DIAGNOSIS

A positive family history of WD is useful when parental consanguinity exists. A recent study from India found consanguinity in 44% WD.

Complete blood count:

- Low hemoglobin due to hemolysis
- Thrombocytopenia/pancytopenia

TABLE 7 Clinical manifestations of Wilson's disease (WD).

System affected	Clinical manifestations
Hepatobiliary	Hepatomegaly (asymptomatic/symptomatic), acute hepatitis, chronic hepatitis, fulminant hepatitis (rare), cirrhosis (compensated/decompensated), acute on chronic liver failure, fatty liver, isolated splenomegaly, cholelithiasis, and hepatocellular carcinoma (rare) Jaundice in WD may be due to: • Hemolysis • Hepatitis (acute/chronic/acute on chronic) • Cholestasis
Neuropsychiatric	Dystonia, tremors, seizures, choreoathetosis, Parkinsonism, dysarthria, drooling, incoordination, gait disturbance, behavioral changes, deteriorating scholastic performance, mood disorders, and psychosis Dysarthria is the most common neurological symptom, seen up to 97% of WD neurological patients. Characteristic facies of WD — Vacuous smile (due to dystonic dropped jaw) (**Fig. 9**)
Musculoskeletal	Arthralgia (predominantly large joint), arthritis, fractures, osteoporosis, osteomalacia, and chondromalacia
Ocular	Kayser–Fleischer (KF) rings, sunflower cataracts (rare; does not hamper vision) KF rings (**Fig.10**) • Bilateral • Occur due to deposition of copper in the Descemet's membrane of cornea • Commonly visible in superior and inferior poles • Confirmed by slit-lamp examination • Present in 95% of patients with neuropsychiatric symptoms of WD • Present in 40–60% of patients with hepatobiliary symptoms of WD • May also be seen in primary biliary cirrhosis, primary sclerosing cholangitis, any cause of chronic cholestasis, multiple myeloma, chronic estrogen intake • Reversible with copper chelation therapy
Renal	Nephrocalcinosis, nephrolithiasis, type 2 renal tubular acidosis, Fanconi syndrome
Hematological	Coomb's negative hemolytic anemia, thrombocytopenia, pancytopenia, coagulopathy
Endocrine	Hypoparathyroidism
Gastrointestinal	Pancreatitis
Cardiovasular	Arrythmias, cardiomyopathy

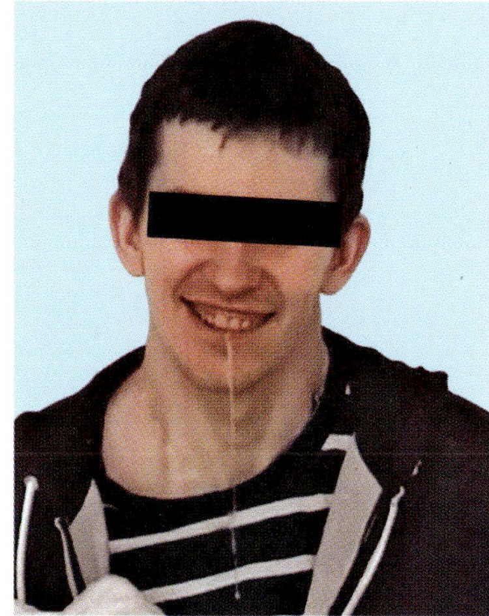

FIG. 9: Vacuous smile with drooling of saliva in Wilson's disease.

Source: Członkowska A, Litwin T, Chabik G. Chapter 10—Wilson disease: neurologic features. In: Członkowska A, Schilsky ML (Eds). Handbook of Clinical Neurology, Volume 142. Netherlands: Elsevier; 2017. pp. 101-19.

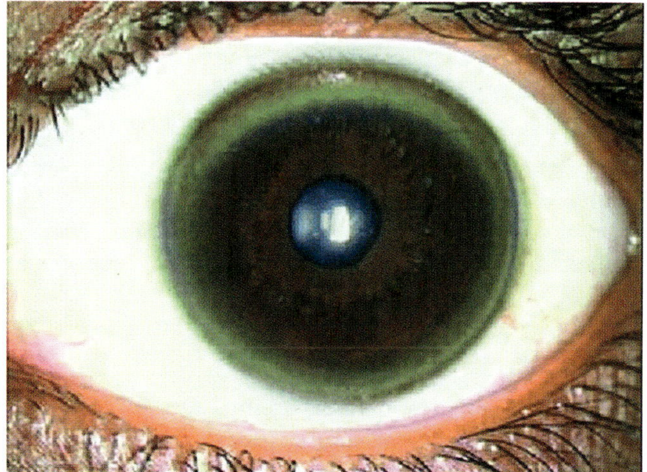

FIG. 10: Kayser–Fleischer ring in Wilson's disease.

Source: Research Gate (2006). Wilson's disease: An update—Scientific Figure [online].

Liver function test:

- Elevated transaminases may be present.
- Low alkaline phosphatase

Serum ceruloplasmin: Normal serum level of ceruloplasmin is 20–40 mg/dL. A low serum level of <15 mg/dL is suggestive of WD, while a level <5 mg/dL is almost diagnostic of WD. The youngest age to test serum ceruloplasmin in order to diagnose WD is 1 year. However, normal values may be seen in up to one-third of WD. Serum ceruloplasmin is usually lower in neuropsychiatric WD compared to hepatic WD.

Falsely low ceruloplasmin levels may be seen in other causes of cirrhosis, malabsorption, and renal disease. Falsely normal ceruloplasmin in a background of WD may be suggestive of an acute inflammation as ceruloplasmin is an acute phase reactant.

Twenty-four-hour urinary copper assay:

- Indirectly estimate of the serum-free copper level
- Sample to be collected in a copper-free container
- The test should be performed before chelation therapy.
- It may be false negative in asymptomatic WD.
- A level >100 µg/24-h is considered highly suggestive of WD.
- *D-penicillamine (DP) challenge test*: If a baseline 24-hour-urinary copper assay reveals a value of 40–100 µg/24-h, a second 24-hour sample may be collected after two 500 mg doses of DP 12 hours apart. It is not recommended now due to high false-positive results.

Kayser–Fleischer rings: Kayser–Fleischer (KF) ring should be looked out for in suspected WD. These are best demonstrated on conventional slit lamp examination.

Serum copper: Serum copper measures the total serum copper (bound copper + "free copper"). About 90% of the serum copper is bound to ceruloplasmin, so with decline of ceruloplasmin, total serum copper decreases.

Serum exchangeable copper: Copper is bound to albumin and other peptides. A value of 15% of relative exchangeable copper has about 100% sensitivity and 100% specificity for the diagnosis of WD.

Hepatic copper estimation: It is gold-standard test for diagnosis of WD. Assessment is done by neutron activation analysis and atomic absorption spectrometry. The normal copper content in liver is <50 µg/g of dry weight, while a level >250 µg/g is diagnostic of WD. The copper level is comparatively high in hepatic WD compared to neuropsychiatric WD. Falsely elevated levels may be seen in chronic cholestasis and in infancy.

Magnetic resonance imaging brain (Figs. 11 A to F): Although the presence of neurocognitive dysfunction with KF ring is sufficient to make the diagnosis of WD, MRI abnormalities in brain are almost universal in those with neurological WD. The characteristic imaging features are enlisted in **Table 8**.

Genetic studies: H1069Q mutation is the most common mutation seen in Western countries but nonexistent in India. p.C271X may be the most common mutation in Western India and p.G1101R may be the most common mutation in Eastern India. Simultaneous analysis for mutations in all 21 exons of *ATP7B* gene can be done using microarray-based tests or next-generation sequencing (NGS).

Modified Leipzig score has been used as a standard diagnostic criterion for diagnosis of WD (**Table 9**).

Histopathology:

- Liver biopsy may reveal vacuolation and fatty change, periportal fibrosis, and macronodular cirrhosis (**Fig. 12**).
- Electron microscopy may reveal dilated tips of cristae of mitochondria with increased intracristal space—tennis racquet appearance.

TREATMENT

Less than 1–2 mg/day of dietary copper is to be taken in WD. Foods rich in copper such as soyabean, nuts, cumin, coriander, cocoa, liver etc., should be avoided at least for the first year of treatment.

Initial phase:

- It aims to reduce serum copper levels to subtoxic threshold. The preferred choice is between chelators (DP or trientine) alone, zinc alone, or a combination of both.
- D-penicillamine is the drug of choice unless the patients develop intolerance, in which case trientine is the preferred drug. DP is given with pyridoxine supplementation.
- *Drug of choice in WD with pregnancy*: Zinc salts
- *Drug of choice for neuropsychiatric manifestations of WD*: Ammonium tetrathiomolybdate (unavailable in India). Additional symptomatic management of neuro-WD shall be continued with these drugs.

TABLE 8 MRI abnormalities in Wilson's disease.

Appearance	Description
Face of giant panda	Normal intensity of red nuclei and lateral portions of substantia nigra pars reticulata with high signal intensity of tegmentum along with hypointensity of the superior colliculus
Miniature panda	Relative hypointensity of the central tegmental tracts (eyes of the panda) with the hyperintensity of the aqueduct opening into the fourth ventricle (nose and mouth of the panda). The superior cerebellar peduncles form the cheeks of the panda
Double panda	Face of giant panda + miniature panda
Others	Central pontine myelinolysis—like abnormalities. Signal changes in basal ganglia, thalamus, and brainstem

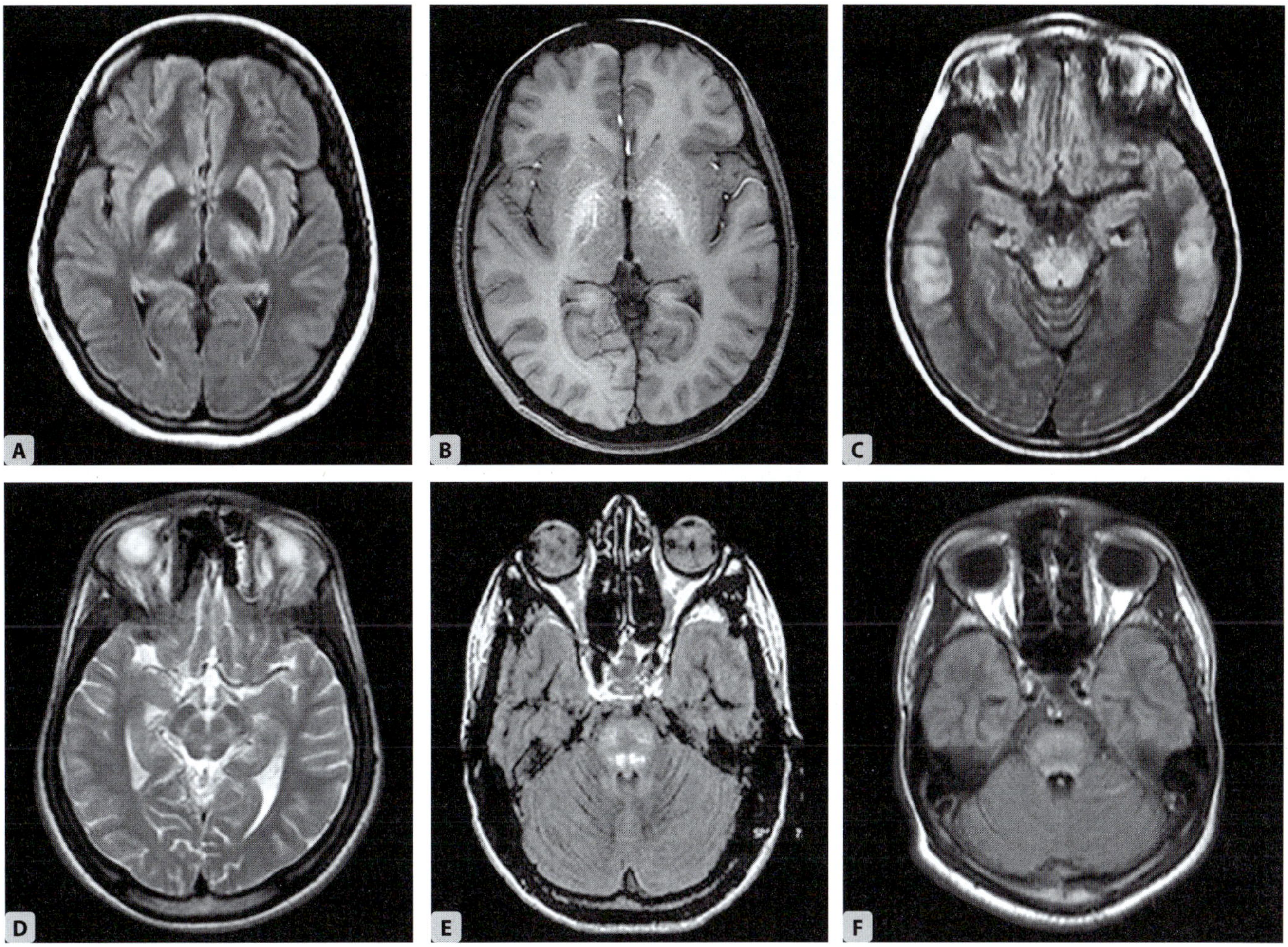

(MRI: magnetic resonance imaging; WD: Wilson's disease)

FIGURES 11 A to F: MRI changes in Wilson's disease. **(A)** Flair axial brain MRI showing hyperintensities in bilateral putamen and thalami with hypointensity of globus pallidi in a patient with neurological manifestations; **(B)** T1W axial brain MRI showing hyperintensity of bilateral globus pallidi in a patient with hepatic form of WD; **(C)** flair axial brain MRI showing hyperintensities in dorsal midbrain and subcortical white matter signal changes in temporal region in a patient with neurological form of WD; **(D)** T2W axial MRI brain depicting "face of giant panda"; **(E and F)** central pontine myelinolysis–like pontine signals changes in WD in flair axial brain MRI.

Source: Aabha N, Sarma MS, Matthai J, Kukkle PL, Devarbhavi H, Sinha S, Alam S, et al. Wilson's disease: Clinical Practice Guidelines of the Indian National Association for Study of the Liver, the Indian Society of Pediatric Gastroenterology, Hepatology and Nutrition, and the Movement Disorders Society of India. J Clin Exp Hepatol. 2019;9(1):74-98.

Maintenance therapy: Lifelong therapy to prevent copper reaccumulation after the patient has been effectively decoppered. Zinc is the drug of choice. DP in low dose is an alternative but patients should be monitored for side effects.

The drug therapy for WD has been enlisted in **Table 10**.

Monitoring therapy for optimal control:

- *For Zinc*: 24-hour-urinary copper <75 μg/day; serum free copper 10–15 μg/dL
- *For DP/trientine*: 24-hour-urinary copper 200–500 μg/day; serum free copper 10–15 μg/dL

Asymptomatic patients: An asymptomatic patient diagnosed to have WD by biochemical or genetic testing should be treated with zinc to prevent symptomatic disease.

Newer therapies: Corrective adenoviral vector–containing human ATP7B DNA is being tried. Cell therapy in an attempt to repopulate the liver with healthy hepatocytes including

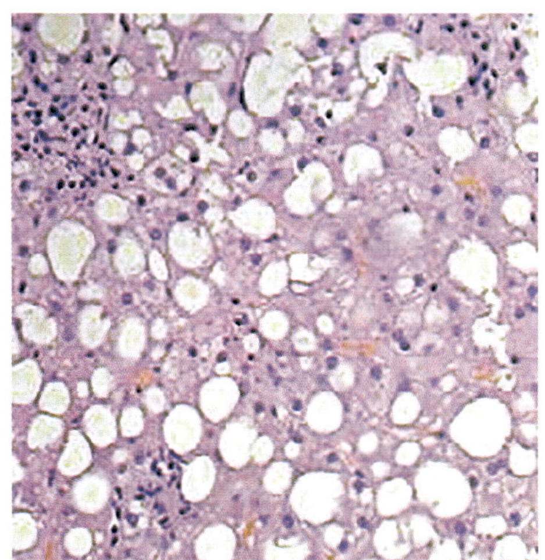

FIGURE 12: Histopathology of liver in WD.

Source: Stättermayer AF, Traussnigg S, Dienes HP, Aigner E, Stauber R, Lackner K, et al. Hepatic steatosis in Wilson disease—role of copper and PNPLA3 mutations. J Hepatol. 2015;63(1):156-63.

TABLE 9 Modified Leipzig score for diagnosis of WD.

Typical clinical symptoms and signs		Other tests	
Kayser–Fleischer rings		**Liver copper** (in the absence of cholestasis)	
Present	2	>250 mg (>4 µmol)/g dry weight	2
Absent	0	50–249 µg (0.8–4 µmol)/g	1
Neurologic symptoms**		Normal: <50 µg (<0.8 µmol)	−1
Severe	2	Rhodanine-pos. granules*	1
Mild	1	**Urinary copper** (in the absence of acute hepatitis)	
Absent	0	Normal	0
Serum ceruloplasmin		1–2 × ULN	1
Normal (>0 2 g/L)	0	>2 × ULn	2
01–02 g/L	1	Normal but >5 × ULN d-penicillamine	2
<0.1 g/L	2	**Mutation analysis**	
Coombs-negative hemolytic anemia		On both chromosomes detected	4
Present	1	On 1 chromosome detected	1
Absent	0	No mutations detected	0
Total Score		**Evaluation**	
4 or more	⟶	Diagnosis established	
3	⟶	Diagnosis possible, more tests needed	
2 or less	⟶	Diagnosis very unlikely	

* If no quantitative liver copper available.

** Or typical abnormalities at brain magnetic resonance imaging.

(ULN: upper limit of normal; WD: Wilson's disease)

Source: Członkowska A, Litwin T, Dusek P, Ferenci P, Lutsenko S, Medici V, et al. Wilson disease. Nat Rev Dis Primers. 2018;4(1):21.

TABLE 10 Drugs used in Wilson's disease.

Drug	Dosage	Mechanism of action	Adverse effects
D-penicillamine	750–15,00 mg/day in two to three divided doses (adults) and 20 mg/kg/day (children) in empty stomach	Promotes urinary excretion of copper	**Early (1–3 weeks):** Fever, rash, lymphadenopathy, thrombocytopenia, proteinuria **Late (3 weeks–3 months):** • Lupus-like syndrome • Goodpasture syndrome • Severe thrombocytopenia, total aplasia • Pemphigus, pemphigoid lesions • Optic neuritis **Very late (after 1 year):** Nephrotoxicity, myasthenia gravis, hepatotoxicity neutropenia, sideroblastic anemia, and hemosiderosis **Direct dose dependent:** • Pyridoxine deficiency • Lichen planus, progeria-like skin changes, D-penicillamine dermopathy Neurological deterioration: Incidence ranges from 10 to 50%
Trientine	750–1,500 mg/day in two to three divided doses (adults) and 20 mg/kg/day (children) in empty stomach	Promotes urinary excretion of copper	• Chelates iron, hence should not be coadministered with iron • Bone marrow suppression • Sideroblastic anemia: Reversible (iron and copper deficiency) • Hemorrhagic gastritis, loss of taste, and skin rash

Continued...

Continued...

Drug	Dosage	Mechanism of action	Adverse effects
Zinc salts	150 mg/day in three divided doses in adults and in children <50 kg, 75 mg/day	Blocks intestinal absorption of copper	• Gastritis • Pancreatitis • Immunosuppression • Bone marrow depression
Ammonium tetrathiomolybdate	20 mg three times a day with meals and 20 mg three times a day in between the meals	Blocks intestinal absorption of copper. Promotes urinary excretion of copper	• Paradoxical worsening • Bone marrow suppression • Hepatotoxicity

TABLE 11 New Wilson index to prognosticate Wilson's disease.

Score	Bilirubin (mg/dL)	INR	AST (IU/L)	WCC (109/L)	Albumin (g/dL)
0	0.5–5.8	0–1.29	0–100	0–6.7	≥4.5
1	5.9–8.7	1.3–1.6	101–150	6.8–8.3	3.4–4.4
2	8.8–11.6	1.7–1.9	151–200	8.4–10.3	2.5–3.3
3	11.7–17.5	2.0–2.4	201–300	10.4–15.3	2.1–2.4
4	≥17.6	≥2.5	≥300	≥15.4	0–2.0

(AST: aspartate transaminase; INR: international normalized ratio; WCC: white cell count)

Source: Nagral, Aabha et al. Wilson's Disease: Clinical Practice Guidelines of the Indian National Association for Study of the Liver, the Indian Society of Pediatric Gastroenterology, Hepatology and Nutrition, and the Movement Disorders Society of India. J Clin Exp Hepatol. 2019;9(1):74-98.

the reconstitution of bile canalicular network may open up new avenues to WD management.

PROGNOSIS

New Wilson's index (NWI) predicts survival in WD (**Table 11**). A score >11 needs liver transplant to survive.

RECOMMENDED READINGS

1. Baker KR, Rice L. The amyloidoses: clinical features, diagnosis and treatment. Methodist Debakey Cardiovasc J. 2012;8(3): 3-7.
2. Pedro L, Pinho R, Marques N. Amyloidosis—A review. Trends Med. 2019;19.
3. Khan MF, Falk RH. Amyloidosis. Postgraduate Med J. 2001;77:686-93.
4. Bissell DM., Anderson KE, Bonkovsky HL. Porphyria. N Eng J Med. 2017;377(9):862-72.
5. Stölzel U, Doss MO, Schuppan D. Clinical guide and update on porphyrias. Gastroenterology. 2019;157(2): 365-81.
6. Thadani H, Deacon A, Peters T. Diagnosis and management of porphyria. BMJ. 2000;320(7250):1647-51.
7. Puy H, Gouya L, Deybach JC. Porphyrias. Lancet. 2010;375(9718): 924-37.
8. Rodriguez-Castro KI, Hevia-Urrutia FJ, Sturniolo GC. Wilson's disease: A review of what we have learned. World J Hepatol. 2015;7(29):2859-70.
9. Członkowska A, Litwin T, Dusek P, Ferenci P, Lutsenko S, Medici V, et al. Wilson disease. Nat Rev Dis Primers. 2018;4(1):21.
10. Taly AB, Prashanth LK, Sinha S. Wilson's disease: An Indian perspective. Neurol India. 2009;57:528-40.
11. Nagral A, Sarma MS, Matthai J, Kukkle PL, Devarbhavi H, Sinha S, et al. Wilson's Disease: Clinical Practice Guidelines of the Indian National Association for Study of the Liver, the Indian Society of Pediatric Gastroenterology, Hepatology and Nutrition, and the Movement Disorders Society of India." J Clin Exp Hepatol. 2019;9(1):74-98.

CHAPTER 19

Poisoning and Drug Overdose: General Principles of Management

Somnath Das, Rina Das

ABSTRACT

This chapter deals with the general management of poisoned patient with history of known or unknown poison. Most of the patients who present at the hospital with history of poisoning are with acute exposure. The success of poison management deals generally with supportive therapy as in most of the cases the antidote is not available.

Specific learning objectives (SLO) of this chapter are:

At the end of the chapter the learners will be able to:

- Define poison, poisoning, poison information center, and antidote.
- Enumerate different poisons.
- Summarize the qualitative descriptions of toxicity.
- Describe the steps of poisoning management in a case of known and unknown poisoning in hospital set-up.
- Identify the difference between the toxic and non-toxic agent-related poisoning.
- Summarize different methods of analytical toxicology.
- Enumerate the laws related to poison.
- Identify the role of a registered medical practitioner in dealing with the medicolegal aspect of poisoning.

The morbidity and mortality of poisoning can greatly be reduced by applying these simple treatment protocols along with revamping the preventive aspects like establishment of poison information center.

"To aquire knowledge, one must study; but to aquire wisdom, one must observe"

—MV Savant

INTRODUCTION

Poison is any substance when introduced into the body causing ill health or death.

Poisoning can be defined as the dose-related effects following exposure to poisons.

Any substance can be a poison, it is only the dose that matters.

The easiest definition of poison in a very simple way is *"anything excess is poison"*. Paracetamol tablet in its usual dose acts to reduce the body temperature, but when taken above the lethal dose can kill the person.

EPIDEMIOLOGY

As per the World Health Organization (WHO) data, in 2012 near about 2 lakh people died worldwide from unintentional poisoning. Accidental poisoning is most common among children whereas deliberate poisoning is prominent among the adults. The Indian data is equally alarming.

An important factor in the increase of self-poisoning is the ready availability of drugs and pesticides. Still today pesticide is the most common form of poisoning that is encountered along with different bites and stings. In the recent times it has become a common practice for several different drugs to be taken at the same time which makes the work of a toxicologist more complicated during the treatment. It can easily be opined that nowadays acute poisoning is a very real medical and social problem in almost all the countries.

POISON INFORMATION SERVICES

The first telephone service giving information on poison was established in Chicago in 1953. It was called the poison control center. Since then, most of the developed and developing countries have started some form of poison information services.

India's first poison information center was established in All India Institute of Medical Sciences in New Delhi. After that another seven institutes have come up with the same type of service for the common people and the medical practitioner. A poison information center provides toxicological information and advice on the management of poisoned patients adapted to the level of the enquirer. For the patients it gives the information regarding the "first aid" and for the healthcare professionals the management protocols with identification of poisons.

CLASSIFICATION OF POISONS

The poisons are classified commonly depending upon their effects on organ system as described in **Table 1**.

TOXICITY RATING OF POISON

Toxins can be located in one of the five toxicity categories based on their toxicity levels (**Table 2**).

LD50: The word LD means lethal dose. LD50 is the amount of toxin given at a time that causes the death of 50% of the test animals. The test animals commonly used are rats and mice.

LC50: The word LC stands for lethal concentration and it usually refers to the concentration of a chemical in air or water.

Remember: LD50 data are mere approximation as in actual scenario, no human experiments have been done.

CLASSIFICATION OF POISONING

Poisoning is basically divided into two groups.

EXPOSURE-RELATED CLASSIFICATION

Acute: Here the person has taken a large quantity of poison at a time or he has taken multiple small quantities within a short period. Onset of the symptoms is rapid.

Chronic: Here the person is exposed to a poison in small quantities over a long period of time. Onset of the symptoms is insidious.

TABLE 1 Classification of poisons.

Corrosive	Acid	**Inorganic:** • Sulfuric acid, hydrochloric acid, and nitric acid **Organic:** • Carbolic acid, oxalic acid, and salicylic acid
	Alkali	• Ammonia, salts of sodium, NAOH and salts of potassium, KOH
Irritants	Inorganic	**Nonmetal:** • Phosphorus and halogen (chlorine, bromine, and iodine)
		Heavy metal: • Arsenic, lead, mercury, iron, copper and thallium
	Organic	**Irritant plant:** • Castor, *Croton*, *Calotropis*, *Abrus*, tobacco, *Digitalis*, and *Capsicum*
		Bites/stings: • Snake, scorpion, spider, bee, and wasp

Continued...

Continued...

Neurotoxic	Cerebral	**Somniferous:** • Opium and other opiates **Deliriants:** • *Datura*, *Cannabis*, and cocaine **Inebriants:** • Alcohol, barbiturates, and benzodiazepines **Psychotropic:** • **Antidepressant:** Amphetamines, TCA, and MAOI • **Neuroleptics:** Phenothiazine and thioxanthine • **Hallucinogen:** LSD and phencyclidine
	Spinal	**Stimulant:** Strychnine **Depressant:** *Gelsemium* and *nux-vomica*
	Peripherally acting	Hemlock and curare
Cardiovascular		**Antihypertensives:** • Nifedipine, amlodipine, enalapril, captopril, and losartan
		Anticoagulants: • Warfarin, acitrom, and LMWH
		Cardiotoxic: • Aconite, *oleander*, *Digitalis*, and quinine
Asphyxiants		• Carbon monoxide, cyanide, methyl isocyanate, and tear gases
Miscellaneous		**Agricultural poison:** • Organophosphorus, carbamates, pyrethroids, cantharides, and organochlorines
		Food poison: • Microbe, mushroom plant, fish, chemical, and botulism
		Pharmaceuticals: • Analgesics, antipyretics, antibiotics, and sedatives
		Substance of abuse: • Yaba and LSD

(LMWH: low-molecular weight heparin; LSD: lysergic acid diethylamide; MAOIs: monoamine oxidase inhibitors; TCAs: tricyclic antidepressants)

TABLE 2 Toxicity rating and dose of poisons.

Toxicity rating	Lethal oral dose in average adult	Examples
Super toxic	<5 mg/kg	Nicotine
Extremely toxic	5–50 mg/kg	Parathion
Very toxic	50–500 mg/kg	Dieldrin
Moderately toxic	500–5,000 mg/kg	Aspirin
Slightly toxic	5,000–15,000 mg/kg	Ethanol
Essentially safe	>15,000 mg/kg	Water

MEDICOLEGAL CLASSIFICATION

Suicidal: When a person, administrator person, himself to end his or her life.

Homicidal: Killing of a man by another human by administering poisonous substance deliberately.

Accidental: Unintentional exposure to poisonous substances.
Occupational: Usually chronic exposure of poisonous substances by professional workers.

MANAGEMENT

While treating the cases of poisoning a physician usually gets two types of patients.

- The first group is having history of poisoning by a specific substance.
- The second group is a case of unknown poisoning.

MANAGEMENT IN EMERGENCY

The procedure of management in both the above groups at the emergency room is basically the same.

At the emergency room we are usually concerned with fixing the *airway, breathing,* and *circulation* as it is called the basic ABC of management.

Fixing the airway: Compromised and threatened airway can easily be identified by the symptoms of dyspnea, air hunger, and hoarseness of voice. Among the signs, stridor, intercostal and suprasternal retractions, tachypnea, and cyanosis are most consistent. Pulse oximetry can be done to measure the oxygen saturation at this stage.

Primary emphasis should be given on removing the upper airway obstruction and maintaining the patency of the airway.

Fixing the circulation: It is always better to establish a vascular access at this stage. The easiest way of assessing the circulatory parameters is to look at the skin and measure the pulse.

- *Skin*: *Look*—for pale flushed cyanosed or normal skin, *feel*—warm, cold, dry, or sweaty skin.
- *Pulse*: Presence of strong weak regular or irregular pulses

MANAGEMENT IN THE WARD

After the process of resuscitation when the patient has entered the hospital ward, the treating physician should assess the initial presentation and take a direct proper history. While taking the history the physician should focus on three important things:

1. *Quick assessment of the potential danger*: The amount of poison ingested, the time passed, and presence of comorbidities. History of current medications and prehospital treatment are also important.
2. *To ascertain the hysterical coma*: Sometimes the patient may pretend to be comatose which is often called a suicide gesture. This is a situation of drawing the attention of the caregivers of the family though there is no real intention of ending one's life. A physician has to be keen enough to differentiate the situation with reality.

   Clinical features that creates suspicion about hysterical coma: The fluttering eyelids, half-awake patients, and inconsistent history of the act. The physician must perform a quick physical examination with particular attention to the breathing, vital signs, and the gag reflex.

   There is a useful technique to identify the situation is to leave the patient's hand directly about his/her face and letting a drop. In cases of psychogenic coma, it drops slowly or at one side rather than obeying the law of gravity and landing on the face. In no way the doctor should humiliate the patient in front of the others.
3. *Differentiate between toxic and non-toxic exposure*: Asymptomatic or mild symptomatic patients not necessarily mean they are good prognosis. There are a whole lot of poisons where the signs and symptoms appear late.

   Though every substance can be poisonous; however, there are a whole lot of substances which when ingested in huge quantity do not show any effects. **Table 3** below shows some of the nonpoisonous substances.

   In order to accept a substance to be nonpoisonous the physician must be sure of:

- The product was placed before him and the level does not contain any warning sign.
- The caregivers are aware of the amount of the ingestion.
- The patient is symptom free after a substantial (usually 24 h) of observation.

The different steps of managing a case of poisoning may be enumerated as follows:

- *Stabilization of the patient*
- *Diagnosing the poison*
- *Elimination of unabsorbed poison*
- *Elimination of absorbed poison*
- *Antidote administration*
- *Psychiatric care*

Sometimes it is very easy to identify that the patient has taken poison depending upon the circumstantial evidence. This is particularly important for the cases of self-poisoning. Doctors must be very much conscious while dealing with patients of age group 15–50 years where apart from head injury the most common cause of impaired consciousness is acute poisoning. It is strongly recommended that the initial management of poisoned patient must be based on clinical assessment as it may be dangerous if delay occurs in order to identify the poison.

STABILIZATION OF THE PATIENT

To stabilize the patient before actual management of poisoning starts the physician has to correct the following parameters.

Correction of hypothermia: Hypothermia is defined as when the body temperature falls below 95° Fahrenheit (F) or 35° Celsius (C). It is essential to use a low reading rectal thermometer to measure the temperature. Hypothermia can be *mild* (between 95°F and 90°F) or *moderate* (between 90°F and 82.4°F) or *severe* (below 82.4°F) (**Box 1**).

TABLE 3 Agents which are nonpoisonous.

Medications	Household items			Nontoxic plants
• Antacids • Calamine lotion • Birth control pills (if single ingestion) • Corticosteroids (if single ingestion) • Mineral oil (unless aspirated) • Oral antibiotics (if overdosage does not happen) • Water-soluble vitamins (excluding iron) • Zinc oxide • Zirconium oxide	• Ashes • Baby products • Ballpoint pen ink • Body conditioner • Bubble bath • Candles • Charcoal • Clay • Cosmetics • Crayons produced • Deodorant • Erasers	• Fabric softener • Felt-tip pens • Highlighting markers • Latex paint • Lipstick • Pencil lead • Petroleum jelly • Pet foods • Plastics • Shaving cream	• Chalk • Silica gel • Starch • Sunscreens • Sweeteners • Thermometer mercury • Toothpaste • Water color paints • White glue	• Spider plant • Snake plant • Rubber tree • Peacock plant • Corn plant

BOX 1 Agents causing hypothermia.

- Antihistamines (diphenhydramine)
- Sedative/hypnotic drug (benzodiazepines)
- Ethanol
- Opioids (drug abuse-morphine)
- Antipsychotic (clozapine)
- Antidepressants (TCAs)

(TCAs: tricyclic antidepressants)

Treatment:

- Passive external rewarming—blankets/sleeping bags.
- Active external warming—hot water bottles, heating blankets, forced air warming.
- Invasive core rewarming—peritoneal dialysis, hemodialysis, gastric or rectal lavage.

However, correction of hypertension, hypoventilation, acidosis, and hyperkalemia usually work as wonder.

Correction of hyperthermia: When the oral temperature of any human being exceeds 102°F we call it hyperthermia. Toxins that cause hyperthermia are enumerated in **Box 2**.

BOX 2 Agents inducing hyperthermia.

- Amphetamines
- Cocaine
- Monoamine oxidase inhibitors
- Strychnine
- Salicylates
- Thyroid hormones
- Anticholinergics
- *Datura*

Treatment: Hydrotherapy or immersion in cold water bath is very effective but can be dangerous in case of elderly patients.

No antipyretic drug like paracetamol is effective.

Correction of hypotension: Hypotension is defined as low blood pressure where the systolic and the diastolic blood pressures respectively are below 90 by 60 mm Hg (**Table 4**).

TABLE 4 Toxin that causes hypotension.

Pharmacological agents	Nonpharmacological agents
• Antihypertensive drugs (α-blockers/CCB/β-blockers) • Disulfiram (ethanol interaction) • Iron • Trazodone, quetiapine, and other antipsychotic agents • Antidepressants	• Cyanide • Carbon monoxide • Hydrogen sulfide • Aluminum or zinc phosphide • Arsenic • Mushrooms (contain pilocarpine)

(CCB: calcium-channel blockers)

Treatment:

- Elevation of the foot end of the bed
- Administration of saline water
- Correction of acidemia

Pharmacological therapy: Dopamine administration—200 mg of dopamine is added with 250 mL of 5% dextrose to make a solution of 800 μg/mL. Infusion may be given at 1–5 μg/kg/min to a maximum of 15–30 μg/kg/min and then titrated.

Noradrenaline administration—8 g of noradrenaline is added to 500 mL of 5% dextrose to make a concentration of 16 μg/mL. It is usually given at the rate of 0.5–1 mL/min and then titrated.

Correction of hypertension: Usually, hypertension is defined as blood pressure above 140/90 mm Hg. It considered severe if the pressure is above 180/120 mm Hg (**Box 3**).

Treatment: Management of hypertension among poisoned patients has to be individualized. Increased blood pressure associated with high dose of different medications ought to be treated differently (**Table 5**).

BOX 3 List of common poisons that cause hypertension.

- Amphetamines
- Anticholinergics
- Cocaine
- MAO inhibitors
- Performance-enhancing products
    - Caffeine
    - Phenylephrine
    - Ephedrine
    - Yohimbine

(MAO: monoamine oxidase)

TABLE 5 Treatment of hypertension and associated symptoms/features.

Hypertension associated with any of the following signs	Treatment
Agitation and anxiety	Lorazepam 2–3 mg IV
Persistent nature	Phentolamine 2–5 mg IV *or* Sodium nitroprusside: 0.25–8 μg/kg/min IV
Excessive tachycardia	Propranolol 1–5 mg IV *or* Esmolol 25–100 μg/kg/min IV *or* Labetalol 0.2–0.3 mg/kg IV
Caution: Do not give β-blockers alone which may paradoxically worsen hypertension as a result of unopposed α-adrenergic stimulation	

Correction of arrhythmia: Arrhythmia in poisoning occurs because of multiple factors involving the change in the homeostasis of the body apart from the direct involvement of the heart. It can result due to hypoxia, metabolic acidosis, or electrolyte imbalance.

Table 6 below gives a glimpse of the common causes of arrhythmia involving toxicity.

Treatment: Treatment of arrhythmia is given below in **Table 7**.

Correction of seizures: Seizure is a very common presentation in poisoned patients especially among the children. Whenever we come across such symptoms, the management should be adequate enough to prevent status epilepticus which is a life-threatening condition.

There is a long list of poisons that cause convulsions which are given below in **Table 8**.

Treatment:

- Intravenous diazepam (10–20 mg in adults; 0.1–0.3 mg/kg body weight in children).
- If convulsion is unresponsive—phenobarbitone sodium (10 mg/kg, may increase up to 100 mg/min to a maximum of 1 g)

TABLE 6 Arrhythmias in different toxicities.

Sinus bradycardia	Beta-blockers, calcium-channel blockers, clonidine, digitalis glycosides, and organophosphates
Atrioventricular block	Beta-blockers, calcium-channel blockers, class 1A antiarrhythmics including quinidine, carbamazepine, clonidine, digital, and lithium
Sinus tachycardia	Beta-agonists, amphetamines, anticholinergics, antihistamine, caffeine, cocaine, pseudoephedrine, and tricyclic and other antidepressants
Wide complex QRS	Class 1A and class 1C antiarrhythmics, phenothiazines, potassium, propranolol, tricyclic antidepressants, lamotrigine, and severe overdose of diphenhydramine
QT-interval prolongation and torsades de pointes	Arsenic, class 1A and class 3 antiarrhythmics, citalopram, lithium, methadone, pentamidine, sertraline, sotalol etc.
Vascular premature beats and ventricular tachycardia	Amphetamines, cocaine, ephedrine, caffeine, chlorinated and fluorinated hydrocarbons, digoxin, aconite, fluoride, and theophylline

TABLE 7 Treatment of arrhythmia.

Cause	Treatment
Electrolyte imbalance ↑K^+ ↓K^+, Mg^{2+}, Ca^{2+}	Correct accordingly
Ventricular arrhythmias	Lidocaine/amiodarone at usual antiarrhythmic doses
TCAs/diphenhydramine/class Ia antiarrhythmic drugs	• Sodium bicarbonate 50–100 mEq • IV bolus infusion
Torsades de pointes	Mg (2 g IV over 2 min) *or* overdrive pacing
Digitalis-induced arrhythmias	Digoxin-specific antibodies
Chlorinated solvents/chloral hydrate/freons/sympathomimetic agents	Propranolol 1–5 mg IV *or* Esmolol 25–100 g/kg/min IV

TABLE 8 Convulsions in different poisonings.

Acute toxicity	Chronic toxicity during withdrawal
• Amphetamines • Antidepressants • Anticholinergics caffeine • Carbon monoxide • Cocaine • Cyanide • Heavy metals • Organophosphates • Strychnine	• Barbiturates • Benzodiazepines • Ethanol • Opiates

- Alternatively, phenytoin (18 mg/kg infusion over 30 min) can be given.

Correction of agitation: Agitation is a condition that is experienced very commonly with patients suffering from chronic toxicity of different substances as well as during the withdrawal symptoms of drugs which are commonly used for abuse.

This condition is aggravated by mental disorder and dyselectrolytemia. Disorientation, irrational behavior, hyperexcitability, hallucinations, and violence are common symptoms that we come across. Common toxins causing agitation are given in **Table 9**.

Treatment:
- Diazepam (oral or IV)
- Lorazepam 2–4 mg intramuscularly (IM) with or without haloperidol 5 mg IM
- Chlordiazepoxide 25–50 mg orally for alcoholics

Correction of dyselectrolytemia: Hyperkalemia, hypokalemia, hyponatremia, and hypocalcemia are the common electrolyte imbalances that are encountered in poisoning cases.

Table 10 shows the lists of drugs which cause the above disorders.

TABLE 9 Common toxins causing agitation.

Acute toxicity	Chronic toxicity (during withdrawal)
• Anticholinergics • Antidepressants • Benzodiazepines • *Cannabis* • Cocaine • *Datura* • Ethanol • Hallucinogens	• Opiates • Ethanol • Barbiturates

TABLE 10 Drugs causing electrolyte imbalances.

Electrolyte imbalances	Drugs causing
Hyperkalemia (potassium level > 5.5 mEq/L)	*Digitalis*, β-2 antagonists, potassium sparing diuretics, fluoride, heparin, nonsteroidal anti-inflammatory drugs
Hypokalemia (potassium level < 3.5 mEq/L)	Chloroquine, hydroxychloroquine, insulin, β-2 agonist, thiazide diuretics, salicylix, loop diuretics, sympathomimetics, and theophylline
Hypernatremia (sodium level > 150 mEq/L)	Lithium, alcohol, mannitol, sorbitol, sodium salts, and colchicine
Hyponatremia (sodium level < 130 mEq/L)	Carbamazepine, chlorpropamide, nonsteroidal anti-inflammatory drugs, biguanides, ACE-inhibitors, and amitriptyline
Hypocalcemia (calcium level < 4 mEq/L)	Hydrogen fluoride, oxalates, ethanol, ethylene glycol, and phenytoin

Treatment: These abnormalities are corrected as given below.

Correction of acid base balance: The diagnosis of acid base disorders is mostly based on arterial blood gas analysis. It must be determined that whether the abnormality is a primary or it is a compensatory one. The acid-base disorder in toxicology is corrected in the same way as in any other case.

DIAGNOSING THE POISON

Poisons are usually diagnosed by two methods.
1. The clinical identification
2. The analytical identification

The clinical identification: Clinically, we can identify poisons by looking at different clues from the patient.
- *The visual clues*: The pupil of the eye is an important organ that can be scrutinized to get an idea about different poisons. It is to be noted that the normal pupillary size is between 3 and 4 mm and the typical conditions. A list of toxins is given below in **Table 11**.
- *The olfactory clues*: There are some drugs that have a distinctive odor which makes it unique. Some of the important examples have been mentioned in **Table 12**.
- *The dermal clues*: There are some poisons that have a dermal manifestation. These manifestations are usually seen in chronic poisoning rather than in acute one (**Table 13**).

The analytical identification: Analytical toxicology is that branch of toxicology which deals in identification of the toxin by laboratory procedure.

Detection of poison can be of two types:
1. Qualitative analysis
2. Quantitative analysis

Qualitative analysis: This includes the bedside tests which include usually the color tests such as:
- Trinder's test for salicylate poisoning

TABLE 11 Toxins having effect on eyes.

Drugs that cause constriction of the pupil	• Benzodiazepines • Barbiturates • Carbonic acid • Nicotine • Opium • Organophosphates
Drugs that cause dilation of the pupil	• Alcohol • Antihistaminic • Amphetamine • Carbon monoxide • Cocaine • *Datura*
Drugs that cause nystagmus	• Alcohol • Barbiturates • Phenytoin

TABLE 12	Drugs/Toxins with special odors.
Garlic	Arsenic, phosphorous, selenium, thallium, and organophosphorus
Sweet/Fruity	Ethanol, chloroform, and nitrites
Bitter almonds	Cyanide
Acrid (pear like)	• Paraldehyde • Chloral hydrate
Rotten eggs	Hydrogen sulfide, mercaptans
Fishy/musty	Zinc phosphide
Solvent/glue	Toluene, xylene
Smoke	Carbon monoxide

TABLE 13	Drugs/Toxins with skin manifestations.
Features	**Poisons**
Dry hot skin	*Datura* poisoning
Diaphoresis	Organophosphates and salicylate poisoning
Cherry pink color of the skin	Carbon monoxide poisoning
Brick red color of the skin	Cyanide poisoning
Blister formation	Barbiturate poisoning
Raindrop pigmentation	Arsenic poisoning
Brown coloration	Bromide and iodide poisoning
Dark pigmentation	Chloroquine and phenytoin poisoning

- Ferric chloride test for phenol phenothiazines or oxyphenbutazone poisoning
- O-cresol test for paracetamol poisoning
- Marquis test for opium poisoning
- Dichromate test for ethanol poisoning

We can get more sophisticated qualitative test using a "thin-layer chromatography".

The quantitative test: Quantitative test for toxin detection is a more sophisticated one which includes:
- Ultraviolet spectrophotometry
- Gas chromatography
- High performance liquid chromatography (HPLC)
- Mass spectrometry (MS)
- The radioimmunoassays
- Atomic absorption spectrophotometry
- Neutron activation analysis

Presence of a small laboratory in every hospital which is dedicated to analytical toxicology is extremely helpful for the management of poison patients.

Biochemical investigations:
- *Hematologic*: Complete blood count (CBC), platelet count, and coagulation profile
  - *Hemolytic anemia*: In lead, nonsteroidal anti-inflammatory drugs (NSAIDs), and quinidine poisoning
  - *Thrombocytopenia*: In aspirin, phenytoin, procainamide poisoning
  - *Coagulopathy*: In snake venoms, warfarin poisoning
- *Liver function tests*: Serum bilirubin, enzymes—aspartate aminotransferase (AST), alanine aminotransferase (ALT), alkaline phosphatase (ALP), and coagulation profile
  - In acetaminophen, sulfonamides, rifampicin, TCA, and INH poisoning
- *Renal functions tests*:
  - In aspirin, lead, barbiturates, alcohol, amphetamines, and copper sulfate poisoning

ELIMINATION OF UNABSORBED POISON

The method also known as decontamination technique is a fast step for reducing the toxic load in the body. Depending upon the route of exposure decontamination process should include.

Decontamination of the eyes:

The steps are:
- Remove contact lens.
- Flush copiously with water or normal saline for 15–20 minutes.
- Use local anesthetic drops.
- Continue irrigation until pH is normal.
- Slit lamp and fluorescein examination.

Decontamination of the skin: Cutaneous absorption of different poison is very common especially for the agricultural substances.

The steps are:
1. Protect yourself and other workers.
2. Remove clothing.
3. Flush with water or normal saline.
4. Use soap and water if oily substance.
5. Chemical neutralization can potentiate injury.
6. Corrosive agents injure skin and can have systemic effects.

Decontamination of lungs in case of inhalation poison:

The steps are:
1. Give supplemental humidified oxygen.
2. *Observe for airway obstruction.*
3. Intubate as necessary.

Decontamination of gut: There are a few methods of decontamination of the alimentary canal. However, all the methods are having its advantages and disadvantages and hence they are not acceptable as a universal regimen for different groups of physicians.

Gastric lavage: Gastric lavage should not be employed routinely in the management of poison patient. When the patient comes within 2 hours of ingestion gastric lavage is more effective. The lavage fluid choice is given in **Table 14**.

The method:
- Prior consent is desirable but not mandatory.
- Patient should be in left lateral position.

TABLE 14 Choice of lavage fluid.

Universal lavage fluid	Water or saline
Oxidizable poisons (vegetable poisons, salicylates etc.)	Potassium permanganate (1:5,000 ratio)
Cyanides	2% sodium thiosulfate
Oxalate	Calcium gluconate
Iron	Deferoxamine (2 g in 1 L of saline water)

- Ideal tube for lavage is lavacuator. Ewald tube can also be used. Ryles tube can only be used for pediatric patients.
- Preferred route of insertion is oral after lubricating the end of the tube with glycerin.
- After the tube has been inserted it should be checked by air insufflation.
- Gastric lavage is carried out with normal saline, if not available, with plain tap water 200–300 mL in each time (pediatrics 10–15 mL/kg body weight) can be used.
- Continue lavage until no particulate matter is seen.
- Keep the first stomach washing for chemical analysis.

Contraindications: The following are the conditions where gastric lavage is not done:

- Corrosive poisoning
- Petroleum compound
- Convulsion
- Patients with gastric surgery or esophageal varices

Catharsis: This method is used for purging the bowel for elimination of poisons.
The usual medications used are:

- Saline catharsis done by magnesium citrate 425 mL/kg or magnesium sulfate 250 mg/kg (around 30 g in case of adult)
- Saccharide catharsis is done by sorbitol citrate. The dose of sorbitol is 50 mL of 70% sorbitol.

Administration of activated charcoal: Out of all the methods that are used for elimination of unabsorbed poison, activated charcoal administration is most likely accepted by almost all schools of physicians. It is usually marketed by different pharmaceuticals company but can be easily prepared at home by burning slice bread directly on fire until it is dark black in color. It can then be crushed and used as an activated charcoal.

The usual dose of activated charcoal is 1–2 g/kg of the body weight and usually administered with water. This compound is highly effective if administered within 1 hour of ingestion.

ELIMINATION OF ABSORBED POISON

Elimination of absorbed poisons is only possible when it is circulating freely in the circulation without being tissue bound. These elimination methods are not frequently administered as they are costly and having their own complications. However, some of the available research data have shown some promise in the process of elimination of toxins by the following methods.

Forced alkaline diuresis: Urine alkalization is a treatment which increases the elimination of some of the poisons which remain in ionic form unchanged. The target pH of the urine should be >7.5 and it is done by the administration of intravenous sodium bicarbonate at a dose of 1–2 mEq/kg infused over 3–4 hours. Urinary flow rate should be >3 mL/min.

To maintain a urinary flow of 500 mL/h bolus dose of furosemide 20 mg intravenous may be required. Potassium replacement has to be done accordingly.

The drugs that can be eliminated by alkaline diuresis are phenobarbitone, barbitone, and salicylates.

Extracorporeal techniques: Hemodialysis, peritoneal dialysis, hemoperfusion, hemofiltration, cardiopulmonary bypass exchange transfusion, and intravenous lipid emulsion all have been tried for elimination of absorbed poison. However, good results have been found in case of hemodialysis and hemoperfusion. The toxins that are easily hemodialysable, having sufficient volume distribution and low fixability with body tissues are lithium, salicylates, phenobarbitone, and theophylline.

ANTIDOTE ADMINISTRATION

Antidotes are therapeutic substances that are used to counteract the toxic actions of poisons. This is to be kept in mind that majority of the poisoning cases get cured mostly by supportive therapies. Specific antidotes are rarely required except for a few.

Antidotes are usually classified into three groups.

1. The mechanical or physical antidotes
2. The chemical antidotes
3. Physiological or pharmacological antidotes

Physicians usually use the pharmacological antidote. A list of these antidotes is given below in **Table 15**.

PATIENT WITH UNKNOWN POISON

Often it is seen that patients come without any history of poisoning; however, the signs and symptoms seem to be highly suspicious of the same. Even sometimes the patient is unconscious and not being accompanied by any attendant. In these situations, it becomes extremely difficult for the treating physician to start the therapy toward any specific poison. In such cases it is preferable to treat the patient in a syndromic approach which is sometimes referred as toxic syndrome.

Sympathomimetic syndrome: The blood pressure and pulse rate are elevated, though with severe hypertension reflex bradycardia may occur. The temperature is often elevated, pupils are dilated, and the skin is sweaty, though mucous membranes are dry. Patients are usually agitated, anxious, or frankly psychotic.

- *Examples*: Amphetamines, cocaine, ephedrine, and pseudoephedrine.

Sympatholytic syndrome: The blood pressure and pulse rate are decreased, and body temperature is low. The pupils are small or even pinpoint. Peristalsis is usually decreased. Patients are usually obtunded or comatose.

TABLE 15 Commonly used antidotes in different poisonings.

Poisons	Antidote	Dose
Acetaminophen	N-acetylcysteine	140 mg/kg. Then 70 mg/kg every 4 h to total of 18 doses over 72 h
Benzodiazepine	Flumazenil	0.1 mg/min infusion to a total of 1 mg
Anticholinergics	Physostigmine	1 g IM or IV
Opioid	Naloxone	2 mg IV, repeated every 0.5–1 min to a total of 20 mg IV
Cyanide	Thiosulfate, nitrite	0.3 g sodium nitrite in 10 mL sterile water IV 25 g sodium thiosulfate IV slow
Iron	Deferoxamine	2 g IM 12 hourly or 10–15 mg/kg/h not to exceed 80 mg /kg/24 h
Organophosphates poisoning	Atropine, oximes	• *Atropine*: Loading dose: 2, 4, and 6 every 5 min • Maintenance: Infusion < 3 mg/h • PAM: 15–30 mg/kg IV to be repeated 6–12 hourly • Infusion: 20–40 mg/kg followed by 5–10 mg/kg/h
Methanol	Ethanol, fomepizole	• Ethanol 50% 1 mL/kg every 2 h for 5 days • Fomepizole 15 mg/kg loading dose followed by10 mg/kg every 12 h for 4 days

- *Examples*: Barbiturates, benzodiazepines and other sedative hypnotics, clonidine and related antihypertensives, ethanol, and opioids.

Cholinergic syndrome: Stimulation of muscarinic receptors causes bradycardia, miosis, sweating, and hyperperistalsis as well as bronchorrhea, wheezing, excessive salivation, and urinary incontinence. Nicotinic receptor stimulation may produce initial hypertension and tachycardia as well as fasciculations and muscle weakness. Patients are usually agitated and anxious.

- *Examples*: Carbamates, nicotine, organophosphates (including nerve agents), and physostigmine

Anticholinergic syndrome: Tachycardia with mild hypertension is common, and the body temperature is often elevated. Pupils are widely dilated. The skin is flushed, hot, and dry. Peristalsis is decreased, and urinary retention is common. Patients may have myoclonic jerking or choreoathetoid movements. Agitated delirium is frequently seen, and severe hyperthermia may occur.

- *Examples*: Atropine, scopolamine, other naturally occurring and pharmaceutical anticholinergics, antihistamines, and tricyclic antidepressants.

NURSING CARE

A successful outcome of poisoning treatment largely depends upon the skill and application of the nursing. Frequent evaluation of the vitals especially in case of unconscious patients must be administered. Attention to prevent the pressure ulcers, exposure keratitis, urinary incontinence, and adequate bronchial toilet will give a better outcome in these patients.

PSYCHIATRIC CARE

As majority of the cases of poisoning are as a result of self-administration of poisons, psychological and psychiatric care is essential for better acute and long-term outcomes.

The role of a psychiatrist is to interview the patient and his or her caregivers to identify the underlying psychiatric illness.

MEDICOLEGAL ASPECTS OF POISONING

LAWS RELATED TO POISONS

Though there are a handful of laws and Indian Penal Codes (IPCs) in relation to poisoning, however, below are three important laws which govern almost all regulations in relation to toxic substances.

1. *Narcotic Drugs and Psychotropic Substances (NDPS) Act*: This was promulgated in 1985. This Act repeals the Opium Act, 1857, the Opium Act, 1878, and the Dangerous Drugs Act, 1930. The Act defines narcotic drug, psychotropic substance, medicinal cannabis, opium, opium derivatives, opium poppy, poppy straw, poppy straw concentrate, *Cannabis* (hemp), *Cannabis* plant, coca derivatives, coca leaf, manufacture, production, preparation, and addict etc.
2. *The Drug Act, 1940*: The purpose of this Act was to regulate import, manufacture, distribution, and sale of drugs such as patent or proprietary medicines, vaccines, sera, toxins, antitoxins, antigen, other biological products such as vitamins, hormones, and drugs commonly used for external or internal consumption.
3. *Pharmacy Act, 1948*: The purpose of this Act is to make better provision for the regulation of the profession of pharmacy and setting up of "Pharmacy Councils".

ROLE OF DOCTOR

- Immediate management is the first and foremost duty.
- Preserve vomitus, urine, stool, and stomach wash samples.
- Preserve suspected food, bottle, paper packets, liquid etc. (i.e., any article which can help in identifying the poison). Noncompliance is punishable under section 201 IPC.
- All the preserved articles must be packed, labeled, signed, sealed, and "police" must be informed to take the sample for necessary action.
- If the doctor is convinced that the nature of poisoning is homicidal or suicidal or the patient dies, he is bound to inform the "police" (S.39 CrPC). *However, for all practical purposes it is advisable to inform the police in all suspected cases of poisoning.*

- If "police" or "court" wants any information about any case of poisoning attended by the doctor, he has to provide it (S.175 CrPC). If he fails to do so, he is liable to be prosecuted (S.202 IPC). So, it is better to preserve all papers and documents.

RECOMMENDED READINGS

1. Pillay VV. Comprehensive Medical Toxicology, 4th Edition. Hyderabad, India: Paras Medical Publisher; 2008. pp. 4-64.
2. Ellenhorn MJ. Medical Toxicology: Diagnosis and Treatment of Human Poisoning, 2nd Edition. Baltimore, USA: Williams and Wilkins; 1997.
3. American Heart Association and International Liaison Committee on Resuscitation. Guidelines 2000 for cardiopulmonary resuscitation and emergency cardiovascular care. Circulation. 2000;(Suppl 8):1-383.
4. Chyka PA. Chapter 10: Clinical Toxicology. United States: McGraw-Hill Education; 2014. pp. 133-57.
5. Satoskar RS, Bhandarkar SD. Pharmacology and Pharmacotherapeutics, 24th Edition. Mumbai, India: Popular Prakashan; 2015. p. 48.
6. Chyka PA, Seger D, Krenzelok EP, Vale JA. American Academy of Clinical Toxicology; European Association of Poisons Centres and Clinical Toxicologists. Position paper: Single-dose activated charcoal. Clin Toxicol (Phila). 2005;43:61-87.
7. Singh S, Wig N, Chuadhary D, Sood NK, Sharma BK. Changing patterns of acute poisoning in adults: experience of a large North-West Indian hospital. (1970-89). J Assoc Physic India. 1997;45:194-7.
8. Richard C. Dart. The 5 Minute Toxicology Consult (5-Minute Consult Series). United Kingdom: Lippincott Williams and Wilkins; 2000. pp. 2-5.
9. Aggrawal A. Forensic Medicine and Toxicology. New Delhi, India: Avichal Publishing Company; 2016. pp. 460-7.
10. Fenton JJ. Toxicology: a case-oriented approach, 1st Edition. Florida: CRC Press; 2002.

CHAPTER 20

Heavy Metal Poisoning

Udas Chandra Ghosh, Manali Chandra

ABSTRACT

We should not take heavy metal poisoning lightly, as it causes health hazards in human life. With the growing of industrial activities along with the pollution, heavy metals enter in human body through food, water and air. Many of these heavy metals are essential to body function in small amounts, e.g., iron, copper, zinc, chromium and manganese. Toxicity occurs when these accumulate in higher doses or inherently toxic heavy metals like lead, arsenic, mercury, and cadmium accumulate in any dose in our body. It causes multiple health hazards involving more or less all systems of the body resulting in different neurological, hematological, cardiac, and hepatic abnormalities. High clinical suspicion with laboratory investigations help to confirm the diagnosis. Treatment is mainly preventive, but some specific treatments help to lead a nearly normal life.

"Toxic metals overload the immune system"

—Anonymous

INTRODUCTION

Heavy metal poisoning is the accumulation of heavy metals in toxic amounts in soft tissues of the body. Many of these heavy metals are essential to body function in small amounts, e.g., iron, copper, zinc, chromium and manganese. Toxicity occurs when these accumulate in higher doses or inherently toxic heavy metals like lead, arsenic, mercury, and cadmium accumulate in any dose in our body.

These metals enter our body through food (including medicines and food containers), water and air. Heavy metal toxicity is becoming more and more relevant for public at large with the growing industrial activities and resulting pollution. Hence, we doctors have to keep this disease in mind, more now, than ever in the past.

This scenario is as much a growing menace in a developing country like India as much it is in rest of the world, if not more. In an all India study published very recently at the end of 2019 (published in The HINDU), the

Central Water Commission found majority of our rivers to be guilty of at least two or more heavy metal contamination. Considering the fact that unfiltered river water is still now an important source of drinking water for majority of Indians, the long-term implications of this study finding are grave. This holds true for most of the states of India and especially for the ones built on banks of rivers like Delhi (by Yamuna) and nine districts of West Bengal (by Ganga).

SOURCES

As mentioned above, most heavy metals enter our body by ingestion or inhalation. To begin with clearing a common misconception about the most common heavy metal detected in water sources tested in India, iron—drinking iron-contaminated water for long-term—does not cause iron toxicity. Iron contamination of water is more of an aesthetic and plumbing issue than a health-related one. In fact, iron toxicity typically presents as acute poisoning in children who might have accidentally ingested a syrup-containing iron. On the other hand, chronic iron toxicities are found commonly in patients requiring frequent blood transfusions, like thalassemia or in primary hemochromatosis patients.

Coming to the hazardous metals, sources of ones like lead, mercury, and cadmium are mostly anthropogenic—industrial activities and vehicles. Lead toxicity, in addition, can also happen from the lead pipes carrying the water to our homes. Children sometimes, accidentally take mouth flakes of wall paintings and toys-containing lead, which may give rise to symptoms of toxicity. In fact, besides lead, polyvinyl chloride (PVC) plastic toys may contain multiple other heavy metals as example cadmium.

Cadmium may come into our body by food, because of the soil in which they are grown. Soil, which is treated with sewage sludge, city wastes, and cadmium-containing fertilizers, transmits the cadmium into its crops, which in turn is transmitted and deposited in our bodies.

Mercury toxicity occurs by inhalation of mercury vapors in industries or by ingestion of fishes-containing organic mercury compounds. Mercury enters from industries handling mercury product like batteries, thermometers, dental amalgams etc., from there into the food chain of edible fishes and from there into our bodies.

Arsenic, on the other hand, has been naturally found in some areas, example the Brahmaputra–Ganges basin for millions of years. Toxicities from the same have been recently noted, though, since the time of shifting of water source from surface water and shallow wells to deep tube wells. Some herbicides and herbal medicines bought over the counter are alleged to contain arsenic too.

CLINICAL FEATURES

Clinical features of heavy metal poisoning depend on:
- Whether exposure is acute or chronic.
- Whether affected person is a child or an adult.
- Type and amount of metal involved.

For example, acute toxicities usually present with acute abdominal symptoms like vomiting, diarrhea, and abdominal pain while features like anemia is a classic sign of chronic metal toxicity. Growth-related problems due to affected bones characteristically occur in children, adults may have sexual problems. The third point of difference is the type of metal involved and this will be dealt in little detail now (**Fig. 1**).

ARSENIC

Acute: As described previously, acute arsenic poisoning presents as acute gastroenteritis (mimics cholera). Characteristic garlicky odor of breath if present, will point toward arsenic. Palpitation in such patients may indicate

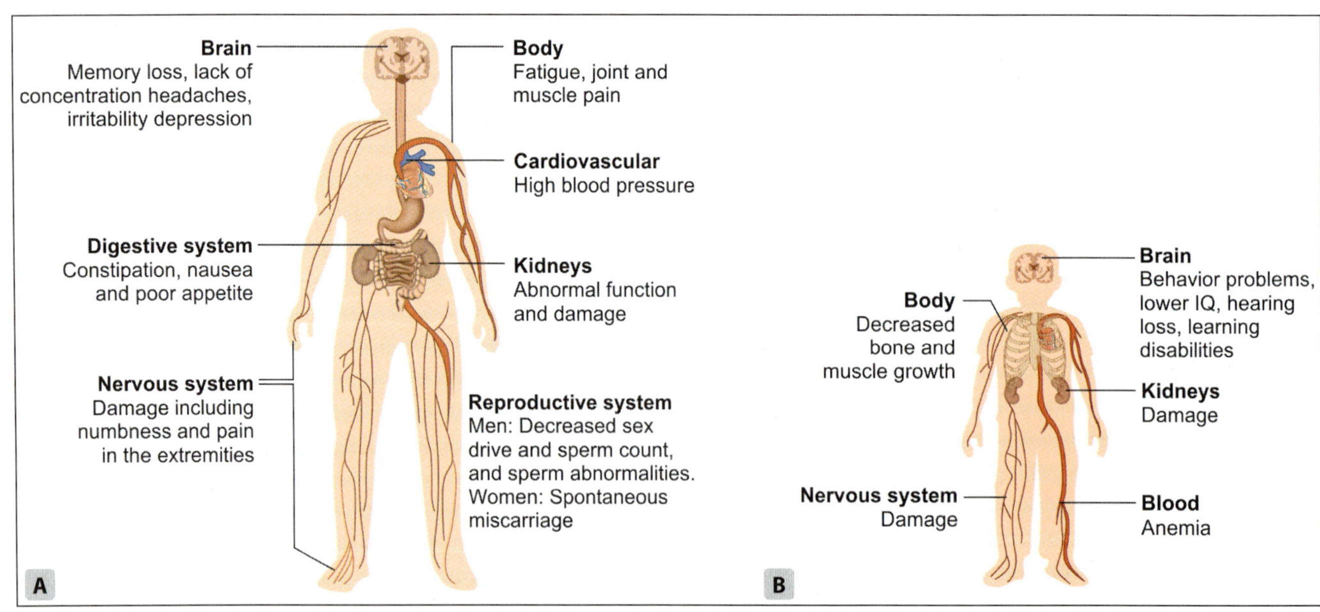

FIGURES 1 A & B: Clinical features of heavy metal poisoning in: (A) Adult; (B) Child.

Source: Tony S. (2020). Symptoms and signs of heavy metal toxicity in your body.

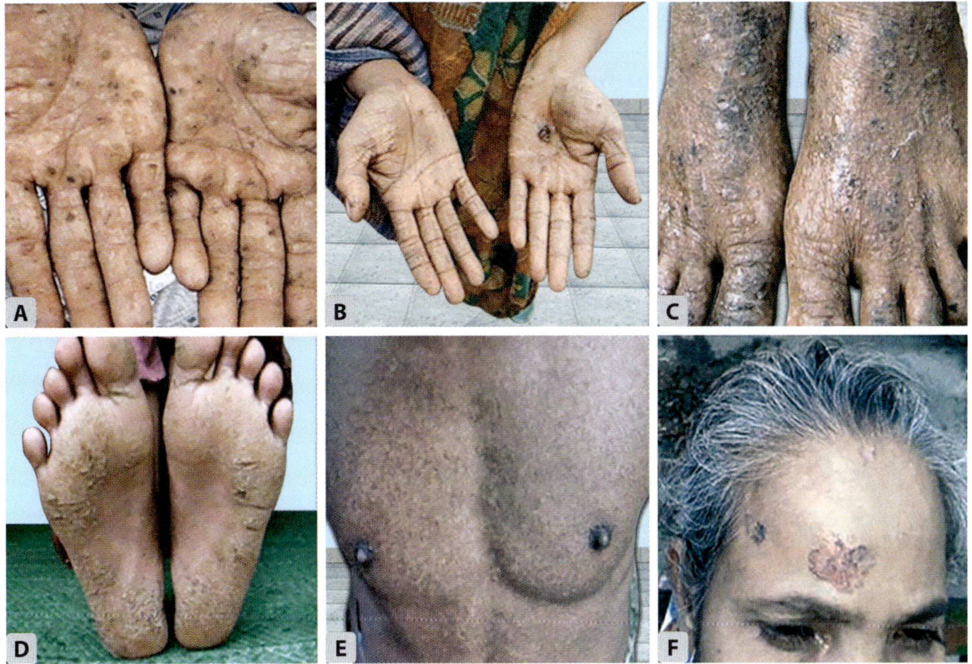

FIGURES 2 A to F: Skin changes in chronic arsenic poisoning patient—(**A and B**) Raindrop pigmentation of palms; (**C and D**) Hyperkeratosis of sole; **(E)** Mottled appearance of skin; **(F)** Skin cancer.

Source: Tony S. (2020). Symptoms and signs of heavy metal toxicity in your body.

life-threatening QTc prolongation. Hematuria and anuria may occur from acute tubular necrosis. Hemolysis may occur.

Chronic: It is chiefly diagnosed from the characteristic skin hyper- and hypopigmentation giving a mottled appearance to palm, sole, extremities affected symmetrically and trunk (raindrop pigmentation) and is one of the earliest manifestations. Hyperkeratosis and scaling usually follow (**Figs. 2 A** to **F**). Inspection of nails may reveal Mees' lines (transverse white striae) (**Fig. 3**).

Other than such changes, skin also runs the risk of being affected by squamous cell cancer arising from hyperkeratotic warts. Cancer of other organs such as kidney, bladder, lung, and liver (the sites of arsenic metabolism and distribution) also occurs.

Chronic arsenic toxicity is a well-known etiology of distal symmetric peripheral neuropathy (sensory and motor both) starting typically with prominent sensory symptoms, like burning of feet and cramping of calves. Like diabetes, early loss of vibratory sensation is a feature of arsenic toxicity as well.

As mentioned above, cardiac arrhythmias especially QTc prolongation can occur with arsenic, a fact that should be kept in mind while prescribing other medications to acute promyelocytic leukemia (APML) patients already on arsenic trioxide therapy.

Vascular complications as severe as gangrene, noncirrhotic portal fibrosis (NCPF) and endocrinal problems like type 2 diabetes mellitus have been noted in chronic arsenic toxicity patients (**Table 1**).

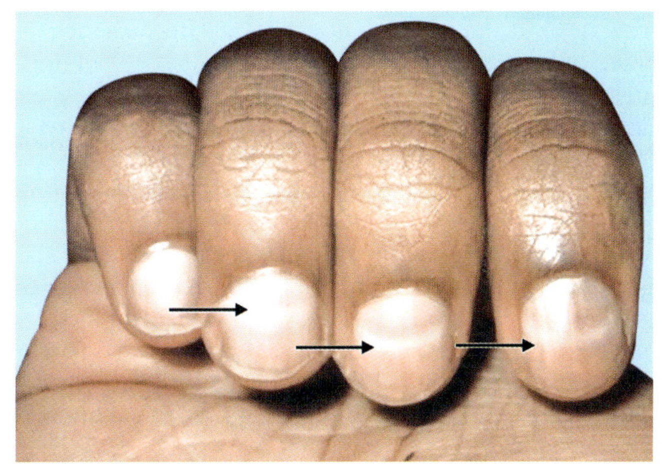

FIGURE 3: Mees' lines.

Source: Cadogan M, Scott K. (2021). Mees lines.

TABLE 1 Arsenic—chief clinical features.

Important heavy metal	Mnemonic	Chief clinical feature
ARSENIC	A-R-S-E-N-I-C	A—Aldrich/Mees' line R—Rain drop pigmentation S—Seizures, delirium E—Excessive pigmentation of palm and sole, exfoliative dermatitis N—peripheral neuritis I—Irregular cardiac arrhythmia, QT prolongation C—Cholera like diarrhea

Diagnosis and treatment: All these clinical features with history suggestive exposure to the metal, like the place they belong to or the profession they are engaged in, will give a strong ground to go for further diagnostic tests.

For recent exposure, 24-hour urinary arsenic is the best test (patient should not take any sea fish 24-hour prior to this sample collection, as organic nontoxic arsenic in sea food will give a falsely elevated result).

For recent past or chronic exposure, hair and nails are the best samples since inorganic arsenic is taken up and bound in these tissues. If nails are analyzed, clippings from all 10 digits (finger or toe) are required.

To treat these patients, decontamination of the skin, gastric lavage, and activated charcoal for acute cases and chelation therapy by parenteral dimercaprol or oral succimer has to be resorted to.

Dose: 5 mg/kg stat intramuscular (IM) followed by 2–3 mg/kg every 4–8 hours for 2 days, then once or twice a day for 10 days. It is better to start the therapy early. Urine should be alkalinized during dimercaprol therapy because the dimercaprol-metal complex dissociates faster in acidic urine and the released metal can damage the kidney.

LEAD

Lead poisoning is the new hypertension (HTN). It is a silent killer. As per a very recent UNICEF report, published this 2020, a third of world's children are poisoned by lead. India accounts for an alarming 275,561,163 of these children. Lead levels in blood of Indian children show that they can lose four intelligence quotient (IQ) points due to lead exposure. This equals to almost $1 trillion of economic potential loss for India and other middle and low income countries suffering from the same malady.

A major contributor to lead exposure is lead acid batteries, the batteries used in ouremergency lights. On top of that, with the surge of solar power, the demand for lead acid batteries is rising in India. Also, lead is found in a lot of commonly consumed Indian foods like garam masala (and not to forget, its recent discovery in a popular brand of instant noodles).

With this reminder of the risk looming around the corner, let us look for the signs and symptoms (**Table 2**) hinting us toward lead toxicity (**Fig. 4**).

TABLE 2 Lead—chief clinical features.

Important heavy metal	Mnemonic	Chief clinical feature
LEAD	A-B-C-D-E-F-G	A—Anemia B—Basophilic stippling C—Colic, constipation D—Dropped foot, peripheral neuropathy E—Encephalopathy F—Facial pallor—earliest sign G—Gum line (Burtonian line)

Acute: Like arsenic, symptoms begin with gastrointestinal (GI) complaints but rather than vomiting and diarrhea, here abdominal pain is predominant, pain which is typically colicky in nature. But what is more classic for lead poisoning is nervous system involvement. Acutely poisoned patients will present with encephalopathy with or without convulsions. Renal dysfunction (resembling Fanconi syndrome with glucosuria, aminoaciduria, and renal phosphate wasting, especially in children) may accompany.

Chronic: Following the lines of acute poisoning, in chronic poisoning (subclinical exposure), the person develops neurobehavioral problems. Children, for whom GI route is the most important site for absorption, show signs of global mental retardation or focal deficits like hearing impairment, motor deficits, and impaired balance; deteriorating school performance is one of the signs. Children may also complain of abdominal pain (lead colic). Adults (inhalational route most important) develop anemia [microcytic hypochromic anemia, with basophilic stippling, 90–95% of lead in blood is sequestered in red blood cells (RBCs)], peripheral neuropathy (typically motor; it was sensory predominant sensory motor neuropathy in arsenic poisoning), tremor, anxiety, depression, and also chronic kidney disease (CKD). CKD from lead resembles hypertensive nephropathy (HTN is a cardiological manifestation of lead toxicity) and chronic urate nephropathy (lead produces hyperuricemia) and hence frequently overlooked. Lead can affect sexual life, decreasing sperm count and can inducing spontaneous abortions (**Fig. 5**).

Diagnosis and treatment: Symptoms of lead poisoning in the background of exposure history should prompt testing blood lead level (BLL), permissible levels being <10 μg/dL in children and <40 μg/dL in adults. If suspicion is high but BLL within range, then test erythrocyte protoporphyrin level.

Chelation therapy to be given in those acutely intoxicated and those with high BLL with symptoms. Dimercaptosuccinic acid (DMSA) and calcium disodium edetate (Ca-EDTA) are the chelators of choice. However, there is clearly no role of chelator in the later case, if exposure is not reduced. Education and reduction of exposure are essential to curb lead toxicity. So much so that if a person is found to have BLL >30 μg/dL, he or she needs to be removed from workplace if that is considered to be the source of exposure.

MERCURY

Mercury and doctors have an intimate relationship. Dental amalgams are used to fill tooth cavities. Mercury comprises 50% of those amalgams—dentists dealing with several patients, filling cavities with such amalgams were thus exposed to substantial amount of mercury vapors, if workplace ventilation was poor. Patients, on other hand, with multiple dental amalgams were inferred to also be poisoned over years by slow erosion of mercury from the tooth amalgam into the gut. However, with improved work place ventilation, doctors are no longer at risk. Also mercury

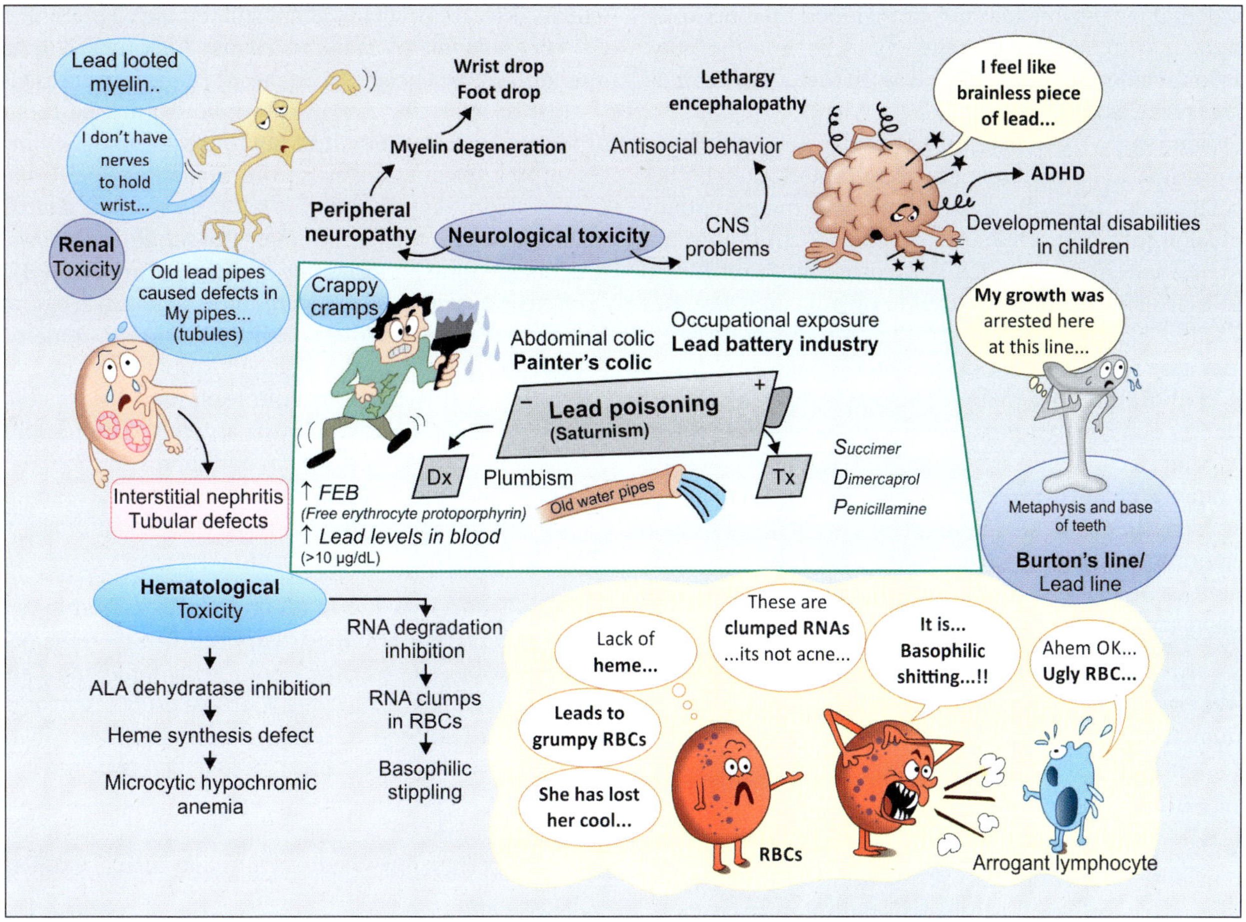

Lead looted myelin..
I don't have nerves to hold wrist...
Renal Toxicity
Old lead pipes caused defects in My pipes... (tubules)
Interstitial nephritis
Tubular defects
Wrist drop
Foot drop
Myelin degeneration
Peripheral neuropathy
Neurological toxicity
Lethargy encephalopathy
Antisocial behavior
CNS problems
I feel like brainless piece of lead...
ADHD
Developmental disabilities in children
Crappy cramps
Abdominal colic
Painter's colic
Occupational exposure
Lead battery industry
Lead poisoning (Saturnism)
Dx
Plumbism
Tx
Old water pipes
Succimer
Dimercaprol
Penicillamine
↑ FEB
(Free erythrocyte protoporphyrin)
↑ Lead levels in blood
(>10 µg/dL)
My growth was arrested here at this line...
Metaphysis and base of teeth
Burton's line/
Lead line
Hematological Toxicity
ALA dehydratase inhibition
Heme synthesis defect
Microcytic hypochromic anemia
RNA degradation inhibition
RNA clumps in RBCs
Basophilic stippling
Lack of heme...
These are clumped RNAs ...its not acne...
It is... Basophilic shitting...!!
Ahem OK... Ugly RBC...
Leads to grumpy RBCs
She has lost her cool...
RBCs
Arrogant lymphocyte

(ADHD: attention-deficit hyperactivity disorder; ALA: aminolevulinic acid; CNS: central nervous system)

FIGURE 4: Pictorial depiction of clinical features with their pathogenesis of lead poisoning.

Source: Creative Med Doses. Lead poisoning: Plumbism/saturnism.

• Abdominal pain
• Constipation
• Lead line (a bluish pigmentation seen at the gum-tooth line)
• Peripheral neuropathy
Irritability
Difficulty in concentrating
Myalgia
Arthralgia

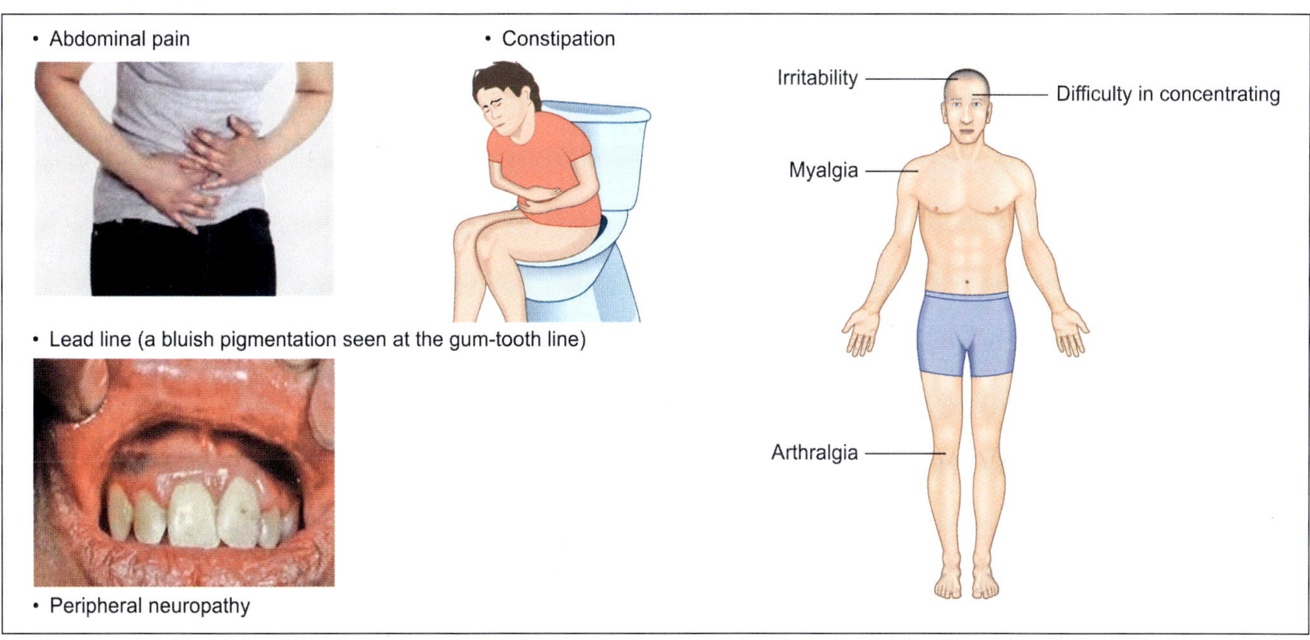

FIGURE 5: Summary of the important clinical features of lead poisoning.

Source: MEDVIZZ. Lead poisoning.

from dental amalgams does not cause blood mercury to be so high so as to cause poisoning. No indication therefore exists for people with already filled tooth cavities to get their cavities re-excavated!

Serious mercury poisoning has been reported instead from eating sea fishes. Inorganic mercury enters water bodies from factories, including those manufacturing essentially medical equipment, like thermometers and mercury sphygmomanometers, which is ingested by the fishes in those water bodies and converted to organic mercury. This now enters human bodies (remember Minamata disease). Similar case happened in 1992 in Kodaikanal, Tamil Nadu, from a thermometer manufacturing factory disposing underprocessed mercury-containing waste in nearby water body. Many local people were admitted with renal failure, a well-known feature of mercury toxicity. Sonbhadra region of Uttar Pradesh, one of the largest reservoirs of coal in India, has mercury in water sources, fishes have increased level of methylmercury, and increased mercury has been found in blood samples of local people (an impending Minamata crisis).

Acute: Acute inhalation in people working where either manufacture or recycling of mercury products is being done, can cause acute shortness of breath, chest pain, severe nausea, stomatitis, conjunctivitis, and dermatitis.

Chronic: Low dose inhalation causes the typical erethism mercurialis, characterized by a change in personality, anxiety, irritability, fearfulness, pathologic shyness, memory loss, insomnia, fatigue, and weakness. A higher dose of exposure produces non-neurological symptoms, like excessive salivation and desquamation as well.

Ingestion of mercury, be it acute or chronic, will produce gastroenteritis and cardiological symptoms—palpitation from arrhythmia, HTN can occur in long-term or hemodynamic collapse and death in case of acute heavy toxicity is a rare occurrence but still remains a possibility in mercury poisoning. Ataxia, visual loss, hearing loss, besides memory loss will accompany chronic ingestion cases also.

Just as mercury crosses the blood-brain barrier and produces such florid central nervous system (CNS) manifestations, it can also cross the placenta. Fetal toxicity ranges from severe features of abnormal neuronal migration and gross fetal anomalies to subtle, but significant neurobehavioral performance decline occurs (**Table 3**).

A historical disease which requires mention is hydrargia (mercurialism) in children. Children exposed to mercury-containing antihelminthics, laxatives (banned now) often presented with irritability, photophobia, and a telltale picture of acrodynia, which was a very painful condition affecting the extremities (due to peripheral neuritis). It was also known as the pink disease because the body acquired a pink discoloration from flushing and morbilliform rash (**Figs. 6 A** and **B**).

Diagnosis and treatment: Mercury is tested in blood and urine. Exposure that ended years ago can be detected by a rise in urine mercury in 24-hour urine following a single test dose of chelating *succimer*. Chronic exposure to organic mercury is diagnosed by testing mercury in hair. Maternal hair for mercury is tested in suspected fetal toxicity.

TABLE 3 Mercury—chief clinical features.

Important heavy metal	Mnemonic	Chief clinical feature
MERCURY	S-Mell-Black-T-E-A	S—Salivation M—Minamata disease B—Black line on gums T—Tremor, intentional E—Erethism A—Acrodynia

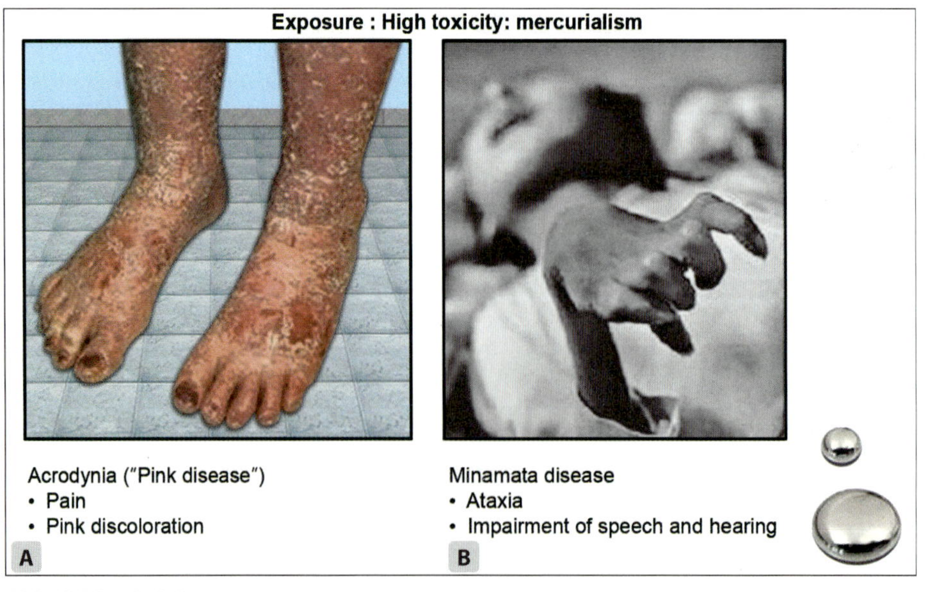

FIGURES 6 A & B: Clinical features of mercury poisoning.

Source: Steemit. Mercury Poisoning.

Just like other heavy metals, acute ingestion of mercury also requires gastric lavage with special benefit from using polythiol (sulfur-containing resins). Chelation is performed in acute cases by dimercaprol, DMSA, or penicillamine. Only N-acetyl penicillamine is used in chronic cases.

CADMIUM

Cadmium levels have been rising steadily in water bodies of India and hence in cereals and grains watered from those very sources. Hence awareness about its clinical features—isn't something we can give a miss! Clinical features include respiratory, GI and renal system.

Acute inhalation (from incineration of plastics, tobacco, and other elements containing cadmium) causes pleuritic chest pain, noncardiogenic pulmonary edema, acute or chronic ingestion produces nausea, vomiting, abdominal cramps, and diarrhea. Renal tubular damage culminates in CKD, osteomalacia, and bone fractures.

OTHER HEAVY METALS

Other heavy metals like aluminum are being associated with Alzheimer's disease of late, while manganese is known to cause Parkinsonian syndrome. Nickel causes allergic reaction, may lead to lung cancer on long-term inhalational exposure. The later is true for chromium and cobalt exposure as well. These heavy metal toxicities are uncommon in India, a high chance of cases being unrecognized and hence unreported remains though.

ROLE OF DOCTORS

- Clinicians should know how to take a good environmental, residential, and occupational history.
- Clinicians should have reasonable understanding of common environment-related illnesses and of the basics of exposure assessment.
- A patient's illness may require assessment regarding his/her ability to perform or continue job/need of short or long-term duty restrictions/if work-related exposure, then assessment of impairment, disability, and eligibility for worker's compensation.
- Clinicians and health centers should have sufficient background to respond to exposures from accidental contamination of air or water from places like factories or as a result of natural disasters, like flood.
- In addition to diagnostic responsibilities, clinicians have an opportunity for preventive care related to occupational and environmental exposures. A patient's exposure when promptly reported by a doctor may require further interventions to prevent future illness for others, say other employees at work site or addressing climate change issues and potential health consequences.

CONCLUSION

Heavy metal toxicity is an important entity. True, it is not as common place as are diabetes and HTN in neither our OPDs nor half as easily spotted in our indoor wards as are chronic liver disease, CKDs, strokes, and congestive heart failures. At the same time, it must be evident to us by now, after reading this chapter, that behind any unexplained anemia, any unknown tingling and numbness of limbs and any chronic crampy abdominal pain, and diarrhea, there might be heavy metal toxicity responsible. It only depends on doctors, how high and consistent; we can keep our suspicions every time we encounter such a case. Suspicion followed by a wise history taking to elicit possibility of any exposure, occupational or environmental, will clinch the diagnosis. Special diagnostic tests are also available to confirm. Treatment with cure is possible, if detected early before permanent damage occurs. However, the biggest challenge lies in preventing the disease in those exposed, who have not yet developed overt symptoms and signs but are at the risk of developing the same anytime in near future. Gradual elimination of the heavy metal from the sources of exposure, using alternative raw materials or changing the occupation will be of help. These measures, it must be said, are by no means easy. And it will take collective effort from the society as a whole to make our country and the world, at large get rid of the burden of heavy metals, and feel light!

RECOMMENDED READINGS

1. Koshy J. (2019). Heavy metals contaminating India's rivers. [online] Available from https://www.thehindu.com/news/national/heavy-metals-contaminating-indias-rivers/article30279681.ece.
2. Indian National Science Academy, New Delhi. (2011). Hazardous metals and minerals pollution in india: Sources, toxicity and management. [online] Available from http://www.insaindia.res.in/pdf/Hazardous_Metals.pdf.
3. National Center for Advancing Translational Sciences. (2017). Heavy metal poisoning. [online] Available from Https://Rarediseases.Info.Nih.Gov/Diseases/6577/Heavy-Metal-Poisoning.
4. World Health Organization. (2019). Exposure to arsenic: A major public concern. [online] Available from https://apps.who.int/iris/bitstream/handle/10665/329482/WHO-CED-PHE-EPE-19.4.1-eng.pdf.
5. Baker BA, Cassano VA, Murray C, ACOEM Task Force on Arsenic Exposure. Arsenic exposure, assessment, toxicity, diagnosis, and management: guidance for occupational and environmental physicians. J Occup Environ Med. 2018;60:e634-e639.
6. National Toxicology Program, US Department of Health and Human Services. (2012). Health effects of low-level lead evaluation.
7. Kosnett MJ, Wedeen RP, Rothenberg SJ, Hipkins KL, Materna BL, Schwartz BS, et al. Recommendations for medical management of adult lead exposure. Environ Health Perspect. 2007;115:463-71.
8. Centers for Disease Control and Prevention (CDC). Very high blood lead levels among adults—United

States, 2002-2011. MMWR Morb Mortal Wkly Rep. 2013;62:967-71.
9. Sullivan M. More evidence of unpublished industry studies of lead smelter/refinery workers. Int J Occup Environ Health. 2015;21:308-13.
10. Magos L. Review on the toxicity of methyl mercury, including its presence as a preservative in biological and pharmaceutical products. J Appl Toxicol. 2001; 21:1-5.
11. Clarkson TW. The three modern faces of mercury. Environ Health Perspect 2002; 110 Suppl 1:11-3.
12. Sue Y. Mercury. In: Hoffman RS, Howland M, Lewin NA, Nelson L, Goldfrank L (Eds). Goldfrank's Toxicologic Emergencies, 10th edition. New York: McGraw-Hill; 2015.
13. WHO. Inorganic mercury. Environmental Health Criteria 118. Geneva: World Health Organization; 1991.
14. Clarkson TW, Magos L, Myers GJ. The toxicology of mercury—current exposures and clinical manifestations. N Engl J Med. 2003;349:1731-7.
15. Landrigan PJ, Baker DB. The recognition and control of occupational disease. JAMA, 1991;266:676-80.
16. Henretig FM, Kirk MA, McKay CA Jr. Hazardous chemical emergencies and poisonings. Reply. N Engl J Med. 2019; 381:393-94.
17. Patz JA, Frumkin H, Holloway T, Vimont DJ, Haines A. Climate change: Challenges and opportunities for global health. JAMA. 2014;312:1565-80.
18. Crowley RA, Health and Public Policy Committee of the American College of Physicians. Climate Change and Health: A Position Paper of the American College of Physicians. Ann Intern Med 2016; 164:608-10.
19. Council on Environmental Health. Global Climate Change and Children's Health. Pediatrics. 2015;136: 992-7.

CHAPTER 21

Genetic Counseling and the Treatment of Genetic Disorders

Rudrajit Paul

ABSTRACT

Genetic tests are becoming an essential part of clinical practice today. The tests include diagnosing a hereditary illness, searching for congenital anomalies, and also finding the specific mutations in cancer tissues for targeted therapy. But a genetic test can have far-reaching consequences for the patient and the family. Hence, proper genetic counseling is essential before such tests. A pretest counseling is necessary to help the patient to understand the concept of genetics and what the test result will mean, not only from medical perspective but also from social, financial, and reproductive points of view. Specialized experts are required and multiple sessions may be necessary. The genetic counselor also helps the patient and family cope with the immediate psychological aftermath of the diagnosis. Physicians, especially of the specialties who advise such tests frequently (like hematology and neurology), should send patients for counseling before the tests. This chapter covers the basic principles of genetic counseling along with the technical details.

The treatment of genetic disorders is now undergoing a sea change with the development of new technology. While common disorders like thalassemia are still mostly treated with conventional methods like regular blood transfusion, a lot of new therapies are in the horizon. This includes enzyme replacement, ribonucleic acid (RNA) silencing, and bone marrow transplant. The recent trial results have been quite encouraging. In oncology, many new drugs have been developed targeting specific mutations in cancer tissues. These offer new hope for relapsed and treatment-refractory cancers. A brief discussion on all these new therapies has been presented and some recent drugs approved for genetic disorders have been described.

"Your genome knows much more about your medical history than you do"

—Danny Hillis

GENETIC COUNSELING

BACKGROUND

Scenario 1: A patient comes to the OPD with recurrent anemia. The doctor finds microcytic hypochromic anemia. There is also history of recurrent joint pain. The doctor suspects sickle cell disease and orders a sickle cell mutation study.

Scenario 2: A young female patient presents with cerebral venous sinus thrombosis. The attending doctor suspects hereditary thrombophilia and along with other tests like protein C level, also orders a factor V Leiden mutation study.

Scenarios like these are quite common. As physicians, we often order a host of tests to reach a diagnosis in our patients. But when we are thinking of a genetic test, we have to stop and think about it a little more, before proceeding. While microbiology or a pathology test can be ordered as and when needed, ordering a genetic test carries a different implication. This is because a genetic test result can have far reaching implications not only for the patient but also the family at large. Thus, before a genetic test is advised, we need to discuss it with the patient and/or the family.

While a kidney biopsy or a blood culture report has health consequences only for the patient, a sickle cell mutation study result or a Huntington's chorea mutation study result can have a different meaning for the whole family. *Should other family members be tested? What is the impact on employment for other family members? What is the implication for health insurance coverage (will a patient with genetic disease get insurance coverage, especially in India where there is no rule to protect preexisting conditions)? Can the patient think of starting a family?* These are some of the questions that crop up when a genetic mutation is discovered. *Also, what does it mean if a genetic test comes negative? Does it mean the patient is free of the disease? Or can it be that there is a new mutation which is not detected by the existing tests?* So, before doing a genetic test, we need something called genetic counseling.

Although the concept of medical genetics and mutation study is slowly becoming popular among the physicians, the need of extensive counseling before those tests is still neglected in India. For example, different genetic tests are done regularly now before treatment of leukemia. But hardly any counseling is done a priori. In this chapter, the author aims to introduce the physicians to the concept of genetic counseling. In the present era of consumer court driven and insurance-based medical practice, this aspect of medical genetics cannot be neglected. Physicians practicing in 2030 or 2040 must make sure that the patient is adequately counseled before any genetic test, to avoid future allegations.

DEFINITIONS

Genetic counseling is a branch of health sciences, which is becoming extremely important with time. Especially, after the mapping of the full human genome (completed in April, 2003), as a host of genetic diseases has been unearthed, the need to explain these diseases to the patients and families has also increased. Recently, the World Health Organization (WHO) has defined genetic counseling as (WHO Genomic resource center):

Genetic counseling is the process through which knowledge about the genetic aspects of illnesses is shared by trained professionals with those who are at an increased risk or either having a heritable disorder or of passing it on to their unborn offspring.

A newer definition, devised by an international task force is (quote):

- Genetic counseling is a communication process, which aims to help individuals, couples and families understand and adapt to the medical, psychological, familial and reproductive implications of the genetic contribution to specific health conditions.

WHO WILL DO IT?

For this purpose, there is need of highly trained professionals called *genetic counselors*. In Europe, to be a genetic counselor, the usual qualification required is a Master's degree in genetics or genetic counseling. People with backgrounds in psychology, nursing or related biological sciences can think of becoming a genetic counselor. The National Health Service (NHS), UK has genetic nurses also. Usually, each country has a board of medical genetics which certifies and registers the counselors.

A genetic counselor has the following jobs:

- To provide information on the inheritance of illnesses
- To address the concern of the families, the patients and also the healthcare providers
- To support the patient and their families, especially after the test result.

According to the European board of Medical Genetics, the counselor is also expected:

- To promote informed choices related to the disease
- To assess and discuss the chances of disease occurrence and recurrence
- To discuss probable ways of prevention including making family planning decisions
- To facilitate access to appropriate healthcare resources including research.

The genetic counselor usually works as a part of a multidisciplinary team in specialized centers. With the number of patients seeking care for genetic conditions on the rise, there is a vast unmet need for these highly specialized professionals. While physicians can supervise the counseling session, physicians cannot act as the primary counselors. The only exception to this is the obstetrician who can act as the primary counselor to the parents for prenatal genetic diagnosis.

PREREQUISITES

The prerequisites for genetic counseling (as discussed by Rantanen E et al. in 2008):

- Appropriately trained professional who understands genetics and the ethical implications
- Relevant and objective information
- Making sure that the counselee understands
- Informed consent
- Psychological support
- *Confidentiality*
- Sensitivity about the familial implications
- Avoiding discrimination in testing
- Ensuring that the counselee makes an autonomous decision.

A proper counseling requires a lot of patience and lengthy discussions, often involving family members, either in groups or separately. Thus, it is impossible to conduct a session of genetic counseling in a busy clinic. This requires a separate visit to a clinic in tranquil settings and the discussion must be unhurried. The counselor has to be empathic and must ensure that the patient and family clearly understand the meaning of the test. *No genetic test can be done without informed consent* and the person(s) must be given sufficient time to come to an autonomous decision (this also includes medicolegal cases).

Any medical specialty can send patients for a genetic test if there is an appropriate clinical history. But usually, the disciplines more involved with these tests include *pediatrics, obstetrics, oncology, and neurology*. With the explosion of new research into the genetics of different human malignancies, the frequency of genetic analysis of tumor tissue has risen astronomically. This will again be mentioned in the last part of this chapter.

COMMON INDICATIONS FOR GENETIC TESTING

- Previous child with some genetic disease
- Family history of an inherited condition
- Follow-up to an abnormal blood test (e.g., newborn screening for cystic fibrosis)
- History of teratogen exposure
- Consanguinity
- Repeated pregnancy losses etc.

TYPES OF GENETIC TESTS

There are various types of genetic tests in clinical practice:

- *Diagnostic testing*: To confirm or refute a diagnosis, e.g., testing for hemochromatosis in a patient with chronic liver disease and diabetes.
- *Predictive testing*: This is done in apparently healthy individuals, if there is a presumed risk of genetic disease, e.g., in cases of familial cancers like BRCA positive breast cancer.
- *Susceptibility testing*: This is done to detect increased or decreased risk of a particular disease in multifactorial conditions, e.g., human leukocyte antigen B27 (HLA-B27) for spondyloarthropathy
- *Pharmacogenetic testing*: This is done if a genetic marker is associated with drug reactions, e.g., for abacavir and HLA-B 57*01
- *Carrier testing*: This is a test to detect a carrier state. Usually, this will have no effect on health of the individual being tested. But it may have implications for the offspring, e.g., thalassemia carrier testing of mother
- *Prenatal testing*: This is done for the fetus during pregnancy, e.g., to detect Down syndrome in advanced maternal age. This test will have tremendous emotional consequences for the parents.
- *Preimplantation genetic diagnosis*: This is done in in vitro fertilization before putting the embryo back into the uterus
- *Medicolegal testing*: This is done for legal purposes like solving paternity contests or tracing deoxyribonucleic acid (DNA) evidence from a crime scene.

As is seen here, the different genetic tests have different consequences. For a diagnostic testing when the patient already has severe symptoms for, say, Wilson disease, the emotional consequences are minimal. But for other types of tests like thalassemia carrier testing, the positive result can have severe emotional setback for the patient and family. The genetic counselor must be aware of the differences in various types of genetic tests while discussing those with the patient.

ROLE OF THE PHYSICIAN

Usually, for diagnostic purposes, it is the physician who advises the test. But sometimes a patient can demand the test on his/her own. For example, if a woman has BRCA-1+ve breast cancer, her daughters can demand the genetic testing to know their future risk. In such patient-initiated testing, the role of counseling (especially discussing the significance of false-negative results) is even more.

Interesting fact: Famous actress Angelina Jolie got herself tested for BRCA1 mutation after her mother died from breast cancer. When she was diagnosed BRCA1+ve, she underwent preventive double mastectomy. [New York Times Op-ed, 2013.]

Since counseling is integral to any genetic test (including karyotyping for leukemia), it may be a good practice to write "counseling followed by testing" whenever advising any genetic study in the prescription.

The physician must also take express consent of the patient before disclosing the result of the test to the family or the employer.

HOW IS THE SESSION CONDUCTED?

Certain points to note: It must be remembered that the patient has the right to waive a counseling session and go straight for the test. However, that should be documented and it must be assessed whether the patient has the mental capacity to take that decision. In cases of institutionalized patients like psychiatric patients, the consent for genetic test must be taken from the legal representative of the patient. In India, this concept of legal representative of a patient is mostly absent. In those cases, it may be a good idea to convene a medical board (including a lawyer) for the decision.

The counseling should be done in a language the patient understands. Since most of the scientific terms are in English, it may be difficult to convert them to local dialects. If needed, the help of pictures and charts should be taken. If the treating physician thinks that a patient is psychologically unstable and may become very depressed following a positive test result, then prior psychiatric evaluation should be done before going for genetic test.

Sessions: Different institutes have different protocols for conducting the sessions. It is not necessary that one person gets just one session before the test. Sometimes, multiple sessions may be required before the person agrees to a test. If a test like whole genome sequencing is required (where multiple findings are possible), then the counseling sessions may be further prolonged. Sometimes, genetic tests are conducted as part of clinical research. In those cases, further discussions about clinical trials may be warranted.

Essentially, genetic counseling involves one or more pretest sessions, communication of test result, one or more posttest counseling sessions and subsequent follow-up.

Pretest counseling: Many counselors first send a video file or leaflets to the patients before the session. This video/reading material gives them a preliminary idea about the concept of genetics and also a taste of what to expect during the session. Then they come to the actual pretest counseling session. This can be conducted by the counselor alone or jointly with a clinical geneticist. Before beginning this session, a written consent is taken. This session is essentially an open-ended one where the patient is explained about genetic tests. Then the patient will decide whether they want to get the test done and if done, whether they want to know the results. *The right of not-to-know is also a valid decision and must be respected.* Usually, the teaching-counseling model is used and the bin framework is used for discussion.

Common themes discussed in pretest counseling are patient's expectations from the test, possible outcomes of the test and the degrees of uncertainty of the results (especially in tests like chromosome microarrays). Also, it is made sure that the patient understands the concepts of genes and inheritance. Relevant family history of the patient is also discussed. Such discussions can include information about family secrets, hidden birth defects, and questions about paternity. Naturally, such information needs to be kept in the strictest confidence.

Sometimes, a person can come for a genetic test by himself/herself due to presence of an inherited disorder or malignancy in the family. In such cases, the ideas and expectations of the patient need to be clarified.

The main aim of this session is to help the patient come to a decision about the testing. The patient must understand what a result may mean for his/her employment opportunities or health insurance. Also, it must be an autonomous decision unaffected by societal or peer pressures. If an agreement is reached about the testing, the counselor may refer the patient to the appropriate laboratory or center. In developed health systems, the counselor would call the laboratory to find out what types of tests are offered and whether the tests are covered by insurance plan. In India, since most health spending is out-of-pocket, such discussions would be meaningless.

The counselor can also direct the patient to some online resources to go through before the test. *Finally, it must also be informed that during genetic testing for one purpose, some incidental findings not related to the disease in question may also be unearthed. These additional findings may be the indicator of a different genetic disease. The patient must also decide whether he/she wants to know those additional results, if any.*

Roughly, a pretest counseling session covers the following topics in this sequence:

- The concept of human cell and the genes
- Inheritance of genetic traits with some idea on penetrance of characteristics
- The concept of genetic testing
- What is a positive and a negative test result?
- Secondary findings in such a test
- The risks (e.g., losing employment) and benefits (e.g., starting early therapy) of a test result
- Reproductive significance of a genetic test result (e.g., chance of passing the disease to children)
- Limitations of genetic testing
- Any other relevant discussion.

The information provided to the patient and family during the pretest counseling should have the following characteristics:

- Honest
- Up-to-date
- Sufficient
- Age-appropriate
- Balanced
- Objective.

Posttest counseling: The posttest counseling can be even more prolonged. In developed health systems where flow of information is structured, the genetic counselor is usually the one person who gets the test results first and who communicates the final test results to the patient or family and also the physician. Now, the final test result can be either positive or negative. If no mutation is detected, the counselor has to discuss the significance of that result, the degrees of uncertainty of genetic tests, and the possibility of new mutations which are not detected by current tests. *In other words, genetic tests cannot "rule out" a disease with certainty*. For example, if checking for thalassemia, a test will only check for the most common mutations. But there are many rare mutations which are not included in the test. So, these rare mutations may not be detected.

If a positive result comes back, the counselor helps the patient and the family to deal with the psychological, economic, social, emotional, and medical dimensions of the disease. The five stages of grief must be addressed (if required, by multiple sessions) and further psychological counseling must be advised if needed. At this point, social support resources like NGOs and online communities may be mentioned. The patient may also want to discuss the need to test other family members. Those family members may be referred for pretest counseling.

This is the point where the family needs to make difficult decisions like aborting a fetus or deciding not to have children. The counselor should support the family during this process.

Is telemedicine an effective way of genetic counseling?

In the post-COVID world, telemedicine will be an important method of communication. The 2017 COGENT trial proved that telephone conversation is an acceptable method of genetic counseling.

TAKE HOME MESSAGES

- Genetic counseling is essential before any genetic study.
- Counseling is not about taking consent for the test. It is about helping the patient to come to a decision about taking the test and also, helping them to decide whether they want to know the results.

- A genetic test result is followed by emotional upheavals and also the time for making difficult decisions. The counselor helps the patient and family through this process.
- A genetic counselor has to be empathic, knowledgeable, and must act in strict confidence.

Thus, as is seen here, genetic counseling is a completely different discipline with its dedicated professionals. Physicians need to develop good liaison with these people for effective patient care.

TREATMENT OF GENETIC DISORDERS

Treatment of genetic disorders is an ever-expanding monograph in itself. "Genetic disorder" is not a homogeneous disorder by any means. It can involve a single system of the body; but mostly, genetic disorders are multisystemic. Treatment, if available, involves targeting the particular metabolic defect and also managing the disabilities arising subsequently. Let's take the example of thalassemia, a common genetic disorder in India. This is primarily a disorder of hemoglobin production. Thus, it requires blood transfusion as the main therapy. But along with that, there is also the need to address other issues like leg ulcers, hypogonadism, iron overload, growth failure, and splenomegaly. These secondary disorders must also be treated. Similarly, in another genetic disorder, hemophilia, the main treatment is factor VIII replacement. But associated care includes orthopedic surgery, treatment of cerebrovascular accident (CVA) etc. Hence, the treatment of genetic disorders requires a multidisciplinary approach in specialized centers.

In this part of the chapter, we will first look at a few novel therapies that have been invented for some select genetic diseases (**Table 1**). Then, we will discuss the general principles of treatment.

Many of the drugs mentioned here will be unfamiliar to the internist today. But in the near future, these drugs will be widely used.

So, as this table makes clear, scientists are trying to tackle the genetic disorders in various ways. Let's look at the basic principles of treatment.

Ribonucleic acid interference: RNA interference is an exciting new technology. The basic principle is that exogenous RNA introduced into a cell will suppress transcription of the targeted gene. Two small RNA molecules, the micro-RNA and the small interfering RNA (siRNA), are useful for this purpose. They cause degradation of the target mRNA inside the cell and thus prevent the faulty protein production. One example is the drug *givosiran*. This is an siRNA which causes degradation of the mRNA for the enzyme ALA synthase in hepatocytes. This causes reduced enzyme activity. Thus, production of porphobilinogen is reduced and attacks of hepatic porphyria are prevented. The drug is given subcutaneously. But how does an siRNA molecule, given subcutaneously, reach the hepatocytes? For this, they are conjugated to GalNAc, which has receptors on hepatocytes.

Antisense oligonucleotide: This technology also uses the same principle of RNA silencing but the pathway used is different. The antisense oligonucleotide is an ssDNA molecule which is complementary to the target mRNA. Binding of the two causes mRNA degradation. One good

TABLE 1 Some new drugs approved by the FDA for genetic disorders over the last few years.

Drugs	Mechanism of action	Disease for which approved
Ivacaftor	CFTR potentiator	Cystic fibrosis
Givosiran	RNA interference therapeutic target for ALA synthase	Acute hepatic porphyria
Voxelotor	Hemoglobin oxygen affinity modulator	Sickle cell disease
Golodirsen	Induces exon skipping in the dystrophin gene	Duchenne muscular dystrophy
Bempedoic acid	Inhibits ATP-citrate lyase	Heterozygous familial hypercholesterolemia
Selumetinib	MAP kinase inhibitor	Neurofibromatosis type I
Risdiplam	Motor neuron directed RNA splicing modifier	Spinal muscular atrophy
Lumasiran	RNA interference therapeutic target for glycolate oxidase	Primary hyperoxaluria type I
Pegvaliase	Pegylated derivative of phenylalanine ammonia-lyase	Phenylketonuria
Patisiran	siRNA that reduces hepatic production of TTR	Hereditary transthyretin-mediated amyloidosis
Migalastat	A pharmacological chaperone that inhibits the enzyme α-GalA	Fabry disease
Lanadelumab	Monoclonal antibody against plasma kallikrein	Hereditary angioedema
Elapegademase	Recombinant ADA	Adenosine deaminase—SCID
Cerliponase alfa	Replacement of the natural enzyme (the drug must be infused directly into the CSF space)	Batten disease
Deutetrabenazine	Vesicular monoamine transporter-2 inhibitor	Huntington's chorea

(ADA: adenosine deaminase; ALA: aminolevulinic acid; CFTR: cystic fibrosis transmembrane conductance regulator; CSF: cerebrospinal fluid; FDA: Food and Drug Administration; MAP: mitogen-activated protein; RNA: ribonucleic acid; siRNA: small interfering RNA; SCID: severe combined immune deficiency; TTR: transthyretin)

example is *mipomersen*. This nucleotide targets the mRNA for Apo-B-100 protein. This reduces LDL production in familial hypercholesterolemia.

Recombinant proteins: Sometimes, a genetic disease causes reduced production of a protein. Then, use of recombinant protein as replacement can be useful. One example is Gaucher disease, where enzyme replacement therapy (ERT) is used as 2 weekly intravenous (IV) infusion, for life. Imiglucerase is the recombinant β-glucocerebrosidase which is used here. This enzyme is deficient in Gaucher disease. Usually, this replacement therapy is highly successful. But the problem with the use of external proteins is the development of antibodies, which can make therapy ineffective.

Bypass pathways: In genetic diseases, sometimes a pathway is blocked due to deficiency of a key enzyme and thus a metabolic process stops. Then, the therapy can be used as a bypass to overcome the metabolic defect. In cystic fibrosis, CFTR mutation causes defective ion transport across membranes due to defective chloride channels. The drug approved for this disease, ivacaftor, causes increased opening of the chloride channels by a nonconventional mode of gating. Thus, it bypasses the transport block.

Bone marrow transplant: Many genetic diseases, especially those involving the hematopoietic system, can be treated permanently by bone marrow transplant. Examples are thalassemia, sickle cell disease etc. Some other diseases which have been successfully treated by this approach are severe combined immunodeficiency and lysosomal storage disorders. The genetic diseases which are associated with deficient production of a protein are best treated by this approach. In a recent issue of the NEJM, there was publication of two cases where CRISPR technology had been used successfully to modify hematopoietic stem cells before autologous bone marrow transplant in Thalassemia. But the diseases like Huntington's chorea, which involve excess production of toxic proteins, are generally not amenable to stem cell therapy.

Monoclonal antibodies: Monoclonal antibodies are also used in some genetic disorders. Lanadelumab is a monoclonal antibody against plasma kallikrein. In hereditary angioedema (mutation in *SERPING1* gene), there is increased kallikrein activity, which, in turn, causes increased bradykinin and increased angioedema attacks. The monoclonal antibody is able to block these attacks.

Any future internist who works with genetic disorders will come across the CRISPR technology. The full form is clustered regularly interspaced short palindromic repeats. This is a gene editing tool that is being developed for human genome modification. Recently, scientists have also used the CRISPR toolkit for RNA editing.

Gene therapy: The basic defect in a genetic disease is defective genes. So, can we directly deliver healthy genes to the cells to replace the defective ones? This seems like stuff of science fiction. But serious intense research is going on to make this a reality.

Over the last 30 years, more than 3,000 clinical trials have been conducted on this therapy. The first approved gene therapy is voretigene. This is used for the autosomal recessive disorder Leber congenital amaurosis. A key step in the visual cycle is conversion of all-trans-retinyl ester to 11-cis-retinol. This is done by an isomerase called RPE65, which is defective in this disorder. The *RPE65* gene is added to an AAV2 vector and the conjugated compound is given by subretinal injection. This therapy has been found to improve vision in many cases. *Just as a genetic test requires counseling, a gene therapy will also require prior genetic counseling.*

CANCER GENETICS AND THERAPY

The genetic change in different malignancies is an area of intense research. Over the last 5 years or so, a lot of new anticancer drugs have been approved, which target specific mutations in cancer tissues. Thus, this type of therapy depends on the presence of specific mutations in the cancer tissue. Let's look at a few examples.

- *Avapritinib*: This drug is used in the treatment of gastrointestinal stromal tumor (GIST) with platelet-derived growth factor receptor alpha (PDGFRA) exon 18 mutation. It is a tyrosine kinase inhibitor.
- *Capmatinib*: This is used in the treatment of nonsmall cell lung cancer (NSCLC) with a mutation that causes mesenchymal-epithelial transition (MET) exon 14 skipping.
- *Pralsetinib*: This drug is also used for NSCLC, but for a different mutation—metastatic RET-fusion positive.

The conventional antineoplastic drugs like carboplatin or ifosfamide will always be there. But with the development of medical genetics, there is development of these new drugs. So, in future, cancer therapy will include genetic study of the tumor and use of drugs based on the mutations detected. Another exciting area of research is gene therapy for cancer. Theoretically, this involves introducing detrimental genes like suicide genes or antiangiogenic genes into the tumor. One clinical trial that is going on is the introduction of *p53* gene into head and neck cancer.

CONCLUSION

Therapy of genetic disorders is undergoing a revolution every year. The internist of tomorrow must be equipped with the knowledge to manage these diseases effectively.

RECOMMENDED READINGS

1. Skirton H, Cordier C, Ingvoldstad C, Taris N, Benjamin C. The role of the genetic counsellor: a systematic review of research evidence. Eur J Hum Genet. 2015;23(4):452-8.
2. Cross D, Burmester JK. Gene therapy for cancer treatment: Past, present and future. Clin Med Res. 2006;4(3):218-27.
3. Patch C, Middleton A. Genetic counselling in the era of genomic medicine. Br Med Bull. 2018;126(1):27-36.
4. Biesecker BB, Marteau TM. The future of genetic counselling: an international perspective. Nat Genet. 1999;22:133-7.

5. Cohen SA, Bradbury A, Henderson V, Hoskins K, Bednar E, Arun BK. Genetic Counseling and Testing in a Community Setting: Quality, Access, and Efficiency. Am Soc Clin Oncol Educ Book. 2019;39:e34-e44.
6. Kenen RH, Smith AC. Genetic counseling for the next 25 years: Models for the future. J Genet Couns. 1995;4:115-24.
7. Agrawal N, Dasaradhi PV, Mohmmed A, Malhotra P, Bhatnagar RK, Mukherjee SK. RNA Interference: Biology, Mechanism, and Applications. Microbiol Mol Biol Rev. 2003;67(4):657-85.
8. Wong E, Goldberg T. Mipomersen (kynamro): A novel antisense oligonucleotide inhibitor for the management of homozygous familial hypercholesterolemia. P T. 2014;39(2):119-22.
9. Lucarelli G, Isgrò A, Sodani P, Gaziev J. Hematopoietic stem cell transplantation in thalassemia and sickle cell anemia. Cold Spring Harb Perspect Med. 2012;2(5):a011825.
10. Amer MH. Gene therapy for cancer: present status and future perspective. Mol Cell Ther. 2014;2:27.
11. Weichselbaum RR, Kufe D. Gene therapy of cancer. Lancet. 1997;349(suppl II):SII10-2.
12. Oliveri S, Ferrari F, Manfrinati A, Pravettoni G. A systematic review of the psychological implications of genetic testing: A comparative analysis among cardiovascular, neurodegenerative and cancer diseases. Front Genet. 2018;9:624.

CHAPTER 22

Human Leukocyte Antigen System in Molecular and Genetic Medicine

Gaurav Sharma, Ajay Kumar Baranwal, Narinder Kumar Mehra

ABSTRACT

The human leukocyte antigen (HLA) system encoded by the major histocompatibility complex (MHC) encompasses several inherent features which distinguishes it from rest of the genome. Candidate gene-based approach as well as genome-wide association studies (GWAS) across worldwide populations have revealed that this highly polymorphic and gene dense region of the human genome has several alleles, some of which are significantly associated with various diseases, although definitive mechanisms of their involvement remain elusive.

In the postgenomics era, remarkable progress has been made in defining the role of HLA system in biology and medicine due primarily to the availability of next-generation sequencing (NGS) platforms permitting identification of alleles at the high-resolution level and the use of solid phase assay systems to identify donor-specific antibodies (DSAs). This has led to an improved understanding of the mechanisms underlying HLA and disease associations on one hand and of improvised HLA matching and antibody detection systems affecting long-term acceptance of the solid organ grafts and hematopoietic stem cell transplantation (HSCT) on the other. Adoption of novel algorithms and molecular approaches could further enhance the translational value of molecular screening tools for: (1) Predicting graft survival and severity of graft-versus-host disease (GVHD) following stem cell transplantation; and (2) Selecting permissible HLA mismatches over nonpermissible mismatches in HSCT and thus avoid GVHD enabling the physician to adopt clinically most beneficial options for achieving long-term acceptance of the graft.

"Natural species are the library from which genetic engineers can work. Genetic engineers don't make new genes, they rearrange existing ones"

—Thomas Lovejoy

MAJOR HISTOCOMPATIBILITY COMPLEX

The MHC exits in almost all animal species as an important biological system whose function is to formally present protein antigens (both exogenous and endogenously derived) to the immune system. It encompasses multiple genetic loci and in humans, the region encodes the HLA that play an overriding role in antigen presentation, thereby orchestrating the adaptive immune responses. Further, the system helps the body to distinguish self from nonself and this leads to the phenomenon of allorecognition. During initial years of the discovery of MHC, skin graft experiments performed on different strains of mice indicated that specific cell surface antigens resulted in immune-mediated rejection of the foreign tissue. Using inbred mice, Peter Gorer (Lister Institute, London) in the early 1930s performed skin exchange experiments and identified four groups of antigens, then designated as I to IV. This was followed by his collaboration with George Snell (Jackson Laboratories, USA) and together they established that the group II antigens encoded genes that attributed to rejection of the transplanted tumors/foreign tissue. These genes were named as "histocompatibility genes" or *H-2* genes by Snell. The Nobel Prize for this work was awarded to Snell in 1980 along with Jean Dausset (France) who described the first human MHC antigen, then called membrane attack complex (MAC) (now recognized as HLA-A2), and Baruj Benacerraf (USA) for proposing the role of MHC in encoding immune response or *IR* genes. Gorer, whose contributions though seminal, could not be considered for the prize because he had unfortunately passed away in 1961 at the young age of 54.

Later, independent studies carried out by Jon vanRood and colleagues at the University of Leiden, Holland and by Rose Payne in USA led to the identification of a diallelic system, 4a and 4b (now called HLA-Bw4 and Bw6). Since then, many other stalwarts contributed to this ever-evolving domain including discovery in 1970 of the third locus, HLA-C and in 1976 of the fourth locus, HLA-DR (or D-related), all of which were later found to be highly polymorphic. In 1974, Rolf Zinkernagel, a Swiss scientist and Peter Doherty, an Australian working together in Canberra, Australia first reported that the MHC antigens were directly involved in T-cell recognition of both foreign (exogenous) as well as endogenous antigens and this led to the description of the phenomenon of *"MHC restriction"* for the first time. The results of their initial experiments were reported in two short and yet momentous letters in *Nature*. They received the 1996 Nobel Prize of Medicine and Biology for their seminal contributions.

The human MHC region is located on the short arm of chromosomes 6 at position 6p21.3, flanking approximately. 4×10^6 nucleotides. It represents the most polymorphic and gene dense region (encoding >252 expressed loci) of the human genome with over ~29,000 HLA alleles having already been identified in the six "transplant relevant loci" distributed in two functionally distinct regions: Class I (HLA-A, B, and C) and class II (HLA-DR, DQ, and DP) and named accordingly (http://www.ebi.ac.uk/imgt/hla/stats.html accessed in March 25, 2021). A high degree of linkage exists among various HLA loci which limits/reduces the possibility of recombination significantly, thus it is inherited en bloc as a haplotype. Each individual carry two HLA haplotypes, inherited one from each parent and resulting in population specific and conserved haplotypes. Of the currently known 28,938 HLA alleles, a large majority (21,040) belong to the class I loci and the remaining 7,898 are class II alleles, of which the large majority are HLA-DR alleles.

ARCHITECTURE OF HLA SYSTEM

The HLA system is characterized by the presence of multiple linked loci including those affecting histocompatibility in transplantation viz. (1) HLA class I (HLA-A, B, C, E, F, and G) spanning ~2MB at the telomeric end, (2) class II (HLA-DR, DQ, DP, DM, and DO) regions spanning ~1MB at the centromeric end, and (3) MHC class III loci genes separating HLA class I and class II genes and including cytokine genes [tumor necrosis factor-α (TNF-α) etc.], complement genes (*C4, C2*, and *Bf*), and several other immunologically important genes, e.g., MIC-A, MIC-B, and heat shock protein genes (**Fig. 1**).

The HLA-A, B, and C of class I and HLA-DR, DQ, and DP alleles of class II loci represent major transplantation elements, matching for which between donor and recipient pairs is critical for achieving long-term graft survival. Theoretically, the haplotypic inheritance results in a probability that: (1) About 25% of siblings will be HLA-identical, i.e., share both parental HLA haplotypes, (2) About 50% of siblings will share one haplotype and will be HLA haploidentical, and (3) About 25% of siblings will be HLA unidentical (histoincompatible) as they will share no parental haplotype.

HLA CLASS I MOLECULES

These are heterodimeric glycoproteins comprised of two polypeptide chains including an MHC region encoded alpha or heavy chain (~45 kDa with ~350 amino acid) and a non-MHC encoded light chain, i.e., ß2-microglobulin (~17 kDa). The alpha chain includes extracellular, transmembrane and intracytoplasmic domains. The extracellular portion is comprised of three globular subdomains of ~90 amino acids each, i.e., α1, α2, and α3. Peptide binding grove is organized by polymorphic αI and α2 domains, while α3 is relatively conserved. As on March 25, 2021, a total of 21,040 HLA class I alleles have been described which include 6,425 at locus A, 7,754 at locus B, 6,329 at locus C, 262 at locus E, 45 at locus F, and 82 at locus G (http://hla.alleles.org/nomenclature/stats.html) (**Fig. 2**).

The major biological role of HLA class I molecules is to present antigen (peptide/epitopes) to CD8+ T cells. Briefly, complex antigen molecules are cleaved into peptides through processing utilizing sophisticated cellular machinery involving transporters, chaperones, peptidases, and housekeeping proteins. Endogenous antigens which are produced within cytoplasm of the antigen-presenting cells (APCs) are processed by HLA class I molecules for presentation to CD8+ cytotoxic T cells.

HLA CLASS II MOLECULES

These are dimer of dimers composed of two glycoprotein chains, α and β, associated noncovalently wherein each chain includes two domains, i.e., α1, α2 and β1, β2, respectively. The peptide binding groove is formed by α1 and β1 domains and represented by high degree of polymorphism. The α2 and β2 domains are membrane

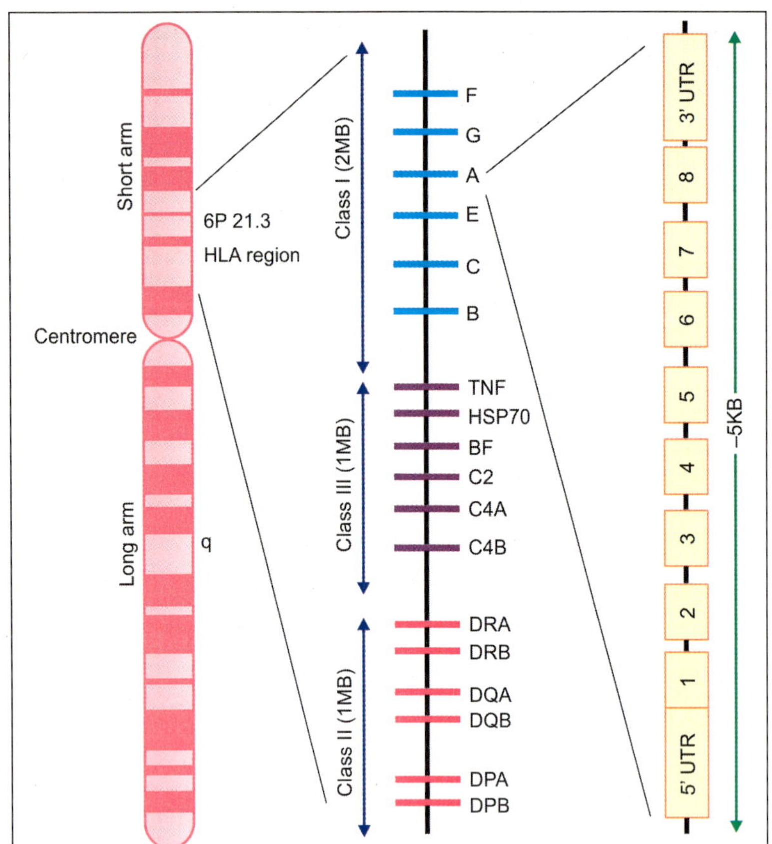

FIGURE 1: Key genetic loci of the human major histocompatibility complex (MHC) reflecting chromosomal location and gene map on the short arm of the chromosome 6 (6p21.3).

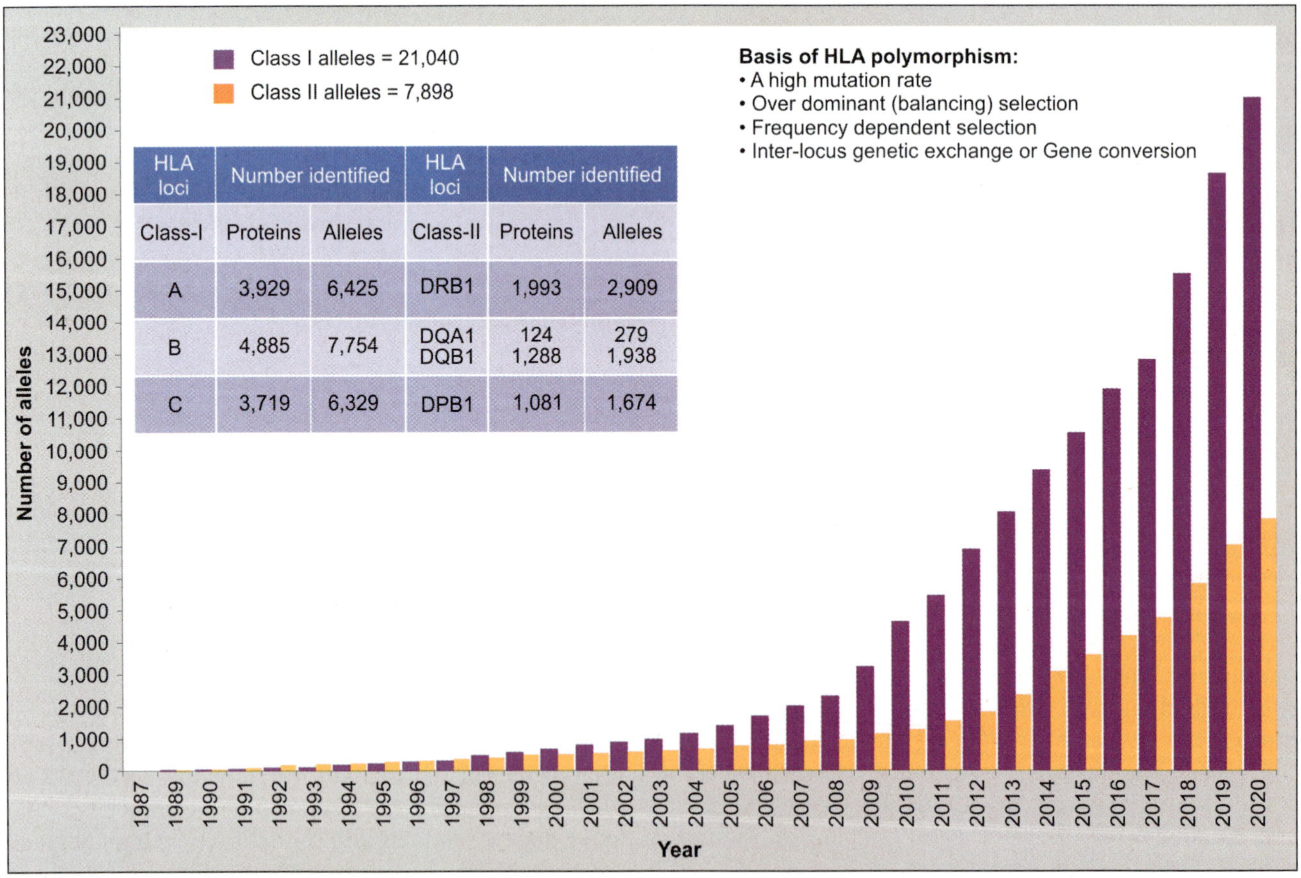

Class I alleles = 21,040
Class II alleles = 7,898

Basis of HLA polymorphism:
- A high mutation rate
- Over dominant (balancing) selection
- Frequency dependent selection
- Inter-locus genetic exchange or Gene conversion

HLA loci	Number identified		HLA loci	Number identified	
Class-I	Proteins	Alleles	Class-II	Proteins	Alleles
A	3,929	6,425	DRB1	1,993	2,909
B	4,885	7,754	DQA1 DQB1	124 1,288	279 1,938
C	3,719	6,329	DPB1	1,081	1,674

Number of alleles (0–23,000); Year (1987–2020)

FIGURE 2: The graph reflecting the total number of human leukocyte antigen (HLA) class I and class II alleles identified since 1987 till March 25, 2021.

Source: EMBL-EBI. (2021). IPD-IMGT/HLA. [online] Available from https://www.ebi.ac.uk/ipd/imgt/hla/.

proximal and are relatively conserved. A total of 7,898 HLA class II alleles have been reported which include 3,621 at DRB locus, 1,938 at DQB1, and 1,674 at the DPB1 locus (http://hla.alleles.org/nomenclature/stats.html).

The HLA class II molecules orchestrate the adaptive immune responses through antigen (peptide/epitopes) presentation to CD4+ve T cells. Briefly, extracellular antigens produced outside the cell (exogenously derived bacterial, viral, and parasitic antigens) or mismatched transplant antigens engulfed by the APCs through phagocytosis or endocytosis are usually processed by the HLA class II molecules for presentation to CD4+ helper T cells. Incidentally, cross presentation (by dendritic cells, macrophages, and B cells) is another way whereby exogenous antigens can be cross presented to CD8+ T cells through HLA class I. Because of its significant biological relevance in health and disease, the HLA system can more appropriately be designated as a "mini genome model" and/or "self-surveillance complex".

We present here the clinical and molecular importance of this system as a significant biomarker for diagnosis and prognosis of several diseases and as a prominent tool for promoting solid organ and HSCT.

HLA AND DISEASE ASSOCIATIONS

First indication for a human disease to be associated with an HLA came in 1973 with a report from UK by Brewerton and colleagues who observed a strong association of HLA-B27 with ankylosing spondylitis. This discovery was followed by a plethora of candidate gene-based studies across different populations leading to identification of several HLA-associated diseases (http://www.hladiseaseassociations.com/). **Table 1** summarizes some of the more prominent associations. These include: (1) Ankylosing spondylitis and related seronegative spondyloarthropathies strongly associated with several molecular subtypes of the *HLA-B27* gene, namely *B*27:02*, *B*27:04*, and *B*27:05* (>90% of patients as compared to 4–6% of healthy controls), (2) An exceptionally strong association of DQB1*06:02 allele with narcolepsy (~90–100% of patients), (3) High occurrence of HLA-DQ2 molecule (HLA-DQA1*05:01-DQB1*02:01) in >90% patients with celiac disease while others carry DQ8 molecule (HLA-DQA1*03:01-DQB1*03:02), (4) Strong association of rheumatoid arthritis (RA) with HLA-DRB1*04 (and its molecular subtypes DRB1*0401, *04:04, *04:05) and other HLA-DRB1 alleles carrying "shared epitopes" of five amino acid motif in DRβ chain (carried by >90% Caucasian and Indian seropositive patients of RA), and (5) Strong association of type 1 diabetes mellitus (T1DM) with HLA-DRB1*03/DQB1*02:01 or DRB1*04/DQB1*03:02 or both these haplotypes (in >90% patients).

DRUG-INDUCED HYPERSENSITIVITIES AND HLA

Development of drug-induced hypersensitivity reactions have also been linked with HLA loci. Key examples

TABLE 1 Prominent human leukocyte antigen (HLA) and disease associations observed across various populations.

Disease	HLA allele/s
Addison's disease	DRB1*03:01-DQB1*02 and DRB1*04-DQB1*03:02
Ankylosing spondylitis	B*27:01, B*27:02, B*27:04, B*27:05
Behçet's disease	B5/B*51, particularly B*51:01
Celiac disease	DQA1*05:01–DQB1*02:01, DQA1*02:01–DQB1*02:02, DQA1*03:01–DQB1*03:02
Crohn's disease	DRB1*07, DRB1*01:03
Graves' disease	DRB1*03:01-DQA1*05:01-DQB1*02:01 and DRB1*04:01-DQA1*03:01-DQB1*03:02
Human immunodeficiency virus (HIV) disease progression	HLA-B*27, B*57 (slow), B*35(Px) (fast)
Multiple sclerosis	HLA-DRB1*15:01on DRB1*15:01-DQA1*01:02-DQB1*06:02
Narcolepsy	DQB1*06:02, DRB1*15:01-DQA1*01:02-DQB1*06:02
Psoriasis vulgaris	C*06
Rheumatoid arthritis	DRB1*01:01, DRB1*01:02, DRB1*04:01, DRB1*04:04, DRB1*04:05, DRB1*04:08, DRB1*10:01, DRB1*13:03, DRB1*14:02 and DRB1*14:06
Scleroderma	DRB1*11:04 and DQB1*03:01, DRB1*15:02 and DQB1*06:01, DQB1*05:01, DRB1*13:02 and DQB1*06:04
Sjögren syndrome	DRB1*03–DQB1*02–DQA1*05:01; DRB1*15–DQB1*06–DQA1*01:02
Systemic lupus erythematosus	DRB1*03:01-DQB1*02:01, DRB1*15:01-DQB1*06:02
Type 1 diabetes mellitus	DRB1*03:01, DQA1*05:01, DQB1*02:01 or DRB1*04:01, DQA1*03:01, DQB1*03:02

include: (1) Abacavir-induced drug hypersensitive reaction in patients of human immunodeficiency virus/acquired immunodeficiency syndrome (HIV/AIDS) is strongly linked to HLA-B*57:01, (2) Allopurinol-induced hypersensitivity is linked specifically to HLA-B*58:01 allele, (3) Dapsone hypersensitivity correlated specifically with HLA-B*13:01, and (4) Carbamazepine-induced Stevens–Johnson syndrome/toxic epidermal necrolysis is specifically associated with HLA-B*15:02. Such reports have helped in developing pharmacological tools for screening of patients who could be at an elevated risk of HLA-associated drug hypersensitivity reactions.

The exact mechanism(s) of many of these observed HLA association with diseases are unknown due to various factors, e.g., (1) linkage disequilibrium in HLA loci complicating identification of the exact locus or their combinatorial effect, (2) possible involvement of non-HLA genes and environmental factors, i.e., multifactorial nature of the diseases, (3) disease specific autoantigens that bind to associated HLA alleles are largely unknown, (4) heterogeneity contributed by several other factors viz. age at onset, other underlying diseases which could be linked as well as therapeutic responsiveness, clinical variability etc.

Nevertheless, various theories have been suggested to delineate the mechanistic insights of these associations: (1) Theory of "mistaken identity" suggesting that the noticeable HLA association could be attributed to an additional unexplored locus in close physical proximity of the observed associated allele (in linkage disequilibrium). This is supported by the observed high degree of linkage in HLA region of multiple genetic loci. (2) The observed HLA allelic association could directly influence disease vulnerability by either antigenic cross-reactivity or mimicry to pathogens ("molecular mimicry") or possible immunogenicity to self-antigens due to anomalous T cell response or immunologically aberrant responsiveness to "altered self" antigens. Additionally, genetic propensity could be attributed to a largely unknown set of other non-HLA genes. For simplicity, we focus our discussion specifically on key aspects of HLA system and their disease association while keeping non-HLA genes beyond the scope of this chapter.

HLA AND EPISTATIC INFLUENCE

In addition to the direct influence of HLA genes, convincing evidence on the cumulative influence of non-HLA genetic variants through epistatic interaction with HLA alleles is evolving, thus adding a further layer to the disease association and complexity. For example there are reports suggesting (1) a cumulative influence of HLA and killer immunoglobulin-like receptors (KIRs) in several diseases including HIV disease progression, (2) an epistatic effect of genetic polymorphisms in *CTLA-4* and *IRF5* genes with HLA susceptibility loci in Systemic lupus erythematosus (SLE), (3) an interactive influence of endoplasmic reticulum aminopeptidase protein 1 (ERAP1) with HLA-B*51 in Behçet's disease, (4) cumulative influence of HLA and ERAP1 in ankylosing spondylitis, and (5) a role of HLA-C and ERAP1 in inflammatory bowel disease.

In the postgenomic era, the focus has shifted from candidate gene-based approaches to more holistic approaches such as GWAS. The latter utilizing advanced technologies further support the evolutionary relevance of HLA system as the most strongly disease-associated genomic region with several infectious and autoimmune diseases as well as tumors. Although the underlying molecular mechanisms of HLA associations are not fully defined, limited progress has been made to unravel a possible causative link. For example, the HLA-DR4 restricted CD4+ T cells that are specific to insulin A chain peptides represented a majority of T cells in the pancreatic lymph nodes of T1DM patients. Similarly, in celiac disease, the undigested proline-rich gluten peptides which are resistant to proteolytic cleavage are transported through the intestinal epithelium, deamidated by tissue transglutaminase in the mucosa and presented through HLA-DQ2 or DQ8 molecules by the APCs. In the lamina propria, these antigens are then recognized by specific CD4+ T cells, resulting in autoimmunity.

More recently, another layer of complexity is being explored which includes polymorphic allele-specific expression of HLA loci. It is hypothesized that variability in HLA expression could potentially affect the strength of immune response. For example, higher expression of autoimmunity favoring HLA alleles could elicit autoimmunity while those of protective alleles could result in strong immune surveillance against tumors through robust antigen presentation. Besides peptide binding, the HLA allele-specific expression could also affect the epistatic cumulative interaction with other molecules, e.g., through interacting with KIRs expressed on natural killer (NK) cells, thus differentially regulating immune responses. To this end, a few genome wide disease associations linked to variable HLA allelic expression have been reported. For example, a higher HLA-C expression with faster progression to AIDS in HIV patients on one side, while adding to vulnerability in Crohn's disease on the other. Similar reports are available for HLA-DP expression and hepatitis B virus (HBV). Evaluating these expression variables in various diseases could unravel the largely unknown mechanisms underlying HLA-linked disease associations.

HLA SYSTEM IN ORGAN TRANSPLANTATION

Initial attempts of renal transplantation date back to 1936, although these were mostly unsuccessful because of lack of proper understanding of transplant immunity and non-availability of immunosuppressive drugs. Experiments in dogs by Simonsen (1953) and Dempster (1953) independently concluded that a humoral mechanism was more likely responsible for allograft failure. Soon, it was recognized that the immunologic barrier needs to be countered for achieving success in renal replacement therapy. Matching donor and recipient for histocompatibility antigens could not only suppress alloimmunity, but also lower the need for immunosuppressive drug dosages. Particularly, an understanding of the molecular structure of HLA by Pamela Bjorkman uncovered the mechanism of antigen presentation and allorecognition. Though the influence of anti-HLA antibodies present at the time of transplantation was observed nearly five decades ago, a better understanding of the importance/relevance of their de novo development post-transplantation is more recent. Additionally, impact of donor-recipient incompatibility of non-HLA molecules on allograft immunity in renal transplants involving HLA matched donors has recently been recognized.

CLINICAL RELEVANCE OF ANTI-HLA ANTIBODIES

The last decade has seen significant advancements in more efficient monitoring of anti-HLA antibodies for detecting antibody-mediated rejection (AMR) and allograft failure. History of blood transfusion, pregnancy, and prior transplantation or other as yet unknown reasons could be attributed for the generation of these antibodies at pretransplant stage. Further, the potential risk factors which can lead to de novo development of DSA include younger age of the patient, molecular mismatch with donor, particularly at HLA class II region, non-compliance of prescribed drugs, and inflammatory insults viz. infections and/or cell-mediated rejection episodes. **Figure 3** summarizes possible risk factors attributable to the development of DSA at pre- and post-transplant level.

It is now clear that a cumulative presence of anti-HLA class I and II antibodies are associated with more frequent rejection episodes in comparison to those with either of these antibodies alone. The development of de novo DSA is considered as the earliest biomarker to predict post-transplant allograft injury resulting in late acute and chronic AMR, and towards transplant glomerulopathy. Plethora of reports suggests that antibodies are generally produced much earlier than the observed upsurge of serum creatinine or rejection episodes. Further, protocol allograft biopsy performed after detection of de novo DSA reveal subclinical AMR disease, thus highlighting the clinical relevance of systematic monitoring of post-transplant HLA-DSA.

INFLUENCE OF NON-HLA ANTIBODIES

In addition to antibodies specific to donor HLA antigens as the major player implicated in AMR, several reports signify the clinical relevance of the presence of non-HLA antibodies in graft rejection. An emerging list of non-HLA antigens has been shown to affect the graft outcome in solid organ transplantation. These include the MICA molecules (MHC class I chain-related molecule A), angiotensin II type 1 receptor (AT1R), vimentin, collagen, cardiac myosin, and K-α1 tubulin. Particularly, humoral response to MICA has been realized as a potential biomarker of AMR. Data from our own centre and of others have revealed a strong association between the occurrence of MICA antibodies (at pre- or post-transplant stages) and adverse graft outcome. Further, the influence of anti-MICA antibodies alone, i.e., in absence of anti-HLA antibodies has been observed both in acute and chronic rejection as well as in hyperacute rejection. Currently, there is lack of consensus with regard to the optimum mean fluorescence intensity (MFI) "cutoffs" for classifying MICA antibodies as clinically relevant. Nevertheless, the risk factor for antidonor MICA antibodies is similar to those involved in HLA sensitization, i.e., pregnancy, blood transfusion, and previous transplantation.

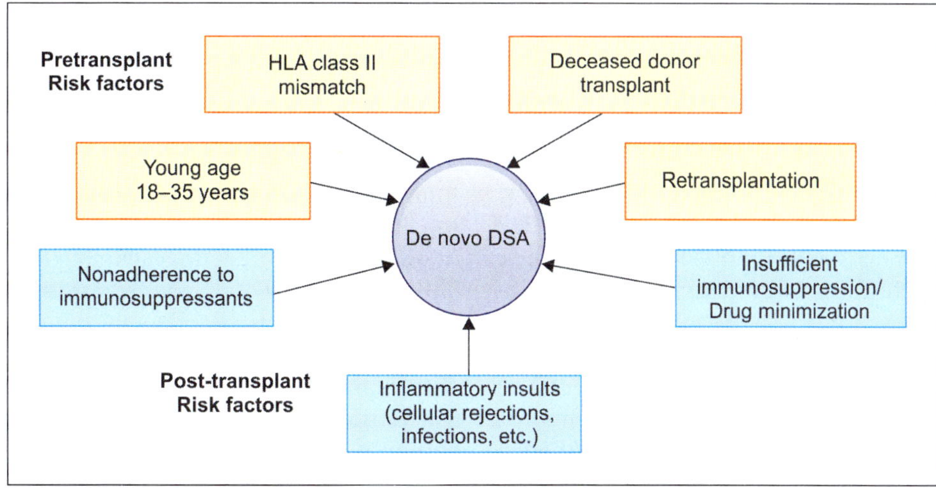

(HLA: human leukocyte antigen)

FIGURE 3: Potential risk factors involved in the development of donor-specific antibodies (DSAs) at pretransplant level (in yellow) and de novo antibodies at post-transplant level (in cyan).

HLA IN HEMATOPOIETIC STEM CELL TRANSPLANTATION

In recent years, the incidence of various malignant and nonmalignant hematopoietic diseases has increased appreciably as a result of improved diagnostic tools including advanced molecular platforms and detection through awareness programs. The treatment of choice for these patients is HSCT, preferably from HLA-identical sibling donors or those from unrelated donor marrow registries that share 10 out 10 alleles in the HLA-A, B, C, DR, and DQ loci (marrow unrelated donor or MUD transplants). Most data indicate that optimal HLA compatibility between donor and the recipient is a prerequisite for obtaining improved graft survival, the limitation being nonavailability of HLA matched/identical donors in most situations. Accordingly, there has been an increasing adoption of HLA mismatched donor strategy by the clinicians and this includes the use of haploidentical or 50% matched donors for transplantation. Although, increasingly improvised strategies are being utilized to maintain and modulate the sensitive immune balance between the recipients and their respective donors, yet the HLA mismatched HSCT considerably increases the risk of allorecognition and development of acute and chronic GVHD over HLA-matched related transplants.

Another highly variable genetic system is the KIRs (comprising of 16 genes with several polymorphic alleles for each gene) present on the surface of NK cells, which regulate their activity through interaction with cognate HLA ligands; particularly HLA-C and HLA-Bw4 alleles. Though evidence is emerging on the potential beneficial effects of KIR-KIR ligand mismatching, particularly in haploidentical HSCT by adopting the post-transplant cyclophosphamide (PTCy) approach, it is not conclusive as yet, due to lack of comparable and population-specific analysis. Nevertheless, it is clear that NK cell reconstitution occurs earlier and that these cells are critical in haplo-HSCT outcomes including relapse and GVHD. Further strategies are needed for selection of donors to optimize NK-mediated antitumor effect and prevention of GVHD. Also, cumulative influence of HLA/KIR genetic axis is yet to be explored in the context of occurrence of GVHD after HLA mismatched HCT.

Since multiple mismatched donors (including HLA haplo-identical) could be available for each patient requiring HCT, the challenge is to select the best for lower allorecognition and minimal risk of GVHD. Recently, an algorithm known as Predicted Indirectly ReCognizable HLA-Epitopes (PIRCHE) has been developed, which theoretically identifies mismatched HLA-derived epitopes, that can possibly be presented by HLA class-I (PIRCHE-I) or HLA class-II molecules (PIRCHE-II). Thus, PIRCHE-I can lead to CD8+ T-cell responses, while PIRCHE-II can stimulate CD4+ T-cell responses. Basically, these computationally predicted peptides are derived from the patient's mismatched-HLA molecules, which can potentially be presented by shared HLA of the donor and recipient leading indirect allorecognition. This algorithm can be utilized to potentially detect well-tolerated (permissible) and detrimental (nonpermissible) HLA-mismatches, thus minimizing the occurrence of the acute and chronic GVHD. Though convincing data has just begun to emerge on these lines, potential clinical utility of these novel approaches is yet to be evaluated in different populations.

More recently, a dimorphism (rs1050458C/T) in the amino acid sequence of exon 1 of HLA-B has been identified that results in the generation of leader peptides containing either methionine (M) or threonine (T). This influences NK and T cell alloimmune responses by modulating the expression of HLA-E. A retrospective analysis done by the Seattle group (USA) involving a very large cohort (33,982 unrelated HCT) showed that HLA-B mismatched HSCT outcomes (particularly GVHD) are influenced by a new paradigm based on the M/T dimorphism of both matched and mismatched alleles between the donors and recipients. Accordingly, the HLA-B leader may be used to avoid risky donor HLA-B mismatches and also identify patients who are at a higher risk of developing GVHD.

Evaluation of the genomic variants at the population level could have a definitive translational value for improvising molecular screening tools for (1) predicting GVHD and its severity; and (2) selecting permissible HLA mismatches over nonpermissible ones in HCT and thus avoid GVHD.

HLA AND BLOOD TRANSFUSION

Human leukocyte antigen alloimmunization brings about some of the serious complications associated with transfusion of blood and blood products. These include febrile nonhemolytic transfusion reactions (FNHTR), immunological platelet refractoriness (IPR), transfusion-related acute lung injury (TRALI), and transfusion-associated graft-versus-host disease (TA-GVHD). Though, leukodepletion practiced by various centers has by far taken care of HLA alloimmunization largely, however antigens displayed by residual cellular components and platelets can potentially induce anti-HLA antibodies and alloreactive T cells.

Febrile nonhemolytic transfusion reaction (FNHTR) and immunological refractoriness to platelets is primarily mediated by the presence of anti-HLA class I antibodies in the recipient reacting against transfused products. The effectiveness of platelet transfusion is assessed most commonly by post-transfusion platelet increment (PI). A PI of $>10 \times 10^9$/L at 1- or 24-hour post-transfusion is considered an adequate response. Platelet refractoriness due to nonimmune etiology will typically have a normal response in platelet count within 1 hour of transfusion, but will often return to baseline within 24 hours. Immunological refractoriness to platelets, unlike that of nonimmune causes, shows little or no increase in platelet count at 1-hour post-transfusion. Immune refractoriness to platelets is primarily associated with alloimmunization either against HLA and/or human platelet antigen (HPA) due to prior exposure from transfusion, pregnancy, or transplantation. HLA alloimmunization as compared to HPA is more commonly implicated as a cause of immune refractoriness to platelets. Anti-HLA antibodies directed against -A and -B antigens are more significant in causing platelet refractoriness than those against -C antigens, as the expression of HLA-A and -B on platelets is much higher than -C.

Various approaches utilized to overcome the immunological refractoriness to platelets include: (1) Transfusion of crossmatch compatible platelets, generally suited for patients that are not highly sensitized. This may have the disadvantage of potential immunization against mismatched HLA antigens; hence avoided for long-term platelet transfusion support. (2) Transfusion of virtually crossmatched platelets based on HLA antibody profile of the patient and not on the degree of HLA matching between patient and the donor. This is more useful for short-term platelet transfusion support. The efficacy of future transfusions is compromised due to the risk of immunizing the patient to the mismatched donor antigens. (3) The third and the most logical approach involves transfusion of selected platelets based on recipient's HLA phenotype and the antibody status as determined through panel reactive antibody screening.

Transfusion-related acute lung injury is known to be associated with the presence of anti-HLA antibodies against both class I and II molecules, as well as neutrophil-specific antibodies in the plasma of both donors and recipients. Use of plasma from male donors and nulliparous or multiparous female donors who are negative for leukocyte-directed antibodies drastically reduces the incidence and severity of TRALI. Similarly, transfusion of leukoreduced cellular blood products reduces the prevalence of TRALI caused by leukocyte antibodies present in the recipient.

Transfusion-associated graft-versus-host disease, a rare and potentially life-threatening complication of blood transfusion, results from the transfusion of immunologically responsive lymphocytes into immunosuppressed recipients. It is seen in 0.1–1% of all transfusions in susceptible recipients. All cellular blood products (red cells, platelet, and granulocyte concentrate) which contain viable immunocompetent T cells have been implicated in TA-GVHD. The risk of TA-GVHD is significantly increased in situations where the donor is homozygous for both HLA haplotypes while the recipient is heterozygous. Owing to the zero HLA mismatch in the direction of host versus graft, donor lymphocytes are not rejected as foreign. However, the HLA mismatch in the direction of graft versus host arising due to homozygous donor, the donor T cells perceive host cells as foreign and react against them. In a nutshell, host immune deficits, component characteristics, and the donor-recipient HLA match status are all thought to play a role in the development of TA-GHVD, although the relative contribution of these individually remains unclear. Evidence of chimerism, i.e., the presence of donor-derived cells, chromosomes or DNA in the blood, and/or affected tissues of the recipient is essential for the definitive diagnosis of TA-GVHD.

CONCLUSION

The human MHC encompasses several peculiar characteristics which differentiate it from other regions of the genome. In various candidate gene-based and GWAS across worldwide populations, alleles of this highly polymorphic gene dense region have been found strongly linked to several infectious and autoimmune diseases, although mechanistic pathways are largely unknown. The postgenomic era has seen significant technological advancements permitting identification of novel alleles at high-resolution level, and this has not only enriched knowledge about HLA and disease associations but has also led to improved organ and stem cell transplant outcomes through enhanced HLA matching and precision in detecting preexisting and post (de novo) transplant DSA. Novel algorithms and molecular approaches have been developed that could translationally improvise prediction of graft survival and severity of GVHD by selecting permissible HLA mismatches in organ and HSCT.

RECOMMENDED READINGS

1. Mallal S, Nolan D, Witt C, Masel G, Martin AM, Moore C, et al. Association between presence of HLA-B*5701, HLA-DR7, and HLA-DQ3 and hypersensitivity to HIV-1 reverse-transcriptase inhibitor abacavir. Lancet. 2002;359(9308):727-32.
2. Hung SI, Chung WH, Liou LB, Chu CC, Lin M, Huang HP, et al. HLA-B*5801 allele as a genetic marker for severe cutaneous adverse reactions caused by allopurinol. Proc Natl Acad Sci USA. 2005;102(11):4134-9.
3. Zhang FR, Liu H, Irwanto A, Fu XA, Li Y, Yu GQ, et al. HLA-B*13:01 and the dapsone hypersensitivity syndrome. N Engl J Med. 2013;369(17):1620-8.
4. Man CB, Kwan P, Baum L, Yu E, Lau KM, Cheng AS, et al. Association between HLA-B*1502 allele and antiepileptic drug-induced cutaneous reactions in Han Chinese. Epilepsia. 2007;48(5):1015-8.
5. Martin MP, Naranbhai V, Shea PR, Qi Y, Ramsuran V, Vince N, et al. Killer cell immunoglobulin-like receptor 3DL1 variation modifies HLA-B*57 protection against HIV-1. J Clin Invest. 2018;128(5):1903-12.
6. Hughes T, Adler A, Kelly JA, Kaufman KM, Williams AH, Langefeld CD, et al. Evidence for gene-gene epistatic interactions among susceptibility loci for systemic lupus erythematosus. Arthritis Rheum. 2012;64:485-92.
7. Kirino Y, Bertsias G, Ishigatsubo Y, Mizuki N, Tugal-Tutkun I, Seyahi E, et al. Genome-wide association analysis identifies new susceptibility loci for Behcet's disease and epistasis between HLA-B*51 and ERAP1. Nat Genet. 2013;45(2):202-7.
8. Cortes A, Pulit SL, Leo PJ, Pointon JJ, Robinson PC, Weisman MH, et al. Major histocompatibility complex

associations of ankylosing spondylitis are complex and involve further epistasis with ERAP1. Nat Commun. 2015;6:7146.
9. Castro-Santos P, Moro-Garcı´a MA, Marcos-Fernandez R, Alonso-Arias R, Díaz-Peña R. ERAP1 and HLA-C interaction in inflammatory bowel disease in the Spanish population. Innate Immun. 2017;23(5):476-81.
10. Kennedy AE, Ozbek U, Dorak MT. What has GWAS done for HLA and disease associations? Int J Immunogenet. 2017;44(5):195-211.
11. Busch R, De Riva A, Hadjinicolaou AV, Jiang W, Hou T, Mellins ED. On the perils of poor editing: Regulation of peptide loading by HLA-DQ and H2-A molecules associated with celiac disease and type 1 diabetes. Expert Rev in Mol Med. 2012;14:e15.
12. Klareskog L, Catrina AI, Paget S. Rheumatoid arthritis. Lancet. 2009;373(9664):659-72.
13. Petersdorf EW, O'hUigin C. The MHC in the era of next-generation sequencing: Implications for bridging structure with function. Hum Immunol. 2019;80:67-78.
14. Bjorkman PJ, Saper MA, Samraoui B, Bennett WS, Strominger JL, Wiley DC. The foreign antigen binding site and T cell recognition regions of class I histocompatibility antigens. Nature. 1987b;329:512-8.
15. Patel R, Terasaki PI. Significance of a positive crossmatch test in kidney transplantation. N Engl J Med. 1969;280:735-9.
16. Wiebe C, Gibson IW, Blydt-Hansen TD, Karpinski M, Ho J, Storsley LJ, et al. Evolution and clinical pathologic correlations of de novo donor-specific HLA antibody post kidney transplant. Am J Transplant. 2012;12:1157-67.
17. Panigrahi A, Gupta N, Siddiqui JA, Margoob A, Bhowmik D, Guleria S, et al. Post-transplant development of MICA and anti-HLA antibodies is associated with acute rejection episodes and renal allograft loss. Hum Immunol. 2007;68:362-7.
18. Dieplinger G, Ditt V, Arns W, Huppertz A, Kisner T, Hellmich M, et al. Impact of de novo donor-specific HLA antibodies detected by Luminex solid-phase assay after transplantation in a group of 88 consecutive living-donor renal transplantations. Transpl Int. 2014;27(1):60-8.
19. Loupy A, Vernerey D, Tinel C, Aubert O, Duong van Huyen JP, Rabant M, et al. Subclinical rejection phenotypes at 1 year post-transplant and outcome of kidney allografts. J Am Soc Nephrol. 2015;26:1721-31.
20. Mehra NK, Siddiqui J, Baranwal A, Goswami S, Kaur G. Clinical relevance of antibody development in renal transplantation. Ann N Y Acad Sci. 2013;1283:30-42.

CHAPTER 23

Electronic Health Records, Artificial Intelligence, and Big Data—Role in Medicine

Rahul Shukla, Ashish Sahani

ABSTRACT

Traditionally, medicine has been reliant on massive amounts of paper-based records. Such records are prone to errors, difficult to store and transmit. With the computer revolution, there has been a rise of electronic health records (EHRs). Such records are fast becoming the norm in healthcare systems. EHRs lead to increase in efficiency, reduction in errors, easy transmission and storage, and better compliance to regulations. There are multiple issues which are faced by medical systems trying to make a leap from paper based to electronic records. In this chapter, we have attempted at giving a broad overview of EHR systems along with case studies and challenges associated with them.

Another two big areas which are changing medicine rapidly are artificial intelligence (AI) and big data. These are new paradigms of computer science which take advantage of recent abundance in digitized structured data to draw insights and make predictive algorithms. AI consists of a set of biologically inspired algorithms that closely mimic the human intelligence. These algorithms when employed in medicine can read images like a radiologist, analyze retinal images like an ophthalmologist, and suggest medications like an expert. In the second half of this chapter, we cover AI in detail and big data briefly.

ELECTRONIC HEALTH RECORD

INTRODUCTION

Electronic health record is a longitudinal electronic record of patient health information recorded from healthcare practitioners in multiple sites where care is provided. An EHR has a unique id and contains the lifetime medical history, behavioral and lifestyle factors, physical examinations, diagnoses, tests, vital signs, immunization dates, allergies, medications, referrals, admissions, and discharge information (**Fig. 1**). In addition to structured data there may exist clinical notes, images of scans, and other such unstructured components. They can have other information like insurance policy coverage of the patient and even data imported from personal wellness devices. EHRs make the patient's medical and other relevant information electronically available.

EVOLUTION

Development of EHR can be divided into two major time periods. In the 1960s and 1970s, academic medical centers started developing their own systems. The first EHR systems were known as clinical information systems. In the mid-1960s, Lockheed developed one such product which has now been acquired by Allscripts. The federal government of United States began using EHR in the 1970s with the implementation of the Vista system at the Department of Veteran Affairs. This was originally known as Decentralized Hospital Computer Program (DHCP). In the 1980s, looking at the commercial potential, industries started developing EHR systems too. The convenience and professionalism brought about by them led to widespread adoption of these systems.

A final report published by Institute of Medicine (IOM) acknowledged and argued the case for using EHR. It has been identified as one of the seven key recommendations for improving patient records. The suggested best way is by converting paper to electronic records. The report also identified the barriers to EHR adoption such as lack of standards, security issues, and cost and suggested private as well as public funding for its development. In 2000, the IOM published a study of medical errors titled "*To Err is Human*" done by humans. They concluded that healthcare would be safer with such systems. IOM has also collaborated on the development of an electronic standards organization, HL7.

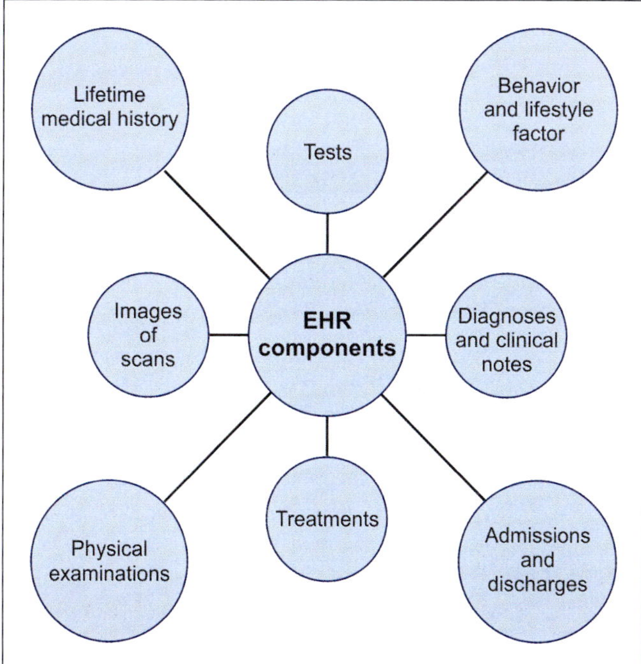

(EHR: electronic health record)

FIGURE 1: The different components of EHR.

ADVANTAGES

Some of the basic benefits of using EHRs are easy access to computerized records and the elimination of errors due to handwriting and illegibility. EHR systems have many potential capabilities. Some particular functionalities hold great promise in improving the quality of care and reducing cost. These are clinical decision support (CDS) tools, computerized physician order entry (CPOE) systems, and health information exchange (HIE).

A CDS system assists the healthcare practitioner in making decisions with regard to the patient's diagnosis and treatment. Some of the functionalities of a CDS system are providing a probabilistically ranked diagnosis based on symptoms, providing suggestive treatment pathways, providing up-to-date information about a drug, cross referencing medication with patient allergy, and alerting about adverse drug interactions and other potential issues. With the continuous growth of medical knowledge, each of these functionalities provides a means for care to be delivered in a much safer and more efficient manner. As adoption of CDS systems increase, one can expect certain medical errors shall be averted and the patient will receive more efficient and safer healthcare.

Computerized physician order entry systems allow healthcare providers to enter information of medicines, laboratory tests, radiological reports, and physical therapy directly into a computer rather than doing so on paper. Electronically storing these information eliminate medical errors caused by handwritten paper records. Studies conducted on medical errors have proved that errors can be reduced up to 55% by using CPOE system alone and it can be further reduced to 83% if coupled with a CDS system which alert about physician errors. Hence, the effectiveness and efficacy of treatment can be improved by using CPOE and CDS jointly.

Health information exchange refers to process of sharing electronic health information between different organizations. This information exchange increases the efficiency of healthcare delivery. By exchanging information in real-time HIE can reduce the repetitive test cost because clinical tests done at another providers location can be accessed by the current healthcare provider. Most of the time, patients get treatment from different doctors and the treatment data is stored locally at provider location. If a patient moves to another clinician then a HIE-enabled system will be very helpful. Patient's health information can be stored at different hospitals, physician's office, specialists, multiple pharmacies, pathology laboratories, and imaging centers. Historically, providers use fax or mail to transfer pertinent information to each other. This is quite inconvenient and inefficient in real time. HIE facilitates the exchange of this information via EHRs, which can result in cost-effective and high-quality care.

A summary of some of the benefits of using EHRs is as follows:

- Quick access to patient records
- Recommends potential treatment options
- Patients have easier access to their medical records easily and are better informed about their health condition
- Improves preventive care
- Lowers mistakes due to handwritten prescriptions and notes
- Update and access patient information in real time
- AI can train over EHRs easily and assist with diagnosis and interpretation of reports
- E-prescribing saves time
- Check automatically for drug-to-drug or drug-to-allergy reactions
- Provides billing and payment tools
- Reduces rejection rates of insurance claims

ADOPTION

Different countries have used different means to promote use of EHR in their healthcare. In the United States, Health Information Technology for Economic and Clinical Health (HITECH) act was enacted in 2009 to promote and expand the use of health information and specific focus was made to promote use of EHR by healthcare providers. As of 2017, nearly 9 in 10 (86%) of office-based physicians have adopted EHRs, and nearly 4 in 5 (80%) had adopted a certified EHR in the US. To modernize its information communication technology (ICT) infrastructure Canada launched an initiative in 2001. In 2015, 91,000 clinicians adopted EHR in their clinic, 91% of Canadians EHR were created.

A national initiative was started by England in 2001 which was called as "National Plan for IT" (NPfIT) for modernizing its healthcare system. Under this initiative, summary of health record was created for 54 million people (96% of the population). In Germany, about 90% of physicians in private practice are using EHR systems. Patient privacy has been given adequate attention in the initiative. The patient can decide to hide or block any entry in the health record.

EHR—EXAMPLE

Cerner Corporation is an American supplier of health information technology (HIT) services, devices, and hardware. Cerner provides service to nearly one-third of US hospitals. They claim to have 650,000 physicians and 2,200,000 nonphysician users. Some features of Cerner EHR systems are scheduling, patient charting, laboratory integration, E-prescribing medicare eligibility verification, audit reporting, medication administration documentation, laboratory and drug alerts, and staff shift planning (**Fig. 2**).

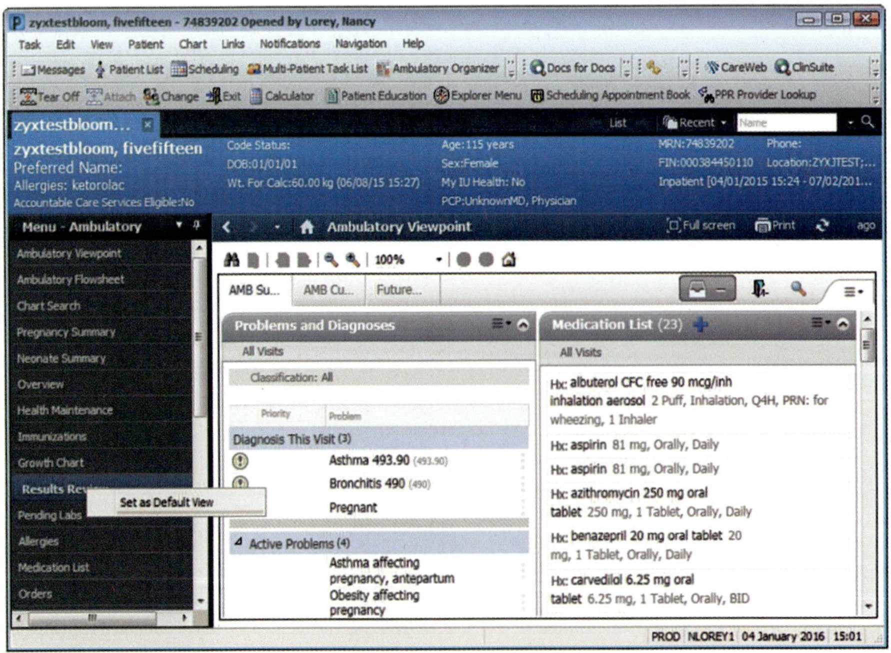

FIGURE 2: Graphical user interface of electronic health record (EHR) from Cerner systems.

Some of the major players in EHR space are Allscripts, Epic systems, Cerner, Meditech and InterSystems. A case study of EHR implementation in the Cambridge university hospital is presented in the e-chapter along with.

EHR—BARRIERS TO ADOPTION

Cost: It is a major hindrance in transferring from traditional paper-based system to EHR as moving to electronic system requires investment in hardware, software, training of staff, converting existing records to electronic record, and good chunk of money to EHR vendors. The cost of EHR systems varies based on the functionality it provides, like if the system handles both clinical as well as administrative functionalities or only clinical one.

After EHR implementation, system requires administrator, maintenance, controller, and support to run system efficiently since the vendors ask for lots of money. The system cost also depends on its type, i.e., if system is purchased, rented, or leased.

Physician resistance: As traditional paper records change to EHR, physicians sometime get frustrated as they are investing more time in documentation process as compared to paper-based data recording. This triggers resistance in physicians to change from traditional system to the new EHR system.

Security and privacy: There is a belief that EHRs have security risk as compared to paper records in non-users which is contrary to evidence. There is an argument from some policy makers that consumers must have some kind of legal protection to their privacy before EHR adoption while others argue that such a move will increase cost and deter adoption. There are some genuine concerns in both patients and physicians regarding data security and privacy; they must be addressed so that resistance to adoption of EHRs may be reduced.

Interoperability: Very few EHR systems allow for easy exchange of clinical data between different healthcare providing facilities such as physician's clinics, hospitals and imaging centers, and pathology laboratories. There is a lack of interoperability standards between different EHR systems. This forces hospitals to stick to their initial choices of EHR vendors and the costs of changing to another EHR system may be prohibitive. This also limits the data sharing capabilities between two hospitals using different EHR systems.

ARTIFICIAL INTELLIGENCE (AI), MACHINE LEARNING (ML), AND DEEP LEARNING (DL)

DEFINITIONS AND INTRODUCTION

Artificial intelligence: It refers to broad classes of theoretical concepts through which intelligent machines or computers can be built. Theoretically, it is possible for AI to achieve or even surpass human level of intelligence.

Machine learning: It is a subset of AI that consists of practical sets of methods in which machines learn from data without being explicitly programmed (**Fig. 3**). Traditionally, software engineering uses human created rules with data to create answers to a problem. Instead, ML uses data and answers to discover the rules behind a problem (**Fig. 4**). Certain classes of ML algorithms called reinforced learning can also evolve with time and improve or adapt themselves as they get exposed to new data.

DEEP LEARNING AND NEURAL NETWORKS

Among the various methods of ML, one method which has stood out is the neural network (NN). As the name suggests, NNs are networks of neurons and is a biologically inspired method. In a biological system, such networks of neurons are responsible for all sensing, control, and emotions of a being. A single neuron is a very simple computing unit. It has dendrites that collect signals from axons of various other prior neurons. There is an addition of all these input signals in the cell body. If this sum crosses a threshold, the neuron is activated and sends out a signal through its axon to other neurons attached to it on the axonic side. The connections between axons and dendrites have chemically controlled gates that can enhance or suppress the signal passing through them. When thousands of such neurons interconnect together in the central nervous system, they can perform complex computations and representations of information. NNs are implemented in a computer through design of mathematical nodes with a closely matching functionality of biological neurons as shown in **Figure 5**. Each of these nodes can take in hundreds of inputs, weigh it by a certain factor, sum it, and then threshold it. By changing the network structure, number of neurons, and weighing factors, computers can represent information just like the human brain. The key idea is that the network variables need not be programmed manually; computers can train on labeled data provided by experts to automatically find out the best network architectures and best weighing factors to perform the best prediction.

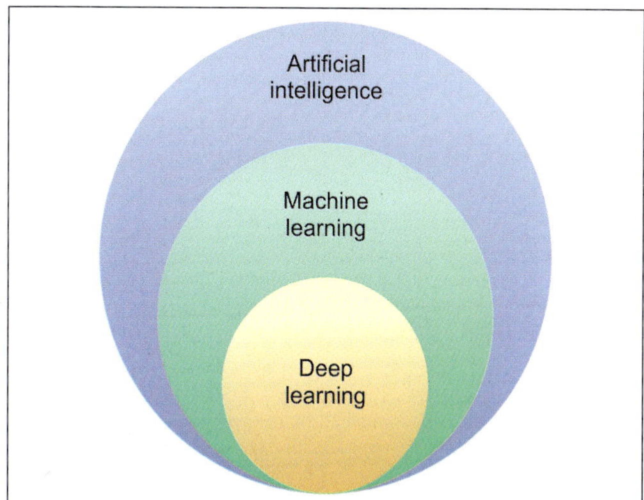

FIGURE 3: A concept diagram explaining the relationships between artificial intelligence (AI), machine learning (MI), and deep learning (DL).

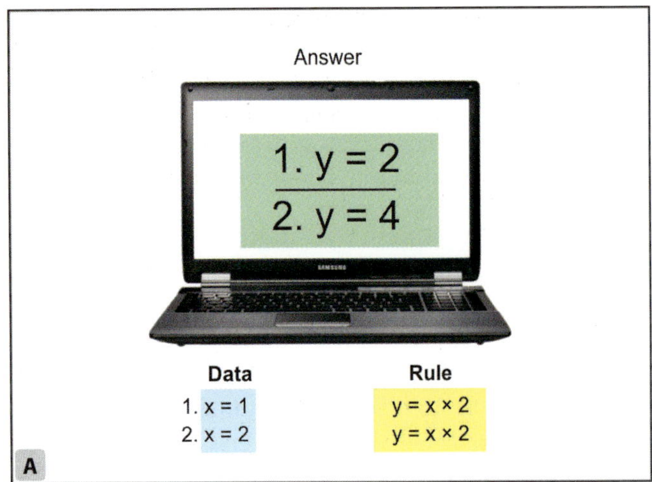

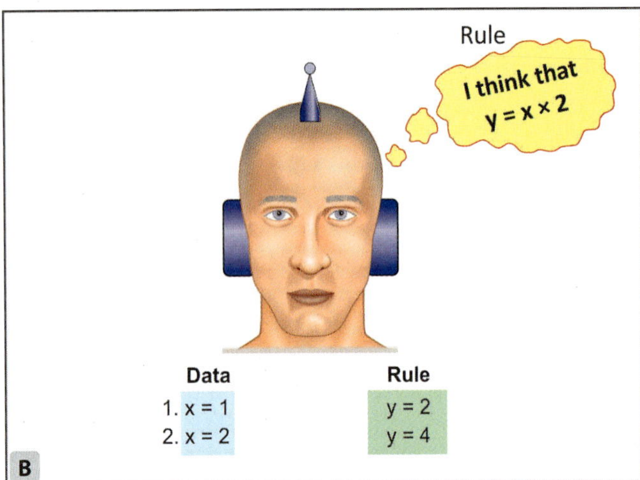

FIGURES 4 A & B: **(A)** In traditional programming, humans discovered the rule from data and communicated to the machine; **(B)** In machine learning approach, machines discover the rules by looking at large sets of data.

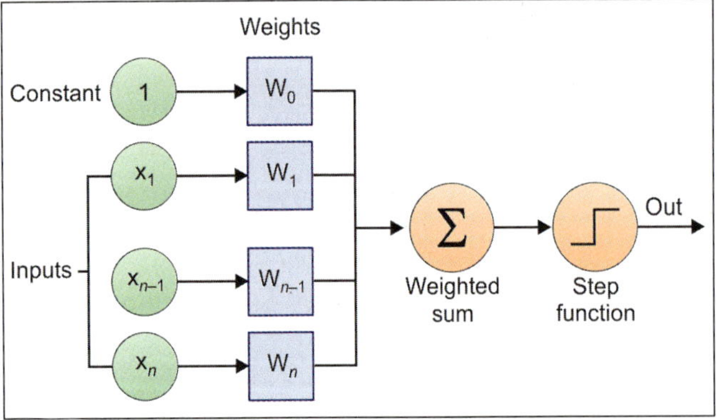

FIGURE 5: Mathematical model of a single artificial neuron (perceptron).

Source: Sharma S. (2017). What the Hell is Perceptron? [online] Available from https://towardsdatascience.com/what-the-hell-is-perceptron-626217814f53.

Neural networks are typically arranged in layers. In most simple arrangements, every neuron of one layer is connected to every neuron of the next layer. There is typically one input layer, few hidden layers, and one output layer. When the number of hidden layers become more than one such network is termed as deep NN and consequently the set of methods employing these are termed as **deep learning (DL)**.

In **Figure 6 A,** functionality of the human brain is shown. Electrical signals from eyes are transmitted to the brain. These signals are fed into a bunch of neurons forming a small NN that are specialized in recognition of objects. The same NN may be able to recognize and differentiate between various different objects. The capability of recognition is brought about by the mathematical operations performed on the signal as it transmits to the NN. The connection strengths between the synapses can be inhibitory or excitatory and these synaptic strengths are trained and retrained through exposure to visual information of different objects over a lifetime.

One of the *primary applications of DL* is in medical imaging. Images are two-dimensional and are typically much larger in size then tabular data. For example, a cancer diagnosis based on biopsy sample analysis may have the following entries: Radius, texture, perimeter, area, smoothness, compactness, concavity, concave point, and symmetry. The same information in the form of an image may have hundred thousand pixels. To get the tabular data out of images, most of the time requires human observation and labeling of the raw image obtained from the machines.

Hitherto, it has been quite impossible to apply deep NN over raw images, as they used to become too large and computationally intensive for current computers to handle. However, recently a class of method called as convolutional neural network (CNN) has gained quite a lot of attraction in medical image analysis.

The key to the operation of CNN is convolution operation, which takes into account the fact that its neighborhood pixels are related to each other. Different convolutional filters are applied on the image to obtain low-level features such as edges and curves contrast in the initial hidden layers right after the input layers. Application of convolution layers spreads out the information contained in the two-dimensional image into a three-dimensional. Another set of layers called a pooling layer used size of the image in the original two-dimensional after application of couple of convolution layers over the image most redundant information is filtered out and only the most essential information is passed through. After this, few layer of traditional fully connected NN are applied. Finally, an output layer takes the final diagnostic decision. Again, the amazing thing about CNN is that we did not program the weights of the convolutional or fully connected layers. These are automatically determined based on the optimization over the labeled data. If we have enough (typically in order of thousands of nodes) labeled images, then CNN can perform surprisingly well and sometimes can surpass human performance. One example of CNN is shown in **Figure 6 B**, where the steps involved in a brain tumor analysis is shown.

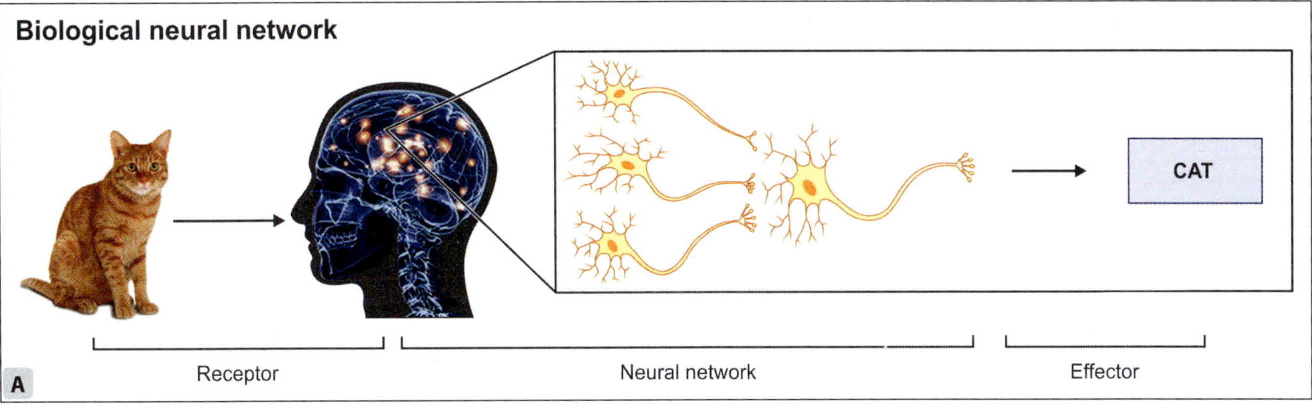

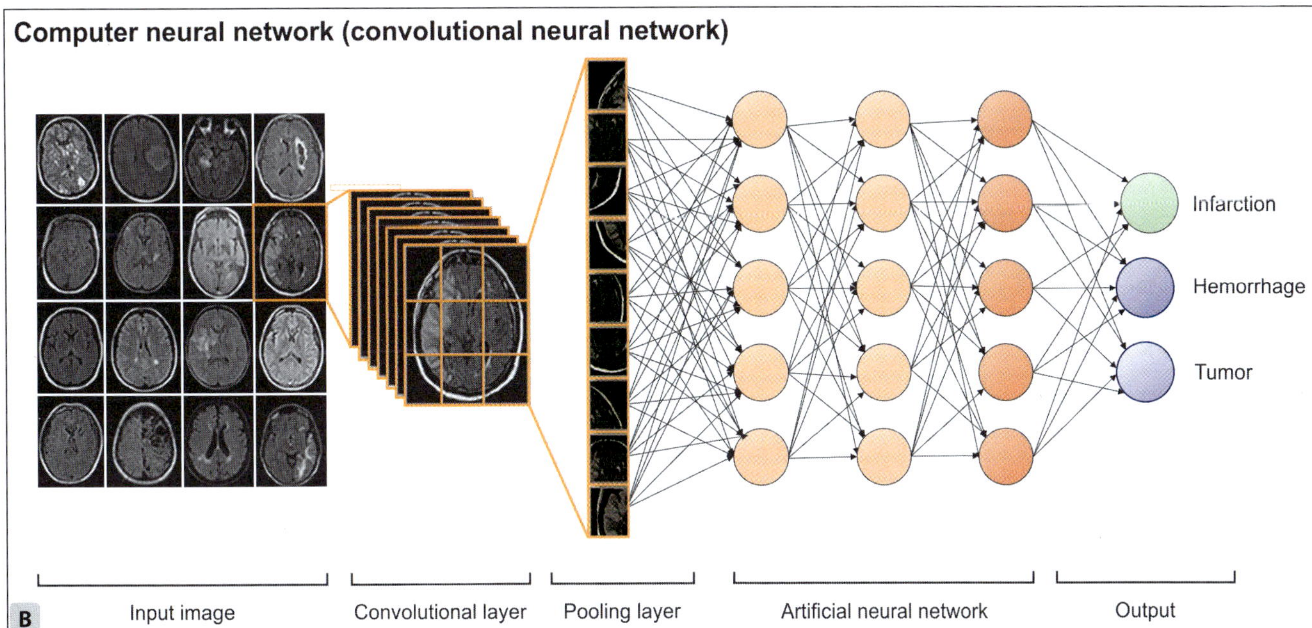

FIGURES 6 A & B: (A) Concept diagram of perception in human brain; **(B)** The basic convolutional neural network (CNN) operating over classifying brain tumor.

Source: Reprinted with permission from Zhu G, Jiang B, Tong L, Xie Y, Zaharchuk G, Wintermark M. Applications of Deep Learning to Neuro-Imaging Techniques. Front Neurol. 2019;10:869.

MODEL PERFORMANCE PARAMETERS

Machine learning and algorithms are applied to broad classes of problems—(1) classification and (2) regression. For example, an algorithm is trying to look at image and find out if it has a tumor or not then it is a classification problem. While if another algorithm is trying to estimate the blood sugar level of a person such an algorithm will be solving a regression problem. Regression performance is characterized by parameters such as mean square error, percentage error correlation and coefficient of determination. Major classes in medicine are classification problems. Here an algorithm has to differentiate between two different classes such as true/false, diseased/healthy, and alive/expired. Here a key table which is used widely is a confusion matrix as shown in **Figure 7**. Different ML models can be built around the same data; some may have a higher false positive rate (FPR) while some may have false negative rate. Many times, there is a tradeoff between sensitivity and specificity. For two different models with similar accuracy, we prefer the model with higher sensitivity. This is to ensure that a patient having a disease is less, likely to be missed. There is another curve which is quite important, specifically when we are comparing different ML models and different decision thresholds in the same model. This is called the receiver operating characteristic (ROC) curve. ROC is the plot of FPR versus true positive rate (TPR). For a particular model, ROC curve can be drawn by varying the decision threshold between 0 and 1. These curves can be drawn on a single graph for different models. A 45° straight line indicates that the model is as good as a coin flip and does not have any predictive value. The area under the curve (AUC) is an indicator of the predictive power of the model as shown in the **Figure 7**.

Area under the curve-receiver operating characteristic curve: The ROC curve shows evaluation metric for binary classification problems. It is a probability curve that is

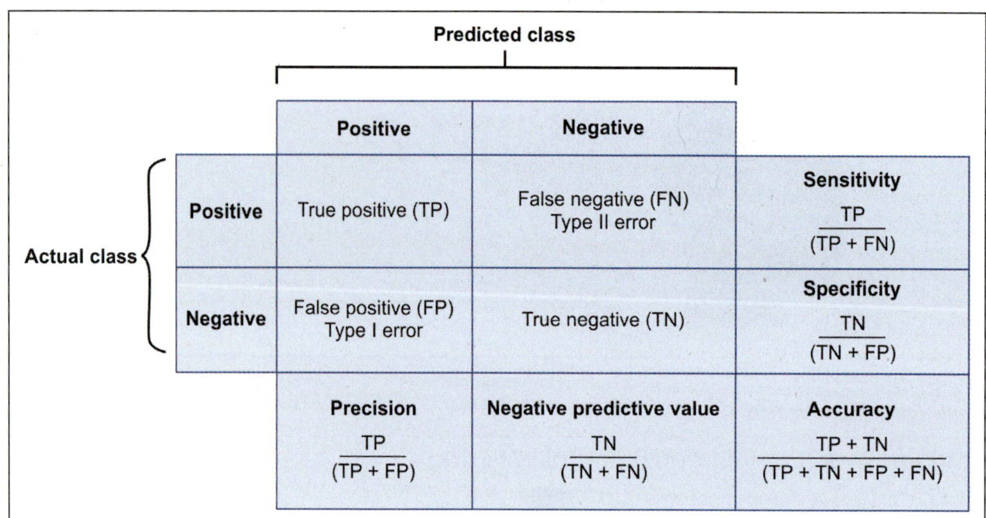

FIGURE 7: Confusion matrix and different classification metrics derived from it.

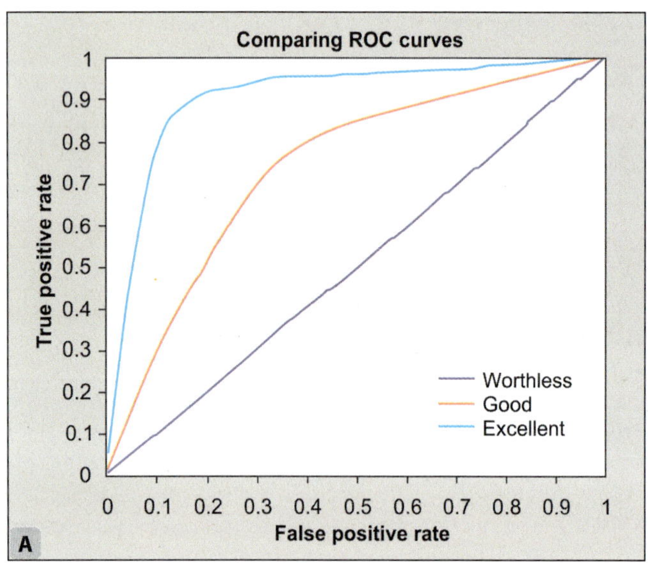

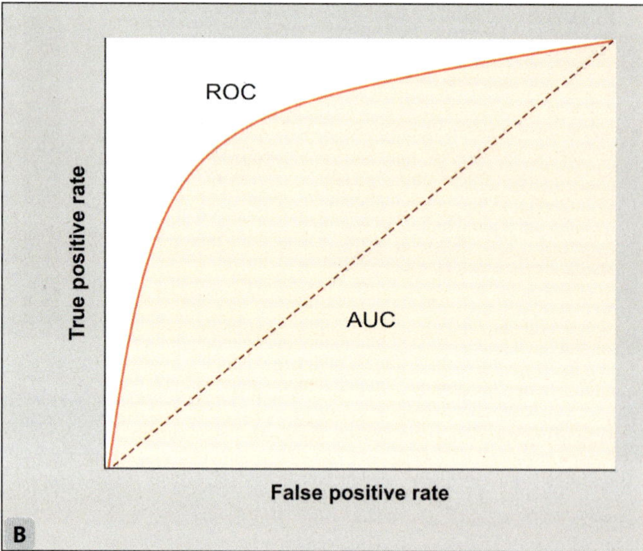

FIGURES 8 A & B: (A) Receiver operating characteristic (ROC) curve for three different models and their relative performance; **(B)** Area under the curve (AUC) calculated from ROC.

plotted between TPR and FPR at various threshold values. The AUC shows the ability of a classifier to distinguish between classes and is used as a summary of the ROC curve. As shown in **Figure 8**, as AUC increases, the model starts performing better. The model ROC depicted by the green line performs best, as its AUC is highest, followed by the red one and worst performing is the blue one.

APPLICATIONS OF AI, ML AND DL

Artificial intelligence in healthcare has gained popularity over the past decade. It is having tremendous impact in improving diagnosis, monitoring, and treatment. Massive quantities of data are generated by high-resolution medical imaging, biosensors, EHRs, and genome sequencing. Today, the amount of data being produced is so large that it cannot be analyzed by humans and traditional software, so this increases the necessity of using current state of art ML, AI, and big data techniques to analyze healthcare data. AI systems promise to better address the increased noncommunicable disease burden, aging population, and low doctor-to-patient ratio problems around the world.

If we look deeper into healthcare delivery, there are serious issues in existing systems, such as large numbers of serious diagnostic errors, treatment mistakes, inefficiencies in the workflow, inadequate time between patients and clinicians, and an enormous waste of resources. Healthcare leaders and computer scientists have asserted that AI has the capability to address all these problems.

Artificial intelligence is performing in many sections of healthcare. Some of them are diagnosing tumors from magnetic resonance imaging (MRI) scans, pneumonia

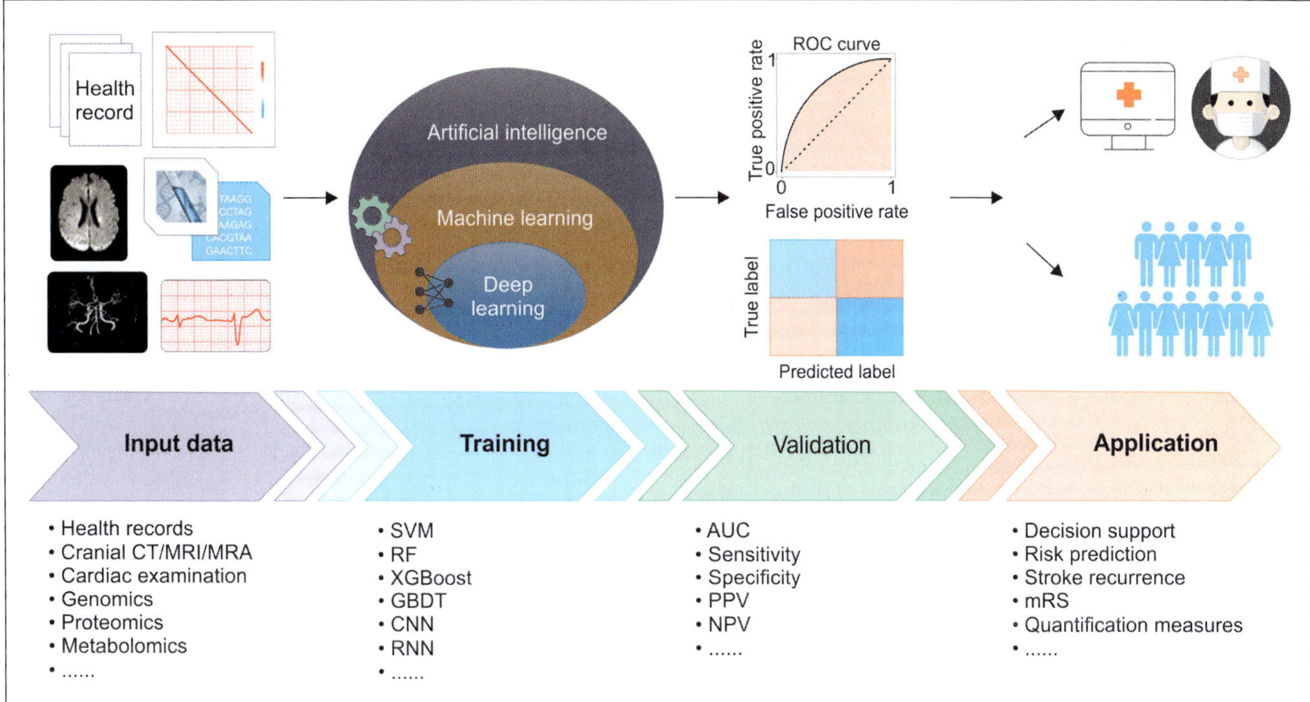

(AI: artificial intelligence; AUC: area under the curve; CNN: convolutional neural network; CT: computed tomography; GBDT: gradient boosting decision tree; MRA: magnetic resonance angiography; MRI: magnetic resonance imaging; mRS: modified Rankin Scale; NPV: negative predictive value; PPV: positive predictive value; RF: random forest; RNN: recurrent neural network; ROC: receiver operating characteristic; SVM: support vector machine)

FIGURE 9: A generalized pipeline of application of AI on any medical dataset is shown.

Source: Reprinted with permission from Ding L, Liu C, Li Z, WangY. Incorporating Artificial Intelligence into Stroke Care and Research. Stroke. 2020;51(12):e351-4.

from X-ray, breast cancer from mammographs, diabetic retinopathy from fundus images, and detecting epidemiology by using EHRs. AI is also useful with medical signals like arrhythmia detection from electrocardiogram (ECG) signals or seizure detection by using physiological signals.

In **Figure 9**, a pipeline of AI systems is shown. First a large amount of data is stored; this is the raw data. The stored data is labeled by a medical expert, like—in MRI scans an expert analyzes the scan and tells if the scan is normal or if a tumor is present in it. Then the ML models are trained; this is based on input data and desired prediction types. After training, the model is validated by presenting it with testing data, which are simply data points that the model has not seen during training. Then the model performance is characterized by methods explained in section titled "Model Performance Parameters".

Even after technical validation, clinical trials are performed before deploying the systems in clinical use. Regulatory bodies such as Food and Drug Administration (FDA) in the USA and Central Drugs Standard Control Organisation (CDSCO) in India are framing and revising rules for regulation of AI-based medical technologies continually. As the technology is evolving rapidly, this is currently a dynamic process.

CASE STUDIES

In recent times, there has been great penetration of AI in multiple clinical domains. It will be quite impossible for us to cover all such applications, but we believe that following interesting examples will help the readers appreciate the amazing impact which AI had on healthcare. There have been examples of publications where DL has been used for interpretation of retinal fundus images, chest X-ray, pathology slides, diagnosing skin cancer, ECG, colonoscopy images, mental health charts, and EHR-derived clinical information. The details of these are given in the **e-chapter** along with.

CHALLENGES FOR AI, ML AND DL

The pace of AI, ML, and DL implementation in the real world is slow. The reasons for this slow usage are many. Some of these are discussed below.

- *Lack of peer-reviewed randomized controlled trials*: Among ML researchers, it is common to publish studies on preprint servers, and many times are claiming groundbreaking results without peer-reviewed evidence. Peer-reviewed evidence is a must in healthcare-related research for the trust and adoption of AI within the wider medical community.
- *Metrics often do not reflect clinical applicability*: The term "AI chasm" had been created to acknowledge the fact that clinical efficacy cannot be only represented by accuracy. Despite its comprehensive use in ML research, "AUC" of a ROC curve is not necessarily the best metric to represent clinical applicability and many clinicians did not feel comfortable in understanding it.

Some papers include sensitivity and specificity but not all of them, positive and negative predictive values. These should also be included in AI-related medical research papers. No single performance measuring parameter captures all the desirable properties, so papers must include multiple performance measuring parameters. Medicine has been traditionally using multiple biostatistical methods such as student t-test and analysis of variance (ANOVA) to derive useful probabilistic conclusions from sparse data. ML researchers typically do not use these tools. However, characterizing the model performance of these tools on test data will instill greater clinical confidence.

- *Unavailability and sparsity of structured data*: Many times, data in medicine is hard to acquire and most of the time researchers have to deal with smaller datasets compared to other fields. Such sparsity of data prevents a data hungry AI algorithm to perform adequately. In addition to this most of the medical data, especially in developing country like India, are still paper based and are unstructured. Unavailability of structured data is one of the biggest impediments to inroads of AI in healthcare.
- *Algorithmic interpretability (black box of AI)*: Machine learning researchers only create a structure of NN, while all its weights and other mathematical functionality is automatic and is based on input data and labels. After the training of big NNs is completed, most of the time it is impossible for the programmer to describe how an algorithm has actually taken a decision and what are the mathematical function and decision pathways which it has followed to arrive at a given conclusion. This is termed as the AI black box. This is not surprising given the fact AI is built based on inspiration from human brain. Just as a person would know how to swim but could be unable to explain the algorithm behind it, AI algorithms are able to make predictions without giving an explanation to it. Such a black box approach can lead to ethical dilemmas and prevent pinning down the responsibility for a wrong action of an AI.
- *Achieving robust regulation and rigorous quality control*: Due to the fast pace of development in this field, a large number of algorithms for different disease detection and prediction keep popping up almost on a daily basis. Many of these algorithms are not trained on sufficient amounts of data or have not followed proper ethical clearance procedures. Many of them report extraordinarily high accuracies without taking in account the sensitivity and specificity aspects. The same stringent regulations that have been applied to medical technologies need to be enforced on AI systems before their deployment. Some governments have already started taking specific steps in this direction.

BIG DATA IN HEALTHCARE

Big data refers to large amount of data that is unmanageable by using traditional software or internet-based platforms. The "big" part of big data is indicative of its large volume. It surpasses the traditionally used amount of storage, processing, and analytical power. Three important dimensions of big data are volume, velocity, and variety. These are also known as three Vs along which big data is growing exponentially. The application of big data analytics in healthcare has a lot of positive and also life-saving outcomes. In essence, big-style data refers to the vast quantities of information created by the digitization of everything that gets consolidated and analyzed by specific technologies. Applied to healthcare, it will use specific health data of a population (or of a particular individual) and potentially help to prevent epidemics and to cure diseases.

The penetration of EHR systems, wearable devices, high-resolution imaging, and 24 × 7 medical monitors are generating huge amounts of data in all three dimensions. In **Figure 10**, some common sources of big data in healthcare are shown. Compared to older data systems, big data comes with bigger challenges in terms of storage, processing, and

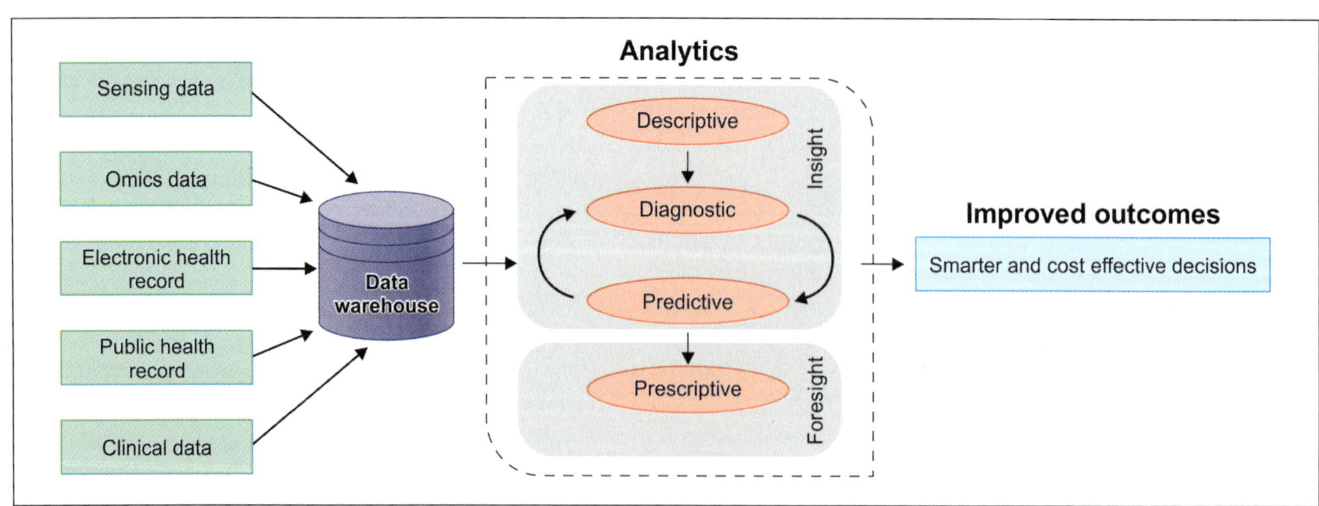

FIGURE 10: Workflow of big data analytics.

Source: Reprinted with permission from Dash S, Shakyawar SK, Sharma M, Kaushik S. Big data in healthcare: management, analysis and future prospects. J Big Data. 2019;6:1-25.

transmission. Many of the older methodology and hardware cannot be directly applied to such high volume and high velocity data.

Big data analytics has lot of life-saving applications and holds great promise to revolutionize healthcare. Health data of population or particular individuals are analyzed by big data analytics and can potentially help to prevent epidemics, cure diseases, and cut down costs. Data is typically stored in large servers called as data warehouses and are analyzed using advanced distributed big data processing software systems such as MapReduce and Hadoop. By using AI and ML, useful information is extracted which leads to smart and cost-effective decision making.

RECOMMENDED READINGS

1. National Institutes of Health National Center for Research Resources. (2006). Electronic Health Records Overview. [online] Available from https://s3.amazonaws.com/rdcms-himss/files/production/public/HIMSSorg/Content/files/Code%20180%20MITRE%20Key%20Components%20of%20an%20EHR.pdf.
2. Bouayad L, Ialynytchev A, Padmanabhan B. Patient health record systems scope and functionalities: Literature review and future directions. J Med Internet Res. 2017;19:e388.
3. Menachemi N, Collum TH. Benefits and drawbacks of electronic health record systems. Risk Manag Healthc Policy. 2011;4:47-55.
4. Office of the National Coordinator for Health Information Technology. (2019). Office-based Physician Electronic Health Record Adoption. [Online] Available from https://dashboard.healthit.gov/quickstats/pages/physician-ehr-adoption-trends.php.
5. Selwyn Jebaraj ASS. Implementing Electronic Health Records in New Zealand : A Critical Appraisal of Literature. Health Inform-An Int J. 2016;5:1-8.
6. CareQuality Commission. (2019). Cambridge University Hospitals NHS Foundation Trust. [Online] Available from https://www.cqc.org.uk/provider/RGT/reports.
7. Boonstra A, Broekhuis M. Barriers to the acceptance of electronic medical records by physicians from systematic review to taxonomy and interventions. BMC Health Serv Res. 2010;10:231.
8. Khalifa M. Barriers to health information systems and electronic medical records implementation a field study of Saudi Arabian hospitals. Procedia Comput Sci. 2013;21:335-42.
9. Ajami S, Bagheri-Tadi T. Barriers for adopting electronic health records (EHRs) by physicians. Acta Inform Medica. 2013;21:129-34.
10. Chollet F. Deep Learning with Python, 1st edition. Shelter Island, New York, United States: Manning Publications; 2017.
11. Zhu G, Jiang B, Tong L, Xie Y, Zaharchuk G, Wintermark M. Applications of deep learning to neuro-imaging techniques. Front Neurol. 2019;10:869.
12. Kelly CJ, Karthikesalingam A, Suleyman M, Corrado G, King D. Key challenges for delivering clinical impact with artificial intelligence. BMC Med. 2019;17:195.
13. Hashmi MF, Katiyar S, Keskar AG, Bokde ND, Geem ZW. Efficient pneumonia detection in chest Xray images using deep transfer learning. Diagnostics (Basel). 2020;10:417.
14. Geras KJ, Wolfson S, Shen Y, Wu N, Kim SG, Kim E, et al. (2017). High-Resolution Breast Cancer Screening with Multi-View Deep Convolutional Neural Networks. [online] Available from https://arxiv.org/pdf/1703.07047.pdf.
15. Wong TY, Bressler NM. Artificial intelligence with deep learning technology looks into diabetic retinopathy screening. JAMA. 2016;316: 2366-7.
16. Ding L, Liu C, Li Z, Wang Y. Incorporating Artificial Intelligence into Stroke Care and Research. Stroke. 2020;51:e351-4.
17. Bejnordi BE, Veta M, van Diest PJ, van Ginneken B, Karssemeijer N, Litjens G, et al. Diagnostic assessment of deep learning algorithms for detection of lymph node metastases in women with breast cancer. JAMA. 2017;318:2199-210.
18. Nature. (2014). High ambition. [online] Available from https://www.nature.com/news/high-ambition-1.16309.
19. Keane PA, Topol EJ. With an eye to AI and autonomous diagnosis. NPJ Digit Med. 2018;40:10-2.
20. Dash S, Shakyawar SK, Sharma M, Kaushik S. Big data in healthcare: management, analysis and future prospects. J Big Data. 2019;6:1-25.

CHAPTER 24

Psychiatric Disorders: Physicians Perspective

Navkiran Sooch Mahajan, Ranjive Mahajan, Deepika Bansal

ABSTRACT

Mental health is an essential component of overall health and the well-being of individuals and communities. Mental illness affects the individual's ability to function, to be productive, to establish and maintain positive relationships, and to experience a state of well-being. About 14% of the global burden of disease has been attributed to neuropsychiatric disorders, mostly due to the chronically disabling nature of psychiatric disorders. Mental disorders can be broadly classified into organic mental disorders and neurodevelopmental disorders, psychotic disorders, mood disorders, neurotic disorders, and substance use disorders. Neurocognitive disorders are those psychiatric disorders that affect people's ability to think and reason due to underlying illnesses. The disorders in this group include delirium as well as disorders of thinking and reasoning caused by such conditions or diseases as traumatic brain injury, infections, organ failure, or Alzheimer's disease (AD).

People suffering from psychotic disorders, for example, schizophrenia generally lack an insight into their illness and suffer from delusions, hallucinations, and disorganized thinking and speech. Mood disorders especially depressive disorders are common and encountered most frequently in general hospital settings leading to significant morbidity. Bipolar affective disorders are severe and lead to significant disability. Neurotic disorders include anxiety disorders which involves anxiety and worrying fearfully and excessively. There is no loss of reality contact and insight is usually present in such disorders, however, they can have long and protracted course. Anxiety disorders include generalized anxiety disorder (GAD), panic disorder, and phobias (extreme or irrational fears of specific things, such as heights). Psychiatric emergencies are also discussed, e.g., such as violent and aggressive patients, and suicidal patients which are seen frequently by physicians.

"The optimist sees the donut, the pessimist sees the hole"

—Oscar Wilde

INTRODUCTION

World Health Organization (WHO) defines mental health as "a state of well-being in which the individual realizes his or her own abilities, can cope with normal stresses of life, can work productively, and is able to make a contribution to his or her community."

Mental illnesses are health conditions involving changes in emotion, thinking, or behavior (or a combination of these). Mental illnesses are associated with distress and/or problems functioning in social, work, or family activities.

Globally prevalence of psychiatric disorders in general population is 10.7%. Psychiatric morbidity is common in the medically ill population ranging from 20 to 67% in general hospital patients. Certain disorders like delirium and depression can adversely affect the underlying medical disorders and worsen their outcomes. Such people have poorer quality of life and shorter life span.

Standard frameworks to uniformly identify and describe psychiatric disorders are ICD-10 (International Classification of Diseases) and DSM-5 (Diagnostic and Statistical Manual of Mental Disorders) and diagnosis are made as per these guidelines.

CLASSIFICATION

Psychiatric disorders can be classified as organic mental neurocognitive and developmental disorders, psychotic disorders, mood disorders, neurotic disorders, and substance use disorders (**Flowchart 1**). The common ones are discussed here.

NEUROCOGNITIVE DISORDERS (ORGANIC MENTAL DISORDERS)

- Cognition includes memory, language, orientation, judgment, conducting interpersonal relationships, performing actions (praxis), and problem solving.
- Cognitive disorders reflect disruption in one or more of these domains and are frequently complicated by behavioral symptoms.
- Cognitive disorders exemplify the complex interface among neurology, medicine, and psychiatry in that medical or neurological conditions often lead to cognitive disorders that, in turn, are associated with behavioral symptoms.

Various types of neurocognitive disorders are given in **Box 1**.

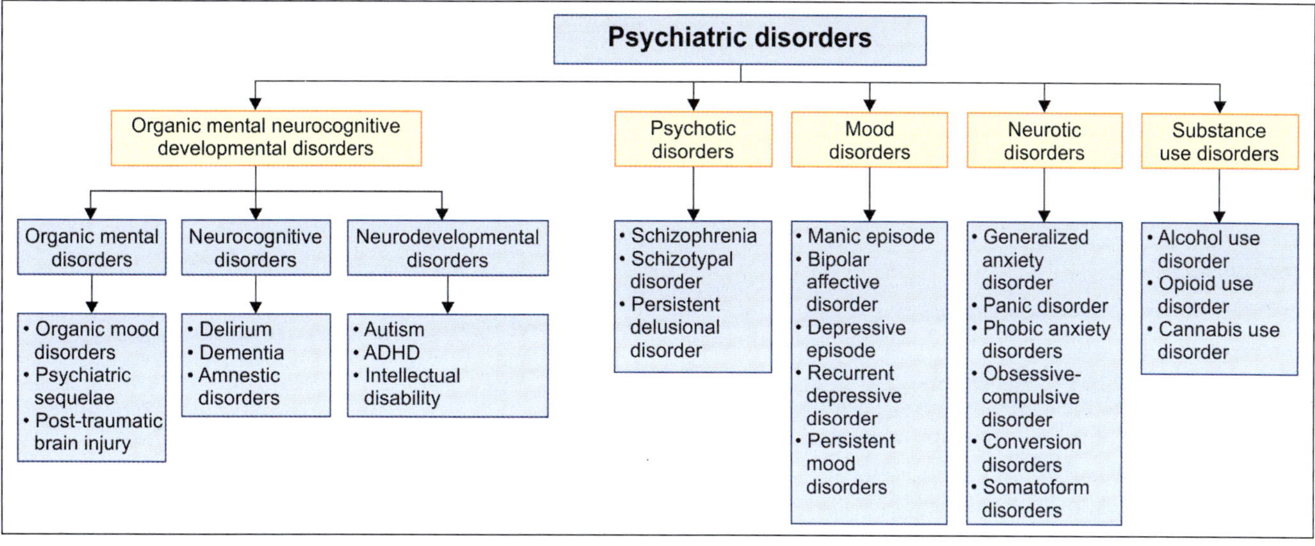

(ADHD: attention deficit hyperactivity disorder)

FLOWCHART 1: Classification of psychiatric disorders.

BOX 1	Types of neurocognitive disorders.
• Delirium	
• Dementia	
• Amnestic disorders	

DELIRIUM

- It is a disturbance in the state of consciousness characterized by confusion, disorientation, restlessness, affective lability, and perceptual disturbances (visual and auditory).
- It occurs with relatively acute onset and is associated with distractibility, short-term memory impairment, and decreased attention span.

Epidemiology:

- Delirium is a common disorder, with most incidence and prevalence rates reported in elderly adults.
- Among elderly emergency department patients, 5–10% have been reported to have delirium. At the time of admission to medical wards, between 15% and 21% of older patients meet criteria for delirium-prevalent cases.
- Delirium occurs in 70–87% of those in intensive care units and in up to 83% of all patients at the end-of-life care.
- Delirium develops in 80% of terminally ill patients.

Causes: The common causes of delirium are given in **Box 2**.

Management:

- Agitated patients must be protected from harm.
- After safety is ensured, a physical and mental status examination should be done.
- Relevant laboratory tests should be performed.
- Identification of cause and its immediate correction should be done.

BOX 2	Common causes of delirium.
• **Infection**	
◦ High-grade fever	
◦ Cerebral malaria	
◦ Septicemia	
◦ Meningitis	
◦ Encephalitis	
◦ Acquired immunodeficiency syndrome	
• **Metabolic disorders**	
◦ Electrolyte imbalance	
◦ Hypo-/hyperglycemia	
◦ Hepatic encephalopathy	
◦ Uremia acidosis	
◦ Porphyria	
• **Endocrinal imbalance**	
◦ Hypothyroidism	
◦ Hyperthyroidism	
◦ Cushing's syndrome	
◦ Addison's disease	
• **Vitamin deficiency:** Wernicke–Korsakoff syndrome	
• **Seizure disorder**	
• **Head injury**	
• **Substance use disorders**	
◦ Alcohol (intoxication/withdrawal)	
◦ Sedatives hypnotics	
• **Drug-induced**	
◦ Anticholinergics	
◦ Sympathomimetics	

- The two major symptoms of delirium that may require pharmacological treatment are psychosis and insomnia. A commonly used drug for psychosis is haloperidol, an antipsychotic drug (refer to **Table 6**).
- Insomnia is best treated with benzodiazepines (BZDs) with short or intermediate half-lives (e.g., lorazepam 1–2 mg at bedtime).

DEMENTIA

- Dementia is defined as a progressive impairment of cognitive functions occurring in clear consciousness (i.e., in the absence of delirium).
- It is an acquired persistent and progressive deterioration in cognitive abilities that impairs the successful performance of activities of daily living.
- Memory is the most common cognitive ability lost with dementia. Global impairment of intellect is the essential feature, manifested as difficulty with memory, attention, thinking, and comprehension. Other mental functions can often be affected, including mood, personality, judgment, and social behavior.
- The disorder can be progressive or static, permanent or reversible.

Epidemiology: The prevalence of moderate to severe dementia in different population groups is approximately 5% in the general population older than 65 years of age, 20–40% in the general population older than 85 years of age, 15–20 in outpatient general medical practices, and 50% in chronic care facilities. Of all patients with dementia, 50–60% have the most common type of dementia, dementia of the Alzheimer's type (AD).

Causes: The causes of dementia are divided into reversible causes and irreversible causes which are given in **Table 1**.

TABLE 1 Common causes of dementia.

Reversible causes	Irreversible causes
• **Neurosurgical causes:** ◦ Subdural hematoma ◦ Normal pressure hydrocephalus ◦ Intracranial tumors ◦ Intracranial abscess • **Infectious causes:** ◦ Meningitis ◦ Encephalitis ◦ Neurosyphilis ◦ Lyme disease • **Metabolic causes:** ◦ Vitamin B12 deficiency ◦ Folic acid deficiency ◦ Niacin deficiency ◦ Hypothyroidism ◦ Hyperthyroidism ◦ Hypoparathyroidism ◦ Hyperparathyroidism • **Others:** ◦ Drugs and toxins ◦ Alcohol abuse ◦ Autoimmune encephalitis	• **Parenchymal brain disease:** ◦ Alzheimer's disease ◦ Pick's disease ◦ Lewy body dementia ◦ Huntington's disease ◦ Parkinson's disease • **Vascular dementia:** ◦ Multi-infarct dementia ◦ Subcortical dementia

Management:

- Donepezil, rivastigmine, and galantamine are cholinesterase inhibitors used to treat mild-to-moderate cognitive impairment in AD. They reduce the inactivation of the neurotransmitter acetylcholine and, thus, potentiate the cholinergic neurotransmitter, which in turn produces a modest improvement in memory and goal-directed thought.
- Donepezil is well tolerated and widely used. Memantine [N-methyl-D-aspartate (NMDA) antagonist] protects neurons from excessive amounts of glutamate, which may be neurotoxic. The drug is sometimes combined with donepezil.
- Clinicians may prescribe BZDs for insomnia and anxiety, antidepressants for depression, and antipsychotic drugs for delusions and hallucinations.

AMNESTIC DISORDERS

The syndrome is defined primarily by impairment in the ability to create new memories. Three variations of the amnestic disorder diagnosis, differing in etiology.

1. Amnestic disorder caused by a general medical condition (e.g., head trauma)
2. Substance-induced persisting amnestic disorder (e.g., caused by carbon monoxide poisoning or chronic alcohol consumption)
3. Amnestic disorder in cases where etiology is unclear.

PSYCHOTIC DISORDERS

Different types of psychotic disorders are given in **Box 3**.

SCHIZOPHRENIA

Kurt Schneider (1887–1967) contributed a description of first-rank symptoms, which, he stressed, were not specific for schizophrenia and were not to be rigidly applied but were useful for making diagnosis and had high predictive value. *Schneider's First Rank Symptoms (SFRS)* of schizophrenia include: Thought withdrawal, thought insertion, thought broadcasting, auditory hallucinations, made feelings, made impulses and acts, somatic passivity (bodily sensations), and delusional perception (normal perception has illogical meaning).

Epidemiology: Schizophrenia affects 1% of the population. Schizophrenia is equally prevalent in men and women. Onset is earlier in men than in women. The peak ages of onset are 10–25 years for men and 25–35 years for women. Unlike men, women display a bimodal age distribution, with a second peak occurring in middle age.

BOX 3	Types of psychotic disorders.
Schizophrenia	
• Paranoid schizophrenia	
• Hebephrenic schizophrenia	
• Catatonic schizophrenia	
• Undifferentiated schizophrenia	
• Residual schizophrenia	
• Simple schizophrenia	
Schizotypal disorder	
Persistent delusional disorders	

Causes: The exact cause of schizophrenia is not known. Various biological theories and psychosocial theories are proposed.

- *Genetic factors*: Schizophrenia has a genetic contribution as reflected by higher monozygotic concordance rate than dizygotic concordance rate. Family studies reveal that first-degree relatives of a schizophrenic patient are at higher risk for genetic inheritability.
- *Biochemical factors*:
  - *Dopamine hypothesis*: It states that schizophrenia is due to a functional increase of dopamine at the postsynaptic receptor.
  - *Serotonin*: Current hypothesis states that serotonin excess as a cause of both positive and negative symptoms of schizophrenia.
  - *Norepinephrine*: A selective neuronal degeneration within the norepinephrine reward neural system could account for anhedonia in schizophrenia.
  - *Gamma-aminobutyric acid (GABA)*: Patients with schizophrenia have a loss of GABAergic neurons in the hippocampus.
  - *Glutamate*: Glutamate has been implicated because ingestion of phencyclidine, a glutamate antagonist, produces an acute syndrome similar to schizophrenia.
  - *Glycine*: Glycine is also implicated in etiology of schizophrenia as there occurs reciprocal regulation of dopamine and glycine in forebrain and glycine is also involved in modulation of glutamate.
- *Neurodevelopmental theory*: It states that patients with schizophrenia are more likely to have history of several neurological and developmental abnormalities such as obstetric complications and later on, have delayed milestones etc.
- *Neuropathological factors*: Abnormalities have been found in cerebral ventricles and limbic system.
- Cultural and social factors and certain medical conditions may also influence symptom formation.

Clinical features:

- *Positive symptoms* of schizophrenia include delusions, hallucinations, disorganized speech, disorganized behavior, catatonic behavior, and agitation.
  - *Delusions* are false, firm, fixed beliefs that are out of keeping with the patient's social and cultural background. Delusions are persistent and organized, and that do not go away even after receiving logical or accurate information. For example, a person who is certain his or her food is poisoned, even if it has been proven that the food is fine, is suffering from a delusion.
  - *Hallucinations* are defined as "a perception without an object." These are unusual sensory experiences or perceptions of things that are not actually present, such as seeing things that are not there, hearing voices, smelling odors, having a "funny" taste in the mouth and feeling sensations on the skin even though nothing is touching the body.
- *Negative symptoms* of schizophrenia include poverty of speech, reduced range of emotions, e.g., feels numb or empty inside, reduced social drive, and interaction; reduced ability to experience pleasure, reduced desire, motivation, and may have poor personal hygiene.
- *Cognitive symptoms* of schizophrenia are impaired attention and impaired information processing.

Subtypes of schizophrenia:

- *Paranoid schizophrenia*: It is persecutory type of schizophrenia. It is the most common form of schizophrenia which includes: Delusion of persecution, reference, jealousy, and hallucinations usually auditory voices that threaten the patient or give commands.
- *Hebephrenic schizophrenia*: It is characterized by marked thought disorder, incoherence, and severe loosening of associations. Delusions and hallucinations are fragmentary. Emotional disturbances (flat or inappropriate affect, silly smiles, or senseless giggling), mannerisms, "mirror-gazing" (for long periods of time), and extreme social withdrawal are present.
- *Catatonic schizophrenia*: It is characterized by psychomotor disturbances which include: Stupor (marked decrease in reactivity to the environment), mutism, excitement, posturing (voluntary maintenance of inappropriate postures), negativism (motiveless resistance to all instructions or attempts to be moved or movement in opposite direction), rigidity, and waxy flexibility (maintenance of limbs and body in externally imposed position).
- *Undifferentiated schizophrenia*: It is a type of schizophrenia that is diagnosed when either features of no subtype are fully present, or when features of more than one subtype are exhibited, and the general criteria for diagnosis of schizophrenia are met.
- *Residual schizophrenia*: The residual schizophrenia is diagnosed after at least one episode has occurred and there are prominent negative symptoms with absence or marked reduction of florid psychotic symptoms such as delusions and hallucinations.
- *Simple schizophrenia*: It is characterized by an early onset (early second decade), very insidious and progressive course, and presence of characteristic "negative symptoms." Delusions and hallucinations are usually absent.

Physical findings:

- *Neurological findings*: Localizing and nonlocalizing neurological signs (also known as hard and soft signs, respectively) have been reported to be more common in patients with schizophrenia than in other psychiatric patients. Nonlocalizing signs include dysdiadochokinesia, astereognosis, primitive reflexes, and diminished dexterity. The presence of neurological signs and symptoms correlates with increased severity of illness, affective blunting, and a poor prognosis.
- *Eye examination*: In addition to the disorder of smooth ocular pursuit (saccadic movement), patients with schizophrenia have an elevated blink rate. The elevated blink rate is believed to reflect hyperdopaminergic activity.
- *Speech*: The inability of schizophrenia patients to perceive the prosody of speech or to inflect their own speech can be seen as a neurological symptom of a disorder in the nondominant parietal lobe. Other parietal lobe-like symptoms in schizophrenia include the inability to carry out tasks (i.e., apraxia), right–left disorientation, and lack of concern about the disorder.
- *Obesity*: Patients with schizophrenia appear to be more obese, with higher body mass indexes (BMIs). This is due to the effect of many antipsychotic medications, as well as poor nutritional balance and decreased motor activity.
- *Diabetes mellitus*: Schizophrenia is associated with an increased risk of type 2 diabetes mellitus (T2DM). This is probably due, in part, to the association with obesity noted previously, but there is also evidence that some antipsychotic medications cause diabetes through a direct mechanism.
- *Cardiovascular disease*: Many antipsychotic medications have direct effects on cardiac electrophysiology. In addition, obesity, increased rates of smoking, diabetes, hyperlipidemia, and a sedentary lifestyle all independently increase the risk of cardiovascular morbidity and mortality.
- *Human immunodeficiency virus (HIV)*: Patients with schizophrenia appear to have a risk of HIV infection that is 1.5–2 times that of the general population. This association is thought to be due to increased risk behaviors, such as unprotected sex, multiple partners, and increased drug use.
- *Chronic obstructive pulmonary disease*: Rates of chronic obstructive pulmonary disease are reportedly increased in schizophrenia compared with the general population.
- *Rheumatoid arthritis*: Patients with schizophrenia have approximately one-third the risk of rheumatoid arthritis that is found in the general population.

Course and outcome:

- Most people get better with treatment. Course is characterized by multiple exacerbations. Total remission is not commonly seen.
- Outcome in schizophrenia is multidimensional including symptoms, social factors, and cognitive functioning of the individual.

TABLE 2 Prognostic factors of schizophrenia.

Good prognostic factors	Poor prognostic factors
Acute or abrupt onset	Insidious onset
Onset >35 years of age (late onset)	Onset <20 years of age (early onset)
Presence of precipitating stressor	Absence of stressor
Good premorbid adjustment	Poor premorbid adjustment
Short duration (<6 months)	Chronic course (>2 years)
Presence of depression	Absence of depression
Predominance of positive symptoms	Predominance of negative symptoms
Good social support	Poor social support or unmarried

- The International Pilot Study of Schizophrenia (IPSS) showed that persons in developing countries including India had a better outcome than those living in developed nations. Untreated schizophrenia likely to result in persistent progressive course.
- Duration of untreated psychosis (DUP) is a prominent prognostic factor. Longer the DUP, worse is the outcome. Various prognostic factors of schizophrenia are given in **Table 2**.

Treatment: The treatment of schizophrenia has two main components:

1. *Pharmacological treatment*:
   - Acute psychotic symptoms require immediate attention. Antipsychotics and BZDs can result in relatively rapid calming of patients.
   - Atypical (or the second generation) antipsychotic drugs, such as risperidone, paliperidone, olanzapine, quetiapine, and aripiprazole, are more commonly used than the older typical (or first generation) antipsychotics such as trifluoperazine and haloperidol due to their extrapyramidal side effects.
   - BZDs such as lorazepam are also effective for agitation during acute psychosis.
2. *Psychosocial treatment*: Apart from medications psychosocial interventions have been found to be effective in treatment of schizophrenia especially after acute phase is treated with medications. These help patients and families cope with the illness and its complications and help prevent relapses.
   - *Electroconvulsive therapy (ECT)* may be indicated for some patients, especially those with marked catatonic or depressed features.
   - *Clozapine* is effective in patients with the most severe psychotic symptoms, as well as in those who had previously responded poorly to other antipsychotics. It also has antisuicidal properties (refer to **Table 6**).

MOOD DISORDERS

Mood can be defined as a pervasive and sustained emotion or feeling tone that influences a person's behavior and colors his or her perception of being in the world. Mood disorders encompass a large group of disorders in which pathological mood and related disturbances dominate the clinical picture.

CAUSES

Biochemical theory:

- Monoamine hypothesis suggests an abnormality in the monoamines, catecholamines (norepinephrine and dopamine), and serotonin system in the central nervous system at one or more sites. Depletion of serotonin may precipitate depression.
- Other neurotransmitters like GABA and neuroactive peptides, particularly vasopressin and endogenous opiates, have been implicated in the pathophysiology of mood disorders.

Genetic hypothesis: Adoption studies show data supporting the genetic basis for the inheritance of mood disorders. Twin studies show concordance rate for monozygotic twins is higher than dizygotic twins in both bipolar patients as well as unipolar depression patients.

Cognitive theory: Depression results from specific cognitive distortion present in persons prone to depression which includes hopelessness, helplessness, and worthlessness.

Psychosocial factors: A long-standing stressful life event and environmental stressors may precipitate mood disorders.

TYPES OF MOOD DISORDER

According to the ICD-10, the types of mood disorders are given in **Box 4**.

MANIC EPISODE

Epidemiology: The life-time risk of manic episode is about 0.8–1%. This disorder tends to occur in episodes lasting usually 3–4 months, followed by complete clinical recovery. The future episodes can be manic, depressive, or mixed.

- *General description*: Manic patients are excited, overtalkative, and frequently hyperactive.
- *Mood, affect, and feelings*: Manic patients can be euphoric and related with an increased sense of psychological well-being and happiness, not in keeping with ongoing events. They can also be irritable.
- *Psychomotor activity*: There is an increased psychomotor activity ranging from restlessness to manic excitement.
- *Speech*: Manic patients are more talkative than usual and may describe thoughts racing in mind and thus develop pressure of speech which at times, may be, difficult to interrupt. Later, flights of ideas (rapidly produced speech with abrupt shifts from topic to topic) may also be present.
- *Perceptual disturbances*: Mood congruent manic delusions are often concerned with great wealth, extraordinary abilities or power.
- *Thought*: Manic patient's thought content includes themes of raised self-confidence and inflated self-esteem.
- *Other symptoms*: Sleep is usually reduced with a decreased need for sleep. Insight is usually absent

BOX 4	Types of mood disorder.
• Manic episode	
• Bipolar mood (affective) disorder	
• Depressive episode	
• Recurrent depressive disorder	
• Persistent mood disorder (including cyclothymia and dysthymia)	
• Other mood disorders (including mixed affective episode)	

BIPOLAR MOOD (OR AFFECTIVE) DISORDER

This disorder is characterized by recurrent episodes of mania and depression in the same patient at different times. They can occur in any sequence.

- *Bipolar I disorder*: Bipolar I disorder is defined as the occurrence of at least one manic or mixed (full mania and full depression simultaneously) episode.
- *Bipolar II disorder*: Bipolar II disorder is defined as an illness course consisting of one or more major depressive episodes and at least one hypomanic episode.

DEPRESSIVE EPISODE

Epidemiology:

- Major depressive disorder has highest lifetime prevalence (almost 17%) of any psychiatric disorder.
- There is 2-fold greater prevalence of major depressive disorder in women than in men. The reasons for the difference are hypothesized to involve hormonal differences, the effects of childbirth, differing psychosocial stressors for women and for men, and behavioral models of learned helplessness.
- The mean age of onset for major depressive disorder is about 40 years.
- Major depressive disorder occurs most often in persons without close interpersonal relationships and in those who are divorced or separated.

Clinical features:

- *General features*: Generalized psychomotor retardation is most common. Classically a depressed patient has a stooped posture, no spontaneous movements, and a down-cast aerated gaze.
- *Mood affect and feelings*: Depressed mood is the key symptom which is present almost throughout the day.
- *Speech*: Depressed patients show decrease in rate and volume of speech, they respond to questions with single words and exhibit delayed response to questions.
- *Perceptual disturbances*: Depressed patient with delusion or hallucination are said to have major depressive disorder with psychotic features. Delusions and hallucinations that are consistent with a depressed mood are said to be mood congruent that include those of guilt, sinfulness, worthlessness, poverty, and failure persecution.
- *Thoughts*: Depressed patients have negative views of world and of themselves. They may have delusion/ideation of hopelessness, helplessness, suicidal

ideations, guilt and shame and are preoccupied with loss of sleep; weakness, and fatiguability.

- *Other symptoms*: Loss of interest in routine activities, physical symptoms such as heaviness of head, body aches, sleep disturbance, and decreased concentration at work may also be present.
- *Somatic syndrome in depression (ICD-10)*: The somatic syndrome is characterized by:
    - Significant decrease in appetite or weight
    - Early morning awakening, at least 2 (or more) hours before the usual time of awakening
    - Diurnal variation, with depression being worst in the morning
    - Pervasive loss of interest and loss of reactivity to pleasurable stimuli
    - Psychomotor agitation or retardation
- *Depression with melancholic features*:
    - Melancholia is one of the oldest terms used in psychiatry, used to refer to a depression characterized by severe anhedonia, early morning awakening, weight loss, and profound feelings of guilt (often over trivial events).
    - Melancholia is associated with changes in the autonomic nervous system and in endocrine functions. For that reason, melancholia is sometimes referred to as "endogenous depression" or depression that arises in the absence of external life stressors or precipitants.
- *Suicidal risk*: Suicidal risk in depressed patients is much more in the presence of following factors:
    - Presence of marked hopelessness
    - Males; age >40 years; unmarried, divorced/widowed
    - Written/verbal communication of suicidal intent and/or plan
    - Early stages of depression
    - Recovering from depression (at the peak of depression, the patient is usually either too depressed or too retarded to commit suicide)
    - Period of 3 months from recovery

RECURRENT DEPRESSIVE DISORDER

This disorder is characterized by recurrent (at least two) depressive episodes (unipolar depression) minimum 2 weeks apart.

PERSISTENT MOOD DISORDER

- *Cyclothymic disorder*: A chronic mood disorder involving numerous episodes of mild depression and mild elation none of which has been sufficiently severe or prolonged to fulfil the criteria for bipolar affective disorder or recurrent depressive disorder (duration >2 years).
- *Dysthymic disorder*: A chronic mood disorder characterized by a depressed mood which is never severe enough to fulfil the criteria for recurrent depressive disorder that lasts most of the time for >2 years.

Comorbid disorders:

- Anxiety
- Alcohol dependence

TABLE 3 Prognostic factors of mood disorders.

Good prognostic factors	Poor prognostic factors
• Acute or abrupt onset • Typical clinical features • Severe depression • Well-adjusted premorbid personality • Good response to treatment	• Comorbid medical disorder • Personality disorder • Alcohol dependence • Double depression (acute depressive episode superimposed on chronic depression or dysthymia) • Catastrophic stress or chronic ongoing stress • Unfavorable early environment • Marked hypochondriacal features, or mood-incongruent psychotic features • Poor drug compliance

- *Other substance-related disorders*: Although manic patients seldom use sedatives to dampen their euphoria, depressed patients often use stimulants, such as cocaine and amphetamines, to relieve their depression.
- *Medical conditions*: Depression commonly coexists with medical conditions, especially in older persons. Some of the physical illnesses commonly associated with depression include epilepsy, poststroke, Parkinson's disease, multiple sclerosis, AD, coronary artery disease, malignancy, and hypothyroidism.

Various prognostic factors of mood disorders are given in **Table 3**.

Course and outcome:

- Bipolar mood disorder has an earlier age of onset (third decade) than recurrent depressive (unipolar) disorder.
- Unipolar depression, on the other hand, is common in two age groups: Late third decade and fifth to sixth decades. Unipolar depression usually lasts longer than bipolar depression.
- An average manic episode lasts for 3–4 months while a depressive episode lasts from 4–6 months.
- With rapid institution of treatment, the major symptoms of mania are controlled within 2 weeks and of depression within 6–8 weeks.
- Nearly 40% of depressives with episodic course improve in 3 months, 60% in 6 months and 80% improve within a period of 1 year. About 15–20% of patients develop a chronic course of illness, which may last for two or more years.

Treatment:

- *Manic episode*: Mood stabilizers and atypical antipsychotics (e.g., lithium carbonate and sodium valproate) are preferred.
- *Unipolar depression*: Antidepressant drugs are the mainstay of the treatment such as selective serotonin reuptake inhibitors (SSRIs) (paroxetine, fluoxetine, sertraline etc.) and serotonin and norepinephrine reuptake inhibitor (SNRIs) (duloxetine, venlafaxine, desvenlafaxine etc.).

Tricyclic antidepressants (TCAs) (imipramine, amitriptyline etc.) are not preferred due to their cardiotoxic side effects.

Benzodiazepines and Z drugs are used to treat insomnia in these patients.

- *Bipolar depression*: Mood stabilizers are the drug of choice. Antidepressants should be used with caution as there is increased risk of switching to manic polarity (refer to **Table 6**).

NEUROTIC DISORDERS

The term *neurosis* has been defined as meeting one or more of the following criteria:

- The presence of a symptom or group of symptoms which cause subjective distress to the patient.
- The symptom is recognized as undesirable (i.e., insight is present).
- The personality and behavior are relatively preserved and not usually grossly disturbed.
- The contact with reality is preserved.
- There is an absence of organic causative factors.

TYPES OF NEUROTIC DISORDERS

Various types of neurotic disorders are given in **Box 5**.

ANXIETY DISORDERS

- Anxiety is the most common psychiatric symptom in clinical practice. Anxiety is a "normal" phenomenon, which is characterized by a state of apprehension or unease arising out of anticipation of danger.
- Anxiety is often differentiated from fear, as fear is an apprehension in response to an external danger while in anxiety the danger is largely unknown (or internal).
- Normal anxiety becomes pathological when it causes significant subjective distress and/or impairment in functioning of an individual.
- There are several disorders within the overall spectrum of anxiety disorders, each with its own characteristic symptoms GAD, panic disorder, social anxiety disorder (SAnD), obsessive-compulsive disorder (OCD), and post-traumatic stress disorder (PTSD)

Etiology: Neurotransmitter dysregulation—NE, 5-HT, GABA and autonomic nervous system activation—locus coeruleus/NE release/limbic system have been implicated in etiology of anxiety disorders.

Symptoms: The symptoms of anxiety are divided into physical and psychological symptoms which are given in **Box 6**.

GENERALIZED ANXIETY DISORDER

Definition: One of the anxiety disorders, where the primary symptoms of anxiety are present at most days for at least several weeks at a time, and usually for several months. The symptoms of anxiety should last for at least a period of 6 months which usually involve elements of:

- Apprehension (worries about future misfortunes, feeling "on edge," etc.)
- Motor tension (restlessness, inability to relax, and trembling)
- Autonomic overactivity (light-headedness, sweating, tachycardia, tachypnea, dry mouth etc.)

Course: This is characterized by an insidious onset in the third decade and a stable, usually chronic course (free floating anxiety) which may or may not be punctuated by repeated panic attacks.

Treatment: Today, first-line treatments include SSRIs (namely fluoxetine, sertraline, paroxetine, fluvoxamine, citalopram, and escitalopram) and SNRIs, venlafaxine as well as BZDs. β-blockers such as propranolol and atenolol are particularly useful in the management of anticipatory

BOX 5 Types of neurotic disorders.

- Generalized anxiety disorder
- Panic disorder
- Phobic anxiety disorders:
  - Agoraphobia
  - Social phobias
  - Specific (isolated) phobias
- Obsessive-compulsive disorder
- Reaction to severe stress, and adjustment disorders:
  - Post-traumatic stress disorder
- Conversion disorder
- Somatoform disorders:
  - Somatization disorder
  - Hypochondriacal disorder
  - Persistent somatoform pain disorder

BOX 6 Symptoms of anxiety.

- **Physical symptoms**
  - *Motoric symptoms*: Tremors, restlessness, muscle twitches, and fearful facial expression
  - *Autonomic and visceral symptoms*: Palpitations, tachycardia, sweating, flushes, dyspnea, hyperventilation, constriction in the chest, dry mouth, frequency and hesitancy of micturition, dizziness, diarrhea, and mydriasis
- **Psychological symptoms**
  - *Cognitive symptoms*: Poor concentration, distractibility, hyperarousal, vigilance or scanning, negative automatic thoughts
  - *Perceptual symptoms*: Derealization and depersonalization
  - *Affective symptoms*: Diffuse, unpleasant, and vague sense of apprehension; fearfulness; inability to relax; irritability; feeling of impending doom (when severe)
  - *Other symptoms*: Insomnia (initial), increased sensitivity to noise, and exaggerated startle response

anxiety (e.g., anxiety occurring before going on stage or before examinations).

PANIC DISORDER

Definition: This is characterized by discrete episodes of acute anxiety with a fear of impending doom. The panic attacks occur recurrently every few days. The episode is usually sudden in onset, lasts for a few minutes, and is characterized by very severe anxiety. Panic disorder can present either alone or with agoraphobia.

Course: The onset is usually in early third decade with often a chronic course.

Treatment: Benzodiazepines (such as alprazolam and clonazepam) are useful in short-term treatment and antidepressants usually SSRIs such as paroxetine are used as maintenance treatment. Beta-blockers do not have much role in panic disorder.

PHOBIAS

Definition: Phobia is defined as an irrational fear of a specific object, situation, or activity, often leading to persistent avoidance of the feared object, situation, or activity.

Types of phobia:
- Agoraphobia (fear of or anxiety regarding places from which escape might be difficult)
- Social phobia (fear of facing certain social situations)
- Specific phobia (excessive fear of a specific object, circumstance, or situation such as claustrophobia—fear of closed spaces, and hydrophobia—fear of water).

The fear is out of proportion to the dangerousness perceived. Patient recognizes the fear as irrational and unjustified (insight is present). This leads to persistent avoidance of the object, situation, or activity.

Epidemiology: Phobias are generally more common in women with an onset in late second decade or early third decade. Typically, the onset is sudden without any apparent cause.

Course: The course is usually chronic with gradually increasing restriction of daily activities. Sometimes, phobias are spontaneously remitting.

Treatment: Benzodiazepines (such as alprazolam and clonazepam) are useful in short-term treatment and antidepressants usually SSRIs such as paroxetine are used as maintenance treatment (refer to **Table 6**).

Individuals with anxiety disorders have various other comorbid medical and psychiatric disorders which are given in **Table 4**.

TABLE 4 Comorbid medical and psychiatric disorders.

Medical	Psychiatric
• Hypertension and other cardiovascular conditions • Gastrointestinal disease • Arthritis • Thyroid disease • Respiratory disease • Migraine headaches	• Substance use disorders • Mood disorders: ◦ Bipolar: 52% ◦ MDD: 60% • ADHD: 47% • Other anxiety disorder: 30%

(ADHD: attention deficit hyperactivity disorder; MDD: major depressive disorder)

OBSESSIVE-COMPULSIVE DISORDER

Obsessive-compulsive disorder is characterized by obsessions, compulsions, or more frequently both. An *obsession* is defined as recurrent and persistent thoughts, urges or images that are experienced as intrusive and unwanted, and that in most individuals cause marked anxiety or distress when the individual fails to resist these thoughts. Common obsessions include contamination, pathological doubt, and need for symmetry. A *compulsion* is defined as repetitive behavior or mental acts that the individual feels driven to perform in response to an obsession or according to rules that must be rigidly applied. It is aimed at either preventing or neutralizing the distress or fear arising out of obsession. Common compulsions include checking, washing, and counting.

Epidemiology: In India, OCD is more common in unmarried males. The average age of onset is late third decade (i.e., late 20s) in India. The life-time prevalence of OCD to be as high as 2–3%.

Course and outcome: Classically thought to have a steady *chronic* course, the longitudinal profile of this disorder can also be *episodic*. A summary of long-term follow-up studies shows that about 25% remained unimproved over time, 50% had moderate to marked improvement while 25% had recovered completely. If untreated, OCD is a chronic illness with a waxing and waning of symptoms.

Comorbid psychiatric disorders: Individuals with OCD have various other comorbid psychiatric disorders as well which are given in **Box 7**.

BOX 7 Comorbid psychiatric disorders.

- **Mood disorders:**
  - Major depression, dysthymia, and bipolar disorder
- **Anxiety disorders:**
  - Panic disorder, generalized anxiety disorder, and social phobia
- **OCD-related disorders:**
  - Body dysmorphic disorder, hypochondriasis, trichotillomania, skin picking disorder, and tic disorders
- **Attention deficit hyperactivity disorder**
- **Oppositional defiant disorder**
- **Personality disorders:**
  - Obsessive-compulsive personality disorder preoccupation with perfectionism, orderliness and rigid control; rigidity, stubbornness, scrupulosity, and over conscientiousness. Typically egosyntonic. No obsessions and compulsions—anxiousavoidant personality disorder borderline personality disorder, and schizotypal personality

(OCD: obsessive-compulsive disorder)

Treatment:
- Pharmacotherapy includes SSRIs which are the first line of treatment.
- Clomipramine, a TCA, is also beneficial (refer to **Table 6**).
- Psychotherapy in the form of ERP (exposure and response prevention) is used to treat OCD.
- A combination of pharmacotherapy and psychotherapy yields the best results.

HOARDING DISORDER

Hoarding was originally considered a subtype of OCD but is now considered to be a separate diagnostic entity.
- Individuals afflicted with this condition have marked difficulties with disposing off items that are deemed to be of little or no value, regardless of their actual values.
- These behavioral difficulties result in accumulation of items that clutter personal living spaces.
- It is commonly driven by an obsessive fear of losing important items that the person believes may be of use at some point in the future, by distorted beliefs about the importance of possessions, and by extreme emotional attachment to possessions.

Epidemiology: Hoarding is believed to occur in approximately 2–5% of the population. It occurs equally among men and women, is more common in single persons, and is associated with social anxiety, withdrawal, and dependent personality traits. Hoarding usually begins in early adolescence and persists throughout the lifespan.

Course: The disorder is a chronic condition with a long course. Patients do not seek treatment as they do not recognize it an illness.

Treatment: Selective serotonin reuptake inhibitors are the drugs of choice. Drug treatment should be combined with psychotherapy (refer to **Table 6**).

POST-TRAUMATIC STRESS DISORDER

- Post-traumatic stress disorder is characterized by recurrent and intrusive recollections of the stressful event, either in *flashbacks* (images, thoughts, or perceptions) and/or in dreams. There is an associated sense of re-experiencing of the stressful event.
- There is marked *avoidance* of the events or situations that arouse recollections of the stressful event, along with marked symptoms of anxiety and increased arousal.
- Usually, it occurs after a terrifying event that involving physical or psychological traumatic event. It may also occur because of witnessing or experiencing a serious harm to other significant persons in life. The symptoms of PTSD may develop, after a period of latency, within 6 months after the stress or may be delayed beyond this period.

Causes: Traumatic events like rape, torture, child abuse, disaster, murder, war etc.

Epidemiology: Lifetime prevalence—8%

Treatment: Multimodal approach for management along with drug treatment (SSRI) is used. EMDR (eye movement desensitization and reprocessing) has been found to be useful.

SOMATOFORM DISORDERS (SD)

Introduction: The term "somatoform disorders" incorporates a variety of diverse clinical presentations of physical symptoms that share the diagnostic prerequisite of absence of a physical etiology to explain emergence of the presenting symptoms. The symptoms tend to be chronic, at times mimic delusional or obsessional features. The diagnosis is valid only in the absence of any other mental or physical disorder or direct effect of a substance that may otherwise explain the symptoms.

Etiology: Precise etiology and pathophysiology of somatization is not known.
- Physiological stimulation or excitement mediated arousal of sympathetic nervous system leads to rise in blood pressure, tachycardia, gastric hypermotility, muscle tension, and pains like tension headaches. Thus, subsyndromal depression and anxiety may have etiological significance.
- Somatic symptoms may be learned illness behavior to dominate or manipulate relationships.
- Developmental theories of early parental separation, traumatic childhood, sexual abuse, presence of somatization in parents, and restrictive parenting are implicated in emergence of SD.

Epidemiology:
- Prevalence rates vary between 0.1% and 6%, depending upon the category and surveyed population. They are not potentially fatal. However, high rates of suicide, side effects related to use of multiple drugs, polypharmacy, and indiscreet drug use merit caution.
- *Gender*: Female to male ratio varies between 2:1 and 10:1 for various categories of SD except hypochondriasis where it is 1:1.
- *Age of onset*: Most cases are present with the history of SD in childhood, adolescence, or early adulthood.

Various types of somatoform disorders are given in **Table 5**.

Management:
- Therapeutic intervention in the form of explaining or educating the patients and their family about the temporal relationship between onset of stress and occurrence of symptoms and that the symptoms do not have a physical correlate is known to help resolution of symptoms.
- *Drug therapy*: Antidepressants and/or BZDs can be given on a short-term basis for associated depression and/or anxiety (**Table 6**).
- Stress management techniques are useful.

CONVERSION DISORDER

It is also known as a functional neurological symptom disorder.

TABLE 5 Types of somatoform disorder.

Somatization disorder	Hypochondriasis (somatic symptom disorder)	Persistent somatoform pain disorder
Clinical presentation: • It requires minimum duration of 2 years for diagnosis. Clinical presentation must include: • Four pain symptoms, related to at least four different sites or functions (common sites of pain are head, back, abdomen, chest, limbs, rectum, and joints. • Two unexplained gastrointestinal symptoms other than pain (like nausea, bloating, diarrhea, indigestion, and intolerance to several foods) • One sexual or menstrual complaint other than pain (like sexual indifference, erectile or ejaculatory dysfunction, irregular menses, excessive menstrual bleeding, and vomiting throughout pregnancy) • One pseudoneurological complaint (like aphonia, paresis or paralysis, hypoesthesia or anesthesia, blindness, or inability to move) • Patients are symptomatic for several years but refuse to accept the medical verdict of absence of any physical illness • Symptoms induce appreciable impairment in functioning	**Clinical presentation:** • Hypochondriasis is defined as a persistent preoccupation with a fear (or belief) of having one (or more) serious disease(s), based on person's own interpretation of normal body function or a minor physical abnormality • Complete physical examination and investigations do not show presence of any significant abnormality • The fear or belief persists despite assurance to the contrary by showing normal reports to the patient • The fear or belief is *not* a delusion but is instead an example of an overvalued idea. The patient may agree regarding the possibility of his exaggerating the graveness of situation, at that time • A preoccupation with medical terms and syndromes is quite common. The patient tends to change the physician frequently, to get investigated again • Duration of the symptoms should be at least 6 months in the absence of any other psychiatric disorders	**Clinical presentation:** • It was previously called as *psychogenic pain disorder*. In this disorder, persistent, severe, and distressing pain is the main feature which is either grossly in excess of what is expected from the physical findings, or inconsistent with the anatomical distribution of nervous system • Preoccupation with pain is common • There is often a precipitating stressful event and secondary gain may be present • Repeated change of physicians *(doctor-shopping)* is common. The affected person often assumes a "sick-role" or an "invalid-role" • This diagnosis is valid only in the absence of other physical condition or other psychiatric disorders

BOX 8 Symptoms of conversion disorder.

- Pseudoseizures
- Impaired coordination
- Paralysis
- Lump in the throat
- Aphonia
- Loss of pain or touch sensation
- Deafness

Clinical presentation: Conversion disorder is characterized by the following clinical features:

- Presence of symptoms or deficits affecting motor or sensory function, suggesting a medical or neurological disorder. The list of possible symptoms of conversion disorder is given in **Box 8**.
- Sudden onset
- Development of symptoms usually in the presence of a significant psychosocial stressor(s)
- A clear temporal relationship between stressor and development or exacerbation of symptoms
- Patient does not intentionally produce the symptoms.
- There is usually a "secondary gain."
- Detailed physical examination and investigations do not reveal any abnormality that can explain the symptoms adequately.

Course and prognosis: This is a complex disorder. Initial presentations remit within a short duration despite nonspecific treatments. However, recurrence is frequent.

Management:

- Management has to be individualized. Some patients remit spontaneously or with resolution of the conflicts. Patients can benefit from antidepressants and antianxiety agents can be used for short-term
- Behavior therapy or psychotherapy is aimed at helping the patient to cope with stress or modify the stress inducing stimuli.
- Avoid BZDs or use only for short duration.

Outcome: Outcome of these disorders can range from mild and transient or severe and chronic. Early treatment, supportive social environment, higher education, absence of ongoing stress, and willingness to accept nonphysical etiology can lead to better prognosis. Psychoeducation and development of good coping skills yield better outcome.

PSYCHIATRIC EMERGENCIES

Emergency psychiatry is a subspecialty of psychiatry that has evolved over the last few decades and is defined as disturbance in thought, mood, and/or action which causes sudden distress to an individual (or to significant others) and/or sudden disability, for which immediate management is required. Thus, the assessment should include an interview, mental status examination, physical and neurological examination, and when necessary, relevant laboratory investigations. Psychiatric history should always be obtained from both the patient and the informant(s).

BASIC PRINCIPLES OF APPROACH

Initial measures: Many a times the patient is uncooperative empathetic, confident, and composed attitude shown by the physician can reassure the patient and relatives. A quiet and secluded room is useful. When necessary, restraints may be needed to hold a patient for proper management. Personal safety should be ensured, and security staff called when necessary. Hospitalization should be considered when necessary.

COMMON TYPES

A psychiatric emergency can be one or more of the following:

- A new psychiatric disorder with an acute onset
- A chronic psychiatric disorder with a relapse
- An organic psychiatric disorder
- An abnormal response to a stressful situation
- Violent and aggressive behavior
- *Iatrogenic emergencies*:
  - Side effects or toxicity of psychotropic medication
  - Psychiatric symptomatology as a side effect
- *Alcohol or drug dependence*:
  - Withdrawal syndrome
  - Intoxication or overdose
  - Complications
- Deliberate harm to self or others.

In this section, we have discussed some common psychiatric emergencies which are important for physicians.

VIOLENT AND AGGRESSIVE BEHAVIOR

Foreshadowing behaviors or warning signs of impending violent behaviors include increased psychomotor activity, clenching of fists and jaw, pacing, slamming doors, banging their fist on a wall, jumpy and easy to startle, sitting on the edge of the chair and clutching the armrest, and verbally abusive patient. Common psychiatric disorders associated with violent behavior are given in **Box 9**.

BOX 9 Common psychiatric disorders associated with violent behavior.

- **Psychosis:**
  - Schizophrenia
  - Delusional disorder
  - Acute psychosis
- **Mania:**
  - First episode
  - Bipolar affective disorder
- Substance use disorder
- **Organic brain disorder:**
  - Postictal states
  - Any systemic condition leading to intracranial pathology and/or delirium
  - As a part of behavioral and psychological symptoms of dementia (BPSD)
- **Personality disorder:**
  - Borderline
  - Antisocial
- Sometimes depression (as murder–suicide)
- Dissociative disorder (transpossession)
- Acute stress reaction
- Adolescents (behavioral problems)

Management of aggressive and violent patient:

- The physician should gather maximum information before facing the patient. Some rapport building exercise like addressing the patient by his name should be tried which will help in making the diagnosis.
- *Pharmacological intervention*: (1) BZDs—lorazepam are a good choice when treating an acute episode of agitation. (2) Neuroleptics—haloperidol 5–10 mg intramuscularly can be repeated every half an hour to one hour till the patient is calm (maximum 15–30 mg/day). Patient should be monitored for extrapyramidal side effects. Yet another approach is to use a combination of injectable haloperidol and promethazine as they can be mixed in the same syringe (**Table 6**).

SUICIDE AND SUICIDAL ATTEMPTS

- Suicide is self-inflicted deliberate self-harm resulting in death with evidence that the person is intended to die.
- Suicidal attempt is self-injurious behavior or unsuccessful suicidal act with nonfatal outcomes.
- Suicidal patient is one who unsuccessfully attempts suicide or demonstrates suicidal ideation, or harbors suicidal intent, or threatens to commit suicide.

Common causes of suicide include depression, schizophrenia, drug dependence, bipolar disorder, adjustment disorder, and personality disorder.

Management of suicidal patients:

Pharmacotherapy:

- BZDs, non-BZD hypnotics, and quetiapine (in low doses) may be given for sleep disturbance and anxiety symptoms.
- Antidepressants are to be given in depression (**Table 6**).
- Lithium may be given when indicated as it has got antisuicidal role.
- Antipsychotics are to be prescribed for psychosis.
- *Electroconvulsive therapy*: It is reserved for severely suicidal, with catatonic, symptoms. It acts faster.

EXTRAPYRAMIDAL SIDE EFFECTS OF NEUROLEPTICS

Acute dystonia: This is an abnormal posture produced by sustained involuntary contraction of muscles of different body parts. It may present as trismus, oculogyric crisis, torticollis, blepharospasm etc. It is a very painful condition and fatalities may occur if the laryngeal muscles are involved. History should be present of taking a neuroleptic/antidopaminergic agent.

Treatment: Treatment consists of antihistaminic like promethazine: 50 mg intravenously/intramuscularly and

TABLE 6 Classification of psychiatric medications.

Drug	Dose-range
Antipsychotic—*typical*:	
• Chlorpromazine	200–1,000 mg/day
• Trifluoperazine	10–30 mg/day
• Prochlorperazine	5–150 mg/day
• Fluphenazine	5–50 mg/day
• Thioridazine	200–800 mg/day
• Pimozide	1–20 mg/day
• Haloperidol	2–20 mg/day
Antipsychotic—atypical:	
• Clozapine	12.5–900 mg/day
• Olanzapine	5–20 mg/day
• Quetiapine	150–800 mg/day
• Paliperidone	1.5–12 mg/day
• Risperidone	2–16 mg/day
• Ziprasidone	40–160 mg/day
• Iloperidone	4–24 mg/day
• Lurasidone	40–160 mg/day
• Amisulpride	300–1,200 mg/day
Antidepressants:	
Cyclic antidepressants:	
• Amitriptyline	50–150 mg/day
• Dothiepin	75–150 mg/day
• Clomipramine	100–200 mg/day
• Nortriptyline	75–100 mg/day
• Amoxapine	200–300 mg/day
• Bupropion	225–400 mg/day
Selective serotonin reuptake inhibitors:	
• Fluoxetine	20 mg/day
• Paroxetine	20 mg/day
• Fluvoxamine	50 mg/day
• Sertraline	50 mg/day
• Citalopram	20 mg/day
• Escitalopram	10 mg/day
Serotonin and norepinephrine reuptake inhibitors:	
• Venlafaxine	75 mg/day
• Duloxetine	60 mg/day
• Milnacipran	30–200 mg/day
	30–200 mg/day
Noradrenaline and specific serotonin antidepressant (NaSSA)	
• Mirtazapine	30 mg/day
Atypical antidepressants:	
• Trazodone	150 mg/day
Benzodiazepines and Z-compounds:	
Long acting:	
• Diazepam	4–40 mg/day
• Chlordiazepoxide	15–40 mg/day

Contiuned...

Contiuned...

Drug	Dose-range
Intermediate acting:	
• Oxazepam	30 mg/day
• Lorazepam	1 mg/day
• Alprazolam	0.25–6 mg/day
• Clonazepam	1–2 mg/day
Short acting:	
• Etizolam	0.25–3 mg/day
• Midazolam	1–5 mg/day
Z-compounds:	
• Zaleplon	5–20 mg/day
• Zolpidem	5–10 mg/day
• Zopiclone	7.5–15 mg/day
Mood stabilizers:	
• Lithium	0.6–1.5 mEq/L
• Valproate	400–1,500 mg/day
• Carbamazepine	200–1,600 mg/day

anticholinergic like benzatropine 1-2 mg intravenously/intramuscularly. Oral drugs should be started after the acute crisis is over. Trihexyphenidyl (6-10 mg/day in divided doses) may be given for this purpose.

Akathisias: It consists of inability to remain seated and is commonly associated with repetitive shifting of weight, pacing, or rocking the trunk when standing. There is an inner sense of restlessness.

Treatment: Propranolol 40-80 mg/day. BZD may be given.

Neuroleptic malignant syndrome: It is uncommon but potentially fatal. It occurs in 0.5% of patients who are on neuroleptics. It is characterized by mental status changes, confusion, disorientation, rigidity, autonomic instability, and temperature dysregulation. Laboratory findings include raised creatine phosphokinase-MM (CPK-MM), increased white blood cells, myoglobinuria, and altered renal function tests.

Management of NMS:

- Discontinue the neuroleptic medication immediately
- Supportive care (intensive care unit care is preferred) with rehydration should be given to manage vitals.
- Dantrolene sodium 2-3 mg per kg intravenously 3-4 times per day or bromocriptine is started with 2.5 mg thrice a day and with gradual increment to maximum daily dose of 60 mg (**Table 6**).
- For management of psychiatric symptoms in such patients after resolution of acute symptoms, depot preparations of antipsychotics and other high potency conventional antipsychotics should be avoided. ECT may be preferred.

STATE OF ACUTE ANXIETY

Anxiety is characterized by a feeling of fear accompanied by somatic signs of autonomic nervous system hyperactivity.

Treatment:
- Provide safe and protective environment and consult physician for medical conditions.
- If any for acute stress, when immediate relief is required, lorazepam is given. Oral BZDs, alprazolam can also be given.
- All cases of panic disorder require proper long-term treatment. SSRIs are the treatment of choice.

TREATMENTS IN PSYCHIATRY

BIOLOGICAL TREATMENTS

Pharmacotherapy (Table 6):
- Antipsychotics
- Antidepressants
- Mood stabilizers
- BZDs and Z-class compounds
- Others

Somatic treatments:
- *Electroconvulsive therapy*: The first biological treatment to be used. It consists of induction of a seizure by a current for 25 second duration to stimulate the brain and alter the neurochemistry. Modified ECT under general anesthesia (GA) is used now which is safe and effective.
- *rTMS (repetitive transcranial magnetic stimulation)*: Noninvasive brain stimulation technique by a strong magnetic field which induces electric current in specific brain areas. It is useful in depression.
- *Vagal nerve stimulation (VNS)*: Use of small implants in neck which stimulate vagus nerve by emitting small periodic currents. It is useful in treatment-resistant depression.
- *Deep brain stimulation (DBS)*: Electrodes are implanted in brain neurosurgically to deliver electric current to specific brain areas to modify neuronal circuit activity. It is useful in treatment-resistant depression and refractory OCD.
- *Transcranial direct current stimulation (tDCS)*: Use of direct current to stimulate brain in noninvasive manner. It is useful in the treatment of depression and anxiety disorders.

PSYCHOTHERAPY

Psychotherapy is a method of intervention, in which a trained professional deliberately establishes a therapeutic relationship to help a person in psychological manner with the goal of removing or reducing symptoms; changing the person's mindset about himself/herself, others and life; improving interpersonal relationships; and personality change.

Types of psychotherapy:
- Psychoanalytic psychotherapy
- Brief psychodynamic psychotherapy
- Group psychotherapy and individual psychotherapy
- Family therapy and couple's therapy
- Dialectical behavior therapy
- Cognitive therapy
- Behavior therapy
- Interpersonal therapy
- Mindfulness techniques

Patients who are suitable for psychotherapy are those who are psychological minded, motivated, emotionally strengthened, and have positive emotional relationship.

Basic principles of psychotherapy include confidentiality, neutral and nonjudgmental attitude of therapist, empathic understanding of patient's inner experiences, and total acceptance of the patient.

PSYCHOSOMATIC DISORDERS

Psychiatric morbidity is very common in patients with medical conditions, with a prevalence ranging from 20% to 67%, depending on the illness. For example, compared with community samples, depressive disorders in the general hospital are more than twice as common, and substance abuse is two to three times as common. Delirium occurs in 18% of patients. Similarly, increased rates are seen in primary and long-term care. It is well established that depression is both a risk factor and a poor prognostic indicator in coronary artery disease. Psychiatric illness worsens cardiac morbidity and mortality in patients with a history of myocardial infarction, diminishes glycemic control in patients with diabetes, and decreases return to functioning in patients experiencing a stroke.

Some psychosomatic disorders: Which require clinical attention include:
- Psychiatric symptoms as a reaction to medical conditions and treatments, e.g., anxiety and depression related to chemotherapy or limb amputation.
- Psychiatric complications of medical conditions and treatments, e.g., depression secondary to interferon treatment.
- Co-occurring medical and psychiatric conditions, e.g., depression in setting of cancer and HIV treatment.
- Psychiatric or psychosocial assessment, e.g., capacity evaluation prior to organ transplantation.
- Classical psychosomatic disorders:
  - Functional gastrointestinal disorders include globus, irritable bowel syndrome, functional diarrhea, noncardiac chest pain etc.
  - Cardiovascular disorders include coronary artery disease, type A personality, hypertension etc.

Treatment of psychosomatic disorders: A major role of psychiatrists and other physicians working with patients with psychosomatic disorders is mobilizing the patient to change behavior in ways that optimize the process of healing. Psychosomatic disorders management schedule should always include psychosocial management strategies regardless of whatever drug treatment they are on. Stress management training for psychosomatic disorders is given in **Figure 1**.

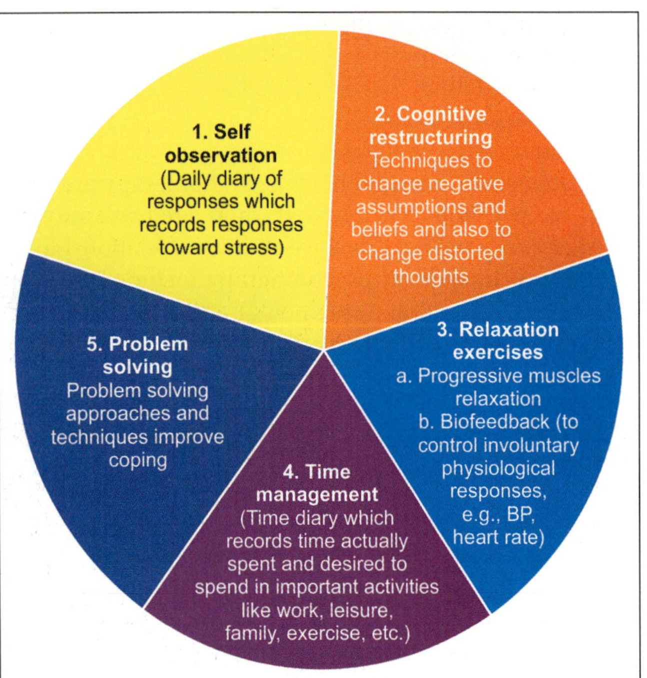

FIGURE 1: Stress management training for psychosomatic disorders.

RECOMMENDED READINGS

1. World Health Organization. (1992). The ICD-10 classification of mental and behavioural disorders: clinical descriptions and diagnostic guidelines. World Health Organization.
2. American Psychiatric Association. Diagnostic and Statistical Manual of mental disorders, 5th edition. 2013.
3. Newman MG, Przeworski A, Fisher AJ, Borkovec TD. Diagnostic comorbidity in adults with generalized anxiety disorder: Impact of comorbidity on psychotherapy outcome and impact of psychotherapy on comorbid diagnoses. Behav Ther. 2010;41:59-72.
4. Lisanby SH, Kinnunen LH, Crupain MJ. Applications of TMS to therapy in psychiatry. J Clin Neurophysiol. 2002;19(4):344-60.
5. Vaingankar JA, Rekhi G, Subramaniam M, Abdin E, Chong SA. Age of onset of life-time mental disorders and treatment contact. Soc Psychiatry Psychiatr Epidemiol. 2013;48(5):835-43.
6. Ketter TA. Diagnostic features, prevalence, and impact of bipolar disorder. J Clin Psychiatry. 2010;71(6):e14.
7. Kroon JS, Wohlfarth TD, Dieleman J, Sutterland AL, Storosum JG, Denys D, et al. Incidence rates and risk factors of bipolar disorder in the general population: A population-based cohort study. Bipolar Disord. 2013;15(3):306-13.
8. Lambert M, Conus P, Cotton S, Robinson J, McGorry PD, Schimmelmann BG. Prevalence, predictors, and consequences of long-term refusal of antipsychotic treatment in first-episode psychosis. J Clin Psychopharm. 2010;30(5):565-72.
9. Sadock BJ, Sadock VA, Pedro R. Psychological factors affecting other medical conditions. In: Sadock BJ, Sadock VA, Ruiz P (Eds). Kaplan Sadock's Synopsis of Psychiatry, 11 edition. Philadelphia: Wolters-Kluwer; 2015. pp. 477-89.
10. Colquhoun DM, Bunker SJ, Clarke DM, Glozier N, Hare DL, Hickie IB, et al. Screening, referral and treatment for depression in patients, with coronary heart disease. Med J Aust. 2013;198:483-4.
11. Barker P. Talking cures: A Guide to the Psychotherapies for Health Care. EMAP Health Care Ltd.; 1999.

CHAPTER 25

Palliative and End-of-life Care

D Thangam

ABSTRACT

The life expectancy of an average Indian is rising over the years. The need for palliative care and end-of-life care in elderly is also on the rise as they suffer from chronic illness more than their younger counterparts. Geriatric patients needing palliative care are different in that they have more comorbidities which can confuse or influence the various aspects of care and decision making, different patterns of expression of various symptoms and, more important, prognostication is difficult due to nonavailability of standard models.

Physicians treating the geriatric patients need to develop skills in determining goals and place of treatment, communication and coordination with the family, various modalities of symptom relief as well as end-of-life care for the patient, and after death care of the family. Effective control of physical symptoms like pain, dyspnea, anorexia, and constipation is vital for providing palliative care. This may also include nonpharmacological methods as well as minor surgical procedures besides medical care alone. Most of this care can be done by physician with some help from the specialists in certain areas. Taking care of chronically ill patient till the end physically, emotionally, and spiritually is a fulfilling job for a physician.

In India with growing need of the palliative care for elderly, we need legal guidelines as well as policy level decisions and dedicated units for providing quality care. This can be achieved only by awareness, skill development, and coordination between government and nongovernment agencies.

"We cannot change the outcome but we can affect the journey"

—Ann Richardson

INTRODUCTION

The population as well as life expectancy across the globe is in increasing trend. In India, the elderly population is steadily growing and is projected to be about 10.7% compared to 8.2% in 2011. India also recorded an improvement in life expectancy at birth, which was 47 years in 1969, growing to 60 years in 1994 and 69 years in 2019. It is also a well-known fact that most of the elderly have chronic illness and multimorbidity which make them disabled, dependent, and bedridden. For these reasons, old age and palliative care go hand in hand. It is estimated that among the adults needing palliative care worldwide, 66–69% are above 60 years of age. Though the death is inevitable consequence of life with or without any chronic disease, there will usually be a time when neither cure nor prolongation of life can be a primary goal. The physician's role in these cases is to provide effective symptom relief and maximize quality of life and that is the essence of palliative care and end-of-life care.

DEFINITIONS

The World Health Organization (WHO) has defined palliative care as *"an approach that improves the quality of life of patients and their families facing the problems associated with life-threatening illness, through the prevention and relief of suffering by means of early identification and impeccable assessment and treatment of pain and other problems, physical, psychosocial and spiritual."* It is appropriate for any type of diagnosis, any stage of a serious illness and importantly, can be provided together with curative treatment.

End-of-life care is a specialized form of palliative care for patients with limited life expectancy. This also provides care and support to family members for coping up of illness of their loved ones and also offers bereavement supports. Hospice is the name given to the institution which provides this sort of care.

PALLIATIVE CARE IN ELDERLY

Though patients of any age and in any stage of illness are eligible for palliative care, the elderly receiving palliative care have certain unique features and requirements. Some of them are:

- *The incidence and death due to cancer increase with age* and thus the need of palliative care also increases with age.
- *Noncancer diagnosis,* which needs palliative care, is also more common in elderly—like dementia, multimorbidity, end-stage cardiac, pulmonary, renal failure, and chronic neurodegenerative diseases resulting in chronic bedridden state. Abnormal health state called frailty can coexist and significantly contribute to any of these illnesses in elderly. It is the demonstrable progressive weakness and deterioration in the overall functional ability unrelated to their comorbidities. They often lack the reserve to tolerate stressors like intercurrent illness, or admission but paradoxically they need frequent hospital admissions.
- Older adults have *different patterns of symptoms* than younger patients including increased frequency of patterns of expression of pain, anorexia, anxiety, and nausea.
- *Prognostication is difficult* due to nonavailability of standard models. They are more likely to be discharged to nursing home or hospice care.
- They are *more likely to have end-of-life consultation* than younger patients, and due to increased incidence of cognitive impairment, surrogate decision- making is also more in this group. This puts more pressure on the physician.

Physicians having elderly clients should have an insight about these issues and instead of exhibiting avoidance behavior when facing such challenge, should try to assist the patients and families using the skills. These skills can be divided into following categories:

- *Determining goals of care*
- *Communication with patients and families*
- *Coordination of care*
- *Symptom control*
- *Coordination of hospice care*
- *After-death care*

UNDERSTANDING THE CARE PROVIDERS

Care providers are the essential part of effective palliative care. Cultural, ethnic, and social differences exist within the communities. In most of the Indian families, the female members of the family, especially the spouse will be the care provider. If the spouse is unavailable, children or other family members take over the responsibility. Minority of them are looked after by paid caregivers too. The family of the terminally ill person is subjected to physical, economical, and emotional stress and they are at increased risk of developing physical illness, depression, and death. So taking the care provider's health into consideration is well justified, as unrelieved stress and burden of care can otherwise result in a breakdown of relationship between the care provider and the patient, potentially spiraling down into situations of neglect, abuse, and worsening health in both parties.

RESPONSIBILITIES OF THE PHYSICIAN

Determining goals of care: This can vary during the course of the disease from prevention, prolongation of life to helping patients to achieve "good death." This should always be done in the presence of or in discussion with patient, family member, or surrogate decision maker. This will not be static and it should be reassessed,

- Whenever there is setback/improvement in patient's condition like new illness/intercurrent illness, unexpected recovery.
- Unresponsiveness to standard treatment, and/or
- When the place of treatment is changed as per patient's wish as in shifting the patient to home care from hospital.

Communication with patients and families: In any patient needing palliative care, family plays an important role. They suffer emotionally, financially as well as spiritually. As discussed above they are the decision makers. The physician should be able to identify the conflicts that arise in the family while taking care of a terminally ill person and take appropriate measures like clearing their doubts, supporting them while taking difficult decisions and arrange professional counseling when needed.

Coordination of care: It is required when more medical and nonmedical specialty care is involved. Good end-of-life care cannot be given by physician alone. It involves besides symptom control, providing nursing care, spiritual, and emotional support for the patient and family. Many of the patients express the desire to be treated at their home. Community-based palliative care delivery is being encouraged and practiced in various parts of the world including India. Here, volunteers after acquiring some basic skills will be taking care of the patients needing palliative care in their area by allocating their time and energy. In southern Indian state Kerala, this has evolved over past 25 years and about 1,400 such organizationally and financially independent units are functioning. The physician has the role of training such volunteers, being the medical in-charge of such units. Various levels of coordination are required locally as well as with the higher level of care centers in case of referral.

Symptom control: This terminology generally refers to the physical symptoms. But in terminally ill patients, the commonly occurring symptoms like pain, dyspnea, and loss of appetite will have strong psychological overlay also. Similarly along with pharmacological approach to the management of symptoms, nonpharmacological methods should be considered. Some of them will be benefitted by the more advanced approach by professionals like neuropsychologists and geriatric psychiatrists in addition to the services offered by the physicians. Surgeons too have the role in palliative care, by doing surgical procedures purely for symptom control and patient comfort. The services of spiritual persons, counselors, and social workers are also used. These modalities are particularly useful in patients and attenders experiencing psychosocial symptoms like anxiety, depression, and insomnia.

Elders express their symptoms in various ways. Those who are cognitively normal and with intact speech can express the symptoms verbally whereas the physician should be able to recognize the nonverbal expression of certain symptoms also. Some of the most common physical symptoms in terminally ill elderly patients irrespective of their underlying illness, are:

- Pain
- Breathlessness and cough
- Nausea and vomiting, anorexia, dysphagia, and constipation
- Anxiety, depression, delirium (very common in those >85 years), and insomnia
- Problems with bladder and bowel control
- Loss of functional capacity and frequent falls.

APPROACH

Systematic approach to symptoms and meticulous clinical examination are very important.

When encountering new problems, causes other than the terminal illness like infection, worsening diabetes, myocardial ischemia, hypothyroidism etc., should be considered. Choice of place for treatment should also be chosen considering the patient's preference. Complete list of symptoms and their characteristics should be listed out. The other factors which should be considered are:

- *Emotional*—fears, grief, worries etc.
- *Social*—about family background and living arrangement
- *Spiritual*—beliefs, regrets etc.
- Awareness about the problem

Pain: It is the most common symptom encountered in terminal illness due to cancer and noncancer conditions. The pain may be the result of disease process itself, due to comorbidities or due to the medical treatments provided. Physician should be aware of the atypical presentation of pain symptoms in elderly. This may include confusion, fatigue, withdrawal, and depression. The assessment by various methods like visual analog scale, numeric rating scale, and face scale can be done. But in persons who are cognitively impaired, the identification and assessment of pain are really a challenging task. The caregiver's observation of patients' change of behavior and facial expression is very important. It could be resistance to changing of position, accompanied by grimacing and screaming; sudden aggressiveness toward the caregiver; development of new undue behavior like inappropriate voiding of urine, motion etc.

Besides pharmacological treatment, simple nonpharmacological measures play a very important role in control of symptoms. For example, in a bedridden patient with terminal neurological illness, simple changing of position of the limb and periodic physiotherapy will relieve musculoskeletal pain to a greater extent. Similarly, simple changes in environment in which the patient is kept would make an enormous change. Some of the examples are, in the case of a patient with nausea, removing a cause of malodor combined with feeding the patient with appropriately cooked favorite meals will offer them some comfort. Providing privacy to the patient combined with bedside commode will help in dealing with constipation.

The following **Table 1** lists some of the most common symptoms which need to be controlled in palliative care medicine.

TABLE 1 Some of the common symptoms and their management.

Symptoms and characteristics	Nonpharmacological treatments	Pharmacological treatments
Pain: • May be the first indicator of local recurrence of cancer, for example, pelvic pain from rectal or gynecological carcinomas • Radicular thoracic or cervical pain may precede leg weakness • Common feature of patients dying from illnesses other than cancer • About 95% of pains are opioid sensitive; the remainder is usually neuropathic in origin, or there may be psychosocial issues exacerbating the pain	• Physiotherapy, heat and cold compressors • The three most important alternate medical therapies: i. Relaxation therapy ii. Music therapy, and iii. Foot massage	• Nonopioids—NSAIDs • Opioids: ∘ Weak opioid: Tramadol—beware of seizures. ∘ Strong opioid: Fentanyl—safe in renal failure ∘ Buprenorphine—long-acting, patches available. ∘ Morphine—oral, parenteral ∘ Adjuvants—pregabalin, antidepressants (neuropathic) ∘ Steroids (nerve compression), bisphosphonates (bone pain), hyoscine (GI pain)
Dyspnea: • Disturbing subjective symptom—common with malignant and nonmalignant conditions • Remains a significant symptom even after disease treatment	• Positioning • Dehumidification of ambient air • Use of fans • Blowing air on face • Soothing environment • Calm reassurance	• Correct anemia • Appropriate management of COPD, CCF, and cardiac arrhythmia • Antibiotics for intercurrent infections • Drainage of pleural effusion • Long-term O_2 therapy on PRN basis • Opioids 1–5 mg oral morphine 4th hourly/SC morphine • Diazepam/Midazolam to anxious patients
Dysphagia: • Common in terminally ill, head and neck cancer, postradiotherapy, degenerative neurological conditions and stroke victims • Predisposes to malnutrition, aspiration • Source of extreme stress and guilt to caregivers	• Positioning, altering texture of food, and safe swallowing techniques • Check for oral hygiene, intact dentures, and dentition	• Artificial and supplemental feeding in appropriate situations: ∘ NG tube feeding ∘ Gastrostomy and jejunostomy ∘ TPN • Stop medications causing dry mouth, treat candida infection, and oral ulcers
Nausea and vomiting: Anorexia-cachexia syndrome usually occurs in end-stage illness due to inflammatory cytokines, altered metabolism leading to protein malnutrition	• Relaxation and massage techniques • Plant-based medications like ginger, orange blossoms • Avoiding malodors • Small, frequent favorite meals	• Hypercalcemia, renal failure, intestinal obstruction, and malignant ascites need specific intervention • Metoclopramide, domperidone—for gastroparesis, emesis sec to liver, heart, respiratory failure, emesis of uncertain etiology • Ondansetron for postradiation therapy, postchemotherapy • Dopamine receptor antagonists—chlorpromazine, haloperidol, and prochlorperazine for bowel obstruction and renal failure • Steroids for intracranial malignancy, liver secondaries • Meclizine for positional vertigo

Continued ...

Continued ...

Symptoms and characteristics	Nonpharmacological treatments	Pharmacological treatments
Constipation: Causes: immobility, medication—opioids and nonopioids, comorbid conditions	Ambulation, dietary changes, hydration, privacy, positioning	• Lactulose, high fiber preparation after good hydration, high-dose polyethylene glycol, enema, and digital evacuation • Oral methylnaltrexone in opioid-induced constipation
Diarrhea: Causes—radiotherapy, malabsorption, stress, antibiotics, and GI bleeding	Dietary modification	• R/O fecal impaction, *Clostridium difficile* infection • If no reversible causes, loperamide, codeine preparations can be tried
Cough: • Nonmalignant causes—postnasal drip, GERD, COPD, LVF, pneumonia, and drug side effects • Malignant—primary and secondaries in lung, pleural deposits	• Lozenges • Cough-assistive devices	• Treatment of the cause: ○ Humidification of O_2 ○ Saline nebulization ○ Low-dose opioids ○ Steroids ○ Radiotherapy
Pressure ulcers: • Immobility leads to—cachexia, incontinence, and malnutrition • Indicator of advanced disease and poor prognosis	• Nursing care • Logroll method of turning	• More focus on relief of pain, odor control, discharge, and comfort • Use of antibiotics (topical metronidazole and sulfasalazine) and antifungal agents when necessary • Charcoal dressing to contain malodor
Delirium: • Very common in sick elderly • Multifactorial in nature • Common causes—underlying cognitive impairment, sensory deficits, dyselectrolemia, infections, and drugs, metabolic abnormalities due to organ failure, malignancies	• Orienting the patient to time and place • Allowing familiar faces with the patient • Avoiding sensory impairment by providing them their glasses and hearing aid • Providing calm environment	• Treatment of reversible causes like hypercalcemia (hydration and pamidronate), using steroids in cerebral metastasis • Short-term low-dose antipsychotics

Role of procedures in palliative care

Symptoms	Procedures
Ascites	• Abdominal paracentesis—simple procedure, no aggressive monitoring required • Endoscopic shunting procedures
Anemia which causes dyspnea, failure, and fatigue Replacement in blood loss	• Blood transfusion • Hospitalization required
Bedridden state: • In terminally ill patient, inoperable urological conditions • Neurodegenerative disorders with mobility issues and cognitive impairment • Management of pressure sore	Continuous bladder drainage (CBD) complications: Chronic renal inflammation, nephrolithiasis, and cystolithiasis, sepsis
Dyspnea	• Thoracocentesis—beware of complications—need for chest tube insertion if necessary • Endobronchial stenting in bronchial obstruction • Tracheostomy
Dysphagia	• Feeding tubes—in advanced neurodegenerative diseases, postradiotherapy strictures, esophageal growth, and disorders • Lead to malnutrition, aspiration pneumonia and repeated admissions • Esophageal stent placement, gastrostomy, and jejunostomy

Continued ...

Continued ...

Symptoms	Procedures
• ***Postrenal failure in cancer cervix*** • ***For respiratory failure patients*** • ***For recurrent arrhythmias*** • ***For pneumothorax/pleural effusion*** • ***For biliary drainage***	• Percutaneous nephrostomy • Home O_2 therapy, BiPAP • Implantable cardioverter • ICD • Endoscopic stent placement
Bone pain	• Multiple metastasis in areas which cannot be immobilized—Depo-Medrol injection • Immobilization of bones where feasible • Surgery in selected cases
Neuropathic pain	• Nerve block in sympathetically mediated pain • Celiac block in pancreatic pathologies
For advanced ovarian cancer	• Debulking surgery reduces tumor burden, reduces ascites, and bowel obstruction also increases survival
In duodenal carcinoma	• Surgical bypass

(BiPAP: bilevel positive airway pressure; CCF: congestive cardiac failure; COPD: chronic obstructive pulmonary disease; GI: gastrointestinal; GERD: gastroesophageal reflux disease; ICD: implantable cardioverter defibrillator; LVF: left ventricular failure; NG: nasogastric; NSAID: nonsteroidal anti-inflammatory drug; TPN: total parenteral nutrition)

SPIRITUAL CARE

Irrespective of previous spiritual beliefs, most of the elderly terminally ill conscious patients seek spiritual help; the physician should be sensitive to the needs of the patients and take appropriate steps in consultation with the family members. This should be the part of the counseling given to the family members.

ACTIVE DYING PROCESS

Care during the last hours of life is another important dimension of palliative care. This is the principle of hospice programs. This needs the coordinated effect of physician, the family members, and caregivers; this also includes what is to be done immediately after the death.

Death generally comes as the result of widespread systemic change rather than the failure of a single system or organ. There will be irreversible decline due to loss of homeostasis and increased catabolic process. The physiological parameters are altered and the individual pharmacokinetic and pharmacodynamic processes are also altered.

Prominent physiological changes and the measures recommended to tackle them are:

- *Altered pharmacokinetics and pharmacodynamics*:
  - Stop nonessential medications, e.g., statins, vitamins, and blood thinners
  - Reevaluate the route of delivery—buccal, rectal, and subcutaneous instead of oral or IV
- *Terminal agitation and delirium*:
  - Stop opioids with potential neuroexcitatory effects, switch over to as and when needed (PRN) dosages of pain relievers
  - Look for and relieve distended bladder, unrelieved pain
  - Benzodiazepines given by buccal or subcutaneous route are highly effective. Neuroleptics may be needed in extreme cases.
  - Nonpharmacological methods like environmental changes, availability of family members at the bedside.
- *Loss of ability to swallow and manage secretions*:
  - Anticholinergic medications if started early will minimize the secretions and the so-called death rattle. Postural drainage rather than suctioning will help in clearing the secretions.
  - Oral diet should be stopped or minimized, IV fluids or tube feeding can be offered to avoid dehydration and to satisfy the family.
- *Irregular breathing and mottled skin*: These are also common changes near death and family should be made aware of this. They should be taught how to identify when death has occurred.

AFTER DEATH CARE

Immediately after death has occurred, physician may be needed to confirm and certify the death, which will also be the right time to arrange all the tubes, catheters to be removed from the patient and to make the body placed in a natural and relaxed position. The family may be encouraged to spend some time with the patient one last time, as much as they desire.

As the definition stated, palliative care includes helping the family and friends to cope up with the situation after the death of their near and dear. This can be done in various ways. In case of the physician being the family physician, frequent phone calls will help. In case of complicated grief, as manifested by intense reactions that do not subside or fluctuate over time, suppressed or postponed reactions, exaggerated or destructive behavior, and lack of awareness of feelings or behavior—identifying and early referral for specialist services can be best done by the physician.

SOME CLINICAL CONDITIONS

PATIENT DIAGNOSED WITH DEMENTIA

These patients need combined geriatric and palliative care approach. In earlier stages, the patient and family should be counseled about the possibility of loss of decision-making capacity by the patient in future and helped regarding advanced care planning. This includes identifying a surrogate decision maker for patient when the disease advances, regarding the medical care of patient, patient's own preference regarding life-sustaining procedures and place of treatment etc., as the disease advances, they may need to help in symptom control like pain, dyspnea, pressure ulcers, and also in feeding and personal care.

Scenario 1: An 80-year-old female, a diagnosed case of vascular dementia was brought with the history of dizzy spells leading to near falls in the past month and patient's refusal of cooperation for personal care by caregiver for the past 1 week. Examination revealed severe anemia with hemoglobin (Hb) of 6.2 g%.

This patient needs basic medical evaluation including cardiovascular and neurological examination to rule out the causes of cerebral hypoperfusion as well as work-up for anemia. Provided the cardiovascular and neurological examination are normal, correction of severe anemia with blood transfusion, correcting the deficient nutrients as well as addressing chronic upper gastrointestinal (UGI) bleed due to aspirin will restore her to previous state of stable health.

Scenario 2: In case, the same patient develops aspiration pneumonia with respiratory failure, as we discussed earlier, the goals of care should be reassessed, such as whether the patient needs hospital admission or home care alone and whether the patient needs to be intubated or ventilated.

PATIENT DIAGNOSED WITH CANCER

Scenario 3: A 75-year-old man was admitted for evaluation of acute right hemiparesis. The evaluation revealed secondaries in brain with primary lung mass. After discussing with the family, further invasive evaluations like biopsy were deferred as per the patient's wish. Patient was sent home on oral steroids and referred to attend nearby palliative care center in case of any new symptoms.

PATIENTS WITH FRAILTY AND MULTIMORBIDITY

As the disease progresses, the goal *also changes.* The persons with severe forms of frailty with scores 4 and 5 along with low albumin and low cholesterol and also patients with more than two chronic conditions (multimorbidity) usually fail to respond to standard treatment and are difficult to be rehabilitated when they develop new illness. These patients are candidates for palliative care which integrates patient's preference, prognosis of the condition, optimal symptom control, and evidence-based approach. There will be a stage when only few essential drugs are given eliminating drugs like statins, platelet inhibitors, supplementary drugs, and drugs used for prevention of osteoporosis from the prescription based on the evidence.

PALLIATIVE CARE—INDIAN SCENARIO

In India, majority of elderly population lives in rural area. They have higher prevalence of disability related to locomotor and visual conditions and have high dependence rates. Poverty is also more in rural areas. The awareness about the existence of palliative care is also not up to the mark among the public and professionals. There is lack of data to estimate the extent of need of palliative care among the noncancerous patients, especially elderly. There is no mention of palliative care for elderly in the National Program for the Health Care of Elderly (NPHCE) launched in year 2010–11.

Being a country with diversity in religion, language, beliefs, and customs, the perspective about final suffering and death is also varied. There are no laws regarding ethical issues in end-of-life care. In India, most of the decision-making is done by family members and doctor rather than the patient himself/herself so that about one-half of the patients seeking cancer treatment are unaware of their problem. Opioid accessibility continues to be a problem for the health providers.

In India, Palliative care centers were established in cancer centers across the country in late 1980s and the early 1990s. The Indian Association of Palliative Care (IAPC) was found in 1994. In November 2012, a strategy for palliative care of India was proposed by expert committee and based on its recommendations, National Programme for Palliative Care (NPPC) was formulated by Ministry of Health and Family Welfare. The program is implemented as part of National Health Mission under the National Programme for Prevention and Control of Cancer, CVD, Diabetes, and Stroke (NPCDCS). It has proposed the palliative care to be provided for elderly also in home set-up, community health centers as well as hospital-based care. There are at present about 500 palliative care centers across India and among them the Kerala model is the popular one.

NEIGHBORHOOD NETWORK IN PALLIATIVE CARE (NNPC)

Palliative care in Kerala, started in 1993 as a civil society organization, ran service linked to a government medical college. Later, it has been evolved into a system of palliative care owned and run by multiple civil society groups, political parties, religious groups, and local governments. It is a program where volunteers from the local community are trained to identify problems of the chronically ill in their area and to intervene effectively with active support from a network of trained professionals. After a brief training session, these volunteers form groups and they make regular follow-up home visits as per palliative care team's instruction, identify and address various nonmedical problems like financial problems, provide respite services for the caregivers, create awareness in community, raise funds etc. They act as a link between medical team and the patient. They do not prescribe or alter prescription. This program has further evolved over a period of time, leading to declaration of palliative care policy by the Government of Kerala in 2008. This has set objectives and has multisectoral approach.

In the state of Tamil Nadu, district level palliative care units have been established in district headquarter hospitals and medical college hospitals as part of noncommunicable disease program (NCD). From the year 2018, community-based palliative services which provide home-based care to the needy patients are started.

CONCLUSION

Taking care of elderly patients and their family till the end of the patient's life and helping them to have a peaceful and respectful end will give an immense sense of fulfillment to the treating physician. Getting oneself equipped with the skills in palliative and end-of-life care apart from curative and preservative treatment skills is worthwhile and rewarding. Provision of conducive environment to advocate the same to needy citizens should be considered by the policy makers.

RECOMMENDED READINGS

1. Central Statistics Office, Ministry of Statistics and Programme Implementation, Government of India. (2011). Situation analysis of the elderly in India. [online] Available from https://www.researchgate.net/publication/274093346_Association_of_Systemic_Diseases_with_Cutaneous_Dermatosis_in_Elderly_Population_Preliminary_Observation_at_a_Rural_Tertiary_Care_Centre/fulltext/55dbd61b08ae9d6594936bc6/Association-of-Systemic-Diseases-with-Cutaneous-Dermatosis-in-Elderly-Population-Preliminary-Observation-at-a-Rural-Tertiary-Care-Centre.pdf.
2. Capel MM. Palliative Medicine for the Older Patient. In: Howard F, Rockwood K, Young J (Eds). Brocklehurst's textbook of geriatric medicine and Gerontology. Philadelphia: Elsevier, Inc.; 2017.pp. 953-63.
3. Tatum P, Talebreza S, Ross JS, Widera E. Palliative care and Special Management Issues. In: Halter JB, Ouslander JG, Joseph G, Studenski, Stephanie S, High KP, Asthana S, Supiano MA, Ritchie C (Eds). Hazzard's Geriatric Medicine and Gerontology, New York: McGraw-Hill Education Medical; 2017.
4. Ogle KS, Hopper K. End-of-Life Care for Older Adults. Prim Care. 2005;32(3):811-28.
5. Santivasi WL, Partain DK, Whitford KJ. The role of geriatric palliative care in hospitalized older adults. Hosp Pract. 2020;48(sup1):37-47.
6. Dunn GP, Martensen R, Weissman D. Chapter 12: Palliative surgery: Definition, Principles, Outcomes assessment. Surgical Palliative Care: A Resident's Guide. Chicago: Cunnif Rixon Foundation; 2009. pp. 137.
7. Sarkar S. Old age and palliative care in Indian scenario. Int J Med Public Health. 2018;8(3).
8. Seamark D, Ajithakumari K, Burn G, Devi PS, Koshy R, Seamark C. Palliative care in India. JR Soc Med. 2000;93(6):292-5.
9. Khosla D, Patel FD, Sharma SC. Palliative care in India: Current progress and future needs. Indian J Palliat Care. 2012;18(3):149-54.
10. Sallnow L, Kumar S, Numpeli M. Home-based palliative care in Kerala, India: the Neighbourhood Network in Palliative Care. Prog Palliat Care. 2010;18(1):14-7.
11. Kumar S. Community participation in palliative care: Reflections from the ground. Prog Palliat Care. 2020;28(2):83-8.
12. Government of Kerala. (2019). Kerala State Policy on Palliative Care 2019. [online] Available from https://palliumindia.org/2020/04/kerala-state-palliative-care-policy-2019.
13. Directorate General of Health Services Ministry of Health & Family Welfare. (2012). Proposal of strategies for palliative care in India (Expert group report). [online] Available from https://palliumindia.org/wp-content/uploads/2020/05/National-Palliative-Care-Strategy-Nov_2012.pdf.
14. Directorate General of Health Services, Ministry of Health & Family Welfare, Government of India. (2019). National Program for Palliative care. [online] Available from https://dghs.gov.in/content/1351_3_NationalProgramforPalliativeCare.aspx.
15. Directorate General Of Health Services, Ministry of Health & Family Welfare, Government of India. (2017). National Programme for Health Care of the Elderly (NPHCE). [online] Available from https://main.mohfw.gov.in/major-programmes/other-national-health-programmes/national-programme-health-care-elderlynphce.

CHAPTER

26 Approach to Older People in Clinical Settings

Prasun Chatterjee

ABSTRACT

Population aging has become a global phenomenon affecting various sectors of the nation including the healthcare system. Catering to the individual needs of the older people and providing them adequate healthcare is a humongous task for the already strained health delivery system. Considering the heterogeneity, existence of multimorbidity and geriatric syndrome and age-related changes in various organ systems, the older people must be assessed by a comprehensive geriatric assessment (CGA) including physical, psychological, functional and socioenvironmental domains to address their health needs. However, detailed assessment is time-consuming and not always pragmatic in usual clinical practice.

To combat this challenge faced by clinicians, the World Health Organization (WHO) has coined a simplified version for assessment which has been termed as "assessment of intrinsic capacity (IC)". IC accesses five domains such as cognition, mobility, vitality, sensory, and psychological aspects of an individual. It is a person-centric assessment and personalized care plan at the community level involving home-based intervention, multidisciplinary care team support for self-management, support for the caregivers and ensures referral and follow-up. The WHO Integrated Care for Older People (ICOPE) package of tools offers an integrated approach to screen and assess IC by the frontline healthcare workers. It would help in referring the older people to the respective specialties, at the earliest to avoid impending functional loss and thereby promoting healthy aging. Hence, the elderly care physicians must be equipped with the knowledge of CGA and ICOPE to effectively manage the healthcare needs of older people.

"The glory of the elderly is their insight to life"

—L G Akita

INTRODUCTION

Population aging is a well-known phenomenon to India considering the demographic shift since last two decades. According to the Longitudinal Ageing Study of India (LASI), there will be over 319 million elderly by 2050, three-fold the number identified by the census in 2011. The decline in birth rate, decrease in child mortality, improvement in medical facilities, implementation of various public health practices such as usage of vaccination, lifestyle modification and success of medical research which invented antibiotics, definite treatment of vascular disease such as hypertension, diabetes, coronary diseases, and the availability of advanced treatment of cancer etc., are a few important factors responsible for this phenomenon.

The primary challenges to population aging in India are economic crisis, social tension, and complex health problems. Predominantly (90%) older people are from unorganized sector, one-third are below the poverty line, and 75% live in rural areas. Thus, catering to the individual needs and providing them adequate healthcare itself is a humongous task for the already strained health delivery system.

Clinician must be aware of why the approach to older people is different from young generation.

SPECIAL FACTORS

Heterogeneity: Elderly population are heterogeneous. The factors responsible for the heterogeneity of health status among older persons are reported to be the accumulation of factors across the life course including health behaviors (e.g., smoking, exercise, and diet), access to healthcare, exposure to physical environments, and exposure to social environments.

Multimorbidity: They have multiple chronic non-communicable diseases such as hypertension, diabetes, and coronary artery diseases together (more than one comorbidity). The presence of multiple coexisting chronic diseases that have less consistency between the pathology and clinical manifestation may pose challenges to the conventional approach. It is difficult to manage as per guidelines which are mostly developed for single disease entity. With multiple coexisting diseases, it becomes difficult and often impossible to assess the severity and manifestation of individual disease and to ascribe functional status to specific disease processes.

Geriatric syndrome: It is a multifactorial condition that is prevalent in older adults and is believed to develop when an individual experience accumulated impairment in multiple systems that compromise their compensatory ability. A spectrum of diseases including loss of vision and hearing, inability to perform the activities of daily living, problems related to mental health and cognition, decreased mobility leading to functional impairment and decreased quality of life has been termed as "geriatric syndrome".

Susceptible to infection: Older people are vulnerable to infections due to weaning immune system.

Age-related changes of various organ system changes complicate it further. They usually suffer from the degeneration of most of the joints, atherosclerotic changes of the vessels, and are at a high risk of malignancy, cognitive impairment, and degeneration of the sensory system (**Table 1**).

Functionality matters the most: The maintenance of functional independence among older people is of high importance as it would help to maintain quality of life and to manage available health resources.

Quality of life: Most distressing symptoms such as pain, dizziness, fatigue, sleep problems, sensory impairment, and gait disorder among older people compromise the quality of life.

Disease-specific approach and treatment would not only be inconclusive but sometimes can be fatal also. For example, treating the consequences of fall without finding and managing the primary cause which may be cardiovascular, neurological, or environmental factors would only give a transient relief to the patient with major complications in the future. As per the WHO global report on falls prevention, people aged 65 years and above fall about 28–35% in each year and this proportion increases

TABLE 1 Age-related changes in older adult.

Physiological changes	
Vision changes	Flattening of the cornea atrophy and increased rigidity of iris discoloration of the lens and loss of elasticity alteration of lens transparency
Hearing changes	• Thickening of ear drums • Loss of high-frequency hearing acuity: Presbycusis
Changes in mouth, sense of taste, and smell	• Loss of teeth • Decrease in mastication strength • Decrease in the number of taste buds • Decrease in saliva production • Decreased sense of smell
Oropharyngeal, gastrointestinal and hepatobiliary changes	• Delayed esophageal emptying • Decreased relaxation of sphincter muscles • Decreased vitamin D and calcium absorption • Reduced motility of stomach • *Liver*: More susceptible to medicine and alcohol-related injury
Cardiovascular changes	• Thickening and stiffening of cardiac tissue • Loss of cardiac conduction system cells • Impaired homeostatic responses • Hypertrophy of the cardiac muscle
Respiratory changes	• Progressive deterioration of respiratory function decreased muscle strength and a stiffer chest wall with reduced compliance • Less ciliary activity in the respiratory tract • Decrease in the alveolar surface and production of surfactant
Endocrine changes	• Decreased insulin production • Increased insulin tolerance in peripheral tissues • Gradual atrophy of the thyroid gland

Continued...

Continued...

Physiological changes	
Musculoskeletal changes	• *Sarcopenia*: loss of muscle mass as well as strength, accelerated by physical inactivity and malnutrition • Replacement of lean body mass by fat and fibrous tissue • Osteoporosis in both sexes, especially accelerated bone loss in women for 5–7 years after menopause • Cartilage destruction in joints
Nervous system changes	• Decreased blood flow to the brain • Fewer cerebral neurons leading to cerebral atrophy with the greatest effect in the frontal aspects • Decrease in neurotransmitters, e.g., acetylcholine slower and weaker reflex responses • Progressive loss of peripheral neurons
Renal and genitourinary changes	• Decreased kidney mass and glomerular filtration rate (GFR) • Reduced bladder elasticity, muscle tone, and capacity • Weakening of the pelvic floor muscles • Enlargement of the prostate in males • Reduced renal functional reserve
Psychosocial changes	
Neuropsychiatric	• Older people take longer to learn new material, but complete learning still occurs • Verbal ability is maintained with age • Psychomotor speed declines • Short-term memory seems to deteriorate with age; long-term memory is preserved • Time taken for memory scanning is longer for both recent and remote memo

as age and frailty level increase. It has been reported that the prevalence of falls in Indian older people ranges from 14 to 53%. The clinicians must carefully elicit the history related to physical symptoms which sometimes could be vague and nonspecific and require further elaboration related to mood, cognition, social history, family history, and history related to mental health. During the decision-making process, the clinician must adhere to a patient-centered approach and the older people along with the family member should participate in decision-making about the future treatment and goal setting, whenever indicated.

Thus, adequate knowledge of various age-related changes in the organs and understanding of geriatric syndromes are necessary for the clinician for managing older adults. So, to effectively address the needs of older people, the approach must be through a CGA which was proposed by Dr Marjorie Warren.

COMPREHENSIVE GERIATRIC ASSESSMENT

It is considered as a multidimensional interdisciplinary diagnostic process focused on determining a frail older person to understand his or her multi-damage medical, psychological, and functional capability to develop a co-ordinated and integrated plan for treatment and long-term follow-up.

- *The domains of comprehensive geriatric assessment* include physical, psychological, functional, and socioenvironmental domains (**Box 1** and **Table 2**).

Functional status includes the basic and instrumental activity of daily living. Another functional scale such as mobility, balance, and fall risk assessment (**Box 2**) is of utmost importance in older people and is mostly neglected by usual clinical practice. Psychological health includes cognitive and socioenvironmental factors such as social network support, environment safety, adequacy, and needs measurement of functional status which is an essential

BOX 1 Domains of comprehensive geriatric assessment.

Comprehensive geriatric assessment

- Comprehensive geriatric assessment (CGA)
  - Multidimensional, diagnostic method
  - Elaborated to identify patient's needs
  - Develop a personalized care plan
  - And improve outcomes of frail older people
- Many different models of care and multiple instruments have been developed and validated over the last 40 years

Domains of comprehensive geriatric assessment

- Majority of CGA tools include similar measurable dimensions, grouped into the four domains:
  - Physical health (traditional history, physical examination, laboratory data, disease-specific severity indicators, and preventive health practices)
  - Functional status (basic and instrumental activities of daily living and other functional scales such as mobility or balance and fall risk assessment)
  - Psychological health (including mainly cognitive and affective status)
  - Socioenvironmental status (such as social networks and supports, and environmental safety, adequacy, and needs

TABLE 2 Screening for problems in older people.

Problem	Screening measure	Positive screen	Positive predictive value	Negative predictive value
Vision	• Do you have difficulty driving, or watching television, or reading, or doing any of your daily activities because of your eyesight?" • Test each eye with Snellen chart	Yes to question and inability to read >20/40 on Snellen chart	0.75	0.89
Hearing	Use audiometer set at 40 dB. Test hearing using 1,000 and 2,000 Hz	Inability to hear 1,000 or 2,000 Hz in both ears or either of these frequencies in one ear	0.75	0.91
Leg mobility	Time the patient after asking: "Rise from the chair. Walk 20 feet briskly, turn, walk back to the chair and sit down"	Unable to complete task in 15 seconds	0.91	0.92

Continued...

Continued...

Problem	Screening measure	Positive screen	Positive predictive value	Negative predictive value
Urinary incontinence	"In the last year, have you ever lost your urine and gotten wet?"— If yes, then ask: "Have you lost urine on at least 6 separate days?"	Yes to both questions	0.86	0.96
Nutrition/ weight loss	"Have you lost 10 lbs over the past 6 months without trying to do so? Weigh the patient	Yes to the question or weight < 100 lb	0.62	0.92
Memory	Three-item recall	Unable to remember all three items after 1 minute	0.60	0.92
Depression	Ask: "Do you often feel sad or depressed?"	Yes to the question	0.71	0.90
Physical disability	Six questions: "... do strenuous activities such as fast walking or bicycling?" "... do heavy work around the house such as washing windows, walls, or floors?" "... go to shopping for groceries or clothes?" "... get to places out of walking distance?" "... bathe, either a sponge bath, tub bath, or shower?" "... dress, such as putting on a shirt, buttoning and zipping, or putting on shoes?	No to any of the questions	0.88	0.77

Source: Adapted from Moore A, Siu AL. Screening for common problems in ambulatory elderly: clinical confirmation of a screen instrument. Am J Med. 1996;100:438-43.

BOX 2 Fall risk assessment.

- Individual with >2 falls is defined as recurrent fall
- It should be subjected to detailed examination using fall risk assessment, also called POMA—performance-oriented mobility assessment
- This employs a series of simple tasks
- Sitting and standing balance, turning, standing without the use of upper extremities for a push-off and balance etc. should be done by a physical therapist

part of the evaluation of older adults. The ability to perform functional tasks can be considered as a comprehensive measure for the overall impact of age-related impairment and health conditions.

Varieties of tools have been proposed and developed to assess the functionality. Some are objective measures of basic activity of daily living which includes toileting, bathing, eating, dressing, continence, transfers, and ambulation should be assessed by Barthel scale (**Box 3**) and the instrumental activity which includes little more complex processes such as cleaning and maintaining the house, managing money, moving within the community, preparing meals, shopping for groceries and necessities, taking prescribed medications, and using the telephone or other form of communication should be assessed by Lawton scale (**Box 4**). However, detailed assessment is time-consuming and not always pragmatic in usual clinical practice.

To combat this challenge faced by the clinicians, the WHO has coined a simplified version for assessment which has been termed as assessment of IC. IC is defined as the combination of all physical and the mental capacity of an individual. The concept of IC relates with healthy aging instead of disease state where it focuses on the assessment of functional capacities across the life course. Considering aging as a continuous trajectory of IC, the WHO ICOPE is an approach to maximize IC and functional ability. It is a person-centric assessment and personalized care plan at community level involving home-based intervention, multidisciplinary care team support for self-management, support for the caregivers, and ensure referral and follow-up (**Fig. 1**).

This model can be practiced in all kinds of healthcare settings from the primary, secondary, or tertiary care levels of healthcare. IC accesses five domains: (1) Cognition, (2) Mobility, (3) Vitality, (4) Sensory, and (5) Psychological aspects (**Figs. 2** and **3**).

CONCLUSION

Older people are not only heterogeneous but also experience age-related changes, multimorbidities, polypharmacy, and geriatric syndromes such as fall, frailty, dementia, depression, and sleep problems. This scenario mandates the clinicians to practice an integrated approach to effectively manage their clients. Elderly care physicians should focus on person-centric care emphasizing the

BOX 3 Barthel scale.

Feeding
0 = UNABLE
5 = Needs help cutting, spreading butter etc., or requires modified diet
10 = Independent

Bathing
0 = Dependent
5 = Independent (or in shower)

Grooming
0 = Needs to help with personal care
5 = Independent face/hair/teeth/shaving (implements provided)

Dressing
0 = Dependent
5 = Needs help but can do about half unaided
10 = Independent (including buttons, zips, laces etc.)

Bowels
0 = Incontinent (or needs to be given enemas)
5 = Occasional accident
10 = Continent

Bladder
0 = Incontinent, or catheterized and unable to manage alone
5 = Occasional accident
10 = Continent

Toilet use
0 = Dependent
5 = Needs some help, but can do something alone
10 = Independent (on and off, dressing, wiping)

Transfers (Bed to chair and back)
0 = Unable, no sitting balance
5 = Major help (one or two people, physical), can sit
10 = Minor help (verbal or physical)
15 = Independent

Mobility (on level surfaces)
0 = Immobile or <50 yards
5 = Wheelchair independent, including corners, >50 yards
10 = Walks with help of one person (verbal or physical) >50 yards
15 = Independent (but may use any aid; for example, stick) >50 yards

Stairs
0 = Unable
5 = Needs help (verbal, physical, carrying aid)
10 = Independent

Scoring and interpretation
Total score: 100
0–20: Total dependency
21–60: Severe dependency
61–90: Moderate dependency
91–99: Slight dependency

BOX 4 Lawton and Brody instrumental activity of daily living.

A. Ability to use telephone
- Operates telephone on own initiative; looks up and dials numbers: 1
- Dial safe well-known numbers: 1
- Answer telephone, but does not dial: 1
- Does not use telephone at all: 0

B. Shopping
- Takes care of all shopping needs independently: 1
- Shops independently for small purchases: 0
- Needs to be accompanied on any shopping trip: 0
- Completely unable to shop: 0

C. Food preparation
- Plans, prepares, and serves adequate meals independently: 1
- Prepares adequate meals if supplied with ingredients: 0
- Heats and serves prepared meals or prepares meals but does not maintain adequate diet: 0
- Needs to have meals prepared and served: 0

D. Housekeeping
- Maintains house alone with occasion assistance (heavy work): 1
- Performs light daily tasks such as dishwashing, bed making: 1
- Performs light daily tasks, but cannot maintain acceptable level of cleanliness: 1
- Needs help with all home maintenance tasks: 1
- Does not participate in any housekeeping tasks: 0

E. Laundry
- Does personal laundry completely: 1
- Launders small items, rinses socks, stockings etc.: 1
- All laundry must be done by others: 0

F. Mode of transportation
- Travels independently on public transportation or drives own car: 1
- Arranges own travel via taxi, but does not otherwise use public transportation: 1
- Travels on public transportation when assisted or accompanied by another: 1
- Travel limited to taxi or automobile with assistance of another: 0
- Does not travel at all: 0

G. Responsibility for own medications
- Is responsible for taking medication in correct dosages at correct time: 1
- Takes responsibility if medication is prepared in advance in separate dosages: 0
- Is not capable of dispensing own medication: 0

H. Ability to handle finances
- Manages financial matters independently (budgets, writes checks, pays rent and bills, goes to bank); collects and keeps track of income: 1
- Manages day-to-day purchases, but needs help with banking, major purchases etc.: 1
- Incapable of handling money: 0

Scoring and interpretation
For Women
0: Low functioning (dependent)
8: High functioning (independent)

For Men
0: Low functioning (dependent)
5: High functioning (independent)

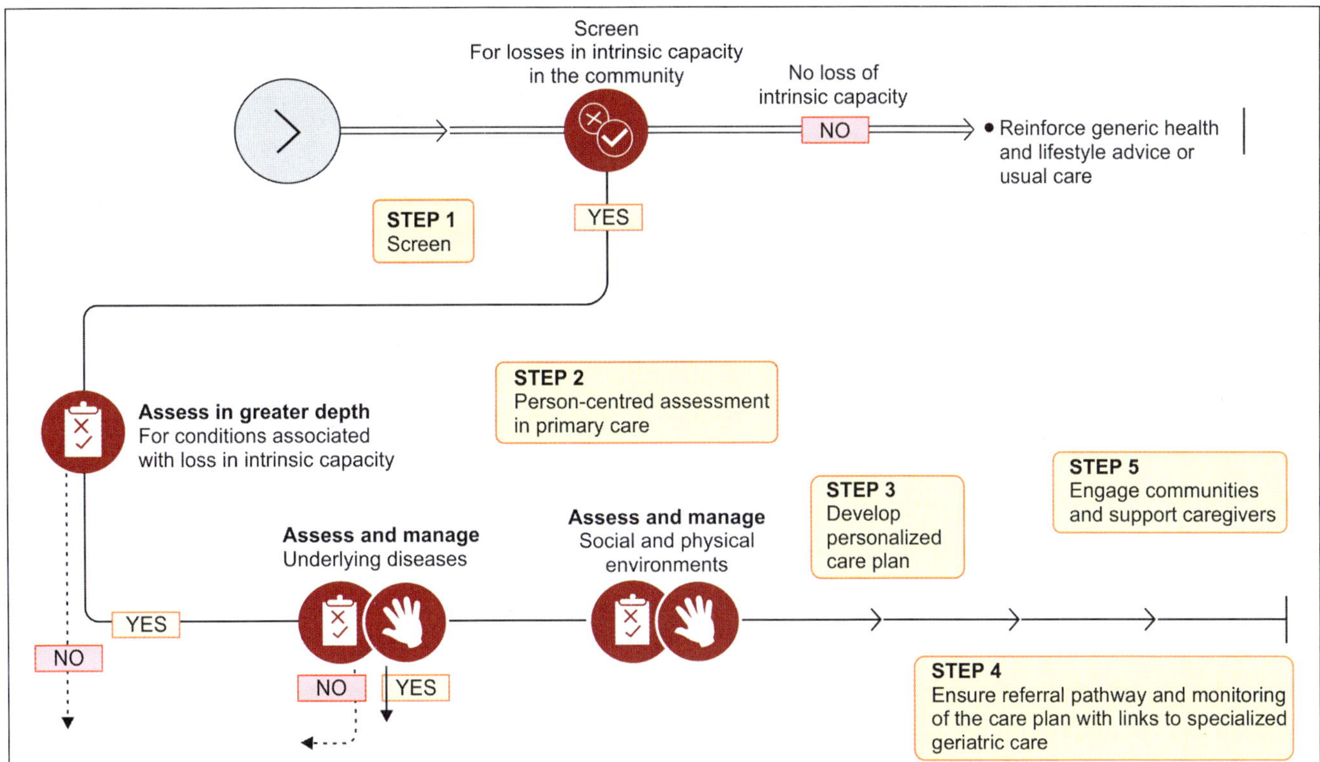

FIGURE 1: Integrated Care for Older People.

Source: Adapted from the Handbook, Guidance on person-centered assessment and pathways in primary care by the WHO.

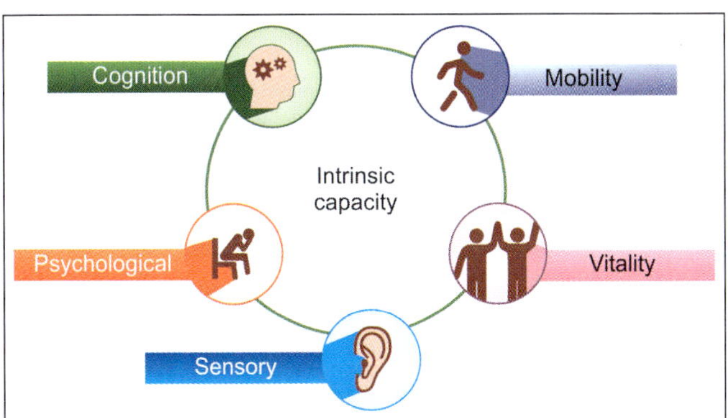

FIGURE 2: Domains of intrinsic capacity.

importance of functional capacity and quality of life in addition to the management of the primary complaints of the patients. Furthermore, they should also facilitate shared decision making with the patient and their care provider.

Comprehensive geriatric assessment with multidisciplinary team to identify medical, psychosocial, and functional capabilities of an older people is mandatory for frail, very elderly (80+) or older people with multimorbidity and people with dementia as it would not be pragmatic to assess every patient with the time-consuming procedure. However, WHO has coined the concept of assessing IC to quickly screen functional deficiency in the following domains: Memory, mood, mobility, vision, hearing, and nutrition. The ICOPE approach is an integrated process to screen and assess IC by the frontline healthcare workers and refer them earliest to the respective specialities with

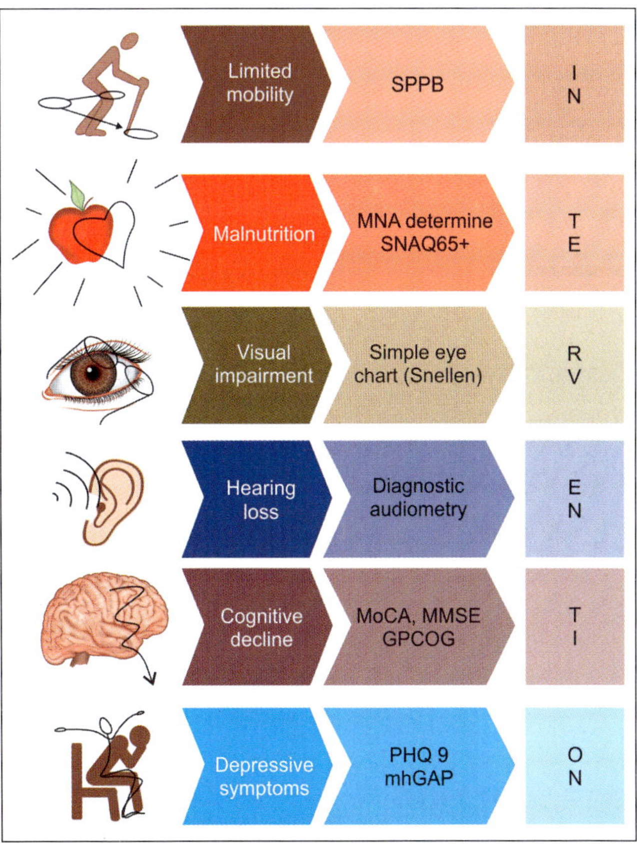

(GPCoG: general practitioner assessment of cognition; mhGAP: mental health gap action program; MMSE: mini-mental status examination; MNA: mini-nutritional assessment; MoCA: Montreal cognitive assessment; PHQ-9: patient health questionnaire-9; SPPB: short physical performance battery)

FIGURE 3: Assessment of intrinsic capacity.

the motto to prevent functional loss and promote healthy ageing for all. Hence, the elderly care physicians should be equipped with the knowledge of CGA and ICOPE to provide holistic care for their client.

RECOMMENDED READINGS

1. Ministry of Health and Family Welfare, Govt. of India. (2021). Longitudinal Ageing Study in India: There will be over 319 million elderly in India by 2050. [online] Available from http://newssimplified.in/health-ministry-launches-longitudinal-ageing-study-in-india/.
2. Ingle GK, Nath A. Geriatric health in India: concerns and solutions. Indian J Community Med. 2008;33(4):214-8.
3. Adhikari P. Geriatric health care in India—Unmet needs and the way forward. Arch Med Health Sci. 2017;5:112.
4. Grigsby JS. The Meaning of Heterogeneity: An Introduction. The Gerontologist. 1996;36(2):145-6.
5. Inouye SK, Studenski S, Tinetti ME, Kuchel GA. Geriatric syndromes: clinical, research and policy implications of a core geriatric concept. J Am Geriatr Soc. 2007;55(5):780-91.
6. Kline KA, Bowdish DM. Infection in an aging population. Curr Opin Microbiol. 2016 29:63-7.
7. Fabbri E, Zoli M, Gonzalez-Freire M, Salive ME, Studenski SA, Ferrucci L. Aging and Multimorbidity: New Tasks, Priorities, and Frontiers for Integrated Gerontological and Clinical Research. J Am Med Dir Assoc. 2015;16(8):640-7.
8. World Health Organization. (2021). WHO Global Report on Falls Prevention in Older Age. [online] Available from http://www.who.int/ageing/publications/Falls_prevention7March.pdf.
9. Dsouza SA, Rajashekar B, Dsouza HS, Kumar KB. Falls in Indian older adults: A barrier to active ageing. Asian J Gerontol Geriatr. 2014;9:1-8.
10. Rubenstein LZ, Stuck AE, Siu AL, Wieland D. Impacts of geriatric evaluation and management programs on defined outcomes: Overview of the evidence. J Am Geriatr Soc. 1991;39(S1):8S-16.
11. Jiang S, Li P. Current Development in Elderly Comprehensive Assessment and Research Methods. Biomed Res Int. 2016;2016:3528248.
12. Moore AA, Siu AL. Screening for common problems in ambulatory elderly: clinical confirmation of a screen instrument. Am J Med. 1996;100:438-43.
13. World Health Organization. (2021). Integrated Care for Older People. [online] Available from https://www.who.int/ageing/health-systems/icope/en/.

CHAPTER

27

Frailty Syndrome

Venugopalan Gunasekaran, Manicka Saravanan Subramanian

ABSTRACT

Frailty syndrome is a state of reduced physiological reserve in various organ systems, which predisposes older adults, even with mild stressors, to adverse outcomes such as hospitalization, morbidity, disability, and mortality. Frail older adults can have variety of clinical manifestations such as unintentional loss of weight, reduced activity or strength or endurance, reduced walking speed, or other nonspecific symptoms making the diagnosis in early stage very challenging. Multiple clinical tools are available to identify frailty. Biomarkers are being tried to detect frailty in early stages. Comprehensive geriatric assessment (CGA) identifies the deficits and helps in making a plan for multidisciplinary intervention. Exercise, nutrition, and correction of underlying diseases are, so far, the proven methods to manage frail older adults. Newer drug therapies are being tried to improve muscle mass and reduce disability.

"Alas, our fraility is the cause, not we! For, such as we are made of, such we be"

—William Shakespeare

INTRODUCTION

Aging is a progressive process associated with decline in structure and function, impaired maintenance and repair systems, increased susceptibility to disease and death, and reduced reproductive capacity. Frailty in older adults is a state of reduced reserve in various organ systems, which predisposes the older adults, susceptible to even the usual internal and external stressors and increases the risk of hospitalization, morbidity, and mortality. Frailty can be considered as an accelerated aging process that happens with different pace in different individuals. The chronological age is not a good determinant of the outcomes/trajectory in older adults. Frailty syndrome can act as a proxy for biological age and its assessment helps in clinical decision-making in older adults.

Approximately, 10% by age 60 years and 25% by age 80 years were found to be frail in various studies. An older adult can be categorized into fit (robust), prefrail, or frail based on frailty assessment scores. The adverse health outcomes such as institutionalization, disability, and death correlate well with the frail category. Frailty syndrome was also found to be associated with increased risk of periprocedural complications, falls, delirium, and cognitive impairment. There is no gold standard investigation to diagnose frailty. It is generally confirmed with CGA and there are lot of well-validated tools available to identify frailty status in older adults with varying sensitivity and specificity. Frailty syndrome typically refers to the physical frailty. The terms such as cognitive frailty and disability are different entities and have relation with frailty syndrome, but should not be used interchangeably.

DEFINITION

Frailty is defined by multiple researchers. Brocklehurst's *model of breakdown* explained that on one side of balance were *assets*: Health, functional capacity, positive attitude, and caregiver support and on other side of balance had *deficits*: Ill health, disability, dependence, and burden on caregivers. In frail older adults, the balance is broken and yielded to the deficit side.

A consensus group defined physical frailty as *a medical syndrome with multiple causes and contributors that is characterized by diminished strength, endurance, and reduced physiologic function that increases an individual's vulnerability for developing increased dependency and/or death.*

MODELS AND SCALES

There are lot of models and scales to define and identify frailty. Two well-described and commonly used models are phenotype model and cumulative deficit model.

PHENOTYPE MODEL

The phenotype model derived from observations of mortality data of two prospective cohorts of Cardiovascular Health Study (CHS), who were followed for 4 and 7 years. Phenotypic or physical frailty was established with five variables: (1) slow gait speed, (2) poor grip strength, (3) unintentional weight loss, (4) low physical activity, and (5) self-reported exhaustion based on Center for Epidemiological Studies-Depression (CES-D) questionnaire, which were associated with predicting institutionalization, morbidity, and mortality in this cohort.

One point was given for each variable and the subjects were divided as robust (0 point), prefrail (1 or 2 points), and frail (3 or more points). The cohort had 7% frail, 47% prefrail, and 46% robust. Observed mortality at 7 years was 43% in frail, 23% in prefrail, and 12% in robust. Though widely used, this model has some limitation such as it does not assess cognitive frailty and cannot be used in activity-restricted patients.

CUMULATIVE DEFICIT MODEL

This model from Canadian Study of Health and Aging (CSHA) is similar to Brocklehurst model. It has 36 questions to measure deficits. Frailty index (FI) is calculated by total number of deficits divided by 36. FI score 0.25 or more is consistent with diagnosis of frailty and FI score 0.6 or more is associated with high risk of mortality and adverse outcomes. This model is inclusive of various deficits, which has accumulated over the years and gives a holistic view and can be used in bed-bound patients. This model tends to overestimate frailty as compared to phenotype criteria. Though widely used, it does not incorporate objective measurement such as gait speed or grip strength.

OTHER SCALES

The Study of Osteoporotic Fractures (SOF) scale uses inability to rise from chair five times without using the arms, weight loss, and reduced energy level. FRAIL scale has five questions on Fatigue, Resistance, Aerobic, Illness, and Loss of weight. Three or more positive responses will be considered as frail. The Gérontopôle Frailty Screening Tool has two-step assessment processes. The Groningen Frailty Indicator (GFI) uses 15 indicators and more than three positive responses will be moderate-to-severe frailty.

PATHOPHYSIOLOGY

The pathophysiology of frailty is not completely known. Various studies have shown associations with failing internal homeostatic systems leading to conceptualization of a model, which could be explained by molecular, physiological, and clinical pathway to frailty. Frailty is associated with rise in inflammatory markers such as interleukin-6 (IL-6), C-reactive protein (CRP), tumor necrosis factor-α (TNF-α), and increased white blood count (WBC) counts and hence considered as proinflammatory state. There is an altered cluster of differentiation cells including $CD8^+/CD28^-$ T cells and $CCR5^-$ T cells resulting in a type I proinflammatory phenotype. These inflammatory cytokines create changes at molecular level, which alter the cellular metabolism. Moreover, the failure of the repair systems and epigenetic mechanisms play a complex role and lead to frailty syndrome. The proinflammatory state affects various systems such as musculoskeletal, endocrine, neurological, cardiovascular, and immunological system resulting in reduction of the dynamic homeostatic response and physiological reserve. The clinical manifestations of frailty are due to failing response of these systems (**Fig. 1**).

Telomeres are repetitive DNA sequences and specialized proteins that are found at the terminal ends of chromosomes and play an important role in frailty. As the cell ages, telomere length reduces to protect the conserved DNA. Translational studies have shown that older adults with shorter telomere lengths died earlier compared to age-matched controls. Senescent cells, which are not able to cope up with the environmental and oxidative stress, get burnt out and manifest as frailty.

The cycle of frailty (**Fig. 2**) explains the plausible pathophysiology. *Sarcopenia* leads to reduced strength

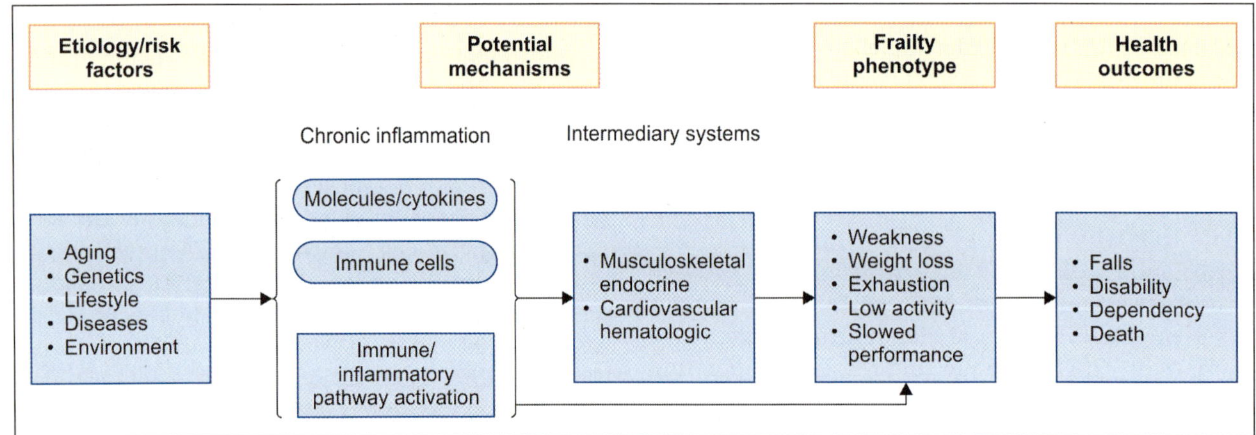

FIGURE 1: Pathophysiology of frailty.

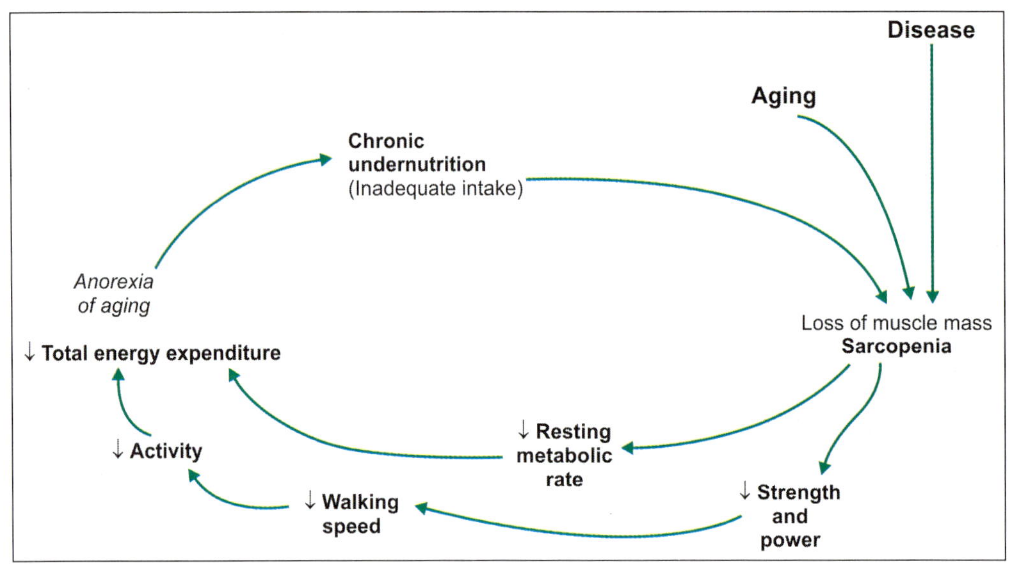

FIGURE 2: Cycle of frailty.

and endurance of the muscles, which manifests as reduced walking speed, poor grip strength, and a state of low physical activity. The reduction in overall energy expenditure reduces nutrition consumption, which further leads to reduced muscle mass. A vicious cycle sets in and manifests clinically as frailty.

Flowchart 1 shows the scheme, which explains the pathophysiology of frailty. It shows that the accumulation of cellular deficits by various mechanisms (genetic, environmental, and epigenetic) affects the physiological reserve in various organ systems. Reduced physical activity and poor nutrition are additive. Any minor stressor can expose the vulnerable state, leading to adverse outcomes and ultimately the person ending up in a vicious cycle. Cumulative deficit model slightly differs from phenotype model by the inclusion of disability and comorbidity in defining frailty.

Frailty should not be confused with disability or comorbidities. Frailty can coexist in a person with disabilities or comorbid conditions and vice versa. Frailty stands out

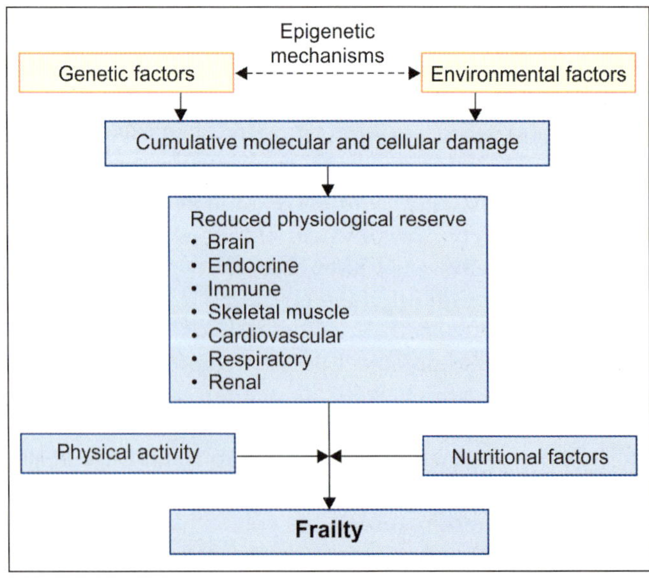

FLOWCHART 1: Scheme representing the pathophysiology of frailty.

from disability or comorbidity by its characteristic feature and reduced ability to regain the homeostatic or functional reserve following a stressor event (falls, hospitalization, illness, infections etc.).

FRAILTY IN ORGAN SYSTEMS

COGNITIVE FRAILTY

This is a heterogeneous condition having components of both physical frailty and decrease in the cognition or cognitive reserve. Though it is potentially reversible, it is often considered to be a precursor to dementia and not a normal age-related decline in cognition. The defining factors of cognitive frailty are:

- Physical frailty with cognitive impairment (CDR0.5)
- Exclusion of Alzheimer's and other dementias

ENDOCRINE SYSTEM

There is an age-related dysregulation of hypothalamic-pituitary-adrenal axis and decreased sensitivity of negative feedback system in higher circulating cortisol levels. When the older person experiences a stressor event (e.g., disease, infection), these higher circulating cortisol levels are sensed as a flight response and get attached to their receptors accelerating the cellular oxidation at cell level and myofibrillar degradation in muscle results leading to muscle loss. Insulin-like growth factor-1 (IGF-1) regulates the gene expression and the enzyme involved in ubiquitin-proteosome pathway. These genes and enzymes have direct and regulatory role in the autocrine, paracrine, and the endocrine activities. Decrease in the levels of IGF-1 with or without the decrease in dehydroepiandrosterone (DHEA) or testosterone results in frailty and sarcopenia. With age, testosterone levels are decreasing, but the bioavailable fraction is available in required quantity. Though testosterone improves muscle mass, replacement studies have not shown effect on mobility and vitality.

With age, the skeletal muscle mass decreases and fat-free adipose tissue increases. There is a complex interplay between visceral adipose tissue, muscle mass, and bone health. The visceral adipose tissue releases proinflammatory mediators promoting insulin resistance and procatabolic state, which accelerates frailty. Advanced aging results in increase in free triiodothyronine (FT3) levels and antithyroid antibodies. Few studies shown that subclinical hyperthyroidism is common with frailty. However, treatment has no effect on the hormonal or frailty status.

IMMUNE SYSTEM

As a part of immune senescence with aging, the T-cell and the stem cell population are decreased. Aging, itself a chronic low-grade inflammatory state, is characterized by elevated immunological markers such as IL-6, CRP, and TNF-α. Along with markers, the elevated cortisol level induces a stress response which induces insulin resistance and inhibits muscle fiber synthesis by Akt-mammalian target of rapamycin (mTOR) activity. The innate immune system also has elevated white cell counts with reduced neutrophil chemotaxis. The slow neutrophil migration may also cause damage to the healthy muscle fibers.

CLINICAL ASSESSMENT

The diagnosis of frailty is by history and clinical assessment. All older adults need to undergo assessment of frailty syndrome as recommended by various geriatric societies (cut-off age varies with societies). The British Geriatric Society (BGS) suggests evaluation of frailty only in older adults with history of fall, incontinence, immobility, delirium, or susceptibility to side effects of medication.

There are lot of scales available for diagnosing frailty. Any well-validated scale can be used for assessment and definitive diagnosis made by geriatrician using basic criteria used in well-defined models. If no proper scales are available for that population, then a CGA can be done to identify frailty and impairment in various domains [activities of daily living (ADL), functionality, physical performance, cognition, depression, nutrition etc.]. Some of the commonly used and validated scales are presented in **Table 1**.

TABLE 1 Common scales for diagnosis of frailty.

Scale	Components/Scoring	Category
FRAIL scale (useful in screening for frailty)	• *Fatigue*—how much of the time during past 4 weeks did you feel tired? (all/most of the time = 1 point) • *Resistance*—do you have any difficulty in walking up to 10 steps without resting? (Yes = 1 point) • *Ambulation*—do you have any difficulty in walking several hundred yards? (Yes = 1 point) • *Illness*—how many illnesses do you have out of list of 11? (5 or more = 1 point) • *Loss of weight*—have you had weight loss of 5% or more? (Yes = 1 point)	0 = Robust 1–2 = Prefrail 3–5 = Frail
Phenotype criteria (well validated, commonly used. The cut-offs may not be applicable for Indian population)	• *Weight loss* (>10 pounds unintentional weight loss in last 1 year) (Yes = 1 point) • *Walking speed* (height and sex-adjusted cut-off) • *Grip strength* (BMI and sex-adjusted cut-off) • *Exhaustion* (CES-D questionnaire) • *Low physical activity* (Minnesota Leisure Time Activity Questionnaire)	0 = Robust 1–2 = Prefrail 3–5 = Frail

Continued...

Continued...

Scale	Components/Scoring	Category
Clinical Frailty Scale (CFS)	• Very fit • Well • Managing well • Vulnerable • Mildly frail • Moderately frail • Severely frail • Very severely frail • Terminally ill	Used for assessing severity of frailty, after initial assessment with other scales
British Geriatric Society	• Gait speed > 0.8 m/s • Timed up and go (TUG) test score >10 seconds • PRISMA-7 questionnaire with a cut-off score 3 or more	Good sensitivity and moderate specificity

(BMI: body mass index; CES-D: Center for Epidemiological Studies-Depression)

BIOMARKERS

Clinical identification of frailty deals with physical manifestation and this occurs after considerable damage has occurred at the cellular level. Biomarkers can be used to identify at early stage and to explain plausible pathophysiological processes. Blood-based biomarkers, tissue-/cell-based biomarkers, and genetic biomarkers are being studied to find a consistent association with frailty in various population groups. Various studies have shown association of frailty with varying levels of hemoglobin, low albumin, WBC, cholesterol level, fibrinogen, transthyretin, retinol-binding protein, TNF-α, IL-6, CRP, IGF-1, testosterone level etc. Relation of sirtuins with frailty is under exploration. Studies have shown that lower circulating levels of SIRT1, SIRT2, and SIRT3 are to be associated with frailty. Newcastle 85+ Study Group has studied a panel of 40 biomarkers of cellular aging, inflammation, hematology, and immunosenescence. Though a correlation between Frailty Index by Biomarker (FI-B) and Frailty Index by Clinical Deficits (FI-CD) was weak in this study, combining FI-B and FI-CD has increased discriminative ability and actually both of them were complementary to each other. Inconsistent results and confounding factors in these studies have precluded any recommendation for biomarker at present.

MANAGEMENT

Comprehensive geriatric assessment involves a holistic, multidimensional assessment of various domains. It may need interdisciplinary team assessment. The impairments in domains are listed and a problem list is made. Steps are taken to correct any reversible conditions and shared decision-making is taken for improving these domains. A reassessment plan to monitor progression is also integral part of CGA. Corrections of reversible medical conditions, avoidance of polypharmacy, and caregiver support can improve quality of life.

NUTRITION

Calorie supplementation to maintain weight and improve nutrition has been studied in various studies. A Cochrane review of 62 trials had shown that protein and energy supplementation had reduced mortality when participants were undernourished [relative risk (RR): 0.79] and small but consistent weight gain, but overall mortality was not reduced. A systematic review and meta-analysis conducted in 2012 involving 36 randomized controlled trials on supplementation of oral high protein nutrition have shown reduced complications [odds ratio (OR): 0.68], reduced admission to hospitals (OR: 0.59), improved grip strength (1.76 kg), and improved weight. There was no data on mortality benefit.

VITAMIN D SUPPLEMENTATION

Restoration of low vitamin D levels activates vitamin D receptor and proper functioning in muscle, bone, and brain and also reduces the negative effect of parathyroid hormone (PTH) on bone. In deficiency state, supplementation of 800–1,000 IU of vitamin D has shown reduction in reduced postural sway, time taken for timed up and go (TUG) and improved lower extremity strength, reduced falls, hip fractures, and mortality.

EXERCISE

A systematic review had shown that multicomponent training interventions of long duration (>5 months), performed three times per week for 30–45 minutes per session, have better outcomes. A Cochrane review looking at physical rehabilitation for older people in long-term care analyzing 67 trials have shown improvement in Barthel ADL index by six points, improved functional independence, improved TUG score, and walking speed (0.03 m/s). Thus, physical rehabilitation as an effective way to reduce disability with few adverse events was proved, but clarity on type and duration of exercise regimen could not be attained. A Cochrane review on 159 trials had shown that group and home-based exercise programs and home safety interventions had reduced the risk of falling, benefitting frail older adults. Same review had shown Tai Chi to be effective in reducing falls.

PHARMACOLOGICAL TREATMENT

Various drugs were tried for treatment of frailty. Angiotensin-converting enzyme (ACE) inhibitors were tried for their presumed effect on skeletal muscle similar to its action in cardiac muscle without any benefit. Anabolic steroids including testosterone and DHEAs had not shown any significant benefit. Growth hormone and IGF-1 supplementation have not produced any beneficial outcome. However, reducing polypharmacy has proven to reduce the unnecessary pill burden and hence adverse outcomes in frail older adults.

Bimagrumab: It is a monoclonal antibody that blocks action of myostatin and has been found to increase muscle mass in humans and increased hand grip strength. But clinical application in frailty and sarcopenia is awaited.

Selective androgen receptor modulator: Selective androgen receptor modulators (SARMs), a class of androgen receptor ligands that have differential activation, have potential of treating frailty and sarcopenia. Various trials are ongoing to assess the clinical utility of this group of drug in muscle mass and function.

CONCLUSION

Identification of frailty and treating reversible causes will improve quality of life in older adults. Identifying frail older adults in their early stage will give us opportunity to prevent disability. When mortality is inevitable, the quality of life and dignity of older adults take precedence in their management plan. Further research is needed for early detection and targeted therapies for frail older adults.

RECOMMENDED READINGS

1. Morley JE, Vellas B, van Kan GA, Anker SD, Bauer JM, Bernabei R, et al. Frailty consensus: a call to action. J Am Med Dir Assoc. 2013;14(6):392-7.
2. British Geriatrics Society (BGS). (2014). Fit for Frailty Part 1: Consensus best practice guidance for the care of older people living in community and outpatient settings. [online] Available from https://www.bgs.org.uk/sites/default/files/content/resources/files/2018-05-23/fff_full.pdf.
3. Fried LP, Tangen CM, Walston J, Newman AB, Hirsch C, Gottdiener J, et al. Frailty in Older Adults: Evidence for a Phenotype. J Gerontol A Biol Sci Med Sci. 2001 Mar;56(3):M146-56.
4. Clegg A, Young J, Iliffe S, Rikkert MO, Rockwood K. Frailty in elderly people. Lancet. 2013;381(9868):752-62.
5. Dent E, Morley JE, Cruz-Jentoft AJ, Woodhouse L, Rodríguez-Mañas L, Fried LP, et al. Physical Frailty: ICFSR International Clinical Practice Guidelines for Identification and Management. J Nutr Health Aging. 2019;23(9):771-87.

CHAPTER 28

Falls in Elderly

Monika Bansal, Jyotirmoy Pal, Purbasha Biswas

ABSTRACT

Falls are among the most serious and common problem faced by the elderly people. It leads to significant morbidity, frequent hospital admissions for them, and sometimes even mortality. There is interplay of multiple factors and situations which lead to recurrent falls. This interaction may be modified by age of the person, associated disease, and the presence of hazards in the surrounding environment. Besides physiological changes in body, change in body composition, neurological and cardiopulmonary changes, other common causes can be postural hypotension, stroke, Parkinsonism, peripheral neuropathy, and orthopedic problems. Falls can be the result of extrinsic risk factors like irregular flooring, poor lighting etc., intrinsic risk factor or a combination of both.

Early identification of fall risk is likely to result in earlier implementation of intervention and to minimize the development of secondary problems such as reduced confidence and activity levels. A comprehensive falls risk factor assessment should be performed for older people who present for medical attention after a fall, those who had more than one fall in the preceding

6 months, or those who have abnormalities of gait or balance. Effective interventions include: (1) health promotion and falls prevention, (2) single interventions, (3) medication review, (4) exercise, (5) home modifications, (6) to improve safety in the home, and (7) to improve safety outside the home. Effective preventive strategies require better understanding of the causes and risk factors for falls among elderly, therefore, a detailed history of all events as well as thorough examination of patient may be helpful.

"The life so short, the craft so long to learn"

—Hippocrates

INTRODUCTION

"A fall is defined as an event which results in a person coming to rest inadvertently on the ground or floor or other lower level" [World Health Organization (WHO), 2007]. Falls of more than two episodes in 6 months is considered as recurrent falls. Recurrent fall is an issue of concern. Two or more falls in 1 month is a red flag sign in elderly and need urgent evaluation. Recurrent falls are a common reason for admission of previously independent elderly persons.

The incidence and severity of falls is most common in 7th and 8th decade. Annually, approximately 35–40% of community-dwelling, generally healthy older persons, in the age 65 years and overpopulation as a whole, fall. The rate of falling increases after 75 years. Though there is high incidence of falls in young children and athletes as well, but there is less concern of serious injuries in them as compared with falls in elderly. This propensity for fall-related injury in elderly persons stems from a high prevalence of comorbid diseases, e.g., osteoporosis and age-related physiological decline, e.g., slower reflexes that make even a relatively mild fall potentially dangerous.

Approximately 5% of older people who fall require hospitalization. Besides cardiovascular, neoplastic, cerebrovascular, and pulmonary causes as a cause of death in elderly, unintentional injuries are the fifth leading cause of death in older adults and falls account for two-thirds of the deaths resulting from unintentional injuries. In addition to physical injury, falls can also have psychological and social consequences. Fear of falling and the post-fall anxiety syndrome are the well-recognized negative consequences of falls. The loss of self-confidence to ambulate safely after falls can result in self-imposed functional limitations.

The reason why elderly people have so frequent falls, we need to understand the change in normal biology and physiology of aging.

PHYSIOLOGY OF AGING

The biological and physiological changes in the body with aging are slow and gradually progressive. These are mentioned below.

BODY COMPOSITION

There is change in body composition with aging as stated in **Table 1**.

- Besides gradual muscle loss of lean tissue and an increase in fat, this loss of lean tissue reflects loss of mass: Total body muscle mass, limb muscle volume, muscle cross-sectional area, and muscle fiber number and area.
- Besides this, bone mineral is lost.

POSTURAL CHANGES

There are significant changes in the posture of the elderly. These are as follows:

- Progressive anterior thrust of the head and extension of the cervical spine.
- Accentuated thoracic kyphosis and straightening of the lumbar spine.
- In the upper limbs, there is increased extension of the arms and scapular protraction at the shoulders is associated with flexion of the elbows.
- Ulnar deviation of the wrists and finger flexion.
- In the lower extremity, there is an increase in hip and knee flexion and a decrease in ankle dorsiflexion.
- There is diminished arm swing and a shorter step length during walking.
- Bony pelvis widens with aging.
- The angle of the femoral neck to the shaft increases, resulting in a valgus deformity of the hips.
- Progressive widening of the standing base is also noted in women, knees can develop varus deformities with narrowing of the standing base.

There is shift in the centre of gravity of the body from just anterior to the first/second sacral level and to shift the plumb line of the body so that it no longer favors extension of the lower extremity joints in relaxed standing. The centre

TABLE 1 Changes in biological functions with aging.

Function	Change with aging
Cardiac output	Decreased
Maximum oxygen consumption	Decreased
Systolic blood pressure (BP)	Increased
Orthostatic tolerance	Decreased
Body water	Decreased
Muscle strength	Decreased
Lean body mass	Decreased
Bone calcium	Decreased
Glucose tolerance	Decreased
Red blood cell (RBC) mass	Decreased
Serum lipids	Increased

of gravity is shifted behind the hip by flexing the knees and this may require the use of ambulatory aid such as a cane. Along with these anatomical changes, there are some physiological effects noted. Increased postural sway occurs with aging. The ability to balance on one leg with either eye closed or open decreases. Righting reflexes decrease and reaction time increases. There are significant differences in quantitative and qualitative walking characteristics differentiating fallers from nonfallers during overground walking at different velocities and during obstacle clearance. Qualitatively, the fallers demonstrated increase knee flexion during both overground walking and the fallers consistently took several small steps immediately prior to the obstacle clearance.

"NORMAL" NEUROLOGICAL CHANGES

To recognize pathological changes in elderly people, it is important to know what is "normal" with aging. Some of the frequently found normal neurological changes with aging are as follows:

- *Eye signs*: Small irregular pupils with diminished reaction to light and accommodation reflex
- Reduced range of movement on convergence and upward gaze and slowed pursuit
- *Motor signs*: Tremor and titubation, short-stepped and broad-based gait with diminished associated movements, poor coordination, atrophy of interossei, and reduced muscle strength
- *Sensory signs*: Reduced proprioception and vibratory sense and increased threshold for light touch and temperature
- *Reflexes*: Appearance of primitive reflexes, absent ankle jerks and diminished other reflexes, and occasionally Babinski's sign
- It should be emphasized that just because a physical finding is normal for an elderly person, it still might have functional significance. For instance, loss of upward gaze is seen in elderly. The normal limit of upward gaze in the young adults is 40–45°, but by eighth decade it is reduced to an average of 16°.
- Mechanical neck problems are of restricted cervical motion and vertical gaze makes it difficult for an elderly person to see wall clocks, exit sign's, and other orienting information.
- In an attempt to compensate for this, the person might lean backwards contributing to imbalance and fall.
- The decline in cognitive function with normal aging tends to be of small magnitude.

CARDIOPULMONARY CHANGES

Cardiac changes that occur with aging include:

- Decreased cardiac reserve
- Contractile function and heart rate
- Blood pressure tends to rise with aging whereas pulmonary function decreases with a decline in vital capacity

However, the main functional deficits secondary to cardiopulmonary system are due to disease and not aging changes.

INACTIVITY

The physical incapacity is more due to inactivity. The principle of "use it or lose it" indicates that the decrease in physiological functioning in the elderly is not solely due to the aging process but is also due to inactivity. If elderly persons initiate an appropriate exercise program they can "lessen" their physiological age as measured by maximum oxygen consumption.

RISK FACTORS FOR FALLS

Because many patients at risk of falling seek neurological consultations, neurologists have opportunities to identify those at greatest risk, document risk factors, and offer interventions that may prevent falls among patients with chronic neurological disease. Risk factors for falls are summarized in **Box 1**.

BOX 1	Risk factors for falls.
General factors:	
• Increased age	
• Living alone	
• Previous falls	
• Use of a cane or walker	
• Acute illness	
• Alcohol	
• Risky behaviors	
Reduced vision:	
• Glare intolerance	
• Altered depth perception	
• Decreased night vision	
• Decline in peripheral vision	
Neurological causes:	
• Seizures	
• Syncope	
• Cerebrovascular accident (CVA)—hemiparesis, sensory, and/or motor function deficits	
• Generalized weakness	
• Alzheimer's dementia, normal pressure hydrocephalous (NPH), or other dementias	
• Parkinson's disease, progressive supranuclear palsy (PSP), and multisystem atrophy (MSA)	
• Vestibular disturbances	
• Diminished sensory awareness for light touch, vibration, and temperature	
• Decline in proprioception	

Continued...

Continued...

Cardiovascular causes:
• Arrhythmias
• Decreased cardiac output
• Outflow or inflow obstruction
• Cardiomyopathy
• Cardiac syncope
• Vasovagal attack
Orthopedic problems:
• Arthritis
• Decreased range of motion and flexibility in lower legs and spine
• Callouses, bunions, and deformities
Decreased hearing:
• Impaired speech discrimination
• Excessive cerumen accumulation
• Loss of high frequency tones
Medications:
• Sedative—hypnotic and anxiolytic drugs
• Tricyclic antidepressants
• Major tranquilizers (phenothiazines and butyrophenones)
• Antihypertensive drugs
• Cardiac medications
• Anticholinergic drugs
• Hypoglycemic agents
• Any medication that is likely to affect balance

Besides changes in physiology and biology of elderly, we need to understand the various precipitating causes leading to falls. Falls may be precipitated by extrinsic or intrinsic causes. Intrinsic factors are those of physiologic origin or falls due to host factors and extrinsic factors are the environmental or related hazards or falls due to environmental factors. Besides these, there are situational factors too which contribute to falls. There is interplay of all these factors which can contribute to recurrent falls in elderly (**Fig. 1**).

EVALUATION

Elderly individuals with falls need evaluation with good history, physical examination, and some investigations.

HISTORY

A single fall is not always a sign of a major problem and an increased risk for subsequent falls. The fall may simply be an isolated event. However, recurrent falls, two falls in a 6-month period, should be evaluated for treatable causes. Elderly patients with known risk factors for falling should be questioned about falls on a periodic basis. Specific inquiry is necessary because of the fears many elderly persons harbor about being institutionalized. An immediate evaluation is required for falls that produce injuries or are associated with a new acute illness, loss of consciousness, fever, or abnormal blood pressure.

- Patient should be asked for any blackout before falling and sensation of giddiness or vertigo preceding fall.
- History of loss of consciousness following fall should be asked from bystanders.
- A thorough history is essential to determine the falling risk factors for falls, impairments that contribute to falls, and the appropriate tripping, but physician must determine if the fall occurred because of an environmental obstacle or another precipitating factor.
- The physician should ask about the activity the patient was engaged in just before and at the time of the fall, especially if the activity involved a positional change.
- The location of the fall should be ascertained.
- It is also important to know whether anyone witnessed the fall and whether the patient sustained any injuries.
- The patient and witnesses or caregivers should be asked in detail about previous falls and whether the falls were the same or different in character.

EXAMINATION

Patient should be examined thoroughly. Vital signs including blood pressure, especially postural (supine, sitting, and standing at 1 min and 3 min) should be checked as well as pulse rate should be monitored. Posture of the patient, gait, spine, hip, or foot deformities should be examined and thorough cardiac and neurological examination should be performed. Patient should be examined for any sustained injuries. Then detailed investigations can be planned according to the clinical assessment made after detailed history and examination. Investigations may vary from blood sugar, serum electrolytes, electrocardiography, Holter monitoring, head-up tilt test, electroencephalography, neuroimaging (CT head/MRI brain), detailed autonomic function tests etc.

ASSESSMENT OF RISK OF FALL

The risk of sustaining an injury from a fall depends on the individual patient's susceptibility and environmental hazards. The frequency of falling depends on the accumulated effect of multiple disorders superimposed on age-related changes. There may be multiple causes for a single fall, and repeated falls may each have a different etiology sometimes. Therefore, it is always better to enquire all events separately if different circumstances. Thus, it is critical to evaluate each occurrence separately. A critical part of the history is a review of medications, including prescribed drugs, over the counter, herbal, and illicit drugs. Red flags are polypharmacy, the initiation of a new drug therapy in the previous two weeks, and the use of any drug.

Usually fall have multiple causes. Sometimes the causes may be reversible, but sometimes not. Nonetheless, a partial positive impact on one or a few causes often makes a major difference in quality of life for the patients and caregivers.

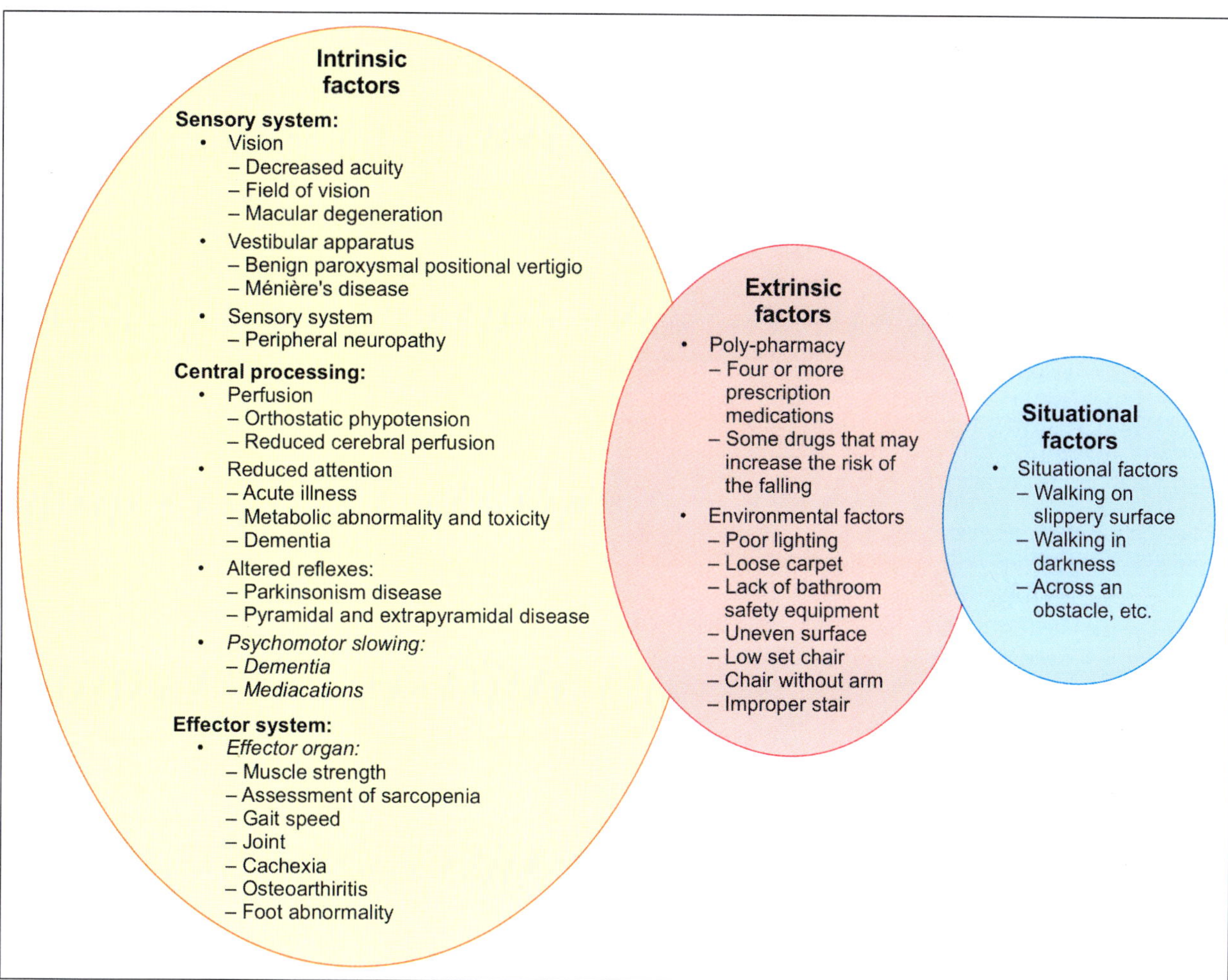

FIGURE 1: **Interplay of various factors leading to fall.**

For the assessment of an individual with falls following methods and scales can be used.

- *A mnemonic* (**I HATE FALLING**) can be used to look for key physical findings in patients who fall or nearly fall. The alphabets signify as follows: I—Inflammation of joints or joint deformity, H—Hypotension, auditory, and visual abnormalities, T—Tremor (Parkinson's disease or other causes of tremor), E—Equilibrium problem, F—Foot problems, A—Arrhythmia, heart block, or valvular heart disease, L—Leg-length discrepancy, L—Lack of conditioning, I—Illness, N—Nutrition (poor; weight loss), and G—Gait disturbance. This mnemonic focuses the physician's attention on common problems that are likely to respond to treatment.
- *Another alternative is the "get-up and go" test.* In this test, the patient is seated in an armless chair placed 3 m (10 ft) from a wall. The patient stands, walks toward the wall (using a walking aid if one is typically employed), turns without touching the wall, returns to the chair, turns, and sits down. This activity does not need to be timed. Instead, the physician observes the patient and makes note of any balance or gait problems (**Video 1**).
- *The Falls Efficacy Scale* was developed by Tinetti et al. It was developed to assess the confidence a person has in performing several activities of daily living (ADL) without falling, in this patient is asked to respond for 10 common life situations on a scale of 1 to 10. 1 being extremely confident and 10 having no confidence at all. Activities like getting in and out of bed, taking a bath or shower, preparing a meal, reaching into cupboards, walking around the house, getting in and out of a chair, answering the door or telephone, doing lighthousekeeping, getting dressed or undressed, and doing simple shopping. A higher score, i.e., a score of 70 or more indicates that patient is afraid of falling. This scale was validated in a sample of community dwelling elderly persons. It has been shown to be reliable and have predictive validity in subsequent studies of similar populations.
- *Morse Fall Scale*: The various factors are mentioned along with the score in brackets (**Table 2**). For interpretation of the scale depending on the score individuals classified as high risk when score is >45, moderate risk when score is 25–45, and low risk when score is <25.

PREVENTION OF FALLS

After thorough history, examination, and detailed risk assessment, it is an important step to plan intervention how to prevent falls at various levels. We need to advise changes

TABLE 2 The Morse Fall Scale for risk of fall in elderly.

Factor	The category in which the person belongs		
History of falling	Yes (0)	No (15)	
Secondary diagnosis	1 (0)	>1 (15)	
Ambulatory aid	Bed rest (0)	Crutches (15)	Furniture (30)
Intravenous access	No (0)	Yes (15)	
Gait	No (0)	Weak (15)	Improper gait (20)
Mental status	Own limit (0)	Overestimation (15)	

TABLE 3 Interventions to prevent falls.

Changes to be done from medical view	• Exercise • Physical therapy assessment • Review all medications by the healthcare provider • Vision examination and correction of vision disorders • Modification of psychotropic medication • Vitamin D supplementation • Nutritional supplements • Psychological interventions • Education of nursing personnel
Changes to be done at home	• Remove throw rugs • Secure carpet edges • Reduce clutter • Remove cords and wires on the floor • Avoid floor wax • Push in the drawers • Check lighting for adequate illumination at night and on the stairs • Install handrails on both sides of the stairwell • Eliminate chairs that are too low to sit in and get out of easily • Keep often used items in cabinets that can be reached easily without using a step stool • Wear well-fitting shoes and slippers with nonskid bottoms
Changes to be done in bathrooms	• Install grab bars in the shower and by the toilet • Use rubber mats in the bathtub and shower • Install a raised toilet seat • Keep drawers closed
Changes to be done outside home	• Repair cracked sidewalks • Install handrails on stairs and steps • Trim shrubbery along the pathway to the home • Install adequate lighting by doorways and along walkways leading to doors

from medical point of view, from altering medications, giving supplements to physical therapy, altering extrinsic factors from making changes at home, bathrooms, outside homes etc. (**Table 3**).

CONCLUSION

Falls are among the most common and serious problems faced by elderly persons. It is associated with considerable mortality, morbidity (from orthopedic injuries to head injuries), reduced functioning, and hospital admissions. Falls generally result from interplay of multiple factors and situations, many of which can be corrected. Therefore, it is very important to understand the exact cause of fall and situations as well as to do fall risk assessment to plan effective intervention strategy for the patient.

ACKNOWLEDGMENT

We are thankful to Dr Subhra Sankar Sen, MBBS, PGY2 Medicine, Midnapore Medical College & Hospital, West Bengal for helping us prepare this chapter.

RECOMMENDED READINGS

1. Tinetti ME, Williams TF, Mayewski R. Fall risk index for elderly patients based on number of chronic disabilities. Am J Med. 1986;80(3):429-34.
2. Downton JH, Andrews K. Prevalence, characteristics and factors associated with falls among the elderly living at home. Aging (Milano). 1991;3(3):219-28.
3. Fleming BE, Pendergast DR. Physical condition, activity pattern, and environment as factors in falls by adult care facility residents. Arch Phys Med Rehabil. 1993;74(6):627-30.
4. Clark RD, Lord SR, Webster IW. Clinical parameters associated with falls in an elderly population. Gerontology. 1993;39(2):117-23.
5. Gillespie LD, Gillespie WJ, Robertson MC, Lamb SE, Cumming RG, Rowe BH. Interventions for preventing falls in elderly people. Cochrane Database Syst Rev. 2003;(4):CD000340.
6. Rubenstein LZ. Falls in older people: epidemiology, risk factors and strategies for prevention. Age Ageing. 2006;35(Suppl 2):ii37-ii41.
7. Beswick AD, Rees K, Dieppe P, Ayis S, Gooberman-Hill R, Horwood J, et al. Complex interventions to improve physical function and maintain independent living in elderly people: a systematic review and meta-analysis. Lancet. 2008;371(9614):725-35.
8. Anderson KE. Falls in the elderly. J R Coll Physicians Edinb. 2008;38:138.
9. Sharif SI, Al-Harbi AB, Al-Shihabi AM, Al-Daour DS, Sharif RS. Falls in the elderly: assessment of prevalence and risk factors. Pharm Pract (Granada). 2018;16(3):1206.

CHAPTER 29

Drug Therapy in Elderly

G Usha

ABSTRACT

Many parameters of physiological changes of aging alter the way a drug acts. Altered drug responsiveness in elderly is due to altered pharmacokinetics and pharmacodynamics. Pharmacokinetics deals with four components, namely, absorption, distribution, metabolism, and excretion. Absorption is not much affected by aging. Drug distribution is determined by body composition, protein binding, and organ blood flow. With aging, body fat increases and total body water decreases. Fat-soluble drugs (lipophilic) get distributed widely and clear slowly whereas water soluble drugs (like digoxin) are distributed less widely. This can lead to misinterpretation of serum drug levels. Hypoalbuminemia in elderly leads to increase in the amount of free-drug levels.

Drugs are metabolized by two types of reaction in the liver. Drugs that undergo phase 1 metabolism (oxidation and reduction) show reduced clearance. In phase 2 metabolism (conjugation), they are not altered with aging. Renal excretion is the primary route of elimination for many drugs and their metabolites. Estimation of creatinine clearance by Cockcroft and Gault equation is essential since serum creatinine is not a reliable indication of renal function in elderly. Drugs primarily excreted by the kidneys have to be avoided or dose adjusted as per the creatinine clearance in patients with altered renal function.

There is not much data available for altered pharmacodynamics in elderly. Altered pharmacodynamics could be due to altered sensitivity to changes in receptors and age-related impaired physiological and homeostatic mechanisms.

Polypharmacy is when the patient is on more than five drugs taken simultaneously. Polypharmacy leads to poor compliance and increased adverse drug reactions (ADRs) which lead to hospital admission, mortality, and morbidity. Prevalence of polypharmacy varies from 5 to 78%.

Compliance is the ability of a person to adhere or comply with prescription. Patients with cognitive impairment, poor vision, swallowing difficulty, and arthritic hands may have poor compliance. A number of interventions can be done to improve the compliance.

Medication-related problems can be due to medication-related errors such as errors in prescription, communication, dispensing, administration, and monitoring. Medication-related adverse drug events can be ADRs, therapeutic failure, and adverse drug withdrawal events. It is estimated that 15–20% admissions are due to ADRs. ADRs could be due to polypharmacy secondary to multiple comorbidities, noncompliance, altered pharmacokinetics, and dynamics ADRs can be of two types, namely: Type A and Type B. Type A is dose-related and type B is idiosyncratic or allergic reaction. Type A is more common in elderly. ADR can be due to drug–drug or drug–disease interaction (D-Dis-I).

Anticholinergic burden is the cumulative effect of using drugs with weak/strong anticholinergic properties leading to central and peripheral effects. This can be assessed by a number of tools. Example: anticholinergic drug scale (ADS) and anticholinergic risk scale (ARS).

Prescription cascade occurs when a new treatment is started for an adverse reaction of a drug, misinterpreting it as a new medical condition.

Quality of prescription is assessed by explicit criteria such as Beers, START (Screening Tool to Alert to Right Treatment), STOPP (Screening Tool of Older Persons' Prescriptions) criteria and implicit criteria like medication appropriateness index (MAI). ACOVE (Assessing Care Of Vulnerable Elders) project not only assesses the inappropriateness of prescription but also other aspects such as patient education, maintenance of records, regular review, and documentation of indications.

Medical reconciliation is a process of identifying the accurate list of all medications a patient is on, comparing with the list of medications prescribed, and making the final list to be followed. Patient and the caregiver are given adequate education on this appropriate prescription. A number of general principles are to be followed while prescribing for the vulnerable elderly population to decrease the morbidity and mortality secondary to inappropriate medication.

"About the only thing that comes without effort is old age"

—Anonymous

INTRODUCTION

Drug therapy in elderly is often a special challenge. Richard Miller's definition of aging as the "process that progressively converts physiologically and cognitively fit healthy adults into less fit individuals with increasing vulnerability to injury, illness, and death" is very useful in understanding how physiological changes observed in elderly makes prescribing medications in elderly challenging. With increasing life expectancy of older persons and declining birth rates along with better healthcare facilities and health awareness, the proportion of elderly has increased dramatically worldwide and will continue to increase for the next 50 years.

The elderly population is increasing worldwide due to increasing life expectancy and declining birth rate along with better healthcare facilities and health awareness. The proportion of elderly has increased dramatically worldwide and will continue to increase for the next 50 years. With increasing number of elderly population it is common to see elderly taking multiple medications over the counter prescription and additional prescribed drugs to treat side effects of medications that they are already on. In India, inappropriate prescription in elderly is found to be very high ranging from 18 to 49% in ambulatory, 25–54% in hospitalized, and 37–67% in nursing home residents. As per the World Health Organization (WHO) statistics, the percentage of elderly is likely to increase from 8% in 2010 to 20% in 2050 in India.

In India, an estimated 50% of elderly people suffer from at least one chronic condition. An average older person uses between three and eight drugs. Hence, prescribing of drugs offers special challenges in elderly.

With the increasing number of older people, it is common to see elderly taking multiple medications over the counter prescription and additional prescribed drugs to treat side effect of medications that they are already on. The average older person uses between three and eight drugs (2003). About 57% patients were on five or more and 19% were on 10 or more drugs. Most of our scientific understanding of therapeutics, clinical pharmacology and pharmacokinetics are based on studies in younger population and hence data with regard to safety of drugs in elderly is based on anecdotal data, clinical impression, and trial and error only.

Prescribing medication is the most frequently employed medical intervention. Creating optimal drug regimens to meet the complex needs of the old require adequate knowledge and careful planning.

ALTERED DRUG RESPONSIVENESS

Altered drug responsiveness could be due to age-related changes in pharmacokinetics and pharmacodynamics. Many parameters of physiological changes of aging alter the way a drug acts.

PHARMACOKINETICS

Pharmacokinetics refers to how the body handles a drug from the time it is ingested to the time it is excreted. This includes absorption, distribution, protein binding, metabolism, and elimination. Each of these processes can vary with age, influenced by genetic factors, individual diseases, environment, and other medications. Changes in renal function have greatest impact on pharmacokinetics.

Absorption: Absorption of drugs is altered by the size of the absorptive surface, gastric pH, splanchnic blood flow, and GI motility but is relatively unaffected by aging as such. However, absorption can be affected by drug–drug and D-Dis-I.

The absorption of substances that are actively transported from the intestinal lumen including some sugars, minerals, and vitamins may be decreased in elderly patients. However, most of the drugs are passively absorbed and major alterations with aging have not been identified.

Distribution: Drug distribution is determined by body composition, protein binding and organ blood flow. The extent of distribution of a drug is determined by its molecular size, lipophilicity, acid/base properties, and binding of the drugs to plasma albumin and tissue proteins. Total body water and body mass decrease with age. Body fat as a percentage of body weight increases with the aging. As a result of these factors, the volume of distribution of water soluble (hydrophilic) drugs is generally decreased and that of fat soluble (lipophilic) drugs is increased. Moreover, changes in volume of distribution can directly affect the loading doses of medications. For many drugs, loading doses will be lower in older individuals compared to younger population.

Example: The volume of distribution of digoxin, a highly water-soluble drug is reduced in elderly as a consequence of reduction in body water and a smaller dose may be needed to provide adequate digitalization and to avoid potential toxicity. The volume of distribution of lipid soluble drugs like lignocaine is increased in old age because of increased body fat leading to increased half-life of the drug. So, this may result in prolonged drug effect and toxicity which may require dosage reduction.

Protein binding: Plasma protein binding may be reduced as a result of reduction in plasma albumin which is the major binding protein or as a result of changes in binding affinity due to aging. This results in an increased free concentration of extensively protein-bound drugs.

In contrast, the concentration of α-1 acid glycoprotein may be increased in the presence of chronic diseases that frequently occur in the geriatric population. This results in the increased binding of drugs such as antidepressants, antipsychotics, and β-blockers which are mainly bound to this protein. Hence, these drugs may be required in higher doses.

Cerebrovascular P-glycoprotein is responsible for the transport of drugs across the blood–brain barrier. Studies have shown that reduced P-glycoprotein activity in the blood–brain barrier is observed with aging. Hence, the permeability across the blood–brain barrier may also be altered in older adults thereby affecting the distribution drugs in the central nervous system.

Metabolism: Hepatic blood flow and liver mass change in proportion to body weight and decrease with aging there is a 40–50% decrease in hepatic blood flow in elderly compared to young. These changes alter the ability of the liver to metabolize the drugs. Drugs are metabolized by two types of reactions:

1. *Phase 1 (oxidation and reduction)*: Drugs that undergo phase 1 metabolism demonstrate reduced clearance with aging.
2. *Phase 2 (conjugation)*: It typically makes the drug biologically inactive and facilitates their excretion. It is not affected by aging.

Elimination: Renal excretion is primary route of elimination of many drugs and their metabolites. Aging is associated with a significant reduction in renal mass and number and size of nephrons. In addition, the glomerular filtration rate, tubular secretion, and renal blood flow decreases with aging. At all ages these three parameters are low in women than men.

The estimation of creatinine clearance serves as a useful screen for renal impairment. Serum creatinine level is an imperfect marker of renal function in elder adults because of reduced muscle mass with advanced age. Normal serum creatinine level does not indicate normal renal function in elderly. Current consensus is to continue to use Cockcroft and Gault equation for renal drug dosing in older adults.

$$\text{Creatinine clearance} = \frac{(140 - \text{age}) \times (\text{actual body weight})}{72 \times \text{Serum creatinine}}$$

For females multiply the result by 0.85.

Where age is in years, actual body weight in kilograms, and serum creatinine in milligrams per deciliter.

Example of medications to be used with caution in older adults with impaired renal functions are digoxin, spironolactone, gentamicin, colchicine, cotrimoxazole, glyburide, and nitrofurantoin.

PHARMACODYNAMICS

In contrast to the changes in pharmacokinetics, fewer data are available on the effect of aging on pharmacodynamics (drug response). Theoretically, altered pharmacodynamics could be due to two basic mechanisms:

1. Altered sensitivity because of changes in the number of receptors or affinity or changes in postreceptor response
2. Age-related impairment of physiologic and homeostatic mechanisms

Older adults are less sensitive to β-agonist and β-blockers and more sensitive to benzodiazepines, warfarin, opioids, and H1 antihistamines.

Homeostatic mechanisms that may become impaired with advanced age include postural or gait instability, orthostatic blood pressure responses, thermoregulation, cognitive reserve, and bowel and bladder function.

POLYPHARMACY

Polypharmacy is a major concern and is often categorized as a geriatric syndrome. Polypharmacy has the following negative aspects as follows:

- Unfavorable adherence
- Accumulated ADR risks
- Unexpected interactions
- Increased risk hospitalization
- Increased risk of medication errors
- Increased cost

Hence, polypharmacy is considered as an independent health-risk indicator.

Five or more simultaneously prescribed drugs are considered as threshold value to define critical polypharmacy. Apart from the mere number of drugs, interaction pattern, and cumulative ADR can add to the problem.

Main cause of polypharmacy is multimorbidity leading to the intake of multiple medications. Medications started for an acute problem continue to be used even after the acute episode is over.

Drug–drug interaction (DDI) and D-Dis-I leading to adverse reactions are common sequences of polypharmacy.

In the context of polypharmacy, the most significant rules are:

- Make a regular reassessment of the patient. Always try to discuss current medications with the patient.
- Try to find the best solution for the individual health situation together with the patient.

To avoid polypharmacy forced reduction of medication numbers in elderly has shown good results. Critical approval of medication schedule allows safe reduction of drugs. In any given situation, risk-benefit ratio needs to be estimated and the drug schedule should be optimized accordingly. Differentiated risk-benefit ratio for the elderly, especially with cognitive decline, is even more difficult.

COMPLIANCE OR ADHERENCE

Adherence is defined as accordance between patient behavior and prescribed therapy. The prevalence rate for nonadherence ranges from 15 to 96%. Since data of nonadherence is difficult to obtain even on well-controlled scientific studies, the range is wide. Nonadherence is higher in asymptomatic diseases [subclinical hypothyroidism (SHT) and dyslipidemia] rather than symptomatic diseases congestive cardiac failure (CCF).

Nonadherence is influenced by complex interplay of factors as given below:

Drug and therapy associated:

- Complexity of therapeutic schedule
- Application route

- Polypharmacy
- Risk-associated with therapy
- Medication package or container

Disease associated:
- Chronicity of disease
- Severity of disease
- Asymptomatic presentation

Patient associated:
- Aging changes (decreased visual acuity)
- Multimorbidity
- Polypharmacy
- Subclinical functional impairment (decreased cognition, swallowing difficulty, and arthritis)
- Educational status

Psychosocial aspects:
- Perception of disease and treatment barriers
- Patient-doctor relationship
- Access to medication or access to health systems
- Social issues such as caregiver support, financial support, and living alone

INTERVENTIONS TO IMPROVE ADHERENCE

- Interventions should be tailored to the individual.
- Most important aspect is assessment of functional and educational status.
- Elder friendly preparations such as small-sized tablets, liquid preparations, suppositories, and transdermal patches
- Avoiding child proof containers, using wide mouth bottles and using clear glass containers
- Keep medication schedule simple, avoid polypharmacy.
- Patient and caretakers' education
- Supervision and assistance by healthcare professionals, technical assistance and guidance in visually impaired, regular home visits, self-reporting service, pill counts, electronics monitoring of medications and health records, and monitoring drug levels
- *Regular medication review*: "Brown Bag review". In this, patient is asked to carry all their medications inside a bag (including the over-the-counter drugs and herbal and their products) and bring it during their consultation for inspection. This provides a good opportunity to assess the patient's understanding and adherence.
- Pharmacological care for older adults is time consuming, hence best done using a team approach.

MEDICATION-RELATED PROBLEMS

Medication-related problems can be due to:
- Medication administration errors
- Medication-related adverse drug events (**Fig. 1**)

MEDICATION ADMINISTRATION ERRORS

It occurs when there is problem in prescription, order communication, dispensing, adherence, and monitoring. Medication administration errors include errors in prescription and lack of awareness of incompatible drugs prescribed by others. Communication regarding right dose, right drug, right route, and right time is important. Dispensing in the correct preparation is essential (tablets, liquids, suppositories etc.) and administering in the correct route is equally important.

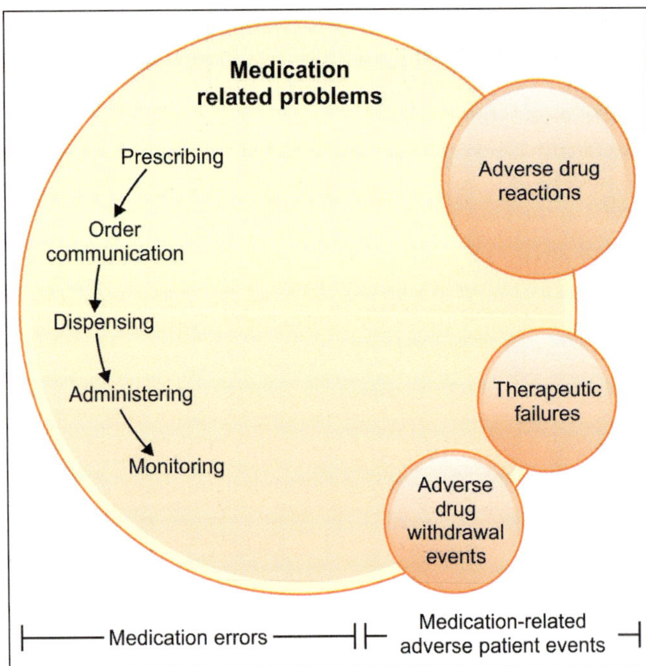

FIGURE 1: Medication related problems.

Monitoring and training of patient, caregiver, and healthcare personnel is essential. Use of barcoded unit dose medications, electronic medication administration records, and scanning patients' identification bracelets will further reduce this medication administration errors.

MEDICATION-RELATED ADVERSE DRUG EVENTS

Adverse drug events (ADE) is defined as injury resulting from the use of a drug.

Three types of ADE are as follows:
1. Adverse drug reaction (ADR)
2. Therapeutic failure (TF)
3. Adverse drug withdrawal event (ADWE)

Adverse drug event: Drug-related morbidity and mortality is an important area to improve quality of medical care and reduce healthcare cost of older population. In a 9-month study period of the ADE, 42 were preventable, <1% were fatal, 4% were life-threatening, and 72% were less serious. In the study, residents using anticoagulants, atypical antipsychotics, diuretics, anti-infective drugs, and antiepileptics were at greatest risk of ADE.

Adverse drug reaction: Any harmful or unwanted effects caused by drugs taken at the correct dosage and frequency. 35% of ambulatory adults experience one or more ADR annually. About 5–10% of hospital admissions are due to ADR. ADR may be due to multiple factors, out of which major factors are polypharmacy due to multiple comorbidities, altered pharmacokinetics, and dynamics and other factors such as prescription errors, lack of awareness of incompatible drug interaction, over-the-counter drugs, herbal drugs with unknown ingredients, and noncompliance of regular medications.

Adverse drug reactions are frequently overlooked in elderly. Diagnosis of ADR is difficult in older people, as the medical personnel may not tend to correlate the symptoms to drugs. More frequently overlooked disorders are depression, cognitive defect, and parkinsonism, all of which can be precipitated or aggravated by drugs. Among the large number of ADRs that are commonly seen, more serious ones are falls and acute confusion.

Diagnosis of ADR is primarily based on meticulous history, establishing temporal relationship between exposure to drugs and clinical manifestation and improvement on withdrawal or dosage reduction. ADRs in elderly often occur during first 1–2 weeks after starting treatment or increasing the dose. However, alteration in serum potassium due to diuretics, angiotensin-converting enzyme (ACE) inhibitors, angiotensin receptor blockers (ARBs), and Tardive dyskinesia due to antipsychotic drugs may take longer time to manifest. Most of the ADRs in elderly are due to the drug's known pharmacological effect, precipitated by drug interactions. Re-challenge is the most powerful diagnostic tool although it is unethical.

Treatment of suspected ADR is by drug withdrawal or reducing the dosage under monitoring. In cases where the patient deteriorates when the dose is reduced, it may be relevant to prescribe an additional drug to achieve therapeutic response.

Minor complaints caused by side effects are usually not a reason for withholding therapy and can be easily handled by reassuring the patient.

Adverse drug reactions can be avoided by choosing safe and effective drugs, applying correct therapeutic principles in prescribing like starting with a small dose, avoiding polypharmacy and frequent monitoring, and patient education. Many drugs are hazardous for long-term treatment to old people due to low margin of safety (low therapeutic index) or elimination reduced due to decreased renal function.

Determination of serum concentration is a valuable tool in geriatric practice for diagnosis of ADR and under-treatment. Hypoproteinemia and hypoalbuminemia in sick old may interfere with the distribution of highly protein-bound drugs. Hence, it may be reasonable to aim at lower half of the recommended therapeutic range when titrating doses for elderly.

Routine serum concentration determination may be appropriate for the following commonly used drugs such as aminoglycosides, digoxin, lithium, and theophylline.

Life-threatening and unusual reactions caused by newly approved drugs should be reported to National adverse drug reaction center. Early recognition of typical diseases as drug induced may save lives.

Adverse drug reactions are classified into two types:

1. *Type A*: Expected unwanted or exaggerated physiological effect of drugs. It is more common in elderly, e.g., β-blocker →bradycardia →syncope.
2. *Type B*: Less common results from idiosyncratic effect unrelated to drugs, e.g., anaphylaxis to penicillin.

Adverse drug reactions can be due to:

- *Drug–drug interaction*: Can lead to ADR by pharmacokinetics and pharmacodynamics mechanism. DDIs are the effect that the administration of one drug has on another drug (**Table 1**).
- *Drug–disease interaction*: Occurs when the underlying disease state makes a patient more susceptible to the unwanted physiological effect of the drug (**Table 2**).

Mantra is "Any new symptom in older adults is a medication side effect until proved otherwise." ADR should always be kept in differential diagnosis for evaluating a new or worsening complaint in the elderly.

ANTICHOLINERGIC BURDEN

Anticholinergic burden refers to the cumulative effects of using multiple medications with either weak or strong anticholinergic properties. Anticholinergic burden results in peripheral adverse effects such as constipation, dry mouth, tachycardia, urinary retention, decreased GI motility, visual disturbances and central effects such as dizziness, sedation, confusion, delirium, cognitive impairment, falls, and physical dysfunction. Therefore, routine assessment of anticholinergic burden should

TABLE 1 Drug–drug interaction and their effect.

Drugs	Interaction	Effect
Antacids interacting with digoxin, isoniazid, and antipsychotics	Interference between drug absorption	Decreased drug effectiveness
Warfarin, oral hypoglycemics, and aspirin	Displacement from binding proteins	Increased effects and risk of toxicity

TABLE 2 Disease-drug interaction and potential ADE.

Disease	Drug	Potential ADE
COPD, bronchial asthma	β-blockers	Bronchospasm
BPH	Anticholinergics	Urinary retention
Constipation	Anticholinergics, CCBs, narcotics	Obstruction, impaction
Peptic ulcer	NSAIDs, steroids, aspirin	Gastritis, UGI bleed
DM	Steroids	Hyperglycemia
HT	NSAIDs, steroids	Uncontrolled hypertension and cardiac failure
Cognitive impairment	Anticholinergics, psychotropics	Worsening

(BPH: benign prostatic hyperplasia; CCBs: calcium-channel blockers; COPD: chronic obstructive pulmonary disease; DM: diabetes mellitus; HT: hypertension; NSAIDs: nonsteroidal anti-inflammatory drugs; UGI: upper gastrointestinal)

be done in routine medication review of patients on polypharmacy.

Recently observed rise in the burden of psychiatric illnesses and the increasing trend for polypharmacy has led to a rise in the increased use of anticholinergic medications.

Older patients are more likely to experience adverse effects due to age-related changes in pharmacokinetics and pharmacodynamics, increased permeability of the blood–brain barrier, and age-related deficit in central cholinergic transmission.

Many older adults suffer from multiple chronic diseases and are commonly prescribed multiple medicines with an anticholinergic property. Anticholinergic burden increases when anticholinergics are prescribed for their anticholinergic effect. It also increases when drugs with anticholinergic side effects are co-prescribed along with these.

Several instruments have been developed and validated to determine the anticholinergic burden, some of which are ARS, ADS, anticholinergic cognitive burden scale (ACB), and drug burden index (DBI).

Of these scales, ADS and ARS scales are found to be more validated.

Anticholinergic drug scale: ADS score of some commonly used drugs (**Table 3**).

Development of country-specific anticholinergic scale for both clinical and research purpose is to be formulated. Anticholinergic burden is a strong predictor of cognitive and physical impairment, especially in the elderly population. It has been linked to an increased rate of falls, decline in cognitive function and memory, decline in activities in daily living, and higher mortality rate.

TABLE 3 ADS score of some commonly used drugs.

S. No.	Drugs	ADS score
1	Alprazolam	1
2	Aripiprazole	3
3	Atenolol	-
4	Captopril	2
5	Cetirizine	-
6	Chlorthalidone	3
7	Cimetidine	1
8	Codeine phosphate	1
9	Colchicine	1
10	Desloratadine	1
11	Diazepam	1
12	Digoxin	1
13	Fentanyl	1
14	Fluvoxamine	1
15	Furosemide	1
16	Hydrocortisone	1
17	Levodopa	-
18	Methylprednisolone	1
19	Metoprolol	-
20	Nifedipine	1
21	Prednisolone	1
22	Quetiapine	-
23	Ranitidine	2
24	Theophylline	1
25	Trihexyphenidyl	3
	Total	

Depending on the scores medications may be stopped or titrated.

PRESCRIPTION CASCADE

Prescribing cascade begins when an ADE is misinterpreted as a new medical condition (**Fig. 2**). An additional therapy may be started for this and the patient is at risk of developing an additional ADE due to this potentially unnecessary treatment. Prescription cascade is a very important aspect in elderly who are likely to be prescribed multiple drugs. Prescription cascade can be prevented only when the healthcare provider carefully considers the relationship between initiation of new drug therapy, adverse problems of that therapy, and the development of new symptoms.

Examples of prescription cascade include:

- Metoclopramide when administered produces extrapyramidal symptoms which are identified as parkinsonism features and patient will be started on levodopa.
- Hydrochlorothiazide therapy increases uric acid levels and precipitates gout for which anti-gout therapy is initiated without considering it to be the side effect of hydrochlorothiazide.
- Nonsteroidal anti-inflammatory drug administration can lead to fluid retention and hypertension for which antihypertensive may be started unnecessarily.

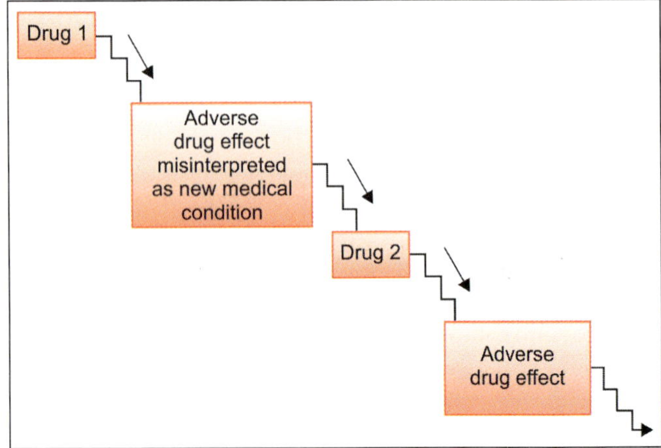

FIGURE 2: Prescribing cascade.

QUALITY OF PRESCRIBING

Optimizing drug therapy means achieving balance between overprescribing of inappropriate therapy and underprescribing of beneficial therapy. Various criteria are developed internationally to assess the quality of medication use in older adults.

- *Beers criteria*: One of the most widely employed criteria for assessment of inappropriate prescribing. Beers criteria was developed in 1991 and revised and updated in 2015. The updated criteria included 40 potentially problematic medications divided into five lists.
  - First and second list—details of potentially inappropriate medication for most of older people or for those with specific conditions
  - Third list—gives list of drugs used with considerable caution.
  - Fourth and fifth list—gives list of clinically important DDI. Lists of medicines to be avoided are used cautiously for people with impaired renal function.

  Beers criteria includes only small fraction of medications implicated in ADE.
- *Assessing Care of Vulnerable Elders*: Acove not only addresses potentially inappropriate medications but also includes the
  - Need to document indication of new therapy
  - Patient education on risks and benefits
  - Need to maintain current medication list in patient records
  - Importance of documenting for response therapy
  - Need for periodic review (annual)
- *STOPP criteria*: STOPP criteria is the screening tool that can detect potential errors in commission.

  Developed initially in 2008, these criteria identified potentially inappropriate prescribing including DDI, D-Dis-I, drugs that increase the risk of fall, and duplicate prescription. Potentially inappropriate medications included in the STOPP criteria have been associated with avoidable ADE leading to hospitalization.

  STOPP-2 version criteria 2014 lists 80 evidence-based potentially inappropriate prescription for older adults and categorizes medication according to organ system. For example:
  - Loop diuretics to be avoided for dependent ankle edema, without clinical signs of cardiac failure.
  - Nonsteroidal anti-inflammatory drugs in the presence of renal failure.
- *START criteria*: START criteria is the screening tool that can detect omission in the therapy of elderly patient.

  This criteria identifies the potential underuse of beneficial medications. As with other criteria this can be used as a guide and not substitute for clinical judgment. For example:
  - Warfarin therapy for chronic atrial fibrillation
  - ACE inhibitor or ARB in diabetic nephropathy.
- *Medication appropriateness index (MAI)*: MAI is another implicit screening tool for assessing the quality of prescription. Details of which is given below:

Item	Score
Is there an indication for the drug?	3
Is the medication effective for the condition?	3
Is the dosage correct?	2
Are the directions correct?	2
Are the directions practical?	1
Are there clinically significant drug–drug interaction?	2
Are there clinically significant drug–disease interaction?	2
Is there unnecessary duplication with other drugs?	1
Is the duration of therapy acceptable?	1
Is this drug the least expensive alternative compare to others of equal utility?	1
Total	**18**

(0: indicates the medication which is inappropriate, 18: indicates maximum appropriateness)

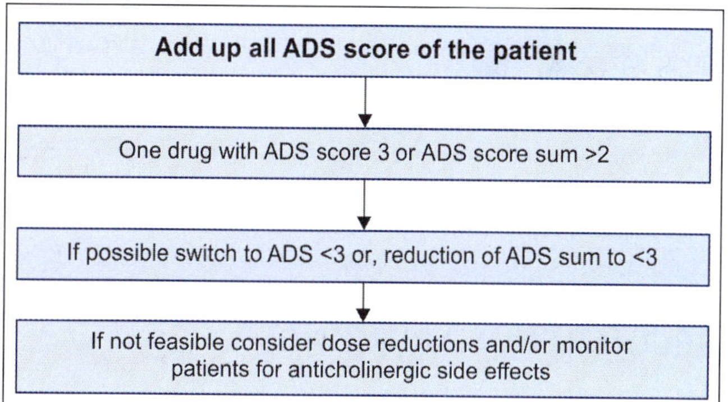

FLOWCHART 1: Steps of reconciliation of drugs.

MEDICATION RECONCILIATION

Medical reconciliation is defined as the process of identifying the most accurate list of all medications that the patient is taking including name, dosage, frequency, and route by comparing the medical records to an external list of medications obtained from a patient hospital or other provider.

This reconciliation is done to avoid medication errors such as omission, duplication, dosing errors, and drug interactions. Patients, physicians, nurses, and pharmacists should be involved in the medication-reconciliation process.

The steps of reconciliation of drugs are shown in **Flowchart 1**.

KEY POINTS

Drug therapy has potential for both helpful and harmful effects in geriatric population. The balance can be achieved by adhering to the following principles:

- Prescribe only for specific and rationale indications

- Know the pharmacology (pharmacokinetics and pharmacodynamics) of the medication in relation to age.
- "Start low and go slow", final dose can be adjusted according to individuals' tolerability. Wait for at least three half-lives before increasing the dose.
- Maintain high index of suspicion regarding drug reaction and interactions (drug-drug and D-Dis-I)
- Monitor for the adverse drug events—an important cause of geriatric syndromes such as falls and acute confusion.
- Slowly taper the medications to prevent/minimize adverse drug withdrawal events.
- Establish clear feasible therapeutic endpoints.
- Simplify the regimen. Once daily or maximum twice daily. Reduce the number of drugs whenever possible.
- Decide on the preferable preparation and route of administration for that patient.
- Large labels on prescription bottles and color coding for visually impaired.
- Physical disability such as tremor, arthritis, and visual problems to be assessed before initiating therapy.
- Health education to the patient and the caregiver
- Social issues such as living alone, cost factor, and caregiver support to be addressed before initiating long-term drugs.
- Careful drug history with regard to regular medications, over-the-counter medications and herbal preparations.
- Periodic review (Brown bag technique) and discontinuation of unnecessary drugs are essential.

RECOMMENDED READINGS

1. Khanna S. Polypharmacy in elderly. In: Sharma OP, Shankar PS (Eds). Management issues in Geriatric care, 1st edition. New Delhi: Rishikul Publication; 2020. pp.148-51.
2. Offerhaus L. Drugs for elderly, 2nd edition. New Delhi: Prentice-hall of India Private limited; 1998. pp. 5-34.
3. Katzung BG. Special aspects of geriatric pharmacology. In: Katzung BG, Marslow SB, Trevor A (Eds). Basic and clinical pharmacology, 12th Edition. New Delhi: McGraw-Hill Education India Pvt. Ltd; 2012. pp. 1151-6.
4. Buxton ILO. Principles of prescription order writing and patient compliance. In: Brunton L, Chabner B, Klollman B (Eds). Goodman and Gilman Pharmacological Basics of Therapeutics, 12th Edition. New Delhi: McGraw-Hill Education India Pvt. Ltd.; 2012. pp. 879-90.
5. Rochon PA, Gill SS, Gurwitz JH. Chapter 24: General principles of Pharmacology and appropriate Prescribing. In: Halter JB, Ouslader JG, (Eds). Hazard textbook of geriatric medicine and gerentology, 7th Edition. New Delhi: McGraw-Hill Education India Pvt. Ltd.; 2017. pp. 401-24.
6. Naples JG, handler SM, Maber RL, Jr., Schmader KE, Hanlon JT. Geriatric Pharmacotherapy and polypharmacy. In: Fillit HM, Rockwood K, Young J (Eds). Brocklehurst's Textbook of Geriatric Medicine and Gerontology, 8th edition. Philadelphia: Elsevier Pvt Ltd.; 2010.pp. 811-2.
7. Oscar A, Cerpeda, Marley JE. Polypharmacy. In: Sinclair AJ, Morley JE, Vellas B (Eds). Pathy's principles and practices of Geriatric Medicine, 5th edition, Volume 1. United States: Wiley-Blackwell; 2012. pp. 154-68.
8. Marcum ZA, Hanlon JT. Inappropriate medication use and medication errors in the elderly. In: Wehling M (Ed). Drug therapy for the elderly. Austria: springer-verlag wien; 2013. pp. 43-9.
9. Burkhardt H. Heterogeneity and vulnerability of older patients, polypharmacy and adherence to pharmacotherapy in the elderly. In: Wehling M (Ed). Drug therapy for the elderly. Austria: Springer-Verlag Wien; 2013. pp. 3-9, 319-29, 313-8.
10. Wehling M. Age-associated general pharmacological aspects. In: Wehling M (Ed). Drug therapy for the elderly. Austria: Springer-Verlag Wien; 2013. pp. 21-34.
11. Slattum PW, Ogbonna EC, Peron EP. Chapter 26: The pharmacology of aging. In: Fillit HM, Rockwood K, Young J (Eds). Brocklehurst's Textbook of Geriatric medicine and Gerontology, 8th edition. Philadelphia: Elsevier Pvt Ltd. pp. 160-5.
12. Steinman MA, Holmes HM. Principles of prescribing for older adults. In: Williams BA, Williams CA, Ahalit C, Conant R, Ritchie C, Chen H, Landefeld S, Yukawa M (Eds). Current diagnosis and treatment, 2nd edition. New delhi: McGraw-Hill Education India Pvt. Ltd.; 2014. pp. 46-57.
13. Gupta YK, Ramachandran S. Pharmacology of aging. In: Sanchetee P (Ed). Textbook of Geriatric Medicine, 1st edition. New Delhi: Paras Medical Publisher; 2009. pp. 51-7.
14. Bennett PN, Brown MJ. General pharmacology. In: Horne T (Ed). Clinical pharmacology, 10th edition. Toronto: Churchill Livingstone Elsevier; 2009. pp. 109-10.
15. Lisibach A, Benelli V, Ceppi MG, Waldner-Knogler K, Csajka C, Lutters M. Quality of anticholinergic burden scales and their impact on clinical outcomes a systemic review. Eur J clin pharmacol. 2020:1-6.
16. Carnahan RM, Lund BC, Perry PJ, Pollock BG, Culp KR. The Anticholinergic Drug scale as a measure of Drug Related Anticholinergic Burden: Associations with Serum Anticholinergic Activity. J clin pharmacol. 2006;46(12):1481-6.

CHAPTER

30

Infections in Elderly

Jyotirmoy Pal, Arkapravo Hati, Tanuka Mandal

ABSTRACT

The risk of infection in elderly has been increased by multiple risk factors, which include preexisting comorbidities, malnutrition, immune senescence, and various social determinants of health. The absence of clinical presentations such as fever, productive cough, and other classic signs in older individuals pose a challenge in the diagnosis of pneumonia. Risk factors for infection caused by resistant pathogens include functional impairment, recent hospitalization, previous antibiotic treatment, the presence of indwelling devices, and severe illness. Hence, it is very important to have an interdisciplinary approach to management. Preventive measures, which diminish the incidence and severity of pneumonia in elderly, include active immunization against influenza and pneumococcus.

Both asymptomatic bacteriuria (ASB) and urinary tract infection (UTI) are the most common reasons for prescribing antibiotics in the community and healthcare settings. Distinguishing between ASB and symptomatic UTI is problematic and many older adults do not present with classical signs of UTI. Human immunodeficiency virus (HIV) infection remains unrecognized in older adults because of the bias that older adults are not at risk and dismissal of clinical clues (frequent pneumonia, weight loss, and progressive cognitive decline) as typical of older age. Increasing age and impaired cellular immunity are the strongest risk factors for herpes zoster; other risk factors include white race, female sex, psychological stress, and physical trauma.

"Wrinkles should merely indicate where smiles have been"

—Mark Twain

PREDISPOSING FACTORS

Infections in elderly adults aged 65 years and more is the primary cause of mortality in majority of cases. In comparison to younger adults, persons belonging to geriatric age group possess certain predispositions to infectious diseases due to several risk factors. Factors which make elderly adults prone to various infections and in turn make them vulnerable to functional disability and increased morbidity and mortality include:

Immune senescence: T cell aging and senescence of the regulatory T cells function; lesser ability of the dendritic cells to stimulate influenza specific CD8+ T cell-mediated cytotoxic response; decrease in natural killer (NK) cells function along with poor expression of receptors such as NKp30 and NKp46; impaired neutrophil migration to the site of infection; weakening of the humoral immunity with age; and drug-induced acquired immunodeficiency (due to prolonged use of steroids and other immunomodulators) are some of the proposed mechanisms.

Comorbid conditions: Comorbidities such as hypertension, diabetes mellitus, chronic pulmonary disease, renal insufficiency, and peripheral vascular disease increase the risk of infection in the geriatric population thereby increasing the mortality and morbidity.

Nutritional deficiencies: Malnutrition in elderly population increases risk of injury and infections. Micronutrients have a role in antibody formation. In frail elderly patients, declination of lean body mass and muscle weakness has been linked with mortality.

- Metabolic disorders, lower socioeconomic status and environmental factors, and poor mental state

RESPIRATORY TRACT INFECTIONS

PNEUMONIA

- It has often been the terminal infectious disease event and one of the leading causes of severe sepsis in geriatric population.
- Adults, 65 years and older, are more susceptible to pneumonia than younger people and the annual incidence of pneumonia in elderly is four times that of younger populations.

Clinical definition: More than and equal to two symptoms + more than and equal to 1 sign + radiological finding from following:

Symptom	Sign	Radiological finding
1. Fever 2. Chill 3. Cough 4. Pleuritic chest pain	1. Hyperthermia/ hypothermia 2. Tachypnea 3. Dullness upon percussion 4. Crackles 5. Wheezing 6. Pleural rub	1. New opacity on chest X-ray not due to other conditions [e.g., congestive heart failure (CHF), vasculitis, pulmonary infarction, atelectasis]

Predisposing factors for pneumonia:

- *Changes in immune system*:
  - Less naïve T cells, more memory T cells
  - Altered T cell distribution (less CD4+, more CD8+)
  - B lymphocyte deficiency
  - Less response to T cell receptor (TCR) stimulation
  - Reduced T cell proliferation
  - Cytokine imbalance [decrease in interleukin-1 (IL-1), IL-2, and interferon (IFN) and increase in IL-4, IL-6, IL-8, IL-10, and tumor necrosis factor (TNF)]
- Reduced barrier function of respiratory tracts due to:
  - Altered mucosal barrier causing increased bacterial adherence
  - Slower/less coordinated ciliary function
- Reduced compliance of chest wall and increased compliance of lungs leading to increased residual volume and decreased forced expiratory volume in 1 second (FEV_1)
- More colonization of respiratory tract with gram-negative bacteria

Pathogenesis:

- Most commonly produced by microaspiration of colonizing flora of oropharynx and sinuses.
- Risk factors of microaspiration:
  - Male gender
  - Dementia
  - Chronic obstructive pulmonary disease (COPD)
  - Antipsychotics and proton pump inhibitor use
- Other sources of infection include:
  - Direct inhalation of infectious agent [tuberculosis (TB), influenza virus, and fungi]
  - Hematogenous spread (especially if *Staphylococcus* pneumonia after a viral influenza infection)
  - Contiguous spread from a subphrenic abscess
  - Iatrogenic contamination via endotracheal tube

Etiology:

- The common agents are *Streptococcus pneumoniae* (20–65%), *Haemophilus influenzae*, gram-negative bacilli, atypical organisms (*Legionella, Mycoplasma,* and *Chlamydophila*), viruses (influenza virus, respiratory syncytial virus, and human metapneumovirus).

Clinical presentation:

- Differs from classical presentation in young population
- Atypical presentation is most common which includes:
  - Exacerbation of chronic disease
  - Altered behavior/mental status
  - Acute functional impairment
  - Loss of consciousness
  - Generalized weakness
  - Anorexia
  - Dehydration
  - Incontinence
- Absences of fever, hypoxemia, or respiratory symptoms do not rule out pneumonia.

Evaluation and prognosis scoring: Risk stratification can be done by both PSI and CURB-65 score but they are not very useful scales for assessing the need for ICU admission as both have certain limitations. Various studies have suggested oxygenation as the best prognostic indicator in older persons.

Other scales like Severity of Community Acquired pneumonia (SCAP), American Thoracic Society/Infectious Disease Society of America (ATS/IDSA), and SMART-COP have been developed for making decision regarding ICU admission. All of them are depicted in **Tables 1** to **5**.

TABLE 1 Pneumonia severity index (PSI).

Patient characteristics	Number of points
Demographic factors	
Age	
Men	Age in year
Women	Age in years-10
Nursing home resident	Age plus ten
Coexisting illnesses (definitions listed below)	
Neoplastic disease	30
Liver disease	20
Congestive heart failure	10
Cerebrovascular disease	10
Renal disease	10
Physical examination findings	
Altered mental status	20
Respiratory rate >30/min	20
Systolic blood pressure <90 mm Hg	20
Temperature <35°C (95°F) or >40°C (104°F)	15
Pulse rate >125/min	10
Laboratory and roentgenographic findings	
Arterial pH <7.35	30
Blood urea nitrogen >30 mg/dL (11 mmol/L)	20
Sodium <130 mmol/L	20
Glucose >250 mg/dL (14 mmol/L)	10
Hematocrit <30%	10
Partial pressure of arterial oxygen <60 mm Hg	10
Pleural effusion	10

Risk class	Criteria
I	• Age <50 years • No existing illnesses or vital sign abnormalities
II	<70 points
III	71–90 points
IV	91–130 points
V	>131 points

Note: Assessment of severity of pneumonia should be done according to the clinical situation, laboratory markers and risk stratification scales. Chances of infection by resistant micro-organisms is increased in severe cases with associated risk factors which require proper assessment and treatment with appropriate antimicrobial therapy.

TABLE 2 Prognostic scales: CURB-65.

A point is assigned for the below mentioned items present	
C	**Confusion**
U	Urea >44 mg/dL (BUN >19.6 mg/dL)
R	Respiratory rate ≥30 bpm
B	Systolic BP <90 mm Hg or diastolic BP ≤60 mm Hg
65	Age ≥65 years old
Score	**Stratification**
0 or 1	Low mortality (0.7–2.1%). Possible outpatient treatment
2	Intermediate mortality (9.2%). Consider hospital treatment
3	High mortality (14.5%). Hospital admission
4–5	Mortality of >40%. Admission. Consider intensive care unit

(BP: blood pressure; BUN: blood urea nitrogen)

TABLE 3 Prognostic scales: Severity of community-acquired pneumonia (SCAP).

Major criteria	Minor criteria
• pH <7.30 (13 points) • Systolic blood pressure <90 mm Hg (11 points)	• C: Confusion (5 points) • U: BUN >30 mg/dL (5 points) • R: Breaths per minute >30 (9 points) • X: Multilobar/bilateral chest X-ray (5 points) • O: PaO_2 <54 mm Hg or PaO_2/FiO_2 <250 mm Hg (6 points) • 80: Age ≥80 years (5 points)

Low-risk: 0–1 (<10 points); intermediate risk: 2 (10–19 points); high risk: 3–4 (>20 points)

(BUN: blood urea nitrogen; FiO_2: fraction of inspired oxygen; PaO2: partial pressure of oxygen)

TABLE 4 Prognostic scales: ATS/IDSA.

ATS/IDSA	
Major criteria	**Minor criteria**
• Septic shock • Need for mechanical ventilation	• Confusion • Urea ≥45 mg/dL • Respiratory rate ≥30 bpm • Systolic blood pressure <90 mm Hg requiring fluid • Multilobar involvement (≥2 lobes) or progression • PaO_2/FiO_2 ≤250 • Leukopenia <4,000/mm^3 • Thrombocytopenia <100,000/mm^3 • Hypothermia (temperature <97°F or 36°C) • Metabolic acidosis • Lactate >3 mmol/L or >27 mg/dL • Hyponatremia • Hyperglycemia in nondiabetic • Alcohol intak

(ATS: American Thoracic Society; FiO_2: fraction of inspired oxygen; IDSA: Infectious Diseases Society of America; PaO_2: partial pressure of oxygen)

TABLE 5 Prognostic scales: SMART-COP

S	Systolic BP <90 mm Hg (2 points)	C	Confusion (1 point)
M	Multilobar affectation (1 point)	O	Oxygenation age-adjusted[b] (2 points)
A	Albumin <3.5 g/dL (1 point)	P	pH <7.35 (2 point)
R	RR age-adjusted[a] (1 point)		
T	Tachycardia ≥125 (1 point)		

- 0–2 points: Low risk for vasopressor support or intensive respiratory support.
- 3–4 points: Moderate risk for vasopressor support or intensive respiratory support.
- 5–6 points: High risk for vasopressor support or intensive respiratory support.
- ≥7 points: Very high risk for vasopressor support or intensive respiratory support.

[a] <50 years: ≥25/min; ≥50 years: ≥30/min.

[b] <50 years: PaO_2 <70 mm Hg or oxygen saturation ≤93% or PaO_2/FiO_2 <333; ≥50 years: PaO_2 < 60 mm Hg or oxygen saturation ≤90% or PaO_2/FiO_2 <250.

(FiO_2: fraction of inspired oxygen; PaO_2: partial pressure of oxygen)

Treatment: Treatment of community-acquired pneumonia in elderly is given in **Table 6**.

Special points in management of pneumonia in elderly:

- Meta-analysis had shown that 7 days antibiotic therapy is enough for treating pneumonia in geriatric population and antibiotic therapy is extended if the organism is *Legionella*, resistant gram-negative bacteria or methicillin-resistant *Staphylococcus aureus* (MRSA), persistent fever >72 hours, persistence of ≥1 criteria of clinical instability, and inadequate initial coverage.
- Treatment failure may occur probably due to resistant microorganism, unusual pathogen, lack in treatment for comorbidity and undiagnosed concomitant disease like neoplasm, and is associated with fivefold increase in mortality.
- Concomitant treatment with proper oxygenation, maintaining fluid balance, correcting electrolyte disturbances if present, adequate glycemic control, prevention of thromboembolic events, and early mobilization.

Prevention:

- Vaccination against pneumococcus and influenza is recommended for all patients aged ≥65 years.
- The 13-valent pneumococcal conjugate vaccine (PCV 13) and 23-valent pneumococcal polysaccharide vaccine (PPV23) are recommended (**Flowchart 1**).
- The medications that potentiate aspiration (e.g., sedatives and antipsychotics) should be avoided.

INFLUENZA

Geriatric population is at more risk than younger population for influenza complications due to presence of comorbidities such as chronic lung disease, congestive cardiac failure, and other metabolic diseases.

Clinical presentation:

- Presentation is often atypical.

TABLE 6 Treatment of community-acquired pneumonia in elderly.

	Scenario	Treatment
Patient without frailty	Outpatient treatment	Amoxicillin/clavulanate or second-generation cephalosporin + Azithromycin or fluoroquinolone
	Inpatient treatment	Amoxicillin/clavulanate or ceftriaxone or cefotaxime or ceftaroline + Azithromycin or fluoroquinolone
	Severe pneumonia	Ceftriaxone or cefotaxime or ceftaroline or ertapenem + Azithromycin or fluoroquinolone ± Linezolid[a] or vancomycin[a] ± Antipseudomonal β-lactam[b] ± Oseltamivir[c]
Patient with frailty	Prefrailty[d]	Amoxicillin/clavulanate or ceftriaxone or cefotaxime or ceftaroline + Azithromycin or fluoroquinolone
	Frail	Ertapenem or Amoxicillin/clavulanate[e] or Ceftriaxone + clindamycin[e]

[a] If there are risk factors for *Staphylococcus aureus*; [b] If there are risk factors for infection by *Pseudomonas aeruginosa;* [c] Assess if influenza is epidemic in the community; [d] Be particularly cautious rating risk factors of microaspiration and multiresistant bacteria; [e] Consider local resistance rates of *Enterobacteriaceae* to amoxicillin-clavulanic and ceftriaxone; and and anaerobes to clindamycin.

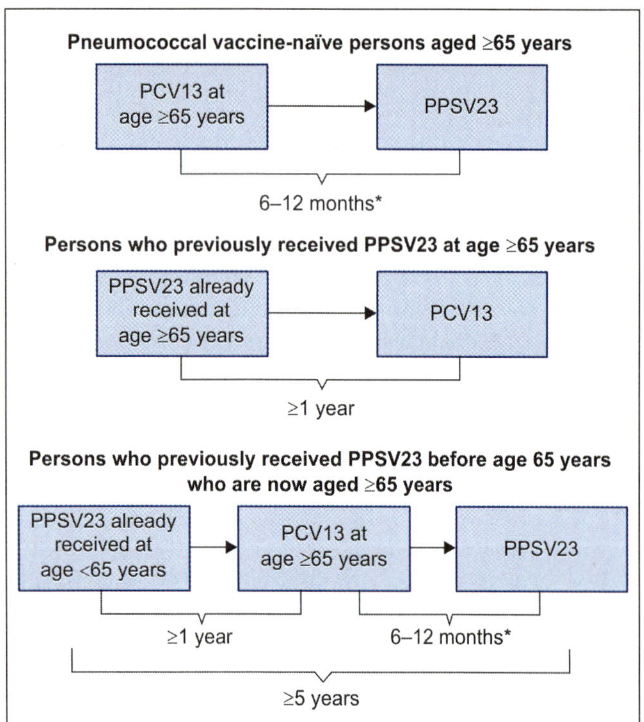

* Minimum interval between sequential administration of PCV13 and PPSV23 is 8 weeks; PPSV23 can be given later than 6–12 months after PCV13 is this window is missed.

(PCV13: 13-valent pneumococcal conjugate vaccine; PPSV23: 23-valent pneumococcal polysaccharide vaccine)

FLOWCHART 1: Sequential administration and recommended intervals for PCV13 and PCV23 for adults aged ≥65 years.

- Common clinical presentations include cough, change in baseline temperature, and exacerbation of chronic conditions [(COPD and congestive heart failure (CHF)].

Diagnosis: Reverse transcription polymerase chain reaction (RT-PCR) is the gold standard for the diagnosis of influenza. **Table 7** shows summary of test characteristics of different diagnostic tests for various respiratory viral pathogens in elderly.

Treatment: Antivirals are mainstay of treatment (**Table 8**).

Vaccination:

- Inactivated influenza vaccine (IIV) is recommended for adults (65 years or more)
- IIV contains components of H1N1, H3N2, and B strain.
- Immune response is poor in elder population, so a high dose *(four times dose than the normal)* inactivated vaccine *[IIV-high dose (IIV-HD)]* has been licensed with same strains. *It is 24% more effective.*
- It has to be administered annually.
- Vaccination of healthcare workers with live attenuated vaccine is useful in preventing outbreaks.

PULMONARY TUBERCULOSIS

- Pulmonary TB is the most common form of TB in the elderly population.
- Extrapulmonary sites are common and include the bones and joints (particularly the spine) and the genitourinary tract.
- Older patients with pulmonary TB can present with typical respiratory as well as systemic symptoms (e.g.,

TABLE 7 Summary of the diagnostic tests for respiratory viral pathogens in elderly.

	Culture	Rapid EIA	DFA/IFA	PCR	Serology
Influenza A	++	+	+	+++	++[a]
Influenza B	++	+	+	+++	++[a]
RSV	+	+/–	+/–	+++	+++

+/– available but poor sensitivity; + fair sensitivity; ++ good sensitivity; +++ optimal sensitivity

[a] Interpretation complicated by vaccination.

(DFA: direct fluorescent antibody; EIA: enzyme immunoassay; IFA: Immunofluorescence assay; PCR: polymerase chain reaction; RSV: respiratory syncytial virus)

TABLE 8 Antiviral therapy of influenza.

M2 proton channel antagonists		Neuraminidase inhibitors		
• **Amantadine (oral)**	• **Rimantadine (oral)**	• **Zanamivir (inhaled)** • May worsen or produce respiratory distress if underlying obstructive disease	• **Oseltamivir (oral)** • Dosing should be based on renal function	• **Peramivir (IV)**
• Only active against influenza A • Current strains are resistant to both, so not used currently		• Active against both A and B strains • 70% effective in prophylaxis • 90% effective as treatment to reduce clinical severity when given within 48 h of symptom onset		• FDA approval on 2015

(FDA: Food and Drug Administration; IV: intravenous)

fever, sputum production, hemoptysis, night sweats, weight loss, and anorexia), a significant number of such patients may manifest atypical complaints or may exhibit minimal pulmonary symptoms.

- Miliary, or disseminated, TB occurs with greater frequency in elderly which is typically associated with an acute or subacute pattern of high, intermittent fever. and clinical evidence of meningeal or serosal involvement.
- Tuberculous meningitis in elderly patients results from reactivation of a primary dormant focus or in association with miliary seeding of infection which may present with a subacute onset of fever, headache, and confusion, and can also manifest with unexplained dementia or obtundation without fever or nuchal rigidity.

Pathogenesis:

- As the T cell-mediated response of the immune system is mainly affected in elderly, dermal reactivity to tuberculin must be evaluated carefully.
- Approximately 90% of cases of TB disease in elderly persons are caused by reactivation of primary infection and immunosenescence or immune dysregulation plays a role in the recrudescence of prior infection.
- However, other comorbidities and age-related diseases (e.g., malignancy and diabetes mellitus), poor nutrition, immunosuppression, chronic renal failure, and chronic hospitalization, contribute to the increased risk of TB in the older population.
- Risk for TB in elderly individuals includes those who are not exposed to *Mycobacterium tuberculosis*, those with latent primary infection that may reactivate, and those who are no longer infected and thus are at risk for reinfection.

URINARY TRACT INFECTIONS

- UTI is the most common infection in geriatric population.
- Second most common infection in hospitalized geriatric population.
- Incidence and prevalence increases with increasing age.

Some definitions: Some important definitions are given in **Table 9**.

Pathogenesis:

- In geriatric population, dysfunction of these defenses occurs, resulting in high rates of ASB.
- Depending on host condition and virulence of organism, ASB can result in urethritis, cystitis, or pyelonephritis.
- In most cases, the infection is ascending, i.e., colonization of organism in periurethral area ascend toward kidney.
- UTI secondary to bacteremia is rare but should be suspected if *Staphylococcus aureus* is isolated in patients without catheterization.

Microbiology:

The etiologic agents are *Escherichia coli* (most common) and other *Enterobacteriaceae* such as *Klebsiella pneumonia*, *Proteus mirabilis*, gram-positive organisms such as *Enterococcus species* and group B and D *Streptococcus*, and rarely *Pseudomonas species*, *Acinetobacter*, *Candida species*, and MRSA.

TABLE 9	Common definitions regarding UTI.
Asymptomatic bacteriuria	Broadly defined as a urinary pathogen isolated in appropriate quantitative counts from a urine culture in adults without genitourinary tract signs or symptoms **In older women:** Two consecutive clean-catch midstream urine samples growing at least 10^5 colony-forming units/mL with no more than two species of microorganisms or a single *catheterized* urine specimen with one uropathogen isolated in a quantitative count $\geq 10^2$ cfu/mL **In older men:** One clean-catch midstream urine samples growing at least 105 colony forming units/mL with no more than two species of microorganisms or a single *catheterized* urine specimen with one uropathogen isolated in a quantitative count $\geq 10^2$ cfu/mL
Pyuria	Presence of ≥10 white blood cells (WBC/mm^3) per high power field (hpf) in a urine specimen
Uncomplicated UTI	Symptomatic bladder infection in immunocompetent women without structural or functional urologic abnormalities
Complicated UTI	Symptomatic bladder infection in adults with structural or functional abnormalities, urinary catheters, or systemic illness
Recurrent UTI	≥3 confirmed urinary tract infections within a 12-month period or ≥2 symptomatic UTIs in a 6-month period following clinical resolution of each infection with antimicrobial treatment
Catheter-associated UTI	Signs or symptoms of a UTI in adults who have an indwelling urethral or suprapubic catheter, perform intermittent catheterization, or in those whose catheters have been removed within the previous 48 h and ≥103 cfu/mL of ≥1 bacterial species in a single catheter urine specimen

(UTI: urinary tract infection)

Diagnosis and management:

- UTI is considered as the most common indication for antibiotic treatment in elderly.
- Antibiotic overuse can lead to negative consequences such as development of multidrug-resistant organisms, unusual side effects (such as *Clostridium difficile* infection), and increased healthcare costs.
- It is a bit challenging to differentiate symptomatic UTI from ASB and treatment of ASB is a common reason for which antibiotics are prescribed.
- Treatment for uncomplicated UTI in older adults is similar to younger individuals.
- It is now recommended to start with nitrofurantoin monohydrate 100 mg twice daily for 5 days, or trimethoprim–sulfamethoxazole 160/800 mg twice daily for 3 days, if local resistance rates do not exceed 20%.
- *E. coli* has shown low resistance to nitrofurantoin; however, other *Enterobacteriaceae* species, which are more common in elderly, may have intrinsic resistance to nitrofurantoin.
- Nitrofurantoin is contraindicated in patients with chronic kidney disease, whose prevalence is increased in older adults.
- Therefore, trimethoprim–sulfamethoxazole should be the preferred empiric oral option for treatment of clinically suspected UTI in older adults keeping in mind the local resistance rates which will guide the empiric antibiotic choices.
- Fluoroquinolones are the most prescribed antibiotics for UTI, but due to their high resistance, they should only be prescribed if sensitivity testing suggests.
- Treatment of ASB is only recommended in older adults prior to transurethral resection of the prostate and any urologic procedures for which mucosal bleeding is anticipated.

OTHER INFECTIONS

HUMAN IMMUNODEFICIENCY VIRUS

- Initial complaints of an undiagnosed elderly person can vary from nonspecific constitutional symptoms to those resembling an acquired immunodeficiency syndrome (AIDS)-defining disease and both normal age-related changes in immune function and poor nutrition may confound the differential diagnosis or contribute to disease progression.
- Although the perception exists that the elderly are not at great risk for HIV disease, data from the national AIDS behavior surveys indicates that 10% of persons over 50 years of age have, at minimum, one risk factor for infection.
- As older patients may not spontaneously report the high-risk behaviors, diagnosis and treatment are delayed compared to younger patients.
- Treatment should begin immediately after diagnosis, regardless of the CD4 cell count.
- A combination regimen is recommended with at least three daily medications, either non-nucleoside reverse transcriptase inhibitor or a protease inhibitor and two nucleoside reverse transcriptase inhibitors considering HIV-1 ribonucleic acid (RNA) viral resistance profile, pre-existing organ system injury, mental illness, or, in the case of abacavir, genetic susceptibility to toxicity.
- Patients should be closely monitored for first several months to ensure suppression of HIV-1 levels and other adverse events, although less frequent monitoring can be done after first 6–12 months in patients who have achieved viral suppression with no active issues and CD4 count more than 350 cells/mL.
- HIV-associated neurocognitive disorders (HANDs) like depression and severe mental illnesses such as psychosis and post-traumatic stress disorder and cognitive dysfunction attributed to cognitive diseases of aging (multi-infarct dementia or Alzheimer's disease)

or from HIV (minor cognitive motor disorder or HIV-associated dementia), and progression to dementia are common in elderly population.

- HIV-infected individuals with hepatitis C coinfection experience more rapid progression of liver cirrhosis and a heighted risk of hepatocellular cancer. Suppression of HIV-1 RNA with ARV treatment slows progression of liver disease among those coinfected with hepatitis C.

HERPES-ZOSTER VIRUS INFECTION

- Herpes zoster is characterized by unilateral, dermatomal pain, and rash (maculopapular or vesicular). Post-herpetic neuralgia (PHN) is pain 90 or more days after rash onset.
- Reactivation may occur after initial recovery from varicella-zoster virus (VZV) infection as cell-mediated immunity wanes in older individuals.
- In immunosuppressed patients, the lesions may cross dermatomes with most lesions developing between dermatomes T1 and L2.
- The ophthalmic (first) division of the trigeminal nerve is affected in 15% of cases and the adjacent dermatomes are affected in 20% of cases, and lesions occasionally cross the midline, especially on the back.

Diagnosis:

- Herpes zoster is typically a clinical diagnosis.
- Identification of herpes zoster may be difficult during the prodrome, but the typical appearance of exanthem aids in diagnosis.
- PCR testing of vesicle or other body fluids is preferred as it is rapid and also highly sensitive and specific (95% and 100%, respectively) for diagnosis.

Management:

- *Antiviral agents* such as acyclovir (800 mg five times a day for 7 days), famciclovir (500 mg every 8 h for 7 days), and valaciclovir (1 g three times a day for 7 days)
- *Analgesics* reduce the acute herpes zoster pain. Mild pain may be managed with acetaminophen or nonsteroidal agents and moderate-to-severe pain usually require treatment with an opioid analgesic.
- *Corticosteroids* may be useful in reducing moderate to severe acute pain unrelieved by antiviral agents and analgesics. They are used to treat VZV-induced facial paralysis and cranial polyneuritis to improve motor outcomes in conjunction with antiviral agents.
- Treatment of postherpetic neuralgia includes use of topical lidocaine patch 5%, gabapentin (100–300 mg at night), pregabalin (50–150 mg daily two to three times a day), tricyclic antidepressants, and opioid and opioid-like analgesics. *Non-invasive treatments* such as transcutaneous electrical nerve stimulation (TENS), percutaneous electrical nerve stimulation (PENS), acupuncture, cold application, and psychological treatments are less effective. *Invasive treatments* such as neural blockade, spinal cord stimulation, and central nervous system drug delivery are given to patients who remain in severe pain and have failed all other therapies.

COVID-19 IN GERIATRIC POPULATION

- The current novel coronavirus disease-2019 (COVID-19) caused by severe acute respiratory syndrome corona-virus 2 (SARS-CoV-2) has been the one of the worst pandemic affecting millions over the world physically (by claiming lives), financially (by lockdown and loss in global economy), and emotionally (by death of near ones and unemployment).
- Evidences and studies shows that elderly are the worst hit among them.

Clinical spectrum: Symptom ranges from mild fever and dry cough to dyspnea and to ARDS leading to death. On top of that, asymptomatic courses are also reported leading to rapid spread of the disease.

Pathophysiology:

- SARS-CoV-2 relies on its spike protein (S) for infectivity.
- Angiotensin-converting enzyme 2 (ACE2) is the cell entry receptor, while TMPRSS2 (serine protease) is required for priming S protein.
- Upon entry, S protein cause internalization and degradation of ACE2 leading to lung damage as ACE2 downregulates the inflammatory effect of angiotensin II.
- In old age, ACE2 is in lower level so there are more severe outcomes.
- Toll-like receptor (TLR) and antigen presenting cell (APC) recognize the strategic segment of the microbe known as pathogen-associated molecular patterns (PAMPs) leading to cytokine mobilization.

Challenges in elderly:

- With age the immune system is disrupted.
- Elderly exhibits "inflammaging"; term which means excessive production of cytokines and inflammation mediators.
- Ciliary function is abnormal in old age.
- Signaling of TLR is impaired in old age leading to aberrant immune response.
- Underlying conditions as cardiovascular diseases, respiratory illness, diabetes, and hypertension.
- Atypical presentation in old age such as delirium, low-grade fever, and abdominal pain complicates the diagnosis.
- Dependence on emotional, physical, and social aspect.
- The elderly patients with different comorbidities and financial and social status are more vulnerable to adverse effects of COVID and are more susceptible to severe COVID.
- An individualized approach is more advisable targeting the infection itself, preexisting disease, and keeping in mind the adverse effects of therapeutic decision in elderly.

RECOMMENDED READINGS

1. Jagger A, Shimojima Y, Goronzy JJ, Weyand CM. Regulatory T cells and the immune aging process: a mini-review. Gerontology. 2014;60(2):130-7.
2. Liu WM, Nahar TE, Jacobi RH, Gijzen K, Van Beek J, Hak E, et al. Impaired production of TNF-alpha by dendritic cells of older adults leads to a lower CD8+ T cell response against influenza. Vaccine. 2012;30(9):1659-66.
3. Hazeldine J, Lord JM. The impact of ageing on natural killer cell function and potential consequences for health in older adults. Ageing Res Rev. 2013;12(4):1069-78.
4. Cabre M, Serra-Prat M, Palomera E, Almirall J, Pallares R, Clavé P. Prevalence and prognostic implications of dysphagia in elderly patients with pneumonia. Age Aging. 2010;39(1):39-45.
5. Chalmers JD, Taylor JK, Singanayagam A, Fleming GB, Akram AR, Mandal P, et al. Epidemiology, antibiotic therapy, and clinical outcomes in health care-associated pneumonia: a UK cohort study. Clin Infect Dis. 2011;53(2):107-13.
6. Hooton TM, Bradley SF, Cardenas DD, Colgan R, Geerlings SE, Rice JC, et al. Diagnosis, prevention, and treatment of catheter-associated urinary tract infection in adults: 2009 International Clinical Practice Guidelines from the Infectious Diseases Society of America. Clin Infect Dis. 2010;50(5):625-63.
7. Huang AJ, Brown JS, Boyko EJ, Moore EE, Scholes D, Walter L, et al. Clinical significance of postvoid residual volume in older ambulatory women. J Am Geriatr Soc. 2011;59(8):1452-8.
8. Rowe TA, Juthani-Mehta M. Urinary tract infection in older adults. Aging health. 2013;9(5):10.2217.
9. Linsk NL. HIV and the elderly. Fam Soc. 1994;75(6):362-72.
10. Kumar P, Sahu D, Chandra N, Kumar A, Rajan S. Aging of HIV epidemic in India: Insights from HIV estimation modeling under the national aids control programme. Indian J Public Health. 2020;64(Supplement):S76-8.
11. Zelenetz PD, Epstein ME. HIV in the elderly. AIDS Patient Care STDS. 1998;12(4):255-62.
12. Nguyen N, Holodniy M. HIV infection in the elderly. Clin Interv Aging. 2008;3(3):453-72.
13. Schmader K. Herpes zoster in older adults. Clin Infect Dis. 2001;32(10):1481-6.
14. Kawai K, Gebremeskel BG, Acosta CJ. Systematic review of incidence and complications of herpes zoster: towards a global perspective. BMJ Open. 2014;4(6):e004833.
15. Abdul Latheef EN, Pavithran K. Herpes zoster: a clinical study in 205 patients. Indian J Dermatol. 2011;56(5):529-32.
16. Schröder C, Enders D, Schink T, Riedel O. Incidence of herpes zoster amongst adults varies by severity of immunosuppression. J Infect. 2017;75(3):207-15.
17. Saadatian-Elahi M, Bauduceau B, Del-Signore C, Vanhems P. Diabetes as a risk factor for herpes zoster in adults: A synthetic literature review. Diabetes Res Clin Pract. 2020;159:107983.
18. Marin M, Harpaz R, Zhang J, Wollan PC, Bialek SR, Yawn BP. Risk Factors for Herpes Zoster Among Adults. Open Forum Infect Dis. 2016; 3(3):ofw119.
19. Saguil A, Kane S, Mercado M, Lauters R. Herpes zoster and postherpetic neuralgia: prevention and management. Am Fam Physician. 2017;96(10):656-63.

CHAPTER 31

Immunology and Vaccination in Elderly

Nandini Chatterjee, Agnibha Maiti, Vikas Gupta

ABSTRACT

As the human body ages, there occurs a decline in innate and adaptive immune responses. This age-related decline and dysregulation of immune response is termed as "immunosenescence" and predisposes the elderly to various infections, cancers, and autoimmune diseases. The elderly individuals also have a state of persistent low-grade inflammation termed as "inflammaging." These age-related changes make vaccinations less effective in the elderly. Hence, it is of utmost importance to employ various strategies to increase the immunogenicity and effectiveness of vaccines administered to the elderly.

It is important to give pneumococcal vaccine and influenza vaccine to all individuals above 60 years. The influenza vaccine is given every year and pneumococcal every 5 years. In addition, herpes zoster vaccine should also be given to the elderly. During high-risk periods with large gathering additional vaccines need to be given to the elderly also. The penetration of vaccination in India is much less than in the western countries for the elderly. Development of regular protocols by institutions and individual physicians will help in its use in larger number of individuals. Now the Coronavirus disease 2019 (COVID-19) vaccination will also become a part of the schedule, especially for the elderly. Those with comorbidities (hypertension, diabetes, cardiovascular disease, and cancer) have greater risk with all these infections and so they are in greater need of vaccination.

"The elderly have so much to offer. They're our link with history"

—John Cusack

INTRODUCTION

The passage of time leads to structural and functional changes in the human body with far reaching consequences at the cellular and molecular levels. The restructuring of the immune system constitutes "immunosenescence." Aging is associated with diminution in adaptive and innate immunity, consequently leading to increase in infections, cancer, and autoimmune diseases in the elderly. There is also a state of persistent low-grade inflammation termed as "inflammaging." Vaccination is less effective and immunogenic in the elderly and it is a challenge to protect them from ailments.

With the predicted doubling of elderly population to nearly 22% in 2050, it is of vital importance to look into these issues.

THE IMMUNE SYSTEM

Protection of the body from microbes and their virulence factors is dependent on the immune system. The prime components of this system are:

- Antigen receptors to recognize pathogens
- Immune memory for rapid response on rechallenges
- Immunologic tolerance to one's own tissues.

The two arms of the immune system comprise:

1. Innate immunity
2. Adaptive immunity

INNATE IMMUNITY

The components of the innate immunity are:

- *Cells*: Dendritic cells (DC), macrophages, natural killer (NK) cells, granulocytes, and epithelial cells
- *Pattern recognition receptors (PRR)*: Toll-like receptors (TLRs), nucleotide oligomerization domain (NOD)-like receptors, retinoic acid-inducible gene (RIG)-like receptors—that identify pathogens.
- *Antimicrobial proteins*: Defensins, cathepsins, and heat shock proteins that are produced by the host in response to insults.
- *Cytokines*: By autocrine, paracrine, or endocrine means, e.g., interleukin-1 (IL-1), IL-6, tumor necrosis factor alpha (TNF-α), IL-12 etc.
- *Complement pathways*
- *Immunity via mucosal surfaces*: -It contains the MALT or mucosa-associated lymphoid tissue which constitutes almost 80% of the lymphoid tissue of the body.

Its functions are: (1) To prevent invasive pathogens from entering, (2) To prevent uptake of foreign proteins, food, and commensals, and (3) To prevent pathologic immune activation. Innate immunity is the first line of defense which recognizes the pathogen-associated molecular patterns (PAMP)-like bacterial endotoxins using the PRRs that may either destroy the pathogen directly or activate the adaptive immunity.

ADAPTIVE IMMUNITY

It comprises of T and B lymphocytes. Both originate from hematopoietic stem cells. The T cells then home to thymus for further maturation. Pool of effector T cells is maintained by new T cell production in the thymus and antigen-driven expansion of virgin T cells into memory T cells in peripheral lymphoid tissues. The CD8 T lymphocytes cause lysis of virus-infected or foreign cells while CD4 T lymphocytes help in development of CD8 and B cells. The B cells express B cell receptor (BCR) for antigens, surface receptor for immunoglobulin G (IgG) molecules, and complement components. On being activated by the antigen-presenting cells (APCs), antibodies are produced.

CONSEQUENCES OF AGING

IMMUNOSENESCENCE

This is characterized by "reorganization" of the immune system. Immunosenescence includes the age-related decline and dysregulated immune responses, leading to poor outcomes of bacterial and viral infections and reduced efficacy of vaccination. In addition to the reduced ability to respond to new antigens, the memory responses in the elderly are also unsustained. Moreover, there is also an increased susceptibility to autoimmunity. The components of immunosenescence are discussed here.

Immunodeficiency: The defect in mounting an appropriate immune response to novel antigens may result in a heightened susceptibility to infectious diseases. This depends on the availability of naïve T cells. Due to the age-related thymic involution, and the consequent decrease of thymic output of naïve CD8+ T-cell reservoir, the body becomes grossly deficient in virgin T cells.

Autoimmunity: Due to thymus involution, there is a decrease in naïve T cells while clonal T cells increase which are activated due to "neoantigens" formed during the aging process. Also, increased CD5+ B lymphocytes in the elderly population contribute to the formation of autoantibodies. Accumulation of end-differentiated effector T cells and homeostatic T-cell proliferation also contribute to increased autoimmunity in the elderly.

Dysregulation of immune system: There is an age-associated decrease in TLR expression by the innate immune cells leading to impaired PRR signaling. The observed downregulation of TLRs and NOD-like receptors (NLRs) with age may contribute to the lack of proper recognition of invading pathogens or the commensal flora. Also, the increase of proinflammatory cytokines is associated with chronic degenerative conditions like dementia, Parkinson's disease, atherosclerosis, type 2 diabetes mellitus (T2DM), and sarcopenia.

INFLAMMAGING

Old age is associated with a duality where a state of chronic inflammation, even in the absence of overt diseases, coexists with a state of immunodeficiency. Elderly individuals develop a chronic low-level inflammation, because of continued exposure to antigens combined with inadequate immune function, increased supply of proinflammatory cytokines by effector memory, and senescent T cells and macrophages. This state of elevated levels of proinflammatory cytokines, acute phase proteins, and clotting factors in steady state has been designated as "inflammaging." It results due to chronic antigen stimulation by repeated clinical and subclinical infections and exposure to other antigens like inhalant allergens, food etc., and to the oxidative stress that involves the production of oxygen-free radicals and toxic products. The accumulation of oxygen metabolites causes damage to various cellular components (lipid membranes, the structural and enzymatic proteins, and nucleic acids), which activate enzymatic and nonenzymatic defense systems, DNA damage, and apoptotic processes.

CHANGES IN INNATE IMMUNITY

Skin and mucous membranes act like frontline warriors for body against pathogens. However, with age, as the skin cell renewal and sweat formation is hampered, along with structural changes in epithelial cells and reduction in number of Langerhans and melanocyte cells, this protective barrier weakens. This results in atrophy of epidermal layer and decline in immune. Changes in the in vivo microenvironment with ageing likely contribute to reduced TNF production by skin macrophages.

DENDRITIC CELLS

Dendritic cells are responsible for the first recognition of pathogens, antigen processing, and regulation of T and B lymphocytes and NK cells. There may be a decrease in the number of plasmacytoid and myeloid DCs with age. Also, the aged DCs show signs of mitochondrial dysfunction, reduced adenosine triphosphate (ATP) turnover, decreased oxidative phosphorylation, and enhanced reactive oxygen species (ROS) production.

NATURAL KILLER CELLS

The NK cells are involved in the elimination of virus-infected or tumor cells. With age there is a redistribution of NK cell subsets as shown by a decrease of CD56 bright cells and an increase of CD56-CD16+ NK cells. The amount of interferon-γ (IFN-γ) secreted by NK cells from the elderly was only 25% of that released by the cells from younger samples. In addition, the decrease in cytokine secretion, there is a decrease in cytotoxicity on a per-cell basis with ageing.

MACROPHAGES AND GRANULOCYTES

In the elderly population, the granulocytes and macrophages exhibit impaired phagocytosis, chemotaxis, presentation of antigens, and production of cytokines, and ROS. Immunosenescence leads to impaired neutrophil migration. Neutrophils also have impaired intracellular bacterial killing due to reduced expression of dehydroepiandrosterone sulfate resulting in decreased superoxide production. Impaired signal transduction responses also result in reduced neutrophil functions in the elderly. Telomeres shorten with age in macrophages leading to a decreased GM-CSF (colony-stimulating factor) but not M-CSF-dependent proliferation of these cells.

T LYMPHOCYTES

Alteration in T cell number as well as function is evident with increasing age. Thymic involution results in decrease in naïve T-cell output that limits the T-cell diversity. Though the naïve CD4+ T-cell compartment is relatively well preserved until seventh decade of life, naïve CD8+ T-cell compartment shrinks. This increases the susceptibility to infections, autoimmune conditions, and malignancy. Further, variations in lymphocyte potassium channels and calcium influx patterns also contribute to these alterations. It also presents a reduction of membrane receptors such as CD28 and CD27 (costimulators important in lymphocyte survival and activation). Persistent cytomegalovirus (CMV) infection is a major factor of T-cell immunosenescence.

B CELLS

The B cell immunosenescence is characterized by alteration in the memory/naïve B cell subsets. There is increase of memory B cells population in the elderly, and naïve B cells can produce IL-10 and TNF-α when stimulated at a lower threshold, indicating that these cells might play a role in the proinflammatory environment in the elderly. Limited available B cell repertoire results in reduced antibody responses in the elderly.

The ability of the immune system is worst, and the risk of infections is the highest in elderly. For the childhood period the vaccination program is well developed. The public awareness is high and so the vaccine coverage is good. However, for the adults and elderly the awareness is low, there are no national guidelines and so the vaccine coverage is poor. One should never miss a chance to vaccinate elderly individuals (**Fig. 1**).

VACCINATION IN THE ELDERLY

The susceptibility to infections, such as influenza virus, meningococcus, pneumococcus, Group B streptococcus, respiratory syncytial virus, and varicella-zoster virus, becomes higher in the older age group. Thus, prevention with existing vaccines or developing new improved vaccines against culprit pathogens is one of the prime strategies to ensure the "healthy aging."

SPECIAL ISSUES

The common issues encountered in geriatric vaccination are due to impaired antibody response because of the following factors: (1) Decreased CD80 expression, (2) diminished opsonization, and (3) deficient TLR-activated

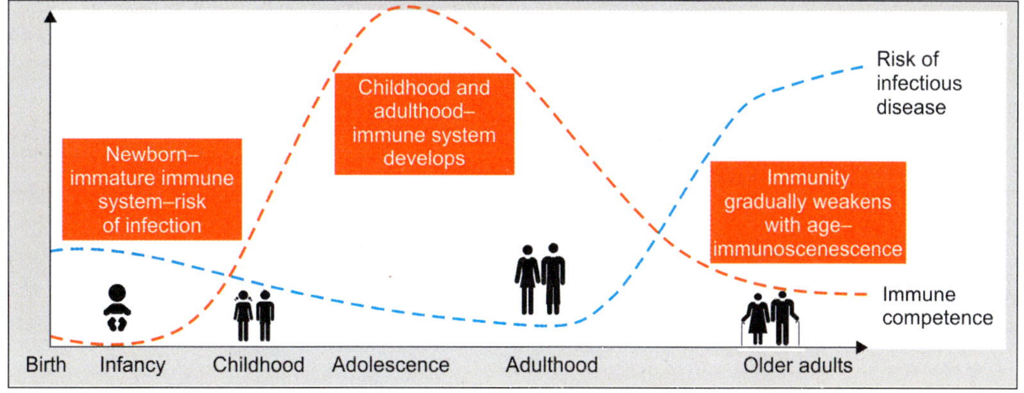

FIGURE 1: Changes in immune competence and risk of infections with age.

cytokine release. Also, there is impaired cellular response due to the following factors: (1) Decreased production of CD4 memory cells, and (2) diminished CD8 lysis.

The most common approaches to improve the effectiveness of vaccines in the elderly include: (1) Increasing the antigenic content per dose, (2) changing the route of administration, (3) giving booster doses, (4) using adjuvants, e.g., flagellin in influenza vaccine enhances immune response by activating TLR5, (5) giving vaccine in the morning, and (6) avoidance of stress.

The use of adjuvants can enhance activation of APCs, cytokine production, and stimulation of B and T cells. Different routes of administration may deliver the antigen to sites rich in APCs, improving its activation and presentation of antigens. The increase in the antigenic dose also encourages the activation of T cells.

VACCINES IN THE ELDERLY

Pneumococcal vaccines: Two types are available: (1) Pneumococcal polysaccharide vaccine (PPSV) 23—contains capsular polysaccharides of 23 serotypes of pneumococcus, and (2) pneumococcal conjugate vaccine (PCV) 13—contains 13 serotypes of pneumococcus.

All adults >65 years, PCV 13 may be given as a single dose, 0.5 mL over deltoid intramuscular (IM). PPSV23 is given as a single dose 1 year after PCV13 IM or subcutaneous (SC). One dose of PPSV23 is to be given to all adults >65 years irrespective of previous immune status. The practice recommendations for use of the two pneumococcal vaccine are given in **Table 1**.

Herpes zoster vaccine: Two types are available: (1) Live attenuated chick embryo vaccine 0.5 mL SC single dose over deltoid. Efficacy is 70%, and (2) the killed herpes zoster vaccine 0.5 mL SC two doses are given 4–6 weeks apart. Efficacy is 90%. All adults older than 50 years should get this vaccine.

Influenza vaccine: Two types are available: (1) Trivalent inactivated influenza vaccine (IIV) and (2) live attenuated influenza vaccine (LAIV). They contain antigen equivalents of influenza A strains H3N2 and H1N1 and influenza B virus. In the people over 50 years, the IIV is recommended annually (0.5 mL IM over the deltoid). Efficacy is 65–70%.

TABLE 1 Schedule of pneumococcal vaccination in elderly individuals.

Individual	Pneumococcal vaccination
Pneumococcal vaccine-naïve persons aged ≥65 years, not previously received pneumococcal vaccine	• One dose PCV13 followed by a dose of PPSV23. PPSV23 should be given 6–12 months after PCV13 • The two vaccines should not be coadministered, and the minimum acceptable interval between PCV13 and PPSV23 is 8 weeks
Previous vaccination with PPSV23 adults aged ≥65 years	• Should receive a dose of PCV13 if they have not yet received it. A dose of PCV13 should be given ≥1 year after PPSV23 • Repeat the dose of PPSV23 every 5 years subsequently

(PCV: pneumococcal conjugate vaccine; PPSV: pneumococcal polysaccharide vaccine)

Booster doses: Tetanus, diphtheria (Td) IM every 10 years after primary immunization. One dose should be substituted by TdaP (addition of acellular pertussis). If no record of childhood vaccination available—two doses of Td 4 weeks apart and one dose of TdaP after 6–12 months.

Vaccines in high-risk groups: Hepatitis A and B, meningococcal vaccine, Hib (*Haemophilus influenzae* type b) vaccine, rabies vaccine, and varicella vaccine are also to be given to high-risk groups.

Vaccines before travel: Special vaccines which are required before travel are the yellow fever, typhoid vaccine, and the hepatitis vaccines. The desirable vaccinations for those going to crowded religious occasions are given in **Table 2**.

Outbreaks: Meningococcal and typhoid vaccines are required during respective outbreaks.

All elderly >50 years with diabetes, chronic obstructive pulmonary disease (COPD), cardiac disease, and kidney disease during pandemic of COVID 19 must be encouraged to take influenza vaccine as well as vaccination against respiratory illnesses (pneumococcal vaccine and Hib vaccine) if not already taken.

TABLE 2 Recommendations for elderly individuals going for pilgrimage.

Vaccine recommendations	Category
Hajj pilgrims	
Meningococcal	Mandatory
Influenza	Recommended
Hepatitis A	Recommended
Hepatitis B	Recommended
Pneumococcal PCV13	4 weeks before travel
Pneumococcal PPSV23	Postreturn
Kumbh mela	
Typhoid	Strong recommendation
Hepatitis A	Strong recommendation
Influenza	Strong recommendation
Measles, mumps, and rubella	Should be up-to-date

(PCV: pneumococcal conjugate vaccine; PPSV: pneumococcal polysaccharide vaccine)

CONCLUSION

The immune system undergoes myriads of changes with advancing age leading to a compromised defense line-up along with a state of chronic inflammation and predisposition to autoimmunity. Thus, older people are vulnerable to infections with poor outcomes and prevention is better than cure. Recommendations have been laid down for specific vaccinations in the elderly though efficacy of immune response is lesser than their younger counterparts.

RECOMMENDED READINGS

1. Ahmed R, Gray D. Immunological memory and protective immunity: understanding their relation. Science. 1996;272(5258):54-60.
2. Dunkelberger JR, Song WC. Complement and its role in innate and adaptive immune responses. Cell Res. 2010;20(1):34-50.
3. Franceschi C, Bonafè M, Valensin S. Human immunosenescence: the prevailing of innate immunity, the failing of clonotypic immunity, and the filling of immunological space. Vaccine. 2000;18(16): 1717-20.
4. Goronzy JJ, Weyand CM. Understanding immunosenescence to improve responses to vaccines. Nat Immunol. 2013;14(5):428-36.
5. Shaw AC, Goldstein DR, Montgomery RR. Age-dependent dysregulation of innate immunity. Nat Rev Immunol. 2013;13(12):875-87.
6. Franceschi C, Capri M, Monti D, Giunta S, Olivieri F, Sevini F, et al. Inflammaging and anti-inflammaging: a systemic perspective on aging and longevity emerged from studies in humans. Mech Ageing Dev. 2007;128(1):92-105.
7. Goronzy JJ, Weyand CM. Immune aging and autoimmunity. Cell Mol Life Sci. 2012;69(10):1615-23.
8. Kottner J, Lichterfeld A, Blume-Peytavi U. Maintaining skin integrity in the aged: a systematic review. Br J Dermatol. 2013;169(3):528-42.
9. Farage MA, Miller KW, Berardesca E, Maibach HI. Clinical implications of aging skin: cutaneous disorders in the elderly. Am J Clin Dermatol. 2009;10(2):73-86.

CHAPTER 32

Cognitive Assessment in Dementia

Parveen Goel, Souvik Dubey, Biman Kanti Ray

ABSTRACT

Dementia is not merely the presence of forgetfulness, but may involve other cognitive domains as well, such as attention, executive function, visuospatial, visuoperceptual, and language. Behavioral problems in dementia needs to be addressed meticulously as it imposes much caregiver burden and at the same time some therapeutic options are available for this issue if used carefully. Cognitive impairment, when it grossly disrupts activities of daily living (ADLs), is considered as dementia. In contrast, single or multidomain cognitive impairment without disruption of ADLs is considered as minimal cognitive impairment (MCI) which according to the presence or absence of memory dysfunction is classified as amnestic or nonamnestic MCI, respectively.

Dementia may be reversible or irreversible dementia. It is important to identify and treat the reversible causes first and foremost. Depending upon the pattern of brain involvement, dementia is divided into cortical and subcortical dementia. Though cortical dementia stems from pure cortical involvement, in advanced stages, subcortical involvement is not unusual.

The same holds true for subcortical dementia, as it predominantly involves subcortical structures; however, late cortical involvement is not rare. Cortical dementia is characterized by the presence of aphasia, agnosia, apraxia, visuospatial, and perceptual impairments. In contrast, classical features of subcortical dementia are attention deficit, executive dysfunction, slow information processing speed, marked perseveration, and presence of pyramidal and extrapyramidal symptoms and signs. In advance stage, sharing of classical features of cortical and subcortical dementia often poses a great challenge in diagnosis of a particular subtype. A debate is ongoing whether lobar functions or network of brain are to be emphasized in routine dementia evaluation.

The backbone of dementia diagnosis is history taking. Cognitive examination must be tailored according to history. In the face of gross attention deficit, examination findings of other cognitive spheres must be carefully interpreted. Mini-Mental State Examination (MMSE) is merely a screening tool for dementia which has certain limitations. Score range is limited and floor and ceiling effects are common. Further, its heavy reliance on language and memory but not executive function limits its scope for frontal lobe assessment. Depression may precede and coexist in dementia leading to further difficulties in diagnosis. Demented brain is very prone to undergo delirious state even in minor metabolic or septic perturbations. Caregiver burden in dementia needs to be addressed carefully and empathetically.

"Aging is not lost youth but a new stage of opportunity and strength"

—Betty Friedan

INTRODUCTION

In 1797, the French psychiatrist, Philippe Pinel coined the term dementia (démence). Dementia is derived from the Latin *de* meaning "out of" and *mens* meaning "the mind". However, dementia is not being "out of one's mind". Dementia is the slow deterioration of mental capacities that is a direct result of a disease process in the brain.

In Diagnostic and Statistical Manual of Mental Disorders, Fifth Edition (DSM-5) (2013), dementia is subsumed under the newly named entity *major neurocognitive disorder (NCD);* however, the term *dementia* is retained for continuity, particularly in the etiological subtypes in which the term is standard. Furthermore, DSM-5 recognizes a less severe level of cognitive impairment, *mild NCD*. The important features of NCDs and the DSM-5 diagnostic criteria are listed in **Boxes 1** and **2**, respectively. The characteristic differences between major and mild NCDs are shown in **Box 3**.

Furthermore, dementia is a complex syndrome with cognitive, behavioral, and functional disturbances (**Fig. 1**). The behavioral and psychological symptoms that can present in dementia are shown in **Figure 2**.

BOX 1	Important features of neurocognitive disorders (DSM-5, APA, 2013).
	• Major NCD, mild NCD, and their etiological subtypes
	• Primary clinical deficit is in the cognitive function
	• Acquired rather than developmental
	• Decline from a previously attained level of functioning
	• Dementia is subsumed under *major neurocognitive disorder*, but the term *dementia* is retained for continuity
	• Individuals with substantial decline in a "single domain" can receive this diagnosis (unlike DSM-IV)
	• Does not necessarily require *memory* to be one of the impaired domains (unlike DSM-IV)

(APA: American Psychiatric Association; DSM-5: Diagnostic and Statistical Manual of Mental Disorders, Fifth Edition; NCD: neurocognitive disorder)

BOX 2	DSM-5 diagnostic criteria.
	• Evidence of significant (for major NCDs)/modest (for mild NCDs) cognitive *decline* from a previous level of performance in one or more cognitive domains based on:
	◦ Subjective concerns about significant (for major NCDs)/mild (for mild NCDs) decline in cognitive function
	◦ A substantial (major NCDs)/modest (mild NCDs) impairment in cognitive performance, preferably documented by *standardized neuropsychological testing*
	• The cognitive deficits interfere (major NCDs)/do not interfere (in case of mild NCDs) with activities of daily living (ADLs)
	• The cognitive deficits do not occur exclusively in the context of a *delirium* (See **Table 1** for differences between dementia and delirium)
	• The cognitive deficits are not better explained by *another mental disorder* (e.g., major depressive disorder and schizophrenia)

(DSM-5: Diagnostic and Statistical Manual of Mental Disorders, Fifth Edition; NCD: neurocognitive disorder)

HISTORY TAKING

History taking key points include:
- Duration
- Symptoms at onset (cognitive/behavioral)
- Progression (sudden/gradual)
- Course (progressive/static/remitting)
- History of gait difficulties
- History of falls
- History of urine/fecal incontinence
- Basic and instrumental ADLs
- Query family or collateral source from prior setting as to "what is normal" for the patient

WHAT ARE COGNITIVE FUNCTIONS

Cognitive functions, also called "*higher mental functions*" are the abilities needed for gathering knowledge, manipulation of gathered information, reasoning, and subsequent planning. These may be localized to specific brain areas, lateralized to dominant or nondominant cerebral hemisphere, or distributed across networks. **Table 2** lists the various dysfunctions arising from the brain lobes, also known as lobar dysfunctions.

BOX 3	Differences between major and mild NCDs.
• Major and mild NCDs exist on a spectrum of *cognitive* and *functional* impairment	
◦ *Cognitive*:	
– For major NCD, performance is typically 2 or more SD below appropriate norms (3rd percentile or below)	
– For minor NCD, performance typically lies in the 1–2 SD range (between 3rd and 16th percentiles)	
◦ *Functional*:	
– For major NCD, ADLs may be completed with assistance or may be abandoned altogether	
– For minor NCD, instrumental activities of daily living (IADLs) may seem more difficult, or requiring extra time and effort or compensatory strategies	
• Changes rather than lifelong patterns	
• Cognitive loss rather than motor or sensory limitations	

(ADLs: activities of daily living; SD: standard deviation; NCD: neurocognitive disorder)

TABLE 1 Differences between delirium and dementia.

Features	Delirium	Dementia
Onset	Abrupt	Insidious (abrupt: stroke)
Course	Fluctuates	Slow decline
Duration	Hours to weeks	Months to years
Attention	Impaired	Intact early
Sleep-wake	Disrupted	Usually normal
Alertness	Impaired	Normal
Orientation	Impaired	Intact in early stage
Behavior	Agitated, withdrawn/ depressed	Intact in early stage
Speech	Incoherent	Word finding problems
Thoughts	Disorganized and delusional	Impoverished
Perceptions	Hallucinations/illusions	Usually intact early

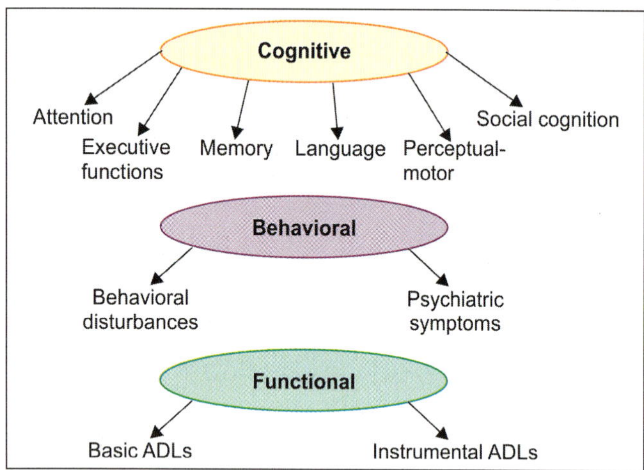

(ADLs: activities of daily living)

FIGURE 1: Dementia is a complex syndrome.

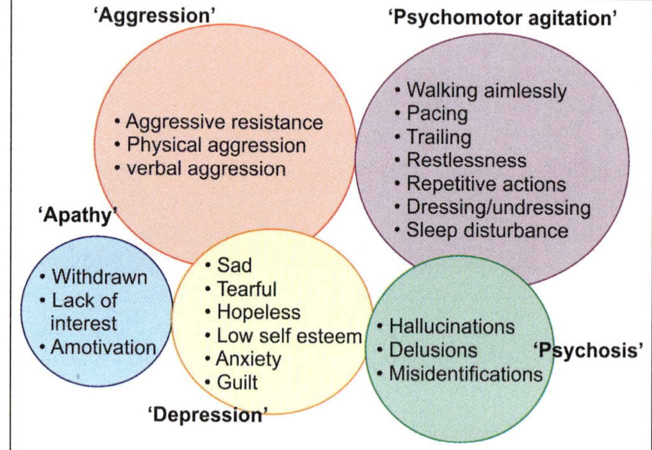

FIGURE 2: Behavioral and psychological symptoms in dementia.

HOW DO WE PERFORM COGNITIVE ASSESSMENT

The DSM-5 lists six cognitive domains of assessment (**Fig. 3**).

Objective cognitive assessment is done using certain multidimensional test instruments as well as specific tests designed for certain functions. The most widely used screening instruments include:

- *MMSE*: This provides a quick assessment for orientation to time and place, attention and calculation, recall, language, praxis, and visuospatial functions.
- *Montreal cognitive assessment (MoCA)*: The cognitive functions assessed include: Visuospatial/executive, naming, memory, attention, language, abstraction, delayed recall, and orientation.
- *Addenbrooke's Cognitive Examination-Revised (ACE-R)*: This provides a quick screening for attention and orientation, memory, fluency, language, and visuospatial functions.
- *Clock Drawing Test* is also widely used as an initial screening instrument—assess visuoconstructional abilities, executive functions, and memory. Scoring: Sunderland's 10-point Scoring.

LANGUAGE ASSESSMENT

Here six key areas of language are assessed:

1. *Spontaneous speech*: Use one of these pictures to elicit spontaneous speech (Cookie Theft picture, Village scene, A scene at a railway station etc.). Assess for the following:
    - Output (present or not)
    - Dysarthric/dysprosodic/aphasic
    - Aphasic speech:
        - Fluent
        - Nonfluent

TABLE 2 Lobar dysfunctions.

Brain lobes	Right cerebral hemisphere	Left cerebral hemisphere	Common/bilateral dysfunctions
Frontal lobe	• Loss of design fluency • Mania-like symptoms • Hyperkinetic behavior	• Loss of letter fluency • Depression like symptoms • Hypokinetic behavior	• Dorsolateral convexity—dysexecutive syndrome • Orbitofrontal—disinhibition syndrome • Medial frontal—apathetic syndrome
Parietal lobe	• Hemineglect • Constructional apraxia • Dressing apraxia • Topographical disorientation	• Apraxia • Central alexia • Acalculia • Components of Gerstmann syndrome	• Contralateral hemisensory loss • Contralateral inferior quadrantanopia • Sensory seizure
Temporal lobe	• Right fusiform—prosopagnosia • Right middle and inferior temporal—general knowledge	• Left fusiform—pure alexia and acalculia • Left middle and inferior temporal—episodic knowledge • Left superior temporal gyrus—pure word deafness or higher order auditory defect, aphasia	• Hippocampal—loss of recent episodic memory • Parahippocampal—anterograde topographic disorientation • Fusiform gyrus—achromatopsia • Superior temporal—cortical deafness
Occipital lobe			**Lesions of primary visual cortex:** • Field defects • Cortical blindness • Denial of blindness and confabulation *(Anton's syndrome)* **Lesions of ventral stream:** • Visual object agnosia • Color vision abnormalities • Prosopagnosia (problem in face identification) • Alexia without agraphia **Lesions of dorsal stream:** • Bálint's syndrome • Defective motion and depth perception (akinetopsia and astereopsis, respectively)

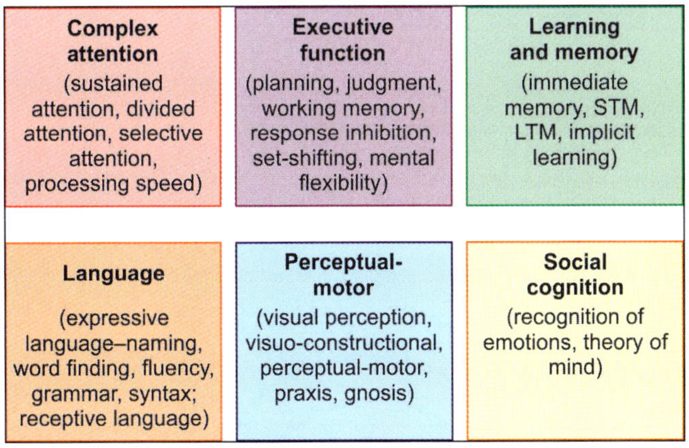

Complex attention (sustained attention, divided attention, selective attention, processing speed)	**Executive function** (planning, judgment, working memory, response inhibition, set-shifting, mental flexibility)	**Learning and memory** (immediate memory, STM, LTM, implicit learning)
Language (expressive language–naming, word finding, fluency, grammar, syntax; receptive language)	**Perceptual-motor** (visual perception, visuo-constructional, perceptual-motor, praxis, gnosis)	**Social cognition** (recognition of emotions, theory of mind)

(DSM-5: Diagnostic and Statistical Manual of Mental Disorders, Fifth Edition; STM: short-term memory; LTM: long-term memory)

FIGURE 3: DSM-5 neurocognitive domains.

- Monophasia
- Paraphasia (phonemic/semantic)
- Neologisms

➢ Automatic speech (old song, rhyme, alphabet, counting etc.)

➢ Emotional speech

2. *Comprehension*:
   ➢ Pointing commands (room, body parts, and articles). Pointing to one, two, three, and four commands.
   ➢ Yes/No responses, e.g., Is this a hotel? Does a stone float on water? etc.
   ➢ Passive possessive construction, e.g., The boy was slapped by the girl. Who got hit?
3. *Repetition*: Repetition of words, phrases, and sentences.
4. *Naming*:
   ➢ Confrontation naming: Colors, body parts, clothing, and parts of objects
   ➢ Spontaneous naming:
   - Category/semantic naming (animals, fruits, kitchen utensils etc.)
   - Lexical/phonemic flexibility (FAS test). Exclude proper nouns, surnames, or morphological variants (e.g., shoe and shoe-maker)

   ➢ Responsive naming (noun, verb, and adjective)
   - Noun: E.g., Where do doctors work?
   - Verb: E.g., What do you do with a cup?
   - Adjective: E.g., How does sugar taste?
5. *Reading*:
   ➢ Reading aloud (letters, words, phrases, sentences, and numbers)

- Reading comprehension (ask something about what is written)
  - *Example*: The boy and the girl walked in the sun.
  - *Ask*: Did the boy go alone? Was it raining when the boy and the girl went for a walk?

6. *Writing*:
   - Copying
   - Writing to dictation (numbers, letters, names of objects, body parts etc.)
   - Spontaneous writing (sentence)

Language disorders:

- *Wernicke's aphasia* (impaired comprehension, paraphasic errors, neologisms, jargon aphasia, repetition, naming, reading, and writing also impaired) (superior temporal gyrus)
- *Broca's aphasia* (spontaneous speech nonfluent, labored, word-finding pauses, dysarthric, reduced output, naming and repetition also impaired, comprehension intact, and insight preserved) (inferior frontal gyrus)
- *Global aphasia* (speech output nonfluent, comprehension impaired, naming, repetition, reading, and writing also impaired) strokes involving the entire middle cerebral artery (MCA) distribution in the left hemisphere (LH)
- *Conduction aphasia* (repetition severely impaired) (perisylvian arcuate fasciculus)
- *Nonfluent transcortical (motor) aphasia* (similar to Broca's aphasia, but repetition intact) (the lesion site disconnects the intact language network from prefrontal areas—anterior watershed zone)
- *Fluent transcortical (sensory) aphasia (features similar to Wernicke's aphasia, but repetition intact) (the lesion site* disconnects the intact core of the language network from other temporoparietal association areas—posterior watershed zone)
- *Anomic aphasia* (impaired naming, word-finding, and spelling) (angular gyrus)
- *Pure agraphia* (left angular gyrus)
- *Pure alexia* (alexia without agraphia) (pure word blindness)
  - Lesions of ventral stream
  - Wernicke's area is intact, but isolated from visual input from both hemispheres

ASSESSMENT OF ATTENTION

- Digit span test [normal is digit forward = 7 ± 2; digit backward (DB) = 6 ± 2]
- Weekdays in reverse (normal: errors = 0, time <7 s)
- Months in reverse (normal: errors = 0, time <24 s)
- Reverse spelling—spell "WORLD" backwards (normal: errors = 0, time < 6 s)
- Serial subtraction test (100–7 series)
- Digit-symbol substitution test
- Processing speed (oral A–Z, normal: time <13 s)
- Line-bisection test (assesses for visuospatial neglect)
- Letter "A" cancellation test

EXECUTIVE FUNCTIONING

- Insight and judgment
- Working memory (*DB, weekdays in reverse, and months in reverse*)
- Visual pattern completion test (**Fig. 4**)
- Repeating loop pattern and spiral (**Fig. 5**)
- Motor Luria test (*fist-edge-palm test*)
- Applause sign (three times clap)
- Trail Making Test (Trail A and B)—visual attention and task switching (**Fig. 6**)
- Verbal fluency (*category/semantic fluency; lexical/mental flexibility*)
- Conceptualization/abstract thinking (*proverbs; similarities*)
- Go-No Go Test (*inhibitory control*)
- Stroop Color and Word Test (**Fig. 7**)
- Conflicting instructions (*sensitivity to interference*)

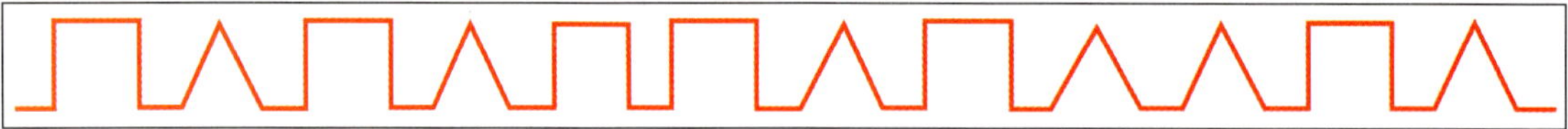

FIGURE 4: Visual pattern completion test.

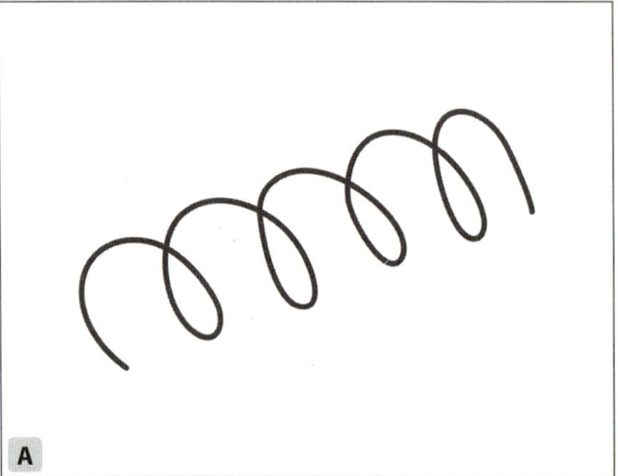

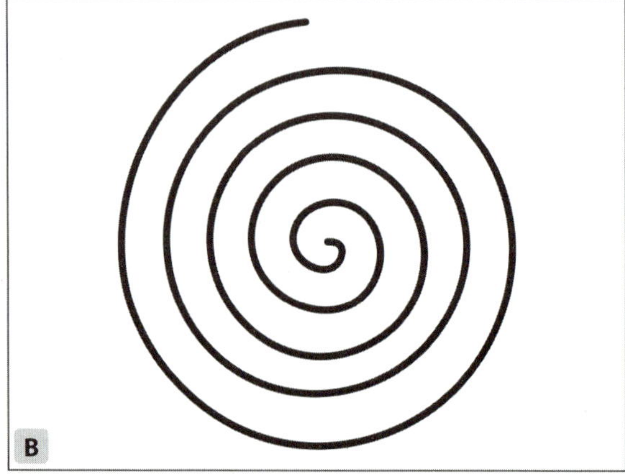

FIGURES 5 A & B: (A) Repeating loops; (B) Spiral.

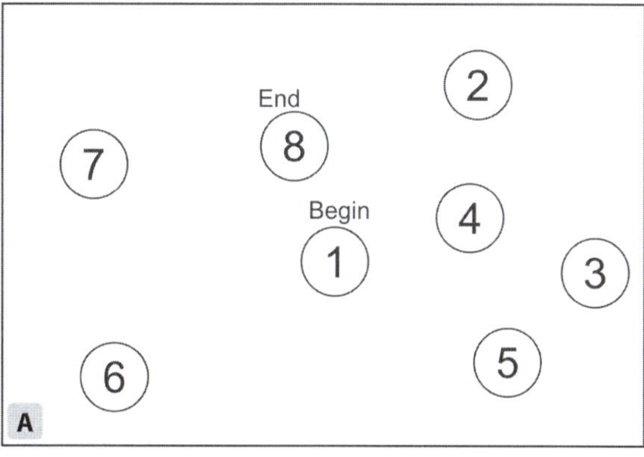

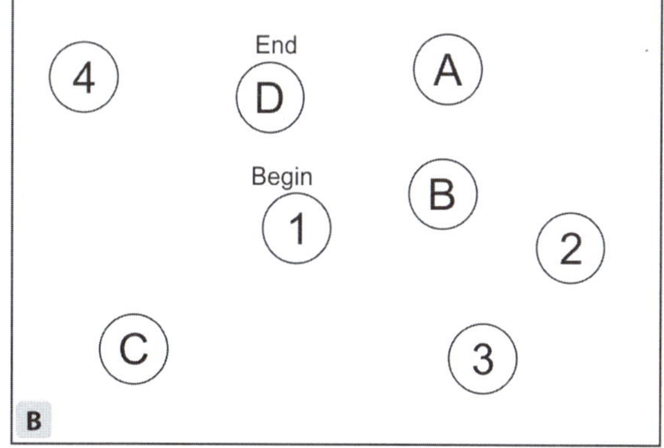

FIGURES 6 A & B: (A) Trail A (practice item); (B) Trail B (practice item).

BLUE	RED	YELLOW	ORANGE
GREEN	BLUE	PURPLE	RED
PURPLE	YELLOW	RED	BLUE
ORANGE	BLUE	YELLOW	RED
RED	GREEN	ORANGE	BLUE
PURPLE	YELLOW	BLUE	ORANGE

FIGURE 7: Stroop Test.

- Proverbs and similarities (*conceptualization and abstract thinking*)
- Environmental dependence (*prehension, imitation, and utilization*)
- Social cognition (*questions on social norms*)
- Battery for executive dysfunction is the *Frontal Assessment Battery* (FAB; *Dubois and Litman, 2000*). It assesses for:
  - Similarities
  - Lexical fluency
  - Motor series Luria test (fist-edge-palm test)
  - Conflicting instructions (sensitivity to interference)
  - Go-No Go (inhibitory control)
  - Prehension behavior (environmental autonomy)

MEMORY ASSESSMENT

- Immediate recall [*digit repetition test (DB); registration of three unrelated words*]
- Recent memory (episodic) (person, place, and time)
- Remote memory:
  - Autobiographical (personal, school, vocational, and family)
  - Semantic (historical facts and general knowledge)
- New learning ability (recall of words at 0, 5, 10, and 30 min)
- Story recall
- Visual memory (using five hidden objects)
- Paired associate learning
- *PGI Memory Test (Prasad and Wig, 1971)* assesses memory based upon 10 subtests:
  i. Remote memory
  ii. Recent memory
  iii. Mental balance
  iv. Attention and concentration
  v. Delayed recall
  vi. Immediate recall
  vii. Verbal retention for similar pairs
  viii. Verbal retention for dissimilar pairs
  ix. Visual retention
  x. Recognition

RELATED CORTICAL FUNCTIONS

- *Apraxia*: To be assessed in descending order of difficulty. Hierarchy of difficulty is:
  Pantomiming → Imitation → Actual object.
  - *Ideomotor*:
    - Buccofacial, e.g., blow out a candle; close your eyes
    - Limb, e.g., salute/namaste/salaam; make a fist; flip a coin
    - Truncal, e.g., stand like a boxer; bow
    - Instruments, e.g., using a stapler, spoon, lock and key, scissors
  - Ideational (*3-step command (MMSE), tasks—toothpaste, letter, sandwich etc.*)
- *Agnosia*:
  - Finger agnosia
  - Visual agnosia (*object agnosia, prosopagnosia, and color agnosia*)
  - Astereognosis (*five objects with eyes closed*)
  - Simultagnosia (*Cookie Theft picture*—**Fig. 8 A**, *Navon hierachical letters*—**Fig. 8 B**)
- Right-left orientation (*identification on self and examiner; cross-commands on self and examiner*)
- Visuospatial and visuoconstructional ability:
  - Dot counting and identifying alphabets (**Figs. 9 A and B**)
  - Copying (*circle, diamond, cross, cube, smoke pipe, and triangle inside triangle*)
  - Drawing to command (*House and flower-vase*)
- Calculation (*verbal rote—simple/complex and written complex*)

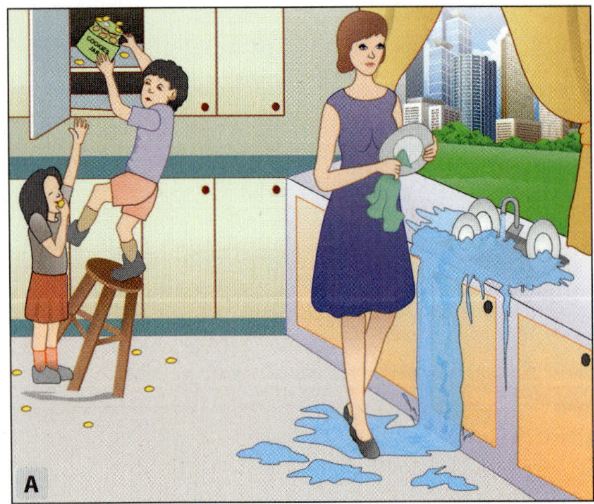

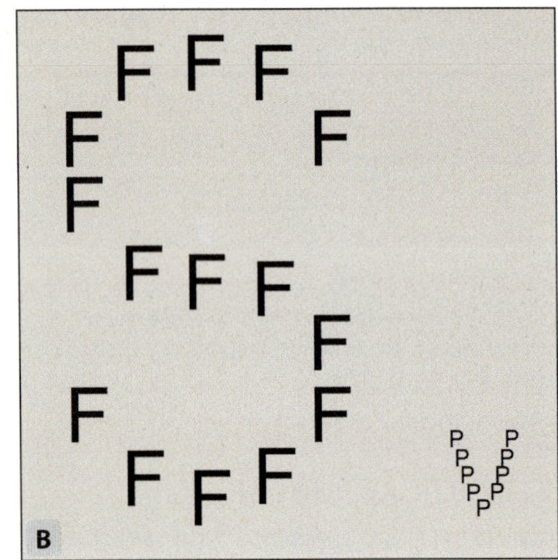

FIGURES 8 A & B: (A) Cookie theft picture; (B) Navon hierarchical letters.

LOBAR FUNCTIONS

Table 2 gives an overview of the lobar functions along with their anatomical substrates. These are described in further detail below.

Occipital lobe:

Disorders of dorsal stream (posterior parietal syndromes):

- *Bálint's syndrome*:
  - Restricted visual attention producing dorsal simultagnosia (modified letter cancellation task, Navon's letters)
  - Optic ataxia
  - Oculomotor apraxia
- Visual disorientation—inability to judge object location, distance, and orientation
- Akinetopsia—defective motion perception
- Astereopsis—defective depth perception

Disorders of ventral stream (occipitotemporal syndromes):

- Visual object agnosia (apperceptive/associative agnosia; optic aphasia)
- Color vision abnormalities
- Prosopagnosia (right fusiform gyrus)
- Pure alexia (alexia without agraphia)
- Ventral simultagnosia (milder) (Cookie Theft picture)

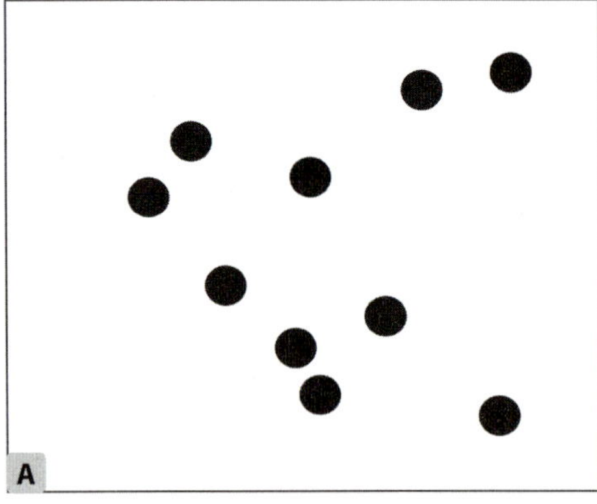

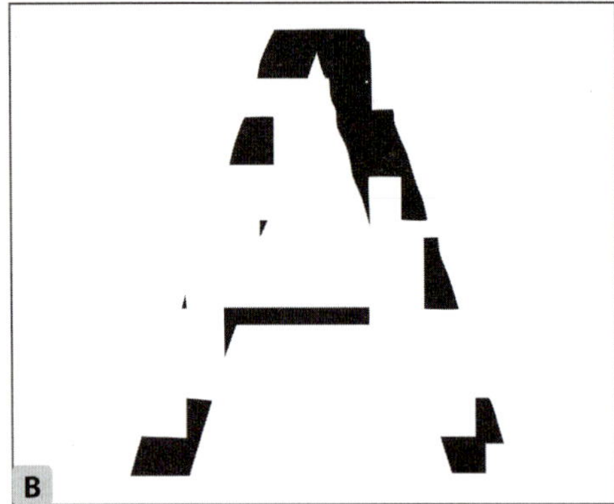

FIGURES 9 A & B: (A) Dot counting; (B) Identifying alphabets.

Lesions of primary visual cortex:

- Field defects:
  - Hemianopia
  - Bilateral quadrantanopia
  - Altitudinal hemifield defect
- *Cortical blindness*: Patient is blind but pupillary reflexes are present and there is macular sparing, i.e., sparing of 5–10 degree of central visual field.
- Anton's syndrome (visual anosognosia—denial of loss of vision)

Parietal lobe:

- *Right parietal lobe*:
  - Cortical sensory loss
  - Left hemineglect (line bisection test and letter cancellation test)
  - Constructional apraxia (overlapping pentagons, Necker cube, and clock face)
  - Dressing apraxia (lack of visuospatial capacity)
  - Topographical disorientation/topographagnosia (locate places on the map)
- *Left parietal lobe*:
  - Apraxia
  - Central alexia
  - Acalculia
- *Gerstmann syndrome (dominant inferior parietal lobule)*:
  - Acalculia
  - Finger agnosia
  - Right-left disorientation; also difficulties with other spatial relationships such as up-down, over-under, and above-below
  - Apraxic agraphia (not associated with alexia)

Temporal lobe:

- *Hippocampus (episodic memory)*:
  - Left—verbal memory
  - Right—visual memory
  - Bilateral lesions—amnesic syndromes
- *Parahippocampus*:
  - Acquisition of novel topographic memories
- *Fusiform gyrus*:
  - Color vision
  - Identification of face
  - Identification of letters and symbols
- *Middle and inferior temporal gyri (anterior temporal lobe)*:
  - Semantic memory and knowledge
- *Superior temporal gyrus*:
  - Heschl's gyrus (anterior) (cortical deafness)
  - Wernicke's area (posterior, area 22) (posterior language disorders)
  - High order cortical areas (middle part) (pure word deafness—can recognize nonverbal sounds)

Klüver-Bucy syndrome (bilateral amygdala):

- Hyperorality (insertion of inappropriate objects in the mouth—an oral tendency or compulsion to examine objects by mouth, eating inappropriate objects—pica; compulsive overeating)
- Hypersexuality
- Blunted emotional reactivity (docility, apathy, placidity, tameness; diminished fear responses or reacting with unusually low aggressiveness)
- Hypermetamorphosis (an irresistible impulse to notice and react to everything within sight)
- *Visual agnosia*: Inability to recognize familiar objects or people
- Short-term memory impairment

Frontal lobe:

Dorsolateral prefrontal—dysexecutive syndrome [Frontal Assessment Battery (FAB)]:

- Planning
- Initiation
- Response inhibition
- Mental flexibility (set-shifting)
- Working memory
- Fluency

Medial prefrontal—apathetic syndrome:

- Lack of initiative and reduced motivation
- Needs prompting to initiate and continue routine activities
- Does not initiate or sustain conversation
- Social isolation

Orbitofrontal areas—disinhibition syndrome:

- Socially inappropriate behavior
- Loss of manners or decorum
- Impulsive, rash, and careless actions

TYPES OF DEMENTIAS

- *Cortical*: Alzheimer's disease, frontotemporal lobar degeneration, and alcoholic encephalopathy
- *Subcortical*: Progressive supranuclear palsy, Huntington's disease, Parkinson's disease, and multiinfarct (white matter) dementia
- *Corticosubcortical*: Lew body disease (symmetrical pathology), corticobasal degeneration (asymmetric pathology), and vascular dementia
- *Multifocal*: Creutzfeldt-Jakob disease (CJD)

Table 3 lists the differences between cortical and subcortical dementia.

TABLE 3 Differences between cortical and subcortical dementia.

Domain	Cortical	Subcortical
Anatomy	Cortical-limbic damage	Frontal-subcortical damage *(basal ganglia, substantia nigra, brainstem etc.)*
Neurological symptoms	Not characteristic	• Profound and characteristic neurological symptoms • PSP *(paralysis of eye movements)* • Huntington's disease *(involuntary jerking movements)* • Parkinson's disease *(rigidity, akinesia, and resting tremor)*
Frontal-executive	Normal until late	Impaired from onset
Episodic memory	Defect in consolidation (impaired delayed recall)	Defective retrieval (recognition yields better results than spontaneous recall—implicit memory preserved), and retrieval by cues
Remote memory	Temporal gradient present	No temporal gradient
Motor memory	Preserved *(not dependent upon hippocampal-diencephalic system)*	Impaired motor skills and motor skill learning
Attention	Spared in early stages	Impaired (deficit in shifting or allocating attention)
Working memory	Relatively mild working memory deficits	Early deficits in all aspects of working memory *(poor digit span)*
Word fluency	More impaired on category fluency than on letter fluency	Severely and equivalently impaired on both (retrieval failure)

Continued...

Continued...

Domain	Cortical	Subcortical
Language	Aphasic features	Normal, except low output and dysarthria
Confrontation naming	Impaired (semantic-based errors). Superordinate errors such as "camel" to "animal"	Relatively spared. Perceptual-based errors such as "pretzel" to "snake"
Praxis	Impaired	Normal
Visuospatial and perceptual abilities	Impaired	Mostly preserved

(PSP: progressive supranuclear palsy)

MILD COGNITIVE IMPAIRMENT

The transitional stage between normal cognitive aging and dementia has been termed mild cognitive impairment (MCI). The core diagnostic criteria for MCI include:

- Subjective cognitive complaints over at least 6 months.
- Objective cognitive impairment (<1.5 SD criteria)
- Essentially intact ADLs.

Mild cognitive impairment can be:

- *Amnestic MCI* characterized by predominant impairment of the memory domain (predominantly episodic memory)
- *Nonamnestic MCI* characterized by:
  - Slight impairment of multiple cognitive domains (multiple-domain MCI)
  - Predominant impairment of a cognitive domain other than memory (single-domain MCI)

TAKE HOME MESSAGES

- One must know cognitive functions and their anatomical substrates.
- Always rule out delirium and psychiatric disorders.
- Rule out reversible causes and treat if found.
- Identify the actual caregiver.
- Always note the handedness.
- History to be documented in detail—formulate appropriate tests as per history.
- Chronological order of cognitive domains involved can be a due to etiological diagnosis.
- Order of tests to be religiously followed—start with attention and language.
- Our final judgment should always be based on social status and education level.
- Formulate a syndromic diagnosis, prognosticate, and choose rational therapy.

ACKNOWLEDGMENT

We are thankful to Dr Subhadeep Gupta, Post Doctoral Trainee, BIN, Institute of Post-Graduate Medical Education and Research, Kolkata for helping us prepare this chapter.

RECOMMENDED READINGS

1. American Psychiatric Association. Diagnostic and Statistical Manual of the Mental Disroders (DSM-5), 5th edition. Washington, DC: American Psychiatric Association Press; 2013.
2. Dubois B, Slachevsky A, Litvan I, Pillon B. The FAB: A Frontal Assessment Battery at bedside. Neurology. 2000;55:1621-6.
3. Folstein MF, Folstein SE, McHugh PR. "Mini-mental state". A practical method for grading the cognitive state of patients for the clinician. J Psychiatr Res. 1975;12: 189-98.
4. Mioshi E, Dawson K, Mitchell J, Arnold R, Hodges JR. The Addenbrooke's Cognitive Examination Revised (ACE-R): a brief cognitive test battery for dementia screening. Int J Geriatr Psychiatry. 2006;21:1078-85.
5. Nasreddine ZS, Phillips NA, Bédirian V, Charbonneau S, Whitehead V, Collin I, et al. The Montreal Cognitive Assessment, MoCA: a brief screening tool for mild cognitive impairment. J Geriatr Soc. 2005;53:695-9.
6. Prasad D, Wig NN. The PGI Memory Scale (PGIMS-PW). Agra: National Psychological Corporation; 1971.
7. Shulman KI, Shedletsky R, Silver IL. The challenge of time: clock-drawing and cognitive function in the elderly. Int J Geriatr Psychiatry. 1986;1:135-40.
8. Sunderland T, Hill JL, Mellow AM, Lawlor BA, Gundersheimer J, Newhouse PA, et al. Clock drawing in Alzheimer's disease. A novel measure of dementia severity. J Am Geriatr Soc. 1989;37:725-9.
9. Hodges J. Cognitive Assessment for Clinicians, 3rd edition. Oxford: Oxford University Press; 2017.
10. Strub RL, Black FW. The Mental Status Examination in Neurology. Philadelphia: FA Davis Company; 1985.
11. Jose J. Cognitive Neurological Examination: A Clinico-anatomical Approach, 2nd edition. Kerala: Neurology Alumni Association of Malabar (NAAM); 2020.

MULTIPLE CHOICE QUESTIONS

To access the multiple choice questions of this Section online, kindly scan the QR code.

CHAPTER 33

Pyrexia of Unknown Origin

OC Abraham

ABSTRACT

This chapter describes the definition, causes, and diagnostic approach to patients presenting with sustained fever where the etiology remains elusive after the initial diagnostic evaluation. Further evaluation is directed toward the identification of potential diagnostic clues (PDCs), which should guide subsequent diagnostic testing. A thorough history and physical examination remain the most important steps in identifying PDCs. Treatment and prognosis of pyrexia of unknown origin (PUO) are dependent on the etiology identified. Empiric treatment should generally be discouraged among such patients.

"If the challenge exists so must the solution"

—Rona Mlnarik

INTRODUCTION

Fever is one of the most common reasons for a medical consultation. Most patients with fever have either *a self-limiting* or *an easily identifiable* condition. The term "PUO or fever of unknown origin" (FUO) refers to a *prolonged febrile illness* where a *clear etiology has not been established despite a comprehensive diagnostic evaluation.* It should be emphasized that it is not the degree or duration of fever, but the lack of a clear etiology is the hallmark of PUO.

DEFINITION

Robert G Petersdorf and Paul B Beeson proposed the most widely quoted and accepted definition of PUO in 1961. In their monograph "Fever of Unknown Origin: Report on 100 Cases," PUO was defined as *fever more than 38.3°C (100.9°F)* on several occasions with a *duration of greater than 3 weeks* and *uncertain diagnosis after 1 week of inpatient hospital investigations.* The cut-off for temperature and duration, though not prospectively validated, was specified to exclude conditions like habitual hyperthermia (see below) and acute self-limited infectious diseases. In 1991, Durack and Street suggested to shorten the duration of investigation to three inpatient days or three outpatient visits. This modification was meant to reflect the advances in diagnostic testing. They also divided PUO (based on host characteristics) into four distinct subclasses as follows:

Classical PUO: Temperature >38.3°C (100.9°F) recorded on several occasions occurring for >3 weeks in spite of investigations on three outpatient visits or 3 days of stay in the hospital or 1 week of invasive ambulatory investigations. Although the list of causes of PUO is quite long and varied, most cases in adults are limited to several dozen possible causes, and more often an atypical presentation of a common disease rather than an unusual disease.

Nosocomial PUO: Temperature >38.3°C (100.9°F) recorded on several occasions in a hospitalized patient who is receiving acute care and in whom infection was not manifest or incubating on admission. Three days of investigations including at least 2 days incubation of cultures is the minimum requirement for this diagnosis. The usual causes of fever in hospitalized adults include nosocomial infections (e.g., catheter-related blood stream infections, ventilator-associated pneumonia, and catheter-associated urinary tract infection), drug fever, transfusion of blood and blood products, deep vein thrombosis, and pulmonary embolism.

Neutropenic PUO: Temperature >38.3°C (100.9°F) on several occasions observed in a patient whose neutrophil count is <500/µL or expected to fall to that level in 1–2 days. This diagnosis should be considered for investigations including at least 2 days of incubation of cultures. Neutropenic fevers are most often due to bacterial, viral, and fungal infections. Patients can have blood-stream infections (from translocation of enteric bacteria into bloodstream or indwelling vascular catheters) or localized infections like pneumonia, cellulitis, enterocolitis etc.

Human immunodeficiency virus (HIV)-associated PUO: Temperature >38.3°C (100.9°F) on several occasions found over >4 weeks or >3 days for hospitalized patients with HIV infection. This diagnosis is considered if appropriate investigations over 3 days, including 2 days of incubation of cultures, reveal no source. Opportunistic infections (OIs) are the most frequent causes of prolonged fever in these patients. The relative frequencies of various OIs depend on the setting. Tuberculosis remains the most frequently diagnosed OI in developing countries. Other common OIs include cryptococcosis, pneumocystis pneumonia, and disseminated histoplasmosis.

CONDITIONS CAUSING PUO

Over 200 causes for PUO have been described in the literature. These causes can be broadly subdivided in four categories: (1) infections (e.g., extrapulmonary tuberculosis, infective endocarditis, brucellosis etc.), (2) malignancies (e.g., lymphomas, renal cell carcinoma etc.), (3) non-infectious inflammatory diseases (NIID) [e.g., systemic lupus erythematosus (SLE), (4) systemic vasculitis, adult onset Still's disease etc.], and miscellaneous causes. Overall, uncommon presentations of common diseases account for most cases. In low- and middle-income countries, infections remain the main cause. In a recent series of 300 patients with classical PUO reported by Rupali et al. from a large teaching hospital in southern India, infections were diagnosed in 48%, malignancies in 22%, NIID in 21%, and miscellaneous causes in 9%. The common infections were extrapulmonary and disseminated tuberculosis (69%) and melioidosis (13%). Other infections were visceral abscesses, infective endocarditis, enteric fever, and disseminated histoplasmosis.

DIAGNOSTIC APPROACH

- Prior to undertaking extensive diagnostic testing, *documenting fever* (multiple recordings of oral temperature >38.3°C or >100.9°F) is essential. The upper limit of the normal oral temperature is 37.7°C (99.9°F). Low-grade fever (oral temperature ≤38.3°C) with no additional diagnostic clues in history and physical examination and absence of ongoing inflammation [erythrocyte sedimentation rate (ESR) and C-reactive protein (CRP) values within normal limits] is mostly due to habitual hyperthermia or chronic fatigue syndrome. Fever patterns are seldom diagnostic.
- Diagnostic evaluation is *aimed at identifying PDCs*, defined as symptoms, signs, and laboratory abnormalities pointing toward a possible diagnosis. This approach is far more efficient than routinely ordering a battery of investigations blindly, which can result in misleading information and waste of resources.
- *A thorough history* (past medical history, intravenous drug use, family history, travel history, sexual history, unusual exposure due to occupation or hobbies, and animal contacts) and physical examination (with specific attention to optic fundus, temporal arteries, lymph nodes, liver and spleen, skin and mucous membranes, and musculoskeletal system) are the essential initial step in identifying PDCs. It is also important to reassess the patient frequently as diseases continue to evolve and PDCs become more evident (e.g., lymph node enlargement in tuberculosis, palpable purpura, or mononeuritis in systemic vasculitis).
- *Initial investigations* usually include complete blood counts, ESR, and CRP, liver and renal function tests, blood cultures (minimum two), HIV serology, chest X-ray ultrasonography of abdomen and pelvis, and antinuclear antibodies (ANA).
- Further evaluation should be guided by PDCs and knowledge of local disease patterns among patients with prolonged fever.
- *When PDCs are misleading or absent*, positron emission tomography using F-18 fluorodeoxyglucose (FDG) as the radiotracer, combined with cross-sectional anatomic information provided by computed tomography (CT) scan (FDG-PET/CT scan) can facilitate anatomical localization of infectious, inflammatory, or neoplastic processes (focally increased FDG uptake), thereby guiding further diagnostic tests. It is very important to understand that an FDG-PET/CT only guides further diagnostic testing, and does not confirm any etiology. A recent meta-analysis by Takeuchi et al. reported the performance characteristics of FDG-PET/CT in patients with classical PUO. Included studies were heterogeneous and had several methodological limitations. According to the authors, the sensitivity was 0.86 [95% confidence interval (CI) 0.81–0.90], specificity 0.52 (95% CI 0.36–0.67), and diagnostic yield 0.58 (95% CI 0.51–0.64). The diagnostic yield was 66% in the series reported by Rupali et al. probably reflecting the high prevalence of infections and neoplasms as leading causes of FUO in their series.
- *Biopsies*: Biopsies (image guided or open) of enlarged or affected organs should be performed for both histopathology and appropriate cultures. Depending on PDCs, this may include lymph node, liver, temporal artery, pleura, peritoneum, or bone marrow biopsy. Bone marrow biopsy should be performed in patients with generalized lymphadenopathy or hepatosplenomegaly, cytopenias, HIV infection, and in areas where enteric fever is endemic.
- A definite diagnosis remains elusive in a varied proportion of patients despite extensive diagnostic evaluation. The prognosis is generally good for this subset of patients, and fever resolves spontaneously with time.

EMPIRIC THERAPY

Every attempt should be made to establish a definite etiology in patients presenting with prolonged fever. An accurate diagnosis is essential for appropriate treatment. Empiric treatment can lead to a false sense of security, and expose patients to expensive and potentially toxic drugs. Tuberculosis is reported to be the most common cause of PUO in studies from India. Empiric antituberculous treatment may be reasonable in our setting if clinical clues are suggestive (e.g., unexplained lymphadenopathy or serous effusions), and further evaluation is not feasible due to lack of access to diagnostic facilities or patient preference due to cost and/or discomfort. Patients on empiric treatment should be followed up carefully to assess therapeutic response, and should be promptly referred for further diagnostic evaluation if fever persists.

CONCLUSION

Prolonged fever remains one of the most challenging problems facing clinicians even today. A definitive diagnosis can be made in most patients with systematic pursuit of PDCs. Empiric therapy is generally discouraged.

RECOMMENDED READINGS

1. Osler W. The study of the fevers of the South. JAMA. 1896;26:999-1004.
2. Petersdorf RG, Beeson PB. Fever of unexplained origin: report on 100 cases. Medicine (Baltimore). 1961;40:1-30.
3. Durack DT, Street AC. Fever of unknown origin--reexamined and redefined. Curr Clin Top Infect Dis. 1991;11:35-51.
4. Kaul DR, Flanders SA, Beck JM, Saint S. Brief report: incidence, etiology, risk factors, and outcome of hospital-acquired fever: a systematic, evidence-based review. J Gen Intern Med. 2006;21(11):1184-7.
5. Zimmer AJ, Freifeld AG. Optimal management of neutropenic fever in patients with cancer. J Oncol Pract. 2019;15(1):19-24.
6. Rupali P, Abraham OC, Zachariah A, Subramanian S, Mathai D. Aetiology of prolonged fever in antiretroviral-naïve human immunodeficiency virus-infected adults. Natl Med J India. 2003;16(4):193-9.
7. Rupali P, Garg D, Viggweswarupu S, Sudarsanam TD, Jeyaseelan V, Abraham OC. Etiology of Classic Fever of Unknown Origin (FUO) among Immunocompetent Indian Adults. J Assoc Physicians India. 2019;67(1): 21-6.
8. Wright WF, Auwaerter PG. Fever and Fever of Unknown Origin: Review, Recent Advances, and Lingering Dogma. Open Forum Infect Dis. 2020;7(5):ofaa132.
9. Affronti M, Mansueto P, Soresi M, Abbene AM, Affronti A, Valenti M, et al. Low-grade fever: how to distinguish organic from non-organic forms. Int J Clin Pract. 2010;64(3):316-21.
10. Mulders-Manders C, Simon A, Bleeker-Rovers C. Fever of unknown origin. Clin Med (Lond). 2015;15(3):280-4.
11. Takeuchi M, Dahabreh IJ, Nihashi T, Iwata M, Varghese GM, Terasawa T. Nuclear Imaging for Classic Fever of Unknown Origin: Meta-Analysis. J Nucl Med. 2016;57(12):1913-9.

CHAPTER

34 Nosocomial Infection

Subhash Todi, Mohuya Bhattacharya

ABSTRACT

Acquiring new infection after hospital admission is termed as nosocomial or hospital-acquired infection. These infections are predominantly related to device use or wound related and can present as ventilator associated, urinary catheter related, central line related, or surgical site infection. Antibiotic associated clostridium difficile infection is also termed as nosocomial infection (NI). Epidemiological data using surveillance definitions have indicated much higher incidence of these infections in developing countries and significantly contribute to increase in mortality and morbidity of hospitalized patients particularly in intensive care unit (ICU). Risk factors include device-related and host-related factors which need to be identified for optimum control of these infections. These infections need to be identified by a constellation of local and systemic features of inflammation and confirmed by appropriate cultures. It is sometimes difficult to differentiate infection from colonization from culture results. Prompt administration of empiric antibiotic based on epidemiological data and removal of devices as source control measures should be undertaken to control the infection. Prevention is the key to control of NI and appropriate hygiene and isolation measures need to be undertaken.

"True prevention is not waiting for bad things to happen, it's preventing things from happening in the first place"

—Dan McPherson

INTRODUCTION

The word "nosocomial" has its origin from two Greek words: nosus (disease) and komeion (to take care of) which means the disease is newly acquired by a person while under medical care. It is an umbrella term which is used to describe infection which is not present during hospital admission but is acquired during hospital stay of the patient. As the incubation period of most of the infections is minimum 48 hours, this term is used to describe new infection occurring after 48 hours of hospital stay or within 48 hours of hospital discharge. Terms like hospital-acquired infection or ICU-acquired infection is used synonymously with NI. This should be distinguished from undiagnosed infection present during admission and detected later during the hospital stay.

Earlier "healthcare associated infection" term was used to describe infection acquired in persons who were recently exposed to healthcare environment, like hospital admission in previous 3 months. The reason to introduce this term was to identify this subgroup of patients who were prone to infection with drug-resistant organism and empirical coverage with broad-spectrum antibiotic was advocated. Over a period of time it was realized that this definition was overly sensitive and has led to widespread overuse of broad-spectrum antibiotic with its attendant problems, moreover these patient population are equally likely to be infected with antibiotic sensitive community-acquired organism, so empirical use of broad-spectrum agent is unwarranted. Due to the above mentioned reason the term "healthcare-associated infection" is abandoned and is no longer in common use.

Nosocomial infections are an increasing problem worldwide as they are usually caused by drug-resistant microorganism and contribute significantly to an increasing burden of mortality, morbidity, hospital length of stay, and economic burden to the patient. This chapter will describe the common NIs encountered in clinical practice highlighting the epidemiology, diagnostic, therapeutic, and preventive aspects.

DEFINITIONS

Common NIs encountered in clinical practice are as follows (**Table 1**):

- Hospital-acquired pneumonia/ventilation-acquired pneumonia (HAP/VAP)
- Catheter-associated urinary tract infection (CAUTI)
- Central line-associated bloodstream infection (CLABSI)
- Surgical site soft-tissue infection (SSTI)
- *Clostridioides difficile* infection

Internationally accepted definition of these infections have been agreed upon to facilitate uniform surveillance and incidence reporting globally. These definitions are predominantly for epidemiological purposes and might be different from clinical diagnosis and subsequent management, which also takes into account clinicians' experience.

EPIDEMIOLOGY

Most of the NIs are related to the use of devices and the incidence increases with increased use and/or increased duration of device use. A standardized nomenclature has been agreed upon for surveillance and comparison purposes which include the number of device days as the denominator to describe the incidence of a particular

TABLE 1 Definitions of nosocomial infections.

Terminology	
CAUTI—symptomatic bacteriuria	Symptoms or signs compatible with urinary tract infection (UTI) (fever, chill, nausea, supra pubic tenderness, abdominal distention, altered mental state, and hypotension) in a patient with indwelling urethral, suprapubic, intermittent catheterization or had urethral, suprapubic, or condom catheters within the past 48 h Plus Culture shows growth of $\geq 10^3$ colony-forming units (cfu)/mL of uropathogenic bacteria
CAUTI—asymptomatic bacteriuria	Asymptomatic patient with indwelling urethral, suprapubic, or intermittent catheterization Plus Culture shows growth of $\geq 10^5$ cfu/mL of uropathogenic bacteria
Hospital-acquired pneumonia (HAP)	Pneumonia that occurs in patients admitted for >48 h in any healthcare facility
Ventilator-associated pneumonia (VAP)	Pneumonia that occurs in patients who are on ventilator for >48 h
CLABSI	Laboratory confirmed bloodstream infection (LCBI)—bacterial or fungal pathogen cultured from one or more blood cultures Or Common commensal organism (e.g., coagulase-negative *Staphylococcus*) identified in two or more blood cultures collected on different days or from different sites Plus No source of infection identified at another site And Features of sepsis: Fever (>38.0°C), chills, or hypotension CLABSI: At least one of the LCBI criteria delineated above Plus Presence of a central venous line for >2 consecutive calendar days
Surgical site infection (SSI)	Infection occurs after surgery in the part the surgery was done and this can involve skin, soft tissue, underlying organ, and implanted material

TABLE 2 **Device-associated infections (DAI).**

Terminologies	Formulae
DAI rate (device-associated infection rate)	Number of DAI cases (sum of VAP, CLABSI and CAUTI cases)/total number of device days (sum of ventilator, central line and catheter days) × 1,000
VAP rate	Number of VAP cases/total number of ventilator days × 1,000
CLABSI rate	Number of CLABSI cases/total number of central line days × 1,000
CAUTI rate	Number of CAUTI cases/total number of catheter days × 1,000
SSI rate	Number of SSI/number of surgeries done × 100
DU ratio	Number of device days/number of patient days
Ventilator utilization ratio	Number of VAP cases/total number of ventilator days
Central line utilization ratio	Number of CLABSI cases/total number of central line days
Urinary catheter utilization ratio	Number of CAUTI cases/total number of catheter days

(CAUTI: catheter-associated urinary tract infection; CLABSI: central line-associated bloodstream infection; DU: device utilization; SSI: surgical site infection; VAP: ventilator-associated pneumonia)

device-related NI (**Table 2**). Incidence of NI is variable worldwide with higher reported incidence and associated mortality and morbidity in developing countries than developed countries. International Nosocomial Infection Surveillance Consortium (INICC) has been publishing data periodically on the incidence of NI in developing countries, including India. Similar data from North America has been published by the Centre for Disease Control-National Health Care Safety Network (CDC-NHSN) previously known as National Nosocomial Infections Surveillance System (NNIS). India specific data has also been reported by INDICAP study. These data can be used a benchmark for audit and quality control. The primary goal of INICC was to establish a global network to reduce the rates of infections associated with healthcare in developing countries. Both NNIS and INICC are surveillance system developed with an intent to identify the trend and magnitude of NIs, identification of risk factors, and bacterial resistance. They periodically publish data related to the attributable mortality and morbidity such as extra length of hospital stay and costs imposed by such infection. The rate of NI from the published data over last 5–18 years remained almost four to five times higher in INICC ICUs compared to NNIS ICUs. INICC analysis involving seven ICUs of India revealed device-associated infection rate varying from 2 to 10 per 1,000 device days.

In general, INICC data has reported average incidence of VAP, CAUTI, and CLABSI as 13.1, 5.07, and 4.11 per 1,000 device days, respectively in medical/surgical ICUs of developing countries for the year 2010–2015. Incidence from North American ICUs reported by NHSN during the same period was 0.9, 1.7, and 0.8 per 100 device days, respectively showing the stark contrast in the incidence of NI rates between developing and developed countries. Attributable (additional) mortality due to NIs was in the range of 25% and 34% and attributable (additional) length of stay was 13 and 10 days for CLABSI and VAP, respectively. In order to minimize morbidity and audit their infection control practices due to NI, each hospital should have a system in place to document their NI rate and compare with similar reported rate from other available national or international benchmark data.

BOX 1 **Risk factors for nosocomial infection.**

Host factors
- Aging population
- Chronic illness
- Immune deficiency state, including human immunodeficiency virus (HIV), steroid, and chemotherapy
- Nutritional deficiency and use of parenteral nutrition
- Hematological malignancy, neutropenia, and bone marrow transplantation
- Loss of skin integrity, as with burns

Device-related factors
- Duration of device in place
- Placed for no definite indication
- Inadequate infection control measure during insertion
- Inappropriate site
- Inadequate adherence of daily bundle of care

RISK FACTORS

Hospitalized patients are vulnerable to NIs. Identifying a target group at high risk and prioritizing infection control practices and surveillance for this group will help in better resource allocation (**Box 1**).

DIAGNOSIS

In general, diagnosis of NI should be suspected on occurrence of any one or more of the following in a patient 48 hours after hospital admission.

- New systemic inflammatory feature like fever
- New local feature of inflammation, e.g., new purulent discharge from wound site, endotracheal suction or sputum turning purulent, cloudy urine, erythema or purulence around a device insertion site like central venous catheter
- Rise in one or more inflammatory biomarker such as white count, C-reactive protein, and procalcitonin
- New changes on imaging such as new infiltrate on X-ray or CT scan and new fluid collection on drain insertion site by ultrasound

Once NI is suspected, diagnosis is confirmed by sending relevant cultures from the clinically suspected areas such as blood, sputum, or urine.

Standard definition to diagnose NI has been published, but in clinical practice many a times all the diagnostic criteria are not met and antibiotics are started on a presumptive basis. Moreover the following confounding features make it difficult to confirm a diagnosis of NI:

- *Differentiating noninfective inflammatory feature from onset of a new infection*, e.g., differentiating fever due to sterile necrotizing pancreatitis from infected necrosis. They may be differentiated if a positive culture from a sterile site like blood or pancreatic tissue by fine-needle aspiration is detected. Certain biomarkers like procalcitonin may distinguish sterile inflammation from an infected one but there can be overlap in the procalcitonin values and literature in this regard is conflicting.
- *Differentiating colonization from infection.* Hospitalized patients particularly in ICU gets colonized with pathogenic organism very early during their stay and growth of such organism from a nonsterile site such as endotracheal suction, drains, and superficial swabs from wounds or burns. Catheter specimen of urine is not indicative of a new infection and should not prompt use of antibiotics. In fact this could be one of the most common causes of undesirable use of antibiotics. Quantitative culture with certain cutoff value of colony count from the bacterial growth has been used to differentiate colonization from infection, but is confounded by prior use of antibiotic and the cutoff values have not been well defined. New polymerase chain reaction (PCR)-based techniques are increasingly utilized for early detection of microorganism from culture specimen but this also can not differentiate colonization from infection.
- *Differentiating new bacterial infection from fungal or viral NI.* Hospital-acquired candidemia and other fungal infection are being increasingly reported in ICU and other immunocompromised patient. Viral infection like reactivation of latent herpes infection or cytomegalovirus infection is also reported in these groups of patients. Procalcitonin values usually remain normal in fungal and viral infections as opposed to bacterial infection.

Due to the above confounding features, development of new unexplained hypotension or new onset organ dysfunction is taken as an important criterion to indicate onset of a new infection in hospitalized patient.

MANAGEMENT

Early suspicion, sending appropriate cultures, empirical use of appropriate antibiotic to cover likely pathogen in appropriate doses, de-escalation if possible once culture results are obtained, stopping antibiotics if alternative diagnosis is confirmed, and appropriate duration of antibiotics are the key principles of antibiotic stewardship.

Empirical choice of antibiotic is mainly dependent on the knowledge of local epidemiology and antibiogram of that institution, if available (**Table 3**). Otherwise national or international guidelines on the use of antibiotics in these infections need to be followed but these may not give desirable results due to increasing incidence of multidrug-

TABLE 3 Choice of empirical antibiotic in suspected nosocomial infection.

Infection	Predominant organism	Preferred treatment
VAP	• Enterobacteriaceae (*Klebsiella pneumoniae, Acinetobacter* species, *Pseudomonas aeruginosa*) • Gram-positive cocci (MSSA and MRSA): In areas with high incidence • Viruses and fungi (for immunocompromised)	Carbapenem or colistin Plus Tigecycline or minocycline Plus Vancomycin or teicoplanin or linezolid (for MRSA)
CLABSI	• Gram-positive cocci (MSSA and MRSA) • Enterococci • Enterobacteriaceae (*K. pneumoniae, Acinetobacter* species, *Escherichia coli*, and *P. aeruginosa*)	Flucloxacillin or cefazolin (MSSA) Vancomycin or, teicoplanin or, daptomycin (MRSA and enterococci) Plus Carbapenem and/or colistin
CAUTI	Enterobacteriaceae (*Klebsiella pneumoniae, E. coli, P. aeruginosa, Proteus* species) Enterococci Fungus (*Candida* in complicated UTI and immunocompromised)	Carbapenem or colistin or fosfomycin Plus Vancomycin or teicoplanin or linezolid (enterococci) Fluconazole or flucytosine
SSI	Polymicrobial (includes anerobic organism, MRSA, Enterobacteriaceae)	Tigecycline, minocycline, doxycycline, and TMP-SMX If drug resistance is suspected: Vancomycin or teicoplanin or daptomycin or linezolid Or BLBLI or carbapenem

(BLBLI: β-lactam/β-lactam inhibitor; CAUTI: catheter-associated urinary tract infection; CLABSI: central line-associated bloodstream infection; MRSA: methicillin-resistant *Staphylococcus aureus*; MSSA: methicillin-sensitive *Staphylococcus aureus*; SSI: surgical site infection; TMP-SMX: trimethoprim-sulfamethoxazole)

TABLE 4 Resistance pattern and choice of antibiotics.

Organisms	Preferred agents
ESBL producing organism	Carbapenems
Carbapenemase producing organism	• For KPC and OXA-48—ceftazidime-avibactam, meropenem-vaborbactam, imipenem-relebactam, cefiderocol, or polymyxins • For metallo-β-lactamases (MBLs)—aztreonam plus ceftazidime-avibactam, cefiderocol, or polymyxins
Carbapenem-resistant *Acinetobacter baumannii*	Polymyxins, minocycline, and tigecycline
Carbapenem-resistant *Pseudomonas aeruginosa*	Ceftazidime-avibactam, ceftolozane-tazobactam, cefiderocol, imipenem-cilastatin-relebactam, and polymyxins

resistant infection in the hospital-acquired infections. In order to avoid overuse of antibiotics, if patient is not in shock or developing new organ dysfunction expeditious use of diagnostics should be pursued to confirm a microbiological diagnosis before starting empirical antibiotic. Due to increasing resistance in bacteria causing NI, tools are available to detect the mechanism of resistance in the bacteria and a working knowledge of antibiotics effective against different resistance mechanism is useful in choosing appropriate antibiotic. Close liaison with the microbiologist is necessary in this regard (**Table 4**).

Prompt removal of devices such as central venous catheters and urinary catheters, if possible, is one of the key management principles apart from early use of appropriate antibiotics in managing these infections. Any empirical therapy should be reassessed 2 or 3 days after its initiation. Antibiotics may be escalated or de-escalated on the basis of report of antibiotic sensitivity tests, though clinical response is sometimes given a priority. Principles of antibiotic stewardship should be followed to optimize the use of precious antibiotics.

PREVENTION

Preventive strategies to reduce NI are as follows:

Environmental cleaning: Environmental and surface cleaning, disinfection, and sterilization are critical to reduce transmission of organisms, reduce transmission from water-containing heater-cooler units, faucets, and water supply system of the patient care area. Surface cleaning at scheduled regular interval is a necessary step to reduce incidence and prevalence of NIs. Disinfection strategies have been published by national and international societies and hospitals should customize and follow these based on resources available.

Standard precaution: It should be followed by all the personnel related to providing care of the patients, including nursing staff, physiotherapist, technicians, and doctors. Component of standard precaution:

- Hand hygiene before and after contact with every patient, regardless of whether gloves are used. In most of the cases, alcohol-based hand rubs are used except in cases of visible soiling and in cases of *Clostridium difficile* infection. In the last two situations soap water-based hand hygiene protocol along with disposable tissue paper for drying of hands are needed. Artificial and long finger nails are prohibited.
- Use of universal precautions such as gloves, gowns, and eye protection in situations in which exposure to blood or body secretions is possible.
- Use of mask (preferably N95) for respiratory hygiene.
- Safe injection practices and safe disposal of needles and sharp instruments in impervious containers.

Isolation precaution: Clearly marked rooms should be available for isolation precaution. In addition to standard precaution, patients are required to be isolated in separate rooms to reduce transmission of certain diseases. This type of segregation is intended to prevent contact, droplet, and airborne spread of pathogens. Contact precaution is required in infection such as methicillin-resistant *Staphylococcus aureus* (MRSA), vancomycin-resistant *Enterococcus* (VRE), *Clostridioides* (formerly *Clostridium*) *difficile*, multidrug resistant gram-negative (MDR-GN) pathogens, where precautions to be taken to minimize environmental contamination. Droplet precaution is to be followed in cases of influenza, diphtheria, and pneumonic plague.

Infection spread by respiratory droplet like Rubella, Mumps, Covid-19, and other Corona virus infection may be prevented by appropriate use of N95 mask. Suspected airborne transmission such as varicella zoster virus (VZV) infection, herpes simplex virus (HSV), measles, and tuberculosis infection should be handled with negative pressure isolation room and using certified respirators. Immunocompromised patients like stem cell transplantation require special isolation area with positive pressure to minimize exposure to invasive fungal infections such as aspergillosis.

Decrease device utilization: All the invasive devices used in each patient needs to be revisited to understand whether they can be removed. Audit of device utilization is a standard practice which may help to reduce infection.

RECOMMENDED READINGS

1. Inweregbu K, Dave J, Pittard A. Nosocomial infections. Contin Educ Anaesth Crit Care Pain. 2005;5(1):14-7.
2. Chalmers JD, Rother C, Salih W, Ewig S. Healthcare-associated pneumonia does not accurately identify potentially resistant pathogens: a systematic review and meta-analysis. Clin Infect Dis. 2014;58(3):330-9.
3. Horan TC, Andrus M, Dudeck MA. CDC/NHSN surveillance definition of health care-associated infection and criteria for specific types of infections in the acute care setting. Am J Infect Control. 2008;36(5):309-32.

4. Dudeck MA, Edwards JR, Allen-Bridson K, Gross C, Malpiedi PJ, Peterson KD, et al. National Healthcare Safety Network report, data summary for 2013, Device-associated Module. Am J Infect Control. 2015;43(3):206-21.
5. Rosenthal VD, Bat-Erdene I, Gupta D, Belkebir S, Rajhans P, Zand F, et al. International Nosocomial Infection Control Consortium. International Nosocomial Infection Control Consortium (INICC) report, data summary of 45 countries for 2012-2017: Device-associated module. Am J Infect Control. 2020;48(4): 423-32.
6. Mehta A, Rosenthal VD, Mehta Y, Chakravarthy M, Todi SK, Sen N, et al. Device-associated nosocomial infection rates in intensive care units of seven Indian cities. Findings of the International Nosocomial Infection Control Consortium (INICC). J Hosp Infect. 2007;67(2):168-74.
7. Edwards JR, Peterson KD, Andrus ML. Dudeck MA, Pollock DA, Horan TC; National Healthcare Safety Network (NHSN) report, data summary for 2006 through 2007, issued November 2008. Am J Infect Control. 2008;36:609-26.
8. Divatia JV, Amin PR, Ramakrishnan N, Kapadia FN, Todi S, Sahu S et al. Intensive Care in India: The Indian Intensive Care Case Mix and Practice Patterns Study. Indian J Crit Care Med. 2016;20(4):216-25.
9. Rosenthal VD, Guzman S, Orellano PW. Nosocomial infections in medical-surgical intensive care units in Argentina: attributable mortality and length of stay. Am J Infect Control. 2003;31(5):291-5.
10. Wang L, Zhou KH, Chen W, Yu Y, Feng SF. Epidemiology and risk factors for nosocomial infection in the respiratory intensive care unit of a teaching hospital in China: A prospective surveillance during 2013 and 2015. BMC Infect Dis. 2019;19(1):145.
11. Kalil AC, Metersky ML, Klompas M, Muscedere J, Sweeney DA, Palmer LB, et al. Management of Adults With Hospital-acquired and Ventilator-associated Pneumonia: 2016 Clinical Practice Guidelines by the Infectious Diseases Society of America and the American Thoracic Society. Clin Infect Dis. 2016;63(5):e61-111.
12. Barlam TF, Cosgrove SE, Abbo LM, MacDougall C, Schuetz AN, Septimus EJ, et al. Implementing an Antibiotic Stewardship Program: Guidelines by the Infectious Diseases Society of America and the Society for Healthcare Epidemiology of America. Clin Infect Dis. 2016;62(10):e51-77.
13. O'Grady NP, Alexander M, Burns LA, Dellinger EP, Garland J, Heard SO, et al. Guidelines for the prevention of intravascular catheter-related infections. Clin Infect Dis. 2011;52(9):e162-93.
14. Klompas M, Branson R, Eichenwald EC, Greene LR, Howell MD, Lee G, et al. Strategies to prevent ventilator-associated pneumonia in acute care hospitals: 2014 update. Infect Control Hosp Epidemiol. 2014;35(8):915-36.

CHAPTER

35

Hospital Infection Control

Gagandeep Singh, Arti Kapil

ABSTRACT

Healthcare facility creates many opportunities for microorganisms to spread between patients, visitors, and healthcare workers. Over the years the medical care has become increasingly complex, with routinely performed invasive procedures that increase the risk of developing healthcare-associated infections (HAIs). Majority of these infections are preventable. Research has proven that infection prevention and control programs can make the experience in healthcare facility safer and affordable for the patients with less suffering. Trained infection prevention and control specialists (including nurses and doctors) oversee the program activities and develop and implement policies. The focus is to implement within the healthcare facility best-practice standards and guidelines. The program has a strong education component that includes training all cadres of healthcare workers. The current chapter deals with policies, team members of hospital infection control committee (HICC), their roles etc. A brief introduction to transmission dynamics of infections and surveillance of different HAIs is also put forth. Finally, we introduce the readers to the concepts of employee health and antimicrobial stewardship.

"A hospital alone shows what war is"

—Erich M Remarque

INTRODUCTION

Healthcare-associated infections are one of the most common complications of healthcare management. Sources of HAIs can be endogenous or exogenous. Endogenous sources are body sites, such as the skin, nose, mouth, gastrointestinal tract, or vagina that are normally inhabited by microorganisms. Exogenous sources are those external to the patient, such as patient care personnel, visitors, patient care equipment, medical devices, or the healthcare environment. HAIs lead to increased morbidity and mortality, length of hospital stay, and overall costs associated with admission to a hospital. A robust infection prevention and control program is vital to offering high quality of healthcare for patients and a safe working environment for the healthcare workers.

The infection control program includes policies on hand hygiene, cough etiquettes, personal protective equipment usage, employee health, environmental hygiene, isolation protocols, antibiotic policy, and stewardship. It also focuses on prevention of HAIs, e.g., ventilator-associated infection, surgical site infections (SSIs), urinary tract infections, intravascular device-related infections etc.

OBJECTIVES

The objectives of a HIC program are to minimize the risk of infection to patients and staff, and to ascertain the roles and responsibilities of key personnel involved in the prevention and control activities, to recommend antibiotic policy for the hospital and identify areas if irrational use of antibiotics and curb irrational use of antibiotics.

INFECTION CONTROL POLICY

The important components of this policy are:

- Monitoring of HAI, microbiological surveillance, investigation and control of outbreaks, if any and monitoring of antimicrobial resistance
- Providing facilities to the hospital staff to maintain good infection control practices
- Conducting ongoing educational/training program for all cadres of hospital staff
- Making provisions for staff health activities
- Having a written document (manual) outlining the various infection control policies and procedures and periodically updating it

INFECTION CONTROL COMMITTEE

The accountability of infection control at any hospital is with the HICC, whose primary duty is to formulate and implement policies to effectively manage infection control issues and outbreaks in hospitals. The policies are implemented under the supervision of HICC which includes the medical superintendent as the chairperson, and the members include professor in charge of the main OT, professor in charge from Microbiology, faculty representatives from each of the clinical departments, representatives from department of hospital administration, and infection control nurses (ICNs). The member secretary is usually a faculty member from department of microbiology or department of hospital administration. The HICC is a body of experts responsible to develop policies and procedures related to infection control in a healthcare setup. It is responsible for implementing agreed policies in order to prevent spread of infection to all areas of the hospital including critical care areas, operation theatres (OTs), Central Sterile Services Department (CSSD) etc. It reviews the incidences and prevalence of "alert" organisms and important infectious diseases, and any outbreaks. It is also responsible for establishing policy and monitoring and control of rational antibiotic usage. The committee prepares and reviews the progress of the annual program of activities. The committee also monitors programs for the education of staff about infection control practices and policies (**Flowchart 1**).

INFECTION CONTROL TEAM

Members of this team include microbiologist, hospital administrator, clinicians (ones who have interest in HIC) and most importantly, the ICNs. This team looks after the surveillance activities and resolving day-to-day issues. It also implements the educational and training programs for the hospital staff. The team also monitors antimicrobial resistance, as well as disinfection and sterilization practices. The team advises on and monitors policies and procedures, liaise with concerned consultants to inform them of suspected cases of notifiable diseases or other significant infections.

MICROBIOLOGIST

The microbiologist is responsible for investigating outbreaks, cross infection, and occupational incidents when indicated. They carry out random surveillance when necessary by applying methods of random surveillance for checking sterilization, disinfection, and environment. They assess the results of antibiotic sensitivity test in order to assess the emergence of resistant microorganisms. The microbiologist also carries out antimicrobial surveillance activity in conjunction with pharmacy for usage of

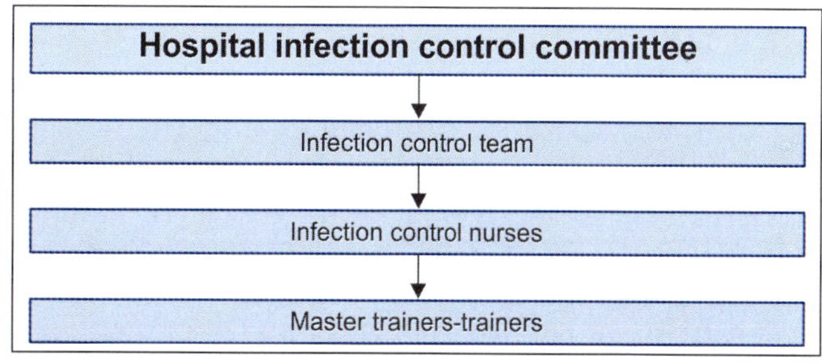

FLOWCHART 1: The structure for infection control program.

restricted usage antimicrobials and to interact with treating consultant(s) or team for effective control of such usage.

INFECTION CONTROL NURSE

The ICNs are members of HICC and Infection Control Team and carry out day-to-day activities of infection control and submit daily reports to infection control officer or the Department of Microbiology. The ICNs regularly visit hospital departments such as clinics, wards, OTs, intensive care units, laboratory areas, kitchen etc. The ICNs liaise with the staff and provide support to all the other healthcare personnel on infection control matters. They also play an important role in identifying potential infection hazards and suggest immediate corrective measures. They are also involved regularly in teaching programs for healthcare workers.

CLINICAL PHARMACOLOGIST

They perform prescription audits and do survey of restricted antibiotics. The clinical pharmacologist coordinates with microbiologists and clinicians for appropriate antibiotic usage, monitoring of antibiotics usage.

HOSPITAL PHARMACIST

The hospital pharmacist shall be responsible for: (1) Obtaining, storing, and distributing medicinal preparations in such a way that infectious agents are not transmitted to the patients; (2) Dispensing antimicrobial agents as per hospital policy and holding all the relevant documentation (regarding potency, incompatibility, and conditions of deterioration); (3) Keeping an inventory of antimicrobial agents distributed to the clinical departments; (4) Provision of data about the usage of all antimicrobials in the hospital to infection control officer/infection control committee, as and when required.

MASTER TRAINER AND TRAINER

They are responsible for implementation of infection control activities at their designated areas. They provide hands-on training to chosen nurses from each area. The infection control team monitors their training effectiveness by interacting with the nurses they have trained. They are required to maintain activity logbook of all their infection control activities. The log is periodically checked by the ICNs or any other member of the HICC.

SALIENT FEATURES OF THE PROGRAM

STANDARD PRECAUTIONS

The standard precautions should be stringently followed at all times. All the healthcare facilities should have an induction program related to infection control practices for every staff member who joins. These trainings should include right methods to perform hand hygiene, cough etiquettes, use of personal protective equipment whenever there is possibility of exposure to infectious material etc.

Hand hygiene is the most important method to prevent transmission of pathogens within a healthcare facility. The hospital administration should ensure adequate supply of soap and water in all patient care areas for handwashing and alcohol-based hand rubs at all patient beds. Alcohol-based hand rubs are frequently used and therefore, have a higher compliance rate. Hand hygiene with soap and water is recommended if hands are visibly soiled and in the setting of *Clostridioides difficile* and Norovirus infections. Audits should be performed at regular intervals to ensure high compliance to hand hygiene at patient care areas. Hand hygiene is recommended before contact with patients, before any aseptic task, after any contact with the patient's body fluid, after patient contact, and after contact with patients' surroundings.

TRANSMISSION-BASED PRECAUTIONS

Organisms vary by size, by how long they survive on surfaces or in the air, and by how they can be transmitted. Example: influenza lasts 1–2 days on surfaces, norovirus up to 7 days, and *C. difficile* up to 7 months. Transmission-based precautions apply to selected patients based on a suspected or confirmed clinical syndrome, a specific diagnosis, or colonization or infection due to epidemiologically important organisms implemented along with standard precautions. *Three major types of transmission-based precautions*:

1. Airborne
2. Droplet
3. Contact

Airborne precautions: These are designed to prevent the transmission of diseases by airborne droplet nuclei (≤5 mm size) or dust particles carrying an infectious agent. These droplet nuclei and particles can travel long distances and remain suspended in the air. If inhaled by a susceptible host, can lead to infection. Patients placed on airborne precautions should be placed in a private room with monitored negative air pressure in relation to surrounding areas. All individuals entering the room should wear N95 masks. Limit movement of patient outside room to medically necessary purposes; if necessary, patient should wear surgical mask and observe cough etiquette. Clinical syndromes that require empiric airborne precautions include vesicular rashes with unknown etiology, rash concerning for measles, or symptoms consistent with tuberculosis.

Droplet precautions: These are used to prevent transmission of large particle droplets generated by coughing, sneezing, and talking. They do not remain suspended in the air for long periods of time or travel long distances (up to 6 feet/2 meters). A susceptible host may become infected if the droplets land on the mucosa of the nose, mouth, or eyes. Patients require isolation in private rooms but not in a negative-pressure room. Individuals entering the room should wear a surgical mask. Limit movement of patient outside room to medically necessary purposes; if necessary, patient should wear surgical mask and observe cough etiquette. Clinical syndromes that necessitate empiric droplet precautions include meningitis and viral respiratory infections.

Contact precautions: These are implemented to prevent spread of epidemiologically significant organisms from an infected or colonized patient to another individual through direct and/or indirect contact. Preferable to place patients in a private room. Healthcare workers should don both gowns and gloves when entering the room. Gowns and gloves should be removed before exiting the room, and hand hygiene should be performed. Clinical syndromes that require empiric contact isolation include acute diarrhea with likely infectious cause, viral respiratory infections in young children, or a draining wound that cannot be covered.

SPECIFIC HEALTHCARE-ASSOCIATED INFECTIONS

Catheter-associated urinary tract infections: Catheter-associated urinary tract infection (CAUTI) is one of the most common HAIs and a leading cause of secondary bacteremia in acute care facilities. Duration of catheterization is the major risk factor for CAUTI. Catheter trauma and catheter obstruction can be precipitating events for CAUTI. Other risk factors for CAUTI: Female sex, severe underlying illness, age greater than 50 years, catheter insertion outside operating room, diabetes mellitus, and renal impairment.

Prevention opportunities: The most important intervention to prevent CAUTI is to avoid use of an indwelling urinary catheter. Other opportunities for prevention include: removal of catheters when no longer indicated, proper education, insertion of catheters under aseptic conditions, using the smallest possible catheter, adherence to hand hygiene, and use of a bundled system of care.

Central line-associated bloodstream infections: Central line-associated bloodstream infections (CLABSIs) have been associated with increased length of hospital stay along with increased costs. A CLABSI is defined as a laboratory-confirmed bloodstream infection (BSI) where a central line was in place for greater than 2 calendar days before the blood culture is drawn, provided that the same BSI is not related to an infection at another site.

Major risk factors: Insertion with less than maximum sterile barriers, placement in an old site via guidewire exchange, heavy cutaneous colonization at the catheter hub, and duration of catheter greater than 7 days.

Prevention: Use and implementation of prevention bundles have been shown to be effective, education of healthcare personnel involved in insertion of central venous catheters (CVCs) as well maintenance and care of patients with CVCs in place has reduced the incidence of CLABSI, checklists have also been used and allow institutions to ensure adherence to infection prevention practices, avoidance of femoral vein catheterization is advised, full sterile barrier precautions are recommended during the insertion of CVCs, exchange of catheter over a guidewire is associated with increased risk for infection, chlorhexidine-based antiseptics allow for prolonged antimicrobial activity on the skin surface after a single application, and use of antiseptic and antimicrobial-impregnated catheters.

Ventilator-associated pneumonia: Ventilator-associated pneumonia (VAP) incidence is difficult to determine as surveillance definitions have changed over the years. VAP used to be defined by clinical, radiographic, and microbiologic criteria, but these signs were neither sensitive nor specific compared to histology.

Ventilator associate events:

- *Ventilator-associated conditions (VACs)*: Deterioration in oxygenation after stable or improving period
- *Infection-related ventilator-associated conditions (IVACs)*: VAC plus temperature or altered white cell count plus new antibiotic
- *Ventilator-associated pneumonia*: IVAC plus positive sputum/BAL microscopy or culture

Mortality of VAP varies based on patient factors. Primary route of infection is by microaspiration of endogenous or exogenously acquired organisms via endotracheal tube leakage around the cuff. Impaired host defenses also play a role. Risk factors and efforts at prevention for VAP have been identified; these include first few days of mechanical ventilation and overall duration of mechanical ventilation.

Prevention: Avoidance of intubation by use of noninvasive positive-pressure ventilation, avoidance of prolonged sedation, daily spontaneous breathing trials, minimization of pooling of secretions above the endotracheal tube cuff, and elevation of the head of the bed to 30–45°.

Surgical site infections: Surgical site infections are considered one of the most common and costly HAIs. A large proportion is considered preventable. Classification of SSIs is based on depth of infection.

- *Superficial incisional infection*: It involves only the skin and subcutaneous tissues. It can often be managed in the outpatient setting.
- *Deep incisional infections*: These involve the fascia and/or muscular layers. These can be further broken down into primary (involves primary incision) or secondary (involves secondary incision).
- *Organ/space infections*: These involve any part of the body opened or manipulated during a procedure, excluding skin incision, fascia, or muscle layers.

Prevention: Guidelines have been well established for the prevention of SSIs.

Guidelines for prevention focus on proper hair removal, glycemic control postoperatively, and maintenance of normothermia. Perform skin preparation in the operating room using an alcohol-based agent, unless contraindicated. Administer a fraction of inspired oxygen during surgery and after extubation in the immediate postoperative period for patients with normal pulmonary function receiving general anesthesia and undergoing endotracheal intubation. Education is the key to prevention within the hospital.

Antimicrobial prophylaxis: Prophylactic antibiotics should be administered within 1 hour prior to incision. Antibiotics should be given prior to the skin incision for cesarean sections. Additional antimicrobial prophylaxis should not be used after the surgical incision is closed in the operating room for clean and clean-contaminated procedures, even if drains are left in place. Prolonged use of antibiotics leads to increased resistance, higher rates of *C. difficile*, and higher rates of acute kidney injury.

Clostridioides difficile infection: *Clostridioides* (formerly *Clostridium*) *difficile* is a well-known hospital pathogen. *C. difficile* infection (CDI) is a leading cause of infectious diarrhea among hospitalized patients. CDI is defined as a case of clinically significant diarrhea or toxic megacolon without other known etiology in which: a stool sample yields a positive result of *C. difficile* toxin; or pseudomembranous colitis is seen on endoscopic examination; or pseudomembranous colitis is seen on histopathologic examination.

The spore-forming nature of *C. difficile* presents challenges for hand hygiene and environmental disinfection practices since spores are resistant to the effects of alcohol. Chlorine-based agents should be used (at least 1,000 ppm available chlorine). Full barrier precautions and hand hygiene are successful interventions to prevent transmission. As mentioned earlier, contact precautions are recommended up to 48 hours after resolution of diarrhea. Effective antimicrobial stewardship is essential along with infection prevention for successful prevention of CDI in hospitals. Restriction of high-risk antibiotics, such as fluoroquinolones, has been successful in stewardship efforts.

IMPLEMENTATION OF PROTOCOLS

Care of equipment, air-conditioning for critical care areas, linen disinfection, biomedical waste management, laboratory safety programs as well as management of blood spills and needle stick injuries should be done according to guidelines established by national and international agencies.

SURVEILLANCE

With an increasing population of immunocompromised patients in acute care and individuals requiring long-term care and the emergence of multidrug resistant (MDR) organisms in healthcare settings, HAIs have become an ever growing challenge. A majority of these HAIs are preventable and effective surveillance systems built into infection prevention and control activities reduce the frequency of these events. Surveillance activities are also useful in monitoring the effectiveness of infection control programs and are required for patient safety.

ANTIMICROBIAL STEWARDSHIP PROGRAM

Antimicrobial stewardship programs (AMSPs) have been established to prevent the emergence of antimicrobial resistance, improve patient outcomes, and reduce costs. Centers for Disease Control and Prevention (CDC) has developed seven core elements for hospital AMSPs to adhere to: leadership commitment, accountability, drug expertise, action, tracking, reporting, and education. It allows for implementation of programs that focus on both pre- or postprescription methods. These programs can be both active (i.e., formulary restriction, preauthorization) or passive (i.e., education, feedback of antimicrobial utilization data). Infection prevention programs can work along with the AMSP to utilize data regarding increasing trends of antimicrobial resistance to form new policies and interventions.

ENVIRONMENTAL SURVEILLANCE

Environmental monitoring of OTs, critical care units, and other patient care areas is not routinely recommended and may be done during an outbreak or after any repair/ maintenance. Additionally, sterilization and disinfection processes should be monitored regularly, drinking water and dialysis water analysis should be done and last but not the least food safety guidelines should be followed.

STAFF HEALTH PROGRAM

Healthcare workers may acquire infections from or transmit infections to patients. In general, healthcare workers who come in contact with patients, body fluids or specimens have a higher risk of acquiring or transmitting infections. The following elements are part of the staff health program:

- *Medical evaluation*: This includes medical examination before placement to ensure that personnel are not placed in jobs that would pose undue risk of infection to them, other personnel, patients, or visitors. Immunization history is important. Periodic evaluations should be done for specific job assignments, for evaluation or work-related problems.
- *Personnel health and safety education*: Education is provided for infection control program so that the staffs understand its rationale and comply with the guidelines.
- *Immunization programs*: Optimal use of vaccines to prevent transmission of vaccine-preventable diseases is advocated to healthcare worker.
- Records are maintained of all accidental HAI acquired by the staff with utmost confidentially.

RECOMMENDED READINGS

1. Damani NN. Basic concepts. In: Damani NN. Manual of Infection Prevention and Control, 3rd edition. Cambridge: Cambridge University Press; 2011.
2. Wilson J. Infection Control in Clinical Practice, 3rd edition. London: Baillière Tindall; 2006.
3. Perry C. Infection Prevention and Control. Oxford: Blackwell Publishing; 2007.
4. 2007 Guideline for Isolation Precautions: Preventing Transmission of Infectious Agents in Healthcare Settings. [online] Available from www.cdc.gov/hicpac/pdf/isolation/Isolation2007.pdfpdf icon.
5. WHO. (2009). WHO Guidelines on Hand Hygiene in Health Care: First Global Patient Safety Challenge: Clean Care is Safer Care. Geneva: WHO. Available from whqlibdoc.who.int/publications/2009/9789241597906_eng.pdf.
6. World Health Organization (WHO). (2007). My 5 Moments for Hand Hygiene. Figure. Retrieved March 16, 2020 from https://www.who.int/gpsc/5may/background/5moments/en/.

CHAPTER

36 Principles of Antibiotic Therapy

George M Varghese, Abi Manesh

ABSTRACT

Antibiotics have saved millions of lives and transformed human health. However, the escalating antimicrobial resistance is threatening the advances in modern medicine. Hence, all physicians must prescribe antibiotics appropriately and judiciously to obtain desired patient outcome and preserve the effectiveness of these lifesaving drugs. This chapter provides insights covering various aspects of choosing antibiotics—pharmacological properties, clinical concerns, and pathogen-related issues. Making an accurate clinical diagnosis is the cornerstone of any effective antibiotic therapy and we also focus in detail on the antibiotic selection in specific clinical syndromes. Also, we discuss recent aspects like de-escalation and modified durations of therapy.

"I think the Internet is the greatest invention in history after antibiotics"

—Jane Haddam

INTRODUCTION

The development and spread of antibiotic resistance which is outpacing the drug discovery jeopardizes the advances in modern healthcare, such as cancer therapy, organ transplant, and advanced intensive care unit (ICU). An estimated 700,000 people die worldwide as a result of drug-resistant infections annually. Antimicrobial resistance (AMR) is projected to result in 10 million deaths and 100 trillion US dollars loss in the global economy annually by 2050. The misuse of antibiotics, the major driver of AMR, is rampant in clinical practice.

Antibiotics are frequently prescribed for nonbacterial causes of illness. For example, use of antibiotics in the management of acute undifferentiated fevers (which could be due to malaria, dengue, chikungunya, typhoid, or scrub typhus) is common practice in India. Even when prescribed for appropriate disease, suboptimal regimens, dosing, or duration may promote the development of AMR. It is essential, therefore, to understand the principles of antimicrobial therapy in order to optimize outcomes and reduce selective pressure on antibiotics. When antibiotic therapy is warranted, current evidence suggests that the goal should be to treat with an effective regimen for the shortest period reasonable to affect a clinical and microbiological cure; this decreases the need for retreatment and the likelihood of developing antibiotic resistance.

Naturally, the first step in this process is to make an accurate diagnosis. Ascertaining the underlying disease process based on the syndrome is necessary in order to decide whether or not it is an illness that would warrant treatment with antibiotics. Empirically treating fever with antibiotics without making an appropriate diagnosis, inevitably ends up treating a broad variety of nonbacterial illnesses in which antibiotics will not only be unhelpful but will also promote future AMR. Treating syndromes such as the common cold, coughs, and bronchitis, which are unlikely to have a bacterial etiology, is of no benefit to the patient and hastens the time when the antibiotics used will no longer be useful because of resistance development.

The appropriate and rational use of antibiotics requires a thorough understanding of the principles of therapy and the current arsenal of antibiotics. Choosing antibiotics for the treatment of an infection, the following factors are important to assist and guide the decision-making process.

CLINICAL FACTORS

PRESUMPTIVE DIAGNOSIS

Making a presumptive diagnosis based on the presenting syndrome is a critical step in choosing the antibiotic regimen, as many diagnoses tend to be associated with a predictable set of pathogens. The clinician should take into account the patient's signs and symptoms, and basic investigations including the chest X-ray, and other imaging studies as appropriate. When choosing to use an antibiotic, there must be at least a strong clinical suspicion, if not solid evidence, that the etiological agent of the illness is bacterial. Many illnesses are nearly always of viral origin (the common cold) while others are most often bacterial (pyelonephritis). The likely etiology or the pathogen that causes the syndrome should be assessed. Additionally, factors such as the age of the patient, their immune status, and presence of comorbidities, and other relevant medical histories should also be considered.

COMORBIDITIES

The choice of antibiotics often depends on the presence of comorbidities, especially the degree of immunosuppression. Human immunodeficiency virus (HIV) infection, corticosteroid or immunosuppressive therapy, chemotherapy, organ transplant, malignancy, or uncontrolled diabetes drastically increases the range of pathogens that could be causing disease and progression to severe disease.

LOCAL RESISTANCE PATTERN

Determining whether the patient is likely to have a community-acquired or hospital-acquired infection is crucial as the set of pathogens and the resistance pattern are clearly different. In addition, the knowledge of local resistance patterns is important which will help in choosing an appropriate antibiotic regimen. A history of the patient's recent antibiotic exposure should be elicited which may determine the possibility of infection with a resistant pathogen. A history of prior infection with resistant pathogens should also be noted.

SEVERITY OF ILLNESS

The severity of illness dictates the need and breadth of coverage of the initial antibiotic regimen. Inappropriate initial antibiotic in patients with severe sepsis is associated with increased risk of mortality. Therefore, in severely ill patients, a broad-spectrum antibiotic regimen to cover suspected pathogens is started and de-escalation is done later guided by microbiologic data. Conversely, a patient with a mild infection may not warrant broad-spectrum antibiotics.

PHARMACOLOGICAL PROPERTIES OF THE ANTIBIOTIC

SPECTRUM OF THE ANTIBIOTIC

After assessing the likely range of pathogens associated with a particular disease syndrome, the choice of antibiotic needs consideration of its spectrum of activity. The antimicrobial activity of an antibiotic can be confirmed by in vitro susceptibility testing. Spectrum of activity of antibiotics against common pathogens is summarized in **Figure 1**.

BACTERICIDAL VERSUS BACTERIOSTATIC

The antibiotics act by destroying the bacterial cell by either preventing cell reproduction or changing a necessary cellular function or process within the cell. Antibiotics are classified into two main categories based on their in vitro effect on bacteria; (1) Bactericidal and (2) Bacteriostatic. Bactericidal antibiotics usually "kill" bacteria and bacteriostatic antibiotics "prevent growth" of bacteria. Although these distinctions are not absolute, bactericidal agents are preferred for serious infections such as endocarditis and meningitis. Based on the mechanism of action, the antibiotics are classified as summarized in **Table 1**.

SITES OF PENETRATION

Choosing an appropriate antibiotic requires knowledge of the distribution and penetration of the drug into different tissue compartments, as well as determination of the patient's most likely site of infection. Important examples of inadequate drug concentration in certain sites include the following:

- *Central nervous system*: First- and second-generation cephalosporins, macrolides, clindamycin, daptomycin, piperacillin-tazobactam, and aminoglycosides tend to have poor penetration and are suboptimal for treatment of meningitis. Third-generation cephalosporins and carbapenems are better choices.
- *Lungs*: Daptomycin is inactivated by surfactant, making it ineffective for pneumonia. beta-lactams and fluoroquinolones are better choices.
- *Urine*: Moxifloxacin and polymyxins does not achieve adequate levels in the urine, making it ineffective for urinary tract infections (UTIs). Levofloxacin and ciprofloxacin are better choices among the fluoroquinolones.

PHARMACODYNAMIC PROPERTY

The two major types of "killing" exhibited by antibiotics are time-dependent killing, where efficacy depends on maximizing the time the antibiotic concentration is above the minimum inhibitory concentration (MIC), and concentration-dependent killing, where efficacy depends on achieving peak concentrations far above the MIC. A third, a mix of both the above phenomena is characterized by the area of the drug concentration curve above the MIC of the organism. Drugs that act via time-dependent killing include beta-lactams and vancomycin; those that act via concentration-dependent killing include aminoglycosides and daptomycin. The mechanism of killing has implications for dosing strategies and is depicted in **Figure 2**. For time-dependent beta-lactams, continuous or prolonged infusion strategies (to maximize time above the MIC) may lead to better outcomes in critically ill patients with resistant organisms. For concentration-dependent aminoglycosides, once-daily dosing strategies are in many circumstances as efficacious and less toxic than traditional q8h dosing. A mixed model will be beneficial for most other antibiotics including polymyxins and fluoroquinolones.

ADVERSE DRUG REACTIONS

Antibiotics, as all other therapies, may be associated with side effects. These side effects vary significantly between, and even within antibiotic classes and are important for the clinician prescribing antibiotics to know. The relative risks and benefits of antibiotic therapy should be weighed prior to prescribing them. Important adverse events of various classes of antibiotics are summarized in **Table 2**.

EMPIRIC ANTIBIOTIC THERAPY

Empirical therapy must often be used in sick patients such as those with severe sepsis, bacterial meningitis, and pneumonia. However, one must consider the whole

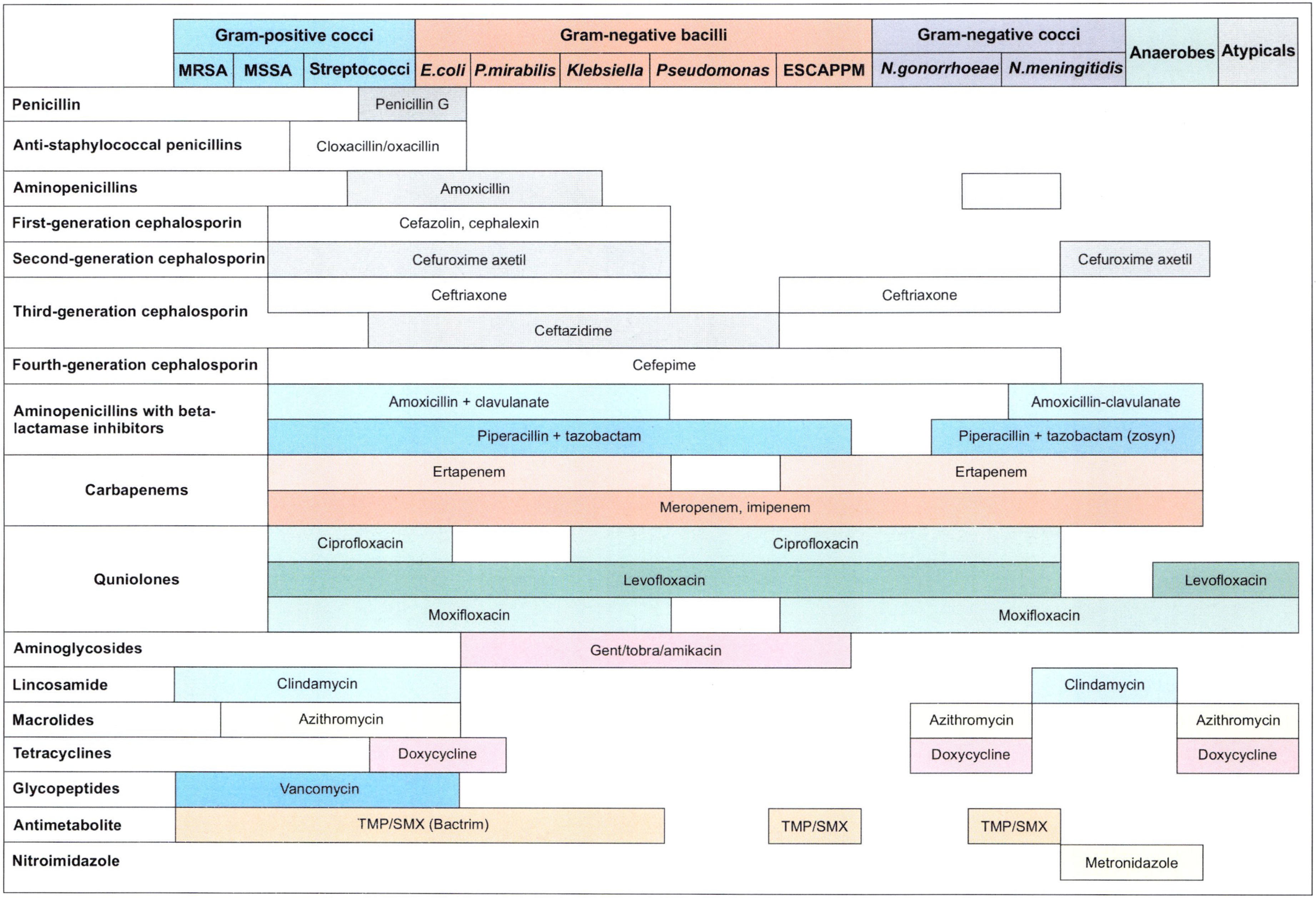

<table>
<tr><th rowspan="2"></th><th colspan="3">Gram-positive cocci</th><th colspan="5">Gram-negative bacilli</th><th colspan="2">Gram-negative cocci</th><th rowspan="2">Anaerobes</th><th rowspan="2">Atypicals</th></tr>
<tr><th>MRSA</th><th>MSSA</th><th>Streptococci</th><th>E.coli</th><th>P.mirabilis</th><th>Klebsiella</th><th>Pseudomonas</th><th>ESCAPPM</th><th>N.gonorrhoeae</th><th>N.meningitidis</th></tr>
<tr><td>Penicillin</td><td></td><td></td><td colspan="2">Penicillin G</td><td></td><td></td><td></td><td></td><td></td><td></td><td></td><td></td></tr>
<tr><td>Anti-staphylococcal penicillins</td><td></td><td colspan="3">Cloxacillin/oxacillin</td><td></td><td></td><td></td><td></td><td></td><td></td><td></td><td></td></tr>
<tr><td>Aminopenicillins</td><td></td><td></td><td colspan="4">Amoxicillin</td><td></td><td></td><td></td><td></td><td></td><td></td></tr>
<tr><td>First-generation cephalosporin</td><td></td><td colspan="5">Cefazolin, cephalexin</td><td></td><td></td><td></td><td></td><td></td><td></td></tr>
<tr><td>Second-generation cephalosporin</td><td></td><td colspan="5">Cefuroxime axetil</td><td></td><td></td><td></td><td colspan="2">Cefuroxime axetil</td><td></td></tr>
<tr><td rowspan="2">Third-generation cephalosporin</td><td></td><td colspan="5">Ceftriaxone</td><td></td><td colspan="3">Ceftriaxone</td><td></td><td></td></tr>
<tr><td></td><td></td><td colspan="5">Ceftazidime</td><td></td><td></td><td></td><td></td><td></td></tr>
<tr><td>Fourth-generation cephalosporin</td><td></td><td colspan="9">Cefepime</td><td></td><td></td></tr>
<tr><td rowspan="2">Aminopenicillins with beta-lactamase inhibitors</td><td></td><td colspan="5">Amoxicillin + clavulanate</td><td></td><td></td><td></td><td colspan="2">Amoxicillin-clavulanate</td><td></td></tr>
<tr><td></td><td colspan="7">Piperacillin + tazobactam</td><td colspan="3">Piperacillin + tazobactam (zosyn)</td><td></td></tr>
<tr><td rowspan="2">Carbapenems</td><td></td><td colspan="5">Ertapenem</td><td></td><td colspan="4">Ertapenem</td><td></td></tr>
<tr><td></td><td colspan="10">Meropenem, imipenem</td><td></td></tr>
<tr><td rowspan="3">Quniolones</td><td></td><td colspan="3">Ciprofloxacin</td><td></td><td colspan="5">Ciprofloxacin</td><td></td><td></td></tr>
<tr><td></td><td colspan="9">Levofloxacin</td><td colspan="2">Levofloxacin</td></tr>
<tr><td></td><td colspan="5">Moxifloxacin</td><td></td><td colspan="5">Moxifloxacin</td></tr>
<tr><td>Aminoglycosides</td><td></td><td></td><td></td><td colspan="5">Gent/tobra/amikacin</td><td></td><td></td><td></td><td></td></tr>
<tr><td>Lincosamide</td><td colspan="3">Clindamycin</td><td></td><td></td><td></td><td></td><td></td><td></td><td colspan="2">Clindamycin</td><td></td></tr>
<tr><td>Macrolides</td><td></td><td colspan="2">Azithromycin</td><td></td><td></td><td></td><td></td><td></td><td>Azithromycin</td><td></td><td></td><td>Azithromycin</td></tr>
<tr><td>Tetracyclines</td><td></td><td></td><td colspan="2">Doxycycline</td><td></td><td></td><td></td><td></td><td>Doxycycline</td><td></td><td></td><td>Doxycycline</td></tr>
<tr><td>Glycopeptides</td><td colspan="3">Vancomycin</td><td></td><td></td><td></td><td></td><td></td><td></td><td></td><td></td><td></td></tr>
<tr><td>Antimetabolite</td><td colspan="6">TMP/SMX (Bactrim)</td><td></td><td>TMP/SMX</td><td></td><td>TMP/SMX</td><td></td><td></td></tr>
<tr><td>Nitroimidazole</td><td></td><td></td><td></td><td></td><td></td><td></td><td></td><td></td><td></td><td></td><td>Metronidazole</td><td></td></tr>
</table>

(MRSA: methicillin-resistant *Staphylococcus aureus*; MSSA: methicillin-susceptible *Staphylococcus aureus*; TMP/SMX: trimethoprim/sulfamethoxazole)

FIGURE 1: Spectrum of activity of antibiotics against common pathogens.

TABLE 1 Different classes of antibiotics.

Bactericidal	
Beta-lactam antibiotics	
Penicillins	
Class/Mechanism	**Drugs**
Penicillin	Penicillin G
	Benzathine penicillin G
	Penicillin V
Aminopenicillins	Ampicillin
	Amoxicillin
Penicillinase-resistant-penicillins	Oxacillin
	Cloxacillin
	Dicloxacillin
Antipseudomonal penicillins	Ticarcillin
	Piperacillin
Cephalosporins	
First-generation	Cefazolin
	Cephalexin
Second-generation	Cefoxitin
	Cefuroxime
Third-generation	Ceftriaxone
	Cefotaxime
	Ceftazidime
Fourth-generation	Cefepime
Other cell wall inhibitors	
Vancomycin	Vancomycin
Beta-lactamase inhibitors	Clavulanic acid
	Sulbactam
	Tazobactam
Carbapenems	Meropenem
	Imipenem (+ cilastatin)
	Doripenem
	Ertapenem
	Aztreonam
Polymyxins	Colistin (polymyxin E)
	Polymyxin B
Deoxyribonucleic acid (DNA) synthesis inhibitors	
Fluoroquinolones	
First-generation	Nalidixic acid
Second-generation	Ciprofloxacin
	Levofloxacin
Third-generation	(Gatifloxacin)
Fourth-generation	Moxifloxacin
	Gemifloxacin

Bacteriostatic	
Protein synthesis inhibition	
Anti-30S ribosomal subunit	
Class/Mechanism	**Drugs**
Aminoglycosides	Gentamicin
	Neomycin
	Amikacin
	Tobramycin
	Streptomycin
Tetracyclines	Tetracycline
	Doxycycline
	Minocycline
	Demeclocycline
Anti-50S ribosomal subunit	
Macrolides	Erythromycin
	Azithromycin
	Clarithromycin
Chloramphenicol	Chloramphenicol
Lincosamide	Clindamycin
Linezolid	Linezolid
Streptogramins	Quinupristin
	Dalfopristin
Other DNA inhibitors	
Metronidazole	Metronidazole
Folic acid synthesis inhibitors	
Trimethoprim/Sulfonamides	Trimethoprim/Sulfamethoxazole (SMX)

picture, including the history, physical findings, presence of leukocytosis, and elevated procalcitonin, rather than each of these features in isolation. Consideration must be given to other factors such as the comorbid conditions, and recent antibiotic exposure in addition to severity of illness. Broad coverage may be necessary in such patients initially. More tailored antibiotics should be chosen once culture and susceptibility data is available. Choices for empiric therapy for common serious infections are given in **Table 3**.

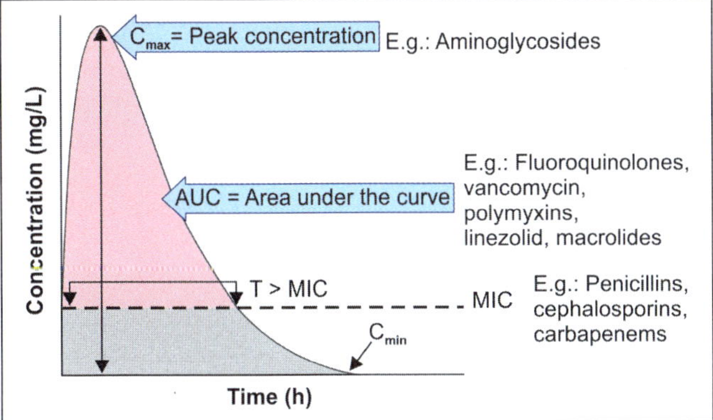

(MIC: minimum inhibitory concentration)

FIGURE 2: The mechanism of killing has implications for dosing strategies.

DEFINITIVE THERAPY AND DE-ESCALATION

The antibiotic regimen should be narrowed once the etiology is identified based on the culture and the susceptibility reports are available. This de-escalation approach is beneficial as it can reduce the cost, toxicities, and emergence of resistance. The targeted regimen of antibiotic therapy reduces the selection pressure and subsequent development of resistance. However, this may not be possible sometimes with concurrent infections in a sicker patient. Whenever possible, a definitive microbiological diagnosis should be obtained in order to tailor therapy to a particular organism, rather than the broader range of possible organisms causing the syndrome. Importantly, finding the exact pathogen, when done by culture, also provides specific antibiotic susceptibilities to be utilized, further allowing for antibiotic optimization.

The need and feasibility for de-escalation should be considered at the bedside every day, especially after day 3 for patients on antibiotics. In high-risk environment like ICUs, tools such as serial procalcitonin measurement can assist in de-escalation decisions. Some of the simple strategies for de-escalation include stopping redundant therapy (multiple antibiotics with the same spectrum of coverage), removing methicillin-resistant *Staphylococcus aureus* (MRSA) coverage when not indicated and discontinuing unnecessary combination therapy. De-escalation happens

TABLE 2 Adverse reactions with different antibiotics.

	Penicillins	Cephalosporins	Carbapenems	Aminoglycosides	Tetracyclines	Chloramphenicol	Rifamycins	Metronidazole	Macrolides/ azalide	Clindamycin	Glycopeptides	Oxazolidinones	Sulfonamides and trimethoprim	Quinolones
Anaphylaxis	++	++	++								+		+	
Nephrotoxicity	+	+	+	++										
Anemia						+						+	+	
Leukopenia	+	+	+			++							+	
Thrombocytopenia	+	+	+			++	+				+	++	+	
Coagulopathy (other than thrombocytopenia)	+	+												
Dermatological toxicity (excluding phlebitis)	++	++	++								+		++	
Neurotoxicity				++				+	++			+		+
Cardiotoxicity									++					+
Hepatotoxicity	+						++							
Musculoskeletal toxicity														
Electrolyte abnormalities	+													
Fever	+	+											+	
Diarrhea	++	++	++		+	+	+		+	++		+	+	+

Note: **+ frequent/severe; ++ frequent and severe.**

TABLE 3 Initial choice of antimicrobial therapy for common infections.

Condition	Likely pathogens	First choice	Alternatives	Comments
		Severe sepsis		
Severe sepsis (community acquired) **Look for common focus:** • **Pyelonephritis** • **Pneumonia** • **Cellulitis** • **Cholangitis**	• Enterobacteriaceae: *Escherichia coli* and *Klebsiella* • *Streptococcus* species • *Haemophilus influenzae* • *Staphylococcus aureus* • *Orientia tsutsugamushi*	• Meropenem 1–2 g IV q8h + doxycycline 100 mg PO BID • To add MRSA cover: ∘ Frequent healthcare contact ∘ Necrotizing pneumonia ∘ Central line in situ ∘ No clinical improvement in 48 h despite therapy ∘ Known colonization with MRSA	Cefoperazone-sulbactam 3 g IV q12h + doxycycline 100 mg PO BID	These patients present with fever and features such as: • Tachypnea and tachycardia • Hypotension • ARDS • Renal failure • Hepatic dysfunction
		Respiratory tract infections		
Acute pharyngitis	Group A ß-hemolytic *Streptococcus* (GABHS)	Amoxicillin 500 mg PO q8h × 7 days	Azithromycin 500 mg PO OD × 5 days	• The large majority are viral and, hence, antibiotic therapy would not be warranted • Supportive treatment (analgesics, antipyretics, and saline gargles) can be given • GABHS infection should receive antibiotics and is suggested by: Fever, tonsillar exudates, lack of cough, and tender cervical lymphadenopathy
Acute epiglottitis	*Haemophilus influenzae*	Ceftriaxone 1–2 g IV OD × 7–10 days		Airway management
• **Ludwig's angina** • **Vincent's angina**	Polymicrobial (oral anaerobes)	Clindamycin 600 mg IV q8h × 2–3 weeks	Amoxicillin-Clavulanate 1,000 mg PO BID	• Airway management • Surgical drainage
Acute bronchitis	Viral	None required		
Acute bacterial rhinosinusitis	• *S. pneumoniae* • *H. influenzae* • *Moraxella catarrhalis*	Amoxicillin 500 mg PO TID × 10–14 days		This is often viral. Antibiotics should be considered if there is fever, facial pain, and purulent nasal discharge
Acute bacterial exacerbation of COPD	• *S. pneumoniae* • *H. influenzae* • *M. catarrhalis*	Amoxicillin 500 mg PO TID × 7 days	• Doxycycline 100 mg PO BID × 7 days • Azithromycin 500 mg PO OD × 3 days	
Community-acquired pneumonia	• *S. pneumoniae* • *H. influenzae* • *M. catarrhalis* • *Legionella*	For inpatient therapy: • Piperacillin-tazobactam 4.5 g IV q8h + Doxycycline 100 mg PO BID	For outpatient therapy: • Amoxicillin 500 mg PO q8h × 5–7 days • Levofloxacin 750 mg PO OD × 7 days	Assess severity based on CURB-65 score: • Score 0 or 1: outpatient therapy • Score 2: inpatient therapy • Score ≥3: ICU therapy

Continued...

Continued...

Condition	Likely pathogens	First choice	Alternatives	Comments
		Respiratory tract infections		
Empyema thoracis	• *S. pneumoniae* • Oral anaerobes	• CP 20 L units IV q4h × 2–3 w eeks	• Piperacillin-tazobactam 4.5 g IV q6h	Chest tube drainage is needed when pleural fluid is: • Frankly purulent or turbid • Nonpurulent, but shows bacteria on Gram stain or culture • pH <7.2
Nosocomial/ ventilator-associated pneumonia	• *E. coli* and *Klebsiella Enterobacter* • *Pseudomonas aeruginosa* • *Acinetobacter* species • *S. aureus*	Colistin 9 MU IV Loading followed by 4.5 MU IV BD × 7 days		Suspect nosocomial/ventilator-associated pneumonia if the patient develops a new fever or leukocytosis with any of the following >48 h after admission/intubation: • New or progressive radiographic infiltrate • Purulent sputum or ET aspirate (for VAP) • Decline in oxygenation
		Cardiovascular infections		
Infective endocarditis (native valve)	Penicillin susceptible (MIC <0.125 μg/mL) *S. viridans*	CP 120–180 L units/day IV × 4 weeks	• Ceftriaxone 2 g IV OD × 4 weeks 2 week regimens: • CP 120–180 L units/ day IV + gentamicin 1 mg/kg q8h IV × 2 weeks • Ceftriaxone 2 g IV OD + gentamicin 1 mg/kg IV q8h × 2 weeks	• 2-week regimen should be used only for uncomplicated cases of native valve endocarditis due to highly penicillin-susceptible *S. viridans* (MIC <0.125 μg/mL) • For patients with penicillin allergy, use vancomycin
	S. viridans with penicillin MIC ≥0.125 μg/mL	CP 240 L units/day IV × 4 weeks + gentamicin 1 mg/kg IV q8h × 2 weeks	Ampicillin 2 g IV q4h × 4 weeks + gentamicin 1 mg/kg IV q8h × 2 weeks	
	Enterococcus	Ampicillin 2 g IV q4h + gentamicin 1 mg/kg IV q8h × 4–6 weeks		
	MSSA	Cloxacillin 2 g IV q4h × 4–6 weeks ± gentamicin 1 mg/kg IV q8h × 3–5 days		Goal trough levels in MRSA endocarditis treated with vancomycin are 15–20 μg/mL
	MRSA	Vancomycin 15 mg/kg IV q12h × 4–6 weeks ± gentamicin 1 mg/kg IV q12h × 3–5 days		
	Culture-negative endocarditis	Ampicillin 2 g IV q4h + gentamicin 1 mg/kg IV q8h × 4 weeks		
Infective endocarditis (prosthetic valve)	MSSA	Cloxacillin 2 g IV q4h × 6 weeks + rifampicin 600 mg PO BID × 6 weeks + gentamicin 1 mg/kg IV q8h × 2 weeks		• Cardiothoracic surgery consultation • Do not add rifampicin until bacteremia has cleared to avoid resistance

Continued...

Continued...

Condition	Likely pathogens	First choice	Alternatives	Comments
		Cardiovascular infections		
Infective endocarditis (prosthetic valve)	MRSA	Vancomycin 15 mg/kg IV q12h × 6 weeks + rifampicin 600 mg PO BID × 6 weeks + gentamicin 1 mg/kg IV q8h × 2 weeks		• Cardiothoracic surgery consultation • Do not add rifampicin until bacteremia has cleared to avoid resistance • Teicoplanin may be used instead of vancomycin (6 mg/kg/12 h × 3 days, followed by 6–10 mg/kg/day)
		Gastrointestinal (GI) and intra-abdominal infections		
Acute gastroenteritis	Viral Enterotoxigenic and enteropathogenic *E. coli*	Antibiotics not indicated		Antibiotics not indicated
Cholera	*Vibrio cholerae*	Doxycycline 300 mg PO × 1 dose	• Tablet azithromycin 1 g PO × 1 dose • Tablet ciprofloxacin 500 mg PO BID × 3 days	Prompt rehydration
Bacillary dysentery	*Shigella* species	None needed for previously healthy patients with mild symptoms	Ciprofloxacin 500 mg PO BID × 3 days in: • Patients with severe symptoms. • Immunocompromised patients	Prompt rehydration
Amoebic dysentery	*Entamoeba histolytica*	Metronidazole 400 mg PO TID × 10 days		
Giardiasis	*Giardia lamblia*	Tinidazole 2 g PO × 1 dose		
Cholangitis/acute cholecystitis	Enterobacteriaceae	Ertapenem 1 g IV OD × 7 days	Cefoperazone-sulbactam 3 g IV q12h	
Spontaneous bacterial peritonitis	Enterobacteriaceae (most often *E. coli*)	Ertapenem 1 g IV OD × 7 days	Piperacillin-tazobactam 4.5 g IV q6–8h	
Secondary peritonitis (bowel perforation)	Enterobacteriaceae Anaerobes (*Bacteroides* species)	Ertapenem 1 g IV OD	• Piperacillin-tazobactam 4.5 g IV q6–8h • Cefoperazone-sulbactam 3 g IV q12h	• Emergency surgery to eliminate source of contamination, reduce bacterial load, and prevent recurrence • Duration: 5–7 days; guided by resolution of clinical signs (fever and leukocytosis) and ability to tolerate oral diet; longer if leukocytosis/left shift and fever are slow to resolve or source control inadequate • If source closed and abdomen cleaned in <12 h, may treat for only 24 h
Intra-abdominal abscess	• Enterobacteriaceae • Anaerobes (*Bacteroides* species)	Ertapenem 1 g IV OD	• Piperacillin-tazobactam 4.5 g IV q6–8h • Cefoperazone-sulbactam 3 g IV q12h	Drainage of abscess

Continued...

Condition	Likely pathogens	First choice	Alternatives	Comments
Gastrointestinal (GI) and intra-abdominal infections				
Amebic liver abscess	*E. histolytica*	Metronidazole 500 mg IV q8h/800 mg PO TID + diloxanide furoate 500 mg PO TID × 10 days		Ultrasound-guided drainage indicated in: • Large abscesses (>10 cm), • Signs of imminent rupture, or • No response to medical treatment
Genitourinary infections				
Acute uncomplicated cystitis in women–dysuria	*E. coli*	Nitrofurantoin 100 mg PO BID × 5–7 days	Ciprofloxacin 500 mg PO BID × 5 days	
Pyelonephritis–uncomplicated (no underlying genitourinary disease)	*E. coli*	Ertapenem 1 g IV q24h × 1 week	Cefoperazone-sulbactam 3 g IV q12h	De-escalate as per susceptibility reports
Complicated UTI (underlying GU disease)/nosocomial UTI	• *E. coli, Proteus,* • *P. aeruginosa,* • *Acinetobacter* species	Meropenem 1–2 g IV q8h × 2 weeks	Cefoperazone-sulbactam 3 g IV q12h	De-escalate as per susceptibility reports
Central nervous system (CNS) infections				
Acute bacterial meningitis (community acquired)	• *S. pneumoniae* • *N. meningitidis*	Ceftriaxone 2 g IV q12h + vancomycin (loading of 25–30 mg/kg IV followed by 22.5 mg/kg) De-escalate once the MIC report is available • PCN MIC <0.1 μg/mL: Step down to CP 20 L units IV q2h • PCN MIC 0.1–1 μg/mL: Step down to ceftriaxone 2 g IV q12h • Ceftriaxone MIC >1 μg/mL: Continue ceftriaxone + vancomycin	Ceftriaxone 2 g IV q12h	Duration:10–14 days Start steroids if: • Cloudy CSF • Bacteria in CSF on Gram's staining, or • CSF WBC count >1,000/mL Dexamethasone 10 mg IV q6h × 4 days; first dose 15 minutes before first dose of antibiotic Steroids should be given before or during the first dose of antibiotics
Brain abscess	• Streptococci (aerobic and anaerobic) • Anaerobes • Enterobacteriaceae	Ceftriaxone 2 g IV q12h + metronidazole 500 mg IV q8h		• Duration: Until resolved • Drainage of abscess (>2.5 cm)
Bone and joint infections				
Acute osteomyelitis	*S. aureus*	Cefazolin 2 g IV q8h	Cloxacillin 2 g IV q4h	• For optimal treatment, microorganism(s) should be identified by blood culture, aspiration, or bone biopsy • Duration: 4 weeks (from initiation or last major debridement) • Can switch to oral therapy (cloxacillin 1 g PO q6h) once clinical improvement occurs

Continued...

Continued...

Condition	Likely pathogens	First choice	Alternatives	Comments
Bone and joint infections				
Chronic osteomyelitis		No empiric therapy		Definitive treatment should be guided by bone biopsy culture and susceptibility studies
Skin and soft tissue infections				
Cellulitis	• *S. pyogenes* • *S. aureus*	Cefazolin 1 g IV. q8h × 7–10 days (until clinical cure)	• Cloxacillin 500–1,000 mg PO q6h × 7–10 days • Cephalexin 500 mg q6h × 7–10 days	No routine role for adding MRSA cover
Furunculosis	*S. aureus*	Cloxacillin 500 mg q6h PO × 7–10 days	Cephalexin 500 mg PO q6h × 7–10 days	
Diabetic foot–mild (localized cellulitis, no or mild systemic symptoms)	*S. aureus*	Cefazolin 1 g IV q8h	• Cloxacillin 500–1,000 mg PO q6h × 7–10 days • Cephalexin 500 mg PO q6h × 7–10 days	
Diabetic foot–moderate-to-severe (limb threatening-severe cellulitis/gangrene/severe sepsis)	Polymicrobial—*S. aureus*, Group A *Streptococcus*, aerobic gram-negative bacilli, and anaerobes	Cefazolin 1 g IV q8h + amikacin 15 mg/kg IV q24h + metronidazole 500 mg IV q8h	• Piperacillin-tazobactam 4.5 g IV q6–8h • Ertapenem 1 g IV OD	Surgical consultation for drainage or debridement
Necrotizing fasciitis	• Group A *Streptococcus* • Occasionally gram negatives or anaerobes	Piperacillin-tazobactam 4.5 g IV q6–8h or meropenem 1 g IV q8h + clindamycin 600 mg IV q8h		• Surgical debridement • Duration: Until clinical cure
Bites (cat, dog, human, and rat)	• *Pasteurella multocida* • *Capnocytophaga* • *Eikenella corrodens* • *Viridans streptococci* • *Spirillum minus* • *Streptobacillus moniliformis*	Amoxicillin-clavulanate 625 mg PO TID	For PCN allergies use trimethoprim-sulfamethoxazole for *Pasteurella* and clindamycin for *Capnocytophaga*	• Duration: 3–5 days • Do not close the wound Consider tetanus/rabies vaccination, as appropriate
Acute undifferentiated febrile illnesses				
Enteric fever	• *S. enterica* serotype Typhi (*S. typhi*) • *S. enterica* serotype Paratyphi A (*S. paratyphi A*)	Azithromycin 1 g PO × 7 days (if MDR and NARST or ciprofloxacin MIC ≥0.125 µg/mL)	• Tablet Co-trimoxazole 1 double-strength tablet PO BID × 14 days • Tablet chloramphenicol 500 mg PO q6h × 14 days • Injection ceftriaxone 2 G IV OD × 10–14 days • Ciprofloxacin 750 mg BID PO × 14 days (only if nalidixic acid susceptible or ciprofloxacin MIC <0.125 µg/mL)	• Nalidixic acid resistant S. typhi (NARST) and/or ciprofloxacin MIC ≥0.125 µg/mL is associated with failure of ciprofloxacin and ofloxacin treatment • Third-generation cephalosporins have higher rates of relapse/clinical failure, and hence they should be given for minimum 2 weeks if used
Scrub typhus	*Orientia tsutsugamushi*	Doxycycline 100 mg PO BID × 7 days	Azithromycin 500 mg PO OD × 3 days	

Continued...

Continued...

Condition	Likely pathogens	First choice	Alternatives	Comments
Acute undifferentiated febrile illnesses				
Leptospirosis	*Leptospira interrogans*	CP 15 L units IV q6h	• Ceftriaxone 1 g IV OD • Doxycycline 100 mg PO BID	Duration: 7 days

(ARDS: acute respiratory distress syndrome; CSF: cerebrospinal fluid; ET: endotracheal; ICU: intensive care unit; IV: intravenous; MIC: minimum inhibitory concentration; MRSA: methicillin-resistant *Staphylococcus aureus*; MSSA: methicillin-susceptible *Staphylococcus aureus*; UTI: urinary tract infection; VAP: ventilator-associated pneumonia; WBC: white blood cell)

TABLE 4 Duration of antibiotic therapy.

Condition	Shorter duration studied	Comparator longer duration studied	Outcome
Community-acquired pneumonia	3–5 days	7–10 days	Outcomes are similar
Ventilator-associated pneumonia	7 days	14 days	Outcomes are similar
Pyelonephritis	7 days	14 days	Outcomes are similar
Gram-negative bacteremias	7 days	14 days	Outcomes are similar
Septic arthritis of small joints	14 days	28 days	Outcomes are similar
Intra-abdominal infections after optimal debridement	3–4 days	10 days	Outcomes are similar

about 10–20% in real world scenario and about 70% in rigorous clinical studies.

ANTIMICROBIAL SUSCEPTIBILITY TESTS

Physicians should be well versed in interpreting antimicrobial susceptibility tests (ASTs). ASTs determine the ability of a particular antibiotic to inhibit the pathogen in vitro. MIC is the most common AST metric used to divide the response to the antibiotic into susceptible, resistant, and intermediate categories. MIC is defined as the lowest concentration of an antibiotic that inhibits visible growth of a microorganism. While the interpretation of the "susceptible" and "resistant" categories is straightforward, the intermediate category infers that the drug can still be used provided it concentrates at the particular site of infection and higher doses can be safely administered.

Certain AST patterns can convey information regarding the mechanisms of resistance present in that pathogen. For example, presence of ceftazidime, cefpodoxime resistance in an Enterobacteriaceae is a surrogate for an extended-spectrum beta-lactamases (ESBLs) production despite first- or second-generation cephalosporin susceptibility. Clinicians must be also aware that the sensitivity report of a pathogen may vary depending on the source of the sample. The interpretive cutoffs for *Streptococcus pneumoniae* are significantly different between meningeal and nonmeningeal isolates.

COMBINATION THERAPY

While the concept of combination therapy is appealing, the benefits are proven only in select circumstances. Synergistic combination of ampicillin with gentamicin is useful in the treatment of enterococcal endocarditis. Combination therapy is the norm in the management of slow growing chronic infections such as tuberculosis and leprosy to mitigate resistance development. However, the benefit of combination therapy in high organism burden situations like sepsis to accelerate pathogen clearance has been unsuccessful. If the empiric therapy has an active antibacterial agent, generally there is no role of adding additional agents. Recently, addition of meropenem to colistin was not found to be beneficial in a large randomized controlled trial for the treatment of carbapenem resistant gram-negative bacteremia.

DURATION OF TREATMENT

The endpoints for antibiotic treatment are largely clinical rather than microbiological. Relatively few infections have been well studied to provide an accurate assessment of the optimal duration of treatment. Shorter regimens are increasingly being attempted and summary of such efforts is given in **Table 4**. Ultimately, clinicians must assess the appropriate duration of treatment for each patient, guided by the data that is available, clinical response, and evidence of the microbiological clearance of the pathogen whenever possible. Increasingly, early switch from intravenous to oral therapy is also encouraged. However, certain caveats should be kept in mind—Is the patient able to tolerate orally? Does the patient have problems with gut absorption? Is the patient safely out of the critically ill stage? Are there sensitive antibiotics with good oral bioavailability available for that pathogen? and Do those antibiotics penetrate well into that particular site?

SOURCE CONTROL

Infections with a clear source such as abscess, central lines, necrotizing fasciitis, and empyema require drainage or removal of the source as promptly as possible. Source control is shown to decrease mortality, reduce the duration of antibiotics, and promote early recovery from the infection.

CONCLUSION

Appropriate antibiotic therapy involves making an accurate diagnosis, determining the need for antibiotic use, understanding the antimicrobial spectrum, dosing strategies, adapting the treatment to host characteristics, and severity. Antibiotic stewardship strategies of using the narrowest spectrum possible, de-escalation, and shortest duration of therapy are not only beneficial to patients but also slow the emergence of resistance.

RECOMMENDED READINGS

1. Slama TG, Amin A, Brunton SA, File TM Jr, Milkovich G, Rodvold KA, et al. A clinician's guide to the appropriate and accurate use of antibiotics: the Council for Appropriate and Rational Antibiotic Therapy (CARAT) criteria. Am J Med. 2005;118(Suppl 7A):1S-6S.
2. Leibovici L, Shraga I, Andreassen S. How do you choose antibiotic treatment? BMJ. 1999;318(7198):1614-6.
3. Spellberg B, Rice LB. Duration of Antibiotic Therapy: Shorter Is Better. Ann Intern Med. 2019;171(3):210-1.
4. McKinnon PS, Davis SL. Pharmacokinetic and pharmacodynamic issues in the treatment of bacterial infectious diseases. Eur J Clin Microbiol Infect Dis. 2004;23(4):271-88.
5. Strich JR, Heil EL, Masur H. Considerations for Empiric Antimicrobial Therapy in Sepsis and Septic Shock in an Era of Antimicrobial Resistance. J Infect Dis. 2020;222(Suppl 2):S119-S131.

CHAPTER

37

Management of Septicemia

Atul K Patel, Ketan Patel

ABSTRACT

Sepsis remains an important reason globally for intensive care unit (ICU) admission and is associated with high mortality. The etiology of sepsis is different in developed and developing countries. Tropical infections such as malaria, dengue, leptospirosis, scrub typhus, and others are additional infections contributing as a cause for sepsis in tropical countries including India. The risk of sepsis with nosocomial multidrug-resistant gram-negative infections is growing in the world. Fungal pathogens are increasingly isolated as a cause of sepsis in the last decade.

History taking and quick physical examination are two indispensable tools in the evaluation, while adequate resuscitation and early appropriate empiric antibiotic therapy are two indispensable tools in the management of sepsis patients. For patients with community-acquired sepsis in India and other tropical countries, ceftriaxone alone or in combination with doxycycline is the initial choice for empiric antimicrobial agents. This combination will cover a few important pathogens responsible for community-acquired sepsis, which include community-acquired pneumonia, leptospirosis, enteric fever, and scrub typhus. Patients with noninfectious causes for sepsis and suspected to have fungal sepsis should undergo specific investigations to arrive at diagnosis and management.

"We try to solve very complicated problems without letting people know how complicated the problem was"

—Janathan Ive

INTRODUCTION

Sepsis and septic shock are leading causes across the globe for ICU admission and mortality. The intensive care over nations (ICON) audit showed that sepsis accounts for 30% of reasons for ICU admission and is associated with a hospital mortality rate of 35%. The incidence rate of sepsis cases reported 270 per 100,000 person-years [95% confidence interval (CI), 176–412] with an inhospital mortality rate of 26%, this equates to 19.4 million cases and 5.3 million deaths globally each year. Despite advances in the understanding of pathophysiology, diagnostic capabilities including widely incorporating molecular tests, biomarkers, and pharmacotherapy in the form of therapeutic monitoring of antimicrobial agents used for infectious diseases, the incidence of sepsis is rising. Septicemia, a systemic illness caused by bloodstream invasion of microorganisms and their toxins, is replaced by new terminologies such as sepsis, severe sepsis, and septic shock. Most of the available data related to the incidence and outcome of sepsis are from Western countries.

In contrast to Western countries where bacterial sepsis (gram-positive followed by gram-negative bacteria) is the predominant cause of sepsis, Asian countries reported tropical infections such as dengue, malaria, leptospirosis, enteric fever, scrub typhus, and tuberculosis as important causes apart from usual bacterial etiology. Epidemiology of infection (both community and hospital-acquired) contributing sepsis are sparse from India. One single-center study from India reported 6% of all ICU admissions were due to severe sepsis out of which 16% were ICU acquired while another (The INDICAP) study reported prevalence of severe sepsis in 28.3% out of which 20.5% were ICU acquired.

DEFINITION

According to 2016 consensus definitions of sepsis and septic shock (sepsis-3):

- *Sepsis*:
    - Suspected infection and
    - An acute change in sequential organ failure assessment (SOFA) score of ≥2 points consequent to infection
- *Septic shock*:
    - Sepsis
    - Hypotension requiring vasopressor therapy to maintain a mean arterial blood pressure of 65 mm Hg or greater
    - Serum lactate level greater than 2 mmol/L after adequate fluid resuscitation

RISK FACTORS

Important risk factors for sepsis are:

- *Advanced age*
- *Bloodstream infection*: Bacteremia is one of the most important risk factors often associated with systemic consequences and in one study, 95% of positive blood cultures were associated with sepsis or septic shock.
- *Malignancy*: All types of cancer, both hematological and solid organ tumors are associated with a 10-fold increase in the risk of sepsis.
- *Hospitalized patients* with community-acquired pneumonia carry a high risk for severe sepsis.
- *Diabetes and obesity*: Both obesity and type 2 diabetes mellitus are associated with an increased risk of recurrent, nosocomial, and secondary infections that lead to sepsis. Obesity increases the risk of community-acquired pneumonia, biliary disease, cutaneous infections, and aspiration pneumonia during hospitalizations. In ICU, obese patients may have a higher risk of infectious complications that lead to sepsis, ventilator-associated pneumonia, central venous catheter-related infections, and increased mortality compared to normal weight patients.
- *Various genetic disorders* affecting immune response to a pathogen such as defective antibody production, lack of T cells, natural killer cells response, or complements increases susceptibility to infection. Genetic diseases associated with a defect in the innate immune system are also identified as increasing susceptibility to a specific class of microorganisms.
- *ICU admission*: ICU care involving line placements (indwelling catheters, central line, and intubations) increases the risk of nosocomial infection and so therefore of sepsis.
- *Immunosuppressive state* (genetic or acquired by medical treatment) is associated with a higher risk of infections including opportunistic pathogens sepsis and septic shock.
- A *previous hospitalization* also increases the risk of sepsis in the next 90 days. Previous hospitalization and antibiotic treatment alter microbial flora and has been associated with a threefold increased risk of sepsis.
- *Major trauma* and burns are associated with a high risk of sepsis.

ETIOLOGY

Infectious organisms associated with sepsis have changed over time. In Western countries, gram-positive bacteria are most frequently identified in patients with sepsis while the gram-negative bacteria are steadily increasing. Fungal organisms as an etiology of sepsis have increased over the past decade. Despite diagnostic efforts, in approximately half of the cases of sepsis, an organism is not identified (culture-negative sepsis).

Any infecting organism can lead to sepsis, so presentation and management are also variable according to the site of infection, organism type, setting of infection (community or hospital setting). Broadly, sepsis can be community acquired or hospital acquired (arising from hospital or healthcare facility). Nearly 80% of cases are of community-acquired sepsis, with the lung being the most common site of infection (64%) followed by abdomen (20%), bloodstream (15%), and genitourinary tract including kidneys (14%).

Table 1 shows common microbiologic organisms according to the site of infection. This may be variable according to geographic distribution.

In addition to this, in tropical countries like us common bacterial, viral, and parasitic infections can frequently present as community-acquired sepsis, so one should be aware of such organisms, their presentations, and management. Important organisms presenting as sepsis in our context are tabulated in **Table 2**.

APPROACH TO SEPSIS

A general algorithm on approach to sepsis is shown in **Flowchart 1**.

Treatment and resuscitation of patients with sepsis and septic shock should commence immediately with priorities to the identification and control of the source of infection, and its treatment with appropriate antibiotics.

TABLE 1 Common organisms according to site of infection.

Common infection sites	Common microorganisms
Pulmonary	Pneumococcus, *Staphylococcus*, atypical infections such as mycoplasma and legionella, viruses and gram-negative bacteria
Abdominal	Gram-negative organisms, anaerobic organisms, *Enterococcus*, and *Candida*
Skin/Soft tissue	*Streptococcus*, methicillin-sensitive *Staphylococcus aureus* (MSSA), and gram-negatives organisms
Urinary	Gram-negative bacilli and *Enterococcus*
Intravascular catheters	Methicillin-resistant *Staphylococcus aureus* (MRSA), coagulase-negative *Staphylococcus*, *Candida*, and gram-negative bacilli
Central nervous system	Pneumococcus, gram-positive organisms, and *Neisseria*
Endocarditis	MSSA, coagulase-negative *Staphylococcus*, and fungi

TABLE 2 Common pathogens causing sepsis in tropical countries.

Genera	Organism
Viruses	Influenza, dengue, chikungunya, rhinovirus, and Crimean-Congo hemorrhagic fever virus
Bacteria	*Leptospira*, *Salmonella typhi* and nontyphoid *Salmonella*, mycobacteria, *Rickettsia* species (scrub typhus group), and *Burkholderia pseudomallei*
Parasite	*Plasmodia* and *Entamoeba histolytica* (causing liver abscess)

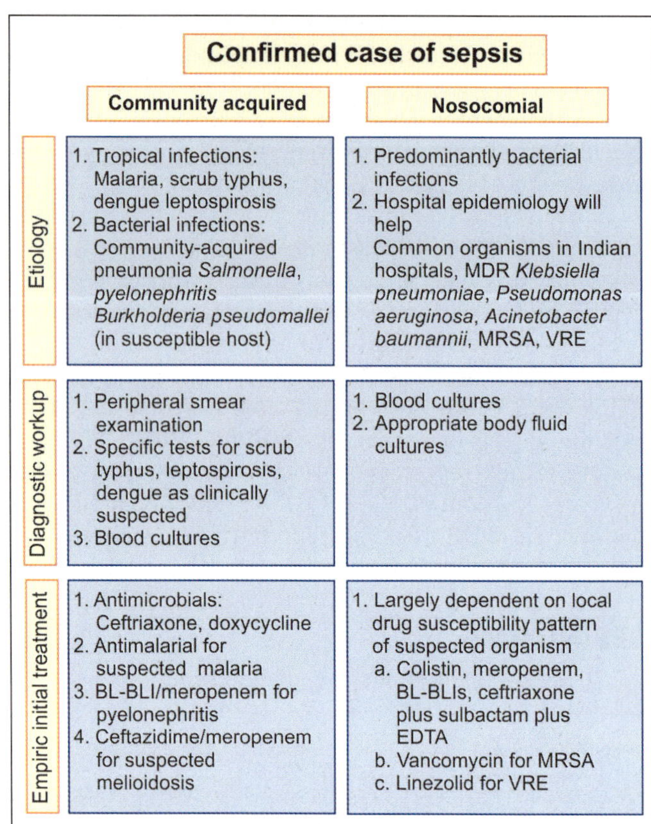

(BL-BLI: beta-lactam-beta-lactamase inhibitor; EDTA: ethylenediaminetetra-acetic acid; MDR: multidrug-resistant; MRSA: methicillin-resistant *Staphylococcus aureus*; VRE: vancomycin-resistant enterococci)

FLOWCHART 1: Etiological diagnostic and empiric antimicrobial treatment for confirmed case of sepsis.

Basic principles of management include:
- Rapid evaluation including history, physical examination, and investigations including blood cultures to arrive at a probable diagnosis.
- Initial assessment and resuscitation to reestablish tissue perfusion and correction of acidosis.
  - Intravenous (IV) fluid, volume replacement if hypotension, and/or elevated lactate
  - Repeat arterial lactate if an initial level is >2 mmol/L
  - *Vasopressor*: If a patient remains hypotensive despite adequate fluid replacement therapy
- Appropriate empiric antibiotic administration
- Source control with intervention for conditions such as bowel ischemia, gastrointestinal perforation, abscesses, necrotizing skin, and soft-tissue infection and implanted devices.
- Other therapy

A quick history and physical examination can give a piece of important information about the possible etiology of sepsis. Clinicians should gather important and relevant history on presentation to identify important risk factors for sepsis (age, diabetes, malignancy, obesity, previous hospitalization etc.). Living in or recent travel history, especially visits to an endemic area for scrub typhus, melioidosis, leptospirosis etc., is very useful for sending appropriate investigations. For inpatients with hospital-acquired sepsis, clinicians should collect information on previous antibiotic use, site of infection, presence of foreign device including central line, and local antibiotic resistant pattern.

A quick *physical examination* for icterus, red eye (conjunctival suffusion), skin rashes and its distributions, presence of eschar, organomegaly, and petechiae can give you a valuable diagnostic clue (**Figs. 1 A** and **B**).

Clinicians should collect appropriate *blood and body fluid cultures* before initiation of empiric antimicrobial therapy. Other diagnostic workup such as radiological assessment of chest and abdomen, biomarkers of sepsis [*procalcitonin (PCT)*], and fungal biomarker (serum beta-D-glucan and serum galactomannan) can be performed after resuscitation and empiric antimicrobial therapy. The clinicians should understand that PCT is not helpful in making a diagnosis of sepsis but is useful in de-escalating antibiotic therapy in patients with community-acquired pneumonia and respiratory tract infections. PCT-guided de-escalation of antibiotics reduces the duration of antibiotic exposure with a trend toward decreased mortality. Serum/bronchoalveolar lavage (BAL) *galactomannan and serum*

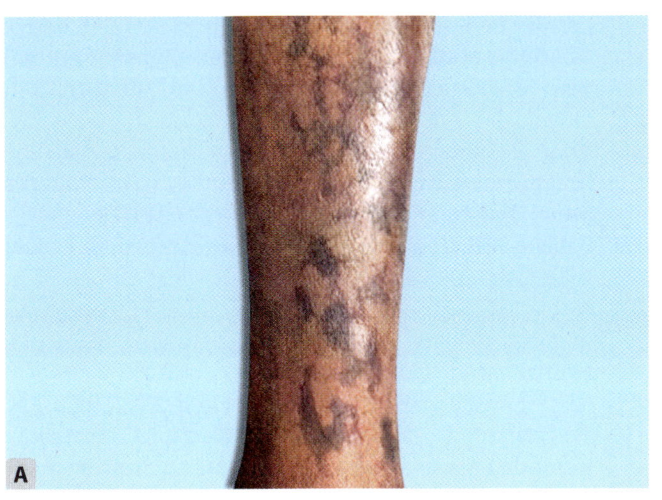

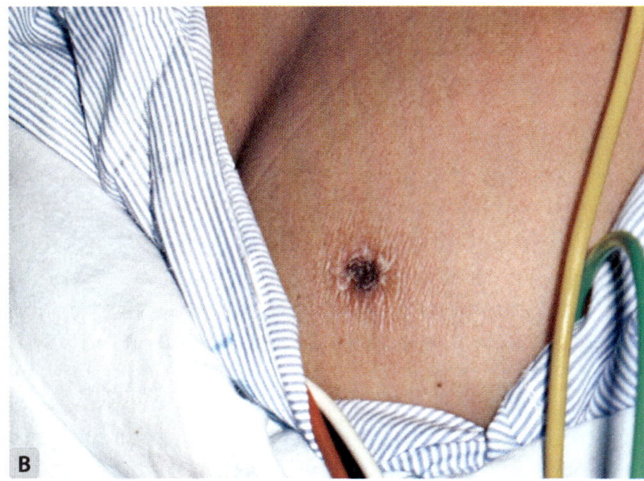

FIGURES 1 A & B: Skin lesions in patients with sepsis (tropical infections). **(A)** Skin erythema with vasculitis skin rashes in a dengue patient; **(B)** Eschar over the right breast of a patient with scrub typhus admitted to intensive care unit (ICU) with septic shock.

beta-D-glucan can be used to detect infections with fungi, especially *Aspergillus* and *Candida* species. Beta-D-glucan is useful in suspected cases of candidemia with negative blood cultures, especially intra-abdominal candidiasis.

Raised lactate concentration remains of prognostic importance for patients with sepsis, and reductions in the concentration of this marker after resuscitation are associated with improved outcomes. It is therefore, important to repeat the measurements of blood lactate to monitor its kinetics and plan further management.

The clinicians should perform appropriate tests to diagnose *noninfectious causes of sepsis* such as acute pancreatitis, myocardial infarction, and systemic vasculitis when clinically suspected. Readers are encouraged to read detailed principles and recommendations of fluid management and vasopressor treatment from the surviving sepsis guide. In general, initial volume replacement should be carefully monitored to avoid volume overload and subsequent complications associated with volume overload.

EARLY ANTIMICROBIAL USE

Appropriate antimicrobial should be administered within 1 hour of sepsis diagnosis. General principle of empiric antimicrobial selection is given in **Flowchart 1**. Delaying antimicrobial therapy is associated with a significant increase in mortality.

One observational study reported a 7% increase risk of death for every hour delay in antimicrobial administration in patients with sepsis having hypotension.

According to Surviving Sepsis Campaign (SSC) guidelines:

- IV antimicrobials should be initiated as soon as possible after the recognition of sepsis (ideally within 1 hour)
- The initial choice should include a broad-spectrum cover (with either a single agent or a combination of agents). For community-acquired sepsis, empiric combination therapy with ceftriaxone along with doxycycline will take care of leptospirosis, scrub typhus, invasive pneumococcal infection, *Salmonella, Shigella enterocolitis*, and methicillin-sensitive *Staphylococcus aureus* (MSSA).
- The antibiotic spectrum should be narrowed when pathogens have been isolated and sensitivities established, or when clinical progress allows it.
- Dosing strategies of antimicrobials should be optimized on the basis of accepted pharmacokinetic and pharmacodynamics principles and liver or renal impairment.
- De-escalation of antimicrobials should be considered daily and at the earliest stage when the clinical situation permits.

In community-acquired viral sepsis, use of antimicrobial is not routinely required unless there is suspicion or high risk for secondary bacterial infection. In the last decades, there has been a significant rise in sepsis due to fungal infection. Empiric antifungal should be considered in a high-risk group such as those who have had total parenteral nutrition, recent broad-spectrum antibiotic exposure, perforated abdominal viscus, or immunocompromised status, or when clinical suspicion of fungal infection is high.

Identifying and early source control is extremely important for the rapid reversal of septic shock. A classic example of this situation is a diabetic patient admitted with obstructive uropathy—pyelonephritis and septic shock. Here, despite the patient is receiving an appropriate antibiotic according to a drug susceptibility of organisms isolated in blood culture, the patient will continue to have features of septic shock (fever, hypotension, and leukocytosis) till the obstructed system is drained with double-J (DJ) stent placement. Rapid improvement in hemodynamic parameters and general clinical features is achieved once the source is drained by surgical intervention. Inadequate source control may lead to worsening organ function and hemodynamic instability despite appropriate resuscitative measures. Other examples of source controls include removal of infected catheter or foreign body, abscess drainage, and removal of infected tissue either through percutaneous drainage or surgery. Identifying a source and its control is critical in sepsis management.

OTHER THERAPIES

Corticosteroids in sepsis: Corticosteroids are not routinely recommended in sepsis. The SSC guidelines recommend against the use of low-dose corticosteroids when fluid resuscitation and vasopressor therapy are adequate in restoring hemodynamic stability. Low-dose corticosteroids, hydrocortisone 200 mg/day IV continuous infusion, or 50 mg bolus every 6 hours administration is recommended in patients with hemodynamic instability despite adequate fluid resuscitation and vasopressor therapy. Results from two meta-analyses showed that low-dose corticosteroids produce either no or a very small reduction in short-term mortality, but the use is associated with more rapid resolution of shock and shorter ICU stay.

OUTCOME

Nearly 25–30% of patients with sepsis and septic shock die from the condition and inhospital mortality is around 40–60%. There has been a drop in mortality due to sepsis and septic shock with an improved management approach that includes early recognition and intervention. Significant postsurvival morbidity led to decreased quality of life, functional disability, and cognitive impairment. Concerted effort needs to be made for improving long-term outcome of patients.

RECOMMENDED READINGS

1. Vincent JL, Marshall JC, Namendys-Silva SA, François B, Martin-Loeches I, Lipman J, et al. Assessment of the worldwide burden of critical illness: the intensive care over nations (ICON) audit. Lancet Respir Med. 2014;2:380-6.
2. Fleischmann C, Scherag A, Adhikari NK, Hartog CS, Tsaganos T, Schlattmann P, et al. Assessment of Global Incidence and Mortality of Hospital-treated Sepsis. Current Estimates and Limitations. Am J Respir Crit Care Med. 2016;193:259-72.
3. Martin GS, Mannino DM, Eaton S, Moss M. The epidemiology of sepsis in the United States from 1979 through 2000. N Engl J Med. 2003;348:1546-54.
4. Singer M, Deutschman CS, Seymour CW, Shankar-Hari M, Annane D, Bauer M, et al. The Third International Consensus Definitions for Sepsis and Septic Shock (Sepsis-3). JAMA. 2016;315:801-10.
5. Agarwal R, Gupta D, Ray P, Aggarwal AN, Jindal SK. Epidemiology, risk factors and outcome of nosocomial infections in a Respiratory Intensive Care Unit in North India. J Infect. 2006;53:98-105.
6. Ghanshani RV, Gupta R, Sood S, Bansal A, Joad SH, Khedar RS. Epidemiology of infections in a medical ICU in India. Intensive Care Med. 2014;40:456-7.
7. Chatterjee S, Bhattacharya M, Todi SK. Epidemiology of Adult-population Sepsis in India: A Single Center 5 Year Experience. Indian J Crit Care Med. 2017;21:573-7.
8. Divatia JV, Amin PR, Ramakrishnan N, Kapadia FN, Todi S, Sahu S, et al. Intensive Care in India: The Indian Intensive Care Case Mix and Practice Patterns Study. Indian J Crit Care Med. 2016;20:216-25.
9. Falagas ME, Kompoti M. Obesity and infection. Lancet Infect Dis. 2006;6:438-46.
10. Netea MG, van der Meer JW. Immunodeficiency and genetic defects of pattern-recognition receptors. N Engl J Med. 2011;364:60-70.
11. Klotz SA, Chasin BS, Powell B, Gaur NK, Lipke PN. Polymicrobial bloodstream infections involving Candida species: analysis of patients and review of the literature. Diagn Microbiol Infect Dis. 2007;59:401-6.
12. Gupta S, Sakhuja A, Kumar G, McGrath E, Nanchal RS, Kashani KB. Culture-Negative Severe Sepsis: Nationwide Trends and Outcomes. Chest. 2016;150:1251-9.
13. Karlsson S, Varpula M, Ruokonen E, Pettilä V, Parviainen I, Ala-Kokko TI, et al. Incidence, treatment, and outcome of severe sepsis in ICU-treated adults in Finland: the Finnsepsis study. Intensive Care Med. 2007;33:435-43.
14. Lam SW, Bauer SR, Fowler R, Duggal A. Systematic Review and Meta-Analysis of Procalcitonin-Guidance Versus Usual Care for Antimicrobial Management in Critically Ill Patients: Focus on Subgroups Based on Antibiotic Initiation, Cessation, or Mixed Strategies. Crit Care Med. 2018;46:684-90.
15. Haydour Q, Hage CA, Carmona EM, Epelbaum O, Evans SE, Gabe LM, et al. Diagnosis of Fungal Infections. A Systematic Review and Meta-Analysis Supporting American Thoracic Society Practice Guideline. Ann Am Thorac Soc. 2019;16:1179-88.
16. Casserly B, Phillips GS, Schorr C, Dellinger RP, Townsend SR, Osborn TM, et al. Lactate measurements in sepsis-induced tissue hypoperfusion: results from the Surviving Sepsis Campaign database. Crit Care Med. 2015;43:567-73.
17. Rhodes A, Evans LE, Alhazzani W, Levy MM, Antonelli M, Ferrer R, et al. Surviving Sepsis Campaign: International Guidelines for Management of Sepsis and Septic Shock: 2016. Intensive Care Med. 2017;43:304-77.
18. Sakr Y, Rubatto Birri PN, Kotfis K, Nanchal R, Shah B, Kluge S, et al. Higher Fluid Balance Increases the Risk of Death From Sepsis: Results From a Large International Audit. Crit Care Med. 2017;45:386-94.
19. Kumar A, Ellis P, Arabi Y, Roberts D, Light B, Parrillo JE, et al. Initiation of inappropriate antimicrobial therapy results in a fivefold reduction of survival in human septic shock. Chest. 2009;136:1237-48.
20. Rochwerg B, Oczkowski SJ, Siemieniuk RAC, Agoritsas T, Belley-Cote E, D'Aragon F, et al. Corticosteroids in Sepsis: An Updated Systematic Review and Meta-Analysis. Crit Care Med. 2018;46:1411-20.

CHAPTER 38

Prevention and Management of Infection in Transplant Recipients

Anupa Thampy, Priscilla Rupali

ABSTRACT

Prevention and management of infections is a key aspect in determining survival in a transplant patient. The three components in management include pretransplant screening for infections and vaccination in the donor and recipient; peritransplant antimicrobial prophylaxis, monitoring of infections, and post-transplant vaccination of the recipient, antimicrobial prophylaxis, and diagnosing infectious syndromes.

Potential etiologies are diverse including nosocomial, community acquired, reactivation of latent infections from the donor and recipient as well as uncommon opportunistic infections of clinical significance only in immunocompromised hosts. Infections in hematopoietic stem cell transplant should be assessed on the basis of risk stratification, period of the transplant and the presenting syndrome of the patient. A differential diagnosis should be generated and evaluation tailored accordingly. Infections in solid organ transplant depend on the epidemiological exposures of the donor and recipient and the net state of immunosuppression of the recipient.

The 1st month post-transplant is complicated by postoperative infections and donor derived infections whereas in later months opportunistic infections take over. Routine tests and serology are usually noncontributory and invasive tests with tissue sent for molecular techniques should be the mainstay for diagnosis. While evaluation is ongoing, therapy for the most likely etiologies should be initiated because delay may compromise the prospects for a successful outcome. Presumptive therapy; however, should not be used as an alternative to a proper assessment and antimicrobial stewardship should be practiced.

"Caution is the parent of safety"

—Anonymous

INTRODUCTION

Constantly evolving immunosuppressives and chemotherapeutics have improved survival in patients undergoing solid and bone marrow transplants (BMTs). Though there is improved survival due to amelioration of underlying disease, this also exposes these patients to the risk of varying infections. Infections are a major cause of morbidity, mortality as well as graft rejection despite prophylaxis, appropriate use of vaccinations, growth factors, and newer antimicrobial drugs. Thus the prevention, diagnosis, and management of infectious diseases are major contributors to a successful transplant.

PRACTICAL ISSUES IN MANAGEMENT

- Inflammatory responses associated with microbial invasion are impaired by immunosuppressive therapy, which results in diminished symptoms and muted clinical and radiologic findings. Rapid progression of infection because of the lack of an appropriate immune response can result in medical emergencies.
- Potential etiologies are diverse including nosocomial, community acquired, and reactivation of latent infections from the donor and recipient. In addition, uncommon opportunistic infections occur only in immunocompromised hosts.
- Tests such as serology which rely on host immune response are not useful in acute infections. Often, invasive diagnostic techniques early in the course of illness may be required to establish a confirmatory diagnosis, but this has to be balanced with the risk of complications that may result from a diagnostic procedure versus institution of empiric antimicrobials.
- The choice of antimicrobial regimens is often more complex than in other patients due to antimicrobial resistance, multiple concomitant pathogens, urgency of therapy, and the frequency of drug toxicities and drug interactions.
- Noninfectious syndromes can mimic infections often leading to inappropriate and unjustified use of antibiotics and antifungals.

TIME PERIOD

- *Pretransplant screening*: To assess risk for development of infections based on type of transplant, recipient immune status, and vaccinate, if required.
- *Peritransplant*: Prevent hospital-acquired infections and start appropriate prophylaxis.
- *Post-transplant*: Vaccination, continuation of antimicrobial prophylaxis in case of rejection or graft-versus-host disease (GVHD) leading to intensified

immunosuppression and maintenance of vigilance for post-transplant infectious syndromes.

EPIDEMIOLOGY

Trends of hematopoietic stem cell transplantation (HSCT) evolved with the first successful transplantation done in India in 1983.

At present, there are 97 transplant centers reporting to the Indian Stem Cell Transplant Registry/Indian Society for Blood and Marrow Transplantation (ISCTR/ISBMT). The most recent report from the registry show approximately 19,000 transplants till now, with a 10% increase every year. India's first organ transplant was conducted in the 1970s (kidney transplant). The number of transplants done annually has been gradually rising. Around 5,000 kidneys, 1,000 livers, and around 50 hearts are transplanted annually in India.

A retrospective study from a South Indian center reported their pattern of infections in 304 allogeneic BMT recipients. There were 415 documented infections which included bacterial (34.9%), viral [42.9%, cytomegalovirus (CMV) in 22.7%], fungal (15.9%, aspergillosis predominantly), and other infections (6.3%) including tuberculosis. The most common bacterial infections were nonfermenting gram-negative bacilli (NFGNB) and *Pseudomonas* in this study, but later studies have shown predominantly *Klebsiella* and *Escherichia coli* isolates. Infection-related 100-day mortality was seen in 14.8%. While fever is the most common syndrome, others such as respiratory infections, diarrhea, and neurological syndromes are seen as well.

A study in patients undergoing allogeneic BMT in South India revealed that 48% of patients undergoing BMT developed diarrhea which was mainly of noninfectious origin in the first 20 days post-transplant. Rotavirus and adenoviruses were found in approximately 12% and 5% of patients, respectively. Bacterial infections in the post transplantation period were found to be more common in India than in developed countries.

Studies in solid organ transplant have revealed lesser frequency of infections in comparison to HSCT. The infections are commonly seen in solid organ transplantation (SOT) in the following decreasing order of frequency multivisceral > intestinal > lung > liver > heart > kidney. In a single center prospective study of 144 renal transplant patients, 50.7% developed infections, with a majority (77.1%) of the infections occurring in the first 6 months. Most common infections were those of urinary tract (34.5%), followed by viral (31.2%), sepsis (15.2%), mycobacterial (9.7%), and fungal (6.2%). CMV accounted for 14.5% and BK virus for 5.5% of total infections.

The two important aspects which affect the pattern of infections in a transplant recipient are the epidemiological exposures of the patient and the microbiome. Microorganisms in tissues and on barrier surfaces are collectively termed the "microbiome" including both commensal flora and acute exposures. The microbiome has a dynamic and regulated interaction with the immune system therefore data has suggested its role in graft rejection as well.

INFECTIONS IN HEMATOPOIETIC STEM CELL TRANSPLANTATION

Hematopoietic stem cell transplantation is performed in patients with functional failure of bone marrow or marrow-derived cells; including aplastic anemia, myelodysplastic syndrome, immunodeficiency syndromes, genetic diseases or hemoglobinopathies; or in hematologic malignancies such as acute or chronic leukemia, multiple myeloma, lymphomas, and myeloproliferative neoplasms. There are two major types of HSCT: Autologous and allogeneic. Autologous refers to the patient serving as his or her own donor. Allogeneic refers to someone else serving as the donor. For allogeneic transplantation, stringent human leukocyte antigen (HLA) matching between donor and recipient is required to minimize the risk for graft rejection and GVHD.

RISK OF INFECTION

It is important to identify the population at high risk for infections and also the magnitude of and period of highest risk in order to predict which patients are most likely to benefit from targeted prophylaxis, diagnostic procedures, and/or preemptive therapy.

The risk of infection is determined by the interaction of the pathogen, environment, organ dysfunction, and net state of immunosuppression (**Fig. 1**).

Risk stratification for infections before, during and after HSCT is shown in **Table 1** and schema of a HSCT is shown in **Figure 2**.

The risk of infections depends on immune recovery and this is best explained by division into three periods. HSCT begins with conditioning regimen (myeloablative or nonmyeloablative) from day 10 to day 0. On day 0, there is infusion of stem cells. Day 7–21 is pre-engraftment period characterized by neutropenia and following this is the postengraftment period.

- *Pre-engraftment period*: From transplantation to neutrophil recovery (neutrophil engraftment), approximately 10–15 days.

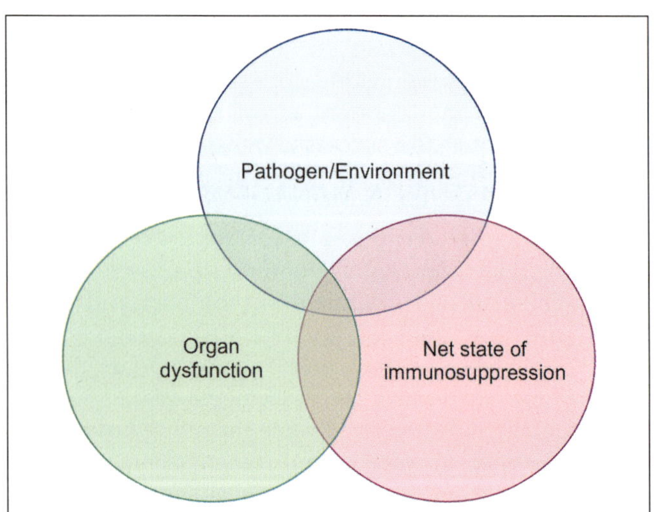

FIGURE 1: Factors affecting infection in hematopoietic stem cell transplantation (HSCT).

TABLE 1 Risk stratification for infections in HSCT.

Risk factor	Intensity of risk	Rationale
Net state of immunosuppression		
• Underlying disease		
◦ AML/aplastic anemia	High risk	
◦ Non first remission malignancy	High risk	
◦ Hemoglobinopathies	Low risk	
• Graft failure	High risk	Intensification of immunosuppression
• Glucocorticoids >1 mg/kg/day	High risk	
• Age > 40 years	High risk	
Graft characteristics		
• Type of transplant		
◦ Allogenic	High risk	Higher risk in allogeneic transplant, especially for herpes and invasive fungal infections because of slower B- and T-cell reconstitution
◦ Autologous	Low-moderate risk	
• Type of allogeneic donor		
◦ Unrelated or mismatched donor	High risk	Slower B- and T-cell reconstitution
• Type of stem cell graft		
◦ Peripheral blood	Low-moderate risk for early but higher for late infections	Early neutrophil engraftment, more chronic GVHD
◦ Bone marrow	Moderate risk for early and late	Slightly delayed neutrophil engraftment with moderate risk of GVHD
◦ Cord blood	High risk for early but low risk for late infections	Delayed neutrophil engraftment but less GVHD
• Type of conditioning		
◦ Myeloablative	High risk	Severe mucositis and longer neutropenia
◦ Reduced intensity	Low risk	
◦ Organ dysfunction		
◦ Severe mucositis	High risk	
◦ Renal, liver, and lung failure	High risk	
◦ Skin barrier disruption by central venous catheter	High risk	
◦ GVHD grade II-IV	High risk	Intensification of immunosuppression

(AML: acute myeloid leukemia; GVHD: graft-versus-host disease; HSCT: hematopoietic stem cell transplantation)

Source: Adapted from Wójtowicz A, Bochud P-Y. Risk stratification and immunogenetic risk for infections following stem cell transplantation. Virulence. 2016;7(8):917-29.

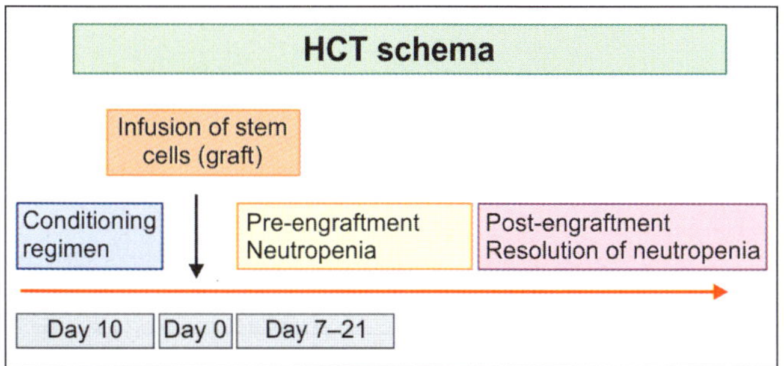

FIGURE 2: Schema of a hematopoietic stem cell transplantation (HSCT).

Courtesy: Dr George Alangaden, Division of Infectious Diseases, Henry Ford Hospital, Detroit, Michigan, USA.

Both innate immune cells [phagocytes, dendritic cells, and natural killer (NK) cells] and adaptive immune cells (T and B cells) are absent. This period is also associated with skin and mucosal barrier disruption. The duration of neutropenia is 7–10 days after autologous HSCT, 10–15 days after allogeneic HSCT using an ablative conditioning regimen, and only 5–7 days using a nonablative conditioning regimen.

- *Early postengraftment period*: From neutrophil recovery to day 100.

The innate cells, including neutrophils, monocytes, and NK cells are the first to recover. Full recovery of NK cell counts is typically achieved within 1–2 months

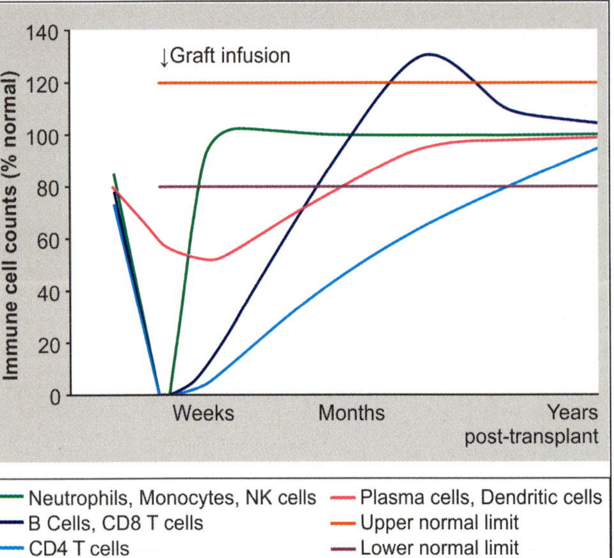

FIGURE 3: Immune recovery in hematopoietic stem cell transplantation (HSCT) postmyeloablative conditioning. Neutrophils, monocytes, and natural killer (NK) cells are the first to recover and attain steady levels within weeks post-transplant. CD8+ T cells and B cells complete recovery in about 2–8 months and CD4+ T cells slowly recover over 1–2 years.

Source: Adapted from Storek J. Immunological reconstitution after hematopoietic cell transplantation—its relation to the contents of the graft. Expert Opin Biol Ther (Informa). 2008;8:583-97.

following HSCT. This is followed by increasing numbers of CD8+ T cells, which takes about 2–8 months to reach subnormal levels.

- *Late postengraftment period*: After day 100.

There is recovery of B cells and CD4+ T cells during this period. Restoration of full humoral immune competence requires reconstitution not only of naïve B cells, but of memory B cell pool as well. Thus in the absence of GVHD, recovery of total B cell numbers can be demonstrated within 6 months post-transplant, recipients remain predisposed to infections from encapsulated bacteria and viruses for at least 1 year post-transplant. CD4+ T cells take 1–2 years to recover (**Figs. 3** and **4**).

The timeline for immune recovery and infections change with GVHD as there is an intensification of immunosuppression. Please note below immune recovery postmyeloablative conditioning and timeline for infections post HSCT.

The common infectious syndromes in HSCT patients include neutropenic fever and bacteremia, mucositis, pneumonia and pulmonary infiltrates, diarrhea, central nervous system syndromes including encephalitis and meningitis, skin rash, hemorrhagic cystitis, hepatitis and cytomegalovirus infections. These clinical conditions are discussed in detail in the e-chapter.

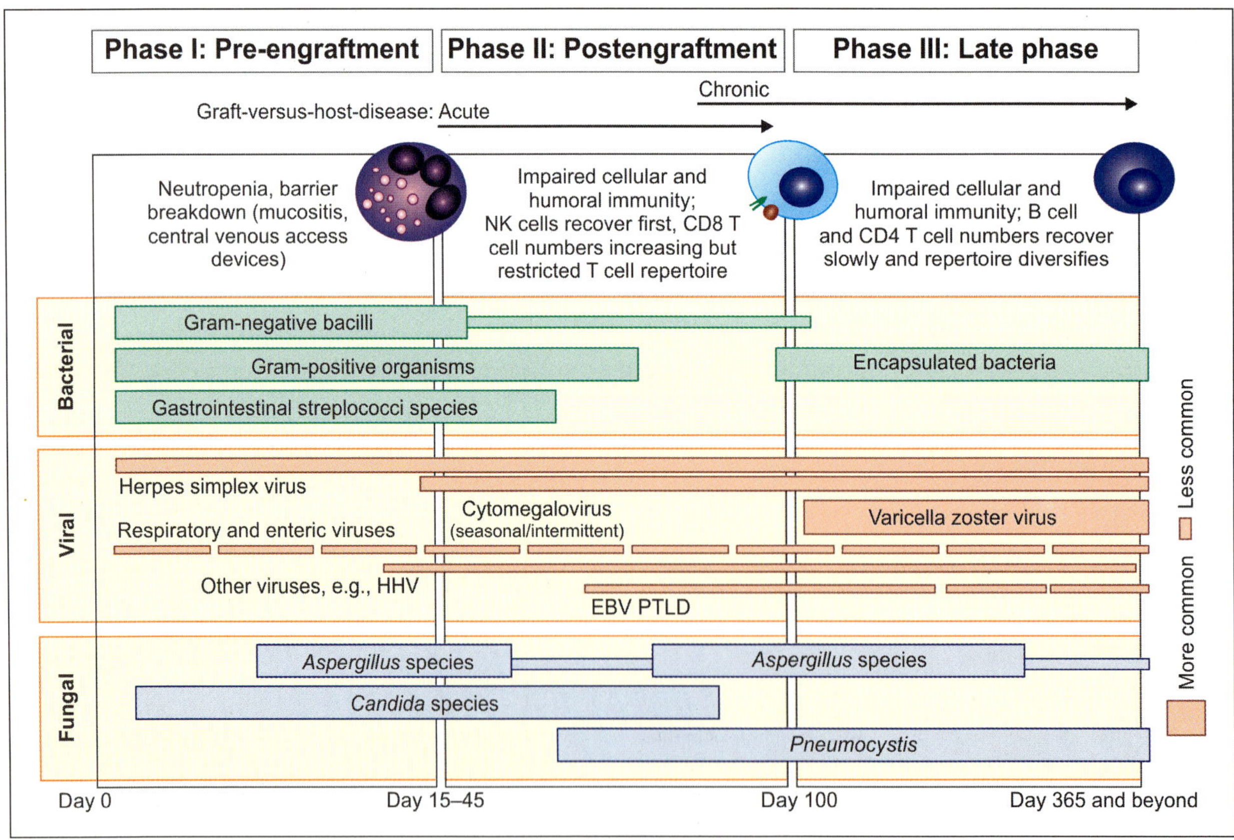

(EBV: Epstein–Barr virus; HCT: hematopoietic stem cell transplantation; HHV: human herpes virus; NK: natural killer; PTLD: post-transplant lymphoproliferative disease)

FIGURE 4: Phases of infections among allogeneic HCT recipients.

Source: Adapted from Tomblyn M, Chiller T, Einsele H, Gress R, Sepkowitz K, Storek J, et al. Guidelines for preventing infectious complications among hematopoietic cell transplantation recipients : a global perspective. Biol Blood Marrow Transplant. 2009;15(10):1143-238.

Prevention:

Pretransplant evaluation: The pretransplantation evaluation is designed to prevent infections by excluding unsuitable donors and by defining specific infection control policies and antimicrobial prophylaxis. The laboratory testing and evaluation in the donor and recipient is illustrated in **Table 2**.

Antimicrobial prophylaxis for HSCT encompasses antiviral, antibacterial and antifungal prophylaxis given to ameliorate risk of developing infection before, during, and after HSCT (refer **Table 3**).

INFECTIONS IN SOLID ORGAN TRANSPLANTATION

As immunosuppressive agents and graft survival have improved, infection and malignancy have become the main barriers to disease-free survival after organ transplantation. The rate of infections in the initial 3 years after kidney transplantation is 45.0 per 100 patient-years of follow-up and rank second as the cause of the death in patients with SOT.

Potent immunosuppressive regimens have led to improved survival in SOT. In addition, improved diagnostic testing has led to earlier diagnosis of opportunistic infections and thus early optimization of appropriate antibiotic therapy.

TABLE 2 Pretransplant evaluation in donor and recipient in HSCT.

Tests and evaluation	Donor	Recipient
History, review of systems, and physical examination	+	+
Dental and ENT evaluation	-	+
Chest X-ray	+	+
Pathogen-specific testing		
CMV IgG	+	+
Hepatitis B (HBsAg, anti-HBsAg, anti-HBc) ± viral load	+	+
Hepatitis C (IgG)	+	+
HIV-1, -2 antibodies	+	+
RPR or VDRL or a *Treponema pallidum* antibody test	+	+
VZV IgG	+	+
HSV IgG	-	+
EBV (VCA IgG)	+	+
Toxoplasma gondii IgG	+	+
SARS-CoV-2 PCR on nasopharyngeal swab specimen	+	+
Staphylococcus nasal culture	-	-

(CMV: cytomegalovirus; EBV: Epstein–Barr virus; ENT: ear, nose, and throat; HBc: hepatitis B core; HBsAg: hepatitis B surface antigen; HIV: human immunodeficiency virus; HSCT: hematopoietic stem cell transplantation; HSV: herpes simplex virus; IgG: immunoglobulin G; PCR: polymerase chain reaction; RPR: rapid plasma regain; SARS-CoV-2: severe acute respiratory syndrome coronavirus 2; VCA: viral capsid antigen; VDRL: venereal disease research laboratory; VZV: varicella zoster virus)

Source: Adapted from Hamadani M, Craig M, Awan FT, Devine SM. How we approach patient evaluation for hematopoietic stem cell transplantation. Bone Marrow Transplant. 2010;45(8):1259-68.

TABLE 3 Antimicrobial prophylaxis in HSCT recipients.

Organism	Pre-engraftment period	Postengraftment period
Antibacterial prophylaxis	Most centers in India advocate no antibacterial prophylaxis due to drug resistance among gram-negative bacilli	Oral penicillin for prophylaxis against *Streptococcus pneumoniae* to continue till all immunosuppressives discontinued
	Fluoroquinolones are used in some centers	
Antiviral prophylaxis		
HSV	Acyclovir from preconditioning till engraftment	Acyclovir to be continued till at least 1 year post-transplant or in case of GVHD till all immunosuppressives discontinued
VZV/Zoster		
CMV (prefer to use preemptive therapy over prophylaxis)	Letermovir	Letermovir till week 14
Antifungal prophylaxis		
Candida	Fluconazole	
Mold aspergillosis/ mucormycosis	Posaconazole	In case of GVHD and steroid dose >1 mg/kg/day for greater than 3 weeks Posaconazole till immunosuppressives discontinued
Pneumocystis		Cotrimoxazole usually for 6 months, longer in case of GVHD
Toxoplasmosis		Double strength cotrimoxazole till immunosuppressives discontinued

(CMV: cytomegalovirus; GVHD: graft-versus-host disease; HSCT: hematopoietic stem cell transplantation; HSV: herpes simplex virus; VZV: varicella zoster virus)

Source: Adapted from Taplitz RA, Kennedy EB, Bow EJ, Crews J, Gleason C, Hawley DK, et al. Antimicrobial prophylaxis for adult patients with cancer-related immunosuppression: ASCO and IDSA Clinical Practice Guideline Update. J Clin Oncol. 2018;36(30):3043-54.

TIME LINE OF INFECTIONS

The post-transplant course can be roughly divided into three time periods related to the risks of infection by specific pathogens (**Fig. 5**):

1. Early period post-transplant: 1st month
2. Intermediate period: 1–6 months
3. Late period: > 6 months

This is a reflection of changing risk factors over time: Surgery/hospitalization, immunosuppression, emergence of latent infections, and community exposures.

FIRST MONTH AFTER TRANSPLANTATION

The two major causes of infection in all forms of SOT during the 1st month are pre-existing infection in the donor or recipient and infectious complications of the transplant surgery and hospitalization.

Infectious complications related to surgery:

- Surgical site (wound infections)
- *Aspiration pneumonitis*: Bacterial aspiration pneumonia with nosocomial organisms. Seen commonly in lung transplantation and in association with prolonged intubation and sedation.
- Central line-associated bloodstream infections (CLABSIs): Bacteremia and candidemia
- *Urinary tract infections*: Bacterial and candidal cystitis or pyelonephritis associated with urinary catheter. Highest risk is seen in kidney transplants.
- Cholangitis with associated candidemia/bacteremia. Seen in liver transplants.
- Superinfection of ischemic or injured graft tissues (e.g., anastomotic suture lines) and anastomotic site leaks.
- Infected fluid collections (e.g., hematomas, lymphoceles, pleural effusions, and urinomas)
- *Clostridium difficile* colitis
- *Peritonitis*: Commonly seen in liver transplants

Donor-derived Infections: Donor-derived infections may be reactivation of latent or subclinical active infection in the donors at the time of transplantation. Unexpected donor-derived infections occur in <1% of grafts and may manifest as a cluster of infections among recipients of organs from a common donor. HIV and hepatitis virus transmission occurs because the donor had presumably been infected during the weeks prior to death since the antibody tests for these viruses were negative during

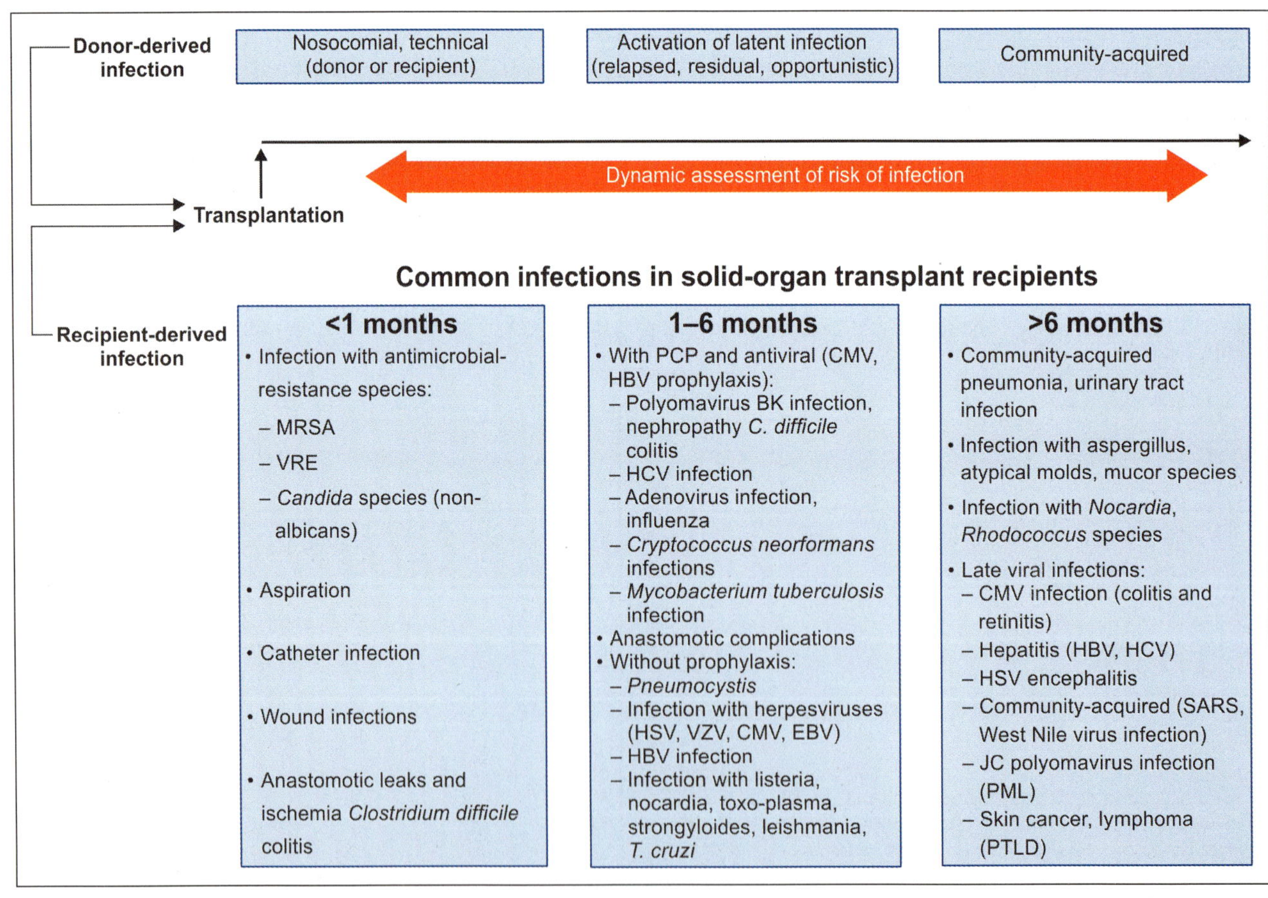

(HBV: hepatitis B virus; HIV: human immunodeficiency virus; HSV: herpes simplex virus; LCMV: lymphocytic choriomeningitis virus; MRSA: methicillin-resistant *Staphylococcus aureus*; PCP: *Pneumocystis carinii* pneumonia; PML: progressive multifocal leukoencephalopathy; PTLD: post-transplantation lymphoproliferative disorder; SARS: severe acute respiratory syndrome; SOT: solid organ transplantation; VRE: vancomycin-resistant enterococci; VZV: varicella zoster virus)

FIGURE 5: Phases of infections among SOT patients.

Source: Adapted from Fishman JA. Infection in solid organ transplant recipients. N Engl J Med. 2007;357(25):2601-14.

the pretransplant donor screening. Infections, such as tuberculosis and histoplasmosis, developing in the first month is almost always donor derived.

Recipient derived viral infections such as hepatitis B virus and hepatitis C virus may reactivate in the first month. But recipient-derived tuberculosis, nontuberculous mycobacteria, histoplasmosis, or toxoplasmosis tend to emerge more than a month after transplantation.

1–6 MONTHS AFTER TRANSPLANTATION

This is the period where there is highest risk as the effect of immunosuppression is maximal. There is significant geographic and institutional variation in the type of infections reflecting differences in local epidemiology, varying immunosuppressive strategies, and specific antimicrobial prophylaxis in the post-transplant period. The differential diagnosis of infectious syndromes is illustrated in **Table 4**.

Fungal infections (**Fig. 6**)*:* In SOT, the most common fungal pathogens include *Candida* and *Aspergillus* species, followed by *Cryptococcus neoformans* and endemic mycoses. Candidal infections are usually seen in the early post-transplant period.

Invasive aspergillosis is seen 1–6 months post-transplant and is associated with mortality varying from 20–50%. The highest risk is seen in lung transplant patients with colonization rates exceeding 25%. Invasive infections in the lung approach 6% overall and include tracheobronchitis, anastomotic infections, invasive pulmonary (32%), and disseminated (22%) infections. *Aspergillus* infections in other organ transplants vary; in livers (1–9.2%), hearts (1–14%), kidney (0.7–4%), and pancreas. In general, the serum galactomannan antigen assay does not perform well in solid organ transplant recipients and diagnosis by microbiological cultures or histopathology in tissue or bronchoalveolar lavage (BAL) galactomannan is preferred. Cryptococcal infections are seen usually 1 month post-transplant with the highest risk in liver and kidney transplants.

Treatment of fungal infections may be complicated by drug interactions and immune reconstitution syndromes seen with recovery or reduction in immunosuppression.

TABLE 4	Differential diagnosis of infectious syndromes between 1 and 6 months post-transplant.
Perioperative and nosocomial infections	*Clostridium difficile* colitis
	Residual pneumonia,
	Technical issues (e.g., anastomotic leaks, empyema, cholangitis, and infected hematoma)
Reactivation of viral infections	CMV, HSV, herpes zoster (VZV), EBV, and HHV-6 or 7
	BK polyomavirus
	Relapsed hepatitis (HBV and HCV)
Community or nosocomially-acquired viral infections	Adenovirus
	Influenza and parainfluenza
	Respiratory syncytial virus
	Metapneumovirus
Opportunistic infections	*Pneumocystis jirovecii*
	L. monocytogenes and *Nocardia* species
	Aspergillus species and *Cryptococcus species*
	Endemic fungi: Histoplasmosis
	Tuberculosis and nontuberculous mycobacteria
	Parasites: Toxoplasmosis, leishmaniasis, strongyloidiasis, and *Cryptosporidium*

(CMV: cytomegalovirus; EBV: Epstein–Barr virus; HBV: hepatitis B virus; HCV: hepatitis C virus; HHV: human herpesvirus; HSV: herpes simplex virus; VZV: varicella zoster virus)

Source: Adapted from Fishman JA. Infection in Organ Transplantation. Am J Transplant. 2017;17(4):856-79.

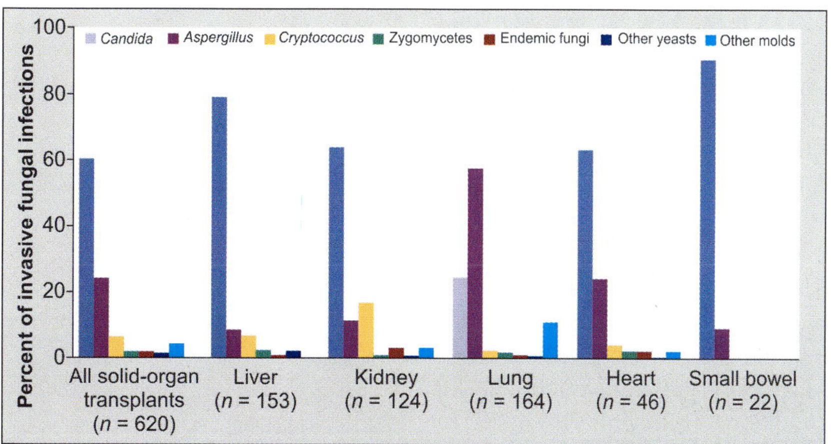

FIGURE 6: Incidence of invasive fungal infections in SOT. Infection due to *Candida* species is most common in all groups. Cryptococcal infection is more common in liver recipients and *Aspergillus* infection in lung recipients.

Source: Adapted from Fishman JA, Gonzalez RG, Branda JA. Case records of the Massachusetts General Hospital. Case 11-2008. A 45-year-old man with changes in mental status after liver transplantation. N Engl J Med. 2008;358:1604-13.

An attempt should be made to establish a definite microbiological diagnosis using invasive techniques, if required. The choice of antifungal should reflect the expected pathogen, penetration into the site of infection avoiding potential for drug interaction.

Cytomegalovirus infection: CMV replicates in all transplanted organs and vessels in fibroblasts, epithelial, endothelial, and other parenchymal cells. It is the most common opportunistic infection in kidney transplant recipients, occurring in 8% of patients.

The primary risk factor for CMV infection or disease is the CMV serostatus of the donor/recipient pair.

- CMV D+/R–: Highest risk
- CMV D+/R+: Moderate risk
- CMV D-/R+: Moderate risk
- CMV D-/R–: Low risk

*Clinical features (**Box 1**)*: Diagnosis of CMV infection or disease is done using nucleic acid testing (NAT)/PCR. There are no widely accepted PCR thresholds that differentiate between past exposure to CMV, CMV infection, and tissue-invasive CMV disease. Clinical judgment must be used when evaluating PCR results. All patients may not demonstrate viremia thus histopathologic examination and immunohistochemistry of biopsied tissue may be necessary to diagnose tissue-invasive CMV disease.

Treatment:

- CMV viremia with no symptoms: The antimetabolite is stopped and CMV PCR is repeated after 1 week. Antiviral is added if there is continued evidence of active CMV replication as evidenced by increase in CMV copies by 2 log values with weekly PCR.
- CMV disease:
  - Antimetabolite to be stopped
  - Antiviral: IV ganciclovir for 3 weeks followed by oral valganciclovir 900 mg OD for 1–3 months.

BK virus nephropathy: BK polyomavirus is a ubiquitous virus with a worldwide seroprevalence of approximately 80–90%. Among kidney transplant recipients, reactivation of latent infection or transmission of new infection via the donor kidney can lead to viruria in 25–30%, viremia in about 12%, and allograft nephropathy (demonstration of virus or virus components in allograft tissue) in 1–10%. Graft loss in BK virus nephropathy (BKPyVAN) is almost 50%.

Clinical manifestations include asymptomatic viruria, viremia, and/or a slow progressive rise in serum creatinine. Rarely BKPy can present with ureteric ulceration and stenosis. The incidence of BKPyVAN is highest in the first 2–6 months post-transplant, but it can occur even years after transplant.

Screening and diagnosis: Screening with quantitative plasma BKPyV PCR (i.e., viral load) and preemptive reduction in immunosuppression for patients with clinically significant BKPyV viremia prevents progression to BKPyVAN in the majority of patients.

- Screening is recommended monthly for the first 6 months following transplant, then every 3 months until 2 years post-transplant, and then annually till 5 years post-transplant. A viral load >10,000 copies/mL has a high positive predictive value for BKPyVAN.
- Whenever renal allograft dysfunction occurs, an allograft biopsy should be performed. The biopsy shows intranuclear basophilic viral inclusions and positive immunohistochemistry suggests BKPyVAN.

Treatment: There is no accepted treatment for BKPyVAN other than reduction in the intensity of immune suppression for those with sustained viral loads. Low-dose cidofovir may be tried and variable response is noted.

BOX 1 Clinical manifestations of CMV infection in SOT recipients.

Direct effects

- Asymptomatic viral shedding and/or seroconversion
- Acute viral syndrome—mono-like illness (fever and myalgia)
- Leukopenia, thrombocytopenia, and fever
- Pneumonitis
- Infection of allograft
  - Hepatitis
  - Pneumonitis
  - Nephritis
  - Myocarditis
  - Pancreatitis
- Infection of native tissues
  - Retina
  - Gastrointestinal tract
  - Pancreas
  - Encephalitis
- Adrenalitis and insufficiency

Indirect effects

- Bacterial and fungal infection
- Activation or accelerated infection of other viruses (HCV, EBV, HHV-6, and HSV)
- Allograft injury and rejection
- Oncogenesis and proliferative syndromes
  - EBV-associated PTLD
  - Accelerated atherogenesis (cardiac)
  - Bronchiolitis obliterans (lungs)

(CMV: cytomegalovirus; EBV: Epstein–Barr virus; HCV: hepatitis C virus; HHV-6: human herpesvirus 6; HSV: herpes simplex virus; PTLD: post-transplant lymphoproliferative disease; SOT: solid organ transplantation)

Source: Adapted from Fishman JA. Infection in Organ Transplantation. Am J Transplant. 2017;17(4):856-79.

MORE THAN 6 MONTHS POST-TRANSPLANT

Most patients are receiving stable and reduced levels of immunosuppression during this period. Usual infectious syndromes seen during this period are:

- Community-acquired infections:
  - Including pneumonia due to respiratory viruses, pneumococcus, and legionella foodborne gastroenteritis
  - Mold infections may be related to occupation or leisure activities
- Late CMV disease may occur in patients who received valganciclovir prophylaxis for the first 3–6 months post-transplant.
- EBV-related post-transplant lymphoproliferative disease (PTLD): This either presents in the first year or 5–7 years after transplant.
- Low- or high-grade rejection may require intensification of immunosuppressive therapy, thus leading to a high risk for opportunistic infections including pneumocystis carinii pneumonia (PCP), cryptococcosis, nocardiosis, molds, and JC virus-associated PML.

The pretransplant evaluation of donor and recipient can help in preventing infections postoperatively. Antimicrobial prophylaxis given peri and post transplant can help in prevention of infections. The protocol for this is given in e-chapter in detail. The schedule for immunization of transplantation patients is also given in detail in the e-chapter along with.

RECOMMENDED READINGS

1. Shah CA, Karanwal A, Desai M, Pandya M, Shah R, Shah R. Hematopoietic stem-cell transplantation in the developing world: experience from a center in Western India. J Oncol. 2015;2015:710543.
2. Saikia TK. Blood and bone marrow transplantation in India: Past, present, and future. Indian J Med Paediatr Oncol. 2020;41(3):308.
3. George B, Mathews V, Srivastava A, Chandy M. Infections among allogeneic bone marrow transplant recipients in India. Bone Marrow Transplant. 2004;33(3):311-5.
4. Kang G, Srivastava A, Pulimood AB, Dennison D, Chandy M. Etiology of diarrhea in patients undergoing allogeneic bone marrow transplantation in South India. Transplantation. 2002;73(8):1247-51.
5. Hamdeh S, Abdelrahman AAM, Elsallabi O, Pathak R, Giri S, Mosalpuria K, et al. Clinical approach to diarrheal disorders in allogeneic hematopoietic stem cell transplant recipients. World J Hematol. 2016;5(1):23-30.
6. Arai S, Lee LA, Vogelsang GB. A Systematic Approach to Hepatic Complications in Hematopoietic Stem Cell Transplantation. J Hematother Stem Cell Res. 2002;11(2):215-29.
7. Hamadani M, Craig M, Awan FT, Devine SM. How we approach patient evaluation for hematopoietic stem cell transplantation. Bone Marrow Transplant. 2010;45(8):1259-68.
8. Sriperumbuduri S, Kalidindi K, Guditi S, Taduri G. Declining trend of infections in renal transplant recipients in a tertiary care hospital from India. Indian J Transplant. 2017;11(3):143.
9. Fishman JA. Infection in Organ Transplantation. Am J Transplant. 2017;17(4):856-79.
10. Taplitz RA, Kennedy EB, Bow EJ, Crews J, Gleason C, Hawley DK, et al. Antimicrobial prophylaxis for adult patients with cancer-related immunosuppression: ASCO and IDSA Clinical Practice Guideline Update. J Clin Oncol. 2018;36(30):3043-54.
11. Cho SY, Lee HJ, Lee DG. Infectious complications after hematopoietic stem cell transplantation : current status and future perspectives in Korea. Korean J Intern Med. 2018;33(2):256-76.
12. Wingard JR, Hsu J, Hiemenz JW. Hematopoietic stem cell transplantation : an overview of infection risks and epidemiology. Infect Dis Clin North Am. 2010;24: 257-72.
13. Tomblyn M, Chiller T, Einsele H, Gress R, Sepkowitz K, Storek J, et al. Guidelines for preventing infectious complications among hematopoietic cell transplantation recipients: a global perspective. Biol Blood Marrow Transplant. 2009;15(10):1143-238.
14. Rubin LG, Levin MJ, Ljungman P, Davies EG, Avery R, Tomblyn M, et al. 2013 IDSA Clinical Practice Guideline for Vaccination of the Immunocompromised Host. Clin Infect Dis. 2014;58:309-18.
15. Karuthu S, Blumberg EA. Common infections in kidney transplant recipients. Clin J Am Soc Nephrol. 2012;7:2058-70.
16. Wójtowicz A, Bochud PY. Risk stratification and immunogenetic risk for infections following stem cell transplantation. Virulence. 2016;7(8):917-29.

CHAPTER 39

Adult Vaccination

V Ramasubramanian, Madhumitha R, Murali Narasimhan

ABSTRACT

Mankind has faced tremendous challenges in the management of infections. With the advent of clean drinking water, sanitation, and childhood vaccinations, the burden of infectious diseases has come under reasonable control. In spite of childhood vaccinations, adults suffer from vaccine-preventable diseases (VPDs). Adults too need vaccinations as part of boosters for certain childhood vaccinations. Moreover, age-related infections, comorbidities, and viral mutations are also indications for vaccinating adults. Vaccines not only prevent infections; they decrease absenteeism and improve work productivity. They can also decrease cardiovascular and cerebrovascular events (influenza vaccine), prevent cancers (hepatocellular carcinoma and cervical cancer), decrease antimicrobial resistance, and can also help in disease eradication (smallpox and polio). Unfortunately, there are several barriers which have to be overcome in India, lack of awareness foremost.

All adult physicians need to understand the fundamental principles of immunization, various types of vaccines, indications, administration methodology, dose schedule, adverse events, and contraindications. Vaccine recommendations can change with time and frequent updates are essential.

An Adult Vaccine Clinic is recommended in all hospitals to improve access to vaccines for the public. Setting up one is not difficult, but ensuring cold chain maintenance and data management should be paramount.

As vaccines for coronavirus disease-2019 (COVID-19) already in the market, every doctor should understand the importance of vaccinations for adults and fight against vaccine hesitancy.

"Vaccines are the tugboats of preventive health"

—William Foege

INTRODUCTION

Infections have been the scourge of human civilization from time immemorial. Infectious diseases account for about 25% of all deaths across the globe. Since the advent of the smallpox vaccine, vaccines have played a significant role in preventing infections. Universal childhood immunization programs have had a significant impact on morbidity and mortality of serious infections that disproportionately affect children. In fact, vaccines have been quintessential in improving longevity and quality of human life. But many childhood VPDs are now found among adults. Certain vaccines require boosters to sustain protection in adults. In recent years, there has been an increased attention on routine immunization of adults due to a large burden of VPDs.

Though after the introduction of the National Childhood Immunization Program, there has been a dramatic decrease in VPDs in India, they still contribute to a disproportionately high share of globally reported cases of diphtheria (60%), Japanese encephalitis (44%), and tetanus (40%). The National Centre for Disease Control has reported 2,679 epidemic outbreaks of diseases such as measles, varicella, food poisoning, and acute diarrheal diseases in 2017. The same report also pegs carcinoma cervix cases at 97,000 with 60,000 deaths and human papillomavirus (HPV) positivity rate of 12% on random testing of women. In spite of a paucity of data, the burden of VPDs in India is high. To ensure control of VPDs in adults, we need to ensure that adults too receive booster doses of childhood vaccines and certain other vaccines based on their age, comorbidities, and lifestyle.

UNDERSTANDING IMMUNIZATION

Immunization is the act of artificially inducing immunity or providing protection against a disease either by active or passive method.

Active immunization results when the immune system produces antibodies in a recipient who is exposed to a killed or weakened form of the disease organism through vaccination. The primary immune response is by inducing B-cell proliferation, antibody response, and T-cell sensitization. In an event of subsequent exposure to the vaccine-directed specific organism, it results in a secondary response that causes increased proliferation of B cells and formation of antibodies. This secondary response protects the individual from developing the disease. Active immunity is expected to be long lasting.

Passive immunization occurs when a person receives antibodies (globulin product) to a disease rather than producing them through his or her own immune system.

This provides a transient immunity for a specific exposure. Most common examples of a passive immunization include the transplacental transfer of maternal antibodies to the fetus and immunoglobulin injections for specific postexposure prophylaxis.

Immunizing agents include vaccines, toxoids, and antibody-containing preparations from human or animal donors.

- *Vaccine*: A suspension of attenuated live or killed microorganisms (bacteria, viruses, or fractions thereof)
- *Toxoid*: A modified bacterial toxin that has been rendered nontoxic but retains the ability to stimulate the formation of antitoxin.
- *Immunoglobulin*: A sterile solution containing antibody from human blood for intramuscular administration. It is primarily indicated for protection of immunodeficient persons and for passive immunization against measles and hepatitis A. Intravenous immunoglobulin (IVIG), a specialized preparation for intravenous administration is primarily indicated for replacement therapy in immunoglobulin G (IgG) deficiency, treatment of Kawasaki disease, Guillain-Barré syndrome, and idiopathic thrombocytopenic purpura.
- *Specific immunoglobulin*: Obtained from disease-specific high-antibody donor pools, e.g., hepatitis B immunoglobulin (HBIG), varicella-zoster immunoglobulin (VZIG), rabies immunoglobulin (RIG), and tetanus immunoglobulin (TIG).

VACCINE TYPES

The World Health Organization (WHO) groups vaccines into four types. Each vaccine group is defined according to the kind of agent employed to trigger the immune system to react.

1. *Live attenuated vaccine (LAV)*:
   i. Tuberculosis [Bacillus Calmette-Guérin (BCG)]
   ii. Oral polio vaccine (OPV)
   iii. Measles
   iv. Yellow fever
2. *Inactivated (killed antigen)*:
   i. Whole-cell pertussis (wP)
   ii. Inactivated poliovirus vaccine (IPV)
3. *Subunit (purified antigen)*:
   i. Acellular pertussis (aP)
   ii. *Haemophilus influenzae* type b (Hib)
   iii. Pneumococcal conjugate vaccine (PCV7, PCV10, and PCV13)
   iv. Hepatitis B (HepB)
4. *Toxoid (inactivated toxins)*:
   i. Tetanus toxoid (TT)
   ii. Diphtheria toxoid

Apart from the basic antigenic components, a vaccine may include stabilizers, preservatives, and adjuvants.

- *Suspending fluid*: This frequently is sterile water or saline, but it may also be a complex fluid, containing small amounts of proteins or other constituents derived from the medium or biologic system in which the immunizing agent is produced (serum proteins, egg antigens, and cell culture-derived antigens).
- *Preservatives*: These components of vaccines are used either to (1) inhibit or prevent bacterial growth in viral culture or the final product or (2) to stabilize the antigen. They include specific antibiotics, thiomersal, formaldehyde, or phenol derivatives. Allergic reactions may occur if the recipient is sensitive to any of these additives.
- *Stabilizers*: Vaccine stability is the key to efficacy. Stabilizers such as $MgCl_2$ for OPV, $MgSO_4$ for measles, lactose-sorbitol for chickenpox, and sorbitol-gelatin for measles, mumps, and rubella (MMR) are used to protect the delicate antigen from degradation during storage. This is especially important if the chain of cold storage cannot be guaranteed during shipping of a vaccine. Correct choice of stabilizer depends on the antigen, and omitted or improperly chosen stabilizers can lead to vaccines that lose their potency and become ineffective.
- *Adjuvants*: Inactivated antigen vaccines and subunit vaccines (e.g., toxoids and HepB vaccine) generate a relatively weak immune response and require properly formulated "helpers" called adjuvants to provide robust and long-lasting immunity. The most common adjuvant used in human vaccines is alum, which comprises particles of insoluble aluminum salts.

WHY DO ADULTS NEED VACCINES

- Protection from some childhood vaccines can wear off over time and adults are prone to these infections (e.g., diphtheria, tetanus, and pertussis).
- Viruses can mutate over time (influenza) and earlier vaccines can become ineffective.
- The immune systems weaken over time, putting adults at higher risk for VPDs as they age (e.g., influenza and invasive pneumococcal disease).
- Adults with certain comorbidities or immunocompromising conditions resulting from drugs or illnesses like human immunodeficiency virus (HIV) or systemic lupus erythematosus (SLE) are more likely to develop complications from certain VPDs (e.g., shingles and pneumococcal infections).
- Adults who contract infections such as measles, mumps, pertussis, or influenza can infect infants who may not yet be fully immunized or adults who are immunocompromised.
- Vaccination can significantly reduce healthcare costs for adults. It is estimated that adult vaccination costs are significantly lower than cost of long-term intake of drugs used in the secondary prophylaxis of noncommunicable diseases like statins.
- Preventing VPDs can indirectly contribute to improved work productivity and reduced absenteeism at work.
- Vaccinations can have additional benefits.
- Influenza vaccines have been reported to reduce risk of heart attacks by 19–45% and pneumococcal vaccination was associated with a significant reduction in the risk of coronary syndrome in adults above 65 years of age.
- Conjugated pneumococcal vaccines have shown promising results in terms of reducing antibiotic

resistance by slowing the spread of resistant pneumococcal serotypes (19A) and also by averting disease occurrence and the resultant hospitalization which may entail antibiotic use.

- Dual vaccination with influenza and pneumococcal vaccines is effective in protecting elderly people with chronic illness from developing complications associated with respiratory, cardiovascular, and cerebrovascular diseases reducing intensive care admissions.
- HPV vaccination could reduce the burden of cervical cancer which is the second most common cancer in India and the most common cause of death due to cancer.

GENERAL PRINCIPLES

Administering vaccine to adults should involve an assessment of the risks of disease, decision on whom to vaccinate, the benefits and risk associated with vaccination and also ensuring appropriate storage and handling of vaccine, administering vaccines, and maintaining vaccine records. Adult vaccine indications can also be decided on age, lifestyle, occupational, and health factors **Figure 1**.

The Advisory Committee on Immunization Practices gives annual recommendations on adult vaccinations (**Table 1**).

Before you vaccinate adults, consider their "H-A-L-O"!

What is H-A-L-O?

As shown below, It's an easy-to-use chart that can help you make an initial decision about vaccinating a patient based on four factors–the patient's Health conditon, Age, Lifestyle, and Occupation. In some situations, though, you can vaccinate a patient without considering these factors. For example, all adults need a dose of Tdap as well as annual vaccination against influenza, and any adult who wants protection against hepatitis A or hepatitis B can be vaccinated. Note that not all patients who mention one or more H-A-L-O factors will need to be vaccinated. Before you make a definitive decision about vaccinating your patient, it's important that you refer to the more detailed information found in the Immunization Action Coalition's "Summary of Recommendations for Adult Immunization," located at www.immunize.org/catg.d/p2011.pdf or the complete vaccine recommendations of the Centers for Disease Control and Preventions' Advisory Committee on immunization Practices (ACIP) at www.cdc.gov/vaccines/pubs/ACIP-list.htm.

How do I use H-A-L-O?

Though some H-A-L-O factors can be easily determined (e.g., age, pregnancy), you will need to ask your patient about the presence or absence of others. Once you determine which of the factors apply, scan down each column of the chart to see at a glance which vaccinations are possibly indicated.

H-A-L-O checklist of factors that indicate a possible need for adult vaccination

	Health factors									Age factors	Lifestyle factors							Occupational or other factors			
Vaccine	Pregnant	Certain chronic diseases	Immunosuppressed (including HIV)	History of STD	Asplenia	Cochlear implant candidate/recipient	Organ transplant (for stem cell transplant, see ACIP's General Recommendations on Immunization)	CSF leaks	Alcoholism		Born outside the US	Men who have sex with men	Not in a long-term mutually monogamous relationship	User of injecting or non-injecting drugs	International traveler	Close contact of international adoptee	Cigarette smoker	College students	Healthcare worker	Certain lab workers	Adults in institutional settings (e.g., chronic care, correctional)
HepA		✓										✓		✓	✓	✓				✓	
HepB		✓	✓	✓							✓	✓	✓	✓	✓				✓		✓
Hib		✓	✓		✓																
HPV (females)										Through 26 years											
HPV (males)			✓							Routine through 21 years: Risk based 22–46 years		✓									
IPV															✓					✓	
Influenza	Annual vaccination is recommended for all adults ---▶																				
Meningococcal		✓			✓										✓			✓		✓	
MMR			?							Routine 1 dose if born after 1956; second dose for some					✓			✓	✓		
PCV13		✓	✓		✓	✓	✓	✓		65 years and older (if not previously vaccinated)											
PPSV23		✓	✓		✓	✓	✓	✓	✓	65 years and older							✓				✓
Tdap	A single dose is recommended for all adults; pregnant women should receive Tdap during each pregnancy ---▶																				
Varicella	Completion of a 2–dose series is recommended for non-pregnant adults through age 59 years who do not have evidence of immunity to varicella ---▶																				
Zoster										60 years and older											

? = Vaccination may be indicated depending on degree of immunosuppression

(CSF: cerebrospinal fluid; HepA: hepatitis A; HepB: hepatitis B; Hib: *Haemophilus influenzae* type b; HIV: human immunodeficiency virus; HPV: human papillomavirus; IPV: inactivated poliovirus vaccine; MMR: measles, mumps, and rubella; PCV13: 13-valent pneumococcal conjugate vaccine; PPSV23: 23-valent pneumococcal polysaccharide vaccine; STD: sexually transmitted disease; Td: tetanus and diphtheria; Tdap: tetanus, diphtheria, and pertussis)

FIGURE 1: HALO checklist for Vaccination.

Source: www.immunize.org www.vaccineinformation.org

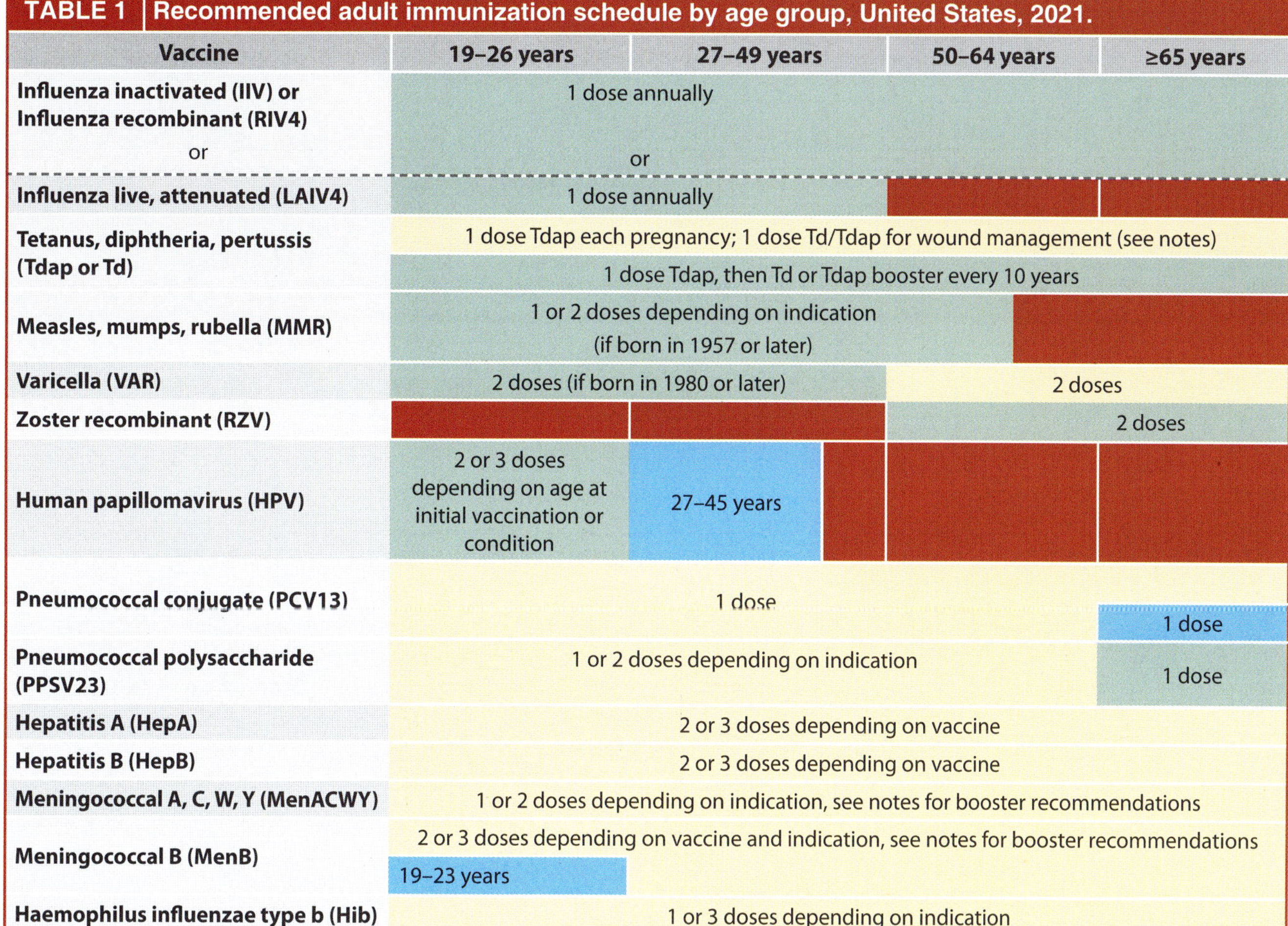

TABLE 1 Recommended adult immunization schedule by age group, United States, 2021.

Vaccine	19–26 years	27–49 years	50–64 years	≥65 years
Influenza inactivated (IIV) or Influenza recombinant (RIV4) or	1 dose annually or			
Influenza live, attenuated (LAIV4)	1 dose annually			
Tetanus, diphtheria, pertussis (Tdap or Td)	1 dose Tdap each pregnancy; 1 dose Td/Tdap for wound management (see notes) 1 dose Tdap, then Td or Tdap booster every 10 years			
Measles, mumps, rubella (MMR)	1 or 2 doses depending on indication (if born in 1957 or later)			
Varicella (VAR)	2 doses (if born in 1980 or later)		2 doses	
Zoster recombinant (RZV)			2 doses	
Human papillomavirus (HPV)	2 or 3 doses depending on age at initial vaccination or condition	27–45 years		
Pneumococcal conjugate (PCV13)	1 dose			1 dose
Pneumococcal polysaccharide (PPSV23)	1 or 2 doses depending on indication			1 dose
Hepatitis A (HepA)	2 or 3 doses depending on vaccine			
Hepatitis B (HepB)	2 or 3 doses depending on vaccine			
Meningococcal A, C, W, Y (MenACWY)	1 or 2 doses depending on indication, see notes for booster recommendations			
Meningococcal B (MenB)	2 or 3 doses depending on vaccine and indication, see notes for booster recommendations 19–23 years			
Haemophilus influenzae type b (Hib)	1 or 3 doses depending on indication			

Recommended vaccination for adults who meet age requirement, lack documentation of vaccination, or lack evidence of past infection.

Recommended vaccination for adults with an additional risk factor or another indication.

Recommended vaccination based on shared clinical decision-making.

No recommendation/Not applicable.

Source: https://www.cdc.gov/vaccines/schedules/downloads/adult/adult-combined-schedule.pdf

Further information and booster recommendations: https://www.cdc.gov/vaccines/schedules/hcp/imz/adult.html

ROUTE

Most adult vaccines are administered intramuscularly or subcutaneously, usually in or over the deltoid muscle.

Deltoid intramuscular injections should be administered at the midpoint of the muscle, 2-3 fingers width below the acromion process (**Fig. 2**). Correct needle length should be used, which depends on weight and sex. The Centers for Disease Control and Prevention (CDC) recommends needle lengths of 5/8 inch for individuals <60 kg, 1 inch for individuals 60–70 kg, 1.0–1.5 inch for women 70–90 kg and men 70–118 kg, and 1.5 inch for women >90 kg and men >118 kg.

Subcutaneous injection should be given with a 23–25-gauge needle with a needle length of 5/8 to 3/4 inch.

In general, gluteal administration of vaccines should be avoided for standard immunizations.

VACCINE COADMINISTRATION

Most vaccines can be administered simultaneously at different sites without compromising efficacy.

- Live virus vaccines should either be administered on the same day or subsequent immunization with live virus vaccines should be delayed 1 month to avoid any concerns of impaired immune response.
- Immunoglobulins should not be administered along with live virus vaccines because the passively administered antibodies can interfere with the vaccine response (this limitation does not apply to inactivated vaccines or oral polio and yellow fever vaccines).

The recommended method of storage, preparation, and route of administration of each vaccine should be followed precisely as per the package insert description.

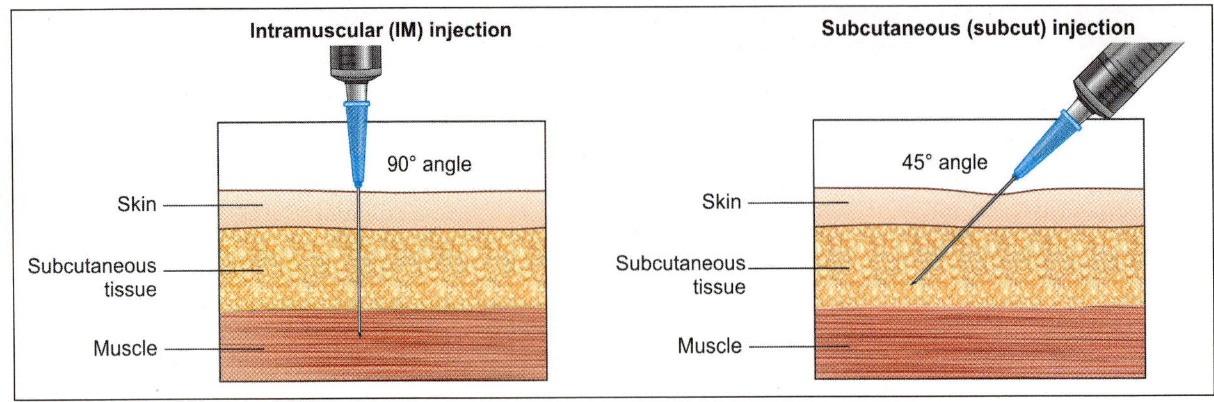

FIGURE 2: Intramuscularly or subcutaneously administration of vaccine.

SCHEDULE

The features of vaccines used in adults are given in **Table 2** and the suggested schedule for adult vaccine in India is given in **Table 3**.

Adverse events: Most vaccines are safe to administer, causing only minor side effects. Many vaccines and toxoids cause side effects such as fever, local reactions at the site of injection, or even serum sickness-like reactions. These adverse reactions can be caused by the immunogenic moiety in the vaccine or by trace amounts of antibiotics, preservatives, stabilizers, and residual animal proteins (**Table 4**). These side effects are not considered true contraindications to vaccination.

The following are *not* contraindications to immunization:

- Current or recent mild illness, with or without low-grade fever
- Current or recent antibiotic therapy
- Previous mild-to-moderate local tenderness, redness, swelling, or fever <40.5°C after any vaccination
- Egg allergy
- Family history of adverse reactions to immunization

The situations when certain vaccines are contraindicated are given in **Table 5**.

VACCINES FOR SPECIAL SITUATIONS

TRAVEL

There are country-specific immunization requirements for both travel and work permits.

Commonly considered vaccines for travelers include measles and rubella containing vaccines, polio vaccines, and boosters for tetanus and diphtheria (Td). In addition, travelers to specified areas or seasonally can take yellow fever, influenza, typhoid, rabies, Japanese encephalitis, hepatitis A and B, polio, and meningococcal vaccines (**Fig. 3**).

HEALTHCARE WORKERS

The desirable schedule for vaccine of healthcare workers is given in **Table 6**.

PREGNANCY

Recommendations for vaccine use in pregnancy are based on disease burden and severity for mothers and infants. For all women who have had their childhood immunizations vaccines recommended include tetanus, diphtheria, and pertussis (Tdap) and inactivated influenza vaccine during the third trimester. The flu vaccine can be given during any trimester if there is an outbreak of influenza. In general, all live virus vaccines are contraindicated in pregnancy except yellow fever vaccine which is recommended if risk due to international travel is high.

HUMAN IMMUNODEFICIENCY VIRUS

Adults with HIV who meet age requirement and who lack documentation of immunization should receive Td/Tdap, annual influenza, PCV13, PPSV23, and HepB and may be considered for MMR and varicella vaccination (if CD4 cell count ≥200 cells/µL). Zoster vaccine should not be given. If specific risk factors are present, Hib, hepatitis A, and meningococcal conjugate vaccine-4 (MCV4) should be considered. Women younger than 27 years should receive HPV vaccine.

IMMUNOCOMPROMISED

Immunocompromised persons are more susceptible to the adverse effects off live vaccines. Their response to inactivated vaccines may also be poor. All routinely indicated vaccines for HIV should be given before planned immunosuppression, if possible. Influenza, Td/Tdap, and pneumococcal vaccines are strongly advised. The household contacts of patients with immunocompromised conditions should be immunized appropriately including the yearly influenza vaccine to reduce the risk of exposure to immunocompromised persons.

POSTEXPOSURE IMMUNIZATION

Passive prophylaxis with specific immunoglobulins can be given after exposure. However, some vaccines can also be given after confirmed exposures. Measles vaccine given within 6 days of exposure may prevent the manifestations of the illness. Varicella vaccine too may prevent the spread

TABLE 2 Vaccine adminstration.

Vaccine	Dose	Route	Site	Needle size
Diphtheria, tetanus, and pertussis (DTaP, DT, Tdap, Td)	0.5 mL	IM	Deltoid muscle	22–25-gauge, 1 to 1½"*
***Haemophilus influenzae* type b (Hib)**	0.5 mL	IM	Deltoid muscle	22–25-gauge, 1 to 1½"*
Hepatitis A (HepA)	≤18 years: 0.5 mL ≥19 years: 1.0 mL	IM	Deltoid muscle	22–25-gauge, 1 to 1½"*
Hepatitis B (HepB)	≤19 years: 0.5 mL ≥20 years: 1.0 mL	IM	Deltoid muscle	22–25-gauge, 1 to 1½"*
Human papillomavirus (HPV)	0.5 mL	IM	Deltoid muscle	22–25-gauge, 1 to 1½"*
Live attenuated influenza vaccine (LAIV)	0.2 mL (0.1 mL in each nostril)	Intranasal spray	Intranasal	NA
Inactivated influenza vaccine (IIV); 3 years and older	0.5 mL	IM	Deltoid muscle	22–25-gauge, 1 to 1½"*
Measles, mumps, and rubella (MMR)	0.5 mL	SC	Fatty tissue over triceps	23–25-gauge, ⅝"
Meningococcal serogroups A, C, W, Y (MenACWY)	0.5 mL	IM	Deltoid muscle	22–25-gauge, 1 to 1½"*
Meningococcal serogroup B (MenB)	0.5 mL	IM	Deltoid muscle	22–25-gauge, 1 to 1½"*
Pneumococcal conjugate vaccine (PCV)	0.5 mL	IM	Deltoid muscle	22–25-gauge, 1 to 1½"*
Pneumococcal polysaccharide vaccine (PPSV)	0.5 mL	IM	Deltoid muscle	22–25-gauge, 1 to 1½"*
		SC	Fatty tissue over triceps	23–25-gauge, ⅝"
Inactivated poliovirus vaccine (IPV)	0.5 mL	IM	Deltoid muscle	22–25-gauge, 1 to 1½"*
		SC	Fatty tissue over triceps	23–25-gauge, ⅝"
Varicella (VAR)	0.5 mL	SC	Fatty tissue over triceps	23–25-gauge, ⅝"
Zoster (Zos)	Shingrix 0.5 mL	IM	Deltoid muscle	22–25-gauge, 1 to 1½"*

*When giving intramuscular injections, a ⅝" needle is sufficient in adults weighing <60 kg; a 1" needle is sufficient in adults 60 to 70 kg; a 1 to 1½" needle is recommended in women weighing 70 to 90 kg and men weighing 70 to 118 kg; a 1½" needle is recommended in women weighing >90 kg or men weighing >118 kg.

(IM: intramuscular; NA: not applicable; SC: subcutaneous)

Source: Immunization action coalition. Administering Vaccines to Adults: Dose, Route, Site, and Needle Size. [online] Available from http://www.immunize.org/catg.d/p3084.pdf.

TABLE 3 Recommended adult immunization schedule.

Vaccine	Schedule	Comments
Tetanus/Diphtheria	Every 10 years	One dose of Tdap at anytime
MMR	Two doses at least 1 month apart	After 1 year of age
Varicella	Two doses 4–8 weeks apart	
Hepatitis B	Three doses at 0, 1, and 6 months	Check antibody titer 4–8 weeks after third dose. >10 IU is protective
Hepatitis A	Two doses at 6 months to 1 year apart	Lifelong immunity
HPV	• Less than 15 years—0 and 6 months • 15 years and over—three doses—0, 1, and 2 months or 6 months depending on vaccine used	Bivalent and quadrivalent vaccines available
Influenza	• Annual	As soon as the new batch for the year is released

Continued...

Continued...

Vaccine	Schedule	Comments
Pneumococcal	• Adults > 65 years—PCV13 followed by PPSV23 after a year • Adults 19–64 years with comorbidities—PPSV23 • Adults 19–64 years who are immunocompromised—PCV13 followed by PPSV23 after 2 months and repeat q5yrs	• PCV13—conjugate 13-valent vaccine • PPSV23—polysaccharide 23-valent vaccine
Meningococcal	One dose only	• Conjugate 4-valent (A, C, W, and Y) and type B strain available • Polysaccharide vaccine also available
Zoster	Recommended for all adults over 60 years (can be given over 50 years)	• Live vaccine one dose • Subunit vaccine two doses, 6 months apart • Currently both unavailable in India
Typhoid	Conjugate vaccine one dose	• Effective for 10 years, maybe longer
Japanese encephalitis (JE)	Two doses 3–4 weeks apart	• For travelers to JE endemic areas provided their expected stay is for a minimum period of 4 weeks • Subunit vaccine unavailable in India
Rabies	• Pre-exposure prophylaxis (PrEP)—0 and 7 days • Postexposure prophylaxis (PEP) 0, 3, 7, and 28 days • In persons who have already received PrEP or earlier PEP—0 and 3 days	• Rabies immunoglobulin or monoclonal antibody recommended for category 3 bites for all unvaccinated persons
Yellow fever	One dose is effective lifelong	• Indicated for yellow fever endemic Sub-Saharan Africa and South America • Second dose after 10 years if risk is very high

(HPV: human papillomavirus; MMR: measles, mumps, and rubella; PCV13: 13-valent pneumococcal conjugate vaccine; PPSV23: 23-valent pneumococcal polysaccharide vaccine; Tdap: tetanus, diphtheria, and pertussis)

TABLE 4 Adverse events.

Reaction	Management
***Localized*:** • Soreness, redness, itching, or swelling at the injection site	• Apply a cold compress to the injection site • Give an analgesic or antipruritic medication
***Psychological*:** • Fright, presyncope, and syncope	Reassure recipient. Ask them to lie flat. Loosen any tight clothing and maintain open airway. Apply cool, damp cloth to patient's face and neck. Keep them under close observation until full recovery
***Anaphylaxis*:** • Skin and mucosal symptoms such as generalized hives, itching, or flushing; swelling of lips, face, throat, or eyes. Respiratory symptoms such as nasal congestion, change in voice, sensation of throat closing, stridor, shortness of breath, wheeze, or cough • Gastrointestinal symptoms such as nausea, vomiting, diarrhea, and cramping abdominal pain • Cardiovascular symptoms such as collapse, dizziness, tachycardia, and hypotension	• Emergency medical protocol • H1 antihistamines: These relieve itching and hives only; they do not relieve upper or lower airway obstruction, hypotension, or shock. Diphenhydramine (e.g., Benadryl) oral, 12.5 mg/5 mL liquid, 25 or 50 mg tablets • Epinephrine 1.0 mg/mL aqueous solution (1:1,000 dilution)

Source: Adapted from Immunization Action Coalition. Medical Management of Vaccine Reactions in Adults in a Community Setting [online].

of infection in exposed individuals if administered within 3–5 days of exposure. Hepatitis A and B vaccines are also used for postexposure prophylaxis. Rabies vaccine along with RIG is indicated after suspected animal bites.

AUTOIMMUNE RHEUMATIC DISEASES

Despite varying degrees of immunocompromised state in patients with autoimmune inflammatory rheumatic diseases (AIRDs), the response to vaccinations is adequate although in some cases it may be blunted. Ideal time to vaccinate a person with AIRDs is when the disease is stable. Long-term stable low-dose corticosteroid therapy (defined as prednisolone <20 mg/day for >14 days) either alone or in combination with low-dose nonbiological oral immune modulating drugs like methotrexate <25 mg/week or azathioprine <3 mg/kg per day is not considered sufficiently

TABLE 5 Contraindications to vaccination.	
Contraindications	**Recommended action**
Previous anaphylactic reaction to a specific vaccine	Avoid revaccination with the specific vaccine
Previous anaphylactic reaction to neomycin or streptomycin	Avoid measles, mumps, and rubella (MMR) vaccine
Immunocompromised adults	Avoid all live virus vaccines
Household members of immunocompromised patients	Avoid oral polio (can cause vaccine-induced polio in the immunocompromised)
Pregnant women	Avoid all live virus vaccines

Source: 1. American College Physicians Task Force on Adult Immunization and Infectious Diseases Society of America. Guide for Adult Immunization. Philadelphia: American College of Physicians; 1994.

2. Centers for Disease Control and Prevention. Prevention and Control of Influenza: Part II, Antiviral Agents Recommendations of the Advisory Committee on Immunization Practices (ACIP). Morb Mortal Wkly Rep. 1994;43:1-10.

3. Gershon AA, Gardner P, Peter G, Nichols K, Orenstein W. Quality Standards for Immunization. Clin Infect Dis. 1997;25:782-6.

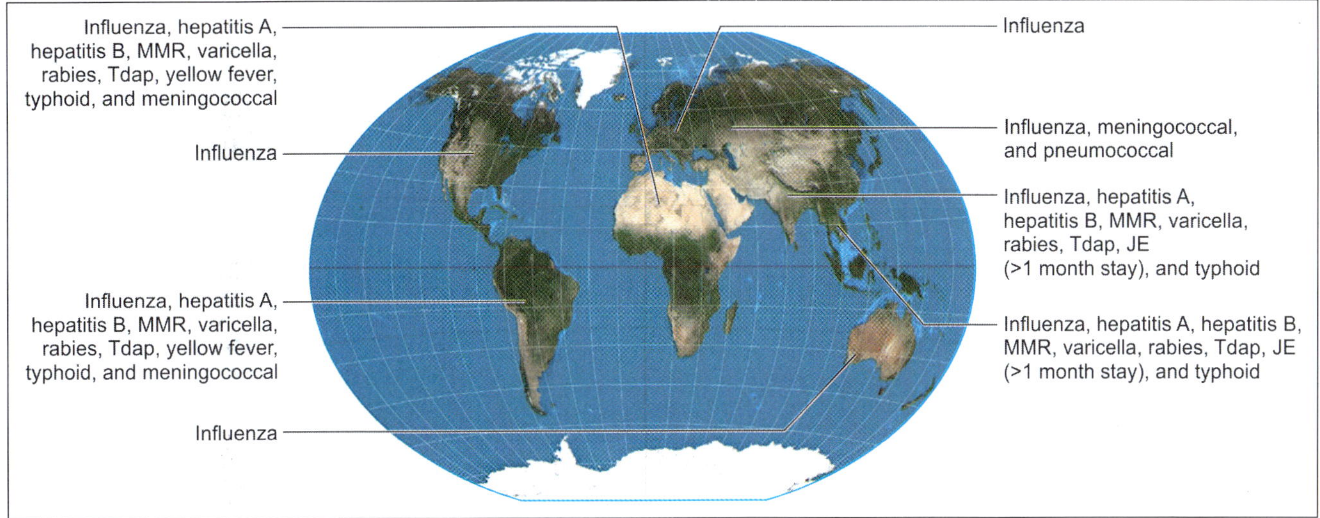

(JE: Japanese encephalitis; MMR: measles, mumps, and rubella; Tdap: tetanus, diphtheria and pertussis)

FIGURE 3: Destination travel vaccine recommendations.

TABLE 6 Healthcare worker vaccination.	
Vaccine	**Recommendations in brief**
Hepatitis B	If no documented evidence of a complete HepB vaccine series, or no serologic evidence of immunity or prior vaccination then give A 3-dose series (dose #1 now, #2 in 1 month, #3 approximately 5 months after #2) intramuscular Anti-HBs serologic test 1-2 months after the final dose, if antibody level (anti HBS) >10 IU, no further booster dose recommended
Influenza	Give 1 dose of influenza vaccine annually. Give inactivated injectable vaccine intramuscularly or live attenuated influenza vaccine (LAIV) intranasally
MMR	If no documented history of vaccination or serological evidence of immunity, give 2 doses of MMR , 4 weeks apart. Give SC
Varicella (chickenpox)	For HCP who have no serologic proof of immunity, prior vaccination, or history of varicella disease, give 2 doses of varicella vaccine, 4 weeks apart. Give SC
Tetanus, diphtheria, pertussis	Give a dose of Tdap as soon as feasible to all HCP who have not received Tdap previously and to pregnant HCP with each pregnancy. Give Td boosters every 10 years thereafter. Give IM
Meningococcal	Give 1 dose to microbiologists who are routinely exposed to isolates of *N. meningitidis* and boost every 5 years if risk continues. Give MCV4 IM; if necessary to use MPSV4, give SC

(HCP: healthcare personnel; IM: intramuscular; MCV4: meningococcal conjugate vaccine-4; MMR: measles, mumps, and rubella; MPSV4: meningococcal polysaccharide vaccine-4; SC: subcutaneous; Td: tetanus and diphtheria; Tdap: tetanus, diphtheria and pertussis)

immunosuppressive and these patients can receive the vaccine. Live vaccines, especially zoster vaccine, should not be used or used with high caution when we are considering biologic therapy or tofacitinib. Influenza and pneumococcal vaccine may be given at the same visit at two different sites. Rituximab therapy and abatacept lead to significantly decreased responses.

When long-term immunosuppressive medications such as high-dose corticosteroids, azathioprine or cyclophosphamide, and biologicals are contemplated vaccines should be given before the initiation of therapy. Indicated vaccines include influenza, pneumococcal, and hepatitis B.

VACCINES FOR COVID-19

For any pandemic to be controlled, the infection needs to have a diagnostic test, absence of animal reservoirs, and the availability of a vaccine. These three prerequisites are present for COVID-19. Some vaccines have been licensed and a few more are in the pipeline. At present these vaccines are only licensed for adults. For the first time, mRNA platform has been introduced for COVID vaccines. Several other technologies have been utilized for vaccine production. They have all been proved to be very safe and significantly effective (**Fig. 4**).

Strategy	Company	Reported efficacy[1]	Storage	Number of doses
Messenger RNA	Moderna	94%	–20°C, 4°C (1 month)	2 4 weeks apart
	BioNTech/Pfizer	95%	–70°C	2 3 weeks apart
	Curevac	Phase 3 ongoing	4°C	2 4 weeks apart
DNA	AnGes-Osaka University	Phase 3 ongoing	Room temperature	2 2 weeks apart
	Zydus Cadila	Phase 3 ongoing	Room temperature	3 4 weeks apart
Viral vector	AstraZeneca/ Oxford (ChAd)	70% (up to 90%?)	4°C	2 4–12 weeks apart
	Gamaleya Institute Sputnik (Ad5, Ad26)	91.4%	4°C	2 3 weeks apart
	CanSinoBio (Ad5)	Phase 3 ongoing	4°C	1
	Johnson & Johnson Janssen (Ad26)	66%[3]	4°C	1
Protein	Novavax	89.3%[2,4]	4°C	2 3 weeks apart
	Medicago	Phase 3 ongoing	4°C	2 3 weeks apart
Inactivated virus	Sinopharm	79%[2]	4°C	2 3 weeks apart
	Sinovac Biotech	Phase 3 ongoing	4°C	2 2 weeks apart
	Bharat Biotech	81%[5]	2–8°C	2 4 weeks apart

[1] Efficacy in preventing symptomatic cases in the vaccine group as compared to the placebo group.
[2] The results haven't been published yet.
[3] 57% efficacy for the South Africa variant, and 85% protection against severe disease.
[4] 95.6% efficacy for the original variant, 85.6% versus the British variant and 60% versus the South African.
[5] Interim results not yet published.

FIGURE 4: Salient features of currently available COVID-19 vaccines.

Soruce: Coronavirus vaccine tracker. New Your Times/European Comission. Coronavirus vaccines strategy as updated on March 2021.

SETTING UP AN ADULT VACCINE CLINIC

Even though there have been marked improvements in immunization rates in adults in the last few years in India, uptake of vaccines in adults is suboptimal. Barriers to immunization of adults include:

- Missed opportunities during contacts with healthcare providers in offices, outpatient clinics, and hospitals.
- Lack of vaccine delivery systems and access to adult vaccines in the public and private sectors that can reach adults in different settings (e.g., the workplace).
- Patient and provider fears about adverse events following vaccination.
- Provider concerns about efficacy of individual vaccines.

The following are the requisites for setting up an Adult Vaccine Clinic:

- Commitment by institutional leadership
- *Infrastructural requirements*: Located for easy access including the disabled. Should have dedicated space for vaccine storage, examination, and vaccine administration room and space for records maintenance. A sink is warranted.
- *Equipment*: Refrigerator for vaccines, cabinet for records maintenance, medical equipment for emergency response, vaccine administration, telephones, and stationary.
- *Staff requirements*: Clinic manager or coordinator, vaccine nurse, receptionist or secretary, and doctor.
- Standard operating procedure and workflow protocols to ensure cold chain is maintained from the time the vaccine leaves the warehouse till it is received and stored in the clinic.

Healthcare providers who administer vaccines should follow vaccine directives, maintain records, and report adverse events.

It is also vital to maintain permanent immunization records that include:

- The type of vaccine and dose
- The site and route of administration
- The date that the vaccine was administered
- The date that the next dose is due
- The manufacturer and lot number
- The name, address, and title of the person administering the vaccine
- Any adverse events

CONCLUSION

Adult vaccination is still a neglected field in most developing countries including India. The potential impact it can have in reducing VPDs, improving quality of life and its impact on antimicrobial resistance cannot be understated. Understanding the principles and indications of adult vaccines and ensuring access to the community should be encouraged. All physicians should actively offer appropriate vaccines to all adults.

RECOMMENDED READINGS

1. Centers for Disease Control and Prevention. (2013). ACIP Vaccine Recommendations and Guidelines. [online] Available from www.cdc.gov/vaccines/hcp/acip-recs/index.html.
2. Centers for Disease Control and Prevention. (2020). General Best Practice Guidelines for Immunization. [online] Available from www.cdc.gov/vaccines/hcp/acip-recs/general-recs/index.html.
3. Centers for Disease Control and Prevention. (2020). Vaccine Information Statements (VISs). [online] Available from www.cdc.gov/vaccines/hcp/vis/index.html.
4. Centers for Disease Control and Prevention. (2014). Manual for the Surveillance of Vaccine-Preventable Diseases. [online] Available from www.cdc.gov/vaccines/pubs/surv-manual.
5. Centers for Disease Control and Prevention. Travelers' Health. [online] Available from www.cdc.gov/travel.
6. Centers for Disease Control and Prevention. Immunization of Health-Care Personnel Recommendations of the Advisory Committee on Immunization Practices (ACIP). Morb Mortal Wkly Rep. 2011;60:1-45.
7. Muruganathan A, Guha S, Munjal YP, Agarwal SS, Parikh KK, Jha V, et al. Recommendations for Vaccination Against Seasonal Influenza in Adult High Risk Groups: South Asian Recommendations. J Assoc Physicians India. 2016;64(7 Suppl):3-11.
8. Expert Group of the Association of Physicians of India on Adult Immunization in India. The Association of Physicians of India evidence-based clinical practice guidelines on adult immunization. J Assoc Physicians India. 2009;57:345-56.
9. Guidelines for vaccination in normal adults in India. Indian J Nephrol. 2016;26(Suppl 1):S7-14.

CHAPTER 40

Infections Caused by Gram-positive Cocci: *Streptococcus, Pneumococcus*, and *Enterococcus*

Bipanchi Mahanta, Anup Kumar Das

ABSTRACT

Gram-positive bacterial infections in healthcare are becoming increasingly common both in the community and in the hospitals including intensive care units (ICUs). Ours being a highly populous tropical nation, a huge number of antibiotics are consumed rampantly. In the last two to three decades, a growing menace is the emergence of gram-positive infections (GPIs) particularly in ICUs as well as drug resistance. Proper identification of these infections is mandatory with close microbiological assistance because they cause a multitude of infections ranging from soft tissue infections to life-threatening ones. Choosing an appropriate antibiotic is crucial to reduce healthcare cost keeping in mind the rapid growth of resistant organisms in our country coupled with unavailability of novel antibiotics, as well as administrative interventions of regulatory bodies.

In India, gram-positive infections are presently a significant public health concern. They cause a wide variety of infections in multiple organ system, some are life-threatening. Infections by multidrug-resistant gram-positive bacteria are rapidly rising and are associated with high mortality and healthcare costs. Options for treating GPIs are shrinking owing to indiscriminate use of high-end antibiotics and lack of antibiotic stewardship programs. Several novel antimicrobial agents are on the pipeline, but alternate therapies to complement traditional treatment regimens needed.

"Give one well-trained physician of the highest type and he will do better work for a thousand people than ten specialists"

—William James Mayo

INTRODUCTION

The Global Burden of Diseases Study reported that although the mortality due to infections has decreased in the last 30 years, they still remain an important cause of mortality and morbidity. In India, too, infections remain an important health issue. In the last century, the infectious diseases in India were mainly parasitic (malaria and leishmaniasis), viral (measles, poliomyelitis, and others), or bacterial and were mostly confined to children and young age groups. Subsequently, control of viral and parasitic diseases has led to emergence of serious bacterial infections at all age groups, especially in middle-aged and the elderly patients.

Classification, nomenclature, and identification of organisms (*taxonomy*) play a crucial role in providing accurate and timely diagnosis of infectious disease in clinical medicine. Although a large variety of methods are used to establish the identity of these microorganisms—usually two broad categories of such methods are used. These methods establish the genotypic characteristics (genetic makeup) and more elaborate phenotypic characteristics (beyond genetic level). Some benefits of taxonomy and identification of organisms are depicted in **Box 1**. Basically, clinically important bacteria are identified by their varying shape, size, and composition plus structure of the cell wall. The cell wall is a most important constituent of the organism with several implications in clinical therapeutics and prognosis of diseases caused by the organisms. They may occur singly, in groups, in pairs, and with varying shapes—circular (cocci) or rod-shaped (bacilli). The cell wall differences differentiate them further into gram-positive or gram-negative bacteria, which demonstrate gross color difference (deep-blue/purple vs. pink/red, respectively) by a basic staining technique called Gram stain, developed in 1884 by Danish bacteriologist Hans Christian Gram. The bacterial cell is made up of mucin, peptidoglycan, and mucopeptides, which are responsible for its rigidity.

BOX 1	Importance of identifying an organism in clinical medicine.
• Establishing association with a disease/diseases	
• Treatment and its outcome associated with specific organisms	
• Epidemiological data	
• During outbreaks and track them	
• Gain knowledge about antibiotic resistance, their pattern, and mechanisms of resistance	
• Recognition of new or emerging organisms	
• Shift in disease patterns associated with specific pathogens	
• Updating taxonomies and thereby evolving methods and knowledge to develop new therapies and strategies to overcome resistance	

The gram-negative cell wall structure is more complex than the gram-positive cell wall (**Fig. 1**). Features of gram-positive bacteria which distinguish them from other bacteria are shown in **Box 2**. Classically, six gram-positive genera are typically pathogenic in humans. Two of these, *Streptococcus* and *Staphylococcus*, are cocci. The remaining are bacilli. Gram-positive bacteria are known to cause several infections which may be life-threatening if not treated and managed properly on time (**Table 1**).

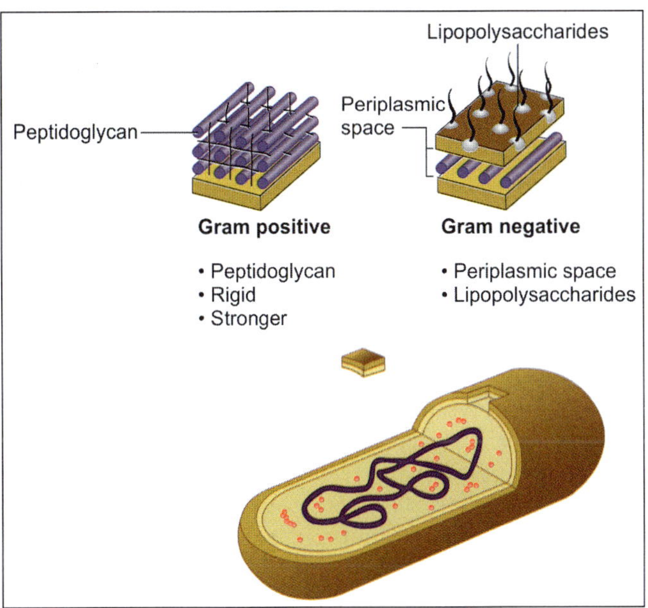

FIGURE 1: Simplified differences in cell wall structure between gram-positive and gram-negative bacteria.

BOX 2	Characteristic features of gram-positive bacteria.

- Absence of an outer membrane
- They have a thin layer of the cytoplasmic lipid layer
- They have a thick peptidoglycan layer
- The peptidoglycan layer has a large quantity of teichoic acid and a thin lipid layer, made up of lipoteichoic acid which plays a major role in bacterial adherence
- The peptidoglycan layer plays a key role in maintaining the rigidity of the cell wall by cross-linking by the assistance of the DD-transpeptidase
- They also have a thin layer of periplasm, as compared to that in the gram-negative bacteria
- Some have a locomotive apparatus, a flagellum that has two basal bodies for support unlike gram-negative which has four basal bodies
- Some have a strong capsule made up of polysaccharides

TABLE 1 Diseases caused by gram-positive bacteria.

Bacterial agent	Diseases
Staphylococcus aureus	Localized and deep skin infections (furuncles, carbuncles, wound infection, cellulitis, and impetigo), pneumonia, endocarditis and septicemia, and musculoskeletal infections such as osteomyelitis and arthritis
Streptococcus pyogenes	Acute pharyngitis or pharyngotonsillitis, impetigo, erysipelas, puerperal sepsis, invasive group A streptococcal disease (necrotizing fasciitis/myositis), streptococcal toxic shock syndrome, acute rheumatic fever, and acute glomerulonephritis
Streptococcus pneumoniae	Community-acquired acute bacterial pneumonia, adult bacterial meningitis, otitis media in children, bacteremia/sepsis, and meningitis
Bacillus anthracis	• Anthrax disease of the pulmonary system (Woolsorter's disease), sepsis which spreads to the gastrointestinal tract causing bowel ulceration and hemorrhagic meningitis • The anthrax disease of the cutaneous layer with pruritic papule lesions and edema, lymphadenopathy, lymphangitis, systemic symptoms of fever, malaise, and headache
Corynebacterium diphtheriae	• Diphtheria, cardiac conduction defects and myocarditis, congestive heart failure, cranial nerve neuritis, and paralysis • Cutaneous diphtheria in wounded or cut skin causing chronic ulcerated nonhealing wounds
Clostridium botulinum	Botulism, visual disturbances (incoordination of eye muscles and diplopia), dysphagia, dysarthria; bulbar paralysis, respiratory paralysis, and cardiac arrest may lead to death
Clostridium tetani	Tetanus
Clostridium difficile	Pseudomembranous colitis
Enterococcus faecium and Enterococcus faecalis	Rarely in healthy persons. Mostly in immune-compromised individuals with wounds and attached devices (respirators, catheters) causing urinary tract infections, bacteremia/sepsis, endocarditis, biliary tract infection, or intra-abdominal abscesses
Listeria monocytogenes	• Listeriosis associated with septicemia and meningitis • Focal and granulomatous skin lesions An asymptomatic vaginal disease spreads to newborns causing flu-like illness and meningitis in the newborn

STREPTOCOCCAL INFECTION

Streptococcal infections in human are caused by a group of gram-positive, nonmotile, nonsporing, catalase negative, facultative anaerobes, nutritionally fastidious, requiring blood or serum for growth—consisting mainly *S. pyogenes, S. agalactiae, S. dysgalactiae* subspecies *equisimilis, S. mitis* group, *S. anginosus* species group, *S. bovis* species group, *S. mutans* species group, *S. salivarius* species group, *S. pneumoniae*, and *Enterococcus.*

STREPTOCOCCUS PYOGENES

Group A (β-hemolytic) *Streptococcus* (GAS) (*S. pyogenes*), commonly causes acute pharyngitis and a variety of cutaneous and systemic infections. Its unique significance stems out from its ability to cause two important nonsuppurative sequelae, namely acute rheumatic fever (ARF) and poststreptococcal glomerulonephritis (PSGN).

Lancefield's classification of β-hemolytic into distinct serogroups in 1933 helped in understanding the epidemiology of streptococcal infections. Most pathogenic strains belong to group A *S. pyogenes.*

Characteristics of *S. pyogenes* are depicted in **Table 2**.

Virulence factors: There are two major groups of virulence factors with (1) somatic components and (2) extracellular/secretory components. The M protein is a major virulence factor that is heat and acid stable. More than 150 serotypes and/or genotypes exist according to antigenic differences. Acquired immunity is based on antibodies against a filamentous macromolecule which is the stable dimer (M protein). In nonimmune hosts, M protein causes antiphagocytosis by inhibiting the activation of alternate complement pathway.

All virulence factors basically act via multiple mechanisms. They retard phagocytosis by polymorphonuclear neutrophils (PMNs) and macrophages, help in adhering to human epithelial surfaces for colonization/attachment by the bacterium, lysis of human fibrin clot by activating plasminogen to facilitate spread of infections, liquefy thick pus thereby causing spread of infection through tissue planes, (cellulitis and necrotizing fasciitis), act as a superantigen-releasing inflammatory cytotoxins causing fever, shock, and tissue damage leading to *Streptococcal toxic shock syndrome* and by leukotoxicity.

Streptolysin O: It is an oxygen labile protein which affects erythrocytes and is toxic to platelets and PMNs. Since it is produced by almost all the strains of *S. pyogenes*, anti-streptolysin O antibodies are an indicator for diagnosing streptococcal infections.

Pathogenicity and clinical features:

Suppurative infections:

Respiratory:
- *Streptococcal sore throat/pharyngitis*: It is the most common bacterial infections caused by GAS, usually affecting children between 5 and 15 years of age (carriage rates up to 15–20%). They adhere to the pharyngeal epithelial cells by fimbriae/pili. Clinical features are summarized in **Table 2**.
- *Scarlet fever*: It is associated with rashes from the second day (upper part of the chest, spreading to the neck, extremities, and other parts). Face, palms, and soles are usually spared. Skinfolds in neck, axilla, groin, and knee appear as red lines called *Pastia's lines.*
- *Clinically*:
  - Scattered petechiae (Rumpel–Leede test of capillary fragility positive)
  - Sand paper skin texture (occlusion of sweat glands) is diagnostic
  - Facial flushing with circumoral pallor

TABLE 2 Important features of *Streptococcus pyogenes.*

Characteristics	Virulence factors (groups)	Clinical features	Complications
• Gram positive • Nonmotile • Nonsporing • Catalase negative • Facultative anaerobes • Nutritionally fastidious, requiring blood or serum for growth	• *Somatic components*: ◦ Hyaluronic acid capsule ◦ Peptidoglycan and teichoic acid ◦ M protein ◦ Adhesion proteins (streptococcal heme-associated protein) ◦ Serum opacity factor ◦ Hair like pili (fimbriae) • *Extracellular/Secretory components*: ◦ Hemolysins – Streptolysin O – Streptolysin S ◦ Pyrogenic exotoxin (erythrogenic, Dick, scarlatinal toxin ◦ Streptokinase ◦ Deoxyribonuclease ◦ NADases ◦ Hyaluronidase ◦ C5a peptidase	• *Usual incubation period*: 2–4 days • *Symptoms*: Starts abruptly with malaise, feverishness, headache, nausea and vomiting and pain abdomen • *Signs*: ◦ Redness, edema and lymphoid hyperplasia of posterior pharynx, enlarged hyperemic tonsils, patchy tonsillopharyngeal exudates, enlarged tender lymph nodes at the angle of mandible ◦ In infants, rhinorrhea, low grade fever, and more protracted course maybe seen. In absence of suppurative complications, fever subsides in 3–5 days	• Otitis media • Quinsy • Ludwig's angina • Adenitis • Peritonsillar cellulitis • Abscess • Retropharyngeal abscess • Cervical lymphadenitis • Mastoiditis • Acute sinusitis • Rarely, pneumonia, meningitis, intracranial brain abscess and thrombosis of intracranial venous sinuses

- Small palatal hemorrhagic spots
- Coated tongue, but extensive desquamation follows for weeks
- Severe form presents with septicemia and toxemia often complicated with jaundice and rarely, hydrops of gallbladder

- *Dermatological infections*:
  - *Streptococcal pyoderma/impetigo*: Begins as a papule in the exposed areas (lower extremities and face), rapidly evolving to vesicles surrounded by erythema, pustule which breaks in 4–6 days to form thick crust. It heals as a depigmented area (*ecthyma)*.
- *Erysipelas*: It is common in extremes of age groups causing superficial cutaneous dermatitis and lymphangitis begins as a localized erythematous lesion (brilliant salmon red) with advancing well-demarcated red margins. It involves the facial malar regions (butterfly appearance) and also the lower extremities.
- *Cellulitis*: Acute skin and subcutaneous inflammation, usually following burns and wounds. It causes local inflammation. Systemic manifestations include fever, chills, and malaise (in contrast to erysipelas), lesion is flat, less demarcated and more erythematous.
- *Necrotizing/gangrenous fasciitis*: Infection of deeper subcutaneous tissue and fascia (rapidly spreads leading to gangrene). Starting as mild erythema, rapidly evolves to dusky/purplish skin bullae containing yellow/hemorrhagic fluid. By 4th to 5th day, frank gangrene develops, followed by extensive sloughing. *Fournier gangrene* is a type of gangrenous fasciitis. Occurs frequently in diabetic patients.
- *Myositis and myonecrosis*: Clinically resembles necrotizing fasciitis.
- *Toxic shock syndrome* (**Table 3**): Clinically, it begins with influenza-like presentation for 1–2 days. Later, they might develop necrotizing fasciitis or myonecrosis (second phase) with tachycardia, tachypnea, and persistent fever. In patients with necrotizing fasciitis or myonecrosis increasing severe pain at the site of infection occurs. In the third phase, they develop shock and multiorgan failure.

Nonsuppurative poststreptococcal sequelae:

Acute rheumatic fever:

Etiopathogenesis: ARF can follow untreated GAS (strains 1, 3, 5, 6, 14, 18, 19, and 24) pharyngitis in individuals who may be genetically susceptible to a delayed nonsuppurative squeal. It is common in school going children in developing countries.

This condition is rare in streptococcal skin infection. This indicates the requirement of the rich lymphoid tissue in pharyngeal site or a lack of rheumatogenicity among the pyoderma strains of GAS. Several theories have been implicated in causing ARF. Streptolysin S or O both can cause tissue injury.

Pathology: Initially, fragmentation of collagen fibers, lymphocytic infiltration, fibrinoid deposition occurs, followed by appearance of characteristic myocardial Aschoff nodules (perivascular focus of inflammation with an area of central necrosis surrounded by rosette of large mononuclear and giant multicellular cells with an owl eyed or a caterpillar/serrated nucleus called "Anichkov monocytes"), leading to pancarditis. A thickened rough area frequently seen in the left atrium or mitral valve called *MacCallum patch*. Valvular lesions show leaflets and chordae having small verrucae, with subsequent thickening of valves, shortened chordae, fused valve commissures, and stenosis as healing occurs. Joint lesions are characterized by fibrinous exudate and serous effusion without residual joint damage (**Table 3**).

TABLE 3 Features and tissue injuries in ARF and toxic shock syndrome.

Clinical manifestations	Modes of tissue injury	Modes of tissue injury
ARF and toxic shock syndrome	**ARF**	**Toxic shock syndrome**
ARF: Major manifestations: • Polyarthritis/fleeting joint pain (75%) • Carditis (40–50%) • Chorea (15%) • Subcutaneous nodules (3–5%) • Erythema marginatum (3–5%) Minor manifestations: Fever, arthralgia, leukocytosis, raised ESR and CRP **Toxic shock syndrome:** Sudden onset shock and organ failure occurring in extremes of age groups usually with comorbidities. Organisms may invade deeper tissue or blood stream during surgery or invasive procedures or any condition causing breach of barrier	• Antigen antibody complexes localized to tissue injury • Serum sickness like reaction • Autoimmune phenomenon (antibody to collagen), inflammation in the subendothelial matrix and perivascular connective tissue • Anticardiac antibodies (M protein shares antigenic determinants with cardiogenic myosin, sarcolemma membrane protein, synovial, and articular cartilages) • During active rheumatic carditis, CD4 cells and CD4: CD8 cells are increased in heart valves/peripheral blood • Enhanced IL-1 and -2 production (M protein and pyrogenic exotoxins can act as superantigens)	• Pyrogenic exotoxins act as super antigens, cause fever, enhance susceptibility to endotoxins and suppress IgM synthesis, resulting in TNF-α, IL-1β and IL-6 secretion (proinflammatory cytokine). Fragments of M protein and SSA also act as superantigens • Noncytokine-mediated shock syndrome might occur due to cysteine proteases produced by group A *Streptococcus* that releases bradykinin, causing vasodilatory shock

(ARF: acute rheumatic fever; CRP: C-reactive protein; ESR: erythrocyte sedimentation rate; IgM: immunoglobulin M; IL: interleukin; SSA: streptococcal superantigen; TNF-α: tumor necrosis factor)

TABLE 4 Diagnostic procedures for Streptococcal infection.

Specimen	Microscopy	Rapid diagnostic test kits	Serology	Typing	Bacitracin sensitivity
Throat swab, pus swab, exudates, and serum for post-streptococcal nonsuppurative infections	Presumptive diagnosis by detection of gram-positive cocci in chains seen on direct smears	To detect streptococcal group A antigen from throat swabs	Detection of ASO titer higher than 200 Todd unit is indicates prior streptococcal infection. High levels are usually found in ARF (low titer in PSGN). Conversely, anti-DNAase B and antihyaluronidase tests are reliable in detection of streptococcal pyoderma	MTR protein-based typing done for epidemiological typing	Using bacitracin disk

(ARF: acute rheumatic fever; ASO: antistreptolysin O; MTR: methionine synthase; PSGN: poststreptococcal glomerulonephritis)

TABLE 5 Drugs used for prevention of ARF.

Agent	Dosage	Route	Duration
Penicillin V	Children <27 kg—250 mg Children >27 kg—500 mg	Oral	Two to three times/day for 10 days
Amoxicillin	50 mg/kg	Oral	Once daily for 10 days
Benzathine penicillin	Children <27 kg—60,000 U Children >27 kg—1.2 million U	IM	Once
For individuals allergic to penicillin			
Cephalosporins	Variable	Oral	10 days
Clindamycin	20 mg/kg/day divided in three doses	Oral	
Azithromycin	12 mg/kg	Oral	Once daily for 5 days
Clarithromycin	15 mg/kg in divided doses	Oral	Twice daily for 10 days

(ARF: acute rheumatic fever; IM: intramuscular)

Poststreptococcal glomerulonephritis: PSGN causing glomerulonephritis (edema, hypertension, hematuria, and proteinuria) is a delayed sequelae of pharyngeal or cutaneous infection with nephritogenic strains of GAS (pyoderma associated—2, 49, 53-55, 57, and 59-61, and pharyngitis associated—1, 4, 12, and 25). In the tropics, skin infections are more relevant in development of PSGN.

Pathogenesis: Possibly due to antigenic cross-reactions between glomerular membrane and cell membranes of GAS, or immune complex deposition.

DIAGNOSIS OF STREPTOCOCCAL INFECTION

Diagnosis of streptococcal infection is by demonstration of antibodies (nonsuppurative infections) or the organism (suppurative infections). Different streptococcal diseases are diagnosed differently (**Table 4**).

TREATMENT

Usually, penicillin or amoxicillin is given by mouth for 10 days in sore throat. One injection of long-acting penicillin (benzathine) can be given instead. People who cannot take penicillin can be given erythromycin, clarithromycin, or clindamycin by mouth for 10 days or azithromycin for 5 days. Cellulitis is often treated without doing a culture. In this situation, we can use antibiotics that are effective against both streptococci and staphylococci (such as dicloxacillin or cephalexin). Serious streptococcal infections (necrotizing fasciitis, endocarditis, and severe cellulitis) require penicillin, given intravenously, sometimes with other antibiotics plus surgical intervention. Invasive GAS needs aggressive treatment.

Duration of therapy is dependent upon the following factors in general for any infection:

- The etiology of infection (the pathogen)
- The severity of infections (e.g., cystitis vs. meningitis)
- The pharmacokinetic/dynamics of the antibiotic
- Host factors (immunocompetency and neutropenia)
- Severity of host inflammatory response as measured by a biomarker, e.g., serum procalcitonin

PREVENTION

Only indication is for prevention of ARF. Any one of following drug dosage schedule is recommended (**Table 5**). Other disease causing streptococcal isolates and their clinico-microbiological characteristics are shown in **Table 6**.

STREPTOCOCCUS PNEUMONIAE (PNEUMOCOCCUS)

It is a leading cause of pneumonia and bacterial meningitis in children <2 years of age. Without any apparent foci of infection, diagnosed by positive blood cultures, (referred to as *"primary bacteremia"*). Globally, 189,937 deaths were attributed to the pneumococcus.

Characteristics, virulence factors, and mechanism of virulence in pneumococci are shown in **Table 7** and

TABLE 6 Other Streptococci commonly isolated from human infection.

Species	Lancefield antigen(s)	Hemolytic reaction(s)	Clinical manifestations
Streptococcus agalactiae	B	B and γ	Pyogenic, cause chorioamnionitis, puerperal sepsis, neonatal sepsis, meningitis
Streptococcus dysgalactiae subspecies equisimilis	C and G	B	Pyogenic, cause respiratory infections, cellulitis and septicemia
Streptococcus mitis group	Not detectable	A	Cause subacute bacterial endocarditis
Streptococcus anginosus species group	A, C, F, and G	α, β, and γ	Pyogenic
Streptococcus bovis species group	D	A and γ	Causes endocarditis
Streptococcus mutans species group	Not useful for differentiation	α, β, and γ	Dental caries and endocarditis
Streptococcus salivarius species group	Not useful for differentiation	A and γ	Infrequent opportunistic infections in immunocompromised hosts

TABLE 7 Virulence factors in pneumococci and mechanism of virulence.

Pneumococcal constituent	Mechanism of virulence
Capsular polysaccharide	Prevents phagocytosis and activate complement
Cell wall polysaccharide	Stimulates inflammation through strong complement activation and cytokine release
Pneumolysin	Primary pore forming toxin that causes both epithelial and endothelial damage, activates complement and cytokines
PspA	Inhibit phagocytosis—blocks activation and deposition of complement
PspC	Inhibit phagocytosis—binds factor H
PsaA	Mediates adherence
Autolysin	Causes bacterial disintegration
Neuraminidase	Supports adherence

TABLE 8 Some characteristics of pneumococci.

Epidemiology	Characteristics	Risk factors	Clinical features
• Causes more morbidity and mortality in LRTIs compared to all other organisms combined (*Haemophilus influenzae*, respiratory syncytial virus) • Risk groups <5 years and > 65 years	• Gram positive, capsulated, α-hemolytic, lanceolate diplococci, catalase negative, bile soluble and optochin sensitive with > 92 serotypes identified by capsular typing • Spreads by droplet infection • Seasonal variability, especially common in winters and cold seasons	Extremes of age, immunocompromised states, malignancies, chronic lung disease, infection with high virulence strain, superadded respiratory viral infection (by quorum sensing it can transfer genetic material from one strain to the other by horizontal gene transfer mechanisms)	Otitis media, sinusitis, lower respiratory tract infections (trachea, bronchi, and lungs), empyema by direct extension. Pneumococcal bacteremia leading to distant infections (heart, peritoneum, and joints). Commonly endogenous, but exogenous infection can occur, with highly virulent strains

(LRTIs: lower respiratory tract infections)

epidemiology and clinical features in **Table 8**. The sequence of pathogenesis is shown in **Table 9**.

COLONIZATION

Most pneumococcal symptomatic infections follow a period of asymptomatic colonization that usually begins by 1 year of age.

POSTCOLONIZATION PROGRESSION

Some strains behave as colonizers and while others progress to invasive diseases. Colonizing strains are cleared by alveolar macrophages and by complement in blood vessels and lung, resulting in lower incidence of invasive disease. Less common colonizers are invasive and are resistant to killing by macrophages and complement. Hence, knowledge of locally prevalent strains is important in preparation of region-specific cocktail vaccine strains.

HOST DEFENSE MECHANISM

Interplay of host complement system, preexisting antibodies, and phagocytic activity are vital after initial colonization.

TABLE 9 Sequence of events leading to pneumonia by pneumococcal infection.

Sequence	Pathology
Colonization	Symptoms follows a period of asymptomatic colonization (begins in the 1st week of life, peaks to 70–100% by 1 year of age, persist through 2nd and 3rd years, then gradually declines). Additionally, local inflammation caused by rhino or influenza viruses helps migration of bacterial cells in epithelium and endothelium
Progression from colonization	Capsular serotype 6A, 6B, 9N, 19F, and 23F are colonizers and while 14, 5, 1, 7F, 18C, 8, 38, and 33F others progress to invasive diseases colonizing strains resist nonopsonic phagocytosis, but cleared by alveolar macrophages and complement in blood vessels and lung, resulting in lower incidence of invasive disease. Invasive serotypes more resistant to killing by macrophages and complement
Host defense mechanism	Anticapsular antibodies appear after 5–8 days of infection and fever spontaneously resolves
Pneumonia	Lobar and bronchopneumonia if disease progresses pneumococci activates complement, generates cytokine production and upregulate receptors on vascular endothelium

TABLE 10 Treatment plan for pneumococcal infections.

Invasive pneumococcal disease	Noninvasive pneumococcal disease
Lobar/bronchopneumonia, meningitis, sepsis, bacteremia, osteomyelitis, and septic arthritis	Acute bronchitis, sinusitis, and otitis media
Broad-spectrum antibiotics, including IV, are prescribed before culture sensitivity is received to stop spread of infection and cause complications. May require hospital stay and sometimes ICU care	May not need treatment, but antibiotics are prescribed to prevent complication in most cases. Community-acquired respiratory tract infections may not need hospitalization
Penicillin and quinolone-resistant pneumococcal pneumonia is increasing	
• Surgical or other speciality consultations may be necessary in certain invasive pneumococcal infections	
• Local antibiogram important	

PNEUMONIA

Streptococcus pneumoniae are the major cause of lobar and bronchopneumonia. In presence of *predisposing factors* (e.g., superadded viral infections, compromised respiratory tract clearance disorders, chilling, anesthesia etc.), the bacteria multiplies, penetrates the bronchial mucosa, and spreads into the lung along the peribronchial tissues and lymphatics. Toxemia follows diffusion of the capsular polysaccharide into blood and tissues. Bronchopneumonia is almost always a secondary infection, and also commonly associated with chronic bronchitis where the copious respiratory secretions aid in pneumococcal invasion.

Meningitis is the most serious infection that occurs usually secondary to other pneumococcal infections.

TREATMENT

The basic principles of therapy are given in **Table 10**.

- Prompt diagnosis and antibiotic administration
- Continuation of treatment at least till host completes the healing process
- Drainage of infection in closed spaces

Drugs and challenges in treatment: Local antibiogram is the mainstay of treatment. Multidrug resistance (MDR) in streptococcal infection is rising.

The prevalence of drug-resistant *S. pneumoniae* (DRSP) has been reportedly increasing in India. Macrolide resistance in pneumococci in 2015 in India was 32% (19–47%). In Western countries, resistance is highly prevalent with beta-lactams (penicillins: 13.8–41.8%, cephalosporins <1–29.9%), macrolides (20–40%), clindamycin (21.8%), trimethoprim-sulfamethoxazole (TMP-SMX) (25–45%), and tetracyclines (25.9%), whereas resistance against fluoroquinolones (<1–2%) is low but increasing. The 2007 Infectious Diseases Society of America/American Thoracic Society (IDSA/ATS) guidelines recommend that respiratory fluoroquinolones (moxifloxacin, gemifloxacin, or levofloxacin), or a beta-lactam alone or in combination with a beta-lactamase inhibitor (high-dose amoxicillin or amoxicillin-clavulanate) along with doxycycline are to be used in areas with >25% infection rate with "high-level" macrolide-resistant *S. pneumoniae*. In meningitis, vancomycin or meropenem may be necessary if there is no response to ceftriaxone 2 g bid.

PREVENTION

Prevention of pneumococcal disease outweighs the risks by vaccination (**Table 11**). Vaccination is the mainstay for preventing pneumococcal invasive infections. Currently two strains are approved for vaccination.

1. *Pneumococcal polysaccharide vaccine 23 (PPSV23)*: It consists of capsular material from 23 pneumococcal types. It is recommended for all adults >65 years, independent of any prior vaccination.

TABLE 11 Vaccination for control of pneumococcal infection.

Indications	Recommendation	Types of vaccines
• All immunocompromised adults >19 years age • Functional or anatomic asplenia • Immunocompetent adults with CSF leaks or cochlear implants	• Sequential two-dose regimen with a dose of PCV13 followed by PPSV23 8 weeks later • Primary immunization with three doses of PCV13 at 2–6 months of age or two doses between 7 and 11 months, each receiving a booster dose at 12–15 months of age	• PPSV23: Consists of capsular material from 23 pneumococcal types. It is recommended for all adults >65 years, independent of any prior vaccination • PCV13: Containing polysaccharide material from 13 pneumococcal types, covalently linked to a nontoxic protein

(CSF: cerebrospinal fluid; PCV13: pneumococcal conjugate vaccine 13; PPSV23: pneumococcal polysaccharide vaccine 23)

2. *Pneumococcal conjugate vaccine 13 (PCV13)*: It contains polysaccharide material from 13 pneumococcal types, covalently linked to a nontoxic protein.

ENTEROCOCCUS

ENTEROCOCCUS SPECIES

These gram-positive facultative anaerobic bacteria are commonly oval in shape, but can assume various other patterns (singles, pairs, short chains, or long chains). They are grouped under group D *Streptococcus*.

Clinically, two species are more important: *Enterococcus faecium* and *Enterococcus faecalis*. Besides these, other enterococci isolated from human infection are *E. gallinarum, E. durans, E. avium, E. raffinosus, E. pallens, E. gilvus, E. cecorum, E. malodoratus, E. italicus, A. sanguinicola, E. mundtii, E. casseliflavus, E. dispar, E. hirae, and E. pseudoavium.*

They are commensals of the gastrointestinal (GI) tract (~10^{12} bacteria/g of colonic content). They dominate the gut microbiota of hospitalized patients receiving broad-spectrum antibiotics. Enterococci are most important cause of endocarditis and also urinary infection.

Enterococci are naturally resistant to various antibiotics. Consumption of broad-spectrum antibiotics and increase of pH by administration of proton pump inhibitors facilitate their over growth.

PATHOGENESIS

From the gut they enter lymphatics and bloodstream. Virulence factors of enterococci (cytolysin/hemolysin) are capable of lysing eukaryotic or prokaryotic cells. Several surface proteins, pili on surface, and polysaccharides are important pathogenic determinants.

CLINICAL MANIFESTATION (BOX 3)

BOX 3 Enterococcal diseases.

- Bacteremia and endocarditis
- Urinary tract infection
- Meningitis
- Intra-abdominal and pelvic infection
- Neonatal infection
- Skin, soft tissue, and other infection

Bacteremia and endocarditis: Bacteremia without endocarditis is a common hospital-acquired infection. A frequent source is the GI or genitourinary tract, after surgical intervention, intravenous, or indwelling catheter. It can infect both native and prosthetic heart valves. The most common complication of bacterial endocarditis is heart failure and cerebral embolism (mortality rate 11–35%).

Urinary tract infection: Enterococcal urinary tract infection (UTI) is mostly associated with indwelling catheter, instrumentation, and anatomical abnormality of urinary tract. *E. faecium* accounts for the majority. To differentiate UTI from asymptomatic colonization, isolation of a significant bacterial count (>105 cfu/mL) in culture is essential. It is frequently associated with prostatitis and epididymitis in elderly males.

Meningitis: It is uncommon, but occurs as hospital-acquired infection in children undergoing central nervous system (CNS) surgeries. Community-associated spontaneous meningitis occurs in patients with comorbidities such as diabetes, malignancies, and immunosuppressive conditions.

Intra-abdominal and pelvic infections: Being commensals of the GI and genitourinary tract, enterococci can act as endogenous source of abdominal/pelvic infections.

Neonatal infections: Neonates often acquire infection during vaginal delivery from the birth canal. Clinically, they present with localized infection or necrotizing enterocolitis. Outbreaks of neonatal sepsis with *E. faecium* have been documented in premature neonates.

Skin and soft tissue infections: Decubitus ulcers, diabetic foot, and soft tissue abscesses are usually associated with enterococcal infections.

TREATMENT AND CHALLENGES

The main hurdle for treating enterococcal infections is their intrinsic resistance to many antibiotics. Bactericidal therapy is required for optimal cure in endocarditis, which is usually impossible by monotherapy (**Table 12**).

β-lactams plus an aminoglycoside (gentamicin and streptomycin) is the choice of treatment regimen for most enterococcal infections, especially endocarditis. But high-level resistance (HLR) to aminoglycosides, especially gentamicin has been documented since 1983.

TABLE 12 Treatment of non endovascular infections with β-lactam and glycopeptide-sensitive enterococci.

Disease	Suggested antibiotics	Dosage and duration (with normal renal and liver functions)
Bacteremia	Ampicillin or	9–12 g daily IV in divided doses q4–6h for 14 days
	Penicillin G or	18–30 million units IV daily in divided doses q4–6h for 14 days
	Vancomycin	30 mg/kg daily IV in divided doses for 14 days
Meningitis	Ampicillin or	2 g q4h IV for 14 days
	Penicillin G plus	4 million units q4h IV for 14 days
	Gentamicin	2 mg/kg loading dose, followed by 1.7 mg/kg IV q8h
UTI	Nitrofurantoin	100 mg PO q6h for 5 days
	Fosfomycin	3 mg PO single dose
	Amoxicillin	875 mg to 1 g PO q12h for 5 days

Relative resistance to β-lactam antibiotics over 16 times the minimal inhibitory concentration (MIC) has been documented. The most potent activity is observed with aminopenicillins (e.g., ampicillin and ureidopenicillins), penicillin G, and imipenem. Since high doses of ampicillin can achieve plasma concentration of >150 mg/L, this suggests that isolates with ampicillin MIC > 64 mg/L might be successfully treated with doses of 18–30 g/day or in combination with β-lactamase inhibitors like sulbactam.

Most cephalosporin antibiotics are ineffective against enterococcal infections since the first and second generations are intrinsically resistant. But ceftriaxone/cefotaxime with ampicillin is recommended for treatment of endocarditis produced by strains of *E. faecalis* exhibiting HLR to all aminoglycosides. The rationale behind is that low concentration of an aminopenicillin can partially delay bacterial cell wall synthesis. The addition of cefotaxime can produce bacterial cell wall insufficiency, thus producing the bactericidal synergistic effect in *E. faecalis*, but not in *E. faecium*.

The two glycopeptides vancomycin and teicoplanin currently in use inhibit the last steps of peptidoglycan synthesis in bacterial cell wall. Vancomycin-resistant enterococci (VRE) are reportedly in up to 80% strains of *E. faecium*. The mechanism of resistance is an altered peptidoglycan synthesis pathway. The recommended treatment regimen for VRE includes linezolid, high-dose ampicillin, daptomycin, nitrofurantoin, fosfomycin (UTI), doxycycline, chloramphenicol, gentamicin, and streptomycin (combination therapy) (**Flowchart 1**).

During the last decade, 11 antibiotics with main activity against gram-positive microorganisms have received international regulatory approval, i.e., ceftobiprole, ceftaroline, telavancin, oritavancin, dalbavancin, tedizolid, besifloxacin, delafloxacin, ozenoxacin, omadacycline, and lefamulin. Some more are in the pipeline in different phases of clinical trials (**Table 13**). Novel approaches such as antibody use and phage therapy should be examined in the future in conjunction with traditional treatment.

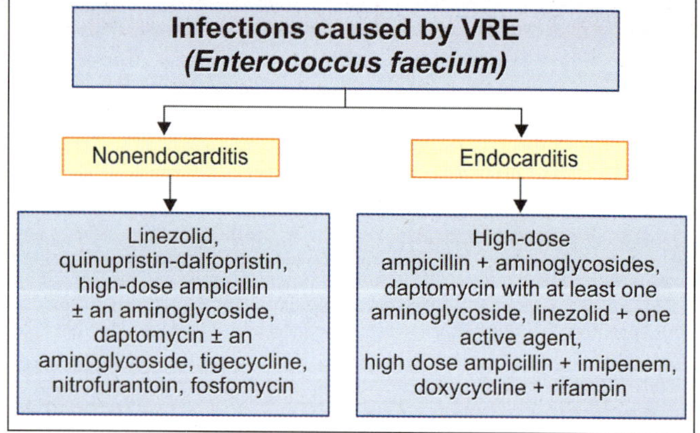

(VRE: vancomycin-resistant enterococci)

FLOWCHART 1: Treatment of endocarditis showing different types of resistance.

Summary of some antibiotics with activity against streptococci with filed or are currently in Phase III and II clinical trials in (New Drug Application category):

- Iclaprim for vancomycin-intermediate and vancomycin-resistant, and macrolide-, quinolone- and trimethoprim-resistant strains
- Cethromycin for ketolide telithromycin-resistant *S. pneumoniae*
- Solithromycin for pneumonia
- Contezolid (MRX-1) for penicillin-resistant and penicillin-intermediate *S. pneumoniae*, and VRE
- Contezolid acefosamil (MRX-4) for VRE
- Lascufloxacin for *E. faecalis*, *S. pyogenes*, *S. agalactiae*, and penicillin-resistant *S. pneumoniae*
- Nemonoxacin (Taigexyn®) for multidrug-resistant *S. pneumoniae* and vancomycin-resistant pathogens
- Zabofloxacin (DW-224a) for *S. pyogenes, E. faecalis*, and *S. pneumoniae*
- Razupenem for penicillin-resistant *S. pneumoniae* and VRE
- Radezolid (RX-1741) for *S. pneumoniae* and enterococci
- Alalevonadifloxacin (WCK2349) for *S. pneumoniae*
- Avarofloxacin (JNJ-Q2 or acorafloxacin) for fluoroquinolone-resistant *S. pneumoniae*

ANTIBIOTIC RESISTANCE IN INDIA

Amongst important GPIs, *Staphylococcus aureus, Streptococcus pneumoniae*, and enterococci are developing resistance (responsible for a global challenges, significant public health burden, and healthcare cost, but nowhere is it as stark as in India), **Table 14**. The overall burden of resistance is hard to assess for the general population but is likely focused on neonates and the elderly (high-risk and vulnerable groups). It is estimated that 58,000 neonatal deaths are attributable to sepsis caused by drug resistance

TABLE 13 Newer antibiotics in the pipeline.

Antibiotic	Class of antibiotic	Spectrum against	Phase of clinical trial
Cethromycin	Ketolide	Telithromycin-resistant *Streptococcus pneumoniae*	III
Contezolid (MRX-1)	Oxazolidinone	Penicillin-resistant and penicillin-intermediate *Streptococcus pneumoniae*, and VRE	III
Contezolid acefosamil (MRX-4)	Oxazolidinone	VRE	III
Lascufloxacin	Fluoroquinolone	*Enterococcus faecalis*, *Streptococcus pyogenes*, *Streptococcus agalactiae*, and penicillin-resistant *Streptococcus pneumoniae*	III
Nemonoxacin (Taigexyn®)	Nonfluorinated quinolone	Multidrug-resistant *Streptococcus pneumoniae* and vancomycin-resistant pathogens	III
Razupenem	Carbapenem	Penicillin-resistant *Streptococcus pneumoniae*, VRE	II
Radezolid (RX-1741)	Oxazolidinone	*Streptococcus pneumoniae* and enterococci	II
Avarofloxacin (JNJ-Q2 or acorafloxacin)	Fluoroquinolone	Fluoroquinolone-resistant *Streptococcus pneumoniae*	II
KBP-7072	Tetracycline	*Streptococcus pneumoniae* strains that exhibit higher minocycline MIC and beta-lactam resistance	I
Teixobactin	Teixobactin	VRE	I
TP-271	Fluorocycline	*Streptococcus pneumoniae* and *Streptococcus pyogenes*	
MGB-BP-3	DNA minor groove binder	*Streptococcus pneumoniae*, VRE	I

(DNA: deoxyribonucleic acid; MIC: minimum inhibitory concentration; VRE: vancomycin-resistant enterococci)

TABLE 14 Few reports of resistance pattern in gram-positive infections (GPIs) in India.

Antibiotic	Resistance over the years	Resistance/Rise in rate
Gentamicin	2008 to 2013	33%
Third-generation cephalosporin		73–83%
Fluoroquinolones		57–73%
Carbapenems	2002 to 2009	2–52%
Vancomycin		11%
Penicillins		4% total resistance + multidrug resistance (MDR), 10% were intermediately resistant

to first-line antibiotics each year. High rates of methicillin-resistant *Staphylococcus aureus* (MRSA) in clinical isolates from various studies in India have been documented, with rates as high as 54.8% (ranging between 32 and 80%) recorded. GPIs, especially MRSA infections, are associated with high mortality rates in India, both in the hospitals and ICUs.

The crude infectious disease mortality rate in India today is 416.75 per 100,000 persons (calculations based on World Bank data and the Global Burden of Disease, 1990) and is twice the rate prevailing in the United States when antibiotics were introduced (roughly 200 per 100,000 persons). However, resistance in 2014 to two older antibiotics—ampicillin, 5% and cotrimoxazole, 4%—is decreasing, possibly because of a decline in consumption of these two drugs.

Multidrug resistance leads to increased mortality and morbidity, ICU admissions, complications, use of multiple antibiotics, and increased overall length of hospital stay.

The main stimulus to the increasing resistance is *injudicious overuse of antibiotics*. Total of 76% of the overall increase in global antibiotic consumption between 2000 and 2010 was attributable to BRICS countries, (Brazil, Russia, India, China, and South Africa). By 2010, India was the world's largest user of antibiotics. Rapid economic growth and rising incomes, availability of over-the-counter (OTC) drugs without improvements in water, sanitation, and public health has a role to play in this antibiotic (mis)use. Infection control in hospitals is poorly monitored and needs improvement. Even in tertiary care Indian hospitals have shown high prevalence of overall healthcare-associated infections in spite of receiving antibiotics. Lack of access to healthcare by a large section of population also increases OTC unprescribed and inappropriate use of antibiotics.

The problem of resistance is exacerbated by *availability of many fixed-dose combinations* i.e., often without scientific or medical rationality or evaluation is also a contributor to resistance development, especially by quacks. Undergraduate and postgraduate teaching should stress upon antibiotic stewardship and principles of infection treatment. Other factors such as discharge of antimicrobial wastes into environment by pharma companies, growing use of antibiotic use in animals/poultries and their consumption, as well as in food products like milk or honey etc., can facilitate increasingly resistant bacterial environment. There are at present no regulatory laws to address these issues in India which have important bearing on bacterial infection, all of which contribute to resistance by gene transfer mechanism.

CONCLUSION

Gram-positive infections are increasing in India, especially in the healthcare and ICU setting. The emerging drug resistance, leading to difficult-to-treat and challenging infections is reaching alarming proportion by vancomycin-intermediate *Staphylococcus aureus* (VISA), vancomycin-resistant *Staphylococcus aureus* (VRSA), VRE, and other multidrug-resistant organisms. Increasing resistance rates to macrolides, fluoroquinolones, beta-lactams, and other antibiotics commonly administered to combat gram-positive bacteria are of great concern.

The prevalence of resistance is bound to increase with increased irrational use of antibiotics. Steps such as restricting usage of antibiotics and antibiotic stewardship programs need to be enforced strictly. But the reasons of such drug resistance is multifactorial and needs policy making at local, regional, national, and international levels. The most important step, however, is the increased push towards research and development (R&D) for development of newer antibiotics against the gram-positive bacteria with novel targets as we have not developed new antibiotics in nearly two decades except linezolid and related oxazolidinones in 2000, and daptomycin and related lipopeptides in 2003.

RECOMMENDED READINGS

1. Laxminarayan R, Chaudhury RR. Antibiotic Resistance in India: Drivers and Opportunities for Action. PLoS Med. 2016;13(3):e1001974.
2. Ghanshani R, Gupta R, Gupta BS, Kalra S, Khedar RS, Sood S. Epidemiological study of prevalence, determinants, and outcomes of infections in medical ICU at a tertiary care hospital in India. Lung India. 2015;32(5):441-8.
3. Van Boeckel TP, Gandra S, Ashok A, Caudron Q, Grenfell BT, Levin SA, et al. Global antibiotic consumption 2000 to 2010: an analysis of national pharmaceutical sales data. Lancet Infect Dis. 2014;14(8):742-50.
4. Bate R, Tren R, Mooney L, Hess K, Mitra B, Debroy B, et al. Pilot Study of Essential Drug Quality in Two Major Cities in India. PLoS ONE. 2009;4(6):e6003.
5. Ghafur A. The Chennai Declaration: a solution to the antimicrobial resistance problem in the Indian subcontinent. Clin Infect Dis. 2013;56(8):1190.
6. Chawla K, Gurung B, Mukhopadhyay C, Bairy I. Reporting emerging resistance of *Streptococcus pneumoniae* from India. J Global Infect Dis. 2010; 2(1):10-4.
7. CDDEP. (20211). Antibiotic Resistance. [online] Available from https://resistancemap.cddep.org/AntibioticResistance.php.
8. Cherazard R, Epstein M, Doan T-L, Salim T, Bharti S, Smith MA. Antimicrobial resistant *Streptococcus pneumoniae*: prevalence, mechanisms, and clinical implications. Am J Ther. 2017;24(3):e361-9.
9. Harnett G. Treatment of community-acquired pneumonia: a case report and current treatment dilemmas. Case Rep Emerg Med. 2017;2017:5045087.
10. Department of Health and Family Welfare. (2016). National Treatment Guidelines for Antimicrobial Use in Infectious Disease, National Centre for Disease Control, Directorate General of Health Services, Ministry of Health and Family Welfare, Government of India, (Version 1.0, 2016). [online] Available from http://pbhealth.gov.in/AMR guideline7001495889.pdf.
11. *Koulenti D, Xu E, Song A, Sum Mok IY, Karageorgopoulos* DE, Armaganidis A, et al. Emerging Treatment Options for Infections by Multidrug-Resistant Gram-Positive Microorganisms. Microorganisms. 2020;8:191.
12. Bennet JE, Raphael D, Blaser MJ. Principles and Practice of Infectious diseases, 8th edition. Philadelphia: Saunders; 2015.

CHAPTER 41

Staphylococcal Diseases

Smarajit Banik, Amit Kumar Adhikari, Indranil Sen

ABSTRACT

Staphylococcus is a genus of gram-positive bacteria in the family Staphylococcaceae. *S. aureus* (nares) and *S. epidermidis* (nares and skin) are common commensals, but also have the greatest pathogenic potential. Surface proteins, enzymes, large polysaccharide capsule, protein A, membrane-damaging toxins, and exotoxins are few of the virulence factors. *S. aureus* causes superficial skin, deep organ infection, and toxin-induced disease such as toxic shock syndrome and food poisoning.

The bacteria become resistant to antibiotic either by not allowing the antibiotic to reach its target at a high enough concentration or modify/bypass the target that the antibiotic acts on. Emergence of antibiotic resistance has led to constant search for newer antibiotics. Identification of methicillin-resistant *S. aureus* (MRSA) and subsequently vancomycin-resistant *S. aureus* (VRSA) has brought in use of novel antibiotics such as daptomycin, tedizolid, telavancin, dalbavancin, oritavancin, quinupristin, and dalfopristin. Removal of foci of infection and addition of culture-specific antibiotics often in combination remains the best bet on treatment.

"Don't forget, the bacteria watch us from the other end of microscope"

—Stanislaw J Lec

INTRODUCTION

Staphylococcus is a genus of gram-positive bacteria in the family. Staphylococcaceae—"staphylo"—meaning a "bunch of grapes" and "*coccus*"—spherical bacterium. This name was coined in 1880 by Scottish surgeon and bacteriologist Alexander Ogston according to their microscopic appearance. Over the years at least 30 species of staphylococci have been recognized by biochemical analysis, in particular by deoxyribonucleic acid (DNA)-DNA hybridization. Up to 11 of these can be isolated from humans as commensals. *S. aureus* (nares) and *S. epidermidis* (nares and skin) are common commensals, but also have the greatest pathogenic potential. *S. saprophyticus* (skin, occasionally) is also a common cause of urinary tract infection. *S. haemolyticus, S. simulans, S. cohnii, S. warneri,* and *S. lugdunensis* can also cause infections in human.

GROUPING

Traditionally they were divided into two groups on the basis of their ability to clot blood plasma (the coagulase reaction). *S. aureus* and *S. intermedius* are coagulase positive. All other staphylococci are coagulase negative. Catalase (ability to breakdown hydrogen peroxide to water and oxygen) test is useful to distinguish staphylococci (catalase positive) from enterococci and streptococci (catalase negative).

IN HEALTH AND DISEASE

The bacterium has been extensively studied over the years due to its frequent association with infections in several organ systems. Interestingly, the same virulent organism is a part of the commonly occurring commensal in humans. Approximately, 50% of the human population are carriers of *S. aureus*, with 20% as continuous carriers and 30% as intermittent carriers. How the bacterium switches gear to attack the host still remains a question to be answered in totality.

Study of *Staphylococcus* has opened new frontiers in microbiology. Be it the study of the components of the cell wall, the various transcription factors, the enzymes produced by bacteria, or study of mechanism of antibiotic resistance, *Staphylococcus* has often served as the prototype gram-positive bacterium. The bacterium is even credited for serendipitous discovery of antibiotic as the original Petri dish on which Alexander Fleming of Imperial College London observed the antibacterial activity of the *Penicillium* fungus was growing a culture of *S. aureus*.

VIRULENCE AND PATHOGENESIS

Staphylococcus aureus expresses many potential virulence factors. These are grouped according to their role in the disease process. While some are similar to other pathogenic bacteria, others are unique to the organism:

- Surface proteins that promote colonization of host tissues (fibrinogen- and fibronectin-binding proteins);
- Invasins that promote bacterial spread in tissues (kinases, leukocidin, hyaluronidase, deoxyribonuclease, lipase, and staphylokinase);
- Surface factors that inhibit phagocytic engulfment (large polysaccharide capsule and protein A);
- Biochemical properties that enhance their survival in phagocytes—carotenoids and catalase production;
- Immunological disguises (protein A and coagulase);
- Membrane-damaging toxins that lyse eukaryotic cell membranes (hemolysins, leukotoxin, and leukocidin);
- Exotoxins that damage host tissues or otherwise provoke symptoms of disease [staphylococcal enterotoxin A-G, toxic shock syndrome toxin (TSST), and exfoliative toxin];
- Inherent and acquired resistance to antimicrobial agents.

For the majority of diseases caused by *S. aureus*, pathogenesis is multifactorial, so it is difficult to determine precisely the role of any given factor.

SPECTRUM OF DISEASE

So many virulence factors make the bacterium one of the most lethal organisms. It has got the ability to invade a variety of tissue to different extent causing a spectrum of disease condition. *S aureus* commonly causes superficial skin lesions such as boils, styes, and localized abscesses but can also cause deep-seated infections such as osteomyelitis and endocarditis. *S. aureus* causes food poisoning by releasing enterotoxins into food. *S. aureus* causes toxic shock syndrome by release of superantigens (TSST-1) into the blood stream. *S. saprophyticus* is one of the causes of urinary tract infections, especially in girls. *S. aureus* is a major cause of nosocomial infection of surgical wounds and along with *S. epidermidis* causes infections associated with indwelling medical devices and implants.

ANTIBIOTIC RESISTANCE

Another arsenal which makes this bacterium such an enigmatic entity is antibiotic resistance. Mechanism of antibiotic resistance is as varied as its virulence factors.

The bacteria become resistant to antibiotic either by not allowing the antibiotic to reach its target at a high enough concentration or modify/bypass the target that the antibiotic acts on.

Stopping the antibiotic from reaching its target:

- Pump the antibiotic out from the bacterial cell (tetracycline and fluoroquinolones)
- Decrease permeability of the membrane
- Destroy the antibiotic. There are bacterial enzymes that can inactivate antibiotics, e.g., penicillinase and extended-spectrum beta-lactamase (ESBL)

Modify or bypass the target of the antibiotic:

- *Camouflage the target*: Changes in the composition or structure of the target or add different chemical groups to the target structure
- Express alternative proteins, e.g., different penicillin (PCN)-binding proteins due to acquiring of resistance gene *mecA* by MRSA
- *Reprogram target*: Sometimes bacteria can produce a different variant of a structure it needs. For example, vancomycin-resistant bacteria make a different cell wall compared to susceptible bacteria.

Emergence of antibiotic resistance has led to constant search for newer antibiotics to deal with the resistant strains, but unfortunately the bacteria seems be to be always one step ahead in the game and now we face a grave situation of dealing with pandrug-resistant bacteria resistant to all known antibiotics. New guidelines take into consideration the antibiotic resistance pattern to formulate recommendations likely to give best result in most situations.

TREATMENT

GENERAL PRINCIPLES OF THERAPY

Staphylococcal infections both by prototype organism *S. aureus* and the group coagulase-negative *Staphylococcus* are a source of concern for their ubiquitous nature, morbidity, and emerging resistance to existing antimicrobial agents. Management should be individualized depending upon the site of infection, susceptibility of the organism as determined by various drug-sensitivity tests and local hospital protocol, and also clinical profile of the patient.

Elimination of the source of infection is an often followed practice, but it is of not much help because approximately 20% of healthy persons are persistent carriers of *S. aureus* and 60% are intermittent carriers. Colonization rates are increased in hemodialysis patients, illicit injection drug users, surgical patients, and patients with insulin-dependent or poorly controlled diabetes. Hence, priority to be focused on elimination from local site like removal of indwelling prosthetic devices such as central venous catheter, incision and drainage of suppurative collections, and correct and repeated handwashing.

CHOICE OF ANTIMICROBIAL AGENTS

Penicillin G was the first antibiotic used in staphylococcal infections in the early 1940s; however, resistance to it emerged due to production of beta-lactamase or penicillinase in a matter of few decades. Nowadays, <5% of hospital isolates are sensitive to PCN. But recent publications have shown a tendency of rise of PCN-sensitive *S. aureus* (PSSA). This gives a distinct advantage because the time above minimum inhibitory concentration (MIC) is much more for PCN compared to other antibiotics due to long half-life and it targets a narrower spectrum than cephalosporins. Still there doubts regarding its widespread operational efficacy because most laboratories use the rapid chromogenic beta-lactamase test rather than polymerase chain reaction (PCR) methods which are not very sensitive in detecting PSSA strains.

Penicillin-resistant strains are treated by semisynthetic penicillinase-resistant penicillin (SPRP) such as the prototype but obsolete methicillin and rarely used nafcillin or oxacillin. In patients with PCN allergy, cephalosporins and carbapenems may be used. In such methicillin-sensitive strains, first-generation cephalosporins are noninferior to higher generations even proving superior to some molecules like ceftazidime.

Only after a year of its introduction there emerged **resistant strains to methicillin** and its incidence is increasing encompassing other SPRP and cephalosporins also. This has led to a new entity of organism named as MRSA. They develop resistance by producing PCN-binding protein 2 which has lower affinity to PCN from the *mecA* gene part of a genomic island called *SCCmec*. The efficacy of the drug varies because resistance in MRSA may be constitutive (expressed in all cells of a population) or heterogeneous (seen only in a proportion of the population). Vancomycin or daptomycin is recommended as the drug of choice for invasive MRSA. Alternatively, linezolid, ceftaroline, telavancin, and trimethoprim-sulfamethoxazole (TMP-SMX) may be used. For skin and soft-tissue infections, newer drugs such as tedizolid, oritavancin, and dalbavancin may be used. Community-acquired MRSA (CA-MRSA) isolates often maintain susceptibility to tetracyclines (tetracycline, doxycycline, minocycline, and tigecycline) and TMP/SMX. Clindamycin susceptibilities vary geographically. If the isolate is erythromycin resistant, must confirm clindamycin susceptibility with D-test.

Resistance to vancomycin has also emerged. Initially there was increase in MIC in strains isolated in different geographical regions. In 1997, a strain with reduced susceptibility known as vancomycin-intermediate *S. aureus* (VISA) was isolated from Japan. They have a thick cell wall which traps the molecule and prevents it from reaching target site. In 2002, fully resistant strain VRSA was isolated. These organisms had *vanA* gene which produces a different cell wall peptide to which the molecule cannot bind.

Antibiotics for vancomycin-resistant organisms: *Daptomycin*, a parenteral bactericidal agent, is used in treatment of bacteremia and soft-tissue infections, but not in respiratory infections as it is neutralized by lung surfactant. It disrupts the cell membrane. But resistance to this molecule has also been reported in form of increased MIC. Patients need to be monitored for rhabdomyolysis and eosinophilic pneumonia.

Linezolid is bacteriostatic and inhibits protein synthesis. It has similar bioavailability in oral and parenteral form. After prolonged therapy, there have been instances of thrombocytopenia, neutropenia, lactic acidosis, and peripheral or optic neuropathy. Tedizolid, another oxazolidinone, is used as single daily dose both as oral or parenteral form. But data on its efficacy for treatment of deep-seated infections is limited.

Ceftaroline, a fifth-generation cephalosporin, has bactericidal action against MRSA strains for nosocomial pneumonia, skin, and soft-tissue infections.

Telavancin, a parenteral lipoglycopeptide derivative of vancomycin, is used for complicated infections. It is active against VISA strains but its use is limited because of nephrotoxicity. Dalbavancin and oritavancin are long-acting parenteral lipoglycopeptide used on once weekly basis for skin and soft-tissue infections. But there is no data on invasive infections yet.

The *parenteral streptogramin* antibiotic quinupristin/dalfopristin display bactericidal activity against MRSA and VISA strains. But there have been instances of serious infusion site reactions with them. Tigecycline, a broad-spectrum minocycline analog, is bacteriostatic and has activity against soft tissue as well as intra-abdominal infections, but not against invasive infections. Rifampicin may be used as an adjunctive agent in prosthetic device-related infections and osteomyelitis.

CHOICE ACCORDING TO CLINICAL SYNDROMES

Bacteremia: Remove foci of infection whenever possible; remove implicated venous catheter, if present, but may occur without apparent focus or entry site. Evaluate if without focus for endocarditis by transthoracic echocardiography or transesophageal echocardiography mycotic aneurysms or other deep infection, e.g., abscess, or any spinal involvement (discitis, vertebral osteomyelitis, and epidural abscess).

- *Treatment*:
  - *Preferred*: Oxacillin 2 g intravenous (IV) q4h and nafcillin 2 g IV q4h
  - *Alternatives*: For nonlife-threatening PCN allergy: Cefazolin 2 g IV q8h

    Consider oxacillin/nafcillin desensitization for life-threatening type 1 PCN allergy (hives/anaphylaxis).
- *Severe beta-lactam allergy*: Vancomycin 15 mg/kg IV q12h and daptomycin 6–8 mg/kg IV q24h
- *MRSA*:
  - *Preferred*: Vancomycin 15 mg/kg q8–12h. Consider loading dose for severe infections: 25–30 mg/kg.
  - *Alternatives*: Daptomycin 6 mg/kg IV daily. Food and Drug Administration (FDA) approved for *S. aureus* bacteremia and right-sided endocarditis, preferred in most instances; some experts recommend higher doses 8–10 mg/kg daily for severe infections. Quinupristin/dalfopristin 7.5 mg/kg IV q12h, TMP/SMX 5 mg/kg IV q8–12h, and ceftaroline 600 mg IV q8h.
- *Duration of therapy*: For bacteremia, 28 daysw is the standard course of therapy. Short-course therapy, 14 days only if the following criteria met:
  - Endocarditis is ruled out by transthoracic echocardiogram (TTE) ± transesophageal echocardiogram (TEE)
  - No implanted prostheses (e.g., prosthetic valves, cardiac devices, or arthroplasties)
  - Blood cultures drawn 2–4 days after the initial cultures were negative, the patient defervesces within 72 hours of appropriate therapy
  - No evidence of metastatic infection
  - No comorbidities such as diabetes, liver or advanced renal disease, and immunosuppression

Endocarditis and native valve: Consult cardiac surgery if the patient has persistently positive blood cultures, evidence of heart failure, or ongoing embolic disease. Evaluation especially recommended if vegetation >10 mm, new heart block, worsening heart failure, and persistent fevers.

- *MSSA, native valve, and left-sided involvement*:
  - *Preferred*: Nafcillin 2 g IV q4h or 3 g IV q6h or oxacillin 2 g IV q4h or 3 g IV q6h, cefazolin 2 g IV q8h
  - *Alternatives*: If highly PCN-allergic, consider allergy consultation or desensitization as beta-lactam therapy preferred. If a history of rash or minor reactions, use cefazolin, vancomycin 15 mg/kg IV q8–12h, and daptomycin 8–10 mg/kg IV q24h. However, if brain abscesses present, nafcillin or oxacillin favored rather than cefazolin.
- *MSSA, native valve, and right-sided involvement*:
  - *Preferred*: Oxacillin or nafcillin 2g IV q4h
  - *Alternative*: Daptomycin 6 mg/kg IV q24 for 2 weeks, ciprofloxacin 750 mg PO twice daily plus rifampin 300 mg PO twice daily for 28 days, if isolate proven susceptible to both agents.
- *MRSA, native valve, and right- or left-sided involvement*:
  - *Preferred*: Vancomycin 15 mg/kg IV q12h
  - *Alternative*: Daptomycin ≥8 mg/kg IV daily for 6 weeks

Endocarditis and prosthetic valve: Transesophageal echocardiogram is recommended for all cases to evaluate for significant perivalvular abscess, leak, or if other valves involved.

- *MSSA, prosthetic valve*: Oxacillin or nafcillin 2 g IV q4h for ≥6 weeks plus gentamicin 1 mg/kg IV q8h (or 1.5 mg IV q12h) for first 2 weeks plus rifampin 300 mg PO q8h for ≥6 weeks after blood cultures have cleared; confirm susceptibility to all agents.
- *MRSA, prosthetic valve*: Vancomycin 15 mg/kg IV q12h for ≥6 weeks plus gentamicin 1 mg/kg IV q8h (or 1.5 mg IV q12h) for first 2 weeks plus rifampin 300 mg PO q8h for ≥6 weeks after blood cultures have cleared; confirm susceptibility to all agents.

Soft-tissue infections: Surgical drainage for any collection. For cutaneous abscess, incision and drainage may be sufficient. But recent randomized controlled trial (RCT) suggested better outcomes if clindamycin or TMP/SMX were used in addition to incision and drainage. Antibiotics indicated for severe/rapidly progressive infections, signs and symptoms of systemic illness, diabetes or other significant immunosuppression, advanced age, location of abscess in an area where complete drainage is difficult, lack of response to initial incision and drainage, necrotizing fasciitis, and extensive abscess-associated cellulitis.

- *Treatment*: Vancomycin 15 mg/kg IV q12h, daptomycin dose is 4 mg/kg IV daily, clindamycin 600 mg IV q8h, ceftaroline 600 mg IV q12h, linezolid 600 mg IV q12h, tedizolid 200 mg IV q24, and TMP/SMX 8–12 mg/kg (based on TMP) divided dosing q6h.
- *Oral regimens*:
  - *MSSA*: Cephalexin 500 mg PO four times a day, dicloxacillin 500 mg PO four times a day, clindamycin 300–450 mg PO three times a day, doxycycline 100 mg PO twice daily, and amoxicillin/clavulanate 875 mg PO twice daily.
  - *MRSA*: Clindamycin 300–450 mg PO three times a day, TMP/SMX 1–2 DS tablets PO twice daily, doxycycline 100 mg PO twice daily, minocycline 100 mg PO twice daily, and linezolid 600 mg PO twice daily.
  - Duration of therapy depends on the extent of disease, usual range 5–10 days.

Pneumonia: Consider MRSA pneumonia in any patient with severe community-acquired pneumonia (CAP) [e.g., intensive care unit (ICU) admission, necrotizing/cavitary disease, and empyema] pending sputum or blood culture results.

- *Treatment*: Vancomycin 15 mg/kg IV q12h, linezolid 600 mg IV/PO q12h, clindamycin 600 mg IV or 300–450 mg PO q8h, and telavancin 10 mg/kg IV q24h.
- Drain or proceed with thoracic surgical consultation for empyema. Duration of therapy is 7–21 days course, depending on severity; many cases of ventilator-associated pneumonia can be treated for 8 days; necrotizing pneumonia usually requires longer courses ≥14 days; and bacteremic pneumonia, at least 14 days.

Osteomyelitis: Drainage and debridement of devitalized bone should be done, if possible.

- *Treatment*:
  - *MSSA*:
    - *Preferred*: Nafcillin 1.5–2 g IV q4–6h or continuous infusion, oxacillin 1.5–2 g IV q4–6h or continuous infusion, cefazolin 1–2 g IV q8h, and ceftriaxone 2 g IV q24
    - *Alternatives*: Vancomycin 15–20 mg/kg IV q12h, daptomycin 6–8 mg IV q24, linezolid 600 mg IV/PO q12h, levofloxacin 500–750 PO daily + rifampin 600 mg PO daily, and clindamycin 600–900 mg IV q8h
  - *MRSA*:
    - *Preferred*: Vancomycin 15–20 mg/kg IV q12h
    - *Alternatives*: Daptomycin 6–8 mg/kg IV q24h, TMP/SMX 4 mg/kg (TMP component) twice daily ± rifampin 600 mg once daily, linezolid 600 mg PO/IV q12h, clindamycin 600 mg IV q8h, and levofloxacin 500–750 PO daily + rifampin 600 mg PO daily.
- *Duration*: For 6–8 weeks with additional 4–12 weeks, especially if osteomyelitis of long-standing nature or if complete debridement not achieved.

Meningitis:

- *MSSA*: Nafcillin or oxacillin 2 g IV q4h.
- *MRSA*:
  - *Preferred*: Vancomycin 15–20 mg/kg IV 12 hours (consider loading dose 25–30 mg/kg).
  - *Alternatives*: Linezolid 600 mg IV q12h [limited data for meningitis but has good central nervous system (CNS) penetration] and TMP/SMX 5 mg/kg (TMP component) q8–12h.

Refractory infection: Consider intrathecal, vancomycin, 5–20 mg daily for 14 days.

Central nervous system shunt infection: Remove the device. Replace only when cerebrospinal fluid (CSF) cultures repeatedly sterile.

Brain abscess, subdural empyema, and epidural abscess:

- Consult neurosurgery urgently for drainage.
- *MSSA or MRSA*: Choices as above except cefazolin for MSSA given poor CNS penetration.
- *Duration*: For 4–6 weeks.

Toxic shock syndrome: Remove focus of staphylococcal colonization or infection; stabilize blood pressure with fluids, or vasopressors.

- *MSSA*: Oxacillin or nafcillin 2 g IV q4h plus clindamycin 600 mg IV q8h.
- *MRSA*: Vancomycin 15–20 mg/kg IV q12h plus clindamycin 600 mg IV q8h (if susceptible) or linezolid 600 mg IV/PO q12h.

RECOMMENDED READINGS

1. Moreillon P, Que Y-A, Glauser MP. *Staphylococcus aureus* (including staphylococcal toxic shock). In: Man-dell GL, Bennett JE, Dolin R (Eds). Mandell, Douglas, and Bennett's Principles and Practice of Infectious Diseases, 6th edition. Philadelphia: Elsevier Churchill Livingstone; 2005. pp. 2321-51.
2. Resman F, Thegerstrom J, Mansson F, Ahl J, Tham J, Riesbeck K. The prevalence, population structure and screening test specificity of penicillin-susceptible Staphylococcus aureus bacteremia isolates in Malmo, Sweden. J Infect. 2016;73:129-35.
3. Papanicolas LE, Bell JM, Bastian I. Performance of phenotypic tests for detection of penicillinase in Staphylococcus aureus isolates from Australia. J Clin Microbiol. 2014;52:1136-8.
4. Gu B, Kelesidis T, Tsiodras S, Hindler J, Humphries RM. The emerging problem of linezolid-resistant Staphylococcus. J Antimicrob Chemother. 2013;68(1):4-11.
5. Daum RS, Miller LG, Immergluck L, Fritz S, Creech CB, Young D, et al. A Placebo-Controlled Trial of Antibiotics for Smaller Skin Abscesses. N Engl J Med. 2017;376(26):2545-55.
6. Talan DA, Mower WR, Krishnadasan A, Abrahamian FM, Lovecchio F, Karras DJ, et al. Trimethoprim-Sulfamethoxazole versus Placebo for Uncomplicated Skin Abscess. N Engl J Med. 2016;374(9):823-32.

CHAPTER

42

Gram-negative Pathogens and Infections

Rajeev Soman, Umang Agrawal

ABSTRACT

Gram-negative infections are a major cause of morbidity and mortality. The various syndromes that they cause pose immense challenges in diagnosis and testing in the laboratory. Optimal interpretation of the tests and fashioning treatment requires an in-depth understanding of resistance mechanisms, pharmacology of the available antibiotics, and combinations. Source control by surgical means is an important part of the treatment. Stewardship principles include the assessment of the true pathogen as against the colonizing organisms, appropriate choice of the antibiotic, optimizing pharmacokinetic/pharmacodynamic (PK/PD) considerations, de-escalation, adequate infection control measures in the hospital.

"...if human numbers increase, the rate of infection also increases"

—William H McNeill

INTRODUCTION

Gram-negative bacterial infections are associated with various clinical syndromes, ranging from septic shock, intra-abdominal infections, genitourinary infections to skin, and soft tissue infections. Some of the clinically important organisms include *Klebsiella, Pseudomonas, Acinetobacter,* and *Enterobacter* species. They pose immense treatment challenges due to developing resistance and dwindling armamentarium against them.

PATHOGEN AND TRANSMISSION

ENTEROBACTER

Enterobacter belongs to the *Klebsielleae* tribe of the family *Enterobacteriaceae.* This organism is motile, capsulated, ferments lactose, and produces mucoid colonies. Important clinical species include *E. cloacae* and *E. aerogenes.*

ACINETOBACTER

Acinetobacter is an aerobic, catalase-positive, oxidase-negative gram-negative *Coccobacillus.* This organism is an important cause of nosocomial infections. The ability of *Acinetobacter* species to survive for weeks on surfaces like sinks, faucets, humidifiers etc. within the hospital environment leads to prolonged outbreaks. Regional spread is facilitated by patient and staff movement between healthcare facilities. This is further facilitated by improper hand hygiene practices and failure to disinfect mobile medical equipment.

PSEUDOMONAS

Pseudomonas comprises of a large group of aerobic, nonsporing, gram-negative bacilli, motile by polar flagella and does not ferment lactose. It is commonly transmitted through water (including distilled water) and is an important cause of nosocomial infections. It may be associated with infections associated with hot tubs, contaminated contact lens solution, and device-associated infections.

KLEBSIELLA

Klebsiella belongs to the *Klebsielleae* tribe of the family *Enterobacteriaceae.* This organism is short, plump, nonmotile and produces large, dome-shaped highly mucoid colonies on ordinary media. With the exception of *K. ozaenae* and *K. granulomatis,* all other species of *Klebsiella* ferment lactose (**Flowchart 1**). It is capable of surviving on the hands of healthcare workers. This property of *Klebsiella* makes this organism a notorious cause of nosocomial infections like hospital-acquired pneumonia, surgical site infections (SSIs), catheter-related blood stream infections (CRSBI), and others.

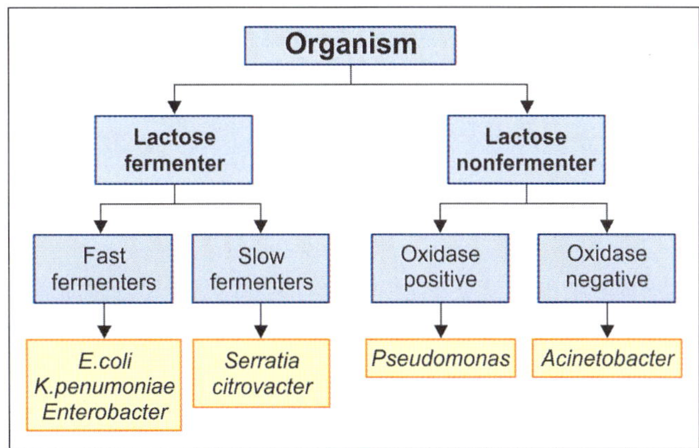

FLOWCHART 1: Classification of gram-negative bacteria on the basis of lactose fermentation.

MECHANISMS OF RESISTANCE

A single organism may produce drug resistance through multiple mechanisms. Optimum detection may be facilitated by phenotypic drug susceptibility testing methods like E-test or VITEK-2 or by sophisticated methods like microbroth dilution (especially for colistin resistance). Newer commercial genetic diagnostic modalities like Xpert Carba are also useful in understanding some of these mechanisms of resistance and direct antimicrobial therapy.

The predominant mechanism of antibiotic resistance in case of lactose fermenters is by production of beta-lactamase enzymes. These may include:

- **Extended-spectrum beta-lactamases (ESBLs)** which confer resistance against penicillin, cephalosporins (first, second, and third generation), and aztreonam, predominantly by hydrolysis. They however do not destroy cephamycins (cefoxitin, cefotetan etc.). Organisms producing these enzymes remain susceptible to the beta-lactam (BL) and beta-lactamase inhibitor (BLI) combination (e.g., piperacillin-tazobactam, cefoperazone-sulbactam) and carbapenems, at least in vitro.
- **Carbapenemases** (encoded by the *KPC, NDM, and OXA* genes) confer resistance to carbapenems. NDM is a particularly notorious cause of carbapenem resistance in India.
- **Antibiotic resistance through AmpC** (enzyme) may be mediated by chromosomes (e.g., in SPICE group of organisms) or by plasmids (horizontal transfer of resistance). In the SPICE group of organisms (*Serratia, Pseudomonas*, Indole-positive *Proteus* species, *Citrobacter* and *Enterobacter* species), the *AmpC* gene exists in a repressed state. On exposure to BL antibiotics, this gene gets "derepressed," produces enzyme, and destroys the BL. Thus, despite the exhibition of in vitro susceptibility to BL (like cephalosporins and penicillins), in vivo resistance to these antibiotics may be seen on prolonged use. In patients with severe infections with a high bacterial burden or those infections requiring prolonged antibiotics, carbapenems or non-BL group of antibiotics are preferable for therapy despite in vitro results showing susceptibility to cephalosporins.
- Over the past few years, the supposedly "rare" polymyxin resistance has emerged in these organisms, further limiting therapeutic options. This resistance may be chromosomally mediated (*mgrB* gene) (especially in *K. pneumoniae)* or plasmid-mediated (*mcr-1* gene).

NONLACTOSE FERMENTERS

Pseudomonas predominantly demonstrates antibiotic resistance through porin channels and efflux pumps. It may also cause resistance due to beta-lactamase production, the clinically important mechanism mediated by the *VIM* gene, which produces a metallo-beta-lactamase enzyme. Multidrug-resistant *Pseudomonas* is an important clinical problem in the Indian intensive care units (ICUs) with limited therapeutic options.

Acinetobacter, an important cause of ventilator-associated pneumonias (VAPs) in the Indian ICUs, demonstrates antibiotic resistance predominantly by the production of beta-lactamases. However, the genes encoding these beta-lactamases are different from the ones produced by *Enterobacteriaceae*. For instance, avibactam, a second generation BLI, is not effective against the OXA enzymes produced by *Acinetobacter*. This organism exhibits good susceptibility to sulbactam and relatively lower rates of resistance to minocycline compared to other carbapenem-resistant organisms. Some strains may also exhibit resistance to polymyxin.

CLINICAL SYNDROMES

These organisms may cause a variety of clinical syndromes. A summary of these has been provided in **Table 1**. A few of these syndromes are discussed here.

VENTILATOR-ASSOCIATED PNEUMONIA

Ventilator-associated pneumonia is a type of pneumonia that develops ≥48 hours after endotracheal intubation. It is important to differentiate this condition from ventilator-associated tracheobronchitis (VAT) which is defined as presence of fever (>38°C) ≥48 hours after endotracheal intubation, with new or increased sputum production or positive culture of tracheal aspirates, but no radiographic infiltrate or evidence of pneumonia and no other recognizable cause of fever. VAT represents a continuum between respiratory tract colonization and VAP. It is unclear if VAT warrants treatment. Some studies have

TABLE 1 Clinical syndromes.

Organism	Clinical syndromes
Klebsiella	• Liver abscess • Pneumonia • Blood stream infections • Urinary tract infections
Pseudomonas	• Hospital-acquired pneumonia • Ventilator-associated pneumonia prosthetic valve endocarditis • Necrotizing enterocolitis • Keratitis • Malignant otitis externa • Ecthyma gangrenosum • Device-related infections
Enterobacter	• Nosocomial infections (pneumonia, wound infections, urinary tract infections, prosthetic joint infections, and meningitis) • Neonatal meningitis and sepsis
Acinetobacter	• Nosocomial infections (ventilator-associated pneumonia, CRBSI, wound infections) • Post-trauma • Urinary tract infections

(CRBSI: catheter-related blood stream infection)

showed reduced incidence of VAP if VAT is treated, but some showed no difference. Clinical judgment based on the patient's condition is important to make this decision.

One method which may be useful in differentiating colonization from infection is the colony count of the respiratory tract isolate. In general, for a particular respiratory tract organism to be considered clinically significant, the colony count of the endotracheal, bronchoalveolar, fluid, and the protected specimen brush (PSB) isolate should be more than 10^5, 10^4, and 10^3, respectively. It must be noted however that these colony count cut-offs are useful "rule-out" tests for VAP. They however carry a poor positive predictive value for the diagnosis of VAP.

CATHETER-RELATED BLOOD STREAM INFECTION

A patient having an intravascular line is said to have CRBSI when the differential time to positivity (time difference between the growth detection in blood drawn from catheter hub and that detected in the blood drawn from periphery) of ≥2 hours. Resistant gram-negative bacteria are important causes of CRBSI in the Indian setting, leading to high morbidity and mortality. In case of established CRBSI, catheter removal is ideal. However, in situations where that is not possible, antibiotic lock therapy may be employed in addition to systemic antibiotics to manage this infection. It is important to know that hemodynamic instability, evidence of exit site infection, growth of *Staphylococcus aureus* or *Candida albicans*, and presence of implants or presence of septic emboli are important absolute indications of catheter removal.

CATHETER-ASSOCIATED UTI

Infectious Diseases Society of America (IDSA) defines catheter-associated urinary tract infection (CAUTI) as the presence of symptoms or signs compatible with UTI with no other identified source of infection along with $\geq 10^3$ colony-forming units (cfu)/mL of ≥1 bacterial species in a single catheter urine specimen or in a midstream-voided urine specimen from a patient whose urethral, suprapubic, or condom catheter has been removed within the previous 48 hours.

DEVICE-ASSOCIATED INFECTIONS

Surgical site infections postlaparoscopy or arthroscopy are commonly associated with *Pseudomonas*/NTM infections. This may be because *P. aeruginosa* is known to contaminate diluted, exposed, decanted, and reused solutions of quaternary ammonium compounds which are used to sterilize these devices. Same holds true for cardiac stent-related infections. Strict infection control practices like avoiding reuse of single-use devices and thorough sterilization of scopes in ortho-phthalaldehyde solutions followed by complete drying would go a long way in preventing these complications.

SURGICAL SITE INFECTIONS

Surgical site infections are a common cause of healthcare-associated infection. The Centers for Disease Control and Prevention (CDC) defines SSI as infection related to an operative procedure that occurs at or near the surgical incision within 30 days of the procedure or within 90 days if prosthetic material is implanted at surgery. An effective infection control program can reduce the incidence of SSI by 40%. Employing antimicrobial prophylaxis, good hand hygiene, use of gloves, patient decolonization, and skin disinfection may help reduce the incidence of this complication.

POSTNEUROSURGICAL INFECTIONS

Neurosurgical infections, secondary to poor infection control practices, may have catastrophic implications. Organisms like *Pseudomonas, Acinetobacter* etc. persist in hospital environment such as water facilities, saline solution used for flushing procedures, disinfectants, and medical devices. Improper hand hygiene and inadequate disinfection practices predispose to neurosurgical infections with these organisms, which are generally multidrug resistant. Poor penetration of systemic antibiotics into the cerebrospinal fluid (CSF) further worsens the prognosis. Tenets of management include device removal, use of systemic and intrathecal antibiotics, and frequently prolonged duration of treatment. This prolongs hospital stay, adds to costs, toxicities, and increased morbidity and mortality.

INTRA-ABDOMINAL INFECTIONS

Intra-abdominal infections occur due to disruption or inflammation of the gastrointestinal tract. These infections are generally polymicrobial, caused by endogenous gut microbiota including fungal pathogens and anaerobes. Nosocomial infections secondary to intra-abdominal procedures (biliary stenting, peritoneal dialysis, laparoscopic/open abdominal surgery etc.) may also occur. Prior antibiotic therapy and healthcare exposures may alter the gut microbiota, eventually leading to infections with drug-resistant organisms. Important organisms associated with intra-abdominal infections include *Escherichia coli, Klebsiella* species, *Enterobacter, Pseudomonas, Enterococcus, Streptococcus,* and *Candida* species. The treatment regimen for these infections should include an agent with a good anaerobic cover for *Bacteroides fragilis.*

LIVER ABSCESSES

Klebsiella pneumoniae may cause different types of liver abscesses. One variety may be the multifocal pyogenic liver abscesses caused as a part of a polymicrobial flora and is generally associated with hepatobiliary and colonic diseases. A second form of community-acquired, single, monomicrobial liver abscess called *Klebsiella* liver abscess (KLA) may be seen in infection with hypervirulent, hypermucoviscous form of this organism. This form of liver abscess generally occurs in the absence of a primary hepatobiliary disease and has a high potential of metastatic spread leading to meningitis, brain abscesses, and endophthalmitis. In laboratory, it may be identified on culture plates by the string test.

MANAGEMENT

Source control, use of antibiotics, and good infection control practices form the important cornerstones of management of these infections.

SOURCE CONTROL

This is the most important modality of management for gram-negative infections. Adequate drainage of abscess and removal of offending agent (line, device etc.) have paramount importance in achieving optimum outcomes. There are several reasons for that:

- *Inoculum effect*: Due to the high bacterial load, once acted upon by the antibiotic, cells lyse and release beta-lactamases in the abscess milieu leading to hydrolysis of the BL antibiotic. This leads to reduced concentrations of BL antibiotic in the milieu which further promotes drug resistance.
- *Poor vascular supply*: Abscesses are associated with poor vascular supply. As a result, antibiotic penetration into the abscess is hampered leading to poor outcomes.
- *Biofilm formation*: Certain bacteria (like *Pseudomonas*, NTM infections etc.) can form biofilms on an intravascular/prosthetic device. Biofilms comprise of a thick peptidoglycan matrix secreted by the organisms which prevent antibiotic penetration. Within these biofilms, the organisms may lie dormant for a long time in view of limited nutrient supply. Owing to these reasons, antibiotic penetration is compromised, exposure to suboptimal antibiotic concentrations promotes drug resistance, and the dormant bacteria escape antibiotic activity since most antibiotics work against dividing bacteria. This causes recurrence of infection.

ANTIBIOTICS

Multiple antibiotic options are available for gram-negative infections including third- and fourth-generation cephalosporins, quinolones, aminoglycosides, tetracyclines, carbapenems, BL with BLI combinations, colistin etc.

Empiric choice depends on the local epidemiology, history of prior antibiotic exposure, site of infection, severity of illness, and the concomitant drugs being given. Directed choice depends on the susceptibility profile of the organism, cost, toxicity, biofilm-producing ability of the bacteria and whether adequate source control has been achieved. De-escalation strategies depend on the clinical response of the patient to the therapy, site of infection, and adequacy of source control. Local treatment strategies (nebulized antibiotics, antibiotic lock therapy, and antibiotic bead insertion in implant-associated infections) may be warranted in case of inadequate source control due to any reason.

Illustrative case: A 68-year-old male, a case of carcinoma pancreas, underwent Whipple's procedure in 2018. Two years later, he developed metastatic lesions in liver for which he underwent radiofrequency ablation. Fifteen days later, he developed fever and abdominal pain for which he was hospitalized many times and treated with antibiotics. Large liver abscesses were detected later. Pigtail drainage grew carbapenem-resistant *E. coli*. As the gut flora is commonly involved in intra-abdominal sepsis, organisms like *E. coli, Klebsiella, Enterobacter, Citrobacter,* and anaerobes should be kept in mind. In selected situations gram-positive cocci like *Enterococcus* species and *Candida* should also be considered.

Hence, antimicrobials covering both gram-negative and anaerobes should be given and should be chosen according to the most frequently isolated microbes and the local trend of antimicrobial resistance. Previous history of hospitalization and treatment, determine whether non-ESBL, ESBL, CRE (carbapenem-resistant Enterobacteriaceae), or colistin-resistant organisms are expected. In India, ESBL is found to be >50%, therefore empiric third-generation cephalosporins have no role in empiric therapy. Empirically, BL-BLIs like piperacillin-tazobactam or cefoperazone-sulbactam could be used if not previously treated, patient is not immunocompromised, and source control is optimal. Meropenem was advised in this patient as it has a good coverage against gram-negative organisms as well as anaerobes. It was combined with teicoplanin to cover *Enterococcus* species and fluconazole for *Candida* species, although this is not always needed. However as the organism isolated was carbapenem-resistant *E. coli* with meropenem minimum inhibitory concentration (MIC) >16, it would remain ineffective. Teicoplanin and fluconazole were discontinued as there was no isolation of gram-positive organisms or *Candida*. Treatment was changed to high-dose tigecycline. It has high concentrations in the liver, gallbladder, and colon. Since this drug covers anaerobes as well, there was no need to add metronidazole. However, the patient had severe nausea and vomiting and did not tolerate tigecycline. A polymyxin alone is another choice but can be nephrotoxic and has limitations. In general, it has a suboptimal efficacy in clinical trials. The next option is the new BL-BLIs like ceftazidime-avibactam (CAZ-AVI) along with aztreonam, but it is important to know the genotypic profile of carbapenemases. Xpert Carba-R will be able to identify if the organism is producing VIM, IMP, NDM and/or OXA-48. This organism was found to be a NDM + OXA-48 producer. Avibactam is not stable against MBLs. Therefore, metallo-β-lactamase (MBL) will destroy ceftazidime. Aztreonam is stable against MBL but is destroyed by other β-lactamases. However, avibactam can inhibit extended spectrum beta lactamases, AmpC, KPC, and OXA-48 and protect aztreonam. So the choice of antibiotics will be altered and most specific with the genotypic profile of carbapenemases.

INFECTION CONTROL PRACTICES

A large part of the daily infectious diseases ward/ICU work today comprises of nosocomial infections. Good infection control practices including hand hygiene, adequate skin sterilization before invasive procedures, avoiding reuse of single-use devices etc. would go a long way in preventing these infections. A good teamwork comprising of physicians, infectious diseases specialists, microbiologists, surgeons, and the management would ensure optimal patient outcomes.

CONCLUSION

Protocols and guidelines for appropriate use of antibiotics for gram-negative infections in various clinical situations have to be made based on the local epidemiology. Rapid, accurate methods of diagnosis to confirm or exclude an infective cause are needed. The steps to be followed are: to send appropriate specimens for tests, select antibiotics based on the syndrome, guidelines and local epidemiology, fine tune therapy based on microbiologic results, optimize PK/PD considerations, carry out source control, and perform a daily assessment for de-escalation or termination. Clinicians must realize that antibiotics are toxic and expensive to the patient and dangerous to the environment. They should not be used as placebos, antipyretics, or as substitutes for diagnosis.

RECOMMENDED READINGS

1. Kalil AC, Metersky ML, Klompas M, Muscedere J, Sweeney DA, Palmer LB, et al. Management of Adults With Hospital-acquired and Ventilator-associated Pneumonia: 2016 Clinical Practice Guidelines by the Infectious Diseases Society of America and the American Thoracic Society. Clin Infect Dis. 2016;63(5):e61-111.
2. Horan TC, Andrus M, Dudeck MA. CDC/NHSN surveillance definition of health care-associated infection and criteria for specific types of infections in the acute care setting. Am J Infect Control. 2008;36(5):309-32.
3. Hooton TM, Bradley SF, Cardenas DD, Colgan R, Geerlings SE, Rice JC, et al. Diagnosis, prevention, and treatment of catheter-associated urinary tract infection in adults: 2009 International Clinical Practice Guidelines from the Infectious Diseases Society of America. Clin Infect Dis. 2010;50(5):625-63.
4. Mermel LA, Allon M, Bouza E, Craven DE, Flynn P, O'Grady NP, et al. Clinical Practice Guidelines for the Diagnosis and Management of Intravascular Catheter-Related Infection: 2009 Update by the Infectious Diseases Society of America. Clin Infect Dis. 2009;49(1):1-45.
5. Consensus paper on the surveillance of surgical wound infections. The Society for Hospital Epidemiology of America; The Association for Practitioners in Infection Control; The Centers for Disease Control; The Surgical Infection Society. Infect Control Hosp Epidemiol. 1992;13(10):599-605.

CHAPTER 43

Gram-negative Bacterial Infections: Salmonellosis, Shigellosis, Brucellosis, Cholera, and Plague

Dwijen Das, Jacquiline D Shira, Indrajit Debnath

ABSTRACT

Gram-negative bacteria are notorious group of organisms causing multiple infections ranging from trivial to the most serious conditions including gastroenteritis, pneumonia, urinary tract infections, peritonitis, meningitis, and wound or surgical site infections. They have a protective capsule that protects against phagocytosis, an outer membrane that limits penetration of antibiotics, and endotoxins which when released lead to severe symptoms and also add to the dreaded pathogenicity of this group. Certain salient features are peculiar to each organism of this group, which aids in diagnosing the etiologic agent. As such gram-negative infections are often regarded the worst enemies of treating physicians. Enteric fever is one such systemic disease caused by a member of this class—*Salmonella*, which are nonlactose fermenting, facultative, anaerobic, motile rods. *Shigella*, a facultative, anaerobic, gram negative, nonspore forming, nonmotile, and nongas producing bacteria are responsible for causing bacillary dysentery. Brucellosis, a zoonotic disease distributed worldwide and endemic in India is caused by the gram negative, facultative, partially acid fast, unencapsulated, nonsporulating, and intracellular coccobacilli—*Brucella*. *B. melitensis* and *B. suis*. They could be exploited as biological weapons. Cholera, caused by another gram-negative organism *Vibrio cholerae*, characterized by abrupt onset of rice watery diarrhea, and is already infamous for seven global pandemics. Plague/Black Death is a systemic zoonosis caused by the gram-negative bacteria *Yersinia pestis*, which are nonlactose fermenting and facultative anaerobes capable of growth at 4–43°C. This article discusses the common diseases caused by gram-negative organisms, their clinical features, diagnosis, and management.

"In the field of observation, chance favours only the prepared mind"

—Louis Pasteur

INTRODUCTION

Bacteria that do not retain the crystal violet stain and turns red on Gram staining are gram-negative bacteria. They are enclosed in a protective capsule, which helps them to prevent leukocytes from ingesting the bacteria. Under this capsule, they have an outer membrane which protects them from certain antibiotics, e.g., penicillin. When the membrane gets disrupted, endotoxins are released which are responsible for severity of symptoms in a patient infected with gram-negative bacteria. These organisms are responsible causing many serious infections, such as gastroenteritis, pneumonia, urinary tract infections, peritonitis, wound or surgical site infections, and meningitis. In this chapter, we will be describing in brief about some of the important gram-negative bacteria responsible to cause various diseases.

SALMONELLOSIS

ETIOLOGIC AGENT

Salmonella are facultative anaerobic, motile, nonlactose fermenting, and gram-negative rods.

Family: Enterobacteriaceae

Genus: *Salmonella*

Species:

- *Salmonella enterica* (human pathogen): There are six subspecies; sub species *enterica,* sub species *indica,* sub species *arizonae,* sub species *salamae,* sub species *diarizonae,* and sub species *houtenae,* which are further divided into >3,000 serotypes.
- *Salmonella bongori* (animal pathogen)

PATHOGENESIS

Pathogenesis of salmonellosis is presented in **Flowchart 1**.

ENTERIC FEVER

Enteric (typhoid) fever is a systemic disease characterized by fever and abdominal pain. It is caused by dissemination of *S. typhi* or *S. paratyphi.*

EPIDEMIOLOGY

Host: Humans are the only natural host. The disease is more common in young children and adolescents than in adults.

Environment: Lack of proper sanitation, improper treatment of drinking water, and contaminated food favors transmission. The major source of bacterial shedding is through feces and also through urine.

Mode of transmission: Fecal-oral route.

Incidence:

- >100 cases per 100,000 population/year in South Central and Southeast Asia
- 10–100 cases per 100,000 population/year in rest of Asia, Africa, and Latin America
- <10 cases per 100,000 population/year in other parts of the world

CLINICAL COURSE

The incubation period varies from 10 to 20 days.

- *First week of illness*: A rising remittent fever (step ladder pyrexia), headache, malaise, constipation, and sometimes mild nonproductive cough. Relative bradycardia with coated tongue is common findings.
- *Second week of illness*: Patients look toxic, apathetic with sustained high temperature, soft tender splenomegaly, rose spots (2–4 mm in diameter, which are salmon colored, blanching, and maculopapular rash mostly located on the trunk and chest) appear between 7th and 12th day and resolves after 2–5 days without a trace. These spots are caused by bacterial embolization. Centrally coated tongue with peripheral hyperemia and tachycardia are common in this week.
- *Third week of illness*: Patient becomes more ill with a continuous high fever and patients lands up in typhoidal state (a delirious confusional state). Abdominal distension, diarrhea, feeble pulse, rapid respiration, crepitations over lung bases, and weight loss occurs if remains untreated.
- *Fourth week of illness*: If the patient survives, fever, mental states, and abdominal distension slowly improves over a few days.

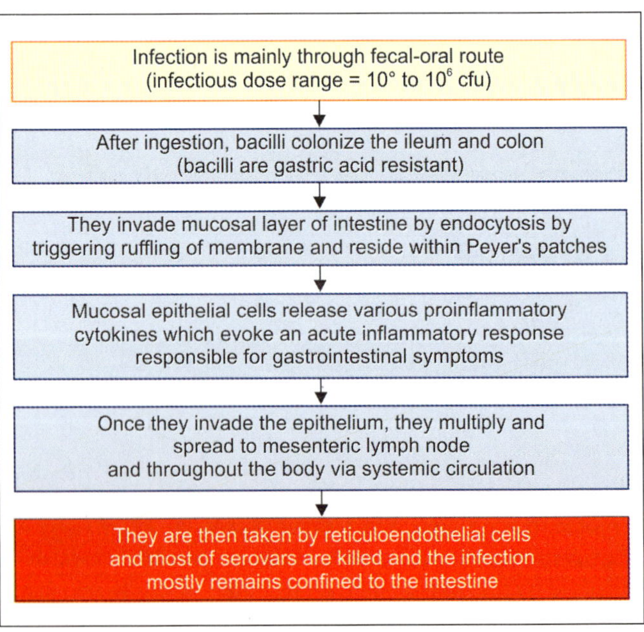

(CFU: colony forming unit)

FLOWCHART 1: Pathogenesis of salmonellosis.

COMPLICATIONS

- *Gastrointestinal*: Intestinal hemorrhage (most common) and intestinal perforation, commonly occurs in the 3rd and 4th week of illness.
- *Neurological*: Meningitis, Guillain-Barré syndrome, neuritis, "muttering delirium", or "coma vigil".
- *Rare manifestations*: Deafness, arthritis, endocarditis, myocarditis, pericarditis, parotitis, nephritis etc.

DIAGNOSIS

- *Culture*: The definitive diagnosis of enteric fever is made from a positive culture.
  - *Blood culture*: Rate of positivity—1st week—>90%, 2nd week—75%, 3rd week—60%, and 4th week—25%
  - *Stool culture*: At the end of 2nd week, positive in 40–50%
  - *Urine culture*: At the end of 3rd week, positive in 30–50%
  - *Bone marrow aspirate culture*: Most sensitive at all stages
- *Serology*:
  - *Widal test*: Has limited sensitivity and specificity in endemic regions.

  Interpretation of Widal test:
    - Significant titer of O antibodies > 100, indicates recent infection or active disease
    - Significant titer of H antibodies > 200, indicates the serotype responsible for the disease.
  - *Typhidot test*: Here immunoglobulin M (IgM) and immunoglobulin G (IgG) antibodies detected separately by enzyme-linked immunosorbent assay (ELISA) method. But this is neither sensitive nor specific.
- *Diazo test*: Detects phenolic compound in urine with a good sensitivity and specificity only in 1st week.
- *Nucleic acid amplification tests (NAATs)* is highly specific test.
- *Leukopenia and neutropenia* are found in 15–25% of cases, whereas leukocytosis is more common in children and in cases with intestinal perforation or secondary infection.

CARRIER STATE IN ENTERIC FEVER

- *Based on site of persistence*:
  - *Fecal carrier*: More common and seen mostly in patients with biliary tract abnormalities.
  - *Urinary carrier*: Seen in patients with urinary tract abnormalities and in countries where urinary schistosomiasis is endemic.
- *Based on duration*:
  - *Convalescent*: Shedding persists up to 3 months.
  - *Temporary*: 3 months to 1 year.
  - *Chronic*: >1 year and is more common in women and in elderly.
- *Diagnosis*:
  - *Screening*: Vi agglutination test to detect Vi antibody.
  - *Confirmation*: Culture from stool, duodenal aspirate, and urine samples.

TREATMENT (TABLE 1)

Uncomplicated cases can be managed at home with oral antibiotic and antipyretics, while patients with persistent vomiting and diarrhea are to be hospitalized.

The initial choice of antibiotic depends on the susceptibility of the *S. typhi* and *S. paratyphi* strains in the area of residence or travel. In Indian subcontinent, patients infected with decreased ciprofloxacin susceptibility (DCS) strains of *S. typhi* and *S. paratyphi* should be treated with ceftriaxone or azithromycin. Ceftriaxone, cefotaxime, and ceftriaxone are effective for treatment of multidrug-resistant (MDR) enteric fever, including that caused by DSC and fluoroquinolone-resistant strains. Antibiotic therapy should be administered for at least 10 days or for 5 days after fever resolution.

PREVENTION

There are three lines of prophylactic measures:

1. *Control of reservoir*:
   - *Control of cases*: Measures include early diagnosis and treatment, disinfection of stool, or urine soiled clothes.
   - *Control of carriers*: Effective treatment of carriers by ampicillin or amoxicillin (4–6 g/day) plus probenecid (2 g/day) for 6 weeks.
2. *Sanitation measures*: Health education, promotion of food hygiene, and purification of drinking water supplies.
3. *Immunization*:
   - *Indications*:
     - Travelling to endemic areas
     - Household contacts
     - People at increased risk (school children)

TABLE 1 Antibiotic therapy for enteric fever in adults.

Drug	Dose (route)	Duration (days)
Empirical treatment		
Ceftriaxone OR Cefotaxime OR Cefixime	2 g/day [intravenous (IV)] 2 g q8h (IV) 400 mg BD (PO)	10–14
Azithromycin	• 1 g/day (PO) or • 1 g on day 1 followed by 500 mg/day (PO) for 6 days	5
Fully susceptible		
Ciprofloxacin	500 mg BD (PO) or 400 mg q12h (IV)	5–7
Azithromycin	1 g/day (PO)	5
Multidrug-resistant and quinolone-resistant		
Ceftriaxone	2 g/day (IV)	10–14
Azithromycin	1 g/day (PO)	5

- *Vaccines*: Two types of typhoid vaccines available presently:
  - i. Parenteral Vi polysaccharide vaccine:
    - Dose: Single dose of 25 µg of Vi antigen intramuscularly or subcutaneously.
    - Booster: Every 2 years
    - Age: Above 2 years of age
  - ii. Typh-oral (oral live attenuated *S. typhi* Ty21a vaccine):
    - Available in lyophilized form, as enteric coated capsule
    - Dosage—given orally on alternate days for three doses
    - Booster: Every 5 years

SHIGELLOSIS

Shigella is the etiologic agent of bacillary dysentery. Bacillary dysentery is an acute bacterial disease manifested by fever, intestinal cramps, frequent passage of bloody mucopurulent stools, and tenesmus.

HISTORY

At the end of 19th century, periodic epidemics of bacillary dysentery occurred in Japan, when Kiyoshi Shiga examined the stools of such patients and isolated bacterium from convalescent patients and not with acute disease. Later the bacterium was named as *Shigella dysenteriae*, the first organism of the genus *Shigella* in the honor of Kiyoshi.

ETIOLOGIC AGENT

Shigella is gram negative, nonspore forming, and facultative anaerobic bacterium, is nonmotile and does not produce gas from sugars, decarboxylate lysine, or hydrolyze arginine.

Family: Enterobacteriaceae

Genus: *Shigella*

Species: Four species, they are:

1. *S. dysenteriae* (serogroup A)—17 serotypes
2. *S. flexneri* (serogroup B)—14 serotypes
3. *S. sonnei* (serogroup C)—1 serotypes
4. *S. boydii* (serogroup C)—20 serotypes

EPIDEMIOLOGY

The annual number of cases of *Shigella* infection have been estimated to be 165 million, with 69% of these cases occurring in children <5 years of age. In developing countries, annual deaths due to shigellosis are 1.1 million. *S. dysenteriae* usually presents in the form of epidemic or outbreak, whereas *S. flexneri* and *S. sonnei* are mainly responsible for endemic disease in developing and developed countries, respectively. *S. boydii* is usually restricted to India and its neighboring countries. In a multicentric study from six Asian countries including China, Vietnam, Thailand, Bangladesh, Pakistan, and Indonesia, *S. flexneri* was found to be the most commonly isolated species (68%) except in Thailand where *S. sonnei* was the most common (84%).

In North-Western India, *S. flexneri* is the predominant serogroup with some temporal shifts in the prevalence of serogroups of *Shigellae*. In Eastern India, *S. flexneri* is again the most prevalent serogroup followed by *S. sonnei, S. dysenteriae, and S. boydii*. In Southern India, *S. flexneri* represents the predominant group with lesser prevalence of *S. sonnei* as compared to Eastern India.

HOST

Humans and primates are the primary reservoir of *Shigella*. It has also been isolated from various other sources such as aquatic bodies, free-living amoebae, insects, birds, and wild animals. The bacterium must pass on from one person to another as it is poorly adapted to survive in environment.

ROUTES OF TRANSMISSION

The primary mode of transmission is through fecal-oral route (as low as 10–100 bacteria). It may be transmitted in the form of contaminated food and water or fomites.

HIGH RISK GROUPS

- Children < 5 years of age
- Older individual > 40 years
- Immunocompromised individuals
- Homosexuals
- Individuals travelling to developing countries

PATHOGENESIS

Pathogenesis of shigellosis is shown in **Flowchart 2**.

CLINICAL MANIFESTATIONS

- Shigellosis evolves through four phases:
  - i. Incubation
  - ii. Watery diarrhea

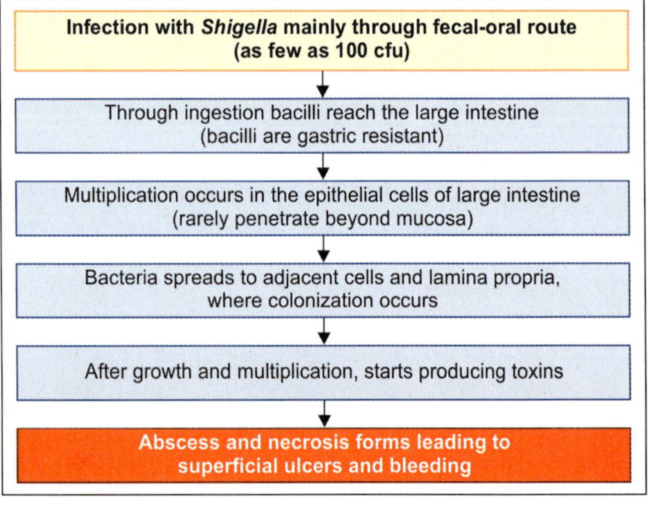

(cfu: colony forming unit)

FLOWCHART 2: Pathogenesis of shigellosis.

iii. Dysentery
iv. Postinfectious phase

- The usual incubation period is 1–4 days.
- Patient initially presents as transient fever, limited watery diarrhea, malaise, anorexia, abdominal discomfort, and vomiting.
- This is followed by passage of bloody mucopurulent stool, abdominal cramps, and tenesmus.
- If left untreated, generally lasts from 1 day to 1 month (average 7 days).

COMPLICATIONS

S—Severe dehydration, febrile seizures (in children), and septicemia
H—Hemolytic uremic syndrome (*S. dysenteriae* I), hyponatremia, hypokalemia, and hypoglycemia
I—Immune complex
G—Glomerulonephritis
E—Ekiri syndrome
LL—Toxic megacolon
A—Reactive arthritis

DIAGNOSIS

- *Gold standard*: Isolation of organism from the stool sample (highest from blood tinged mucous part). Transport medium such as MacConkey agar, *Salmonella-Shigella* Agar, and Hektoen.
- Rectal swabs
- Blood culture (<5% cases)
- *Polymerase chain reaction (PCR)*: Gene coding for invasion plasmid antigen H gene sequence (IPAH)

TREATMENT (TABLE 2)

- Since 1940s, *Shigella* has developed resistance to sulfonamides, tetracycline, chloramphenicol, nalidixic acid, and ampicillin.
- Ciprofloxacin was recommended as the first-line treatment in 1990, but now found resistant to it due to its overuse.
- The World Health Organization (WHO) now recommends ceftriaxone, azithromycin, and pivmecillinam as an alternative to fluoroquinolones.

TABLE 2 Recommended antimicrobials for shigellosis.

Drug	Dose	Comments
First line		
Ciprofloxacin	500 mg BD	To be avoided in children <18 years
Second line		
Azithromycin	1–1.5 g once daily for 1–5 days PO	• Prolong QT interval • Rapid emergence of resistance
Ceftriaxone	50–100 mg/kg (2–4 g daily) once daily for 2–5 days	For inpatient treatment
Pivmecillinam	100 mg QID for 5 days PO	Emerging resistance

BRUCELLOSIS

Brucellosis is a zoonotic disease transmitted to humans under certain circumstances. Its diagnosis is often challenging as it has nonspecific sign and symptoms.

HISTORY

The early history of brucellosis is related to British military in the island of Malta. In 1861, Marston, first differentiated brucellosis from other clinical fevers, and 25 years later Bruce first isolated *Brucella melitensis* as the causative agent for Malta fever.

ETIOLOGIC AGENT

Brucella is gram negative, partially acid fast, unencapsulated, nonsporulating, facultative intracellular rods, or coccobacilli.

Family: Brucellaceae

Genus: *Brucella*

Species:

- *B. melitensis* (sheep, goats, and camels)
- *B. ovis* (sheep)
- *B. abortus* (cattle and buffalo)
- *B. neotomae* (desert rodents)
- *B. suis* (swine)
- *B. ceti* (marine mammals)
- *B. canis* (dogs)
- *B. pinnipedialis* (marine mammals)

EPIDEMIOLOGY

Brucellosis is distributed worldwide and is endemic in India. The true prevalence of brucellosis in human is unknown because of the imprecision in diagnosis and inadequacy in the reporting and surveillance of the cases.

It is transmitted through infected livestock by their contaminated milk and its product, aerosols, through skin wounds etc.

B. melitensis and *B. suis* could be exploited as biological weapon.

POPULATION AT RISK

- *Occupation*: Dairy farmers, cattle ranchers, abattoir worker, and laboratory workers
- Hunters
- Travelers

PATHOGENESIS

Pathogenesis of brucellosis is presented in **Flowchart 3**.

CLINICAL MANIFESTATIONS

- Incubation period—1 week to several months
- Fever, usually occurs at night and with profuse sweating. If left untreated, it shows an undulating pattern (weeks of fever followed by afebrile period, which may relapse)
- Apathy, fatigue, loss of appetite, weight loss, myalgia, headache, and chills

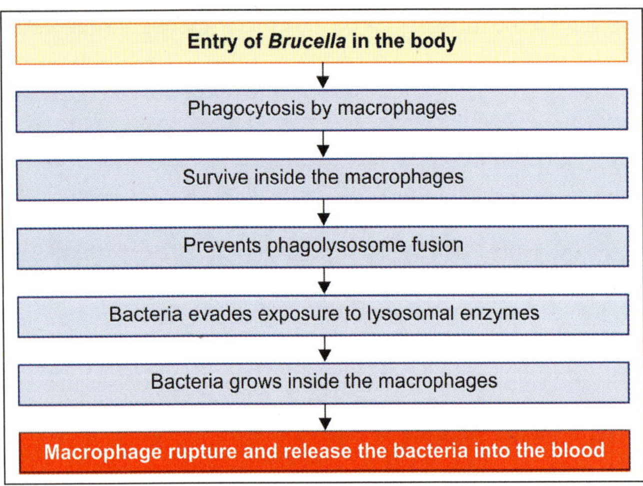

FLOWCHART 3: Pathogenesis of brucellosis.

- Musculoskeletal symptoms and signs like acute monoarthritis typically of hip or knee or polyarthritis, musculoskeletal pain, osteomyelitis (commonly lumbar and lower thoracic vertebrae), and septic arthritis (knee, hip, sacroiliac joint, shoulder, and sternoclavicular joints).
- Respiratory system—pneumonia, empyema, adenopathy, and lung abscess
- Hepatosplenomegaly
- Lymphadenopathy (10–20%)
- Epididymo-orchitis (10%), prostatitis, salpingitis, and pyelonephritis
- Neurological symptoms such as depression, lethargy, and lymphocytic meningoencephalitis
- Endocarditis (1%) affecting mainly aortic valve
- Metastatic abscess
- Fetal loss

LABORATORY INVESTIGATIONS

- Blood or tissue culture—definitive test. *Brucella* is isolated in 50–70% of cases.
- *Serology*:
  - *Brucella agglutination test (BAT)*:
    - In endemic areas titer 1:320–1:640 or higher is considered diagnostic
    - In nonendemic areas a titer of ≥1:160 is considered significant
    - Or a rising titer after 2–4 weeks
  - *Rose Bengal test*: It is a slide agglutination test where a suspension of *B. abortus* smooth cells stained with Rose Bengal dye (pink color) is used. This suspension when mixed with samples containing specific IgG or IgM antibodies agglutinate.
  - Dipstick assay for anti-*Brucella* IgM
  - ELISA for IgM, IgG, and IgA antibodies. ELISA of CSF helps diagnosing neuro-brucellosis.
- *PCR*: It is quicker, more sensitive, and does not pose the threat of biohazard as with culture.
- *Complete blood count (CBC)*: Low or normal leukocyte count with relative lymphocytosis

TABLE 3 Recommended drug regimens for brucellosis.

Dual drug regimens	Doxycycline 100 mg BD for 45 days + streptomycin 1 g for 15 days	Doxycycline 100 mg BD for 45 days + rifampicin 600–900 mg for 45 days	Doxycycline 100 mg BD for 45 days + gentamicin 5–6 mg/kg/day for 15 days
Triple drug regimen	Doxycycline + rifampicin + aminoglycoside (for complicated and poor adherence patients)		
With neurologic diseases	Standard treatment + ceftriaxone for 3–6 months		
For endocarditis	Triple drug regimen for 4–6 months		

- *Cerebrospinal fluid (CSF) analysis*: Hypoglycorrhachia with lymphocytosis. Adenosine deaminase (ADA) may be elevated.

TREATMENT

Table 3 presents recommended drug regimens for brucellosis.

CHOLERA

Cholera is an acute diarrheal disease caused by *Vibrio cholerae* serotype O1 or O139. Previously the term cholera referred to any acute severely dehydrating secretory diarrhea due to infectious or noninfectious cause.

HISTORY

The term cholera has ancient origin and is derived from a Greek word which means "flow of bile". Cholera like diseases have been mentioned in *Sushruta Samhita* in India, but it first gained attention in the year 1817 when first pandemic of cholera occurred from India to several other countries. Later in 1854, English physician John Snow started investigation on cholera after an outbreak in Soho, London. The organism responsible for cholera was discovered twice, first by Filippo Pacini an Italian physician and then by Robert Koch in India in the year 1883.

ETIOLOGIC AGENT

Vibrio cholerae are highly motile, facultative anaerobe, and comma-shaped gram-negative rods. The bacterium has single polar flagellum. It has flagellar H antigen and somatic O antigen.

Family: Vibrionaceae

Genus: *Brucella*

Species: *V. cholerae*

It has >200 serogroups of which only two serogroups are associated with epidemics of cholera, they are:

1. *V. cholerae* O1—2 biotypes:
   i. Classical → Inaba
   ii. El Tor → Ogawa
2. *V. cholerae* O139

EPIDEMIOLOGY

Cholera is responsible for seven global pandemics. The first six occurred between 1817 and 1923, the first six pandemics were most likely caused by *V. cholerae* O1 of classical type and the latest 21st century seventh pandemic of cholera is caused by El Tor type. In October 1992, an unexpected cholera epidemic occurred in Madras, India with subsequent cases being reported along the Bay of Bengal. The new serogroup O139 was responsible for this epidemic.

The natural habitat for cholera is coastal salt water and brackish estuaries. Humans are incidental host, but once infected act as vehicles for spread. Ingestion of contaminated water and food is the most common mode of transmission.

The infective dose for infection is relatively high (water 10^3 to 10^6 and food 10^2 to 10^4) except in conditions where gastric acidity is reduced like hypochlorhydria, those taking antacids, histamine blockers, and gastrectomy.

For unexplained reason, susceptibility to cholera is highest and least in blood group O and AB, respectively.

PATHOGENESIS

Pathogenesis is presented in **Figures 1 A** and **B**.

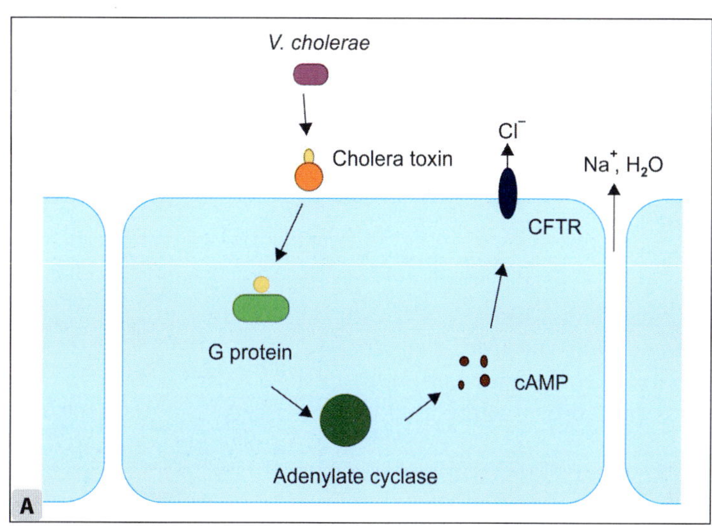

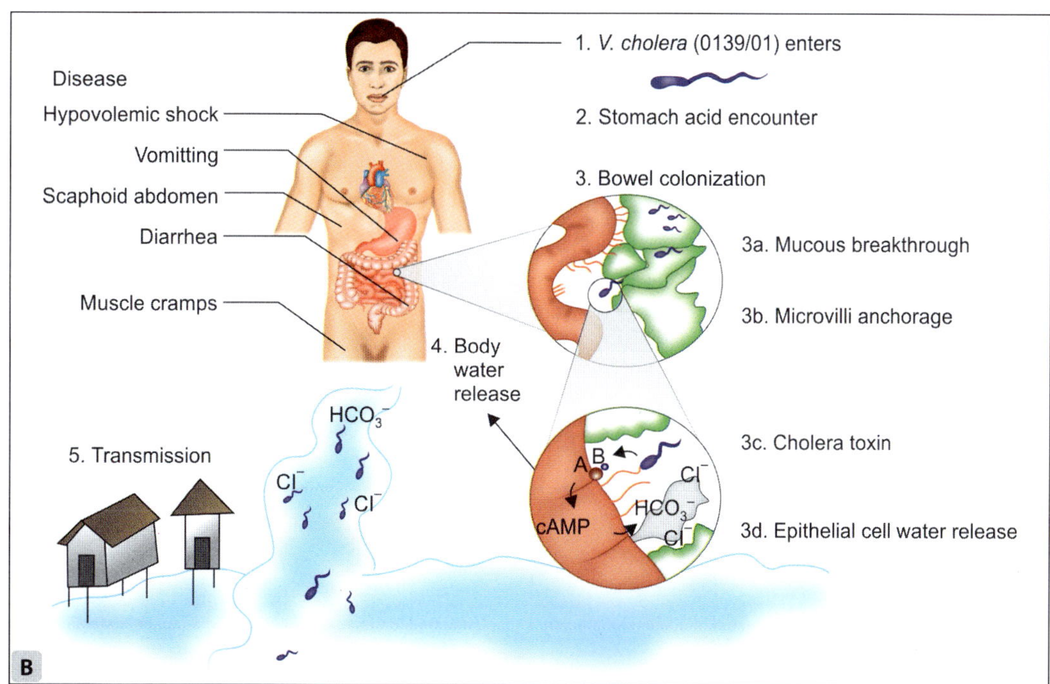

(cAMP: cyclic adenosine monophosphate; CFTR: cystic fibrosis transmembrane conductance regulator)

FIGURES 1 A & B: (A) Molecular image of cholera toxin; **(B)** Steps required for *Vibrio cholerae* to establish disease in the human host.

CLINICAL MANIFESTATIONS

- The hallmark of cholera is the production of watery diarrhea that may vary from mild diarrhea to severe and life-threatening diarrhea (*cholera gravis*).
- The onset is abrupt (incubation period is usually 24–48 h) and is characterized by watery diarrhea without strain, tenesmus, or prominent abdominal pain, followed or sometimes preceded by vomiting. Fever is seen in <5% of cases.
- In severe cases, stool volume may exceed 250 mL/kg in first 24 hours leading to hypovolemic shock, if not replenished with fluid.
- *Stool characteristics*: Nonbilious, grayish, slightly cloudy with flecks of mucus, and fishy in odor (rice watery).
- *Symptoms in relation to volume loss*:
  - Loss of <5% of body weight: Increases thirst
  - 5–10% loss: Postural hypotension, weakness, tachycardia, and decreased skin turgor
  - >10% loss: Weak or absent pulse, oliguria, sunken eyes, wrinkled skin (washerwoman skin), somnolence, and coma.
- *Cholera sicca*: Some patients do not present with diarrhea, but instead have abdominal distension and ileus.
- *Laboratory abnormalities*
- Increase in PCV, total protein
  - Prerenal azotemia
  - Metabolic acidosis with high anion gap
  - Low/normal potassium, sodium, and chloride levels
  - Hyperglycemia (due to high concentration of epinephrine, glucagon, and cortisol stimulated by hypovolemia)
- Acute tubular necrosis leading to acute renal failure.

LABORATORY INVESTIGATIONS

- *Stool culture*: Isolation of organism from stool or rectal swab is the definitive diagnosis. Transport medium is Cary-Blair and selective medium are thiosulfate-citrate-bile salts-sucrose (TCBS) agar or taurocholate-tellurite-gelatin (TTG) agar.
- *Dark-field microscopy*: Highly mobile (shooting star like) which can be inhibited by specific antiserum.
- *Rapid diagnostic tests*: The WHO recommends the use of cholera rapid diagnostic tests (RDTs) with a sensitivity of at least 90% and specificity of 85%.
- PCR test.

TREATMENT

Steps in the management of suspected cholera:

- Assessment for dehydration (**Table 4**)
- *Rehydrate, monitor, and reassess hydration*:
  - Severe dehydration (**Flowchart 4**)
  - Some dehydration:
    - Give oral rehydration solution (ORS) solutions of 2,200–4,000 mL for patients with 30 kg or more or older than 15 years.
    - Reassess every 4 hours
  - No dehydration:
    - Give ORS to take home and take orally as much as they desire.

TABLE 4 Assessment of the diarrhea patient for dehydration.

For interpretation	Symptoms	Signs
Severe dehydration	• Lethargic or unconscious; floppy • Eyes sunken and dry • Tears absent • Tongue very dry • Not able to drink or drinks poorly • Skin pinch goes back very slowly	Two of the following including one sign
Some dehydration	• Restless, irritable • Sunken eyes • Tears absent • Tongue dry • Thirsty, drinks eagerly	Two of the following including one sign
No dehydration		Not enough signs to classify in any

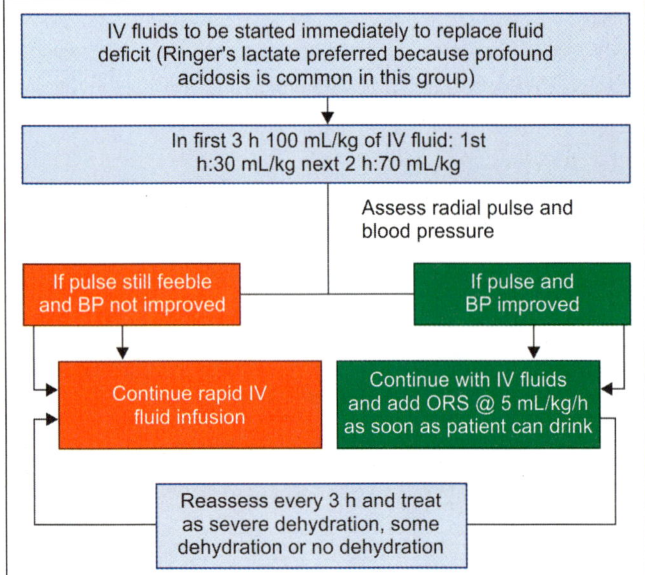

(BP: blood pressure; IV: intravenous; ORS: oral rehydration solution)

FLOWCHART 4: Treatment of severe dehydration.

- *Maintain hydration*: Infusion to be stopped if going on and continue with ORS. Requirement differs from person to person but average requirement in first 24 hours is 200 mL/kg.
- *Oral antibiotics to patients with severe dehydration*: It is seen that addition of antibiotics reduces the severity and duration of diarrhea.
  - Doxycycline—300 mg single dose
  - Cotrimoxazole—960 mg BD for 3 days
  - Azithromycin—1 g single dose
  - Ciprofloxacin—500 mg BD for 3 days
- Feed the patient

PLAGUE

Plague is a systemic zoonosis caused by *Yersinia pestis*.

ETIOLOGIC AGENT

Yersinia species are gram negative, nonlactose fermenting, and facultative anaerobes capable of growth at temperature ranging from 4 to 43°C.

Family: Enterobacteriaceae

Genus: *Yersinia*

Yersinia pestis, the causative agent for plague has emerged from the gut pathogen *Yersinia pseudotuberculosis* shortly after the first epidemic.

Biovars: Three biovars:

1. Antiqua
2. Mediaevalis
3. Orientalis

PATHOGENESIS

Pathogenesis of plague is presented in **Flowchart 5**.

EPIDEMIOLOGY

Plague, also known as "Black Death", is one of the greatest killers known to mankind. Worldwide, 12,503 cases were reported with 843 deaths over a period of 5 years (2004–2009). It was mainly confined to 16 countries of Africa (highest—97%), Asia, and America.

Reservoir: Wild rodents

Vector: Rat flea (**Fig. 2**)

CLINICAL MANIFESTATIONS

Bubonic plague:

Route: Bite of rat flea.

Incubation period: 2–6 days.

This is characterized by fever, malaise, dizziness, and painful regional lymphadenitis near flea bite. Lymph nodes are tender with boggy consistency with an underlying hard core. Most common site of bubo is inguinal, other sites include crural, axillary, and cervical. Untreated case may disseminate to cause secondary pneumonic plague and meningitis.

Mortality:

- Untreated: 50–90%
- Treated: 10–20%

Pneumonic plague:

Route: Aerosol inhalation.

Incubation period: 1–7 days.

This is characterized by sudden onset fever, headache, myalgia, vomiting, and dizziness. Cough with scanty sputum production, dyspnea, chest pain, and hemoptysis typically arises after 24 hours.

Mortality:

- Untreated: 100%
- Treated: 50%

Primary septicemic plague: This usually occurs secondary to bubonic/pneumonic plague. Around 10–25% of patients may present with septicemia, hypotension, and shock without preceding lymphadenopathy.

Mortality: 20–25%.

Others uncommon presentations of plague are meningitis (<6%) and plague pharyngitis.

DIAGNOSIS

Specimen: Bubo aspirate, bronchoalveolar lavage fluid or sputum, and blood.

- *Wayson stain*: Appears bipolar with a closed safety pin appearance.
- *Culture*: Done only in biosafety level III laboratory.
- *F1 antigen* detection by immunofluorescence.
- *Serology*: Antibodies appear by 2nd week.
- *Molecular method*: Most sensitive method which targets gene coding F1, pesticin gene.

TREATMENT

Antibiotic therapy for plague has been depitcted in **Table 5**.

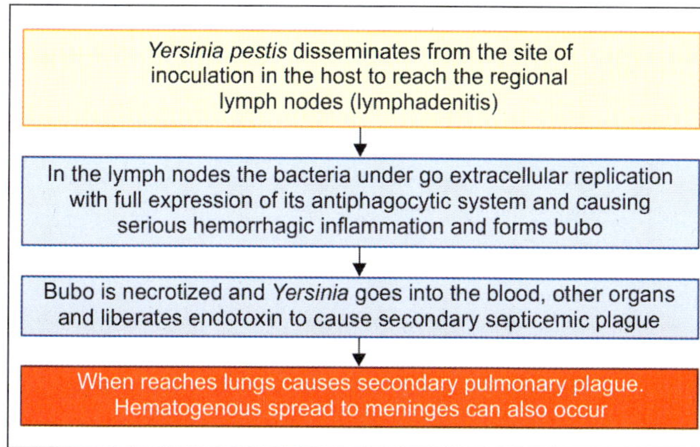

FLOWCHART 5: Pathogenesis of plague.

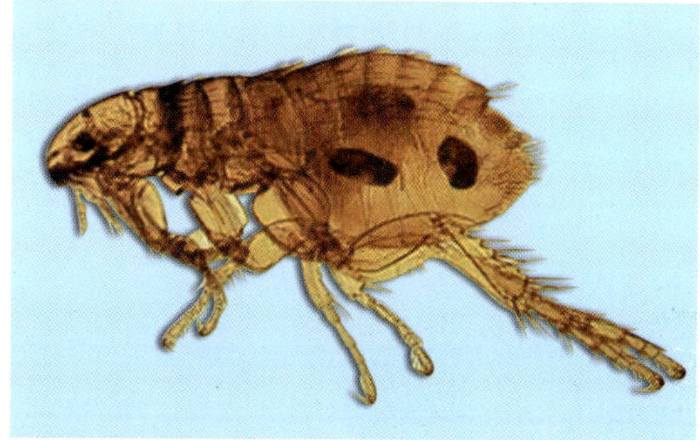

FIGURE 2: Rat flea.

TABLE 5 Antibiotic therapy for plague.

Drug	Dose (route)	Duration (days)
Streptomycin#	Adults: 1g q12h (IM) Child: 15 mg/kg q12 h (IM)	10–14
Gentamicin§	Adults: 5 mg/kg q24h (IM/ IV) Child: 5 mg/kg q24h (IM/IV)	10–14
Other effective drugs are: Levofloxacin, ciprofloxacin, moxifloxacin, doxycycline, chloramphenicol		

#Streptomycin is the parenteral treatment of choice for plague.

§Gentamicin is preferred over streptomycin by some experts because of wide adverse reaction profile of streptomycin.

PREVENTION

- *Postexposure prophylaxis*: Antimicrobial prophylaxis for a duration of 7 days, recommended for household, hospital other close contact (contact with a patient at <2 m) with persons with untreated pneumonic plague.
  - *Levofloxacin*:
    - Adult and child > 50 kg—500 mg q24h PO
    - Child < 50 kg and >6 months of age—16 mg/kg q12h PO (maximum 250 mg/dose)
  - *Alternatives*: Ciprofloxacin, doxycycline, and tetracycline
- *Pre-exposure prophylaxis*: The WHO recommends using vaccine only for prevention of an anticipated outbreak. Vaccine used is Sokhey's modification of Haffkine vaccine:
  - Two doses are given subcutaneously, 4 weeks apart
  - Booster—after 6 months
  - Contraindication—infants <6 months

RECOMMENDED READINGS

1. Pegues DA, Miller SI, Salmonellosis. In: Jameson J, Fauci AS, Kasper DL, Hauser SL, Longo DL, Loscalzo J (Eds). Harrison's Principles of Internal Medicine, 20th edition. New York: McGraw-Hill Education; 2018. pp. 1173-9.
2. Mogasale V, Maskery B, Ochiai RL, Lee JS, Mogasale VV, Ramani E, et al. Burden of typhoid fever in low-income and middle-income countries: a systematic, literature-based update with risk factor adjustment. Lancet Glob Health. 2014;2(10):e570-80.
3. Jenkins C, Gillespie SH, *Salmonella* infections. In: Cook GC, Zumla AI (Eds). Manson's Tropical Diseases, 22nd edition. Philadelphia: Saunders Elsevier; 2008. pp. 931-6.
4. Sastry AS, Bhatt KS. Enterobacteriaceae II: *Salmonella*. In: Sastry AS, Bhatt S (Eds). Essentials of Medical Microbiology, 2nd edition. New Delhi: Jaypee Brothers Medical Publishers (P) Ltd. ; 2019. pp. 330-9.
5. Taneja N, Mewara A. Shigellosis: Epidemiology in India. Indian J Med Res. 2016;143(5):565-76.
6. Sansonetti PJ, Bergounioux J. (2018). Shigellosis. In: Jameson J, Fauci AS, Kasper DL, Hauser SL, Longo DL, Loscalzo J (Eds). Harrison's Principles of Internal Medicine, 20th edition. New York: McGraw-Hill Education; 2008. pp. 1180-3.
7. Dupont HL. *Shigella* species (bacillary dysentery). In: Mandell GL (Ed). Principles and Practice of Infectious Diseases, 6th edition. Churchill, Livingstone: Elsevier; 2005. pp. 2655-9.
8. Young EJ. (2005). *Brucella* species. In: Mandell GL (Ed). Principles and Practice of Infectious Diseases, 6th edition. Churchill, Livingstone: Elsevier; 2005. pp. 2669-72.
9. Waldor MK, Ryan ET. Cholera and other vibrioses. In: Jameson J, Fauci AS, Kasper DL, Hauser SL, Longo DL, Loscalzo J (Eds). Harrison's Principles of Internal Medicine, 20th edition. New York: McGraw-Hill Education; 2018. pp. 1186-91.
10. Seas C, Gotuzzo E. (2005). *Vibrio cholerae*. In: Mandell GL (Ed). Principles and Practice of Infectious Diseases, 6th edition. Churchill, Livingstone: Elsevier; 2005. pp, 2536-42.
11. WHO. (2020). Management of the patient with cholera. [online] Available from https://www.who.int/topics/cholera/publications/WHO_CDD_SER_91_15/en/.
12. Achtman M, Zurth K, Morelli G, Torrea G, Guiyoule A, Carniel E. Yersinia pestis, the cause of plague, is a recently emerged clone of *Yersinia pseudotuberculosis*. Proc Natl Acad Sci USA. 1999;96(24): 14043-8.
13. Prentice MB. Plague and other Yersinia infections. In: Jameson J, Fauci AS, Kasper DL, Hauser SL, Longo DL, Loscalzo J (Eds). Harrison's Principles of Internal Medicine, 20th edition. New York: McGraw-Hill Education; 2018. pp. 1200-8.
14. Prentice MB, Rahalison L. Plague. Lancet. 2007; 369(9568):1196-207.
15. Sastry AS, Bhatt KS. Enterobacteriaceae I: tribe Yersinieae. In: Sastry AS, Bhatt S (Eds). Essentials of Medical Microbiology, 2nd edition. New Delhi: Jaypee Brothers Medical Publishers (P) Ltd.; 2019. pp. 325-7.

CHAPTER 44 Tetanus, Botulism, and Other Clostridial Infections

Priyam Batra, KVP Saikiran, Rama Chaudhry

ABSTRACT

Anaerobic bacteria are a part of the normal flora/microbiota specially of the mucosal surfaces and thus cause various infections whenever there is a breach in the mucosal barrier leading to leak of the indigenous flora into sterile normal sites. We have witnessed a variety of anaerobic infections in the past decades, yet handling specimens, cultivation, and identification has been a challenge.

Some infections like those caused by *Clostridium tetani* and *C. botulinum* have limited role in early laboratory diagnosis as their diagnosis is mainly clinical. Both these diseases are because of intoxication resulting in neurological effects yet their clinical pictures are different as they target their respective different cells in the central nervous system (CNS). The clinical picture and laboratory diagnosis of *C. difficile* is different as it is a complication of continuous or long-term antibiotic treatment that leads to antibiotic associated diarrhea and colitis that may be further complicated with toxic megacolon, perforation, and sepsis. Hence, diagnosing these diverse clinical conditions is a challenge and having a thorough knowledge on these aspects would help in early diagnosis of these conditions and better early patient management.

"Neglect is a major reason for some of the most painful experience we suffer in life"

—S Adelaja

INTRODUCTION

- The genus *Clostridium* comprises of anaerobic gram-positive spore forming (bulging) bacilli belonging to phylum Firmicutes.
- They are present ubiquitously in soil, decaying matter, intestines of humans and animals.
- They can be present as commensal or can also be pathogenic causing varied range of diseases including skin and soft tissue infections, myonecrosis, food poisoning, and diarrhea.
- *Clostridioides difficile* can cause diarrhea, pseudomembrane colitis; *Clostridium tetani* can cause tetanus; *C. botulinum* causes botulism (infant/food/wound/inhalational); *C. perfringens* can cause gas gangrene and food poisoning.
- Patient's history (mode of injury—road traffic accident/soiled wound) and examination (deep seated abscess/site of infection in proximity to mucosal surfaces/presence of gas or crepitus/foul smelling discharge) can indicate a possible underlying anaerobic infection.
- Being anaerobes, they require media providing lower redox potential for their growth.
- In addition, transport of the samples requires protection from exposure to atmospheric oxygen and can be done via transport media containing reducing agents or in CO_2 vials.
- Robertson's cooked meat (RCM) medium can be used for transport as well as for culture of anaerobes. The glutathione and unsaturated fatty acids present in the meat particles provide reduced environment for the anaerobic bacteria to grow. Further, proteolytic species change the color of the meat particles to black while it remains pink in case of saccharolytic species.
- The anaerobic conditions can be maintained by the use of anaerobic jars (McIntosh and Fildes' anaerobic jar); or anaerobic glove box with mixture of gases (80% nitrogen, 10% hydrogen and 10% carbon dioxide); or by using gas pack systems; or prereduced anaerobically sterilized (PRAS) media.
- The general algorithm followed in laboratory diagnosis is shown in **Flowchart 1**.

TETANUS (CLOSTRIDIUM TETANI)

INTRODUCTION

Clostridium tetani, causative agent of "tetanus"—a persistent tonic spastic skeletal muscle disease with derangement in autonomic nervous system. It is an obligate anaerobic, gram-positive bacillus with terminal spherical spore. It is ubiquitous in nature, widely distributed in manure soil, intestine of animals, hospital environment etc.

Tetanus was well known since ancient times described by Egyptians and Greeks. Active immunization with tetanus toxoid was described by Behring and Kitasato.

EPIDEMIOLOGY

In developing countries, although the incidence rates are decreasing in recent times, yet tetanus has a mortality

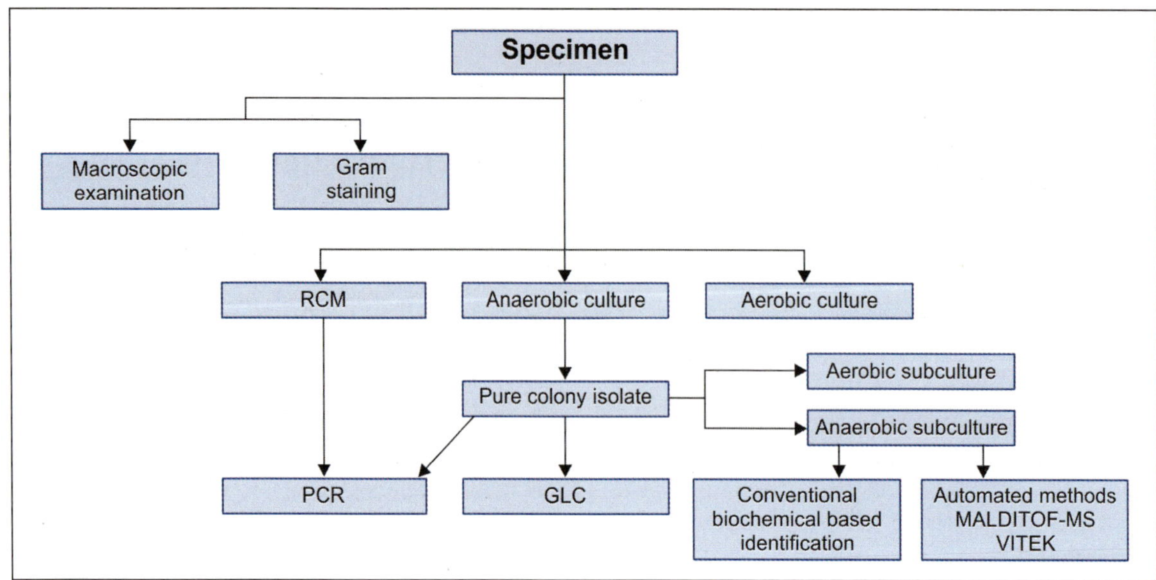

(GLC: gas liquid chromatography; MALDITOF-MS: matrix-assisted laser desorption ionization-time of flight mass spectrometry; PCR: polymerase chain reaction; RCM: Robertson's cooked meat)

FLOWCHART 1: Laboratory diagnosis of anaerobic culture samples.

rates of 28/100,000 with neonatal infection causing 40% of tetanus cases. Widespread immunization of infants and pregnant mothers have reduced the incidence to a larger extent.

Mode of Transmission of *C. tetani* spores is given in **Table 1**.

TABLE 1 Mode of transmission of spores of *Clostridium tetani.*

By injuries	By aseptic procedures
• Punctured wounds • Superficial abrasions • Road traffic accidents	• Surgeries • Following abortions • In neonates: Unhygienic delivery practices, umbilical stump infection, and inadequately immunized mother

VIRULENCE

Clostridium tetani produces two exotoxins (zinc dependent matrix metalloproteinases category) — tetanospasmin and tetanolysin. The characteristics of both these toxins is given in **Table 2**.

Mechanism of action: The mechanism of action tetanus toxin (tetanospasmin) is shown in **Figure 1**.

Clinical Manifestations: Incubation period is 3–21 days, after that the disease manifests early phase which later progresses to advanced disease and autonomic hyperactivity. The various clinical features of the various stages of the disease and the various complications seen is given in **Table 3**. The various diseases which can have similar manifestations is given in **Table 4**.

TABLE 2 Characteristics of tetanospasmin and tetanolysin toxins.

Tetanospasmin (or tetanus toxin)	Tetanolysin
• Causes disease manifestations and toxin is neurotoxic in nature • It is oxygen stable, heat labile toxin encoded on a plasmid that is present in all toxigenic strains • Toxin is a 151 kDa polypeptide chain cleaved to produce heavy chain (involves binding to cell surface receptors) and light chains (presynaptic inhibition of transmitter release) joined by a disulfide bond • It is antigenic, can be toxoided with loss of virulence, and hence used for vaccine preparation	• It is a heat labile and oxygen labile hemolysin • It is of uncertain importance in the pathogenesis of tetanus

LABORATORY DIAGNOSIS

Tetanus is diagnosed clinically. Laboratory testing provides supportive evidence for confirmation. The various methods for diagnosis are given in **Table 5**.

MANAGEMENT

Stabilization: At presentation:

- Management of ventilation and airway
- Get immunization history
- Diphenhydramine (50 mg, IV)/benztropine (1–2 mg, IV) administration for ruling out dopamine-blocking agent causing dystonic reaction.
- For controlling spasms and to decrease rigidity: diazepam 5 mg increments/lorazepam 2 mg increments.

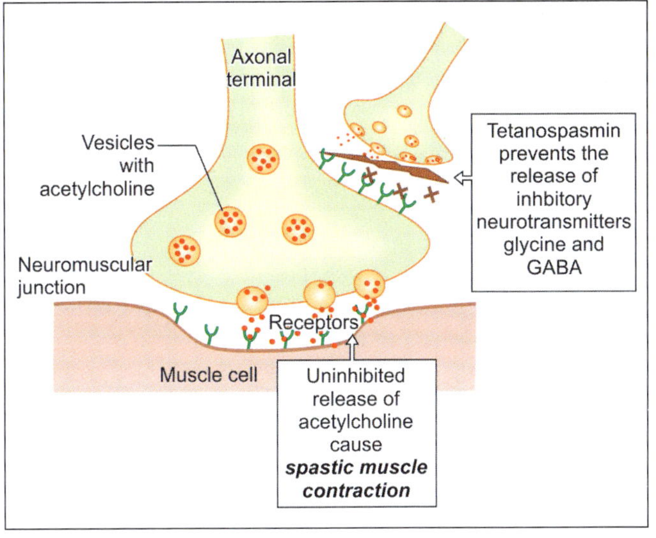

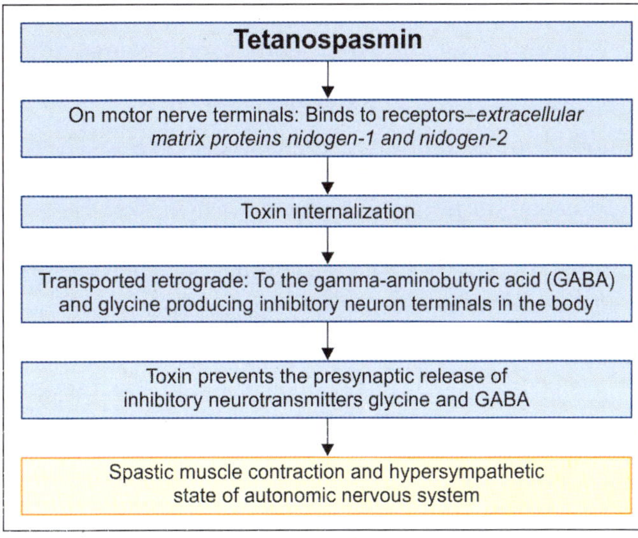

FIGURE 1: Mechanism of action of tetanospasmin at the level of neuromuscular junction.

TABLE 3 Clinical manifestations and complications of tetanus.

Early disease	Advanced disease	Autonomic hyperactivity	Complications
• Incubation period: 3–21 days • Trismus or locked jaw (masseter rigidity): First symptom • Muscle stiffness • Back pain • Difficulty in swallowing • Neonates: Feeding difficulty and apnea	• Generalized painful muscle spasm • Descending spastic paralysis • Deep tendon reflexes are exaggerated • Limb extremities generally unaffected	Maximal during the second week of severe disease: • Hypertension • Tachycardia • Intestinal stasis • Sweating • Increased tracheal secretions • Acute renal failure etc.	• Risus sardonicus: Sustained abnormal spasm of the facial muscles→grinning • Opisthotonos position: Generalized spastic contraction of the extensor muscles→Abnormal body posture • Respiratory muscles spasm: Airway obstruction

TABLE 4 Differential diagnosis of tetanus

Symptom	Differential diagnosis
Trismus	• Dental pathology • Hypercalcemia • Temporomandibular disease
Spasms	• Intracranial lesions/hemorrhages • Strychnine poisoning • Drug induced dystonic reactions (e.g., phenothiazines, metoclopramide)
Neck stiffness and rigid abdomen	• Meningitis/encephalitis • Rabies • Muscle spasm
Dysphagia	• Acute pharyngeal disease • Peritonsillar abscess
Neonatal tetanus	• Sepsis • Meningitis • Convulsions

TABLE 5 Methods of laboratory diagnosis of *Clostridium tetani*.

Gram staining	Gram-positive bacilli with terminal and round spores: *Drum stick appearance*
Culture	• Clinically has no significance because a positive culture does not indicate whether the organism contains the toxin-producing plasmid • Robertson cooked meat broth: They are asaccharolytic but proteolytic organisms hence turn the meat particles black and produce foul odor • Blood agar: Produces characteristic swarming growth incubated under anaerobic conditions, at 37°C for 24–48 h
Toxigenicity test	Can be done as: • Mouse inoculation test in vivo • Hemolysis inhibition test in vitro

Management at first 24 hours (early):

- Human-tetanus immunoglobulin (Ig) administration 500 U, IM/pooled immune globulin administered IV alternatively
- Administer diphtheria-tetanus (DT) vaccine 0.5 mL/ diphtheria-pertussis-tetanus (DPT) vaccine (0.5 mL) at different site intramuscularly
- Metronidazole 500 mg, IV, 6 hourly for 7–10 days
- If spasms lead to airway compromise, do tracheostomy
- Benzodiazepines for controlling spasms

Management over next 2–3 weeks (intermediate):

- Labetalol 0.5–2 mg/min or morphine 0.5–1 mg/kg/h continuous infusion for treating sympathetic hyperactivity
- Saline resuscitation in case of hypotension
- Begin prophylactic heparin
- Maintain benzodiazepines until spasms diminish substantially. Then taper over 14–21 days.

Management next 2–6 weeks (convalescent stage):

- Begin physical therapy when spasms terminate
- Another dose of DPT/DT vaccine at discharge
- 4 weeks after the second, third and last dose of toxoid is to be given

IMMUNITY WANING

Waning of tetanus immunity happens with aging according to recent serologic analysis. The seropositivity was noted to go down to 28% by 70 years of age whereas 6 to 39 year aged individuals have around 80% protective antibodies. Therefore tetanus diphtheria toxoid (Td) booster is recommended for all adults every 10 years.

BOTULISM

Botulism comes from "botulus" in Latin which means sausage. It refers to an outbreak that occurred back in the 19th century in a town in Southern Germany, where hundreds of patients developed poisoning characterized by paralytic illnesses which was found related to sausage.

- Botulism can be of different types—foodborne, infant, wound and rarely may also be caused by inhalation.
- Due to its association with food poisoning, foodborne botulism can present in outbreaks while the other types of botulism present as sporadic cases.

CLOSTRIDIUM BOTULINUM

- *C. botulinum* is a gram-positive anaerobe.
- It produces a botulinum toxin that causes flaccid paralysis that results in botulism.
- It is present ubiquitously and as a saprophyte in soil, manure, fruits and vegetables.
- *C. botulinum* has been divided into four phenotypic groups (I to IV) and seven toxinotypes A to G.
- The I and II *C. botulinum* groups cause human disease while group III causes botulism in animals. Group I has been known to produce A, B, and F toxin while group II produces B, E, or F toxin.
- Though one strain produces one type of toxin, multiple toxin producing strains have also been reported.
- Other *Clostridial* species like *C. butyricum* (type E toxin) and *C. baratii* (type F toxin) can also cause botulism.

BOTULINUM TOXIN

- 150–165 kDa
- Zinc-dependent metalloproteinase
- Most potent and most lethal toxin known in nature
- Category A bioterrorism agent as per the Centers for Disease Control and Prevention (CDC)
- The toxin consists of a 100-kDa heavy chain which is linked via a disulfide bond to a 50-kDa light chain.
- Heavy chain helps in binding of this toxin to the presynaptic surface of the cholinergic neurons and its translocation.
- The light chain interacts with the proteins like synaptosomal associated protein (SNAP) 25, syntaxin, vesicle-associated membrane protein and prevents fusion of acetylcholine vesicle with the presynaptic membrane.
- Inhibition of fusion of these vesicles prevents release of acetylcholine in the neuromuscular junction leading to flaccid paralysis (**Fig. 2**).

PATHOGENESIS

- Pathogenesis of foodborne botulism differs from that of infant and wound botulism.
- Ingestion of the preformed toxin can cause foodborne botulism.
- While infant botulism results from ingestion of the spores.
- Wound botulism is caused following inoculation and germination of spores at the site of injury followed by production of toxin.

CLINICAL MANIFESTATIONS

Foodborne botulism:

- Symptoms can begin as soon as 6 hours but usually after 18–36 hours consumption of contaminated food containing the preformed toxin.
- Homemade canned foods are often the implicated source.
- The cases may be sporadic or occur in small outbreaks.
- The symptoms include nausea and vomiting, pain abdomen, diarrhea, dryness of mouth and descending flaccid paralysis.

Infant botulism:

- Following ingestion of spores in food or honey by an infant of <12 months age, that germinate releasing toxin and its manifestations results in infant botulism.
- The clinical manifestations include weakness, difficulties in feeding, irritability, weak cry, constipation, generalized weakness, poor muscle tone, and floppy neck giving a typical picture of a "**Floppy child**".

Wound botulism:

- The signs and symptoms are similar to foodborne botulism including double vision, drooping of eyelids,

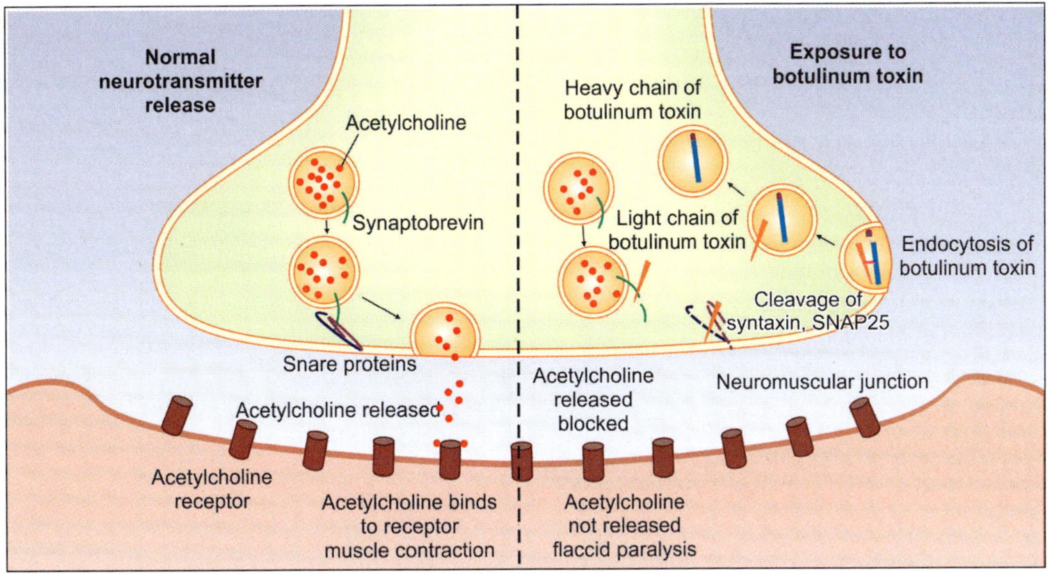

FIGURE 2: **Mechanism of action of *Clostridium botulinum* infection.**

mouth dryness, difficulty in swallowing, and muscle weakness, except that there are no gastrointestinal symptoms.

- Difficulty in breathing and paralysis develop in severe cases.

Uses of botulinum toxin:

- Botulinum toxin has been exploited and used in highly diluted form in the cosmetic industry.
- In addition, it has also been used in treatment of various neurological disorders like cervical dystonia, blepharospasm, chronic pain syndromes etc.

LABORATORY DIAGNOSIS

Botulism can be a life-threatening condition. Typical clinical features can aid in the diagnosis of the patient. Suspected food articles, feces, wound swabs, and tissue can be used for diagnosis.

Gram staining and culture:

- They are gram-positive bacilli with subterminal oval spores.
- Culture can be performed on brain heart infusion (BHI) blood agar and egg yolk agar and requires incubation under anaerobic conditions.
- Colonies of group I on blood agar are 2–6 mm in diameter with irregular margin and a raised center and have a narrow zone of hemolysis. While group II colonies are 1–3 mm, translucent to semiopaque with a narrow zone of hemolysis. The margins are a bit irregular and lobate, the surface is matt and a mosaic structure in oblique light may be noted.
- The lipase activity can be demonstrated by presence of the iridescent sheen on and around colonies on egg yolk agar.
- Further identification may be done conventionally or by automated platforms.

Toxin demonstration:

- Mouse bioassay:
  - The laboratory mice are injected by the diluted sample by an intraperitoneal injection. In case the sample contains the toxin, the mouse develops muscle weakness, respiratory failure, and other signs of botulism within a day postinoculation.
- *Enzyme immunoassays*: Enzyme-linked immunosorbent assays (ELISAs) are also available for detection of botulinum toxin. They are the commonly used immunoassays for detection of the botulinum toxin.

Molecular detection:

- Detection of the *BoNT* genes by conventional or a multiplex polymerase chain reaction (PCR) assay provide sensitive and specific mode of diagnosis as compared to culture and mouse bioassay.
- However, a PCR can only indicate the presence of gene and cannot comment on the activity of the gene product or toxin.

MANAGEMENT

- Botulism can be a life-threatening condition hence prompt treatment is important.
- Symptomatic treatment and extensive supportive care including intubation and mechanical ventilation may be needed in case of respiratory distress and paralysis.
- Cleaning and debridement of the wound in case of wound botulism may be needed.

Botulinum antitoxin:

- The antitoxin can bind to the circulating botulinum toxin and prevent its binding.
- Though it can prevent further deterioration of the symptoms, it cannot reverse the effects of already bound toxin. Hence early administration of the antitoxin becomes crucial.

- Heptavalent botulinum antitoxin:
  - Equine origin
  - Approved by the Food and Drug Administration (FDA) in 2013
  - Consists of antibodies against all toxin types, except type H
  - Because of the equine origin, there is a risk of sensitization to equine proteins and anaphylaxis
  - Not approved for use in infants
- Human botulinum immune globulin
  - Approved by FDA in 2003
  - Can be used in infants

CLOSTRIDIODES DIFFICILE INFECTION

Definition: *Clostridiodes difficile* infection (CDI), a distinct colonic disease, is generally associated with prolonged duration of hospitalization caused by the overuse of antimicrobials leading to disruption of composition and functionality of normal colonic flora along with CDI. However, *C. difficile* accounts for only one-forth of the cases of antibiotic associated diarrhea, the others being caused by infection with *Staphylococcus aureus* or *Klebsiella oxytoca* or due to disruption of the normal colonic epithelium.

ETIOLOGY AND PATHOGENESIS

C. difficile, a gram-positive spore bearing obligate anaerobe, has the following risk factors implicated in its causation (also given in **Box 1**). A flowchart of the CDI is given in **Flowchart 2**.

BOX 1 Risk factors for development of *Clostridium difficile* infection.

- Antibiotic exposure
  - Number of antibiotics
  - Duration of antibiotic therapy
- Type of antibiotic
  - Highest risk: Clindamycin, Fluoroquinolones, and second and third generation cephalosporins
  - Moderate risk: Penicillin, macrolides, beta lactam/beta lactam inhibitor combination, carbapenems, vancomycin, and metronidazole
  - Lowest risk: Aminoglycosides, tetracycline, trimethoprim, sulfonamides, and rifampin
- Use of proton pump inhibitors and histamine type 2 blockers
- Patient age: Elderly at increased risk
- Prior hospitalization and duration of hospitalization
- Long-term care residency
- Severity of underlying illness
- Abdominal surgery and nasogastric tube insertion

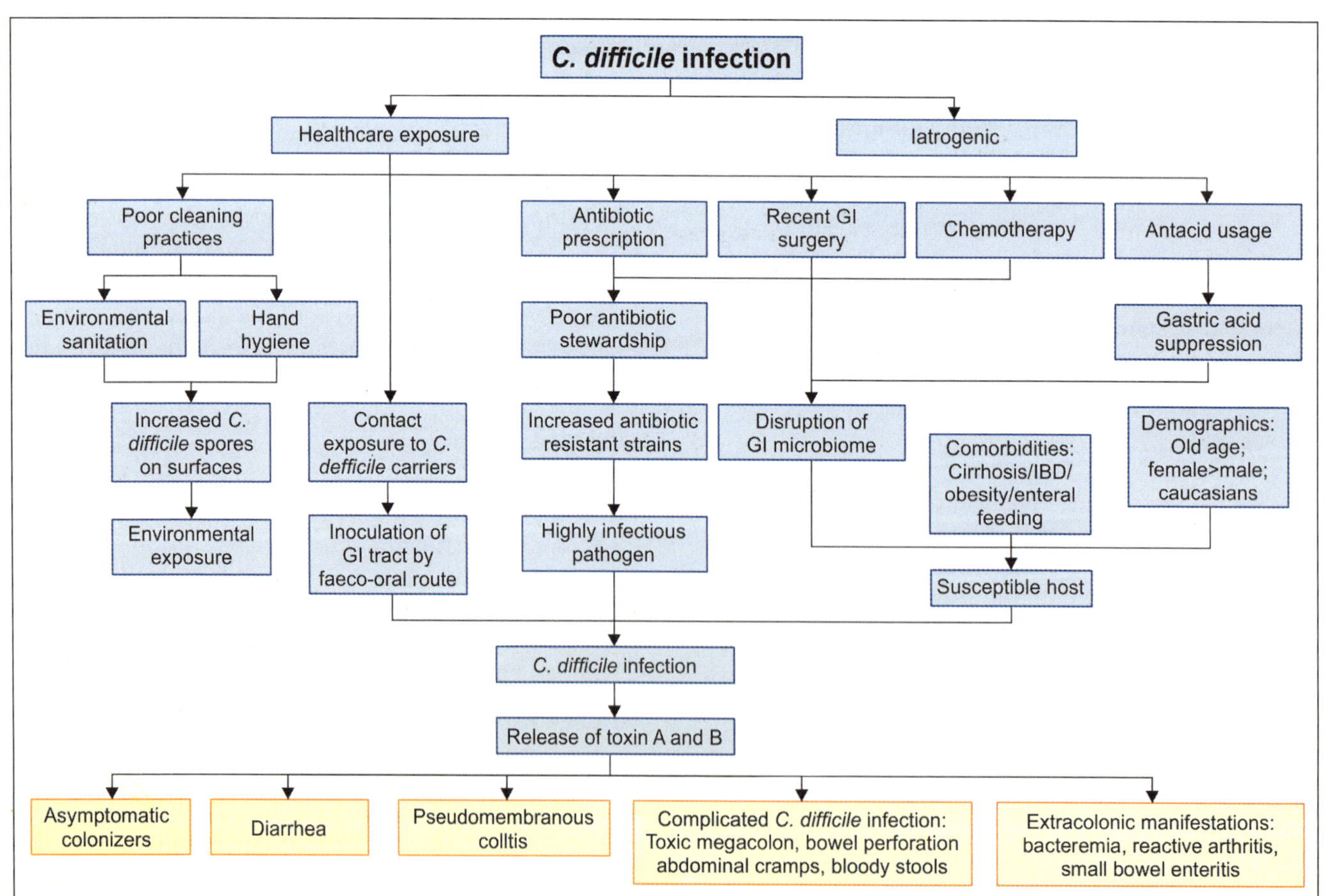

FLOWCHART 2: Profile of Clostridium difficile infection.

- *Prolonged hospital stay*: It is found in the nature specially in that of the hospital and chronic care facilities. However, <10% cases have also been seen to be from the community.
- *Prolonged antimicrobial usage and colonization resistance*: The excessive antibiotic intake disrupts the normal colonic gut flora which disrupts the gut homeostasis and the colonization resistance of *C. difficile*. The presence of normal gut microbial flora maintains colonization resistance by competition for nutrients, occupancy of the niches, antimicrobial peptide production, and host immune system signaling. The class of drugs being implicated in the causation of CDI are enlisted in **Box 1**.
- *C. difficile* sporulation, germination, and toxin production:
  - Spores (resistant to alcohol-based hand rubs) are ingested from hospital environment
  - Germination in the gut due to primary bile acids such as taurocholic acid. Bile acid analogues may have preventive role in germination
  - They produce toxins such as toxin A (enterotoxin) and toxin B (cytotoxin), which cause disruption of the epithelial cells
  - Binary toxin related to *C. perfringens* iota toxin→ produced by NAP1/B1/027 strains
  - **Figure 3** illustrates the mechanism of action of the toxins.
- Host immune response may determine the outcome of the infection.
  - Persons developing strong IgG response to toxin A become asymptomatic carriers.
  - Persons with inadequate IgG response to toxin A develop disease.
  - Infants do not develop symptoms despite having CDI as they lack the toxin receptors on mucosa. These receptors develop later in life.
- *Other risk factors*: Include older age, underlying illness, intestinal surgery, use of electronic rectal thermometers, and antacid treatment.
- *Recurrent CDI*: Conditions predisposing to recurrent CDI include—
  - Pathogen characteristics: Infection with NAP1/BI/027 *C. difficile* strain due to increased antibiotic resistance (especially quinolone resistance), presence of additional binary toxin, presence of deletion mutation in the *tcdC* gene leading to overproduction of ToxB, and increased ability to sporulate thus increasing the ability to spread in the healthcare system
  - Inability to restore the gut microbiota

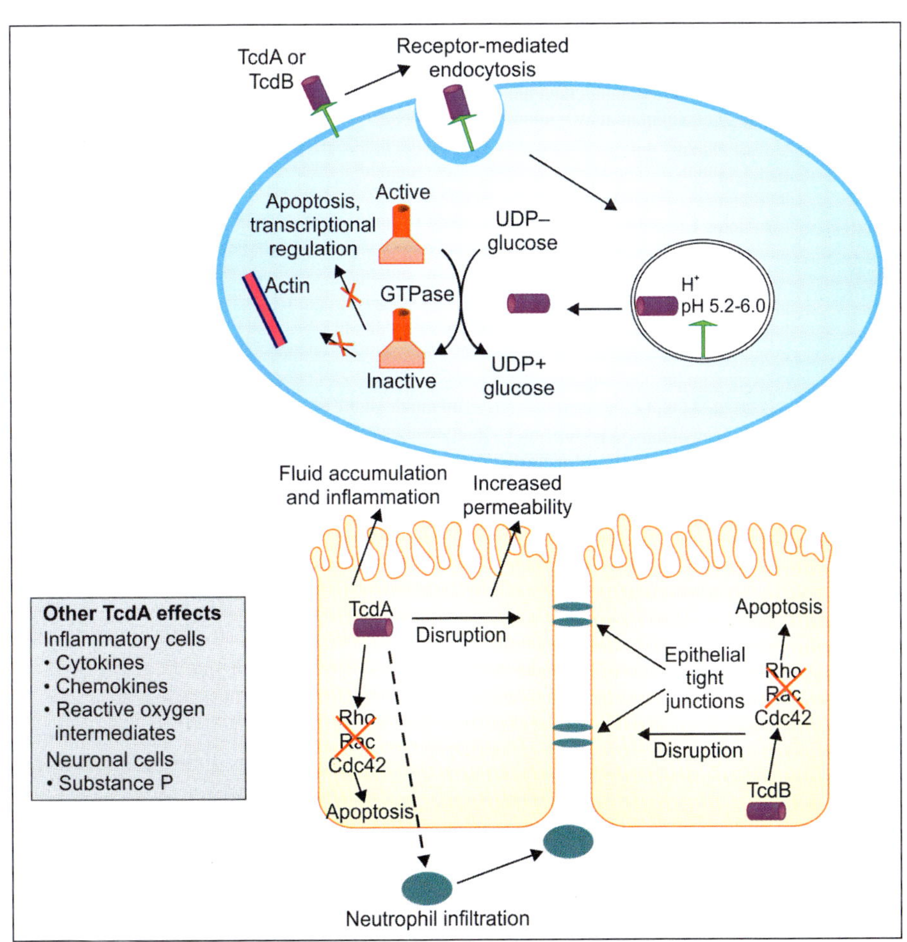

FIGURE 3: Mechanism of action of *Clostridium difficile* toxins.

CLINICAL MANIFESTATIONS

- *Diarrhea*: Most common manifestation, up to 20 bowel movements per day. Characterized by soft, not formed to watery or mucoid consistency of stool and characteristic odor. Often associated with fever (28% cases), abdominal pain (22% cases), and leukocytosis (50% cases) with leukemoid reaction.
- *Adynamic ileus*: This is seen on X-ray in ~20% cases and is characterized by cessation of passage of stool and unexplained leukocytosis (>15,000 WBC/μL).
- *Pseudomembranous colitis*: There is colitis which is associated with the formation of pseudomembrane composed of necrotic leukocytes, mucus, fibrin, and cellular debris. It attaches to the underlying mucosa and is seen as a whitish yellow plaque approximately 1–2 mm in size. But at times, the size may be large enough to spread over the entire colonic mucosa.
- *Complicated CDI*: This is characterized by leukocytosis (>25,000/mm), hypoalbuminemia, and elevated serum creatinine. May be associated with toxic megacolon (acute dilatation of colon >6 cm), intestinal perforation, and acute peritonitis.

LABORATORY DIAGNOSIS

Criterion for confirming diagnosis: A combination of clinical criteria, i.e.,

- Diarrhea characterized by ≥3 unformed stools in 24 h for ≥2 days with no other identifiable cause plus
- Toxin B detected in the stool by ELISA or PCR or genexpert
- Presence of pseudomembranes in the colon.

Stool culture: Involves anaerobic culture of stool samples at 37°C for 24–48 hours using *C. difficile* selective media such as cycloserine cefoxitin fructose agar (CCFA). *C. difficile* may be present as gut colonizer, therefore simultaneous detection of toxin production is more important.

Toxin demonstration: Toxin detection is done using the following methods:

- *Cell culture cytotoxicity assay*: Dilutions of supernatants of the stool are placed on the cell culture lines and incubated for 24–48 hours. This is followed by observation for cell rounding. Neutralization with *C. difficile* or *C. sordelli* antitoxin is performed to confirm that the rounding is due to *C. difficile* toxin. This test is very specific but lacks sensitivity. Not cost effective.
- Stool ELISA for toxin A detection or toxins A and B detection.
- *Stool ELISA/latex agglutination test for detection of glutamate dehydrogenase (GDH)*: GDH antigen is present in *C. difficile* strains (**Flowchart 3**). This test is very sensitive but lacks specificity.
- Stool ELISA for toxin B detection or toxins A and B detection.
- *PCR for C. difficile toxin A as well as B*: This is sensitive as well as specific test.

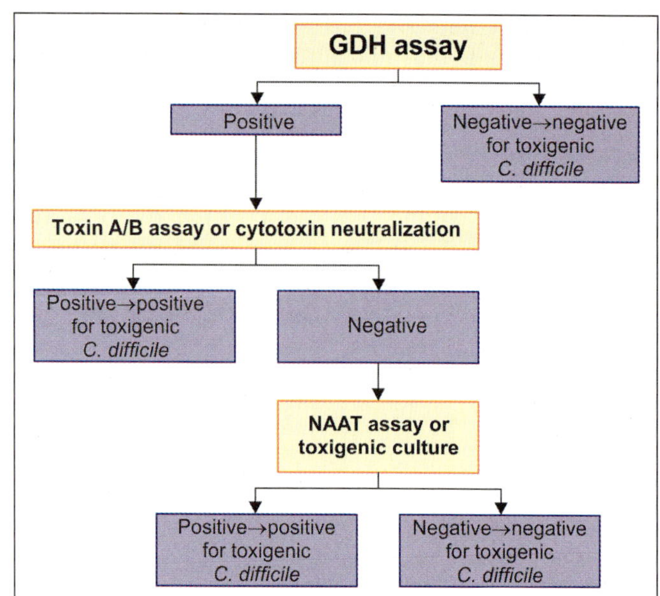

(*C. difficile*: *Clostridium difficile*; GDH: glutamate dehydrogenase)

FLOWCHART 3: Laboratory diagnosis of *C. difficile* infection using three test algorithm.

- *Genexpert*: For the detection of toxigenic strain of *C. difficile* and also the *C. difficile* NAP1/BI/027 strain.

Colonoscopy or sigmoidoscopy: It is highly specific if pseudomembranes are present; lack sensitivity in the absence of the same.

A flowchart for the diagnosis of CDI is given in **Figure 3**.

TREATMENT

The primary goal of successful treatment is cure of the patient symptoms and the secondary goal is prevention of recurrent CDI. It has been seen that *C. difficile* persists in the stool of majority of the patients despite successful treatment for 6 weeks or more. Therefore, there is no need of repeat stool testing after treatment as a "test of cure". The treatment can be summarized as given in **Table 6**.

PREVENTION

Prevention of *C. difficile* spore transmission can be achieved by:

- *Prevention of C. difficile transmission to the patient*: By following regular hand hygiene practices (using soap and water for hand wash as alcohol-based hand rubs do not kill *C. difficile* spores) and following standard precautions which includes regular wearing of gloves.
- Removal of *C. difficile* spores from the environment by using bleach for cleaning.
- Judicious use of antimicrobials specially clindamycin, fluoroquinolones, cephalosporins, and aminoglycosides.
- *Preventing development of CDI despite acquisition of C. difficile spores*: This involves the use of *C. difficile* vaccines, monoclonal antibodies directed against *C. difficile* toxins, and use of probiotics. However, this approach is under investigation.

TABLE 6 Treatment recommendations for *Clostridium difficile* Infection (CDI).

Clinical definition	Supportive clinical data	Recommended treatment[a]
Initial setting, non-severe	Leukocytosis with WBC count ≤15,000 cells/mL and serum creatinine <1.5 mg/dL	• VAN 125 mg given 4 times daily for 10 days, OR • FDX 200 mg given twice daily for 10 days • If above agents unavailable: MTX 500 mg 3 times a day for 10 days
Initial episode, severe	Leukocytosis with WBC count ≥15,000 cells/mL and serum creatinine >1.5 mg/dL	• VAN 125 mg given 4 times daily for 10 days, OR • FDX 200 mg given twice daily for 10 days
Initial episode, fulminant	Hypotension or shock; ileus; megacolon	• VAN 500 mg 4 times a day by mouth or by nasogastric tube • If ileus is present, add rectal instillation of VAN with intravenous VAN 500 mg every 8 hours
First recurrence		• VAN 125 mg given 4 times daily for 10 days if metronidazole was used in the first episode, OR • Use a prolonged tapered and pulsed VAN regimen if the standard regimen was used for the initial episode, OR • FDX 200 mg given twice daily for 10 days if VAN was used for the initial episode
Second or subsequent recurrences		• VAN in a tapered and pulsed regimen, OR • VAN 125 mg given 4 times daily for 10 days followed by rifaximin 400 mg 3 times daily for 20 days, OR • FDX 200 mg given twice daily for 10 days, OR • Faecal microbiota transplantation

[a] If delayed response is observed, then extending the treatment duration to 14 days should be considered.

(FDX : fidaxomicin, MTX: Metronidazole; VAN: vancomycin; WBC: White Blood cells)

ACKNOWLEDGMENT

We are thankful to Dr Swati Khullar, senior resident, department of microbiology, AIIMS, New Delhi for helping us prepare this chapter.

RECOMMENDED READINGS

1. World Health Organization, United Nations Population Fund & United Nations Children's Fund (UNICEF). Maternal and Neonatal Tetanus Elimination by 2005: Strategies for Achieving and Maintaining Elimination. New York: UNICEF; 2000.
2. McQuillan GM, Kruszon-Moran D, Deforest A, Chu SY, Wharton M. Serologic immunity to diphtheria and tetanus in the United States. Ann Intern Med. 2002;136(9):660-6.
3. Bennett JE, Dolin R, Blaser MJ. Mandell Douglas and Bennett's Principles and Practice of Infectious Diseases, 9th Edition. Netherlands: Elsevier; 2019.
4. Centers for Disease Control and Prevention. Tetanus surveillance—United States, 2001–2008. MMWR Morb Mortal Wkly Rep. 2011;60(12):365-9.
5. Expanded programme on immunization. The global elimination of neonatal tetanus: progress to date. Wkly Epidemiol Rec. 1993;68(38):277-82.
6. Bruggemann H, Baumer S, Fricke WF, Wiezer A, Liesegang H, Decker I, et al. The genome sequence of Clostridium tetani, the causative agent of tetanus disease. Proc Natl Acad Sci USA. 2003;100(3):1316-21.
7. Matsuda M. The structure of tetanus toxin. In: Simpson LL (ed). Botulinum Neurotoxin and Tetanus Toxin. San Diego: Academic Press; 1989. pp. 69-92.
8. Centers for Disease Control and Protection. (2018). Recommended Immunization Schedule for Children and Adolescents Aged 18 Years or Younger, United States, 2018. [online] Available from https://www.cdc.gov/vaccines/schedules/ downloads/child/0-18yrs-child-combined-schedule.pdf.
9. Lindström M, Korkeala H. Laboratory Diagnostics of Botulism. Clin Microbiol Rev. 2006;19(2):298-314.
10. Chaudhry R. Botulism: a diagnostic challenge. Indian J Med Res. 2011;134(1):10-2.
11. Joshy L, Chaudhry R, Chandel DS. Multiplex PCR for the detection of Clostridium botulinum & C. perfringens toxin genes. Indian J Med Res. 2008;128(2):206-8.
12. Jousimies-Somer HR. Wadsworth-Ktl anaerobic bacteriology manual. Star Publ.; 2002.
13. Harrison's Principles of Internal Medicine. 19th edition. McGraw-Hill Education; 2015.
14. Chaudhry R, Sharma N, Gupta N, Kant K, Bahadur T, Shende TM, et al. Nagging Presence of Clostridium difficile associated diarrhoea in North India. J Clin Diagn Res. 2017;11(9):DC06-9.

CHAPTER 45

Influenza Viruses Including H1N1

S Anuradha

ABSTRACT

Influenza is an important acute respiratory illness that has seasonal outbreaks world-wide. Influenza outbreaks and pandemics have scourged mankind for centuries. Influenza is caused by influenza viruses, chiefly influenza A viruses. These viruses undergo antigenic rearrangements called antigenic drifts and shifts that have importance in pathogenesis of the disease. Most often it is a mild disease in adults and children. In a subgroup of high-risk individuals influenza has serious clinical manifestations that can be life-threatening. Effective neuraminidase (NA) inhibitor drugs like oseltamivir are the cornerstone of management of influenza. Strict personal protection recommendations are also crucial in the prevention of infection. Influenza vaccination is recommended annually for prevention of infection. Global surveillance for influenza is the key to successful monitoring of the disease patterns.

"Influenza is something unique. It behaves epidemiologically in a way different from that of any other known infection"

—Sir Christopher Andrewes

INTRODUCTION

Influenza is a common illness that presents as an acute respiratory infection. It is caused by the Influenza viruses and is also referred to as the "flu" in common parlance. Indeed, in most adults, influenza is a mild disease and most people recover completely from uncomplicated influenza. However, in a subgroup of at-risk people, influenza can be a serious, life-threatening disease. Globally, there are an estimated about 3–5 million cases of severe illness, and about 290,000–650,000 respiratory deaths associated annually with influenza. Seasonal influenza outbreaks from 2010 to 2018 were associated with an estimated 4.3–23 million clinic visits, 140,000–960,000 hospital admissions, and 12,000–79,000 deaths annually in the United States. Influenza has a worldwide distribution and has definite seasonal peaks of outbreaks.

EPIDEMIOLOGY

The Agent: Influenza is caused by the influenza viruses—types A, B, C, and D belonging to the family Orthomyxoviridae. Influenza viruses are enveloped, segmented ribonucleic acid (RNA) viruses (**Fig. 1**).

Influenza type C viruses do not cause severe outbreaks or pandemics and influenza D viruses are not known to cause illness in humans. The most clinically relevant are the influenza A viruses. These viruses have important surface proteins called hemagglutinin (HA) and NA and are divided into various subtypes based on these. There are 16 HA and 9 NA subtypes with different hosts like avian species, pigs, horses, dogs etc. Among influenza A viruses in causing disease in humans, subtypes H1N1 and H3N2 are currently circulating globally. Usually, the influenza viruses circulate in specific hosts—avian influenza, swine influenza etc. Sometimes these influenza viruses are able to switch over from one to another host causing outbreaks in humans.

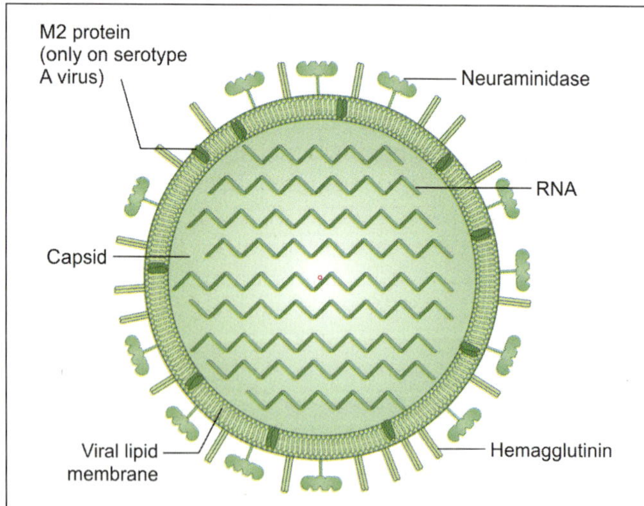

Influenza A and B viruses have 2 surface glycoproteins: hemagglutinin, which is necessary for the virus to attach to host-cell membranes, and neuraminidase, an enzyme involved in viral penetration and release of virus from infected cells

(RNA: ribonucleic acid)

FIGURE 1: Structure of the influenza virus.

Source: NCDC, MOHFW.

A characteristic rearrangement of HA and NA proteins is seen among the influenza viruses. The antigenic drift is a gradual, continuous change in HA and NA proteins that is of great relevance to the mankind. Due to this, the antibodies produced to previous strains are rendered ineffective and frequent updating of the influenza virus vaccine components are necessitated. Yearly epidemics occur in human populations with ever emerging new strains. A highly dramatic event is the phenomenon of antigenic shift. This involves an abrupt and rapid antigenic change that results in a virus with a novel HA or NA antigen. Such new viruses are capable of infecting large proportion of the world's population causing major pandemics.

During the 20th century, pandemics occurred in 1918 [influenza A (H1N1)]—The Spanish Flu, 1957 [Influenza A (H2N2)]—the Asian Flu, and 1968 [Influenza A (H3N2)]—Hong Kong Flu. Recently in April 2009, the influenza A (H1N1) virus emerged to cause an influenza pandemic—Swine Flu in more than 40 years. H1N1, which reached pandemic status in June 2009 also affected India severely. Between 2010 and 2017, 114,667 cases and 8,543 deaths due to H1N1 were recorded from India with a case fatality rate of 7.5%. The states of Maharashtra, Gujarat, Rajasthan, Delhi, and Karnataka together accounted for nearly 68% of all cases reported from India.

Host factors: Influenza affects all ages and genders. The incidence of disease is higher in extremes of age—the very young and old people. The reservoir of infection for seasonal influenza are human hosts and the symptomatic case or a subclinical case is the source of infection and transmission. The usual incubation period in adults is 1–2 days with a period of communicability of 3–5 days and up to 7 days in young children. The peak viral shedding occurs on the first day of symptoms in the cases. Certain populations are considered at high risk for infection and severity (**Box 1**).

Seasonality: India witnesses two peaks of seasonal influenza—in January to March and again post monsoon from August to October. In the US, influenza activity typically occurs during October through May.

Transmission: Influenza spreads easily, with rapid transmission noticed in crowded areas like schools and nursing homes and residential care facilities. When an infected person coughs or sneezes, the infectious droplets are dispersed and can spread up to 1 meter. The virus can also be spread by contaminated hands and fomites.

CLINICAL FEATURES

Uncomplicated influenza is characterized by acute onset of symptoms such as fever, headache, myalgia, chills, nasal congestion, arthralgia, abdominal pain, and nonproductive cough. There is usually accompanying weakness, malaise, rhinorrhea, fatigue, and sore throat. There can also be chest pain, diarrhea, and vomiting.

In adults, influenza can present with more serious complications like:

BOX 1 Persons at high risk of complications.

- Children aged <5 years, and especially aged <2 years
- Adults aged ≥65 years
- Persons with chronic pulmonary (including asthma), cardiovascular (except hypertension alone), renal, hepatic, hematologic (including sickle cell disease) or metabolic disorders (including diabetes mellitus).
- Neurologic and neurodevelopment conditions [including disorders of the brain, spinal cord, peripheral nerve, and muscle such as cerebral palsy, epilepsy (seizure disorders), stroke, intellectual disability (mental retardation), moderate to severe developmental delay, muscular dystrophy, or spinal cord injury]
- Persons with immunosuppression, including that caused by medications or by HIV infection
- Women who are pregnant or postpartum (within 2 weeks after delivery)
- Children and adolescents through 18 years who are receiving aspirin- or salicylate-containing medications and who might be at risk for experiencing Reye syndrome after influenza virus infection
- Persons with extreme obesity (i.e., body mass index ≥40 kg/m^2)
- Residents of nursing homes and other chronic care facilities

- Parotitis
- Bronchitis
- Sinusitis
- Pneumonia
- Myocarditis and pericarditis
- Myositis and rhabdomyolysis
- Invasive bacterial coinfection
- Toxic shock syndrome due to *Staphylococcus aureus* or *Streptococcus pyogenes*
- Precipitation of acute cardiovascular events (e.g., cardiac failure, myocardial infarction, heart failure, and cerebrovascular accident)
- Acute kidney injury and acute renal failure
- Encephalopathy and encephalitis

The disease has been categorized into three categories based on severity of symptoms for easy recognition and triage by the Ministry of Health and Family Welfare Government of India guidelines (**Table 1**). In addition to assigning prognosis, these categories also help in diagnostic and therapeutic recommendations for these patients.

DIAGNOSIS

The majority of cases of human influenza are clinically diagnosed. The symptoms and signs of influenza in the setting of an outbreak or during expected influenza activity are sufficient for making a diagnosis. Testing for influenza in all suspected patients is not recommended. Many respiratory viruses like rhinovirus, parainfluenza virus, and respiratory syncytial virus can present with influenza-like illness and it is difficult to clinically distinguish between these viral agents. The Government of India guidelines recommend testing for influenza only in category C patients. However, the clinician may test for influenza if the

TABLE 1	Influenza categorization according to severity.
Category A	***Uncomplicated/Mild:*** • Symptomatology: Patients with mild fever and cough/sore throat with or without body aches, headache, diarrhea, and vomiting
Category B	***Uncomplicated but severe symptoms/high-risk groups:*** • B1: In addition to all the signs and symptoms mentioned under Category A, if the patient has high-grade fever (≥102°F) and severe sore throat • B2: In addition to signs and symptoms of Category A, patient has one or more of these risk factors: ◦ Age ≥65 years ◦ Pregnancy (including up to 2 weeks postpartum) ◦ Infants and children aged ≤5 years (especially <2 years of age) ◦ Chronic respiratory disease ◦ Chronic heart, kidney, liver, or neurological disease ◦ Diabetes mellitus ◦ Blood disorders (including hemoglobinopathies) ◦ Persons with immunosuppression (including HIV/AIDS and use of long-term (≥2 weeks) corticosteroids, post-transplant patients) ◦ Extreme obesity (body mass index ≥40 kg/m^2) ◦ Malignancy
Category C	***Complicated:*** In addition to the above signs and symptoms of Category A and Category B, if the patient has one or more of the following: • Symptoms: ◦ Breathlessness ◦ Hemoptysis ◦ Altered mental status ◦ Somnolence and poor feeding (in children) ◦ Seizures ◦ Decreased urine output ◦ Persistence or worsening of initial symptoms beyond 72 h ◦ Worsening of underlying chronic conditions like diabetes mellitus, chronic kidney disease etc. • Sign: ◦ Tachypnea ◦ $SpO_2 < 90\%$ ◦ Hypotension ◦ Reduced urine output ◦ Cyanosis

(AIDS: acquired immunodeficiency syndrome; HIV: human immunodeficiency virus)

Source: MOHFW, GOI, NCDC guidelines.

clinical presentation or epidemiological setting is unusual or atypical.

The collection of appropriate respiratory samples and appropriate laboratory diagnostic tests are mandatory to establish a definitive diagnosis. Proper collection, storage, and transport of respiratory specimens is the essential first step for laboratory detection of influenza virus infections.

Nasopharyngeal specimens are the preferred specimens. If nasopharyngeal specimens are not available, nasal and throat swab specimens can be collected. It is better to test both these combined together over single specimens from either site (particularly over throat swabs) to increase the detection. *For hospitalized patients, endotracheal swabs or bronchoalveolar aspirates where applicable can also be collected. There is no role of testing* specimens from nonrespiratory sites such as blood, plasma, serum, cerebrospinal fluid, urine, and stool.

The preferred tests are the rapid molecular assays (i.e., nucleic acid amplification tests) over rapid influenza diagnostic tests (RIDTs). The reverse transcription polymerase chain reaction (RT-PCR) is the recommended preferred assay. Respiratory specimens should ideally be collected as early as possible (ideally <4 days after illness onset when influenza viral shedding is highest) in persons without lower respiratory tract disease and tested as soon as possible.

The RT-PCR tests are most sensitive and specific and have a rapid turn-around time. Serological tests are not recommended for Influenza diagnosis.

TREATMENT

ANTIVIRAL TREATMENT

Whom to treat? It is recommended that treatment with antiviral agents should be started as soon as possible in patients with Category B and C disease. This includes:

- All patients hospitalized with influenza
- All outpatients of any age with severe or progressive illness
- All outpatients with high or severe risk category
- Children younger than 2 years and adults ≥65 years
- All pregnant women and those within 2 weeks postpartum

All patients with influenza in category A need not be treated with antiviral drugs. Individualized decisions may be taken in specific cases by treating physicians.

When to start treatment? Antivirals agents should be started as soon as possible preferably within 48 hours. In many instances, presumptive treatment may be started pending the availability of laboratory results, especially in the category C patients.

Drug, dose, and duration: Neuraminidase inhibitors are the preferred agents for the treatment of influenza including H1N1 influenza. A single NA inhibitor should be started—oseltamivir, zanamivir, and peramivir are the agents available globally. Depending on availability, one of these can be started. Oral oseltamivir is the agent recommended and available in India. Doses higher than those recommended and combination of agents are not recommended. The doses of oseltamivir recommended are summarized in **Table 2**.

GENERAL MANAGEMENT

- Treatment is recommended for a minimum of 5 days, but can be extended until there is satisfactory clinical improvement in specific situations such as immunocompromised states.
- Corticosteroids should not be used routinely, unless indicated for other reasons (e.g., asthma and other specific conditions); as it has been associated with prolonged viral clearance, immunosuppression leading to bacterial or fungal superinfection.
- All currently circulating influenza viruses are *resistant* to adamantane antiviral drugs (such as amantadine and rimantadine), and these are therefore not recommended for monotherapy.

For patients who are not at high risk, *symptomatic treatment* is advised. They are advised home stay in order to minimize the risk of infecting others in the community. Antipyretics like paracetamol to reduce fever, warm fluids, and nasal decongestants, steam inhalation, and throat lozenges may be advised for symptomatic relief. Patients should monitor themselves for any worsening of clinical status and should report to the hospital at the earliest sign of deterioration. Clinicians must educate the patients for any such warning signs.

Patients hospitalized with category C disease should be managed with standard protocols for intravenous fluids, oxygen therapy, mechanical ventilation, inotropes if needed, and antibiotics for superadded bacterial infections. Standard protocols of infection control must be strictly followed within the hospital wards and intensive care units to prevent nosocomial spread to other patients and healthcare workers.

TABLE 2 Dose of oseltamivir.

Weight-based	Age	Dosage
<15 kg	1–5 years	30 mg bid for 5 days
15–23 kg	5–8 years	45 mg bid for 5 days
24 to <40 kg	8–12 years	60 mg bid for 5 days
>40 kg	>12 years	75 mg bid for 5 days
	Infants (<1 year)	
<3 months*	12 mg bid for 5 days	
3–5 months	20 mg bid for 5 days	
6–11 months	25 mg bid for 5 days	

*In preterm infants the dose may be modified from 1 to 3 mg/kg/dose bid oseltamivir is also available as a syrup (6–12 mg/mL). If needed dose and duration can be modified as per clinical condition.

Source: MOHFW, GOI, NCDC guidelines.

PREVENTION

CHEMOPROPHYLAXIS

Postexposure prophylaxis with antiviral agents can be considered in special circumstances by clinicians. These include:

- For adults and children aged ≥3 months who are at very high risk and for whom influenza vaccination is contraindicated or unavailable.
- For healthcare workers and adults and children aged ≥3 months who are unvaccinated and are household contacts of a person at very high risk of complications from after exposure to influenza.

Oseltamivir in full dose should be administered within 48 hours of the exposure and continued for 7 days.

VACCINATION

Vaccination is the most effective way to prevent influenza. Very safe and effective vaccines are available for use against influenza.

World Health Organization (WHO) recommends annual vaccination for prevention against influenza for:

- Pregnant women at any stage of pregnancy
- Children aged between 6 months to 5 years
- Elderly individuals (aged >65 years)
- Individuals with chronic medical conditions
- Healthcare workers

The Clinical Practice Guidelines of 2019 of the Indian Chest Society and the National College of Chest Physicians of India provide a detailed consensus-based document on the vaccination strategies developed for adults in India. As per these guidelines, the recommendations for influenza vaccination are summarized in **Tables 3** and **4**.

TABLE 3 Recommendations for influenza vaccination in India.

Proposed vaccination timings	Cities
April to May	Delhi, Lucknow, Kolkata, Dibrugarh, and Pune
September to October	Srinagar, Chennai, and Vellore

TABLE 4 Recommended vaccination schedules for India.

Age group (years)	Influenza vaccine recommendations
18–49	One dose IIV/LAIV annually: The choice of the vaccine is based on the discretion of the doctor and patient while vaccinating people in this age group
>50	One dose annually: Vaccination is strongly recommended

(IIV: inactivated influenza vaccine; LAIV: live attenuated influenza vaccine)

BOX 2 Recommended composition of influenza vaccine (2020–2021) WHO.

Quadrivalent influenza vaccines	Trivalent influenza vaccines
It is recommended that quadrivalent influenza vaccines for use in the 2020–2021 Northern Hemisphere influenza season contain the following:	It is recommended that trivalent influenza vaccines for use in the 2020–2021 Northern Hemisphere influenza season contain the following:
Egg-based vaccines:	
• An A/Guangdong-Maonan/SWL1536/2019 (H1N1)pdm09-like virus	• An A/Guangdong-Maonan/SWL1536/2019 (H1N1)pdm09-like virus
• An A/Hong Kong/2671/2019 (H3N2)-like virus	• An A/Hong Kong/2671/2019 (H3N2)-like virus
• A B/Washington/02/2019 (B/Victoria lineage)-like virus	• A B/Washington/02/2019 (B/Victoria lineage)-like virus
• A B/Phuket/3073/2013 (B/Yamagata lineage)-like virus	
Cell- or recombinant-based vaccines:	
• An A/Hawaii/70/2019 (H1N1)pdm09-like virus	• An A/Hawaii/70/2019 (H1N1)pdm09-like virus
• An A/Hong Kong/45/2019 (H3N2)-like virus	• An A/Hong Kong/45/2019 (H3N2)-like virus
• A B/Washington/02/2019 (B/Victoria lineage)-like virus	• A B/Washington/02/2019 (B/Victoria lineage)-like virus
• A B/Phuket/3073/2013 (B/Yamagata lineage)-like virus	

The composition of the influenza vaccine for the year 2020–2021 as recommended by the WHO for Northern Hemisphere is summarized in **Box 2**.

NONPHARMACOLOGICAL INTERVENTIONS

The most effective strategy to mitigate the impact of a pandemic is to reduce contacts between infected and uninfected persons, thereby reducing the spread of infection. Social distancing measures like contact tracing, isolation, quarantine, school and workplace measures, and avoiding crowding may be employed in measured capacities depending upon the need. All those who are ill must isolate themselves at home to reduce transmission. Hand hygiene reduces the load of virus on the hands and is an important intervention that should always be recommended. Improved respiratory etiquette and the use of face masks in community settings during influenza epidemics and pandemics are also useful. More severe epidemics and pandemics call for harsher restriction measures like travel restrictions, school and workplace closures etc.

CONCLUSION

Influenza is a common respiratory illness that affects large populations in the world. Usually, it is a mild disease but in specific risk groups it can be serious with fatal consequences. Influenza outbreaks occur annually globally and major antigenic variations can cause large pandemics. NA inhibitors are the drugs of choice for treatment and must be instituted at the earliest. Most critical is prevention of influenza with annual vaccination recommendations. It is also very important to stress on isolation, cough etiquette, hand hygiene, and social distancing measures.

RECOMMENDED READINGS

1. Uyeki TM, Bernstein HH, Bradley JS, Englund JA, File TM, Fry AM. Clinical Practice Guidelines by the Infectious Diseases Society of America: 2018 Update on Diagnosis, Treatment, Chemoprophylaxis, and Institutional Outbreak Management of Seasonal Influenza. Clin Infect Dis. 2019;68(6):e1-e47.
2. Centers for Disease Control and Prevention. Disease Burden of Influenza. [online] Available from https://www.cdc.gov/flu/about/burden/index.html.
3. Chatterjee P, Seth B, Biswas T. Hotspots of H1N1 influenza in India: analysis of reported cases and deaths (2010–2017). Trop Doct. 2020;50(2):166-9.
4. H1N1 Technical Guidelines. National Center for Disease control, MOHFW, GOI. [online] Available from https://www.ncdc.gov.in/index1.php?lang=1&level=1&sublinkid=409&lid=359.
5. Kulkarni SV, Narain JP, Gupta S, Dhariwal AC, Singh SK, Macintyre CR. Influenza A (H1N1) in India: Changing epidemiology and its implications. Natl Med J India. 2019;32:107-8.
6. World Health Organization. Influenza. [online] Available from https://www.who.int/influenza/en/
7. Dhar R, Ghoshal AG, Guleria R, Sharma S, Kulkarni T, Swarnakar R, et al. Clinical practice guidelines 2019: Indian consensus-based recommendations on influenza vaccination in adults. Lung India. 2020;37:S4-18.
8. World Health Organization. (2019). Global Influenza Programme. Non-pharmaceutical public health measures for mitigating the risk and impact of epidemic and pandemic influenza. [online] Available from https://apps.who.int/iris/bitstream/handle/10665/329438/9789241516839-eng.pdf.

CHAPTER

46

RNA Virus Infections

Sajithkumar R

ABSTRACT

Ribonucleic acid (RNA) viruses produce various infections in humans ranging from simple catarrhal type to paralytic variants. These viruses tend to have specific tropism for organ systems. Most of them are self-limited and resolve by themselves. But serious infections like Ebola have significant mortality. They are all highly infectious but vaccines are available against some of them. The following RNA virus infections are discussed in this chapter (1) Measles (2) Rubella (3) Mumps (4) Ebola, and (5) Enteroviruses (poliomyelitis, ECHO, and Coxsackie viruses). The pathogenesis, clinical details, and brief epidemiology are discussed.

"The environment is changing and so are the viruses"

—Steven Magee

MEASLES

Measles is an acute febrile exanthematous illness caused by rubeola virus belonging to the genus *Morbillivirus* of the family Paramyxoviridae. It is usually described as a childhood disease with high infectivity rates. Because of the widespread measles vaccination in children, it is not commonly seen in children now. Adult measles is a serious illness characterized by upper and lower respiratory symptoms like running nose, sore throat, cough associated with conjunctivitis, and tracheobronchitis. The characteristic pattern of popular eruptions occurring usually on the fifth day of fever gives it the name of fifth day fever colloquially. Measles is distributed globally.

Even though measles was known to occur for many centuries, the first scientific description was by Pannum (1846), who described the details of an epidemic that happened in the Faroe Islands. The attempts to grow the virus in human renal tissue culture cells from 1954 resulted in the live measles vaccine that was licensed in 1963. This vaccine which has been included in universal immunization in the 21st century has led to a significant decline in childhood measles.

ETIOLOGY

Measles viruses are pleomorphic spheres with a diameter of 100–250 nanometers. The inner nucleocapsid is composed of protein and 4.5 kilodalton single-stranded RNA. There are two surface projections (peplomers)—conical hemagglutinin and dumbbell-shaped fusion peplomer. There are six structural proteins. The large protein, polymerase protein, and the nucleoprotein are complexed with RNA. The M protein and two glycoproteins H and F are associated with the membrane envelope. Of these the F glycoprotein is responsible for the fusion of the virus with the host cell.

PATHOLOGY

The incubation period of measles is between 10 and 14 days. The infection occurs through the lining epithelium of the nostrils or any part of the respiratory tract. Local replication leads to release of new viruses and viremia associated with infection of reticuloendothelial cells and leucocytes. Secondary viremia is associated with involvement of all parts of the respiratory system with edema and ciliary loss in the epithelial cells. The infection by measles virus leads to typical cytopathic effects, characterized by increased refractility, and formation of multinucleated giant cells with intranuclear inclusions.

Koplik's spots are described as pathognomonic of measles. Described by Koplik in 1896, they are bluish gray spots on a red velvety base appearing in the buccal mucosa opposite the second molar. They are likened to the appearance of sprinkled common salt crystals on a red velvet. They usually appear on the third day of febrile illness, persist for a variable period and slough off as the skin eruptions appear.

By the fourth or fifth day, the viremia is reduced and the papular eruptions are thought to be due to a hypersensitivity phenomenon.

Neurons, astrocytes, oligodendrocytes, and vascular endothelium are also infected by the measles virus. This has been postulated as a cause for acute encephalitis as well as the late onset neurological complications.

CLINICAL MANIFESTATIONS

The illness begins as a nonspecific prodrome of fever, coryza, running nose, and conjunctival congestion. Koplik's spots soon appear. The classic description of measles is the papular eruption which starts on the fourth or fifth day. Initially the discrete papules appear near the hairline on the forehead and progresses caudally to involve the trunk and extremities on subsequent days in that order. The papules will be discrete pinhead shaped in the beginning. By the time new areas are involved the lesions that appeared on the previous day coalesce together and disappear in the same sequence in which they appeared. The transformation of the eruptions takes around 5 days, so that by the 10th day of fever, most papules would have been converted to brownish desquamation. It may take a few more days for these to clear. Permanent cutaneous discoloration practically never happens in measles. By the time the eruptions disappear, fever also subsides in uncomplicated measles.

COMPLICATIONS

Measles is associated with significant short-term reduction in immunity. Coupled with the disruption of ciliary function by the virus, this leads to various complications. The complications can be grouped into immediate, intermediate, and late.

The virus has a tendency to involve the cells of respiratory and nervous system. However in the majority of individuals, measles is associated with secondary bacterial infections in and around the respiratory tract. Immediate complications are bacterial infections mostly caused by gram positive cocci. These include sinusitis, pharyngitis, laryngitis, tracheobronchitis, bronchiolitis, pneumonia, and even empyema. Bacterial conjunctivitis and otitis are also seen. Patients will develop corresponding symptoms depending on the diseases. Acute encephalitis usually manifests during convalescence with reappearance of fever associated with headache, drowsiness, seizures, and loss of consciousness. Encephalitis is thought to occur only in one out of thousand infections and most of them recover without any serious sequelae. Since the virus isolation from central nervous system is not successful, it is presumed that measles encephalitis is more of a hypersensitivity phenomenon. Demyelination, gliosis, and perivascular cuffing and infiltration with macrophages are described. Occasional cases of hepatitis have also been reported.

The fall in immunity is associated with reactivation of dormant infections like tuberculosis or herpes zoster. The diagnosis of tuberculosis must be considered in all patients having persistent respiratory symptoms. Recurrent infections of the trachea bronchial tree leads to development of bronchiectasis. This etiopathogenesis is likely in many cases of adult bronchiectasis following childhood infections.

The late complication of subacute sclerosing panencephalitis (SSPE) is not common, but reported.

Atypical measles is a more severe form of measles where the eruptions may appear peripherally, maybe urticarial, vesicular, and hemorrhagic. The patient may have high fever, interstitial lung infiltrates, pleural effusion, and hepatitis. Because of the bleeding into the lesions that appear black in color, this is also referred to as black measles. Hypersensitivity against measles antigen is supposed to be the underlying pathology. This is more common in those who had received a killed measles vaccine in the past.

Attenuated measles is measles in a modified form because of the immunity in persons who have either received a vaccine, had measles in the past, or received immunoglobulins (Igs) through breast milk or passive immunization. The manifestations tend to be milder and short lasting in these individuals.

Severe measles has been reported in immunosuppressed individuals like those with malignancies, radiation or chemotherapy, HIV infection, and malnutrition. They may not develop the classical manifestations like skin eruptions, Koplik's spots etc., but tend to have more of respiratory symptoms, particularly interstitial pneumonia. High mortality ranging from 40% to 70% have been reported in this group.

Measles during pregnancy, unlike rubella does not cause any significant congenital anomaly in the fetus. However incidence of respiratory complications are more in pregnant women.

DIAGNOSIS

Measles is mostly a clinical diagnosis and no test is recommended. Diagnostic test is usually required when the clinician is not familiar or when other differential diagnoses are considered. Leukopenia is the usual pattern in blood smear. Except in patients with severe viral pneumonia, virus isolation is not attempted as it is difficult in most instances. A sensitive reverse transcription polymerase chain reaction (RT-PCR) is available but not usually done. Patients in the 2nd week will have IgM antibodies that can be picked by enzyme-linked immunosorbent assay (ELISA). ELISA test is available in most places and can be useful.

TREATMENT

Patient with measles must be isolated and treated as per symptoms. They may require antipyretics for fever, antihistamines, and decongestants for upper respiratory symptoms. Antibiotics are indicated only when bacterial superinfection is suspected. Bacterial infections are usually caused by gram positive organisms and azithromycin is a preferred choice in such instances. Prophylactic antibiotics are not recommended. Vitamin A supplementation has been advised in children to decrease the severity of measles.

PREVENTION

Active immunization with live attenuated measles vaccine has been accepted universally now. It is recommended to be given at the age of 9 months through intramuscular route. Considering the possibility of interactions with passively transmitted maternal antibodies, another dose is recommended after 15 months of age. In many countries the second dose is given along with mumps and rubella components in measles, mumps, and rubella (MMR) vaccine. About 95% of immunized persons in general develop sufficient immunity. Live measles vaccine is not recommended for pregnant women and children with severe immunodeficiency. However, measles vaccine is given even for children with HIV, unless severely immunosuppressed.

Even after contact with a case of measles, vaccine can be administered for prevention in the first few hours. This is useful in case accidental exposure is identified early, except in pregnant and immunosuppressed persons, as the incubation period for measles vaccine virus is 7 days only, compared to 10 days for measles virus.

RUBELLA

Rubella (German measles) is an acute exanthematous fever in children and adults caused by rubella virus. Rubella virus belongs to the Togaviridae family. The clinical illness is mild and transient, however occurrence in pregnancy leads to fetal infections and consequent birth defects. Rubella was recognized from 19th century. However it was Gregg (1941) who reported the link with birth defects.

ETIOLOGY

Rubella virus is spherical in shape, has short surface projections and has a diameter of about 60 nm. The 30 nm size nucleocapsid has a helix of protein and RNA. Even though closely related to *Alphaviruses*, rubella virus does not require a vector for transmission. Transmembrane glycoproteins E1 and E2 and C, the capsid protein are the major structural polypeptides. The virus is relatively unstable and inactivated by heat, lipid solvents, and ultraviolet (UV) light. They are grown in rabbit kidney cells. The spread is via droplets from respiratory secretions. Patients are infective from 10 days before the onset of eruptions to about 15 days after the onset. Infants with congenital infection shed the virus for many months, even after developing high titers of neutralizing antibodies.

PATHOGENESIS

The incubation period is reported as 12–23 days. As much as 1 week before the onset of illness, virus has been demonstrated in leukocytes. As in measles, primary viremia is followed by development of hypersensitivity that is thought to play the major role in development of skin eruptions.

Various mechanisms have been postulated for the lesions in congenital rubella. Mitotic arrest of the cells because of viral infection leads to retarded organ maturation. Angiopathy leading to placental and fetal vasculitis, tissue necrosis, chromosomal breakage, and production of a growth inhibitor are other postulated causes for the congenital anomalies.

CLINICAL FEATURES

The classical manifestations of rubella are maculopapular skin eruptions and lymphadenopathy. The eruptions start from the face and spreads to the rest of the body and may disappear within a few hours. Occasionally they may persist for 3–5 days. Few patients have associated nasal congestion, nasal discharge, and conjunctivitis. The cervical lymph nodes are the most commonly affected with a predilection for posterior auricular and suboccipital nodes. Splenomegaly also occurs occasionally. Fever is usually present on the first day only. Petechial lesions on the soft palate (Forchheimer spots) is seen but nor pathognomonic of rubella. Many infections tend to be subclinical.

COMPLICATIONS

Unlike measles, rubella infection in nonpregnant individuals is rarely associated with any complication. Mild arthralgia or arthritis can occur, rarely in women. Rarely, hemorrhagic manifestations are reported caused by thrombocytopenia and vascular damage, likely to be immunologically mediated. Thrombocytopenia tends to persist for weeks or months. Thrombocytopenic purpura may be the only manifestation in children. Mild encephalitis and hepatitis has been reported rarely.

Congenital Rubella: Rubella infection during pregnancy, particularly the first trimester, leads to fetal death, premature delivery, and many congenital birth defects. The younger the fetus is, the more severe disease it develops ranging from 65% to 85% in the first 2 months to <10% in the next 3 months. Fetal infection in the 3rd month of fetal life leads to a chance of developing defects to the tune of 30–35%. After the second trimester, the risk is significantly reduced. Deafness, congenital heart disease, cataract, glaucoma, and mental retardation are the major manifestations. Low birth weight, microcephaly, myopia, and retinopathy may also be observed. Patent ductus arteriosus and pulmonary stenosis are the most common cardiac defects. Hepatitis and pneumonitis are also reported with small frequency.

Many studies have suggested that congenital rubella is an ongoing illness with manifestations appearing or progressing even at school going age. Insulin-dependent diabetes mellitus detected later has been associated with occurrence of human leukocyte antigen DR3 (HLA-DR3) in those with congenital rubella syndrome. High titers of neutralizing antibodies persist for many years and subsequently lose them.

DIAGNOSIS

As a mild exanthematous febrile illness, the disease may be confused with infectious mononucleosis, mild measles, scarlet fever, erythema infectiosum etc. Peripheral blood examination may reveal leukopenia. Routine blood counts may not be helpful and specific tests are necessary for diagnosis. Virus can be isolated from throat swabs, synovial fluid, or urine. But the technique is quite cumbersome. Amniotic fluid has been positive for viruses in cases of congenital rubella. Even though tests like hemagglutination are very specific, currently ELISA test for IgM and IgG is the most convenient and popular test used. If rubella IgM is detected in the serum of newborn, it is conclusive evidence of transplacental infection.

TREATMENT

Because the clinical illness is mild, no specific drug is indicated. Symptomatic and supportive therapy using antipyretics and antihistamines may be given in select instances.

PREVENTION

Because of the significant chance for congenital infection, immunization against rubella is recommended before puberty in all persons. The live attenuated vaccine has been in use from 1969. In India, this is incorporated in the MMR vaccine given after 15 months of age. A booster dose may be given before puberty. The vaccine may occasionally cause fever, adenopathy, and arthralgia. Since the vaccine virus can cause fetal infection, it is advised that women be advised not to become pregnant at least for 3 months after the vaccine has been administered.

MUMPS

Mumps is an acute infection of multiple glands in the body. It is a benign and self-limited disease more common in children and adolescents. Though parotid swelling with parotitis is the most common manifestation, patients may develop pancreatitis, encephalitis, orchitis, oophoritis, or myocarditis

ETIOLOGY

Mumps virus belongs to the Paramyxoviridae family and genus *Rubulavirus.* The virion is irregular spherical in shape with a diameter of 200 nm. The envelope has various glycoproteins with neuraminidase, hemagglutinin and cell fusion capabilities. Viral antigen (V) is also found in this layer. The helical nucleocapsid is a single-stranded RNA with capsid proteins surrounding it. The capsid proteins include RNA polymerase enzyme and also hosts the soluble (S) antigen. There is only one serotype of mumps virus known. Antibodies to S antigen appear first, followed by those against V antigen.

PATHOGENESIS

In human cell lines, mumps virus produces rounding of cells, intracytoplasmic eosinophilic inclusions, or syncytia formation. The virus is transmitted by droplets that spread by direct contact or through fomites. Prolonged contact during the prodromal phase or first few days leads to maximum number of infections. The virus that infects the respiratory tract epithelium spreads to other organs after a small period of viremia.

Parotid glands that are the most commonly affected, develop diffuse interstitial edema with serofibrinous exudate that contains predominantly mononuclear leucocytes. Necrotic debris accumulates in the salivary ducts and salivary epithelium undergoes degenerative changes. Involvement of the testis leads to polymorphonuclear infiltration with occasional interstitial hemorrhage. Increased build-up of pressure inside a solid tunica can lead to compromised vascular supply and consequent pressure infarcts. When severe, germinal epithelium can undergo atrophy which may lead to hyalinization, fibrosis, and atrophy, even though rare. The central nervous system involvement is mostly by postinfectious process and has been quoted as the most common form of aseptic meningitis. Demyelination around the veins, perivascular cuffing, and an increase in microglial cells are observed.

CLINICAL FEATURES

The incubation period is usually 14–18 days, extending up to 4 weeks. Following a nonspecific prodrome of mild fever, malaise, headache, anorexia, patient feels pain in front of the ear associated with tender swelling of the parotids. This is usually unilateral to start with but involving both parotids in >60% cases. Maximum size of the swelling is noticed by third or fourth day, by which it usually elevates the earlobe upward and outward. The angle of the mandible will be obliterated by the swelling. Trismus (difficulty in opening the mouth) is seen in around 50% cases. The Stenson's duct that drains the saliva from the parotids is usually inflamed. This can be appreciated by inspection of the buccal mucosa. An erythematous ring is seen around the orifice of the Stenson's duct. Citrus fruits and juices may exacerbate the pain. After the swelling has reached its peak, fever usually subsides. The swelling is gradually reduced and may take a week or two to disappear.

Involvement of submandibular and sublingual salivary glands occur in about 10% cases. Except the swelling, they do not cause much trouble. Presternal edema is seen in patients who develop submandibular sialadenitis. This is attributed to accumulation of lymph due to blockage of drainage.

Central nervous system involvement is in the form of encephalitis. Meningeal symptoms like headache, vomiting, and neck stiffness may occur at any stage with or without fever and sometimes unrelated to parotid swelling. Some patients develop early disease due to viral invasion, while others have a late, postinfectious demyelinative pattern. Convulsions, loss of consciousness, abnormal movements, and paresis have also been reported. Cerebrospinal fluid (CSF) study reveals lymphocytic pleocytosis in majority of cases with mildly elevated CSF protein values. Low CSF sugar values (hypoglycorrachia) are reported in around 30% patients. Few patients can have neutrophilic reaction in CSF, in whom it may be confused with bacterial meningitis. Occasional patients may develop transient deafness and vertigo. Cerebellar ataxia, facial palsy, transverse myelitis, and Guillain-Barré syndrome have been reported rarely.

Epididymo-orchitis develops mostly in postpubertal males and is the most common extrasalivary gland manifestation. This is usually unilateral and rarely bilateral. Majority occurs during the 1st week, even though it can happen without parotitis as well. It is a very painful condition associated with swelling, warmth, and tenderness of the testicle and redness of the scrotal skin. The testicles may swell up to four times the normal size. Fever may be present in severe cases and may last for less than a week. Very rarely testes may undergo atrophy. Anxiety about sterility or impotence is a major concern in patients with mumps orchitis. However, the risk of sterility is only for those who develop bilateral testicular atrophy following orchitis. Bilateral disease is rare and still rare is atrophy in both testes. Therefore the chance of occurrence of sterility following mumps is very uncommon. Oophoritis can occur in postpubertal women with mumps. Fever, nausea, and abdominal pain are usual in such patients.

Joint involvement following mumps is a rare sequelae. Monoarticular arthritis or migratory polyarthritis has been described. This may occur 1 or 2 weeks after the onset of parotitis and may last up to 6 weeks. The process usually resolves without any residual effects.

Pancreatitis is another associated feature of mumps, which can be independent of parotitis as well. Severe epigastric pain, vomiting accompanied by tenderness are the features. Abnormal electrocardiograms with prolongation of PR intervals, ST segment depression, and inverted T waves are observed but frank myocarditis is rare. Prostatitis, mastitis, hepatitis, thyroiditis, thrombocytopenia are also recognised associations. There is no significant linkage between mumps and pancreatitis, even though diabetes is occasionally attributed to childhood mumps.

Other than the above associations, mumps usually does not lead to any complications and is mostly a self-limited disease.

DIAGNOSIS

The diagnosis of mumps is mostly clinical based on a history of exposure. No specific test is recommended. Peripheral blood examination reveals leukopenia with relative lymphocytosis. Serum amylase level is elevated with parotitis and remains elevated for weeks. Elevation in pancreatic lipase must lead to suspicion of pancreatitis. The CSF study will reveal features of aseptic meningitis as described above.

Definitive diagnosis of mumps is by IgM ELISA demonstrating serial elevations in titer between acute and convalescent sera. Isolation of virus from saliva is possible from 2 to 3 days before and 4 to 5 days after the beginning of parotid swelling. However, this is not used as a diagnostic modality.

TREATMENT

Symptomatic and supportive therapy using analgesics and antipyretics will relieve the symptoms in the majority of patients. Frequent saline gargles is recommended to maintain oral hygiene and to reduce inflammation of the salivary ducts and glands.

Management of orchitis is by proper scrotal support using a tunneling cloth bridge avoiding elastic compression of the scrotum. Anti-inflammatory drugs and occasionally high-dose steroids as single shot will relieve the pain. Adrenocorticotropic hormone (ACTH) has also been advised in severe cases. Anesthetic blockade at the level of spermatic cord with local anesthetics is recommended for severe pain. Surgical decompression by cutting open the tunica vaginalis testes capsule has been recommended for severe cases to relieve the pressure within.

PREVENTION

Isolation of the affected person is the best option to prevent the spread of disease. Active immunization with live attenuated virus vaccine produces protective antibody levels in >95% persons and is maintained for 10–15 years. In India combined MMR vaccine is given at 15 months of age. A booster in adolescence (12–14 years) is good for better adult immunity. Mumps vaccine is not recommended in immunosuppressed persons, pregnant women, and those with severe febrile illnesses.

EBOLA

Ebola virus and Marburg virus are *Flaviviruses* belonging to the order Mononegavirales that cause severe hemorrhagic fever with very high mortality. Ebola virus was first identified in 1976 in Zaire and Sudan, where they caused two unrelated epidemics where 88% and 53% patients died, respectively. The most recent outbreak in Congo (2020) led to the death of 2,299 persons out of 3,481 persons affected. The disease has since been reported in various parts of the world. Zaire subtype virus was identified in 1977. The Reston subtype was identified in Reston, Virginia among cynomolgus monkeys imported from Philippines. Italy had cases in 1992, and USA in 1996. These clusters were also associated with very high transmission rates among hospital staff also. Parenteral inoculation with contaminated equipment in hospitals and laboratories has been reported to be efficient and associated with increased mortality. The skin of these patients is thought to harbor the viruses in fibroblasts and contact with skin even after death is considered dangerous. Airborne infection is also possible, though not efficient. Exposure to nonhuman primates or infected cases is present in almost all cases.

ETIOLOGY

The Ebola virus has an elongated structure with 80 nm diameter and around 970 nm long. The envelope is studded with glycoprotein spikes. The nucleocapsid contains a single-stranded negative sense RNA of 4.2 kilodalton size. Four different subtypes of Ebola viruses are known. These are Zaire, Sudan, Cote d'Ivoire, and Reston.

PATHOGENESIS

The viremia occurs before the clinical disease and persists till antibodies appear later in the course. There is a deficient response to interferon induction and extensive damage to lymphoid tissues. Focal necrosis in the liver is common. Cytokines are activated extensively while inflammatory cell infiltrates are minimal. The virions have been identified in the eye (anterior chamber) and semen for several weeks.

CLINICAL FEATURES

After an incubation period ranging from 2 to 19 days, fever sets in accompanied by severe myalgia and headache. Nausea, vomiting, abdominal pain, diarrhea, chest pain, and cough are the other symptoms. Photophobia, jaundice, lymphadenopathy, and conjunctival congestion are also seen. Somnolence, delirium, or coma sets in rapidly. Bleeding manifestations occur soon, manifesting as petechiae, echhymoses, and hemorrhages around injection sites. A maculopapular or hemorrhagic rash is seen in the trunk by the end of first week. Death occurs as a result of shock, multiorgan dysfunction, disseminated intravascular coagulation, extensive bleeding, or renal and hepatic failure. Recovering patients may have arthralgia, recurrent hepatitis, transverse myelitis, uveitis etc.

DIAGNOSIS

Diagnosis is usually suspected with an epidemiologic linkage. Leukopenia, thrombocytopenia, and grossly elevated transaminase levels are seen. Antigen detection or PCR positivity is the most sensitive diagnostic tool. Virus culture and IgM ELISA are also helpful in the first and second weeks, respectively.

TREATMENT

No specific antiviral therapy is available. Convalescent plasma from recovered persons has been tried with doubtful benefit. Supportive and symptomatic treatment is advised. Careful maintenance of hydration and correction of coagulation abnormalities using heparin in disseminated intravascular coagulation (DIC) are helpful in most cases. Infection control precautions, quarantine, and proper disposal are key factors in reducing transmission.

PREVENTION

Vector-derived vaccines using vesicular stomatitis virus (rVSV-ZEBOV) that codes for viral proteins have been found to be useful in preventing the spread. Zabdeno (Ad26.ZEBOV) and Mvabea (MVA-BN-Filo) vaccines have been authorized for use now and given as two doses. US FDA approved the vaccines in 2019. After that Burundi, Central African Republic, the Democratic Republic of the Congo, Ghana, Guinea, Rwanda, Uganda, and Zambia have also approved the vaccine. These have been used in the Republic of Congo in 2020. Ring vaccination to cover susceptible individuals is the recommended strategy during outbreaks.

ENTEROVIRUSES

Enterovirus infections are present worldwide, more commonly in children. The enteroviruses found in the human gastrointestinal tract have been divided into subgroups viz. polio viruses, Coxsackie viruses (group A and B), echo viruses. They belong to the big family of picornaviruses, so named from words that suggest very small RNA virus. They are single-stranded RNA viruses that are approximately 30 nm in diameter and nonenveloped. There are more than 72 serotypes.

POLIOMYELITIS

Poliomyelitis infection, known to affect humankind from time immemorial, is a disease with wide spectrum ranging from mild febrile illness with no sequelae to a severe paralytic variant with involvement of spinal or brainstem nuclei. The disease is usually sporadic although epidemics have been reported. Poliomyelitis used to be a common childhood infection in India with reported incidence of around 200 cases per million population and around 90% of children developing antibodies by age 5 in the previous century. By extensive immunization strategies, the world is moving toward elimination of poliomyelitis from humankind. The polio eradication activities were started in 1988, when wild polio virus was endemic in 125 countries, and 1,000 children used to be paralyzed every day. By 2003, there was a 99% reduction and as of 2021 Pakistan and Afghanistan are the only countries reporting wild poliovirus infections with fewer than 40 cases. India was declared polio free in 2014.

ETIOLOGY

The poliomyelitis virus is a picornavirus. Three pathogenic types are identified viz. 1, 2, and 3 of which Type 1 was the most common. The virus infects only primates. The virus enters the body through ingestion of fecally contaminated material. Host cell susceptibility to infection is mediated by specific membrane receptor proteins. 2–3 days after entry, the virus localizes in the mucosal M cells, Peyer's patches, and mesenteric nodes. Thereafter primary viremia occurs enabling spread of virus to pharynx, peritonsillar tissues, and cervical lymph nodes. The virus is secreted in the intestines and upper respiratory tract for a period of up to 6 weeks. Excretion to intestine and fecal shedding continues longer. The second viremia that ensues later ensures dissemination of virus to central nervous system, heart, and skin, where necrosis and inflammatory reactions are seen. The anterior horn cells of the spinal cord and nuclei in medulla are swollen and congested. Chromatolysis and pericellular infiltration lead to total destruction of neurons. In the central nervous system, other parts like midbrain, substantia nigra, thalamus, and hypothalamus may also be involved. CSF studies reveal early polymorphonuclear and later lymphocytic predominance and moderate elevation in protein level.

Serotype-specific immunity to enteroviral infections is well recognized. IgM antibodies are produced as early as 1–3 days. IgG antibodies appear after the first week and may persist for months. Passive administration of IgG at the onset of clinical illness has been shown to reduce excretion of viruses from the pharynx and intestine but does not influence the central nervous system changes. Mucosal immunity mediated by IgA antibodies has been suggested as important following oral ingestion of wild type or vaccine virus. Antibodies against polioviruses has been demonstrated in colostrum and milk of immune women. These may also interfere with orally administered vaccine viruses.

CLINICAL FEATURES

Poliomyelitis is common below 15 years of age including infants. The incubation period ranges from 2 days to 2 weeks. All over the world approximately 95% infections are completely asymptomatic. Undifferentiated febrile illness, muscle pain, or diarrhea occurs in almost all patients. The second phase is manifested as neurological illness. In nonparalytic form, features of meningeal irritation are seen, but subsides within a week. In paralytic polio spinal, bulbar, or combined involvement can be seen. Initial symptoms of diffuse muscle cramps and fasciculations are followed by rapid onset of weakness. Paralysis sets in within a few hours. Paralysis is typically unilateral and tends to recover to some extent with time. Totally affected neurons do not recover while others may recover partially, so that a combination of both is usually seen. When the lower cranial nerves are involved, dysarthria, dysphonia, and dysarthria can occur. Apneic spells, transient hypertension, circulatory collapse, and rarely acute pulmonary edema may occur with involvement of RAS (reticular activating system). Recovery of the partially affected neurons leads to gradual improvement, often accompanied by hypertrophy of the unaffected parts.

DIAGNOSIS

Various other enteroviruses can produce similar illness. If the child is unimmunized and develops classical features, CSF study is recommended. The virus can be isolated from feces and rectal swabs and cultured in primate cell lines. PCR studies also help in distinguishing the serotypes. High titers of IgM antibodies are also demonstrable in serum. Toxic neuropathies, Guillain–Barré syndrome, and acute motor neuronopathy are included in immediate differential diagnosis. Nerve conduction studies may be needed in such cases. Muscle weakness due to acute intermittent porphyria may also cause confusion but can be diagnosed by urine porphobilinogen elevation.

TREATMENT

Complete bed rest, analgesics, and supportive care is all that is needed. Feeding by nasogastric tube and ventilation support may be required in bulbar forms. Restricted activity of the affected muscles and application of local heat is advisable. Active physiotherapy can be instituted later. Axial skeletal abnormalities, asymmetric hypertrophy of muscles, and contractures need to be addressed by relevant surgical interventions or physiotherapy later.

PREVENTION

As appreciated by now, poliomyelitis is a preventable disease. International involvement by various agencies are leading close to elimination, except in some pockets. Two types of polio vaccines are available. Killed (Salk) vaccine was the first to be discovered. The new variant developed from viruses grown in monkey kidney cell cultures is administered subcutaneously in four doses 2 months, 4 months, 6–18 months, and 4–6 years after birth. The trivalent oral polio vaccine (OPV) that is extensively used all over the world is given in multiple doses as per Expanded Program on Immunization or Universal Immunization Program. The first dose is now given on Day 1 followed by three doses at 4–6 week intervals. The first booster is given 1 year after the fourth dose. Under the current program, fractionated inactivated polio vaccine (IPV) is given along with the second and third dose viz. 6 weeks and 14 weeks. Under the Pulse Polio Program, all children below the age of 5 years are given additional doses every year to complete the elimination strategy. This is given irrespective of previous immunization history.

ECHO VIRUSES

Enteric cytopathogenic human orphan (ECHO) viruses cause a spectrum of illnesses in humans ranging from mild febrile episodes to aseptic meningitis. The virus is spread through the feco-oral route. The usual incubation period is 2–5 days. Nonspecific fevers, infections of the upper respiratory tract, diarrhea, pneumonia, myocarditis, and aseptic meningitis are the common manifestations. There is no specific treatment or vaccines. Improvement in sanitation and avoiding contact with flies and contaminated food are suggested as preventive measures.

They also cause the acute hemorrhagic conjunctivitis (AHC) with an incubation period of 24–72 hours. Infection is acquired through contaminated hands and fomites. Bilateral conjunctivitis with irritation of the eyes usually subsiding in a few days is the manifestation. Occasional patients may develop neurological complications with asymmetric flaccid paralysis affecting the limbs or cranial nerve palsies.

COXSACKIE VIRUSES

These viruses belonging to the family of picornaviruses were discovered from the village by name Coxsackie near New York in 1948 by Dalldorf. They are a set of about 30 immunologically distinct types grouped as Coxsackie A and B viruses. They infect humans by the feco-oral route and produce various illnesses like respiratory infections, hand, foot, and mouth disease, herpangina, carditis, meningitis, or flaccid paralysis. The involvement of pleura by Coxsackie virus type B leads to pleurodynia—also called as Bornholm's disease. This is usually accompanied by severe pain and may lead to complications like pleural effusion, pericarditis, myocarditis, hepatitis, orchitis etc. Both A and B type Coxsackie viruses may be the cause for myopericarditis, cardiomyopathy, or constrictive pericarditis. Coxsackie type B has also been associated with congenital infection leading to congenital heart diseases.

Hand, foot, and mouth disease caused by various subtypes of Coxsackie virus type A is a vesiculobullous exanthematous fever of children but spreading to adults also. Superficial vesicles develop in the palms, soles, and buccal mucosa. This is a self-limited disease which heals without any scar formation or other sequelae. No specific treatment or vaccine is available.

RECOMMENDED READINGS

1. Bennett JE, Dolin R, Blaser MJ (Eds). Mandell, Douglas, and Bennett's Principles and Practice of Infectious Diseases, 9th edition. Elsevier; 2019.
2. Spec A, Escota GV, Chrisler C, Davies B. Comprehensive Review of Infectious Diseases, 1st edition. Elsevier; 2019.
3. World Health Organization. (2019). Global Polio Eradication Initiative investment case 2019–2023. Geneva (WHO/POLIO/19.06). [online] Available from https://polioeradication.org/wp-content/uploads/2019/08/Polio-InvestmentCase-Report-20190819.pdf.
4. World Health Organization. (2014). Ebola and Marburg virus disease epidemics: preparedness, alert, control and evaluation. [online] Available from https://apps.who.int/iris/bitstream/handle/10665/130160/ WHO_HSE_PED_CED_ 2014.05_eng.pdf?sequence=1.

CHAPTER 47

DNA Viruses: Herpes Simplex, Varicella Zoster, Epstein–Barr Virus, Cytomegalovirus, and Human Papillomavirus

Jaya Chakravarty, Shubham Gupta, Aakash Rai

ABSTRACT

Herpesvirus family contains various deoxyribonucleic acid (DNA) viruses which are known to cause latent infection and reactivate when the host is immunocompromised. Herpes simplex virus type 1 (HSV-1) and type 2 (HSV-2) both are known to cause mucocutaneous infections and central nervous system (CNS) infections with permanent sequelae and death, if not treated. HSV can also cause neonatal HSV infection which also has high mortality. Varicella zoster virus causes two manifestations; primary infection can cause chicken pox while reactivation causes herpes zoster. Both the manifestations can be prevented by appropriate vaccination.

Epstein–Barr virus (EBV) causes infectious mononucleosis (IM) and it is also associated with various lymphoproliferative disorders and malignancy. Substantial mortality and morbidity due to cytomegalovirus (CMV) infection can be seen in immunocompromised individuals. It can be a primary infection or a secondary infection due to reactivation or reinfection. Transmission can occur via multiple routes such as sexual exposure, close contact, blood or tissue exposure, occupational exposure, and perinatal exposure. Most common presentation in immunocompetent host is CMV mononucleosis.

Human papillomavirus (HPV) is the most common sexually transmitted disease and is associated with various malignancies such as cervical, penile, anal, and vulvovaginal cancers. Vaccination of adolescents and regular screening for cervical cancer should be done to prevent cervical cancer.

"An inefficient virus kills its host. A clever virus stays with it"

—James Lovelock

HERPESVIRUSES

The herpesvirus family contains numerous species of DNA viruses that infects humans and animals. There are eight herpesviruses which infect humans: HSV types 1 and 2, varicella-zoster virus (VZV), CMV, EBV, human herpesvirus 6 (HHV-6), HHV-7, and Kaposi's sarcoma virus or HHV-8. These viruses establish latent infections which can persist indefinitely with periodic activation.

TABLE 1 Subfamilies of family *Herpesviridae*.

Subfamily	Duration of replication/ cytopathology	Sites of latency	Species
• **Alphaherpesviridae**	12–18 h/cytolytic	Neurons	• Human herpesvirus 1 (herpes simplex virus 1) • Human herpesvirus 2 (herpes simplex virus 2) • Varicella-zoster virus
• **Betaherpesviridae**	>24 h/cytomegalic	Glands and kidneys	• Cytomegalovirus (CMV)
	>24 h/lymphoproliferative	T cells	• Human herpesvirus 6 • Human herpesvirus 7
• **Gammaherpesviridae**	Variable/lymphoproliferative	B cells	• Epstein–Barr virus (EBV) • Human herpesvirus 8

Genome of herpesvirus consists of linear double stranded DNA (dsDNA) surrounded by icosahedral capsid and lipid envelope. Between capsid and lipid layer, there is tegument which contains various proteins.

Family *Herpesviridae* is divided into three subfamilies based on physical, biochemical, and genetics properties (**Table 1**).

HERPES SIMPLEX VIRUS

Herpes simplex virus type 1 and HSV-2 cause infections of mucocutaneous surfaces, the CNS, and visceral organs. HSV subtypes share 50% genomic homology and 80% proteome homology. Type-specific regions unique to HSV-1 and HSV-2 used to develop serological assays to distinguish between these two.

PREVALENCE

Herpes simplex virus type 1 infections are more common than HSV-2 and around 90% adults have antibodies to HSV-1 by fifth decade of life. Antibodies to HSV-2 are not detected routinely until puberty.

Prevalence of HSV-2 is higher in developing countries. Studies suggest that prevalent HSV-2 infection increases the risk of human immunodeficiency virus (HIV) infection by seven to nine times. It is more frequently reactivated and transmitted in persons coinfected with HIV-1.

TRANSMISSION

Transmission of HSV infection occurs from contact with persons who have active ulcerative lesions or with persons who have no clinical manifestation and shedding HSV from mucocutaneous surfaces. Rate of shedding is highest during initial years and immunosuppressed patients shed HSV at higher frequency.

PATHOGENESIS

After exposure to HSV at mucosal surfaces or abraded skin sites, virus enters into epidermal and dermal cells and replication of virus therein followed by infection of sensory and/or autonomic nerve endings and then transported intra-axonally to the nerve cell bodies in ganglia. During initial phase of infection, viral replication occurs in ganglia and contiguous neural tissue. Virus then spread to other mucocutaneous surfaces through centrifugal migration of infectious virions via peripheral sensory nerves. In 30–40% of primary HSV-2 infections, there can be HSV viremia. Trigeminal ganglia is most commonly affected followed by inferior and superior cervical ganglion in HSV-1 while sacral ganglia in HSV-2.

After resolution of primary disease, infectious HSV cannot be cultured from the ganglia; however, neuronal infection (presence of viral DNA) persists in ganglionic cells at site of initial infection.

CLINICAL MANIFESTATIONS

The clinical manifestations and course of HSV infection depend on site involved, age, immune status, and the antigenic type of the virus. Primary HSV infections are frequently accompanied by systemic signs and symptoms, have longer duration of symptoms and virus isolation from lesions, involve both mucosal and extramucosal sites as compared with recurrent episodes. The incubation period ranges from 1 to 26 days (median, 6–8 days). Both viral subtypes can cause genital and orofacial infections, and is clinically indistinguishable. Genital HSV-2 infection is twice as likely to reactivate and recurs 8–10 times more frequently than genital HSV-1 infection. Conversely, orolabial HSV-1 infection recurs more frequently than orolabial HSV-2 infection.

Mucocutaneous lesions: Gingivostomatitis and pharyngitis (involving hard and soft palate, gingiva, tongue, lip, and facial area) are the most common clinical manifestations of HSV-1 infection and commonly seen among children and young adults. Other cutaneous lesions that can be seen are herpetic whitlow, herpes gladiatorum, eczema herpeticum, and erythema multiforme.

In HSV-1 reactivation, recurrent herpes labialis is the most common clinical manifestation with asymptomatic virus excretion, intraoral mucosal ulcerations, or herpetic ulcerations on the vermilion border of the lip or external facial skin.

Primary genital herpes is characterized by fever, headache, malaise, and myalgias with local symptoms such as pain and discharge. Widely spaced bilateral lesions in various stages on external genitalia are characteristic. The cervix and urethra are involved in >80% of women with first-episode infections.

Occasionally, there can be endometritis and salpingitis in women and prostatitis in men.

COMPLICATIONS

Ocular lesions: Herpes simplex virus type 1 is more common to infect eye and severe conjunctivitis is the most common manifestation. There can also be HSV keratitis or chorioretinitis can be seen in neonates or in patients with HIV infection.

Central and peripheral nervous system:

Herpes simplex virus encephalitis: It is more common in children and young adults due to neurotropic spread from the periphery via the olfactory bulb or via latent HSV-1 infection reactivation and present with acute onset of fever and focal neurologic symptoms and signs, especially in the temporal lobe. In cerebrospinal fluid (CSF), there is leukocytosis (lymphocytic), increased protein and red blood cell (RBC) due to hemorrhagic necrosis. Brain biopsy is gold standard for HSV encephalitis. Polymerase chain reaction (PCR) for HSV DNA in CSF is highly sensitive and has replaced biopsy. Antibodies to HSV in CSF and serum increase in most cases of HSV encephalitis, generally after 10 days. Antivirals like acyclovir decreases mortality, if initiated early. Acyclovir intravenous (IV) (30 mg/kg/day in three divided doses) should be given to suspected patients until the diagnosis is confirmed or an alternative diagnosis is made. Even with therapy, neurologic sequelae and recurrences are common, especially among patients >50 years of age.

Herpes simplex virus meningitis: It is an acute, self-limited disease lasting 2–7 days. HSV is the most common identified cause of recurrent lymphocytic meningitis (*Mollaret's meningitis*). In frequent recurrences of HSV meningitis, daily antiviral therapy reduces the frequency of recurrence. *Autonomic dysfunction*: It is seen especially in sacral region. Other neurological manifestations can be transverse myelitis, Guillain-Barré syndrome, Bell's palsy, and cranial polyneuritis.

Visceral infections: It is due to viremia, and multiple-organ involvement is common. It can manifest as HSV esophagitis (distal esophagus is commonly involved), HSV pneumonitis, herpetic tracheobronchitis, and hepatitis and rarely as monoarticular arthritis, adrenal necrosis, idiopathic thrombocytopenia, and glomerulonephritis.

Immunosuppression is risk factor for dissemination to other visceral organs such as adrenal glands, pancreas, small and large intestine, and bone marrow.

Neonatal herpes simplex virus infections: Neonates have the highest frequency of visceral and/or CNS infection. Risk is highest when mother is recently infected and is usually acquired perinatally from contact with infected genital secretions at delivery. It may also be acquired postnatally through contact with individuals having orolabial HSV-1 infection or nosocomial transmission, 30–50% are due to HSV-1 and 50–70% are due to HSV-2. Without treatment, the mortality rate is 65% and antivirals have decreased mortality rate to ~15%.

DIAGNOSIS

Staining of scrapings from base of lesion with Wright's, Giemsa's (Tzanck preparation) or Papanicolaou's stain detects giant cells or intranuclear inclusions of HSV. This method has got low sensitivity (<30%) and does not differentiate between HSV and VZV infections.

Best method is detection of virus, viral antigen, or viral DNA in scrapings from lesions. HSV DNA detection by PCR is the most sensitive laboratory technique for detecting mucosal or visceral HSV infections and is the recommended test for laboratory confirmation of a diagnosis. This can also differentiate between HSV-1 and HSV-2. Culture is indicated when antiviral sensitivity testing is required.

TREATMENT

Viral DNA polymerase inhibitors like acyclovir and its congeners famciclovir and valacyclovir are mainstays of therapy. IV acyclovir is the treatment of choice for HSV encephalitis and neonatal herpes. Valacyclovir offers greater bioavailability than acyclovir and thus can be administered less frequently. For newly acquired genital HSV infection during pregnancy, acyclovir (400 mg TDS) or valacyclovir (500–1,000 mg BD) for 7–10 days is recommended. Daily acyclovir and valacyclovir reduces the frequency of HSV reactivations among HIV-positive persons. Once-daily valacyclovir (500 mg) has been shown to reduce transmission of HSV-2 between sexual partners.

VARICELLA-ZOSTER VIRUS

It is a double-stranded, enveloped DNA virus. It causes two clinically distinct forms of disease: Varicella (chickenpox) and herpes zoster (shingles). Primary infection results in the diffuse vesicular rash of varicella, or chickenpox while reactivation of latent VZV typically results in a localized skin infection known as herpes zoster, or shingles.

CHICKENPOX

It is highly contagious, with secondary household attack rates of >90% and is transmitted by aerosolized droplets from nasopharyngeal secretions or by direct cutaneous contact with vesicle fluid from skin lesions. Manifestations are more severe in pregnant women, adults, and immunosuppressed (malignancy, steroid use or immunosuppressive therapy, HIV infection, or solid organ transplantation). Incubation period is 11–20 days and infectivity starts from 48 hours prior to the onset of rash until skin lesions have fully crusted.

Clinical manifestations: It typically starts with fever, malaise, pharyngitis, and loss of appetite followed by the development of a generalized vesicular rash within 24 hours. Rashes are pruritic, appears in successive crops in centripetal distribution. The lesions begin as macules that rapidly become papules followed by characteristic vesicles. Children may have increased incidence of secondary group A streptococcal skin and soft-tissue infection. Immunosuppressed host can include ongoing development of crops of vesicles over weeks, large and hemorrhagic skin lesions, pneumonia, or widespread disease with disseminated intravascular coagulation.

Complications: Encephalitis, hepatitis, and pneumonia are the most serious complications of VZV infection. Two distinct forms of encephalitis occur usually toward the end of the first week of the exanthem—acute cerebellar ataxia and diffuse encephalitis. Acute cerebellar ataxia mostly occurs in children and is generally followed by complete recovery. Diffuse encephalitis most often occurs in adults and is characterized by delirium, seizures, and focal neurologic signs. It is associated with approximately 10% mortality rates and long-term neurologic sequelae in up to 15%.

Reye syndrome is also reported in children due to use of aspirin. It typically presents with nausea, vomiting, headache, excitability, delirium, and combativeness with frequent progression to coma.

Pneumonia: Varicella pneumonia typically develops insidiously within 1–6 days after the rash has appeared with symptoms of progressive tachypnea, dyspnea, and dry cough. Risk factors are cigarette smoking, pregnancy, immunosuppression, and male sex. It is characterized by impaired gas exchange leading to progressive hypoxemia. Chest radiographs shows diffuse bilateral infiltrates. Prompt administration of IV acyclovir has been associated with clinical improvement. Overall mortality is between 10 and 30%.

Hepatitis: Affects immunosuppressed hosts including transplant recipients and HIV patients; the outcome is frequently fatal.

Treatment: Individuals at high risk for complications such as unvaccinated adolescents, adults, pregnant women, and immunocompromised hosts should be given antiviral therapy like valacyclovir (1 g thrice daily) or acyclovir (800 mg five times per day) for 5–7 days to reduce the severity of symptoms and/or reduce the risk of complications.

Prevention: Two doses of live attenuated vaccine can be part of universal vaccination, but it is particularly important to immunize people who have close contact with people at high risk for severe disease (e.g., healthcare workers and family contacts of immunocompromised people). Vaccine can be given as postexposure prophylaxis to those who had a significant exposure within the last 5 days and are eligible for varicella vaccine. Passive immunization with varicella-zoster immune globulin is indicated for susceptible individuals after a significant exposure if they are ineligible for varicella vaccine but are at high risk for severe infection and/or complications and can receive immunoprophylaxis within 10 days of exposure.

HERPES ZOSTER

Herpes zoster, also known as shingles, results from reactivation of latent VZV that gained access to sensory ganglia during varicella. During the initial phase of varicella, the virus infects the nasopharyngeal lymphoid tissue followed by viremia and appearance of rash. Once the rash develops, the virus, present in skin vesicles, infect nerve endings in skin and move retrograde along sensory axons to establish latency in neurons within the regional ganglia. During reactivation virus spread, antegrade down the sensory nerve to the skin and cause the typical rash. Patients with herpes zoster can transmit VZV, causing chickenpox. The most common risk factor for herpes zoster is age, other risk factors are HIV, iatrogenic immunosuppression in patients undergoing transplant, rheumatologic or cancer therapy. Herpes zoster is characterized by a painful, unilateral vesicular eruption, which usually occurs in a restricted dermatomal distribution. The thoracic and lumbar dermatomes are most commonly involved. Prodromal pain may precede the rash by 2–3 days.

Complications:

Postherpetic neuralgia: Approximately 10–15% patients, especially those above 60 years, have significant pain persisting for 90 days after the onset of rash.

Herpes zoster ophthalmicus: It is potentially sight-threatening condition due to involvement of the ophthalmic division of the fifth cranial nerve. It starts with headache, malaise, and fever. Unilateral pain or hypesthesia in the affected eye, forehead, and top of the head may precede or follow the prodrome. Then the typical rash occurs, at the same time hyperemic conjunctivitis, uveitis, episcleritis, and keratitis may also occur. Early treatment prevents progressive corneal involvement and potential loss of vision.

Acute retinal necrosis: It starts with blurring of vision which later progresses to painful loss of vision.

Ramsay Hunt syndrome (herpes zoster oticus): It is due to reactivation of latent VZV in the geniculate ganglion. It causes ipsilateral facial paralysis, ear pain, and vesicles in the auditory canal or on the auricle. Other features may be ipsilateral altered taste perception and tongue lesions, hearing abnormalities, lacrimation, and vestibular disturbances (vertigo).

Other neurological complications are aseptic meningitis, encephalitis, peripheral motor neuropathy, myelitis, Guillain–Barré syndrome, stroke syndromes, and secondary infections. Recurrent herpes occurs in 1–6% more in women and immunosuppressed.

Treatment and prevention: Antivirals acyclovir (800 mg five times daily), valacyclovir (1,000 mg three times daily), or famciclovir (500 mg three times daily) should be given within 72 hours of presentation or if new lesions are appearing. Steroids may be given in those with severe manifestations, e.g., acute retinal necrosis and Ramsay Hunt syndrome. Amitriptyline, gabapentin, or pregabalin can be used for postherpetic neuralgia. There are two types of vaccines, a recombinant glycoprotein E vaccine and a live attenuated vaccine which decreases the risk of developing herpes zoster and postherpetic neuralgia. It is recommended in those above the age >60 years and those ≥50 years old who are planning immunosuppressive therapy (e.g., transplant patients and chronic autoimmune disease), should be given zoster vaccination provided vaccination can be completed within a certain period of time prior to immunosuppression.

EPSTEIN–BARR VIRUS

Epstein–Barr virus is the primary agent of IM, persists asymptomatically for life in nearly all adults, and is associated with many malignancies. Reactivation disease is not a prominent issue with EBV, in contrast to other common herpesviruses.

PREVALENCE

Infectious mononucleosis is usually a disease of young adults. In developing countries, EBV infects children at an early age, and IM is uncommon. In developed countries, infection with EBV is often delayed until adulthood, and IM is more prevalent.

TRANSMISSION

Epstein–Barr virus is spread by contact with oral secretions from asymptomatic adults to infants and among young adults by transfer of saliva during kissing. Transmission by less intimate contact, transfusion, and bone marrow transplantation is rare.

CLINICAL MANIFESTATION

In infants and young children, most EBV infections either are asymptomatic or present as mild pharyngitis with or without tonsillitis. In contrast, ~75% of infections in adolescents present as IM. IM in the elderly often presents with nonspecific symptoms, including prolonged fever, fatigue, myalgia, and malaise.

The incubation period for IM in young adults is ~4–6 weeks. A prodrome of fatigue, malaise, and myalgia may last for 1–2 weeks before the onset of fever, sore throat, and lymphadenopathy. Fever is usually low-grade and is more common in the first 2 weeks of the illness; however, it may persist for >1 month.

Lymphadenopathy and pharyngitis are more prominent during the first 2 weeks of the illness, while splenomegaly is more prominent during the second and third weeks. Lymphadenopathy usually affects the posterior cervical nodes, but may be generalized. A morbilliform or papular rash, usually on the arms or trunk, develops in ~5% of cases.

COMPLICATIONS

Meningitis and encephalitis are the most common neurologic manifestations. There can also be cranial nerve palsies, Guillain–Barré syndrome, acute transverse myelitis, peripheral neuritis, and autoimmune hemolytic anemia (Coombs-positive, with cold agglutinins directed against the RBC antigen).

Death though rare can occur most often due to CNS complications (usually during first 2 weeks), splenic rupture (more common among males), upper airway obstruction (due to hypertrophy of lymphoid tissue in the tonsils or adenoids), or bacterial superinfection.

Other rare complications associated with acute EBV infection include hepatitis, myocarditis or pericarditis, pneumonia with pleural effusion, interstitial nephritis, genital ulcerations, and vasculitis.

Acute EBV infection has also been associated with non-specific antibody responses, may also include rheumatoid factor (RF), antinuclear antibody (ANA), anti-smooth muscle antibody (SMA), antiplatelet antibodies, and cryoglobulins. IM has been associated with red cell aplasia, severe granulocytopenia, thrombocytopenia, pancytopenia, and hemophagocytic lymphohistiocytosis.

Epstein–Barr virus has been associated with lymphoproliferative disease and has been described in patients with congenital or acquired immunodeficiency. Oral hairy leukoplakia with lesion containing EBV DNA is an early manifestation of infection with HIV in adults.

Chronic active EBV infection is very rare, affected patients have an illness lasting >6 months with elevated levels of EBV DNA in the blood; high titers of antibody to EBV; and evidence of organ involvement, including hepatosplenomegaly, lymphadenopathy, and pneumonitis, uveitis, or neurologic disease.

Epstein–Barr virus is associated with several malignancies including gastric carcinoma (most common EBV-associated malignancy), Burkitt lymphoma, anaplastic nasopharyngeal carcinoma, Hodgkin lymphoma (especially the mixed-cellularity type), non-Hodgkin lymphoma, lymphomatoid granulomatosis, angiocentric nasal natural killer (NK)/T-cell lymphoma, T-cell lymphoma, and CNS lymphoma.

DIAGNOSIS

The white blood cell count is usually elevated and peaks at 10,000–20,000/μL during the second or third week of illness. Lymphocytosis is usually demonstrable, with >10% atypical lymphocytes. CD8+ T cells predominate among the atypical lymphocytes. Low-grade neutropenia and thrombocytopenia are common during the first month of illness. Liver function test (LFT) is abnormal in >90% of cases (aminotransferases and alkaline phosphatase are mildly elevated; bilirubin is elevated in ~40% of cases).

Heterophile test: For the diagnosis of IM in children and adults, a titer of ≥40 is diagnostic of acute EBV infection in a patient who has symptoms compatible with IM and atypical lymphocytes. It is positive in 40% of patients with IM during the first week and in 80–90% during the third week. These antibodies usually are not detectable in children <5 years of age, in the elderly, or in patients presenting with symptoms not typical of IM.

Monospot test for heterophile antibodies: It is more sensitive (75%) and specific (90%) than the classic heterophile test and EBV-specific serologies.

About 90% of cases of IM are due to EBV, other causes of heterophile-negative mononucleosis include CMV (most common), HIV, toxoplasmosis, HHV-6 infection, rubella, and lymphoma.

Epstein–Barr virus-specific antibodies: It is required only in patients with suspected IM who have a negative heterophile test. Immunoglobulin M (IgM) viral capsid antigen (VCA) antibodies are highly suggestive of acute EBV infection, while immunoglobulin G (IgG) VCA antibodies persist for life and are a marker of EBV infection.

Detection of Epstein–Barr virus deoxyribonucleic acid, ribonucleic acid, or proteins: It is valuable in demonstrating the association of the virus with various malignancies such as CNS lymphoma and lymphoproliferative diseases.

TREATMENT

Therapy for IM consists of supportive measures, with rest and analgesia. Prednisone (40–60 mg/day for 2–3 days, with tapering over 1–2 weeks) has been used for the prevention of airway obstruction in patients with severe tonsillar hypertrophy, for autoimmune hemolytic anemia, for hemophagocytic lymphohistiocytosis, and for severe thrombocytopenia. Glucocorticoids have also been administered to rare patients with severe malaise and fever and to patients with severe CNS or cardiac disease. Acyclovir has been used for EBV-induced hemophagocytic lymphohistiocytosis.

In post-transplantation EBV lymphoproliferative diseases immunosuppressive therapy should be reduced.

CYTOMEGALOVIRUS

Cytomegalovirus infection in the immunocompetent host is generally asymptomatic or may present as a mononucleosis syndrome, but can be fatal in immunocompromised patients, especially among transplant recipients and HIV. Infection of pregnant women, even if asymptomatic, is occasionally associated with the syndrome of congenital CMV in newborns with long-term sequelae.

Secondary infection can be due to reactivation of latent CMV or reinfection (**Flowchart 1**). Reactivation of CMV may occur at any time during the life of the human host, but risk is higher in the setting of systemic immunosuppression. Titers of CMV-specific IgG do not appear to predict the risk of reactivation in immunocompetent hosts. The bulk of CMV-related disease in immunocompetent hosts is related to primary infection.

TRANSMISSION

Cytomegalovirus has been cultured from multiple sites, including urine, blood, throat, cervix, semen, stool, tears, and breast milk. Transmission can occur via various sites (**Table 2**).

CYTOMEGALOVIRUS MONONUCLEOSIS

A syndrome resembling IM is the most common presentation of symptomatic CMV infection in immunocompetent adults. Classic mononucleosis is an illness characterized by significant, often protracted fevers and lassitude in setting of absolute lymphocytosis and atypical lymphocytes. When the patient with symptoms and signs of classic IM is heterophile negative, then the most likely etiology is CMV infection.

Cytomegalovirus mononucleosis can be accompanied by dermatologic manifestations in approximately one-third of patients including macular, papular, maculopapular, rubelliform, morbilliform, and scarlatiniform eruptions.

COMPLICATIONS

Gastrointestinal: Cytomegalovirus colitis is almost always secondary to the reactivation of latent infection in

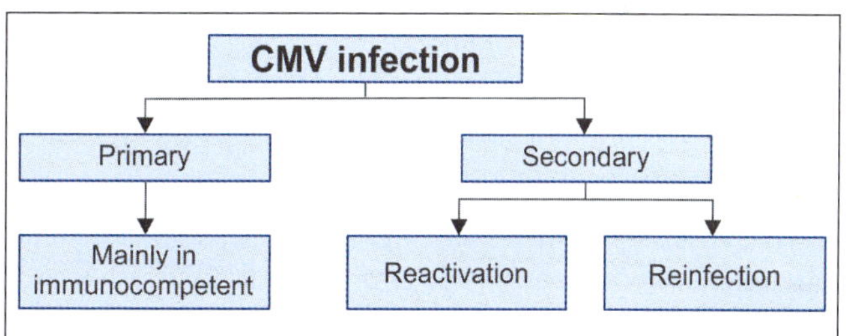

(CMV: cytomegalovirus)

FLOWCHART 1: Infection, latency, and reactivation.

TABLE 2 Transmission of CMV through various exposures.

Sexual exposure	Supported by evidence that seroprevalence rates are higher among patients with multiple sexual partners or history of prior STDs
Close contact	Seroconversion is well described among family members and children in daycare centers. Contacts are probably exposed to virus shed from the upper respiratory tract and urine
Blood or tissue exposure	Transmission of CMV following transfusion of blood products and transplantation of organs from seropositive donors is well documented
Occupational exposure	Healthcare workers may also be exposed, but the actual risk of seroconversion among susceptible individuals appears to be low.
Perinatal exposure	Neonates and infants may be infected with CMV in utero during maternal viremia, during exposure to secretions in the birth canal, or postnatally from breast milk

(CMV: cytomegalovirus; STDs: sexually transmitted diseases)

immunosuppressed patients. CMV colitis in the immunocompetent host can occur in the setting of primary infection. Diarrhea, fever, and abdominal pain are common presenting symptoms. Subclinical transaminitis is the most common finding in immunocompetent patients; elevations of alkaline phosphatase and total bilirubin are less typical.

Neurologic manifestations: Cytomegalovirus infection has been associated with numerous neurologic sequelae in the immunocompetent host.

Encephalitis: Although rare, encephalitis is a serious potential complication of CMV infection, and should be considered in the differential diagnosis of unexplained encephalitis.

Guillain-Barré syndrome: CMV-related Guillain-Barré syndrome is typically associated with the development of antibodies to ganglioside GM2, although the exact role of these antibodies remains unresolved.

Other manifestations: Brachial plexus neuropathy, diffuse axonal peripheral neuropathy, transverse myelitis, Horner's syndrome, and cranial nerve palsies.

Ocular manifestations: Cytomegalovirus retinitis is a well-known presentation in patients with advanced immunosuppression from HIV infection. It causes painless loss of vision in HIV patients with CD4 count <50/μL. Frequency of anterior uveitis due to CMV infection is increasing among immunocompetent patients.

Cardiovascular manifestations: Pericarditis and myocarditis have been described in immunocompetent patients with acute CMV infection; direct causality has not been clearly demonstrated.

TREATMENT

Among patients with symptomatic CMV infection, especially the mononucleosis syndrome, the illness is generally self-limited, with complete recovery over a period of days to weeks. Antiviral therapy is not usually indicated.

Currently, there are several agents available for the systemic therapy of CMV infection in immunosuppressed, including ganciclovir, valganciclovir, foscarnet, and cidofovir.

HUMAN PAPILLOMAVIRUS

Papillomaviruses are double-stranded, icosahedral, and nonenveloped DNA viruses that constitute the papillomavirus genus of the Papillomaviridae family. There are more than 200 types of HPV, which can be subdivided into cutaneous or mucosal categories based upon their tissue tropism. Anogenital HPV is the most common sexually transmitted infection globally. HPV infection is associated with an increased risk for HIV acquisition.

TABLE 3 Human papillomavirus (HPV) genotypes and tissue tropism.

Disease	HPV type
Cutaneous warts	
Common and plantar warts	1, 2, and 4
Flat wart	3 and 10
Butcher's wart	7 and 2
Bowen's disease	
Genital	16
Extragenital	2, 3, 4, and 16
Epidermodysplasia verruciformis	2, 3, 5, 8, 9, 10, 12, 14, 15, and 17
Condylomata acuminata	6 and 11
Squamous intraepithelial lesions	
Low grade	16, 31, 6, and 11
High grade	16, 31, 52, and 18
Oropharyngeal cancer	16
Anal cancer	16
Respiratory papillomatosis	6 and 11

NATURAL HISTORY

Most HPV infections, including those with carcinogenic HPV genotypes, typically resolve within 12 months. However, carcinogenic HPV infections that persist beyond 12 months increase the likelihood of precancerous or cancerous lesions, although not all persistent infections progress.

Human papillomavirus can enter a latent state. Additionally, there is evidence of cervical viral reactivation in some populations, including women with HIV and older women.

DISEASE ASSOCIATION

Human papillomavirus DNA is detected in almost all cases of cervical cancer, with HPV-16 accounting for approximately 50% of cases and HPV-18 for 20%. It is also associated with vulvar, vaginal, anal, oropharyngeal, penile cancer, and recurrent respiratory papillomatosis besides genital and nongenital warts.

GENOTYPES AND TISSUE TROPISM

Different HPV types have a propensity to infect different body sites and are thus associated with different diseases (**Table 3**).

PREVENTION OF CERVICAL CANCER

Pap smear is done for screening of cervical cancer. It should start at 21 years of age, and done every 3 yearly, between 21 and 29 years of age. Between 30 and 65 years, PAP test and HPV DNA cotesting every 5 year or PAP smear every 3 years.

The World Health Organization (WHO) recommends that the primary target of HPV vaccination programs is females aged 9–14 years. There are three types of vaccines:

1. Bivalent vaccine (CERVARIX) protects against HPV-16 and -18, given at 0, 1, and 6 months and approved for females of 9–25 years age.
2. Quadrivalent vaccine (GARDASIL) protects against HPV type 6, 11, 16, and 18, given at 0, 2, and 6 months and approved for both males (prevents genital wart and anal cancer) and females (prevents genital warts, cervical cancer and anal cancer) of 9–26 years.
3. Nine-valent vaccine (GARDASIL-9) protects against HPV type 6, 11, 16, 18, 31, 33, 45, 52, and 58, given at 0, 2, and 6 months.

RECOMMENDED READINGS

1. Looker KJ, Elmes JAR, Gottlieb SL, Schiffer JT, Vickerman P, Turner KME, et al. Effect of HSV-2 infection on subsequent HIV acquisition: an updated systematic review and meta-analysis. Lancet Infect Dis. 2017;17(12):1303-16.
2. Looker KJ, Magaret AS, Turner KME, Vickerman P, Gottlieb SL, Newman LM. Global estimates of prevalent and incident herpes simplex virus type 2 infections in 2012. PLoS One. 2015;10:e114989.
3. Gnann JW Jr, Whitley RJ. Herpes Simplex Encephalitis: an Update. Curr Infect Dis Rep. 2017;19(3):13.
4. Dunmire SK, Verghese PS, Balfour HH Jr. Primary Epstein-Barr virus infection. J Clin Virol. 2018;102:84-92.
5. Dunmire SK, Hogquist KA, Balfour HH Jr. Infectious mononucleosis. Curr Top Microbiol Immunol. 2015;390:211-40.
6. Mansfield SA, Dwivedi V, Elgharably H, Griessl M, Zimmerman PD, Limaye AP, et al. Cytomegalovirus immunoglobulin G titers do not predict reactivation risk in immunocompetent hosts. J Med Virol. 2019;91: 836-44.
7. Choi JA, Kim KS, Jung Y, Park HY, Park CK. Cytomegalovirus as a cause of hypertensive anterior uveitis in immunocompetent patients. J Ophthalmic Inflamm Infect. 2016;6:32.
8. Nangle S, Mitra S, Roskos S, Havlichek D. Cytomegalovirus infection in immunocompetent adults: Is observation still the best strategy? IDCases. 2018;14: e00442.
9. Maglennon GA, Doorbar J. The biology of papillomavirus latency. Open Virol J. 2012;6:190-7.

CHAPTER 48

Other Virus Infections: Chikungunya, Hantavirus, Nipah Virus, and Zika Virus

Gaurav Gupta, Manasvini Bhatt, Ashutosh Biswas

ABSTRACT

Chikungunya fever (CHIKF) is an acute febrile illness typically accompanied by rash and severe, debilitating and often chronic arthralgia. Chikungunya virus (CHIKV) is an arthropod-borne *Alphavirus* transmitted by *Aedes aegypti* mosquitoes. The typical distribution of CHIKV has been observed in Africa and Southeast Asia. Outbreaks of chikungunya disease have also occurred in Europe, Islands in the Indian and Pacific Oceans, and subsequently in the Americas. Previously, the large outbreak occurred in 2006 and this was seen as reemergence of the virus in India. In August 2016, another large outbreak was reported from New Delhi and the National Capital Region, which resulted in around 14,656 clinically suspected cases. There was no direct mortality reported but yes, few cases especially in elderly population had a fatal outcome. Signs and symptoms begin abruptly with fever, maculopapular rash, malaise, and polyarthralgia. The majority of infected individuals is symptomatic and about 5–15% of the cases may be asymptomatic. There is no antiviral drug approved for treatment of CHIKV infection and supportive management has to be initiated in all the cases which depend on the phase and duration of the illness.

Hantaviruses belong to family Bunyaviridae, which is acquired through inhalation of aerosols or dust particles contaminated with virus-containing rodent excreta. The two important acute febrile clinical syndromes associated with hantavirus infection are hemorrhagic fever with renal syndrome (HFRS) in Asia and Europe and hantavirus pulmonary syndrome (HPS). Hantaan (HTN) viruses were first isolated in Korea in 1978, present in striped field mouse, *Apodemus agrarius*. HTN viruses are responsible for HFRS in China, eastern Russia, and Korea. Dobrava-Belgrade virus (DOBV) was present in *Aedes flavicollis* which is reported to cause severe HFRS in Balkans countries. The clinical hallmarks of HFRS are fever, thrombocytopenia, and acute renal dysfunction pathologically typical of acute interstitial nephritis. The mortality rate in severe HFRS is around 5% caused by HTN or Dobrava viruses, one-third during the shock phase and the remaining two-thirds with renal failure and pulmonary edema. HPS is much more severe form in comparison to HFRS, which begins with a febrile prodrome and followed by a rapid increase in pulmonary vascular permeability and shock. There is no recommended drug for treatment of hantavirus infections. However, in vitro and in vivo studies suggest anti-hantaviral property with ribavirin but remain ineffective in management of HPS. Supportive therapy including careful fluid management, electrolyte balance, and hemodynamic measure is the best possible measures to decrease the mortality.

Nipah virus is highly fatal and emerging zoonotic paramyxoviruses that infect humans directly or indirectly from animals. Nipah virus was first identified in Malaysia and Singapore in 1998–1999 during outbreaks of severe encephalitis in farmers who were in direct contact with sick pigs or their contaminated tissues. Since the emergence, the virus has reappeared in parts of India and Bangladesh with a mortality rate of 60–70%. Large fruit bats of *Pteropus* genus are the natural host and reservoir of Nipah virus. Presumably, pigs may become infected after consumption of partially bat eaten fruits that are dropped in pigsties. The virus causes severe acute encephalitis and the illness may manifest with self-limiting influenza-like symptoms and/or severe respiratory distress. Nipah infection primarily involves the blood vessels leading to vasculopathy and vasculitis resulting in perivascular cellular infiltration, inflammation, and necrosis. There is no definite treatment or vaccination for protection from infection either for animals or humans. Hence, the mainstay management is limited to supportive care, including rest, hydration, and treatment of underlying symptoms. Patient isolation and barrier nursing should be practiced.

Zika virus (ZIKV) was first identified in Zika forest, Entebbe, Uganda in 1947 in a caged rhesus monkey. Later in 1952 in Uganda and the United Republic of Tanzania, it was reported in humans too. This virus is mostly mosquito-borne and the infection usually presents with minimal or no signs and symptoms and usually goes unnoticed or labeled with undifferentiated tropical fever. Neurotropic nature is the reason to worry as a subset of cases may end up with Guillain–Barré syndrome (GBS), neuropathy, myelitis, and congenital Zika syndrome (CZS). *Aedes aegypti*, *Aedes polynesiensis*, and *Aedes albopictus* are the most potential vectors responsible for the transmission of ZIKV infection. ZIKV infection should be suspected in patients reporting with symptoms among those individuals who travelled to areas with ongoing transmission during the 2 weeks preceding the onset of illness. The infection mimics dengue and chikungunya during the acute infection phases and imperative to differentiate between the infections. There is no definite treatment approved yet for ZIKV infection. Hence, the mainstay of management is limited to supportive care, including rest, hydration, and treatment of underlying symptoms.

- Chikungunya and Hantavirus infections are given in detail in the printed book and in the E-book.
- The abstracts of Nipah virus and Zika virus are given in the printed book and in the E-book.
- The detail write up of Nipah virus and Zika virus is available in the E-book only. The interested reader should go to the E-book. The MCQ's of all four are given together in sequence.

"Science is organized knowledge. Wisdom is organized life"

—Immanuel Kant

CHIKUNGUNYA

INTRODUCTION

Chikungunya fever is an acute febrile illness typically accompanied by rash and severe debilitating and often chronic arthralgia. CHIKV is an arthropod-borne *Alphavirus* transmitted by *A. aegypti* mosquitoes and was first identified in Tanzania in 1953. Since then it is reported all over the African continent and later in 1960, outbreaks in Southeast Asian countries like India, Sri Lanka, Thailand, and Malaysia. The name chikungunya is inspired from an African language and means "that which bends up" or "stooped walk" because of the debilitating nature of disease. The resurgence of this viral infection is seen in past few decades, which have a huge economic and social impact due to lack of any approved antiviral or vaccines.

VIROLOGY

Chikungunya virus is a member of Togaviridae family, genus *Alphavirus*. The virus is 70 nm in diameter in an icosahedral symmetry which comprises repeating units of envelope glycoproteins (E1 and E2), the capsid (C), positive-sense single stranded RNA virus, and host-derived lipid bilayer. The genome encodes nonstructural proteins and structural proteins.

EPIDEMIOLOGY

History and emergence: Since its first outbreak in 1952, several outbreaks have been reported. The typical distribution of CHIKV is observed in Africa and Southeast Asia. Although outbreaks of chikungunya disease have also occurred in Europe, Islands in the Indian and Pacific Oceans, and subsequently in the Americas. Most outbreaks occur during the tropical rainy season and abate during the dry season. Several major outbreaks were observed in 2004 in Kenya and in 2005 La Réunion Islands. The virus soon was transmitted to several Islands in Indian Ocean and then to India, Sri Lanka, Malaysia, and Thailand. **Figure 1** shows the geographical distribution of endemic CHIKV and its primary vectors, *A. aegypti*, and *Aedes albopictus*.

India: The first case reported in India was isolated in Calcutta in 1963 and subsequently it is reported in several

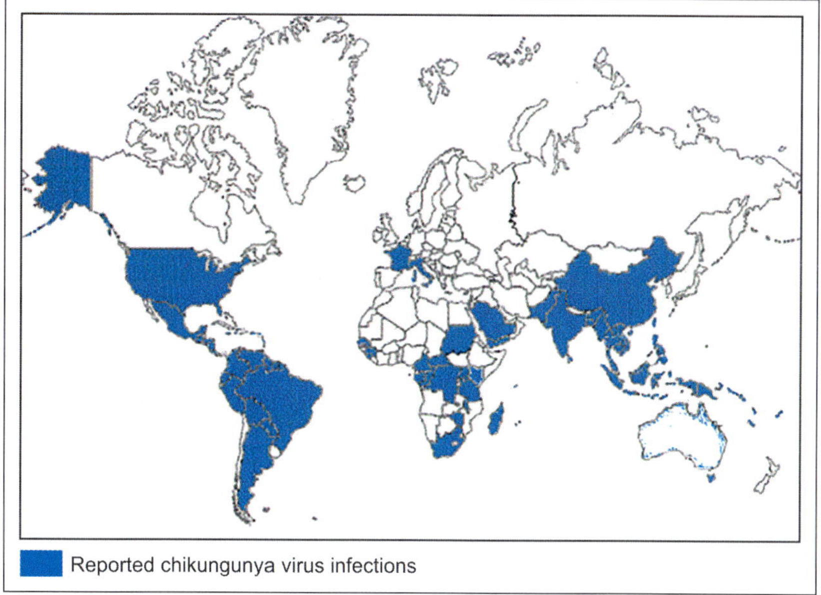

FIGURE 1: Geographical distribution of endemic chikungunya virus and its primary vectors, *Aedes aegypti* and *Aedes albopictus*.

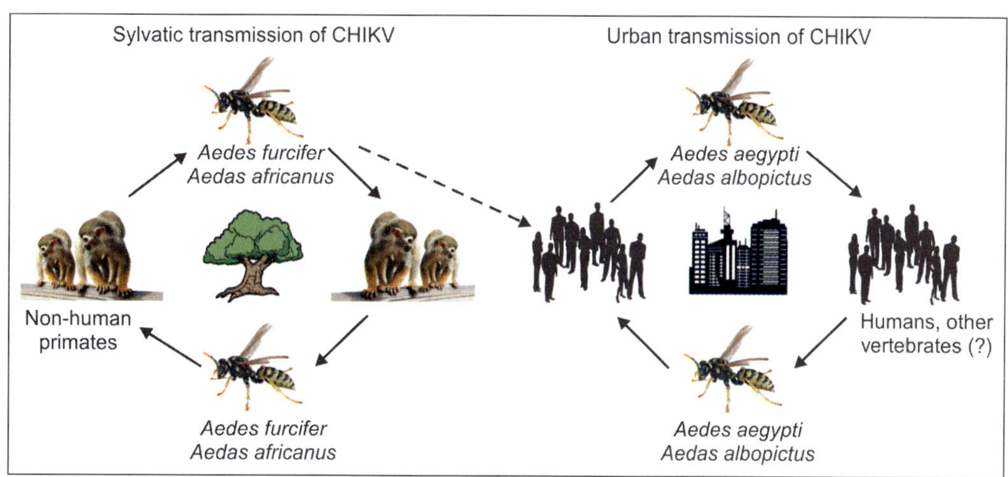

FIGURE 2: Transmission cycle of chikungunya virus (CHIKV).

parts of central and southern India. The major outbreak was observed in 2006 and considered as reemergence of the virus in India. Since then the disease has reappeared in 16 states/UTs and during 2015 outbreak 27,553 clinically suspected cases were reported. In August 2016, another large outbreak was reported from New Delhi and the National Capital Region, which resulted in around 14,656 clinically suspected cases. There was no direct mortality reported whereas few cases especially in elderly population had a fatal outcome.

Vector-borne transmission: Chikungunya is transmitted by the mosquito vectors *A. aegypti* and *A. albopictus*. They bite primarily during the daytime and these mosquito vectors are also capable of transmitting *Zika virus, Dengue virus*, and yellow fever. Nonvector-borne transmission is not significant such as blood transfusion, breast feeding, and occupational exposure to potentially infectious material in healthcare settings and sexual transmission. CHIKV has not been detected in breast milk, and transmission of CHIKV via breastfeeding has not been reported. **Figure 2** shows diagrammatic representation of transmission cycle of CHIKV.

Till now are three lineages of CHIKV with distinctive genotypic and antigenic characteristics have been identified. The largest phylogenetic group East/Central/South African (ECSA) was isolated during 2004–2006 epidemics in Indian Ocean. The other two lineages are Asian and West African. There are two natural cycles identified in transmission of CHIKV, one is sylvatic cycle affecting primates and mosquitoes and the other one is an urban cycle affecting humans and mosquitoes. The sylvatic cycles maintain the virus via enzootic infections in wild primates and *Aedes* in the forests. The epidemics are mostly occurring due to spillover of enzootic infection in person working in forests or nearby localities and subsequent passage of the virus to urban and suburban places with *Aedes* vector. Another way of spread occurs via infected air travelers who are in the asymptomatic period of incubation (usually 1–4 days).

PATHOGENESIS

The infection starts with the bite of mosquito to the skin and the viral replication takes place in the susceptible cells including macrophages and fibroblasts. The virus disseminates in the body via lymphatic and hematogenous routes. Patients with CHIKF typically develop viremia within two days of infection, and the virus directly invades and replicates within the joints. The virus directly infects the synovium, tenosynovium, and muscle, leading to immune response and production of proinflammatory mediators and recruitment of leukocytes. This leads to extensive infiltration of inflammatory cells macrophages and monocytes, and proinflammatory chemokines and cytokines. Due the immune response, the individual complains of myalgia and arthralgia. Typically, infectious virus is cleared from the circulation within days and from joints within a couple of weeks. In recent times, the atypical manifestation such as hemorrhage, hepatitis, myocarditis, ocular disease, and neurological disorders is also observed. The most vulnerable groups are neonates, elderly, and individuals with comorbidities.

In the chronicity, up to 60% of individuals may develop CHIKV-induced arthritis. There may be a persistent viral replication and a persistent inflammatory response [especially interleukin-6 (IL-6), IL-8, and monocyte chemoattractant protein 1 (MCP-1)] within the synovial fluid leading to inflammatory arthritis.

CLINICAL MANIFESTATIONS

Signs and symptoms begin abruptly with fever, maculopapular rash, malaise, and polyarthralgia. Following an incubation period of 3–7 days (range 1–14 days), the clinical symptoms start and the acute illness usually lasts for 7–10 days. The majority of infected individuals is symptomatic and about 5–15% of the cases may be asymptomatic. **Table 1** describes the three stages of the disease.

ACUTE STAGE

Fever: Acute infection starts with high grade fever and severe arthralgia, this may be accompanied by rash for a period of 1–7 days. The fever is abrupt, high grade with intermittent chills and lasts for 2–3 days and the fever may return for 1–2 days after a gap of 4–10 days, this is known as "saddle back" fever curve.

Arthralgia and arthritis: Arthralgia is a prominent feature of acute CHIKV infection, usually bilateral and symmetrical in about 70% of cases. Arthralgia involves distal joints more than proximal joints and is associated with morning stiffness. The predominant joint involvement is ankle, wrist, and small joints. Migratory polyarthritis with periarticular edema was reported in almost 70% of cases in recent outbreaks.

Cutaneous manifestations: Skin manifestations have been reported in 40–75% of patients. The most common cutaneous manifestation is macular or maculopapular rash reported in 40–70% of patients which usually starts 3–4 days or later after onset of illness and lasts for 3–7 days. The rash starts from the limbs and trunk, may involve the face, and is patchy or diffuse in nature. The rash is associated with pruritus in about 25–50% of patients.

Other clinical manifestations: Additional clinical manifestations in acute phase of illness may include headache, myalgia, facial puffiness, red eyes, and nausea. Neonates are at risk of severe infections and mostly have neurologic complications. **Table 2** describes the clinical manifestations of acute chikungunya disease.

The most common laboratory abnormalities are lymphopenia, thrombocytopenia, and mild elevation in hepatic transaminases and creatinine level.

CHRONIC STAGE

Usually, 10–15% of patients those who have severe CHIKF progress to subacute or chronic phase. Patients may continue to have chronic inflammatory polyarthritis, tenosynovitis, plantar fasciitis, and frozen shoulder.

LABORATORY DIAGNOSIS

In a suspected case of CHIKV infection, laboratory diagnosis of CHIKV depends on the day of the illness and the availability of the test. The diagnosed can be confirmed with either real-time reverse transcription polymerase chain reaction (RT-PCR) or chikungunya serology or combination of both.

TABLE 1 Stages of chikungunya disease.

Stages of disease	Characteristics
Acute stage (<3 weeks)	Fever with inflammatory arthralgia/arthritis, accompanied by other nonspecific symptoms, e.g., myalgia, headache, and rash
Subacute stage (3 weeks–3 months)	Occurs in ~50% of patients and involves persistent joint pain
Chronic stage (>3 months to years)	Occurs in a small proportion of patients. In most, it involves various musculoskeletal features; some (5–10%) have chronic inflammatory rheumatism

TABLE 2 List of clinical manifestations of acute chikungunya disease.

Typical	Infrequent	Atypical
• Fever • Arthralgia • Backache • Headache • Rash	• Stomatitis • Oral ulcers • Hyper-pigmentation • Exfoliative dermatitis	• Acute encephalopathy • Meningoencephalitis • Guillain–Barré syndrome • Iridocyclitis and retinitis • Myocarditis • Acute hepatitis • Acute respiratory failure • Acute renal failure

In a suspected patient with duration of illness 1–7 days, a RT-PCR for detection of CHIKV RNA is preferred for a virus detection. A negative RT-PCR result should be followed by CHIKV serologic testing via enzyme-linked immunosorbent assay (ELISA) or indirect fluorescent antibody (IFA).

In a suspected with duration of illness >8 days, a CHIKV serologic testing via ELISA or IFA should be performed. A positive result establishes a diagnosis of CHIKV infection. Immunoglobulin (Ig) M anti-CHIKV antibodies can be detected as early on 5th day and may persist for several weeks to 3 months. IgG antibodies begin to appear about 2 weeks following onset of symptoms and persist for years. **Table 3** describes the case definition of suspected and confirmed chikungunya case. **Table 4** describes the differential diagnosis of acute and chronic CHIKV disease.

TREATMENT

There is no antiviral drug approved for treatment of CHIKV infection and supportive management has to be initiated in all the cases which depend on the phase and duration of the illness. **Table 5** describes the treatment options according to stages of chikungunya disease.

ACUTE STAGE

Treatment of acute phase of disease comprises supportive care with rest, fluids, and antipyretics (e.g., acetaminophen). Hospitalization is not frequently required and needed only in infants, older adults, or immunocompromised patients with organ-threatening disease.

SUBACUTE STAGE

In some patients, arthralgia persists in the postacute phase (between 1 month and up to the end of the third month after onset of infection). These patients require a prolonged analgesic (e.g., acetaminophen) and nonsteroidal anti-inflammatory agents (NSAIDs) are recommended for duration of 2–3 weeks of duration. In cases with arthralgia or arthritis, tendinitis, or bursitis, especially with clinical

TABLE 3 Case definition of suspected and confirmed chikungunya case.

Suspected case	A patient fulfilling only the clinical criteria (described below)
Confirmed case	A patient meeting both the clinical and laboratory criteria
	Clinical criteria: Acute onset of fever and severe arthralgia/arthritis with or without skin rash and residing or having left an epidemic area 15 days prior to onset of symptoms
	Laboratory criteria: At least one of the following tests done in the acute phase of illness
	Direct evidence: Virus isolation/presence of viral RNA by RT-PCR
	Indirect evidence: • Presence of virus specific IgM antibodies in single serum sample collected in acute or convalescent stage • Fourfold increase in IgG values in samples collected at least 3 weeks apart. Cases are to be categorized for the purpose of epidemiological reporting

(Ig: immunoglobulin; RT-PCR: reverse transcription polymerase chain reaction)

TABLE 4 Differential diagnosis of acute and chronic chikungunya virus (CHIKV) disease.

Acute CHIKV disease	Chronic CHIKV disease
• Dengue fever • Malaria • Leptospirosis • Rickettsial disease • Reactive arthritis • Acute rheumatic fever • Zika virus	• Seronegative rheumatoid arthritis • Reactive arthritis • Systemic lupus erythematosus

TABLE 5 Treatment options according to stages of chikungunya disease.

Drug class	Drug	Acute stage	Subacute stage	Chronic stage
Analgesics	Acetaminophen (<4 g/day for adult)	+	+	+
	Antineuropathic drugs	–	±	+
Anti-inflammatory drugs	Oral NSAIDs including aspirin	–	+	+
	Topical NSAIDs	–	+	+
	Oral corticosteroids	–	±	+
	Intra-articular corticosteroids	–	±	+
Disease-modifying antirheumatic drugs	Methotrexate	–	±	+
	Hydroxychloroquine	–	±	±
	Sulfasalazine	–	±	+
	Leflunomide	–	±	+
	Biological agents	–	–	+
Physical treatment		+	+	+

(+: indicated; ±: restricted indication; –: not indicated)

and radiological of severe synovitis and joint swelling and persistent elevation of inflammatory markers, a short course of oral prednisone 10–20 mg daily for 5 days and then tapered over 10 day is recommended.

CHRONIC STAGE

In patients with refractory chronic arthritis (duration >3 months of illness), the treatment should be initiated with disease-modifying antirheumatic drugs (DMARDs). The most common and recommended DMARDs are methotrexate and hydroxychloroquine for the management of chronic arthritis. If the DMARDs are contraindicated or ineffective then immune-modulating biologic agents as etanercept, rituximab, and tocilizumab should be used in management.

PREVENTION

- Mosquito protection measures to avoid mosquito bites include personal protection and environmental control measures.
- Vaccine development—development of a vaccine for prevention of CHIKV infection is underway: A live-attenuated, measles-vectored vaccine expressing CHIKV structural proteins (MV-CHIK), and CHIKV-like particle (VLP) vaccine have demonstrated safety and tolerability.

HANTAVIRUS

INTRODUCTION

Hantaviruses belong to family *Bunyaviridae,* which is acquired through inhalation of aerosols or dust particles contaminated with virus-containing rodent excreta. The important two acute febrile clinical syndromes associated with hantavirus infection are HFRS in Asia and Europe, and HPS. The fundamental mechanism behind the pathogenesis of both HFRS and HPS is an increase in vascular permeability which leads to hypotension, thrombocytopenia, and leukocytosis.

VIROLOGY

Hantavirus viron has spherical shape, with size ranging 80 and 120 nm, single-stranded, negative-sense RNA genomes that are divided into three segments as shown in **Figure 3**. On the basis of their sizes, these RNAs are named as small (S), medium (M), and large (L). All the three RNAs are encapsidated by the nucleocapsid (N) protein to form ribonucleoprotein (RNP). L segment encodes viral polymerase, while M and S segments encode the precursor (GPC) for two viral surface glycoproteins (G1 and G2, or alternatively called Gn and Gc).

EPIDEMIOLOGY

Almost 40 hantavirus species are discovered till now and out of which 22 are considered to be pathogenic.

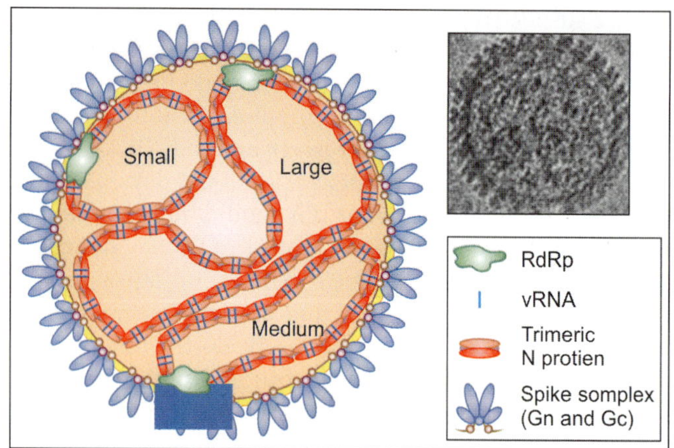

FIGURE 3: Pictorial representation of hantavirus structure, showing three RNAs are encapsidated by the nucleocapsid (N) protein enveloped in a lipid bilayer.

HTN viruses were first isolated in Korea in 1978, present in striped field mouse, *A. agrarius.* HTN viruses are responsible for HFRS in China, eastern Russia, and Korea. DOBV was present in *A. flavicollis* which is reported to cause severe HFRS in Balkans countries. In Europe, *Puumala virus* hosted by *Myodes glareolus* causes a mild form of nephropathia epidemica (NE), a mild form of HFRS. In the both North and South Americas, hantaviruses cause acute respiratory disease called as hantavirus pulmonary syndrome. *Sin Nombre virus* (SNV) which is hosted by deer mice, *Peromyscus maniculatus* is the etiologic agent of HPS in North America. In South America, Andes virus (ANDV) is common cause of HPS and is the only hantavirus spread by human-to-human transmission. *Thottapalayam virus* (TPMV) is the only virus isolated from India, however, very scarce knowledge is available about the natural host and biology of the virus. **Figure 4** shows the global distribution of hantaviruses and the clinical syndrome associated with the viral illnesses.

TRANSMISSION

The most important factor in the transmission of hantaviruses to humans is the interaction between humans and rodent. Each virus species has unique mammal host with its geographical distribution. They get chronically infected and excrete virus in urine, feces, and saliva for weeks to months. The transmission to humans is via aerosol route with virus-contaminated rodent urine or feces.

PATHOGENESIS

The viral infection begins with inhalation of aerosol contaminated urine or feces of rodent. The virus primarily infects macrophages and endothelial cells of the capillaries of the lung and kidney. Hantaviral Gn and Gc surfaces protein use beta-3 integrin receptor to enter endothelial cells, which leads to dysfunction and thus increases vascular permeability and loss of vascular integrity. The viral load is strongly associated

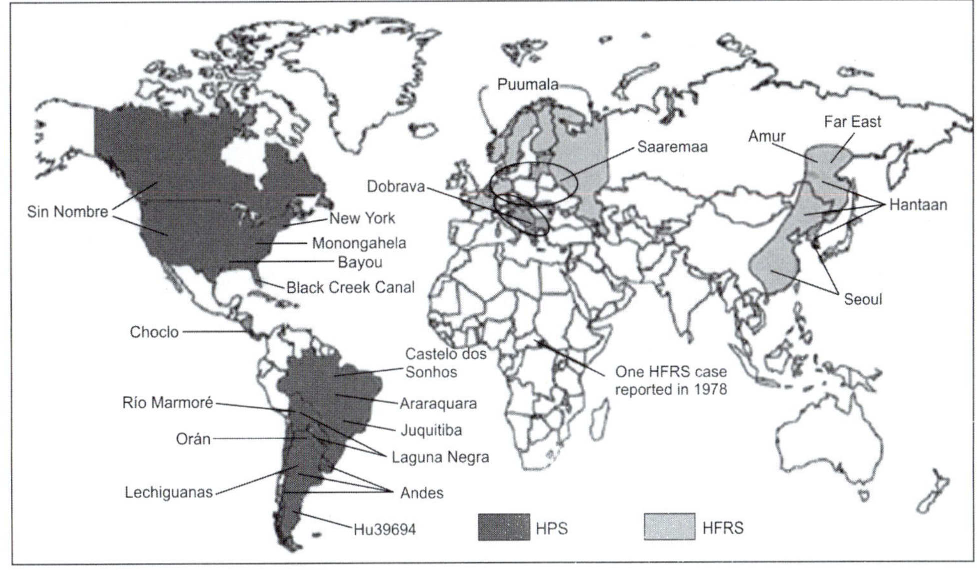

(HPS: hantavirus pulmonary syndrome; HFRS: hemorrhagic fever with renal syndrome)

FIGURE 4: Global geographic distribution of hantaviruses and the clinical syndrome associated with the viral illnesses.

with disease severity in HTN virus, ANDV, and DOBV infections. Vascular endothelial growth factor (VEGF) is a vascular permeability factor which is upregulated by hantaviral infection. The exaggerated immune response due to upregulation of toll-like receptors (TLRs) triggers the release of inflammatory cytokine and type 1 interferon (IFN-1). In HFRS, upregulation of TLR4 leads to overexpression of IFN-beta, tumor necrosis factor (TNF) alpha, and interleukin-6 (IL-6).

CLINICAL MANIFESTATIONS

HEMORRHAGIC FEVER WITH RENAL SYNDROME

The clinical hallmarks of HFRS are fever, thrombocytopenia, and acute renal dysfunction pathologically typical acute interstitial nephritis. The severity of HFRS depends on the infecting species like HTN and Dobrava viruses manifest with severe form of the illness. Classically clinical course can be described in five phases namely, (1) febrile (toxic), (2) hypotensive, (3) oliguric, (4) polyuric, and (5) convalescent. The mortality rate in severe HFRS is around 5% caused by HTN or Dobrava viruses, one-third during the shock phase and the remaining two-thirds with renal failure and pulmonary edema. An incubation period of 2–4 weeks followed by the febrile phase manifests with fever, headache, vomiting, abdominal pain, dizziness, and blurring of vision. In some patients in the febrile phase, petechiae on the palate, erythematous rash in upper body, and conjunctival suffusion can be seen. Leukocytosis usually >20,000/mm^3 with left shift is well appreciated in febrile phase. In the end of febrile phase, clinical shock occurs for about 4–7 days and some of the patients succumb to the severe shock. The patients who survive the shock phase will experience renal failure with its all complications like anuria, oliguria, diathesis, acid-base abnormalities, pneumonitis, hypertension, and pulmonary edema. After the oliguric phase, polyuria begins which is good prognostic indicator but fluid and electrolyte balance is challenging in the phase. The milder forms caused by Puumala virus called as nephropathica epidermica is rarely fatal and mortality is reported in <1% of cases. Seoul virus is associated to mild-to-moderate illness in parts of Eurasia with predominantly hepatic involvement. **Figure 5** shows schematic diagram of hantavirus infection with typical clinical course of HFRS in humans.

HANTAVIRUS PULMONARY SYNDROME

Hantavirus pulmonary syndrome clinical course comprises three phases, (1) prodromal, (2) cardiopulmonary, and (3) convalescent. HPS is much more severe form in comparison to HFRS, which begins with a febrile prodrome and followed by a rapid increase in pulmonary vascular permeability and shock. Hallmark features of prodrome are fever, chills, malaise, myalgias, headache, abdominal pain, diarrhea, and vomiting. The prodrome lasts about 4–5 days, and after that patient develops respiratory symptoms such as cough and dyspnea. Blood investigations may reveal leukocytosis with left shift with or without atypical lymphocytes, mild thrombocytopenia, prolonged activated partial thromboplastin time, mildly elevated aspartate aminotransferase, and lactate dehydrogenase. Here mild renal dysfunction with proteinuria is also appreciated which may worsen with severity of HPS. The respiratory involvement may occur rapidly and may range from mild to diffuse interstitial pulmonary edema. The case-fatality ratio for caused by North American and South American hantaviruses, SNV, and ANDV range from 30 to 50%.

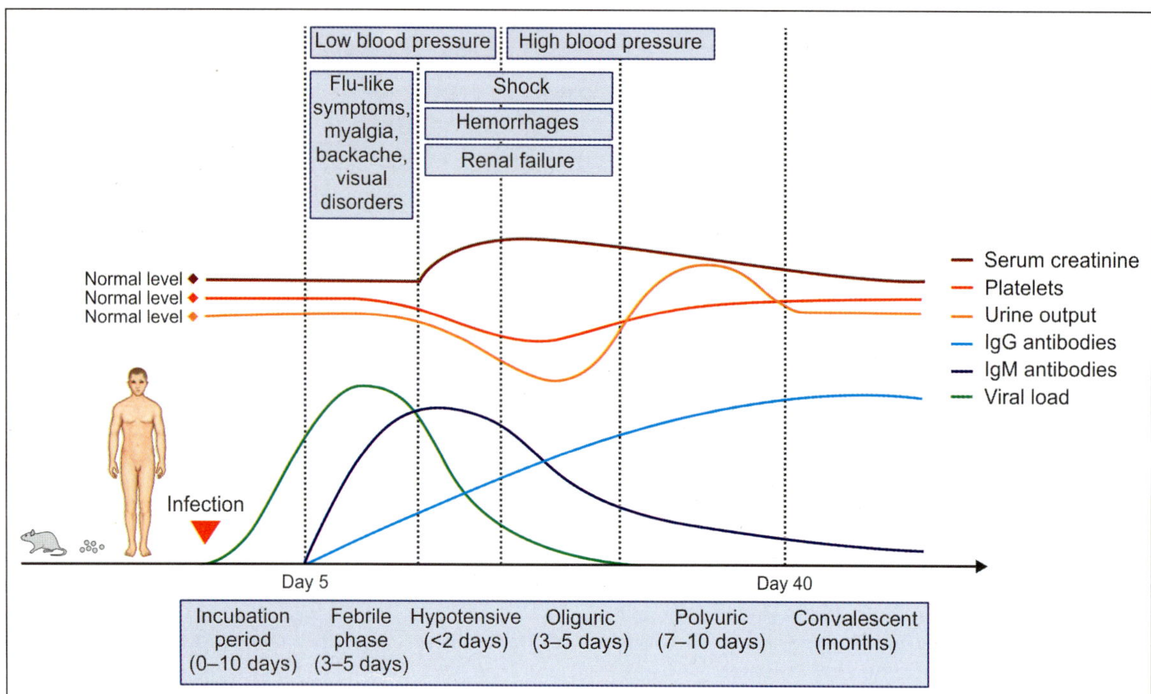

FIGURE 5: Schematic diagram of hantavirus infection with typical clinical course of hemorrhagic fever with renal syndrome (HFRS) in humans.

LABORATORY DIAGNOSIS

Most of the patient of HFRS and HPS will have leukocytosis, thrombocytopenia, increased hematocrit, proteinuria, and azotemia.

SEROLOGY

Serologic methods are preferred for the diagnosis of either human or rodent hantavirus infections in most laboratories. By the time, symptoms are evident, patients will have detectable antihantavirus IgM and/or IgG class of antibodies. Therefore, diagnostic assays including enzyme-linked immunosorbent assays (ELISAs), strip immunoblot tests (SIAs), Western blot, indirect immunofluorescence (IFA), complement fixation, and hemagglutinin inhibition, and plaque reduction neutralization tests may be used to detect antibodies to hantavirus antigens. A high level of anti-N IgM is usually corroborating with the onset of symptoms in hantaviral disease. Antibody against the Gn and Gc are not much useful in diagnostic purpose.

POLYMERASE CHAIN REACTION

Hantavirus genome is possible to detect by nested reverse-transcriptase polymerase chain reaction (RT-PCR) using whole blood or serum during the early stages of pulmonary disease.

A pan-hantavirus RT-PCR targeting the L segment of viral genome is used to detect known set of viral species.

PREVENTION

RODENT CONTROL

The most effective way to decrease the occurrence of hantaviral diseases is to decrease the interaction between rodents and humans. CDC recommends for rodent-proofing of houses, minimal food availability for rodents, and careful disposal of dead rodents.

VACCINES

Approved vaccines for HFRS in China and Korea: China has implemented a widespread preventive measure in its all the provinces with Hantavax®, a formalin-inactivated vaccine prepared by HTN virus growth in suckling brain mouse. A vaccination schedule of three doses at 0 days, 15 days, and 1 year is followed as a part of National expanded Program on Immunization.

Virus-like particles vaccines: In regard to the safety issues with inactivated whole virus vaccine, membrane bound immune-stimulating molecule CD40 ligand (CD40L) and granulocyte macrophage colony-stimulating factor (GM-CSF) are incorporated in HTN virus S and M segments. A high neutralizing antibody titer in mice was observed after two doses of virus-like particles (VLPs).

Virus-vectored recombinant vaccines: This is a chimeric molecular vaccine developed by incorporation of HTN virus S and M segment into vaccinia virus (VACV). Initial testing in Syrian hamster with two doses concluded that the vaccine protected all of infected hamsters with either HTN virus or SEO virus. Phase 1 and 2 trials results were encouraging with HTN virus neutralizing antibodies in about 72% of VACV-naïve subjects but the further research was stopped due to preexisting VACV immunity.

Nucleic acid-based molecular vaccines: DNA vaccine was developed to enhance the CD4+T cell response, the vaccine encodes HTN virus Gn and lysosomal-associated membrane protein 1 (LAMP1). A vaccination schedule of three doses enhances immune response over 6 months in mice population. These vaccines are still in developing phase and have promising potential for prevention of hantavirus infection.

TREATMENT

Hantavirus treatment is described based on the timing of drug administration in clinical course of the disease. The available armamentarium is either experimental or inadequate efficacy and is administered either as postexposure prophylactic or as a therapeutic measure.

The indication of therapeutic is either onset of clinical course or detection of virus by serology or RT-PCR. There is no recommended drug for treatment of hantavirus infections. However, in vitro and in vivo studies suggest anti-hantaviral property with ribavirin but remain ineffective in management of HPS. Supportive therapy including careful fluid management, electrolyte balance, and hemodynamic measure is the best possible to decrease the mortality.

RIBAVIRIN

The drugs demonstrate protection in lethal HPS animal models at a dose of 100 mg/kg without toxicity. Clinical trial concluded in HFRS, ribavirin administered postexposure (i.e., prior to the onset of the symptoms) reduces both morbidity and mortality. In contrast, in HFRS caused by PUUV infection it did not alter the outcome. In patients with HPS, once the cardiopulmonary phase sets in there is no role of ribavirin.

FAVIPIRAVIR

A pyrazine derivative initially popular for anti-influenza properties but this compound also demonstrates antihantavirus in vitro activity. A dose of 100 mg/kg of favipiravir reduced the detection of ANDV RNA in blood and lung.

LACTOFERRIN

Lactoferrin prevents HFRS in vivo suckling mouse model, at a dose of 40 and 160 mg/kg when administered prior to virus challenge.

1-BETA-D-RIBOFURANOSYL-3-ETHYNYL-(1,2,4)

ETAR is a nucleoside analog with antiviral activity against HTN virus and ANDV in vitro. In mice model postexposure of HTN virus, 12.5 mg/kg or 25 mg/kg ETAR for 15 days significantly increased the survival.

VANDETANIB

The increased microvascular endothelial cell permeability occurs in response to overt expression of VEGF-A in response to ANDV infection. Thus, vandetanib, a tyrosine kinase inhibitor targeting VEGF-receptor 2 (VEGFR2) and prevents phosphorylation of VEGFR2 and thus decreases the degradation of VE-cadherin. Hamster model has been treated with 10 and 25 mg/kg/day 5 days before ANDV challenge and showed increase in survival.

CORTICOSTEROIDS

Clinical trials have evaluated the role of corticosteroids in patients with HPS and concluded that either oral or intravenous administration does not alter the outcome.

CONCLUSION

Hantaviral disease occurs in endemic and epidemic forms usually in natural rodent. Both HFRS and HPS hantaviruses are transmitted by wild rodents. These clinical syndromes offer a narrow window to initiate the counter measures to combat the viral infection and timing of treatment is a challenge especially in HPS. Newer diagnostic methods such as pan-hantavirus RT-PCR could help in early diagnosis in the patients with subtle clinical signs and symptoms in endemic regions and may change the outcome of the disease. Therefore, a syndromic approach should be developed for endemic areas to deal with hantaviral disease. Vaccination would prevent the spread of infection in the endemic areas.

RECOMMENDED READINGS

1. Rajapakse S, Rodrigo C, Rajapakse A. Atypical manifestations of chikungunya infection. Trans R Soc Trop Med Hyg. 2010;104(2):89-96.
2. Chhabra M, Mittal V, Bhattacharya D, Rana UVS, Lal S. Chikungunya fever: A re-emerging viral infection. Indian J Med Microbiol. 2008;26(1):5.
3. Murhekar M, Kanagasabai K, Shete V, Joshua V, Ravi M, Kirubakaran BK, et al. Epidemiology of chikungunya based on laboratory surveillance data—India, 2016-2018. Trans R Soc Trop Med Hyg. 2019;113(5):259-62.
4. National Health Mission. (2016). National Guidelines for Clinical Management of Chikungunya 2016. [online] Available from https://dhs.kerala.gov.in/wp-content/uploads/2020/06/cgn_11092018.pdf.
5. Chandy S, Mathai D. Globally emerging hantaviruses: An overview. Indian J Med Microbiol. 2017;35(2):165.
6. Hepojoki J, Strandin T, Lankinen H, Vaheri A. Hantavirus structure- molecular interactions behind the scene. J Gen Virol. 2012;93(8):1631-44.
7. Brocato RL, Hooper JW. Progress on the Prevention and Treatment of Hantavirus Disease. Viruses. 2019;11(7):610.

CHAPTER 49

Rabies

Sajithkumar R

ABSTRACT

Rabies, a zoonotic disease transmitted to humans by animal bites, claims thousands of lives all over the world. The virus is maintained in nature in wild animal reservoirs and through domestic animals reach human beings. It is perhaps the only 100% fatal disease. It has variable incubation period. The clinical features are manifestations of limbic encephalitis and brain stem encephalitis. It manifests with hydrophobia, aerophobia, behavioral, and autonomic disturbances. Even though there is no cure for rabies, it is preventable using pre-exposure and postexposure strategies using antirabies vaccine and antirabies immunoglobulin. Antirabies vaccines in use are all purified cell culture vaccines and are safe. Antirabies immunoglobulins are also available as monoclonal antibodies. Proper first aid using immediate washing with soap and water is also important. Attempts are now started to reduce deaths by rabies to zero by 2030.

"Awareness is the greatest agent for change"

—Eckhart Tolle

INTRODUCTION

Rabies is an acute zoonotic viral infection, affecting mammals. It is transmitted to human beings through contact with the saliva of infected animals, causing a fatal disease characterized by progressive encephalitis and death in a short span.

Rabies is present in all continents. Approximately 55,000 people die of rabies all over the world, of which 20,000 are reported from India, every year, amounting to almost one death every 9 minutes. Most Southeast Asian countries like Sri Lanka, Bangladesh, Pakistan, Vietnam, and countries in Africa and South America report high incidence of the disease. A disproportionate increase has also been noted in rural areas and in a young age.

ETIOLOGY

Rabies is caused by an RNA (ribonucleic acid) virus of the genus *Lyssavirus* from the group of rhabdoviruses, so named because of the bullet shape of the virus. The virus is 100–300 nm long and 75 nm in diameter. It is composed of a lipid envelope and the nucleocapsid with a ribonucleoprotein complex constituted by genomic RNA and N, L, and P proteins. In wild animals, it gets adapted through repeated passages and remains as a fixed virus. The virus is secreted through the salivary glands of animals. Domestic dogs and cats are highly vulnerable to die of the disease and account for the majority of transmission to humans. The entry of the virus is mostly through animal bites, and occasionally through open wounds getting contaminated with animal saliva. The virus gets destroyed by heat at 56°C and on exposure to detergents. However, in the body temperature, it may survive for up to 7 days, during which time it gets attached through its surface glycoprotein to a cell into which enters by endocytosis. Local replication in the striated muscles has also been documented. After entry into the neuron directly or through postsynaptic neuromuscular junctions, it is carried in transport vesicles in the axoplasm of the nerve very slowly (at around 3 mm/h) to reach the dorsal root ganglia. The spread to neurons of the brain through synapses results in massive replication and viral budding. The limbic system and autonomic nervous system are selectively involved. From there, it may spread to salivary glands and other tissues.

Vampire bats, jackals, and wolves are recognized carriers of the virus. Aerosol transmission of the virus is reported to occur in dark caves inhabited by vampire bats. Accidental exposure has been reported to occur rarely in laboratories and vaccine production units as well. Human to human transmission is not documented. Viral concentration in human saliva is negligible. It is possible that organ transplantation, particularly corneal transplantation, may transmit the virus to the recipient.

PATHOLOGY

The hippocampus and basal ganglia are the major areas of involvement. Congestion of blood vessels is observed. Severe congestion of the gray matter and white matter with perivascular mononuclear cell infiltration is seen. Perivascular cuffing with monocytes and polymorphonuclear cells, lymphocytic foci, and Babes nodules consisting of glial cells are also described. *Negri bodies are the classical intracytoplasmic inclusion bodies* seen in cases, initially described by Adelchi Negri in 1903, as round or oval inclusions measuring 0.25–27 μm in the cytoplasm of neurons. They are found frequently in the pyramidal cells of Ammon's horn, and the Purkinje cells of the cerebellum. They are seen in the cells of the medulla and various ganglia. Negri bodies are also seen in the nerve cells in salivary glands, tongue, or other organs. Giemsa stain can differentiate rabies inclusions from other intracellular inclusions appearing magenta in color with small dark-blue interior basophilic granules. Negri bodies are seen in approximately 50% of cases and are not highly sensitive. Failure to demonstrate Negri bodies is inconclusive. Focal degeneration in salivary glands, adrenals, lymph nodes, and myocardial cells is demonstrable in patients dying of rabies.

CLINICAL FEATURES

The incubation period in humans is between 3 weeks to 3 months. There are wide variations with shorter (7 days) and very long (extending to many years even) periods. Bites on the head and neck area or multiple bites may present with a shorter incubation period. The earliest manifestation may be fever, malaise, and nonspecific upper respiratory symptoms. Paresthesia, tingling sensation, or stiffness is usually seen in the affected limb or other parts of the body where the animal has bitten. Behavioral problems with alternating attacks of rage and calm periods suggest the involvement of the limbic system. The periods of calmness become shorter and the patient drifts to continuous agitation and violent behavior.

Hydrophobia, the term used synonymously with rabies, is a manifestation of powerful spasm of the pharyngeal, tracheal, and laryngeal muscles, which makes swallowing of liquids extremely difficult. The spasms may get precipitated by any visual, auditory, or tactile stimuli in connection with water or other liquids and may not always be related to swallowing, hence the term "phobia." When water is brought near the patient, powerful spasmodic jerks occur and the patient tries to move away. This is also associated with tonic spasms, usually manifesting initially as stiffness of the affected part of the body. *Generalized tonic spasms* set in within hours and progress with lowering of stimulus threshold.

All manifestations progress over the next few days. A breeze of air over the face or other parts of the body or airflow classically following switching of the fan leads to similar spasms. This is described as aerophobia. Autonomic disturbances like hypertension, tachycardia, and cardiac arrhythmias may occur. *Localized hyperhidrosis*, described as excessive partial sweating on certain parts of the body only, and fasciculations over large muscles are also seen. The patient becomes comatose and usually succumb to the disease within 96 hours. Very rarely, patients have survived over a week or two, with good ventilatory support. Ultimately 100% of patients die due to respiratory paralysis and/or cardiac arrhythmias as a result of bulbar involvement.

Paralytic form of rabies is described more in animals, but can rarely occur in humans as well. Patients develop ascending paralysis starting as paraparesis and progresses to involve the trunk muscles including respiratory muscles. Respiratory system complications like aspiration pneumonia, pneumothorax, and pulmonary edema may precede respiratory arrest.

Rabies must be suspected when patients present with any of the above features and a history of a bite by animals. The differential diagnosis to be considered includes encephalitis due to other viruses, tetanus due to *Clostridium tetani* infection. This has to be differentiated from hysterical reactions, seen commonly after animal bites as well.

INVESTIGATIONS

Usually, no investigation is needed in patients presenting with classical signs and history. The virus can be isolated from cerebrospinal fluid and saliva in the first few days. Neutralizing antibodies can be demonstrated in cerebrospinal fluid (CSF). Polymerase chain reaction (PCR) test can confirm the presence of rabies virus in CSF. Negri bodies may be demonstrable in buccal and corneal smear samples. Rabies-specific immunofluorescence in nerve tissue on skin biopsy is very specific. Tests using fluorescent labeled antibodies [fluorescent antibody test (FAT)] which bind to the viral proteins in infected nerve cells are accepted by World Health Organization (WHO) and other international agencies as confirmatory. Another test recommended by WHO is the direct rapid immunohistochemistry test (dRIT) using streptavidin-biotin peroxidase staining. Serological tests are not useful, as antibodies take longer to develop. Fluorescent antibody neutralization (FAVN) test and rapid fluorescent focus inhibition test (RFFIT) are used to quantify the antibody levels. These are more useful in vaccinated individuals to assess the immune status.

CASE DEFINITION

Clinical case definition: A person presenting with an acute neurological syndrome (encephalitis) dominated by forms of hyperactivity (furious rabies) or paralytic syndromes (dumb rabies) progressing toward coma and death, usually by respiratory failure, within 7–10 days after the first symptom if no intensive care is instituted.

- *Suspect case*: A case that is compatible with the clinical case definition.
- *Probable*: A suspected case plus a history of contact with a suspected rabid animal.
- *Confirmed*: A suspected case that is laboratory-confirmed.

TREATMENT

As stated above, *rabies is associated with 100% mortality*, and no specific lifesaving treatment is available, as of now. Even though various antiviral drugs, interferons, monoclonal antibodies, immunoglobulins, corticosteroids etc. have been used aggressively, there is no reported success with any of these. The patient must be cared in a dark, quiet room with minimum stimulus and minimum handling. The spasms can be controlled with muscle relaxants like benzodiazepines. Proper hydration and nutrition can be maintained with intravenous fluids. Antibiotics may be administered to treat any respiratory infections, as per standard guidelines. The relatives must be counseled with proper information about the prognosis. They must be instructed to use gloves and use soap for handwashing while handling body fluids, even though human to human transmission is not likely.

Very few instances of rabies patients surviving have been reported across the globe. Most of them have been documented in persons who have taken active and passive prophylaxis and still developed the disease. One regimen called "Milwaukee protocol" named after the city where a 6-year-old boy had recovered from Rabies was discussed by Rodney Willoughby Jr et al. (2004). They had used antiexcitatory drugs like ketamine, muscle relaxants like benzodiazepines, and antiviral drugs like amantadine and induced coma in the patient. It is presumed that after some time, the body develops an immune response and succeeds in overcoming the neuronal damage. But success stories are too few to reach any conclusion. Few survivors had long-standing neurological sequelae, yet the regimen is not accepted as standard practice anymore.

PROPHYLAXIS

While rabies is an inevitably fatal disease, it is also a preventable infection. After exposure to the saliva of animals (domestic, stray, or wild) through bites or through wounds or mucous membranes, immediate flushing with soap and running water is to be instituted. The wound should not be explored or expanded and no caustic materials should be applied. Suturing should be deferred or done along with local infiltration of specific antirabies immunoglobulins only.

All wild animal bites and bites by stray dogs and cats must be considered as infective. Any unprovoked bites, multiple bites with lacerated wounds, and bites on highly sensitive areas with dense innervation (e.g., fingertips, genitalia, and mucocutaneous junctions) must be considered as significant. Bites by rodents and birds are not considered as infective. As domestic dogs and cats start shedding the virus in saliva about 4–5 days prior to the onset of clinical rabies in them, it is likely that the animal may not show any behavioral variation at the time of the bite. There is a possibility that they may survive for five more days after the onset of clinical disease. Hence domestic dogs and cats only must be observed under captivity and well maintained for a period of 10 days after the bite. Any deviation from normalcy like aggressiveness, running amok, biting nonliving objects, failure to feed, motor weakness, paralysis, or death during this period must be taken as a red alert.

VACCINATION

Vaccination against rabies can be discussed under two headings:

1. Postexposure prophylaxis
2. Pre-exposure prophylaxis

POSTEXPOSURE PROPHYLAXIS

As soon as a person is bitten by a rabid animal or under the conditions described above, he/she must be started on antirabies immunization. Various types of vaccines and schedules are available. Conventional nerve tissue-derived animal vaccines have been discontinued worldwide. Cell culture vaccines using human diploid cell lines (HDCV), chick embryo, and monkey kidney culture are available. They are administered as intramuscular 5-day schedule (1 mL each on 0, 3, 7, 14, 28 days) or as two site intradermal 4-day schedule (0.1 mL × 2 sites on 0, 3, 7, and 28 days). If the animal under observation survives 10 days, further doses can be stopped or can be converted to the pre-exposure schedule by giving another dose on day 28. It may be noted that there is absolutely no contraindication to rabies immunization, as the disease is 100% fatal. The vaccination should not be withheld because of pregnancy, infancy. In immunosuppressed individuals double the standard dose is recommended. Interchangeability or shift of vaccine types and routes are acceptable but permitted only in cases where the same cannot be followed.

Antirabies immunoglobulin is available as human (HRIG) and equine (ERIG) products. The dose is calculated as 20 and 40 units/kg body weight, respectively. In all stray animal bites, wild animal bites, and bites with multiple lacerations, and in situations where the behavior of the animal suggests active rabies, immunoglobulin must be administered. The current recommendation is to infiltrate as much of the calculated dose as possible locally around the wound and administer the remaining as deep intramuscular injection. Separate syringes and needles must be used for administering vaccine and immunoglobulin. Antirabies immunoglobulin can be administered up to 7 days after the bite, but not later. Passive immunity provided by passive immunization is expected to be available for around 21 days, by which time, active immunization would have led to production of sufficient antibodies in vaccines. Recently introduced rabies monoclonal antibody (RMAb) is described to be able to achieve better central nervous system (CNS) concentrations. Dosage of the RMAb marketed by Serum Institute of India is 3.33 IU/kg body weight.

In the case of repeated exposure after one full course of immunization, immunoglobulins need not be given. Instead, immunity in such instances can be boosted by a 2-day (0, 3) intramuscular or intradermal schedule.

PRE-EXPOSURE PROPHYLAXIS

Rabies infection can be prevented fully by pre-exposure immunization. This is recommended on a voluntary basis for all individuals staying in rabies prone areas. Many developing countries including India may fall under this category, because of the high population of stray animals. It is also recommended in those engaged in vulnerable professions like veterinarians, staff in laboratory handling rabies or related viruses, forest and wildlife department staff, animal keepers, dog trainers, and for those likely to enter dangerous areas frequently like postmen, salespersons, milkmen, newspaper boys etc.

Pre-exposure immunization is done using three dose (0, 7, 28 days) intradermal or intramuscular injections. Routine antibody estimations are not recommended following this schedule. However, persons working in laboratories with live rabies virus and veterinarians and others at permanent risk of exposure are advised to check the levels of neutralizing antirabies antibodies once in 6 months to 2 years. They are required to take a booster dose if the antibody levels fall below 0.5 IU/mL.

CONCLUSION

Even though a dreaded disease, rabies is preventable with proper regular animal vaccination and proper care of wounds. Pre-exposure immunization will prevent infection in susceptible individuals.

World Health Organization along with World Organization for Animal Health and Global Alliance for Rabies Control has declared a global strategic plan "Zero by 30" to end human deaths from dog-mediated rabies by 2030. This includes effective use of human and animal vaccines, motivation, innovation, monitoring, commitment, and sustenance by all countries.

RECOMMENDED READINGS

1. World Health Organisation. (2019). United Against Rabies Collaboration. First annual progress report. Global Strategic Plan to End Human Deaths from Dog-mediated Rabies by 2030. [online] Available from https://www.who.int/neglected_diseases/resources/WHO-CDS-NTD-NZD-2019.04/en/
2. National Guidelines for Rabies Prophylaxis 2019. National Rabies Control Program. Division of Zoonosis Disease Program, National Centre for Disease Control, DGHS, New Delhi. 2019. pp. 1-39.
3. WHO Expert Consultation on Rabies, third report. Geneva: World Health Organization; 2018 (WHO Technical Report Series, No. 1012). Licence: CC BY-NC-SA 3.0 IGO. pp. 3-183.
4. CDC Factsheet. Centers for Disease Control and Prevention, National Center for Emerging and Zoonotic Infectious Diseases (NCEZID), Division of High-Consequence Pathogens and Pathology (DHCPP). [online] Available from https://www.cdc.gov/rabies/index.html

CHAPTER 50

Dengue Fever

Ayan Basu, Bibhuti Saha

ABSTRACT

Dengue is *Aedes* mosquito-borne viral infection. It can cause a wide spectrum of clinical manifestations, from mild undifferentiated fever to hemorrhage, shock, and severe organ involvement due to capillary leakage and hemostatic abnormalities. Management mainly lies on judicious fluids administration as there is currently no antiviral drug for dengue.

"If you think you're too small to make a difference you haven't spent a night with a mosquito"

—African proverb

INTRODUCTION

The World Health Organization (WHO) mentioned dengue as one of the 17 neglected tropical diseases in 2010. Worldwide dengue affects an estimated 100 million people annually with 0.5 million severe cases and 0.02 million deaths. Dengue is endemic in India. In 1945, dengue virus (DENV) was first isolated in India. In 1956, dengue fever (DF) was first reported from Vellore district in Tamil Nadu. In 1963, the first outbreak of dengue hemorrhagic fever (DHF) occurred in Kolkata, West Bengal. In 2019, highest number of dengue cases and deaths were seen in Gujarat (18,219 cases) and Maharashtra (29 deaths), respectively. In the last few years, incidence of dengue is increasing. But case fatality ratio (i.e., number of deaths per 100 cases) has declined from 0.17% in 2018 to 0.05% in 2020 [National Vector Borne Disease Control Programme (NVBDCP)].

EPIDEMIOLOGY

Dengue virus is a member of genus *Flavivirus* under Flaviviridae family. It is a single-stranded enveloped ribonucleic acid (RNA) virus with a diameter of 30 nm. Its genome is composed of an envelope protein (E), a membrane-associated protein (M), three structural protein genes encoding the nucleocapsid of core protein (C), and seven nonstructural (NS) proteins—NS1, NS2A, NS2B, NS3, NS4A, NS4B, and NS5. There are four closely related but distinct serotypes (DENV-1, -2, -3, and-4). Their antigens cross-react with other members in the same genus such as Japanese encephalitis, yellow fever, and West Nile viruses. Based on the phylogenetic analysis of the genomic region in the envelope gene, the following genotypes or subtypes are detected within each serotype: Five genotypes each in DENV-1 and DENV-2, four each in DENV-3 and DENV-4. In endemic areas, the four DENV serotypes can cocirculate because the immunity to one serotype does not give protection from infection by a heterologous serotype.

Dengue is endemic in the tropical and subtropical zones between 30°N and 40°S with temperature range of 25°C ± 5°C and around 80% relative humidity. Every year, an increase in the cases of DF and DHF occurred from July to November. Dengue has a seasonal pattern with increased transmission, usually occurred in the rainy season. However, perennial transmissions are reported from the states of Western and Southern parts of India. Outbreaks occur most frequently in areas where multiple serotypes are simultaneously endemic or sequentially epidemic and infections with heterologous types are frequent. In endemic areas, dengue occurs most frequently in 2–15 years aged children. Severe dengue is usually associated with secondary dengue infection and in primary infection of infants <1 year, born to dengue-immune mothers.

Transmission of dengue occurs by the bite of the female *Aedes* mosquito. *Aedes aegypti* is the main vector in most urban areas in India; however, *Aedes albopictus* is also incriminated in many states. In some countries other species such as *Aedes niveus* and *Aedes polynesiensis* have also been identified as secondary vectors. Female mosquito bites during daytime. Dengue can also be transmitted by blood transfusion, organ transplantation, and vertically from the mothers infected very late in pregnancy.

PATHOGENESIS

In the pathogenesis of DF, host immunity plays an important role. Though the exact immunopathogenesis of different signs and symptoms of DF is still not clear but several mechanisms are proposed to explain the pathogenesis of clinical manifestations, e.g., antibody-dependent enhancement (ADE), cross-reactivity of T cell-mediated antibodies with vascular endothelium, activation of various complements, cytokines, and chemokines. Among these, the most important are ADE and memory T cells in secondary infection, which results in "cytokine storm". They target platelets, vascular endothelium, and different organs which lead to vasculopathy and coagulopathy, which is responsible for hemorrhage and shock.

ADE causing severe dengue is seen in sequential dengue infections. In secondary infection by a different serotype, preexisting antibody (which usually persists for 2–12 months) of the first infection fails to neutralize, but may enhance uptake and replication of virus in mononuclear cells. Some studies showed secondary infection mainly by DENV-2 caused severe dengue. Another example of ADE is severe primary dengue in infants born to dengue-immune mothers. In infants of 4–12 months, maternally derived immunoglobulin G (IgG) antibody falls below neutralization level causing severe disease through ADE.

A study showed that in secondary dengue infections, there is predominant expansion of T cells with low avidity for the current viral serotype but high avidity for a presumed previous serotype. This skewing of the immune response to the previous serotype is known as original antigenic sin, which delays viral control and causes high viremia and severe manifestations. This activation of memory CD4 and CD8+ T cells, sensitized during a previous infection, leads to release of proinflammatory cytokines such as tumor necrosis factor-α (TNF-α) and interferon-γ (IFN-γ) causing tissue damage and plasma leakage.

CAPILLARY LEAKAGE AND SHOCK

In dengue, there is transient disturbance in the function of the endothelial glycocalyx layer and temporary alteration of the characteristics of the fiber matrix of the endothelium. NS1 antigen can selectively bind to heparan sulfate in the glycocalyx layer of microvascular endothelial cells. This facilitates immune complex formation and antibody-dependent complement (C3a and C5a anaphylatoxins) activation causing endothelial damage and microvascular leakage. As a result of plasma leakage there is hypotension, shock, hemoconcentration/rise in hematocrit, hypoproteinemia, pleural effusion, or ascites. It usually occurs on 3rd to 7th day of illness. Activation of T lymphocytes and virus infected monocytes are responsible for increased level of cytokines as seen in DHF/dengue shock syndrome (DSS). Complement also causes vascular leakage and immune modulation leading to a higher viremia.

HEMOSTATIC ABNORMALITIES

It is caused by:

- Vasculopathy
- Thrombopathy—moderate-to-severe thrombocytopenia, impaired platelet function, and sequestration
- Coagulopathy—activation of the coagulation system and fibrinolysis. In the later stages of severe disease—disseminated intravascular coagulation (DIC) occurs
- Bone marrow changes—depression of all marrow elements, with maturation arrest of megakaryocytes during the early phase of the illness, which is reversed after defervescence.

The most consistent finding in dengue is a transient *thrombocytopenia*. The exact underlying mechanism remains unclear. It is multifactorial. Causes of thrombocytopenia are presented in **Box 1**.

In severe dengue, there is activation of the coagulation system and fibrinolysis. Persistently, elevated levels of tissue activator inhibitor levels and an increased thrombin-antithrombin to plasmin-antiplasmin ratio was associated with poor outcomes. There are mild prolongation of prothrombin time (PT) and partial thromboplastin time

BOX 1	Causes of thrombocytopenia.
• Suppression of megakaryocytopoiesis	
• Increased platelet clearance by DENV-induced apoptosis and	
• Antiplatelet antibodies	
• Peripheral sequestration of platelets	

(DENV: dengue virus)

BOX 2	Causes of coagulation abnormalities.
• Due to capillary leakage, various coagulation factors including fibrinogen and other intravascular proteins are lost	
• Prolongation of PT and APTT coincides temporally with maximal vascular leakage	
• In vitro studies showed that virus can bind and activate plasminogen	
• In acute and convalescent serum of dengue patients, cross-reactive antibodies to plasminogen have been demonstrated	

(APTT: activated partial thromboplastin time; PT: prothrombin time)

and reduced fibrinogen. Fibrinogen degradation products however are rarely raised and not to the levels consistent with a classical DIC picture. Causes of coagulation abnormalities are listed in **Box 2**.

CLINICAL MANIFESTATIONS

Patient with DF may be asymptomatic (in majority of cases) or symptomatic and clinical spectrum varies from undifferentiated fever to hemorrhage, shock, and severe organ involvement. Several factors such as age, host's immune status, virus strain, and primary or secondary infection are responsible for varied clinical presentations. Infection with one dengue serotype gives lifelong immunity to that particular serotype.

UNDIFFERENTIATED DENGUE FEVER

Mild-to-moderate fever occurs in primary dengue infection and it is often indistinguishable from other viral infections. Maculopapular rash may/may not appear during febrile period or defervescence. The signs of capillary leakage and hemorrhagic manifestations may be absent.

SEVERE DENGUE FEVER

Severe manifestations are plasma leakage leading to shock and/or fluid accumulation, severe bleeding, and organ impairment. Based on platelet count, hematocrit, capillary leakage, hypotension, and bleeding, DHF has been divided into four grades (**Boxes 3** and **4**). Nonsevere cases may be DF and grade I and II of DHF without significant bleeding. Severe dengue may be grade III and IV of DHF with or without significant bleeding. DHF grade I and II can be severe when significant bleeding or electrolyte and metabolic abnormalities are present. Sometimes, severe bleeding without evidence of capillary leakage or hemoconcentration is seen in DF. Some patients may also present with multiple organ involvement without bleeding and shock. Hepatic, renal, cardiac, pulmonary, and central nervous system (CNS) involvement causes high morbidity and mortality. Unusual atypical manifestations are also seen.

BOX 3	Grading of DF/DHF.
• **DF:** Fever of 2–7 days with ≥2 of following: Headache, retro-orbital pain, myalgia, arthralgia with or without leukopenia, thrombocytopenia and no evidence of plasma leakage	
• **DHF I:** Above criteria plus positive tourniquet test and evidence of plasma leakage. Thrombocytopenia with platelet count <100,000/mm^3 and Hct rise >20% over baseline	
• **DHF II:** Above plus some evidence of spontaneous bleeding in skin or other organs (black tarry stool, epistaxis, gum bleeds) and abdominal pain. Thrombocytopenia with platelet count <100,000/mm^3 and Hct rise >20% over baseline	
• **DHF III (DSS):** Above plus circulatory failure (rapid weak pulse, narrow pulse pressure <20 mm Hg, hypotension, cold clammy skin, restlessness). Thrombocytopenia with platelet count <100,000/mm^3 and Hct rise >20% over baseline	
• **DHF IV (DSS):** Profound shock with undetectable blood pressure or pulse. Thrombocytopenia with platelet count <100,000/mm^3 and Hct rise >20% over baseline	

(DF: dengue fever; DHF: dengue hemorrhagic fever; DSS: dengue shock syndrome; Hct: hematocrit)

BOX 4	Clinical criteria for DF/DHF/DSS.

Clinical features of dengue fever (DF):

An acute febrile illness of 2–7 days duration with ≥2 of the following manifestations: Headache, retro-orbital pain, myalgia, arthralgia, rash, hemorrhagic manifestations

Dengue hemorrhagic fever (DHF):

1. A case with clinical criteria of dengue fever

   Plus

2. Hemorrhagic tendencies evidenced by ≥1 of the following:
   i. Positive tourniquet test
   ii. Petechiae, ecchymoses or purpura
   iii. Bleeding from mucosa, gastrointestinal tract, injection sites or other sites

   Plus

3. Thrombocytopenia (<100,000 cells/mm^3)

   Plus

4. Evidence of plasma leakage due to increased vascular permeability, manifested by ≥1 of the following:
   i. A rise in average hematocrit for age and sex ≥20%
   ii. A >20% drop in hematocrit following volume replacement treatment compared to baseline
   iii. Signs of plasma leakage (pleural effusion, ascites, hypoproteinemia)

Dengue shock syndrome (DSS):

All the above criteria for DHF with evidence of circulatory failure manifested by rapid and weak pulse and narrow pulse pressure (≤20% mm Hg) or hypotension for age, cold and clammy skin and restlessness

TABLE 1 Warning signs and symptoms.

• Recurrent vomiting • Abdominal pain or discomfort • Hepatic dysfunction or hepatomegaly • Palpitation, breathlessness • Decreased urinary output • Minor bleeding from different sites, scanty hemoptysis, hematemesis, hematuria, increase menstrual flow, gum bleeding etc.	• Hypotension • Rapid pulse • Narrow pulse pressure • Cold clammy extremities • Pleural effusion/ascites/ gallbladder edema on imaging • Rapid fall in platelet count • High Hct (>45%)

(Hct: hematocrit)

TABLE 2 Manifestations of expanded dengue syndrome.

System	Unusual or atypical manifestations
CNS involvement	Encephalopathy, encephalitis, febrile seizures, I/C bleed
GI involvement	Acute hepatitis/fulminant hepatic failure, cholecystitis, cholangitis, acute pancreatitis
Renal involvement	Acute renal failure, hemolytic uremic syndrome, acute tubular necrosis
Cardiac involvement	Cardiac arrhythmia, cardiomyopathy, myocarditis, pericardial effusion
Respiratory	Pulmonary edema, ARDS, pulmonary hemorrhage pleural effusion
Eye	Conjunctival bleed, macular hemorrhage, visual impairment, optic neuritis

(ARDS: acute respiratory distress syndrome; CNS: central nervous system; GI: gastrointestinal; I/C: intracranial)

WARNING SIGNS AND SYMPTOMS

Following warning signs and symptoms (**Table 1**) are indicators of severity and disease progression.

EXPANDED DENGUE SYNDROME

Mild-to-severe organ involvement or unusual manifestations may be seen in DF/DHF. Manifestations of expanded dengue syndrome (EDS) are shown in **Table 2**, **Figures 1** and **2**.

Tourniquet test: The test is done by inflating blood pressure (BP) cuff to the midpoint between systolic blood pressure (SBP) and diastolic blood pressure (DBP) and maintains it for 5 minutes. Positive test means ≥10 petechiae per one square inch area over forearm. ≥20 petechiae are usually seen in DHF. During the phase of profound shock, i.e., in DSS, the test may be negative or only mildly positive.

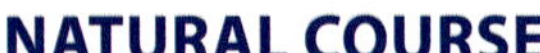

NATURAL COURSE

The clinical course of illness has three phases.

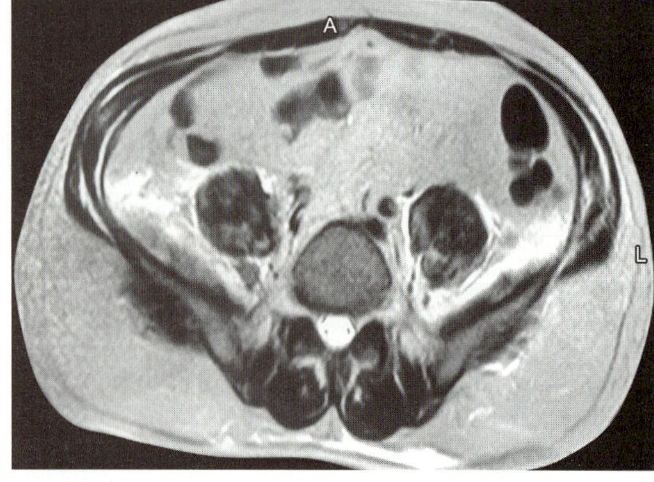

FIGURE 1: Dengue myositis.

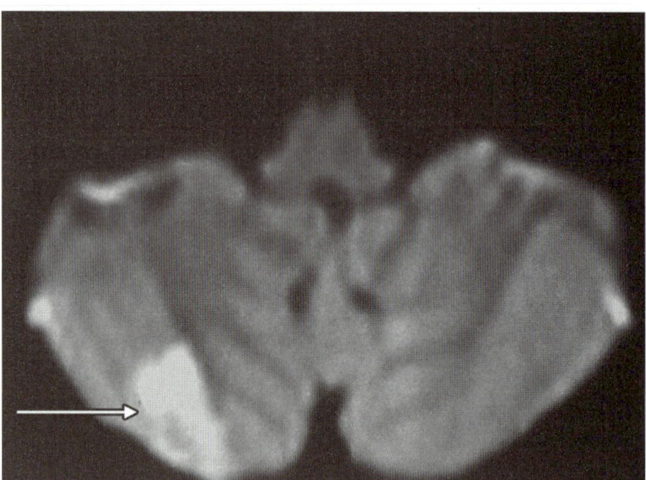

FIGURE 2: Cerebellar infarction.

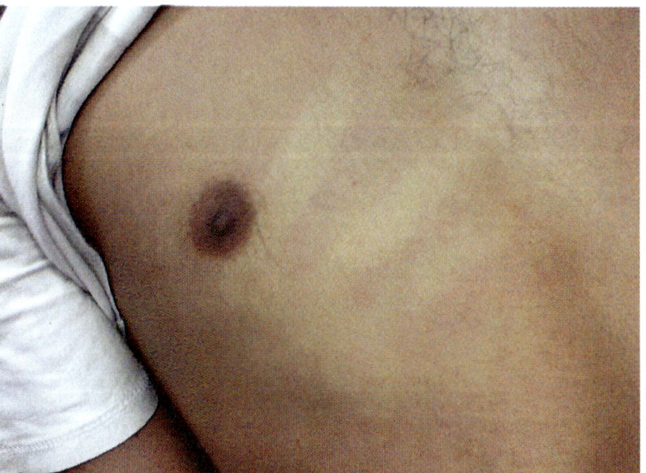

FIGURE 3: Blanchable rash.

FEBRILE PHASE

This phase lasts for 2–7 days, may be biphasic, associated with headache, flushing, and rash. There is retro-orbital, bone, joint, or muscles pain. Different types of skin rashes are seen (**Fig. 3**). Initially, transient, diffuse

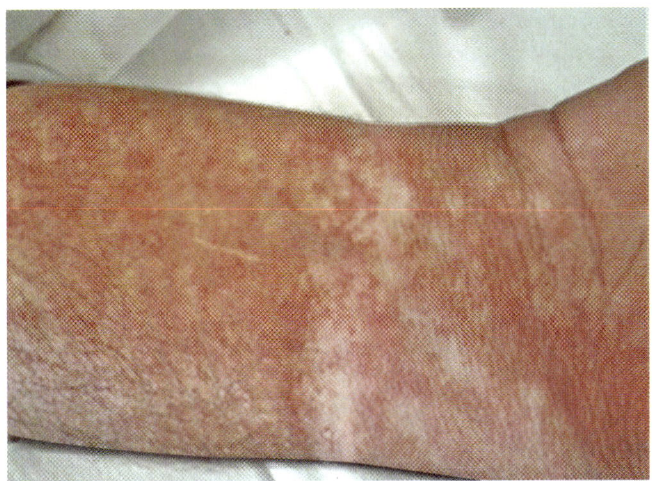

FIGURE 4: White island in red sea.

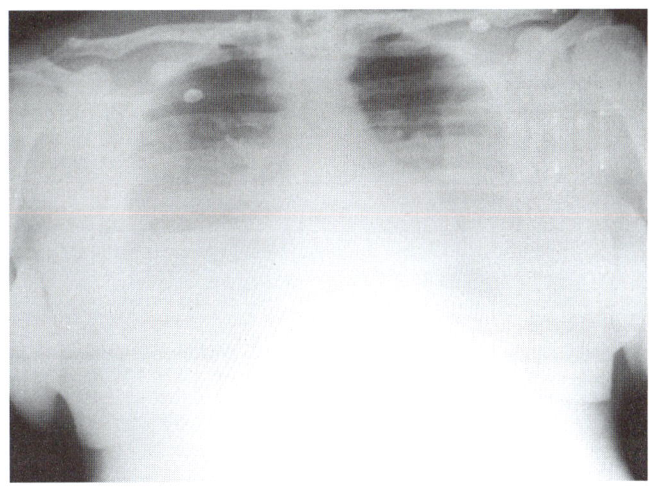

FIGURE 5: Accumulation of fluid in pleural cavity.

flushing, mottling, or fleeting pinpoint eruptions may be seen on the face, neck, and chest. Then a scarlatiniform or maculopapular rash which starts on the chest and trunk and spreads to the face and extremities appears on 3rd or 4th day. There may be itching and dermal hyperesthesia. This generalized rash fades in the later part of febrile period and during defervescence a localized clusters of petechiae may appear over arms, hands, legs, and dorsum of the feet. This confluent petechial convalescent rash is characterized by islands of white (i.e., normal skin) in the sea of red (**Fig. 4**).

CRITICAL PHASE

This phase starts after 3–4 days of onset of fever and usually persists for 36–48 hours. There is plasma leakage which leads to hemoconcentration, hypotension, shock, and accumulation of fluid in pleural (**Fig. 5**) and peritoneal cavity. Abnormal hemostasis leads to severe bleeding. There is also severe organ impairment and metabolic abnormalities.

CONVALESCENT PHASE

This phase usually occurs after 6–7 days of fever and last for 2–3 days. There may be pulmonary edema due to fluid overload, if fluid replacement is excessive.

LABORATORY DIAGNOSIS

Following are the diagnostic tests of dengue.

ELISA-based NS1 antigen tests: During the early stages of infection, a highly conserved glycoprotein—NS1 antigen is abundantly found in the serum of patients. Enzyme-linked immunosorbent assay (ELISA)-based NS1 antigen assay is a useful method for the diagnosis of acute/early infections, i.e., viremic stage (within first 5 days of onset of fever). It is highly sensitive and specific. Because of its specificity, it is useful for differentiating from other flaviviruses.

Immunoglobulin M antibody ELISA: Immunoglobulin M (IgM) antibody capture ELISA (MAC-ELISA) is a simple test that detects dengue specific IgM antibodies in the serum. IgM antibody is usually detectable by 5th day of illness. It may be detectable in some patients as early as 2–4 days of illness, while in others it may not be detectable for 7–8 days after the illness. In primary infections, mostly it becomes undetectable by 60 days but sometimes it may persist for more >90 days. It is specific in distinguishing dengue from other flavivirus infections.

Isolation of dengue virus: Most strains of DENV can be isolated if the sample is taken within the first 5 days of illness. Virus can be isolated from acute phase serum or plasma, washed buffy coat, autopsy tissues, and mosquitoes. But as 7–10 days are required for virus isolation, hence it may not be useful for starting the management in severe cases.

Polymerase chain reaction: Molecular diagnosis is based on reverse transcription polymerase chain reaction (RT-PCR), e.g., one step or nested RT-PCR, real-time RT-PCR or nucleic acid sequence-based amplification (NASBA). In the first 3–5 days of illness (during the febrile phase), RT-PCR techniques that detect DENV RNA in the blood are the most sensitive and specific test.

Immunoglobulin G ELISA: This test differentiates between primary and secondary dengue infections. It also indicates past infection. IgG antibodies rapidly increase in secondary dengue infection (usually titer exceeds 1:1,280).

Serological tests: Several serological tests, e.g., hemagglutination inhibition (HI), complement fixation, and neutralization test are available but are not commonly used.

Rapid diagnostic tests: Rapid diagnostic test (RDT) kits for NS1 antigen and IgM or IgG antibodies that give result within 15–25 minutes are commercially available. However, their accuracy is not known as most of them are not properly validated. Hence, their use is not recommended under the national program. Case definition of dengue is given in **Box 5**.

Presence of other common causes of fever, especially malaria, is to be excluded.

BOX 5 Case definition of dengue.

Probable DF/DHF:

A case compatible with clinical description of dengue fever (see Clinical Criteria) during outbreak

OR

Non-ELISA based NS1 antigen/IgM positive

(A positive test by RDT will be considered as probable due to poor sensitivity and specificity of currently available RDTs)

Confirmed dengue fever:

A case compatible with the clinical description of dengue fever with at least one of the following:

- Isolation of the dengue virus (virus culture +ve) from serum, plasma, leukocytes
- Demonstration of IgM antibody titre by ELISA positive in single serum sample
- Demonstration of dengue virus antigen in serum sample by NS1-ELISA
- IgG seroconversion in paired sera after 2 weeks with 4-fold increase of IgG titer
- Detection of viral nucleic acid by polymerase chain reaction (PCR)

(DF: dengue fever; DHF: dengue hemorrhagic fever; ELISA: enzyme-linked immunosorbent assay; IgM: immunoglobulin M; IgG: immunoglobulin G; NS1: nonstructural protein 1; RDT: rapid diagnostic test)

MANAGEMENT

According to all prevailing guidelines and clinicians' experiences the management of dengue mainly lies on fluids. DF will be cured on its own only if the complications can be prevented. Fluids are the only proven way of treatment and prevention of complication or the development of severe dengue, specifically DHF or DSS.

INITIAL BASIC MANAGEMENT

When a patient presents with fever with relevant clinical features suggestive of DF and same is confirmed by detection of NS1 antigen/IgM antibody by ELISA method, some general principles of managements are followed:

- Categorization of the patient into high-risk group, if applicable.
- Bed rest during the acute phase.
- Adequate fluid intake including oral rehydration solution (ORS), fruit juices, coconut water, milk, and soup along with water. Only plain water should be avoided for electrolyte imbalance.
- Cold/tepid sponging to keep temperature below 38.5°C.
- *Antipyretics*: Aspirin/nonsteroidal anti-inflammatory drugs (NSAIDs) should be avoided since it may cause gastritis, vomiting, platelet dysfunction, severe bleeding, or acidosis. Paracetamol is preferable. In adults, the dose is 500 mg/dose and can be repeated at the interval of 6 hours, depending upon fever and body ache. In children, the dose of paracetamol is 10 mg/kg body weight per dose.
- Antibiotics are not necessary.
- Monitoring for any warning signs or symptoms are utmost important, particularly within 24–48 hours after patients become afebrile for development of complications.
- Looking for mosquito breeding places and prevention of further mosquito bites by using bed nets is essential as it will prevent the transmission of disease.
- *Notification*: For epidemiological purpose of taking control measures.

The WHO proposed the simple form of disease classification of dengue (with or without warning signs) and severe dengue (**Fig. 6**).

The management principle will depends upon the severity of the disease namely severe and nonsevere dengue with less complexity (**Flowchart 1**).

DENGUE WITHOUT WARNING SIGNS

Nonsevere forms of dengue can easily be managed in home by adequate fluid therapy, antipyretics, and nutritional support. Event of vomiting must be actively treated either with antiemetics like ondansetron or by prokinetics like domperidone, so that adequate oral intake of fluid should not be hampered. Careful monitoring of fluid status and danger signs must be carried throughout. More stringent monitoring is essential after the time of defervescence. Regular measurement of platelet count and packed cell volume (PCV) must be done for optimum monitoring and early identification of complication. Home management of nonsevere dengue without warning signs is shown in **Flowchart 2**.

INPATIENT MANAGEMENT

Dengue fever with warning signs and symptoms must be admitted in hospital for optimum management. Severe dengue and also any form of dengue in high-risk group must be admitted for obvious reasons. High-risk group should be monitored carefully rather treated. Regular investigations of platelet count and PCV as well as clinical evaluation are of utmost importance.

Management of dengue fever with warning signs including grade I and II dengue hemorrhagic fever (Flowchart 3): Close monitoring of the patient is most important. When a patient gets admitted in hospital with warning signs or high-risk category, evaluation of complications and assessment of fluid status are done. Daily requirement of maintenance fluid (by Holliday–Segar formula) and ongoing deficit is calculated (**Table 3**). This total amount is divided into intravenous (IV) infusions and ensured oral intake. After 24 hours re-evaluation of fluid status is done and the maintenance fluid is continued in the form of oral fluid and IV infusion.

Total fluid requirement in first day: Maintenance fluid + 5% of ongoing deficit (50 mL/kg).

This total amount of fluid is divided into oral fluid according to the capacity of the patient and the rest is infused in 24 hours. Fluid therapy should be tapered off according to the response and ability of the patient for oral intake or within 24–48 hours whichever is longer.

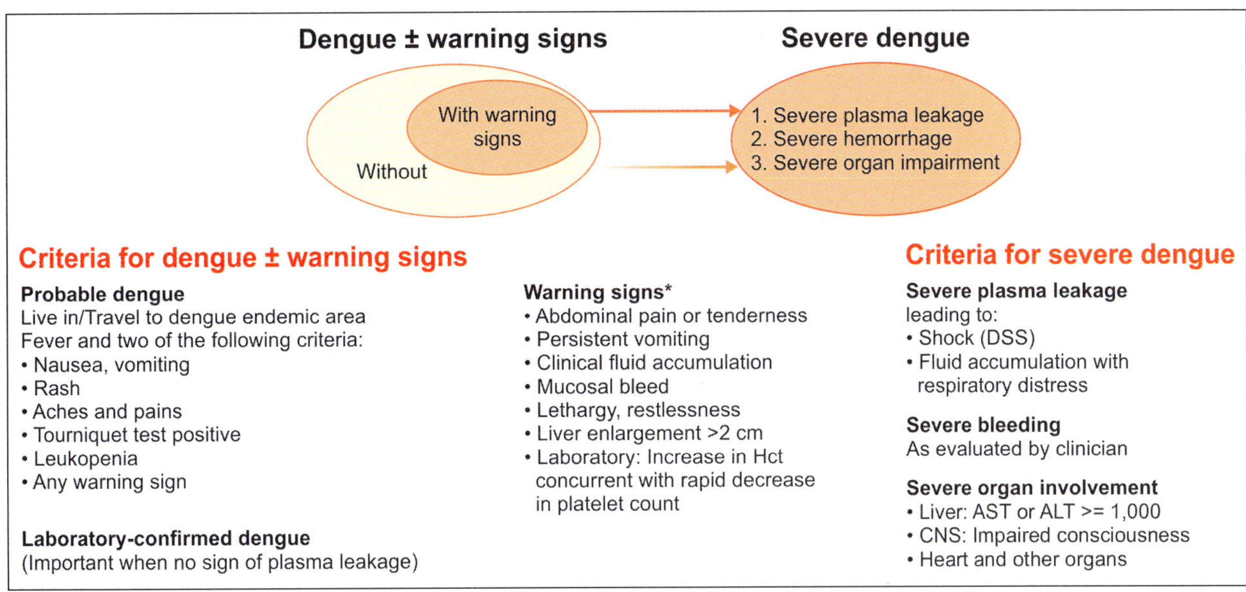

(ALT: alanine aminotransferase; AST: aspartate aminotransferase; CNS: central nervous system; DSS: dengue shock syndrome; Hct: hematocrit)

FIGURE 6: Simple form of disease classification of dengue (with or without warning signs) and severe dengue proposed by World Health Organization.

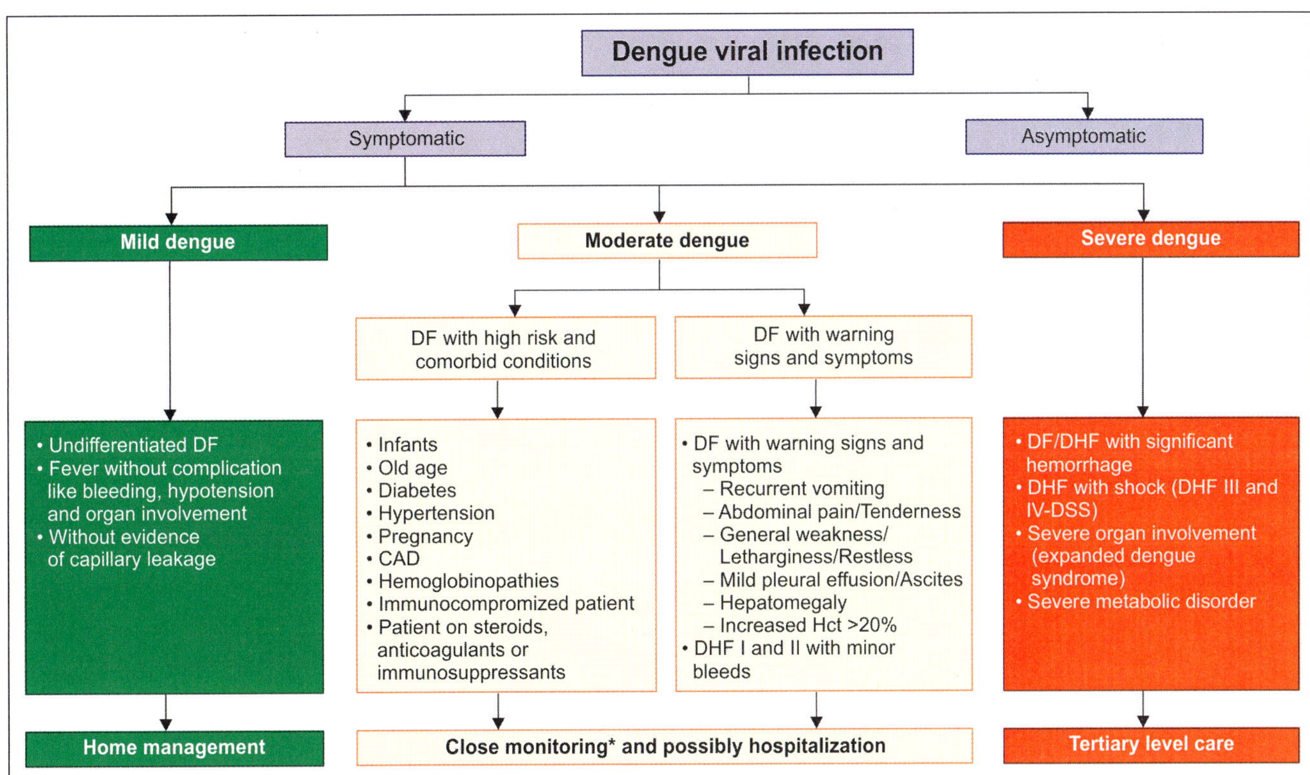

*Close monitoring: Hct, Plt, Hb, fluid intake/output, HR, RR, BP, consciousness.

(BP: blood pressure; CAD: coronary artery disease; DF: dengue fever; DHF: dengue hemorrhagic fever; DSS: dengue shock syndrome; Hb: hemoglobin; Hct: hematocrit; HR: heart rate; Plt: platelet; RR: respiration rate)

FLOWCHART 1: Dengue case classification and management.

Choice of intravenous fluids for resuscitation:

- No clear advantage of colloids over crystalloids in terms of the overall outcome.
- Colloids restore BP quickly and reduce the hematocrit faster than crystalloids in patients with intractable shock and pulse pressure ≤10 mm Hg, but major concerns are impact on coagulation, allergic reaction, and osmotic renal injury in hypovolemic patients.
- *Crystalloids*: Start with NS. Initial large volume may lead to hyperchloremic acidosis which may add to the lactic acidosis. Other is Ringer's lactate.

Outpatient management

During the febrile phase (may last 2–7 days) and subsequent critical phase (1–2 days), your clinic should

- Follow CBCs
- Watch for dehydration
- Watch for warning signs, including decreasing platelet count and increasing hematocrit
- Watch for defervescence (indicating beginning of critical phase)

Advise patient or their family to do the following

Control the fever

- Give acetaminophen every 6 hours (maximum 4 doses per day). Do not give ibuprofen, aspirin, or aspirin-containing drugs
- Sponge patient,s skin with tepid water when temperature is high

Prevent dehydration which occurs when a person loses too much fluid (from high fever, vomiting, or poor oral intake). Give plenty of fluids (not only water) and watch for signs of dehydration. Bring patient to clinic or emergency room if any of the following signs develop:

- Decrease in urination (check number of wet diapers or trips to the bathroom)
- Few or no tears when child cries
- Dry mouth, tongue or lips
- Sunken eyes
- Listlessness, agitation, or confusion
- Fast heartbeat (>100/min)
- Cold or clammy fingers and toes
- Sunken fontanel in an infant

Prevent spread of dengue within your house

- Place patient under bed net or have patient use insect repellent while febrile to avoid infecting mosquitoes that can infect others within 2 weeks
- Kill all mosquitoes in house
- Empty containers that carry water on patio
- Put screens on windows and doors to prevent mosquitoes from coming into house

Watch for warning signs as temperature declines 3–8 days after symptoms began. Return immediately to clinic or emergency department if any of the following warning signs appear:

- Severe abdominal pain or persistent vomiting
- Red spots/patches on skin
- Bleeding from nose or gums
- Vomiting blood
- Black, tarry stools
- Drowsiness or irritability
- Pale, cold, or clammy skin
- Difficulty breathing

(CBC: complete blood count)

FLOWCHART 2: Home management of nonsevere dengue without warning signs.

Source: Centers for Disease Control and Prevention. Dengue Case Management. [online] Available from https://www.cdc.gov/dengue/resources/dengue-clinician-guide_508.pdf.

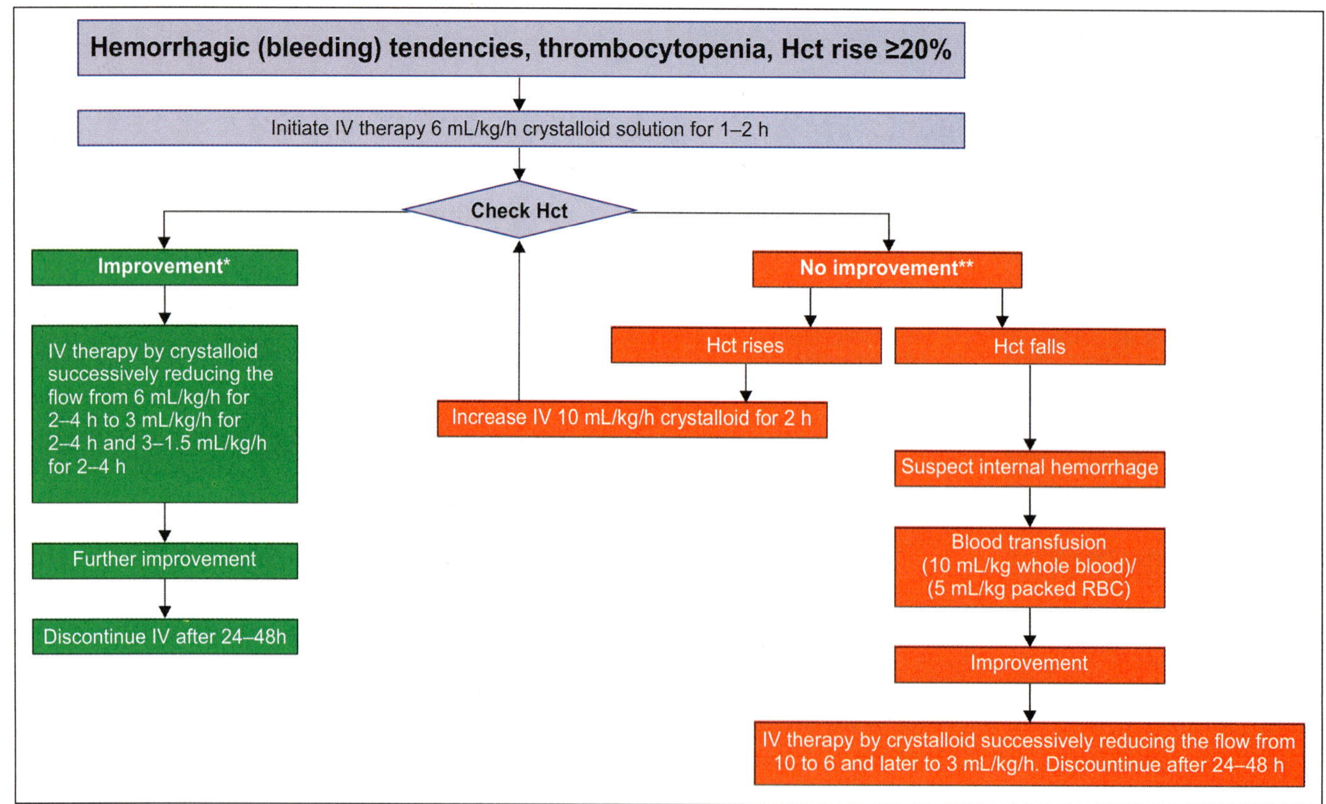

*Improvement: Hct falls, pulse rate and blood pressure stable, urine output rises.

**No improvement: Hct or pulse rate rises, pulse pressure falls below 20 mm Hg, urine output falls.

(Hct: hematocrit; IV: intravenous; RBC: red blood cell)

FLOWCHART 3: Management of dengue fever with warning signs including grade I and II dengue hemorrhagic fever.

TABLE 3	Holliday–Segar formula for calculation of maintenance fluid.
Body weight in kg	**Maintenance fluid in 24 hours**
<10 kg	100 mL/kg
10–20 kg	1,000 + 50 mL/kg body weight exceeding 10 kg
>20 kg	1,500 + 20 mL/kg body weight exceeding 20 kg

MANAGEMENT OF SEVERE DENGUE

- First patient should be admitted in intensive care unit for stringent observation, monitoring, and prompt management.
- Complete investigation must be obtained as early as possible, which includes complete blood counts with PCV, liver function test (LFT), kidney function test (KFT), electrolytes, arterial blood gas (ABG), and coagulation profile [PT/international normalized ratio (INR) and activated partial thromboplastin time (APTT)]. Comparison of blood counts and PCV must be done with the previous one to predict the progress of the disease severity.

Fluid accumulation: Patient may have severe fluid accumulation in pleural and peritoneal cavity leading to respiratory distress and abdominal pain. Respiratory distress must be managed conservatively with oxygenation and even with noninvasive ventilation (NIV) in extreme cases with partial desaturation. Abdominal pain is managed with injection tramadol.

Severe bleeding: Grade of bleeding must be assessed properly, but sometimes gastrointestinal (GI) bleed or intraperitoneal bleed may be difficult to locate. Attempts should be made to control the bleeding. Tranexamic acid is used most commonly. Severe bleeding will require transfusion of platelet at any platelet count. For adults, standard dose is 5–6 units of random donor platelet (RDP) or one unit of single donor platelet (SDP) (contains 3×10^{11} platelets/bag). SDPs are expected to raise platelet count by 30–50,000/µL. For neonates/infants, the dose is 10–15 mL/kg. Prophylactic platelet is indicated at count <10,000/mm^3 in absence of bleeding. Estimation of coagulation profile should be done simultaneously. For an altered coagulation profile, transfusion of fresh frozen plasma or cryoprecipitate is indicated. Re-evaluation must be done after 8–12 hours for the need of repeated platelet transfusion. If the hematocrit drops significantly (>10%), packed red blood cell (PRBC) transfusion should be given at a dose of 5 mL/kg per dose depending upon the intensity of bleeding.

Dengue hepatitis: Mild-to-moderate rise of liver enzymes does not require any special attention. Severe hepatitis with enzyme level >1,000 IU/mL needs monitoring of synthetic function of liver by coagulation profile and albumin. Prevention of GI bleeding by proton-pump inhibitor (PPI), use of lactulose and L-ornithine and L-aspartate may have some protective benefit. Prolonged PT may require vitamin K.

Dengue myocarditis: Both tachyarrhythmia and bradyarrhythmia are observed. Appropriate fluid management with inotrope support is the mainstay of treatment. Heart failure and arrhythmias, if present, are managed appropriately.

Dengue shock syndrome (Flowcharts 4 and 5): Vasopressors are introduced as required.

***When to discharge*:** Criteria for discharge are given in **Box 6**.

FUTURISTIC CONTROL MEASURES

The global population of dengue epidemic and measures that can be developed to control it are given in **Figure 7**.

Directly acting antivirals: They target structural (E protein) and nonstructural (NS5 and NS3) proteins and exert antiviral effects; e.g., doxycycline, ivermectin, balapiravir, recombinant retrocyclin-1, and α-ketoamide and α-methyltransferase inhibitors.

Agents targeting host: These include α-glucosidase inhibitors, lovastatin, heparin and heparan sulfate, kinase inhibitors, INF, viral sensor [retinoic acid-inducible protein I (RIG-I) and toll-like receptor 3 (TLR3)] agonists, D4 dopamine receptor antagonists, chloroquine, amodiaquine, pentoxifylline, and morpholinos. They are active either in animal models or in cell lines. None of them has convincing clinical data.

Host modulators: They inhibit viral replications by host factor deprivation such as ribavirin and mycophenolic acid.

Agents perceived to be active: Critical phase is molecularly triggered by cytokines and interleukins. An agent that reduces the activation and production of cytokines is thought to definitely reduce the inflammatory reaction and thus decrease the disease severity. Corticosteroids and IV immunoglobulin are under trial with conflicting results.

Herbal treatment of dengue: Few studies showed *Carica papaya* leaf extract increases platelet count in dengue patients, but further high-quality human trials are needed to provide scientific evidence for or against papaya leaves.

Predicting recovery: Immature platelet fraction (IPF), which measures reticulated platelets, is an index of thrombopoiesis. The reference range for IPF is 1.1–6.1%. In dengue, IPF is measured to predict the recovery from thrombocytopenia. An IPF value of more >10% predicts recovery of platelet count within 48 hours and indicates that further platelet transfusion is not necessary.

DENGUE VACCINE

A live recombinant tetravalent dengue vaccine *CYD-TDV (Dengvaxia)* developed by Sanofi Pasteur has been licensed in over 20 countries in Latin America and Southeast Asia. It is a formulation of four chimeric yellow

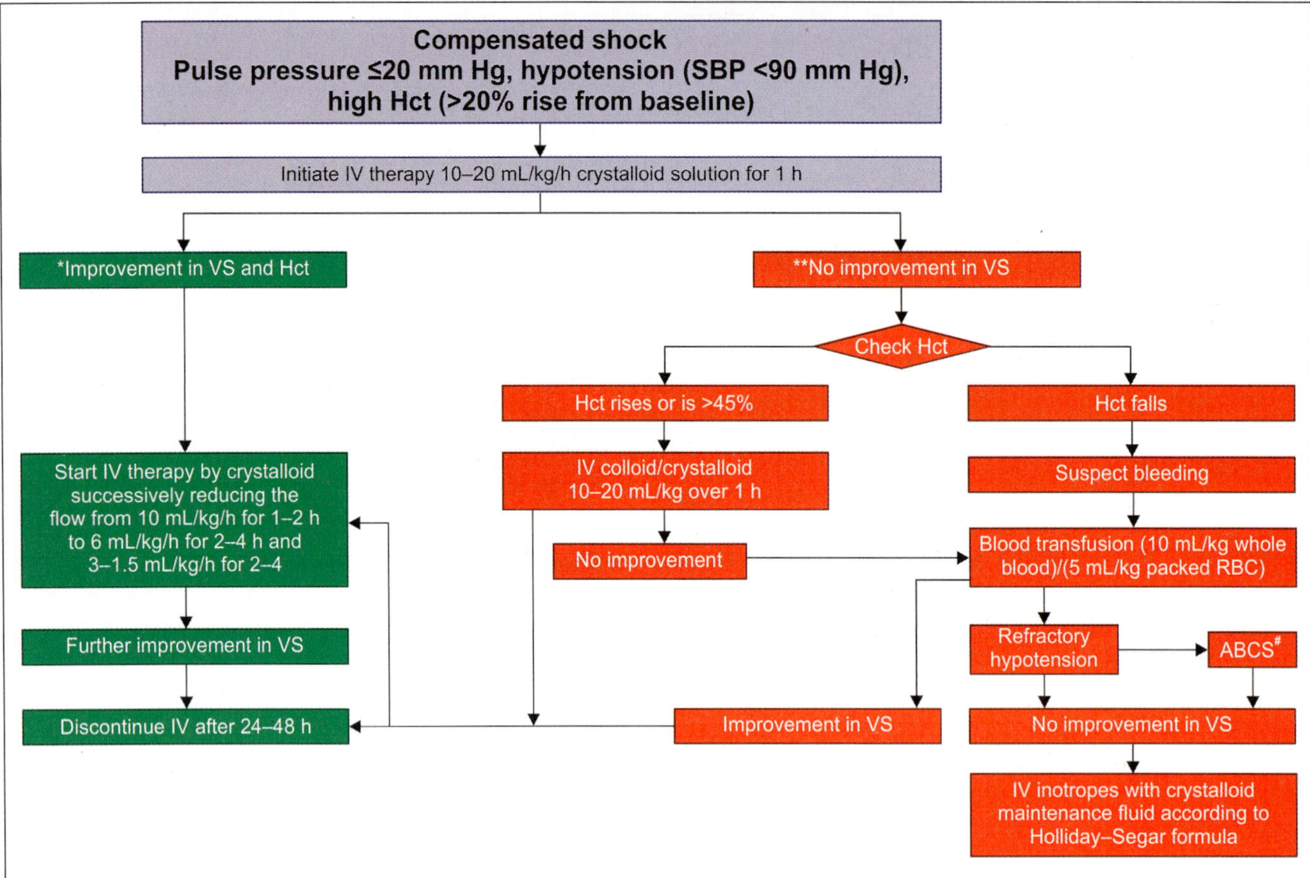

Notes:

Crystalloid: Normal saline, Ringer lactate; Colloid: Dextran 40/degraded gelatin polymer (polygeline)

\# ABCS = Acidosis, Bleeding, Calcium (Na^{++} and K^{+}), Sugar.

* Improvement: Hct falls, pulse rate and blood pressure stable, urine output rises.

** No improvement: Hct or pulse rate rises, pulse pressure falls below 20 mm Hg, urine output falls.

- Unstable vital signs: Urine output falls, signs of shock
- In cases of acidosis, hyperosmolar or Ringer's lactate solution not be used
- Serial platelet and Hct determinations: Drop in platelets and rise in Hct are essential for early diagnosis of DHF
- Cases of DHF should be observed every hour for vital signs and urine output

FLOWCHART 4: Management of patients in compensated shock.

fever 17D-dengue vaccine viruses, where the premembrane and envelope proteins from each of the four DENV types replace the same proteins in a yellow fever 17D backbone virus. Three doses are administered at 0, 6, and 12 months in persons aged 9–45 years who had previous dengue infection and residing in endemic areas. Vaccines in clinical development include TAK-003 (Takeda) and a tetravalent, live-virus vaccine attenuated through directed mutagenesis with a DENV 2/4 chimeric strain (National Institute of Health, licensed to Merck and Butantan).

DENGUE AND COVID COINFECTION

During the ongoing coronavirus disease (COVID) pandemic, many cases of coinfection of dengue and COVID have been observed. Most of them have not caused serious problems though some patients posed serious challenges and deaths have been reported from many states. There are many similarities in signs and symptoms of dengue and COVID. However, respiratory symptoms are more common in COVID. Cytokine storm occurs in both though may be little earlier in dengue. During current outbreak, all fever cases have to be tested for severe acute respiratory syndrome coronavirus-2 (SARS-CoV-2) as per protocol. Dengue patients usually show leukopenia with relative lymphocytosis whereas lymphocyte percentage decreases in COVID with progression of disease.

Thrombocytopenia is common in dengue. False positive rapid tests of dengue has been reported in COVID, hence rapid tests are to be avoided. Dengue patients need liberal fluids whereas conservative fluid management is the rule in COVID, hence cautious decisions have to be taken. Use of steroids is indicated for hypoxic COVID patients—dengue coinfection is not a contraindication. As dengue patients are already having leukopenia and thrombocytopenia, use of tocilizumab should be avoided as it can itself cause

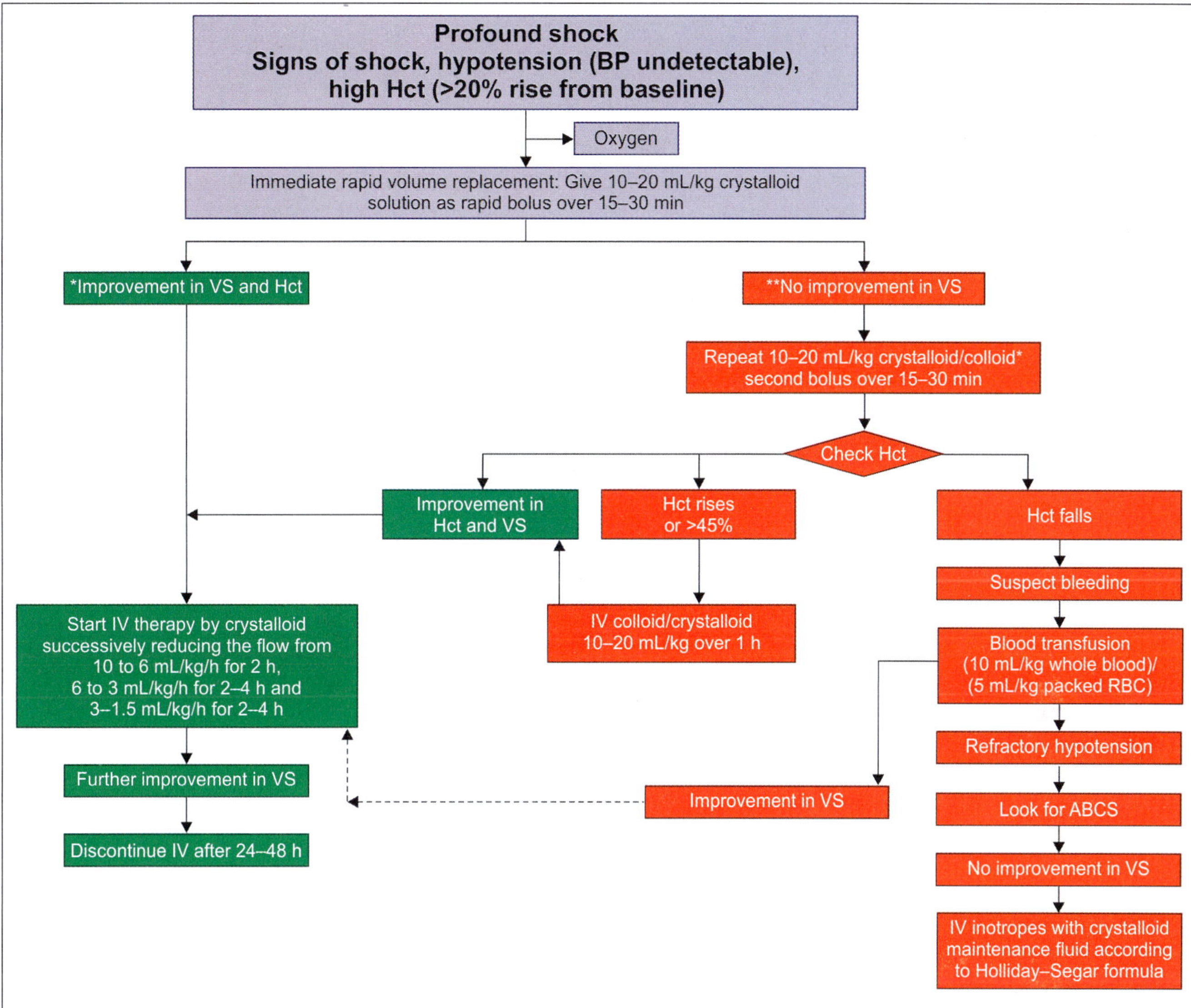

Note:

Crystalloid: Normal saline, Ringer lactate; Colloid: Dextran 40/degraded gelatin polymer (polygeline)

ABCS = Acidosis, Bleeding, Calcium (Na^{++} and K^{+}), Sugar

*Improvement: Hct falls, pulse rate and blood pressure stable, urine output rises.

**No improvement: Hct or pulse rate rises, pulse pressure falls below 20 mm Hg, urine output falls.

FLOWCHART 5: Management of patients in profound shock.

BOX 6	Criteria for discharge of patients.
• Absence of fever for at least 24 h without antipyretic medication	
• No respiratory distress from pleural effusion or ascites	
• Adequate urine output	
• Minimum of 2–3 days after recovery from shock and normal blood pressure	
• Return of appetite	
• Platelet count >50,000/mm^3	

cytopenias. Use of anticoagulants for prophylactic and therapeutic purposes in coinfected patients has to be carefully judged keeping in mind the clinical condition, risk of thrombosis, and bleeding. If there is active bleeding, anticoagulant needs to be discontinued immediately. Multidisciplinary expert team may be formed to manage difficult cases.

CONCLUSION

Dengue is a self-limited viral infection, which is usually cured with time if only the proper fluid therapy is administered. Severity of dengue develops only if the fluid could not be administered satisfactorily and also in some patients with preexisting comorbidity. Advanced management with pressure support medications and blood products including packed cell, plasma, and platelets

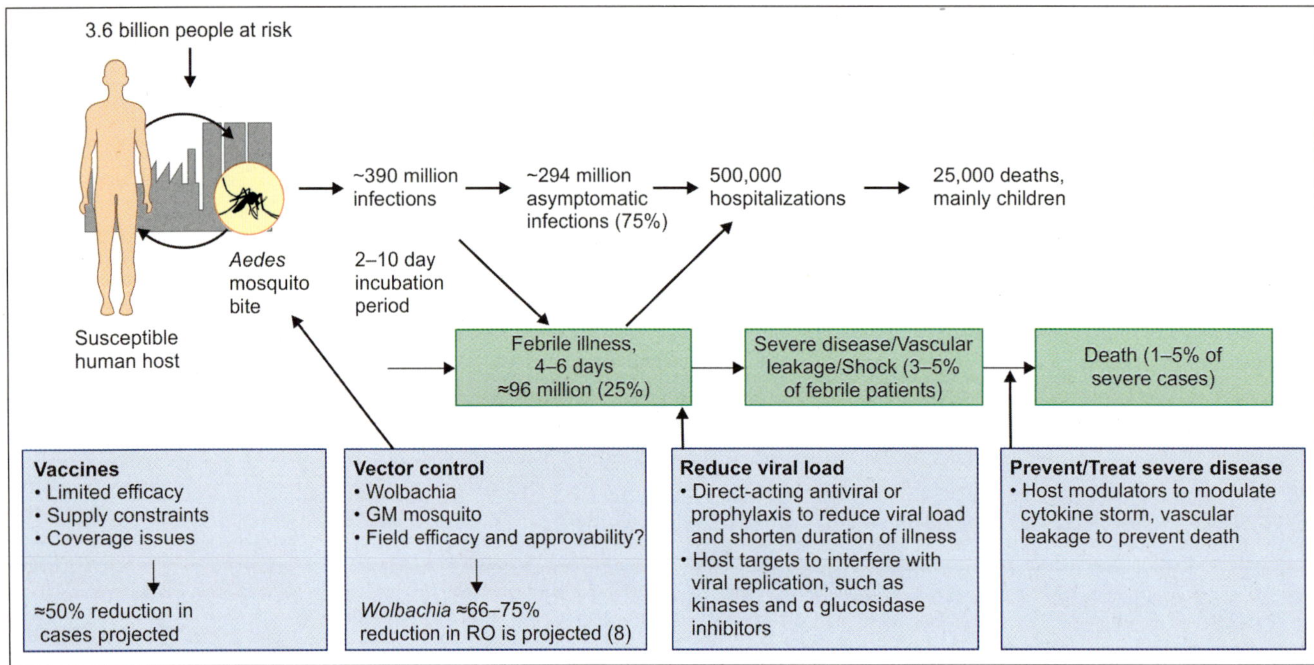

(GM: genetically modified; RO: reverse osmosis)

FIGURE 7: Global dengue epidemic, counter measures, and their impact on the total dengue burden.

may be required in some severe cases. Severe organ damage requires appropriate support. Newer drugs are mostly under trials and do not have any proven efficacy to recommend their use uniformly in all patients. Some newer techniques of predicting severity are also in the horizon. Dengue is treatable and curable in most cases, if managed sensibly. Current COVID pandemic has thrown additional challenges.

RECOMMENDED READINGS

1. WHO. (2015). National Guidelines for Clinical Management of dengue Fever. [online] Available from https://apps.who.int/iris/handle/10665/208893?mode=simple.
2. Yacoub S, Farrar J. Dengue. In: Farrar J, Hotez P, Junghanss T, Kang G, Lalloo D, White N (Eds). Manson's Tropical Diseases, 23rd edition. Amsterdam, Netherlands: Elsevier; 2013. pp. 162-70.
3. Thein S, Aung MM, Shwe TN, Aye M, Zaw A, Aye K, et al. Risk factors in dengue shock syndrome. Am J Trop Med Hyg. 1997;56:566-72.
4. Screaton G, Mongkolsapaya J. T cell responses and dengue haemorrhagic fever. Novartis Found Symp. 2006;277:164-71.
5. Van Gorp EC, Setiati TE, Mairuhu AT, Suharti C, ten Cate HT, Dolmans WM, et al. Impaired fibrinolysis in the pathogenesis of dengue hemorrhagic fever. J Med Virol. 67:549-54.
6. World Health Organization. Dengue: Guidelines for diagnosis, treatment, prevention and control. Geneva: World Health Organization; 2009.
7. Low JG, Ooi EE, Vasudevan SG. Current Status of Dengue Therapeutics Research and Development. J Infect Dis. 2017;215(Suppl_2):S96-102.
8. Fusco DN, Chung RT. Review of Current Dengue Treatment and Therapeutics in Development. J Bioanal Biomed. 2014;S8:1.
9. Briggs C, Kunka S, Hart D, Oguni S, Machin SJ. Assessment of an immature platelet fraction (IPF) in peripheral thrombocytopenia. Br J Haematol. 2004; 126:93-9.
10. Dadu T, Sehgal K, Joshi M, Khodaiji S. Evaluation of the immature platelet fraction as an indicator of platelet recovery in dengue patients. Int J Lab Hematol. 2014;36:499-504.
11. UpToDate. (2020). Dengue virus infection: Prevention and treatment. [online] Available from https://www.uptodate.com/contents/dengue-virus-infection-prevention-and treatment/print?search=dengue vaccine.
12. MoHFW GOI. (2020). Guidelines for management of co-infection of COVID-19 with other seasonal epidemic prone diseases. [online] Available from https://www.mohfw.gov.in/pdf/GuidelinesformanagementofcoinfectionofCOVID19withotherseasonalepidemicpronediseases.pdf.

CHAPTER 51

Human Immunodeficiency Virus Epidemiology and Prevention

BB Rewari, Priyanka Ojha

ABSTRACT

Despite major decline in new human immunodeficiency virus (HIV) infections and acquired immunodeficiency syndrome (AIDS)-related deaths, HIV continues to be a major global public health issue with an estimated 38.0 million people living with HIV (PLHIV) at the end of 2019. Between 2000 and 2019, globally new HIV infections fell by 39% and HIV-related deaths fell by 51%, with 15.3 million lives saved due to antiretroviral therapy (ART). There is a major progress on UN 90-90-90 targets and at the end of 2019, an estimated 81% of PLHIV globally knew their status, 67% were receiving ART, and 59% had achieved suppression of the HIV virus with no risk of infecting others.

India has also shown major gains in controlling the epidemic through an approach focusing on the continuum of prevention, testing, treatment, and care. New infections and AIDS-related deaths have come down by 37% and 26% since 2010, increased access to free ART has changed the perception of HIV from a virtual deaths sentence to a chronic manageable condition.

Combination of prevention and continuum of care remain the pillars for ending AIDS. A lot of focus has been laid by Indian National AIDS Control Programme (NACP) on prevention front to protect 99.78% of population which is still uninfected. However, the decline is plateauing as majority of infections come from key populations (KPs) and their partners and they still have unequal access to prevention and treatment services. So, the prevention focus must address these issues to further reduce new infections. The engagement with communities, use of combination prevention tools, and adoption of newer tools such as HIV self-testing and pre-exposure prophylaxis (PrEP) as well as high level advocacy for political commitment will be key to vision of ending AIDS as a public health problem by 2030.

"An ounce of prevention is worth a pound of cure"

—Anonymous

INTRODUCTION

The terms HIV and AIDS were not known to mankind till around four decades ago. In 1981, it was observed that there is an unusual increase in the incidence of *Pneumocystis carinii* pneumonia (PCP) among men who had sex with men. The first three clinical descriptions of these were published in 5th June 1981 edition of Morbidity and Mortality Weekly Report (MMWR) describing some cases of *Pneumocystis* pneumonia in previously healthy homosexuals from Los Angeles, USA. Soon, cases of PCP were noticed among hemophiliacs also. Similar reports were elicited from France, the Caribbean, and Central America. In the United States, the disease was first labeled "gay-related immune deficiency (GRID)" because homosexual men first exhibited characteristic symptoms. In some areas in Africa, the disease was called "slim" or "slim disease" because of the profound wasting and the association of death with progressive weight loss and diarrhea. In 1982, this illness was named as AIDS. In 1984, a lymphotropic virus was identified as causative agent in USA and France and named as HIV.

Very soon, HIV infection became world's one of the most serious health issue with profound social and economic dimensions. However, with concerted efforts from clinicians, researchers, social scientists, and above all community of PLHIV, the epidemic is finally showing a decline and is becoming more and more manageable with availability of ART, though a vaccine still eludes us.

GLOBAL SITUATION AND PROGRESS

CURRENT STATUS

Over last four decades, >35 million people have died of AIDS worldwide, and another 38 million are currently living with HIV. At the end of 2019, an estimated 38 million (31.6–44.5 million) people were living with HIV globally. In 2019, nearly 1.7 million (1.2–2.2 million) got newly infected with the virus and 0.7 million (0.5–1.0 million) died of AIDS (**Table 1**). This translates to 4,500 new infections every day in 2019, about 59% of which are in Sub-Saharan Africa, about 400 are among children under 15 years of age, and about 4,100 are among adults aged 15 years and older, of whom almost 47% are among women, 31% are among young people (15–24), and 19% are among young women (15–24).

Nearly two-thirds of the all people who are infected with HIV globally live in Sub-Saharan Africa. Next largest

TABLE 1 Global summary of AIDS in 2019.

Number of people living with HIV	**Total**	→	**38.0 million (31.6–44.5 million)**
	• Adults	→	36.2 million (30.2–42.5 million)
	• Women (15+ years)	→	19.2 million (16.4–22.2 million)
	• Children (<15 years)	→	1.8 million (1.3–2.2 million]
People newly infected with HIV in 2019	**Total**	→	**1.7 million (1.2–2.2 million)**
	• Adults	→	1.5 million (1.1–2.0 million)
	• Children (<15 years)	→	150,000 (94,000–240,000)
AIDS-related deaths in 2019	**Total**	→	**690,000 (500,000–970,000)**
	• Adults	→	600,000 (430,000–840,000)
	• Children (<15 years)	→	95,000 (61,000–150,000)

Source: UNAIDS. (2020). 2020 Global AIDS Update—Seizing the moment—Tackling entrenched inequalities to en epidemics. [online] Available from https://www.unaids.org/en/resources/documents/2020/global-aids-report.

TABLE 2 Region wise global HIV and AIDS statistics in 2019.

	Adults and children living with HIV	Adults and children newly infected with HIV	Adult and child deaths due to AIDS
Eastern and Southern Africa	20.7 million (18.4–23 0 million)	730,000 (580,000–940,000)	300,000 (230,000–390,000)
Western and Central Africa	4.9 million (13.9–6.2 million)	240,000 (150,000–390,0001)	140,000 (100,00–210,000)
Middle East and North Africa	240 000 (170 000–400 000)	20, 000 (11,000–38, 000)	8,000 (4,900–1,4000)
Asia and the Pacific	5.8 million (4.3–7.2 million)	300,000 (210,000–390,000)	160,000 (94,000–240,000)
Latin America	2.1 million (1.4–2.8 million)	120 000 (73,000–000)	37000 (23,000–56,000)
Caribbean	330 000 (270 000–400 000)	13000 (8,700–19,000)	6,900 (4,900–10,000)
Eastern Europe and Central Asia	1.7 million (1.4–1.9 million)	170 000 (140,000–190,000)	3,5000 (26, 000–45, 000)
Western and central Europe and North America	2.2 million (1.7–2.6 million)	65000 (49,000–87,000)	12 000 (8,700–19,000)
Global	**38.0 million (31.6–44.5 million)**	**1.7 million (1.2 million–2.2 million)**	**690,000 (500,000–970,000)**

Source: UNAIDS. (2020). 2020 Global AIDS Update—Seizing the moment—Tackling entrenched inequalities to end epidemics [online].

number of HIV infected people live in Asia and Pacific (5.8 million) (**Table 2**).

Certain groups of population are at a much higher risk of acquiring HIV. These are commonly referred to as KPs such as sex workers (SWs), men having sex with men (MSM), transgenders (TG), and people who inject drugs (PWID) (**Fig. 1**).

Globally, 62% of new infections occur among the KPs and their partners. Most countries in Asia and Pacific have a concentrated epidemic with almost 98% of new infection being from KPs and their partners (**Fig. 2**).

GLOBAL PROGRESS

We are now in the fourth decade of the AIDS epidemic. The epidemic has been largely contained from its rapid growth trajectory in early years. It has halted and begun to show reversal in the spread of HIV (in accordance to Millennium Development Goal 6.A) and there is decline in new infections as well as mortality related to AIDS (**Fig. 3**). Efforts are now on to meet the Sustainable Development Goal target 3.3 (SDG 3.3) on ending AIDS as a public health problem by 2030.

Globally, between 2000 and 2019 new HIV infections fell by 39% and HIV-related deaths by 51%. More than 15.3 million lives have been saved due to ART. Similarly, between 2010 and 2019, the new HIV infections in South East Asia reduced by 23.8% and AIDS-related deaths came down by 26.7%, respectively. Similar progress has been seen in India as well and is described in subsequent section.

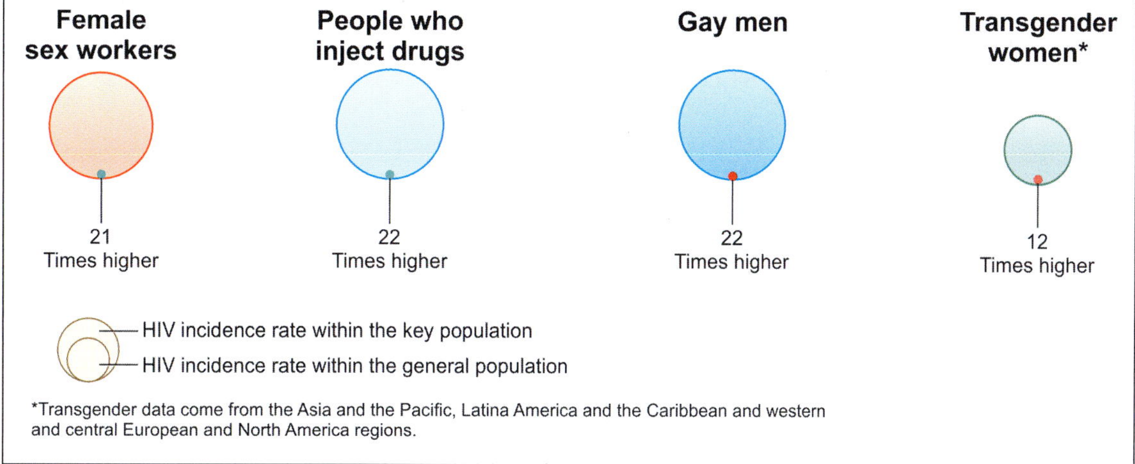

FIGURE 1: Key populations at relatively higher risk.

Source: UNAIDS. (2020). 2020 Global AIDS Update—Seizing the moment—Tackling entrenched inequalities to end epidemics [online].

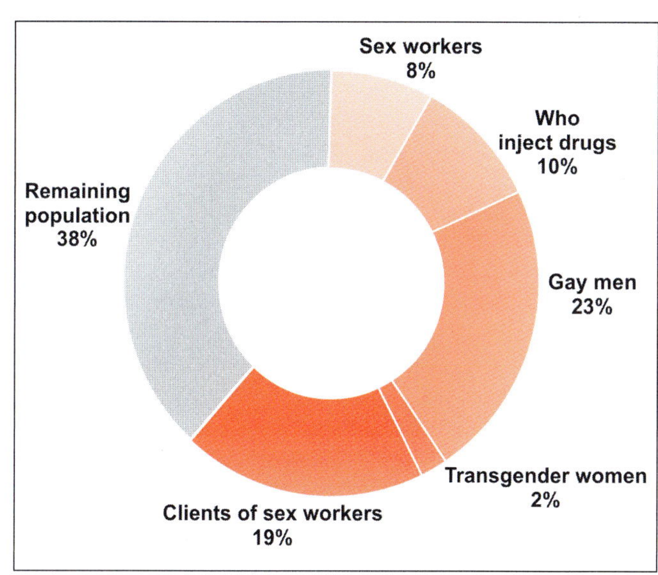

FIGURE 2: Distribution of new human immunodeficiency virus (HIV) infections by key population, global (2019).

Source: UNAIDS. (2020). 2020 Global AIDS Update—Seizing the moment—Tackling entrenched inequalities to end epidemics [online].

There has been major progress on UN fast track targets which aimed, among others, that by 2020, 90% of people infected with HIV should be aware of their status; that 90% of people who were aware of their status should be on treatment; and that 90% of people on treatment achieved viral suppression. As of December 2019, 81% of estimated 38 million know their status, 66% are on ART, and 55% are virally suppressed. The Joint United Nations Program on AIDS/HIV (UNAIDS) has now proposed the 95-95-95 targets by 2025 on similar lines with a view to ending AIDS as a public health problem as part of SDG 3.3 and World Health Organization (WHO) Global Health Sector Strategy on HIV.

HIV IN INDIA

CURRENT SCENARIO

The first few cases of HIV were reported in India in Chennai in 1986. Demographically the second largest country in the world, India has also the third largest number of PLHIV after South Africa and Nigeria.

The national scenario of HIV has been changing over years. After the initial few cases were detected in Chennai among SWs in 1986, the infection started to spread but was mainly confined to five states, i.e., Andhra Pradesh, Maharashtra, Tamil Nadu, Manipur, and Nagaland, initially. The scenario has changed but spread is still heterogenous with nearly 200 districts being high prevalence out of nearly 718 districts in the country.

As per the HIV estimation report 2019, there are an estimated 23.49 lakh PLHIV in India, with an adult (15–49 years) HIV prevalence of 0.22% (0.17–0.29%). This includes nearly 10 lakh women and 80,000 children. There were 69,220 new HIV infections and 58,960 AIDS-related deaths in the year 2019 (**Table 3**).

Overall, the estimated adult (15–49 years) HIV prevalence is 0.22% (higher among males at 0.24%) and has been declining since the peak in 2,000 and stabilizing in recent years (**Fig. 4**).

The epidemic in India is heterogenous and prevalence varies widely among states. Maharashtra is estimated to have the highest number of PLHIV (3.96 lakh), followed by Andhra Pradesh (3.14 lakh), Karnataka (2.69 lakh), Uttar Pradesh (1.61 lakh), Telangana (1.58 lakh), Tamil Nadu (1.55 lakh), Bihar (1.34 lakh), and Gujarat (1.04 lakh) (**Fig. 5**).

Together, these eight states constitute 72% of the total PLHIV estimates in the country. The states of West Bengal, Delhi, Punjab, Rajasthan, Madhya Pradesh, Odisha, and Haryana contribute another 18% of the total PLHIV size. Overall, 90% of PLHIV estimates were from these 15 states (**Fig. 6**).

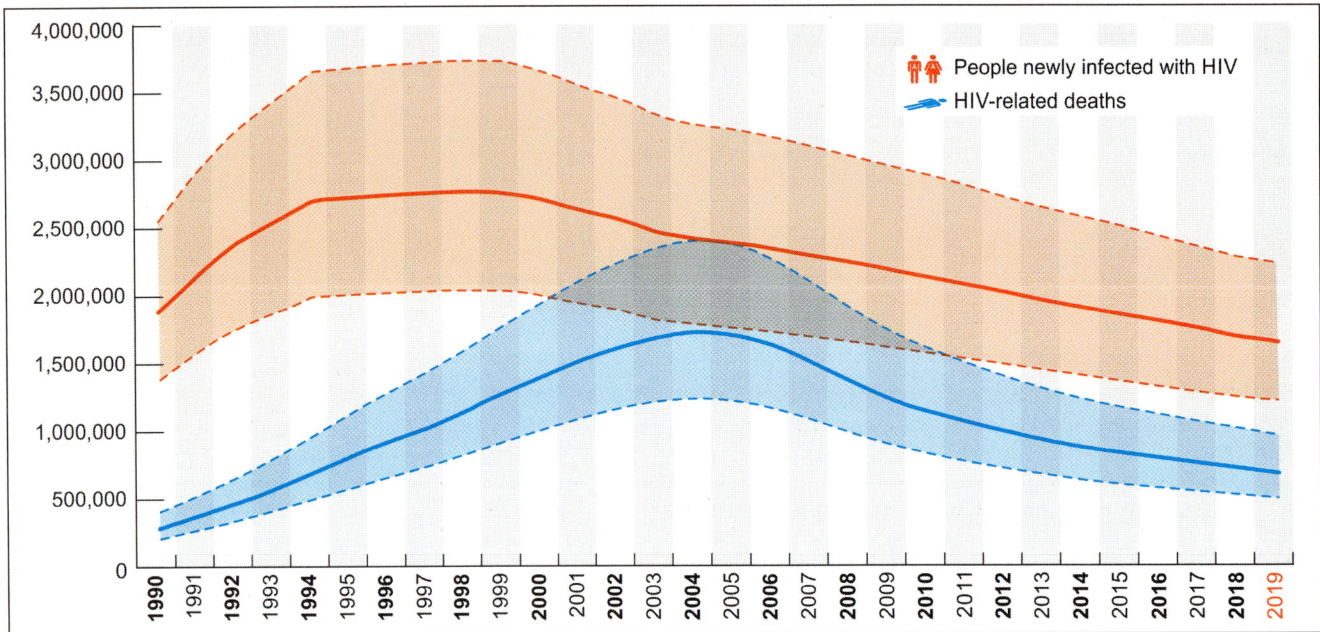

FIGURE 3: Decline in human immunodeficiency virus (HIV) incidence and mortality over time, 2019, global.

Source: UNAIDS. (2020). 2020 Global AIDS Update—Seizing the moment—Tackling entrenched inequalities to end epidemics. [online] Available from https://www.unaids.org/en/resources/documents/2020/global-aids-report.

TABLE 3 Snapshot of the HIV epidemic in India—2019.

Adult (15–49 years) HIV prevalence (%)	Total • Male • Female	0.22 (0.17–0.29) • 0.24 (0.18–0.32) • 0.20 (0.15–0.26)
Number of people living with HIV (lakh)	Total • Children (<15 years)	23.49 (17.98–30.98) • 0.79 (0.58–1.05)
New HIV infections (thousand)	Total	69.22 (37.03–121.50)
AIDS-related deaths (thousand)	Total	58.96 (33.61–102.16)

Source: National AIDS Control Organisation. India HIV Estimates 2019 Report [online].

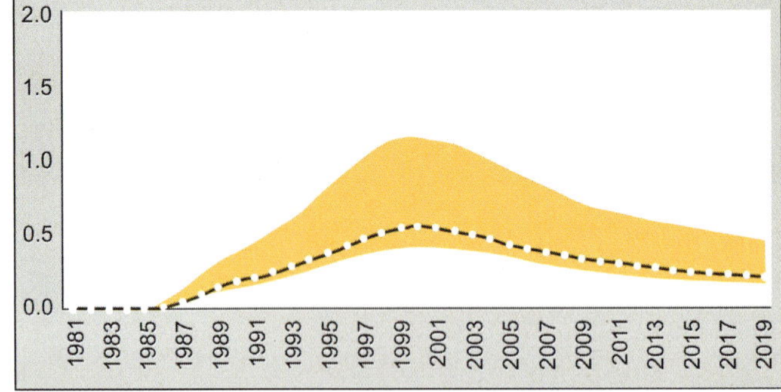

FIGURE 4: Declining human immunodeficiency virus (HIV) prevalence over the years in India.

Source: National AIDS Control Organisation. India HIV Estimates 2019 Report [online].

The epidemic in India is concentrated among high-risk group populations and the prevalence among different high-risk groups is depicted in the **Figure 7**.

The common routes of transmission are unprotected sex—both heterosexual and homosexual, intravenous drug users (IDUs) sharing the needles, transfusion of blood and blood products from infected donor, and vertical transmission from infected parents. Information from persons testing positive for HIV at the Integrated Counseling and Testing Centers across the country shows that 94% of HIV infections are still occurring through heterosexual routes of transmission (**Fig. 8**). Migrants and truckers form the bridge population between high-risk groups such as female sex worker (FSW), MSM, IDU, and TGs and the general population.

PROGRESS

Due to concerted efforts by the NACP on prevention activities as well as scale up of ART, there has been a major decline in new infections and AIDS-related deaths over the years. The HIV incidence has declined from 0.54 in 1995 to 0.05 in 2019 per 1,000 uninfected populations (**Fig. 9**).

In 2019, there were 69,220 estimated new HIV infections that translate into 190 new infections every day and eight new infections every hour. The new infection has declined by 37% since 2010. The decline has been noted in all states/union territories (UTs) except for Tripura, Arunachal Pradesh, Chhattisgarh, and Chandigarh. The state-wise new annual infection is shown in **Figure 10**.

An estimated 58,690 AIDS-related deaths occurred among PLHIV in 2019. The AIDS-related deaths kept on

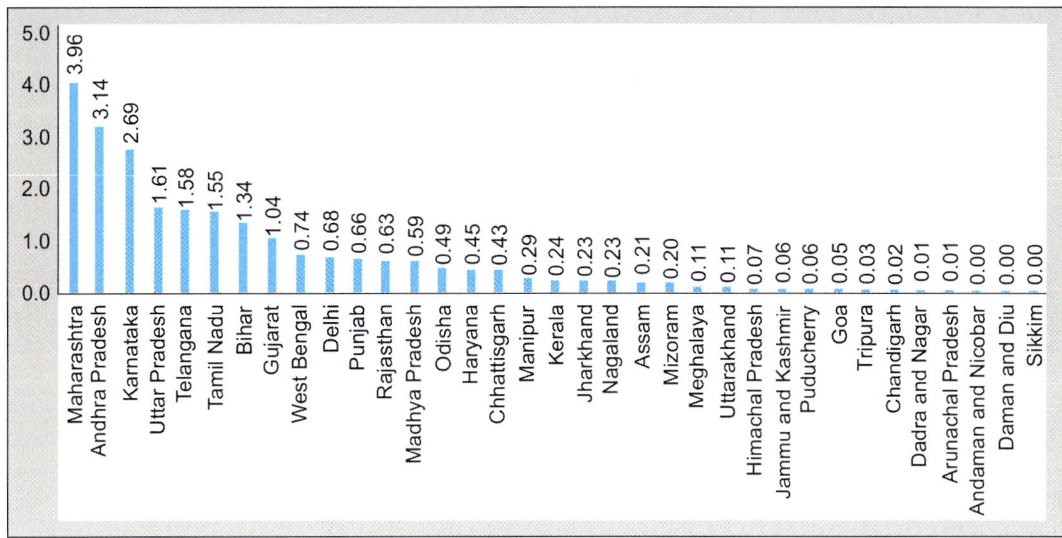

FIGURE 5: State-wise number of estimated people living with human immunodeficiency virus (PLHIV) in India.

Source: National AIDS Control Organisation. India HIV Estimates 2019 Report [online].

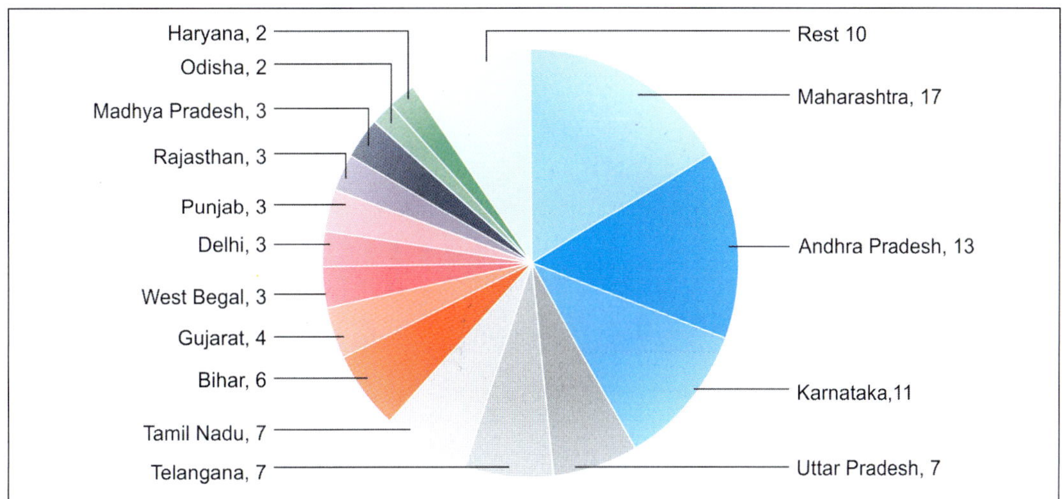

FIGURE 6: Distribution of people living with human immunodeficiency virus (PLHIV) by state/union territory (UT), 2019 (in %).

Source: National AIDS Control Organisation. India HIV Estimates 2019 Report [online].

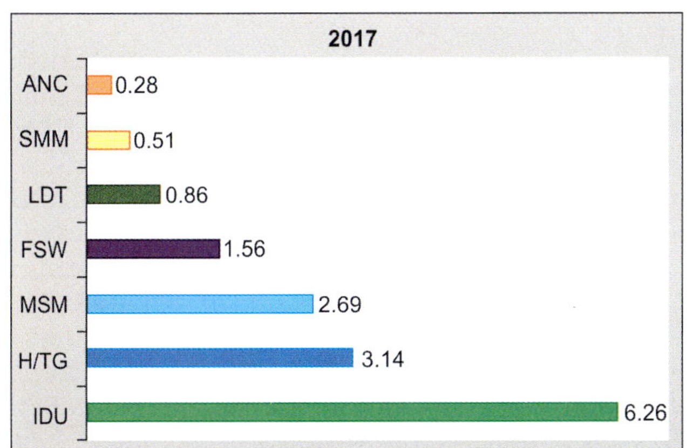

(ANC: antenatal care; FSW: female sex worker; HIV: human immunodeficiency virus; HSS: HIV Sentinel Surveillance; H/TG: *hijra*/transgender; IDU: intravenous drug user; LDT: long-distance trucker; MSM: men having sex with men; SMM: single male migrant)

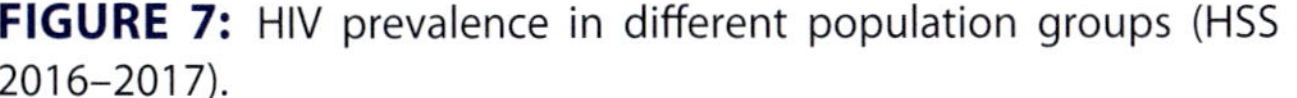

FIGURE 7: HIV prevalence in different population groups (HSS 2016–2017).

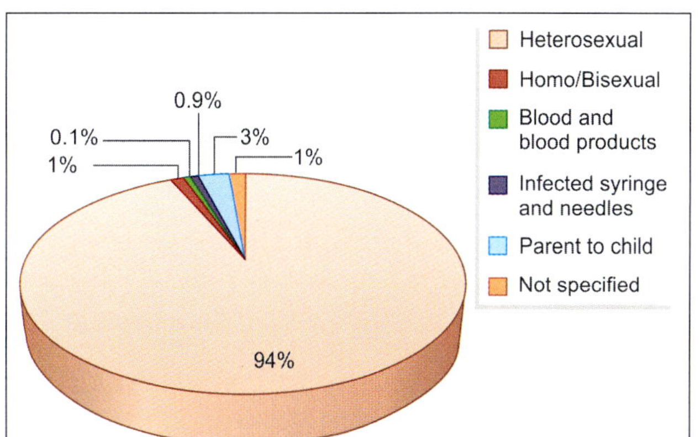

FIGURE 8: Routes of human immunodeficiency virus (HIV) transmission.

Source: NACO SIMS data 2014–2015 (annual report).

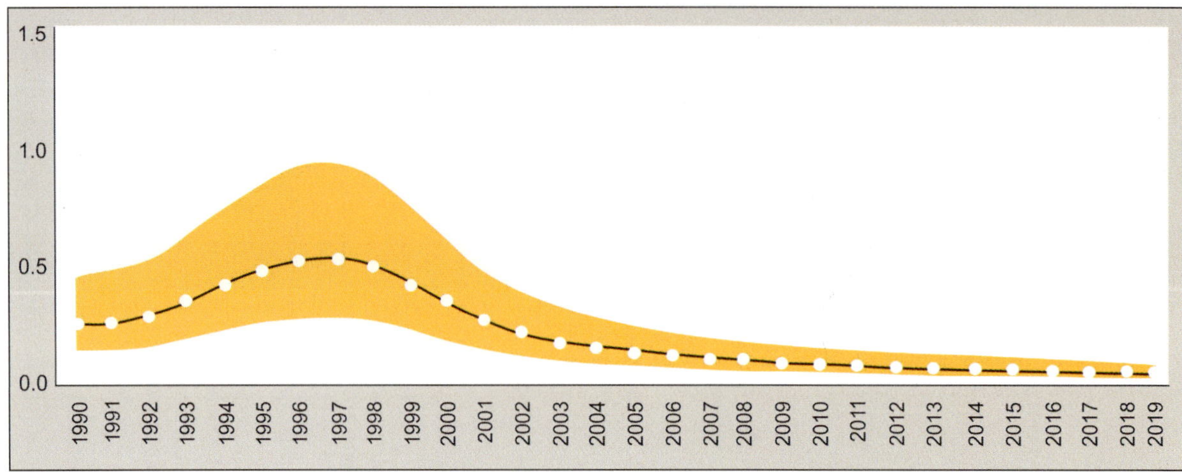

FIGURE 9: Trend of human immunodeficiency virus (HIV) incidence in India, 1990–2019 (per 1,000 uninfected population).

Source: National AIDS Control Organisation. India HIV Estimates 2019 Report [online].

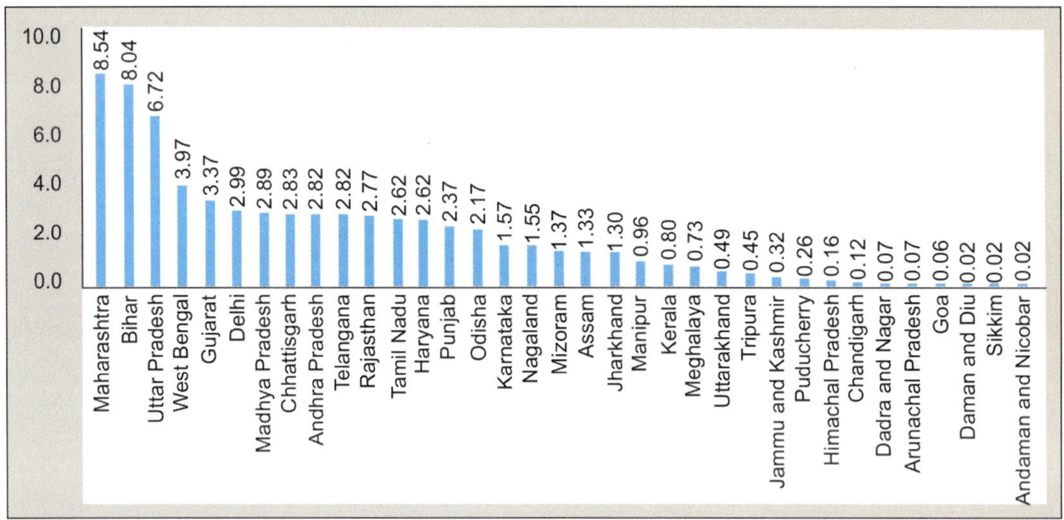

FIGURE 10: Annual new human immunodeficiency virus (HIV) infections by state/union territory (UT), 2019 (in thousand).

Source: National AIDS Control Organisation. India HIV Estimates 2019 Report [online].

increasing till 2005 and then started to decline. Since the peak, the annual AIDS-related deaths have declined by almost 71% (**Fig. 11**).

NATIONAL RESPONSE IN INDIA

Right after detection of first few cases, an AIDS Task Force was set up by the Indian Council of Medical Research (ICMR) and a National AIDS Committee headed by the Secretary, Department of Health. In 1992, the Government of India set up an autonomous body, National AIDS Control Organization (NACO), under Ministry of Health and launched the first NACP-I. The NACP-I was implemented during 1992–1999 with an objective to slowdown the spread of HIV infections so as to reduce morbidity, mortality, and impact of HIV epidemic in the country. In November 1999, the NACP-II was launched with the objective to reduce the spread of HIV infection in India and to increase India's capacity to respond to HIV on a long-term basis, i.e., the focus shifted from raising awareness to changing behavior, decentralization of program implementation at the state level, and greater involvement of non-governmental organizations (NGOs). The NACP Phase III (2007–2012) was launched with the goal to halt and reverse the epidemic in India over the 5-year period. The evolution of the NACP in India is depicted in **Figure 12**.

The NACO has now developed a National Strategic Plan (NSP) for HIV and sexually transmitted infection (STI) (2017–2024): "Paving Way for an AIDS Free India". This NSP will herald the country to the midpoint of the 2030 goals. The critical and investments made now will result in substantive gains towards "Ending of AIDS" as public health problem by 2030.

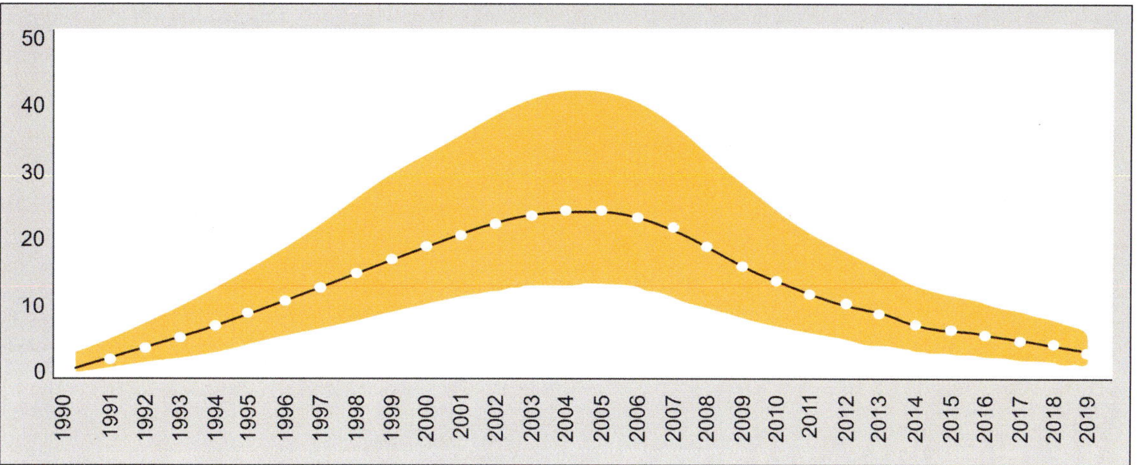

FIGURE 11: Decline in acquired immunodeficiency syndrome (AIDS)-related deaths over the years.

Source: National AIDS Control Organisation. India HIV Estimates 2019 Report [online].

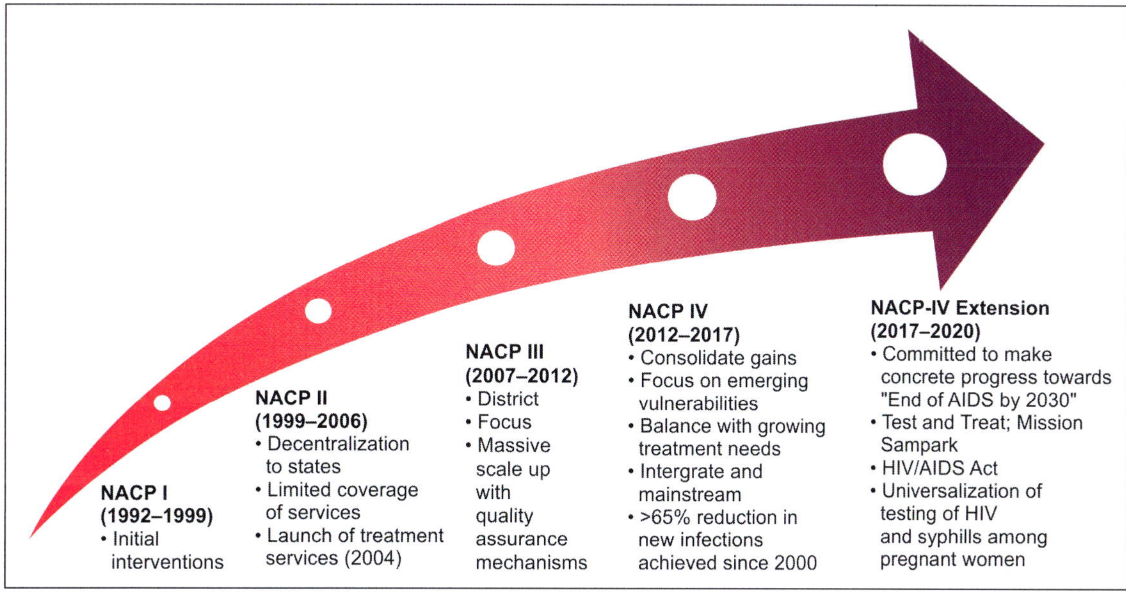

(NACP: National AIDS Control Programme)

FIGURE 12: Evolution of NACP in India.

PREVENTION OF HIV

Prevention of HIV is one of the core components of strategies to combat HIV epidemic. Before understanding various tools for HIV prevention, it is essential to understand the transmission dynamics of HIV—how it spreads from high-risk groups to general population.

TRANSMISSION DYNAMICS

Predominant route of transmission of HIV globally is sexual. Hence, this epidemic spreads as one would envisage in a classical epidemic of sexually transmitted disease (STD). HIV epidemic spreads classically in three waves. In the first wave, HIV infection is seen amongst KPs of SWs, MSM, or IDUs which are also called as core transmitters or core groups. In its second wave, HIV infection reaches the clients of SWs, MSM, or partners of IDUs. When evidences suggest affection of spouses and children of the clients of SWs, the HIV epidemic is understood to have reached its third wave. HIV infection is brought into the low-risk population from the core transmitters through the bridge population, a term used to connote mobile population such as truck drivers and single male member migrants. In some settings, IDUs constitute the first wave which is followed by the SWs and so on. Recently, a fourth wave comprising of adolescents has also been proposed to indicate the severity of the epidemic (**Fig. 13**).

COMBINATION PREVENTION

Combination prevention is a full bag of various approaches that help in preventing new infections and is defined as a rights-based, evidence-informed, and

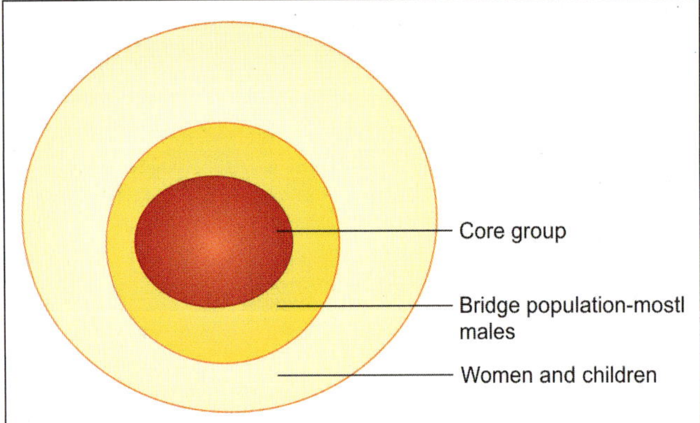

FIGURE 13: A schematic model of waves in the spread of human immunodeficiency virus (HIV) epidemic.

community-owned program that uses a mix of biomedical, behavioral, and structural interventions, prioritized to meet the current HIV prevention needs of particular individuals and communities, so as to have the greatest sustained impact on reducing new infections. These need to be carefully tailored to national and local needs and conditions, i.e., based on current information on the modes of transmission, the populations or groups most at risk of exposure and transmission, and their risk and vulnerability. They include the strategic mix of structural as well as biomedical and behavioral approaches required to meet the needs of those groups (**Fig. 14**). Through structural interventions, these approaches create a more enabling environment for prevention action.

Behavioral interventions: The behavioral intervention strategies to promote individual risk reduction include following:

- HIV testing and risk reduction counseling
- Behavior change communication to promote partner reduction, condom use, uptake of HIV testing and counseling etc.
- HIV education
- Interpersonal communication, including peer education and persuasion
- Social marketing of prevention commodities, cash incentives for individual risk avoidance etc.
- Addressing legal barriers
- Enabling environment

Biomedical interventions:

- Male and female condom provision
- Drug treatment including opioid substitution therapy (OST), needle and syringe provision
- Male circumcision
- Biomedical prophylaxis—antiretrovirals (ARVs) in prevention of mother-to-child transmission (PMTCT) services, ART-"Treat All", postexposure prophylaxis (PEP), PrEP etc.
- Appropriate and accessible STI services, voluntary medical male circumcision (VMMC), and ART for prevention
- Blood safety, standard precautions in healthcare setting etc.

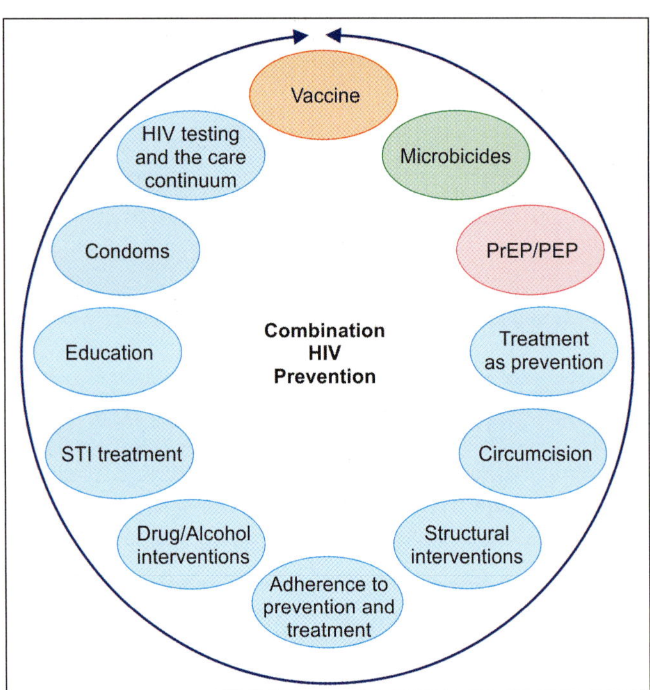

(HIV: human immunodeficiency virus; PEP: postexposure prophylaxis; PrEP: pre-exposure prophylaxis; STI: sexually transmitted infection)

FIGURE 14: Overview of HIV combination prevention modalities.

Some other key preventive tools are listed below.

Pre-exposure prophylaxis (PrEP): The WHO guidelines recommend offering PrEP, with oral tenofovir or tenofovir-containing regimens, to those at substantial risk of HIV infection, defined as an incidence rate of 3 per 100 persons per year or above within specific geographical areas or populations. The newer drugs like cabotegravir also offer opportunity of monthly PrEP option.

- PEP must be provided after an unsafe sexual act/shared needles with potential for transmission followed by evaluation of ongoing risk and provision of PrEP as required.

Harm reduction and medication-assisted treatment (MAT) for KPs: PWID are among the groups most vulnerable to HIV infection. PWID should have access to sterile injecting equipment through needle and syringe programs and those who are dependent on opioids should be offered and have access to MAT inform of methadone or buprenorphine. MAT has been shown to be a highly effective treatment for opioid dependence, reducing injecting behaviors that put PWID at risk for HIV, preventing HIV transmission, and improving retention on HIV treatment.

Voluntary medical male circumcision (VMMC): VMMC reduces female-to-male sexual transmission of HIV by 60%. The WHO and UNAIDS recommend the implementation of VMMC programs in countries with a high HIV prevalence among the general population. VMMC is cost-effective and should be included, alongside behavioral and structural strategies, as part of a comprehensive HIV prevention plan.

Condoms and lubricants: Effective condoms and lubricants use play an important role within the context of HIV prevention and must be integrated with other services as part of an "informed choice" and client-centered approach to prevention.

HIV case finding: Timely and appropriate case-finding activities are critical to ensure focused and timely access to prevention, treatment services for individuals as well as for reducing HIV transmission and achieving epidemic control. Strategies for HIV case finding:

- *Index testing*: Index testing refers to contact tracing or partner notification or partner services and is a critical case-finding strategy.
- *Self-testing*: HIV self-testing (HIVST) is defined by WHO as a process in which a person collects his or her own specimen (oral fluid or blood) and then performs an HIV test and interprets the result, often in a private setting, either alone or with someone he or she trusts.
- *Community-based testing*: Community-based testing services are those offered outside of a health facility within the broader community.
- *Optimized provider-initiated testing and counseling (PITC)*: This includes testing of patients who present with signs or symptoms suggestive of HIV, including signs or symptoms of tuberculosis (TB) and testing of subpopulations of increased risk as identified by behavioral, clinical, or demographic characteristics, or a combination of these such as STI clients, MSM, FSW, or high burden areas.

Prevention for women and PPTCT: PPTCT program is to keep mothers healthy and alive on ART and prevent HIV transmission from the woman living with HIV to her infant through preventing incident infections in women of reproductive potential, prevention of unintended pregnancies among women living with HIV by providing voluntary family planning counseling and services, identifying all pregnant and breastfeeding women (PBFW) living with HIV as early as possible, including through HIV testing services (HTS) at antenatal care (ANC) and provide ART to all those infected with HIV.

Early infant diagnosis: For children born to positive mother.

Preventing and treating STI: Persons with STI are at 2–17 times higher risk of acquiring HIV. Hence, early diagnosis and adequate treatment of STIs are important components of HIV prevention.

PREVENTION FOCUS IN INDIAN NATIONAL PROGRAM

The NACP lays a lot of focus on the prevention component as 99.78% population in the country is still not infected and it is important to keep them negative. There are around 1.6 million most at-risk population and 9 million bridge populations (truckers, migrants, and clients of SWs). The available data shows that around 40% FSW and MSM have STIs, around 40% of IDUs share needles, and there is evidence of higher HIV prevalence among migrants and spouses. To address these issues, the NACP has adopted

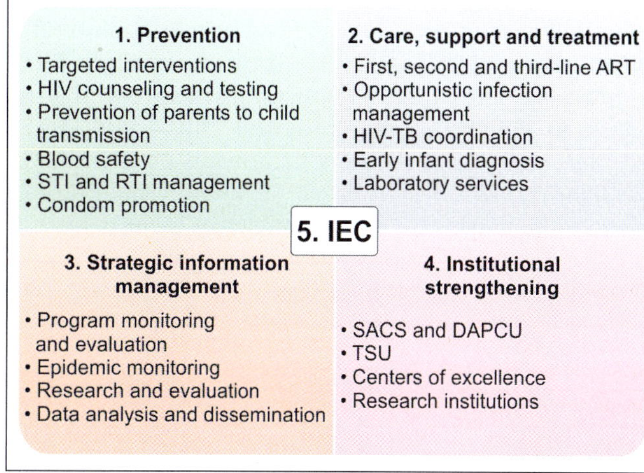

(DAPCU: District AIDS Prevention Control Unit; IEC: information, education, and communication; NACP: National AIDS Control Programme; RTI: reproductive tract infection; SACS: State AIDS Control Societies; STI: sexually transmitted infection; TB: tuberculosis; TSU: Technical Support Unit)

FIGURE 15: Five-pronged strategies under NACP.

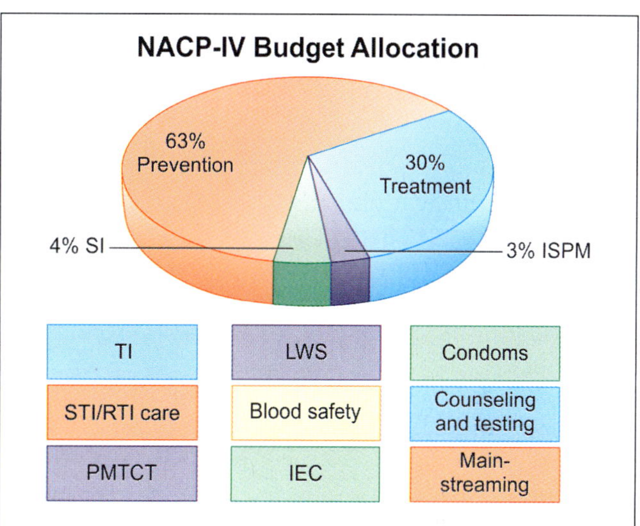

(IEC: information, education, and communication; LWS: Link Worker Scheme; PMTCT: prevention of mother-to-child transmission; RTI: reproductive tract infection; STI: sexually transmitted infection; TI: targeted intervention; SI: Strategic Information; ISPM: Institutional Strengthening and Project Management)

FIGURE 16: Key elements of prevention activities and funding under NACP-IV.

a five-pronged strategy for prevention and control of HIV (**Fig. 15**).

The package of prevention services is summarized in **Figure 16** and includes PPTCT, information, education, and communication (IEC), targeted interventions customized and tailored to the needs of different target groups, KP outreach, behaviour change communication (BCC), condom promotion, needle and syringe exchange, OST, counseling and testing, blood safety, mainstreaming of HIV into other sectors, youth interventions, Link Worker Scheme, and management of STIs and reproductive tract infections (RTIs). Prevention received 64% of the budget under NACP-IV.

To implement these activities NACO works by engaging communities of infected and affected people, community-based organizations, and NGOs through the State AIDS Control Societites (SACS). NACO has also established District AIDS Prevention and Control Units (DAPCUs) in 188 high prevelance districts to provide programmatic oversight through decentralized facilitation, monitoring, and coordination of HIV program activities in the district.

A brief description of some key prevention strategies adopted over the years is given below.

Targeted intervention program: For high-risk population groups including KPs, but also focusing on long distance truck drivers, migrant workers, and people from KPs in the past and their partners. This includes provision of risk reduction measures such as enabling environment, information, condoms, behavior change communication, community mobilization, and treatment for STIs and remains the mainstay of the response under NACP.

Comprehensive sex education: For young people has been an essential part of HIV prevention activities. This included training in life skills such as negotiating healthy sexual relationships as well as accurate and explicit information about how to practice safer sex, counseling on safer sexual behavior through media campaigns, social marketing, peer education, and small group counseling.

Condom promotion: It has been widely implemented as a prevention strategy. Condoms, if used consistently and correctly, are highly effective at preventing HIV infection. Free supply of condoms at strategic locations and hot spots through targeted intervention programs is being widely practiced.

The integrated counseling and testing centers: Help more people to get tested and make them aware of their infection and thereby reducing further transmission of the virus from the infected people.

Needle exchange programs: They have been shown to reduce the number of new HIV infections among injecting drug users. These programs distribute clean needles and safely dispose of used ones, and also offer related services such as referrals to drug treatment centers, provision of OST, and HIV counseling and testing.

Using safe blood and blood products: And implementing blood screening for blood-borne pathogens in all blood banks in India.

The Link Worker Scheme: It implemented to address complex needs of rural HIV prevention, care, and support through identification and training of village level workforce of Zonal Supervisors, Cluster Link Workers and other stakeholders on issues of HIV, gender, sexuality, and sexually transmitted infections.

For PMTCT of HIV: Universal HIV and syphilis screening has been made a part of routine ANC at all Primary Health Centers, Community Health Centers (CHCs), and other secondary and tertiary care facilities for all ANC clients.

Rapid scale of free: It *ART* has also contributed significant reduction in new infections as the transmission from infected partners is reduced due to suppression of viral replication by ART.

Due to these efforts there has been continuous decline in prevalence among FSW and MSM. However, the epidemic has stabilized among IDUs. The trends of HIV prevalence among KPs recorded through the HIV Sentinel Surveillance (HSS) 2003–2011 and Integrated Bio-Behavioral Surveillance (IBBS) 2014–2015 are shown in **Figure 17**.

One key component of NACP is to reduce stigma and discrimination with PLHIV. To address issues related to stigma and discrimination, India has enacted a law, "The Human Immunodeficiency, Virus and Acquired Immune Deficiency Syndrome (Prevention and Control) Act, 2017". The act provides an environment

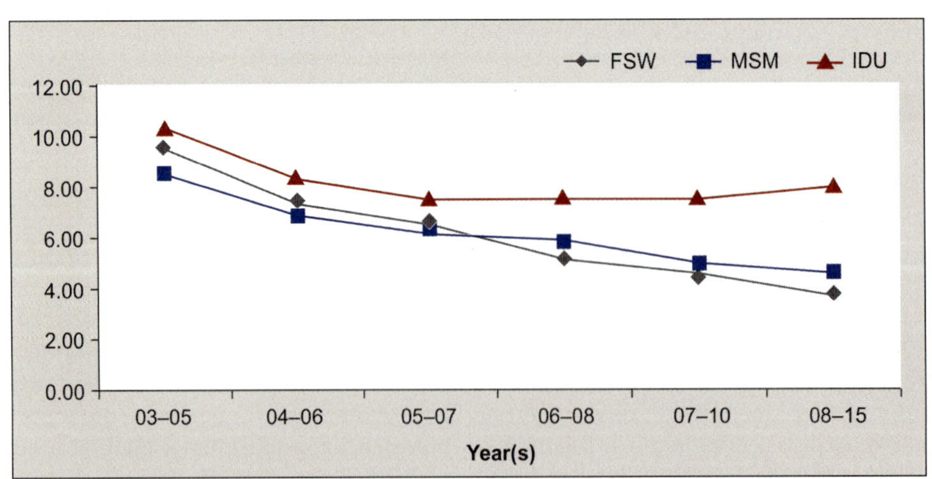

(FSW: female sex worker; HSS: HIV Sentinel Surveillance; IBBS: Integrated Behavioral and Biological Surveillance; IDU: intravenous drug user; MSM: men having sex with men)

FIGURE 17: HIV prevalence trend among key populations, HSS, and IBBS, India 2003–2015.

Source: NACO HSS and IBBS, India 2003–2015.

for enhancing access to healthcare services by ensuring informed consent and confidentiality for HIV-related testing, treatment, and clinical research. It also prohibits disclosure of a person's HIV positive status to his or her partner, by any healthcare provider, except a physician or a counselor. The law specifies certain conditions to be satisfied and circumstances under which a physician or counselor may disclose status to partners. Further, it protects healthcare providers from any criminal or civil action for any disclosure or nondisclosure of confidential HIV-related information made to a partner under the provisions of this law. The act also enlists contexts or settings on which discrimination against PLHIV is prohibited such as: (1) Employment; (2) Educational establishments; (3) Healthcare services; (4) Residing or renting a property; (5) Standing for public or private office; and (6) Provision of insurance.

It was observed during multiple programmatic reviews that while there is overall reduction in new infections nationally, the trends are not uniform across all geographic locations in India and especially among certain subpopulations. Hence, NACO has been promoting certain focused prevention programs in partnership with international and national NGOs. Examples of such initiatives are:

Project Sunrise: That aims to have an accelerated response based on prevention-treatment-care continuum of services among KPs, particularly PWID, in the North-Eastern states of India.

Project Hridaya: That aims to address the capacity building needs and implementation gaps among PWID and their sexual partners in Uttarakhand, Uttar Pradesh, and Bihar.

Project Nirantar: Which is a civil society capacity building initiative among all KPs in Chhattisgarh, Madhya Pradesh, and Odisha.

Linkages Project: That aims to strengthen linkages across the continuum of HIV services for KPs through provision of technical assistance (TA) for promoting the HIV cascade of services in districts of Andhra Pradesh and Maharashtra.

The national program is also planning to impellent some of the newer tools like HIV self-testing and PrEP in the program after some successful pilots.

MOVING AHEAD

The NSP for HIV and STI (2017–2024) envisages that the national response will accelerate HIV prevention in key and at-risk populations to reduce HIV infection through upgrading of the package relevant to specific populations. Efforts will be made to scale-up and modify targeted interventions to address other "at-risk" populations also including outreach through social networks, community-based screening, and specific points of integration with sexual and reproductive health. Expansion of testing and treatment facilities coupled with early detection and retention in care are also important components of preventing further spread of HIV. The five key priorities of the program are shown in **Table 4**.

TABLE 4	Key priorities of National Strategic Plan 2017–2024.
Priority 1	Accelerating HIV prevention in "at-risk group" and key population
Priority 2	Expanding quality assured HIV testing with universal access to comprehensive HIV care
Priority 3	Elimination of mother-to-child transmission of HIV and syphilis
Priority 4	Addressing the critical enablers in HIV programming
Priority 5	Restructuring the strategic information system to be efficient and patient centric

Source: National AIDS Control Organisation. National Strategic Plan, 2017-24. [online].

The HIV in India is on decline and government is committed to end AIDS by 2030 through a multi-pronged strategy involving all partners, civil society, and communities of people infected and affected by HIV and AIDS.

RECOMMENDED READINGS

1. UNAIDS. (2020). 2020 Global AIDS Update—Seizing the moment—Tackling entrenched inequalities to end epidemics. [online] Available from https://www.unaids.org/en/resources/documents/2020/global-aids-report.
2. MOHFW. National AIDS Control Organization (NACO). [online] Available from https://main.mohfw.gov.in/sites/default/files/24%20Chapter%20496AN2018-19.pdf.
3. National AIDS Control Organisation. India HIV Estimates 2019 Report. [online] Available from http://naco.gov.in/sites/default/files/INDIA%20HIV%20ESTIMATES.pdf.
4. National AIDS Control Organisation. HIV Sentinel Surveillance 2016-17 Technical Brief. [online] Available from http://naco.gov.in/sites/default/files/HIV%20SENTINEL%20SURVEILLANCE_06_12_2017.pdf.
5. National AIDS Control Organisation. National Strategic Plan, 2017-24. [online] Available from http://naco.gov.in/national-strategic-plan-hivaids-and-sti-2017-24.
6. World Health Organization. Consolidated Guidelines on HIV Prevention, Diagnosis, Treatment and Care for Key Populations–2016 Update. Geneva: World Health Organization; 2016.
7. Ministry of Law and Justice. The Human Immunodeficiency Virus and Acquired Immune Deficiency Syndrome (Prevention and Control) Act, 2017. [online] Available from http://legislative.gov.in/actsofparliamentfromtheyear/human-immuno-deficiency-virus-and-acquired-immune-deficiency-syndrome.
8. National AIDS Control Organisation. MTA of NACP IV. [online] Available from http://www.naco.gov.in/mid-term-appraisal-mta-nacp-iv.

CHAPTER

52 Management of HIV

Subhasish Kamal Guha, Soumendra Nath Haldar

ABSTRACT

A multidisciplinary approach involving counselors, primary care physicians, human immunodeficiency virus (HIV)/infectious diseases physicians, and various specialists is needed for acute and chronic care of people living with HIV (PLHIV). It involves counseling and diagnosis of HIV, diagnosis and treatment of opportunistic infections (OIs), neoplasms, coinfections, sexually transmitted infections (STIs), and antiretroviral therapy (ART). The standard guidelines for diagnosis of HIV and OIs need to be followed. ART has now become "universal" regardless of degree of immunodeficiency, plasma viral load, and clinical stage of the disease. Fixed dose, coformulated, potent, well-tolerated regimens with potential for harmonization across population groups are preferred nowadays in public health program. The comorbidities should also be taken into consideration while prescribing ART.

The preferred regimen is a combination of two nucleoside reverse transcriptase inhibitors (NRTIs) like tenofovir plus lamivudine (3TC)/emtricitabine with one integrase inhibitor like dolutegravir (DTG). Preparedness counseling of the patient for committing to a life-long treatment is important before starting ART so also is exclusion of common OIs like tuberculosis (TB), cryptococcosis, and *Pneumocystis jirovecii* pneumonia (PCP). In general, all OIs should be treated first, followed by ART initiation. Regular follow-up is needed to assess adherence, identify OIs, side-effects, immune reconstitution inflammatory syndrome (IRIS), and treatment failure. As life span of PLHIV has increased with ART, the noncommunicable diseases such as diabetes, cardiovascular, liver, kidney diseases, malignancies, neurocognitive disorders, substance abuse etc., are emerging as major treatment challenges.

"Education, awareness and prevention are the key, but stigmatisation and exclusion from family is what people suffer the most"

—Ralph Fiennes

ANTIRETROVIRAL THERAPY (ART)

Consequent to access and availability of potent antiretroviral treatment regimens, the natural history of HIV/acquired immunodeficiency syndrome (AIDS) has transformed from an invariably "fatal" disease to a "chronic manageable" infectious illness. HIV-infected persons with sustained viral suppression under effective ART fail to transmit the virus to susceptible population. There has been significant decline in rate of new infection and death due to HIV following decentralization of ART services and augmentation of preventive measures. The UNAIDS has set a new, ambitious but achievable goal of 90:90:90 by 2020, i.e., 90% of PLHIV will know their HIV status, 90% of all people with diagnosed HIV infection will receive sustained ART, and 90% of all receiving ART will have viral suppression. Management of HIV has many facets—counseling, diagnosis and treatment of OIs and neoplasm, chemoprophylaxis and vaccination, ART, treatment of coinfections such as TB, hepatitis B virus (HBV), HCV etc. Treatment strategies also differ in infant, children, and adults. This chapter will focus on the ART in adults and adolescents including pregnant and lactating women, HBV/HCV, and TB coinfections.

Globally, the "test and treat" policy has been adopted for treating HIV-positive individuals as evidences from clinical trials show benefits in terms of reduction in mortality, disease progression to AIDS, incident TB, non-AIDS events, malignancy, and importantly transmission of infection.

Selection of ART regimen should ideally be individualized and based on potency, genetic barrier, side-effects, pill burden, availability of fixed-dose coformulated combination, dosing frequency, drug-drug interaction, and other comorbid conditions. However, in public health programs potent, well-tolerated, fixed-dose coformulated, once daily regimens without significant drug-drug interaction and harmonization across all population groups (adults, adolescents, children, TB, hepatitis, pregnancy, elderly etc.) are usually preferred initial regimens with alternate options (**Table 1**).

Recently, DHHS (Department of Health and Human Services, USA) guideline has recommended a dual-drug regimen of DTG plus 3TC as first-line ART based on two large randomized controlled trials (RCTs) in PLHIV except those with high baseline plasma HIV RNA (ribonucleic acid) ≥ 500,000 copies/mL, HIV/HBV coinfection, and where baseline genotypic NRTI resistance is not known. Treatment response was also poor in patients with CD4

TABLE 1 Preferred first-line antiretroviral regimens for treatment naive HIV patients.

Guidelines	DHHS 2020	BHIVA 2016	WHO 2019	NACO 2020
Recommended first-line antiretroviral regimen	1. BIC + TAF + FTC 2. DTG + ABC + 3TC 3. DTG + FTC/3TC + TAF/TDF 4. DTG + 3TC 5. RAL + FTC/3TC + TAF/TDF	1. NRTI backbone is TDF/TAF + FTC 2. Third agent may be ATV/r, DRV/r, RAL, DTG, EVG/c, RPV	1. TDF + 3TC/FTC + DTG 2. TDF + 3TC/ FTC + EFV	TDF + 3TC + DTG

(3TC: lamivudine; ABC: abacavir; ATV: atazanavir; BHIVA: British HIV Association; BIC: bictegravir; DTG: dolutegravir; DHHS: Department of Health and Human Services, USA; DRV: darunavir; EVG: elvitegravir; c: cobicistat; FTC: emtricitabine; RPV: rilpivirine; NRTI: nucleoside reverse transcriptase inhibitor; RAL: raltegravir; r: ritonavir, TAF: tenofovir alafenamide; TDF: tenofovir disoproxil fumarate)

TABLE 2 Definition of virologic failure and second-line regimens.

NACO 2020	WHO 2019	DHHS 2020
	Virologic failure	
Plasma viral load above 1,000 copies/mL	Plasma viral load above 1,000 copies/mL two measurements after 3 months	Persistent plasma HIV RNA level ≥200 copies/mL
	Second-line regimens	
• *TDF + 3TC + DTG* (previously on AZT/d4T + 3TC + EFV/NVP) • *AZT + 3TC + DTG* (previously on TDF +3TC + EFV/NVP with Hb% > 9 g/dL) • *RAL + LPV/r* (previously on TDF/ABC + 3TC + EFV/NVP with Hb% < 9 g/dL OR all other cases of first-line failure with exposure to more than one NRTI)	• *Two NRTIs + ATV/r or LPV/r* (previously on two NRTI + DTG) • *Two NRTI + DTG* (previously on two NRTIs + EFV) • Alternate second-line regimen *(DRV/r) ± DTG + 1–2 NRTIs* (if possible consider optimization using genotyping)	• *Two NRTIs + boosted PI/INSTI* *INSTI + boosted PI* (previously on NNRTI + NRTI) • *INSTI + 2 NRTI* *Another boosted PI + 2 NRTI* • *INSTI + boosted PI* (previously on boosted PI + 2 NRTIs) *Boosted PI + 2 NRTI* • *DTG + 2 NRTI* (previously on INSTI + 2NRTI)

(3TC: lamivudine; ABC: abacavir; ATV: atazanavir; AZT: azidothymidine; d4T: stavudine; DHHS: Department of Health and Human Services, USA; DTG: dolutegravir; DRV: darunavir; EFV: efavirenz; INSTI: integrase strand transfer inhibitor; NRTI: nucleoside reverse transcriptase inhibitor; NVP: nevirapine; LPV/r: lopinavir/ritonavir; PI: protease inhibitor; RAL: raltegravir; r: ritonavir; TDF: tenofovir disoproxil fumarate)

count ≤ 200 cells/mm^3 with dual-drug therapy. Two-drug regimens may reduce the NRTI-related long-term bone, kidney, and cardiovascular complications and reduce cost of therapy. Another two-drug regimen of DTG + rilpivirine (RPV) among individuals without hepatitis B coinfection, without prior virological failure, without resistance to any of the drug, was associated with durable viral suppression for 2 years, improvement in bone mineral density, and improved kidney tubular function. One attractive option for patients with poor adherence to clinic attendance is monthly intramuscular injections of long-acting combination of cabotegravir (CBG) and RPV after 4 weeks induction period with CBG and RPV orally. It was noninferior to stable, virologically suppressive regimen of NNRTI (nonnucleoside reverse transcriptase inhibitor) or INSTI (Integrase Strand Transfer Inhibitor) or bPI (boosted protease inhibitor)-based regimen without prior virological failure or NRTI resistance mutations at 48 weeks. This regimen is awaiting regulatory body approval and wide availability. Apart from reduction in mortality and morbidity, ART reduces sexual transmission of HIV in patients with suppressed viral load.

During follow-up visits patients are monitored clinically by recording body weight, looking for OI, IRIS, side-effects of ART and concomitant drugs, and measurement of adherence (self-report, pill count). In addition, nutritional and prevention counseling is also re-emphasized during all visits.

Most of the guidelines recommend second-line ART after obtaining the genotypic drug resistance test report of the patient failing the first-line regimen. National AIDS Control Organization (NACO) recommends second-line ART based on data available for resistance of NRTI, NNRTI, and protease inhibitor (PI) in India (**Table 2**). Genotypic drug resistance is to be endorsed in all patients with documented first-line ART failure.

HIV AND PREGNANCY

The objectives are detection of 90% of pregnant women with HIV, access to comprehensive Prevention of Parent-to-Child Transmission (PPTCT) services, diagnosis of ≥90% of HIV-exposed infants, access to antiretroviral (ARV)/ART to 100% HIV-exposed infants, and ≥90% adherence to both mother and infant. World Health Organization (WHO) recommends initiation of ART in all pregnant and breastfeeding women living with HIV, regardless of WHO clinical stage and at any CD4 cell count and continued lifelong. WHO and NACO recommend baseline CD4 count and exclusion of OIs like TB and coinfections, e.g., STI or viral hepatitis B and C. DTG has a very small potential risk for development of neural tube defects and may be started in pregnancy after counseling and explaining the risks as DTG causes faster and greater maternal viral suppression with consequent reduction of maternal-to-child transmission. Efavirenz-based ART should be started instead of DTG in women not willing to take DTG before conception. Patients infected with HIV-2 infection or past exposure to single dose nevirapine should start with TDF (tenofovir disoproxil fumarate) + 3TC with either DTG or LPV/r (lopinavir/ritonavir). If a treatment naïve PLHIV attends first in labor room, tenofovir + 3TC + DTG should be started according to NACO, although DHHS guideline recommends intravenous zidovudine followed by full ART, if HIV RNA is ≥1,000 copies/μL or not known. Cesarean section is indicated in women with obstetric indications only although DHHS recommends routine cesarean section if PVL is ≥1,000 copies/mm^3.

OPPORTUNISTIC INFECTIONS (OIs)

TUBERCULOSIS

World Health Organization data revealed one in every third death in PLHIV is due to TB. The most common OI in India is due to *Mycobacterium tuberculosis*. Treatment of TB should be started immediately followed by ART. If the CD4 count is ≤50 cells/mm^3, ART has to be started within 2 weeks and if it is ≥50 cells/mm^3, it should be initiated within 2–8 weeks when the patient is stabilized on anti-TB treatment. ART initiation is to be delayed for 4–8 weeks in case of TB meningitis to prevent central nervous system (CNS) IRIS. Corticosteroids are recommended in TB meningitis and pericardial disease.

Recently, the WHO has launched recommendation of three "I"s—*Intensified Case Finding, INH Preventive Treatment,* and *Infection Control Practices* for reducing the incidence of TB among HIV-infected subjects. Monitoring for anti-TB drug-associated hepatotoxicity and development of IRIS is very important. Management of latent TB infection is important both in country with low or high burden of TB. The NACO guideline recommends 6 months of daily INH (isoniazid) prophylaxis therapy for all PLHIV post 6 months of ART initiation after ruling out active TB. Studies from low prevalence regions have observed benefit of isoniazid preventive therapy (IPT) in persons with a positive tuberculin skin test (TST), but studies in high burden regions like South Africa and West Africa documented that IPT decreases TB risk regardless of TST or IGRA (interferon gamma release assay).

IPT protects against progression of latent TB infection to active disease, prevents TB reinfection, and augments the effect of ART. Resistance of isoniazid among IPT-exposed persons is similar to background population. The WHO has recently approved newer shorter options for preventive TB treatment. These include 1 month of daily regimen of rifapentine plus isoniazid, to 3-months weekly rifapentine plus isoniazid, 3-months daily rifampicin plus isoniazid, and 4 months of daily rifampicin alone.

CRYPTOCOCCAL MENINGITIS

It is one of the two common causes of meningitis among PLHIV in India, in addition to tubercular meningitis. Confirmation of diagnosis is done by presence of budding yeast cells in cerebrospinal fluid (CSF) or antigen positivity in CSF by enzyme-linked immunosorbent assay (ELISA)/latex agglutination/lateral flow assay. Treatment consists of induction therapy for 1 week with amphotericin B deoxycholate (1.0 mg/kg/day) and flucytosine (100 mg/kg/day, divided into four doses) followed by 1 week of fluconazole 1,200 mg (12 mg/kg/day for children and adolescents, up to a maximum dose of 800 mg daily). Alternate regimens are either amphotericin B or flucytosine with fluconazole 1,200 mg/day for 2 weeks.

After induction therapy, 8 weeks of consolidation therapy with fluconazole 800 mg/day is recommended. Maintenance therapy with fluconazole 200 mg/day is continued till CD4 count raises ≥100 cells/mm^3 and persists for 3 months with sustained viral suppression by ART. ART is deferred for 4–6 weeks following initiation of antifungal therapy. Management of raised intracranial tension is equally important and needs repeated therapeutic lumbar puncture to reduce the CSF opening pressure to ≤20 cm of H_2O or halving the baseline pressure when the pressure is extremely high. Screening of cryptococcal antigen test in serum or plasma is recommended in patients having CD4 ≤ 100 cells/mm^3 and preemptive antifungal therapy in antigen positive patients is recommended to prevent invasive cryptococcal disease. After initiation of ART, monitoring for cryptococcal IRIS is important. Use of corticosteroids is associated with increased mortality in cryptococcal disease.

PNEUMOCYSTIS JIROVECII PNEUMONIA

Typically, the disease presents with subacute onset of dry cough, progressive breathlessness, and low-grade fever. The median CD4 count is <200 cells/mm^3. Physical examination may be normal in initial stage but signs like tachypnea, tachycardia, and diffuse cellophane rales are often observed following exercise and in advanced cases. Cyanosis is a late finding. Chest X-ray reveals bilateral, diffuse, symmetrical interstitial infiltrates. High-resolution computed tomography (HRCT) is sensitive in demonstration of patchy, ground glass opacities. Silver staining of bronchoalveolar lavage (BAL) or induced sputum sample demonstrates the organisms. Serum lactate dehydrogenase (LDH) and β-D-glucan has a high negative predictive value for exclusion.

High-dose cotrimoxazole (15–20 mg/kg of trimethoprim) in 3–4 divided doses is the drug of choice. Alternatives include combination of clindamycin and primaquine. The duration of treatment is 3 weeks followed by secondary prophylaxis with cotrimoxazole double strength tablet once daily. Moderate-to-severe disease (PaO_2 < 70 mm Hg at room air and alveolar-arterial DO_2 gradient ≥ 35 mm Hg) is treated with prednisolone; 40 mg BD from day 1 to 5, followed by 40 mg OD from day 6 to 10 and then 20 mg OD from day 11 to 21.

HISTOPLASMOSIS

It is caused by a dimorphic fungus *Histoplasma capsulatum*, usually in patients with CD4 count ≤ 150 cells/mm^3. Disease spectrum ranges from mild respiratory illness to progressive disseminated histoplasmosis or involving the CNS, gastrointestinal (GI), or cutaneous manifestations. Histoplasma antigen testing in urine or blood has high sensitivity and specificity. Due to limited availability of antigen testing facility, diagnosis is often based on demonstration of fungal bodies (2–4 μm budding yeast cells) in tissue or bone marrow or BAL fluid with compatible clinical background.

The Centers for Disease Control and Prevention (CDC) guideline recommends treatment with injection liposomal amphotericin B 3 mg/kg/day for 2 weeks followed by oral itraconazole 200 mg thrice daily for 3 days followed by 200 mg twice daily for ≥12 months. WHO guidelines recommend itraconazole 200 mg twice daily for 12 months following induction therapy. Therapeutic drug monitoring of itraconazole is recommended and serum level of 1–2 μg/mL is recommended. The WHO recommends initiation of ART as early as possible among people with disseminated histoplasmosis for whom CNS infection is not suspected or proven.

TOXOPLASMA ENCEPHALITIS

In addition to CNS tuberculoma, it is one of the most common causes of ring-enhancing lesion with neurodeficits or seizure in HIV-infected subjects. Diagnosis is usually based on subacute onset of focal neurodeficits with systemic features, multiple ring-enhancing lesions on neuroimaging [magnetic resonance imaging (MRI) with gadolinium contrast or contrast-enhanced CT (CECT)], serological evidence of toxoplasma immunoglobulin G (IgG) positivity, and most importantly response to treatment.

The usual treatment comprises of pyrimethamine, sulfadiazine, and leucovorin. Pyrimethamine is given as 200 mg loading dose on first day followed by 50–75 mg/day subsequently with 4–6 g of sulfadiazine per day in divided doses for 6 weeks depending on clinical response. Chronic maintenance therapy with pyrimethamine (25–50 mg) and sulfadiazine (2–4 g/day) is to be continued till the CD4 count raises ≥200 cells/mm^3 and persists over 6 months. Pyrimethamine plus clindamycin and high-dose cotrimoxazole can be used as alternative regimen with equal efficacy. Clinicoradiological response is evident in most cases of cerebral toxoplasmosis by 2 weeks. Primary prophylaxis for toxoplasmosis is indicated in patients with CD4 count ≤ 100 cells/mm^3. NACO recommends cotrimoxazole prophylaxis in patients with CD4 count ≤ 350 cells/mm^3. Most of the physicians recommend initiation of ART 2–3 weeks following start of anti-toxoplasma therapy.

Routine prophylaxis against fungal or viral infections is not recommended in HIV, some recommend fluconazole prophylaxis against candida and cryptococcal disease and to protect against endemic fungal infections (e.g., histoplasmosis) in patients with CD4 cell count < 50 cells/mm^3. The emergence of resistant candida strains is a realistic concern. Oral valganciclovir prophylaxis is reserved for patients with CD4 count ≤ 50 cells/mm^3 and evidence of past cytomegalovirus (CMV) infection.

HEPATITIS

India has an estimated 39 million HBV carriers and around 6–12 million people are infected with HCV. Chronic HBV affects around 2–8% of PLHIV in India and 15–25% of those in Southeast Asia and Africa. Concurrent or sequential infections with these viruses cause severe and progressive liver disease leading to cirrhosis and hepatocellular carcinoma. Coinfection with HIV causes higher rates of chronicity after acute HBV infection, higher level of HBV DNA (deoxyribonucleic acid) replication and rates of reactivation, reduction of anti-HBe and anti-HBs seroconversion, less spontaneous clearance, higher rates of occult HBV [i.e., detectable HBV DNA positivity in the absence of HBsAg (hepatitis B surface antigen) seropositivity], increased fibrosis, more rapid progression to cirrhosis and hepatocellular carcinoma, higher liver-related mortality, and decreased treatment response compared with persons without HIV coinfection. The HIV-hepatitis coinfected persons show faster CD4 decline, slower CD4 recovery following ART, increased incidence of AIDS and non-AIDS events, increased rate of ARV toxicity, and increased chances of immune reconstitution hepatitis.

Before initiation of therapy, evaluation of HBV disease severity should be done by quantitative HBV DNA assay, alanine aminotransferase (ALT), aspartate aminotransferase:platelet ratio index (APRI), ultra-sonography (USG), HBeAg etc. Tenofovir (TDF/TAF), 3TC, and emtricitabine have activity against both HIV and HBV. The NRTI component of ART must include tenofovir and 3TC/emtricitabine. If ART is changed due to drug resistance or poor adherence, the NRTI backbone of TDF and 3TC has to be continued to suppress the HBV DNA. If TDF/TAF cannot be used, then entecavir is to be added in addition to a fully effective ART, otherwise it may lead to emergence of 3TC resistance against HBV. Discontinuation of an agent with anti-HBV activity as a part of ART may lead to severe hepatocellular injury due to HBV reactivation. All newly diagnosed PLHIV should be tested for HBsAg and Anti-HBs titer and if the anti-HBs titre is <10 IU/L, then vaccination with double dose of recombinant HBV vaccine with four-dose schedule (0, 1, 2, 6 month) is recommended.

Because of common routes of infection, HIV and HCV coinfection is common in certain population group like person with injection drug user, recipients of multiple blood transfusions, men who have sex with men etc. Anti-HCV antibody positive patients with detectable HCV RNA need treatment for hepatitis C. NACO guidelines recommend the screening of all injection drug users, those with history of multiple blood/blood product transfusion, or those with raised liver enzymes (ALT) more than two times the upper limit of normal (ULN) or based on strong clinical suspicion. The direct-acting antiviral drugs (DAAs) have changed the treatment outcome of HCV infection. After clinical and laboratory assessment, DAAs are to be started considering potential drug-drug interactions. In absence of moderate fibrosis or decompensation of liver ART is initiated first, followed by Anti-HCV therapy.

Treatment response is similar to HIV-uninfected persons with sustained virologic response rate of ~95%. The National Viral Hepatitis Control Program guideline recommends use of daclatasvir and sofosbuvir for chronic HCV infection including those with compensated cirrhosis, and velpatasvir and sofosbuvir for decompensated cirrhotic patients. Before initiation of Anti-HCV therapy HBsAg, Anti-HBs, and Anti-HBc antibody (total/IgG) tests should be done to rule out HBV infection. HBV reactivation has been observed in persons with HBV infection during HCV treatment with DAAs. Before initiating HCV therapy, persons with HCV/HIV coinfection and active HBV infection (HBsAg positive) should receive ART that includes two agents with anti-HBV activity. Drug interaction involving DAAs and ARVs needs to be considered in HIV/HCV coinfected patients. The daily dose of daclatasvir has to be increased to 90 mg once daily with efavirenz whereas the dose has to be reduced to 30 mg once daily with atazanavir/ritonavir. The usual dose of 60 mg once daily can be used with DTG.

CONCLUSION

Long-term management of HIV disease continues to be a challenge for healthcare providers. ART is evolving fast with advent of newer classes of drugs and newer drugs in the existing classes. ARV simplification strategy has become popular among physicians as well as patients. With longer survival of PLHIV with potent ART, the noninfective conditions associated with HIV disease such as diabetes, cardiovascular, liver, kidney, neuropsychiatric diseases, and malignancies have emerged as crucial treatment needs which should be managed through multidisciplinary approach.

RECOMMENDED READINGS

1. NACO. (2018). Technical Guidelines on Anti-retroviral therapy, October 2018, Government of India. [online] Available from https://lms.naco.gov.in/frontend/content/NACO%20-%20National%20Technical%20Guidelines%20on%20ART_October%202018%20(1).pdf
2. Guidelines for the use of antiretroviral agents in adults and adolescents with HIV; Department of Health and Human Services. [online] Available from https://clinicalinfo.hiv.gov/sites/default/files/guidelines/documents/AdultandAdolescentGL.pdf
3. WHO. (2018). Updated recommendations on first-line and second-line antiretroviral regimens and post-exposure prophylaxis and recommendations on early infant diagnosis of HIV. WHO Interim Guidelines 2018. [online] Available from https://apps.who.int/iris/handle/10665/277395
4. Saag MS, Gandhi RT, Hoy JF, Landovitz RJ, Thompson MA, Sax PE, at el. Antiretroviral Drugs for treatment and Prevention of HIV Infection in Adults: 2020 recommendations of the International Antiviral Society-USA Panel. JAMA. 2020;324(16):1651-69.
5. BHIVA. Treatment of HIV-1 positive adults with ART 2015 (interim update 2016): British HIV Association Current Guidelines. [online] Available from https://www.bhiva.org/file/RVYKzFwyxpgiI/treatment-guidelines-2016-interim-update.pdf%20accessed%20on%205.1.2019
6. WHO. (2018). The diagnosis, prevention and management of cryptococcal disease in HIV-infected adults, adolescents and children, March 2018. [online] Available from https://apps.who.int/iris/bitstream/handle/10665/260400/WHO-CDS-HIV-18.2-eng.pdf?sequence=1
7. PAHO. (2020). Guidelines for diagnosing and managing disseminated histoplasmosis among people living with HIV April 2020, WHO; PAHO. [online] Available from https://iris.paho.org/handle/10665.2/52304
8. National Guidelines for Diagnosis and Management of Viral Hepatitis, 2018: Ministry of Health and Family Welfare, Government of India. [online] https://www.inasl.org.in/diagnosis-management-viral-hepatitis.pdf
9. Chouchana L, Pariente A, Pannier E, Tsatsaris V, Treluyer JM. Dolutegravir and neural tube defects: a new insight. Lancet Infect Dis. 2020;20(4):405-6.
10. Cahn P, Madero JS, Arribas JR, Antinori A, Ortiz R, Clarke AE, et al. Dolutegravir plus lamivudine versus dolutegravir plus Tenofovir diproxil fumarate and emtricitabine in antiretroviral-naive adults with HIV infection (GEMINI1 and GEMINI 2): week 48 results from two multicentre, double-blind, randomised, non-inferiority, phase 3 trials. The Lancet. 2019;393(10167):143-55.
11. Swindells S, Andrade-Villanueva JF, Richmond GJ, Rizzardini G, Baumgarten A, Masiá M, et al. Long-acting Cabotegravir and Rilpivirine for maintenance of HIV-1 Suppression. N Engl J Med. 2020;382:1112-23.

CHAPTER 53

Coronaviruses and the Epidemics

Mahesh Moorthy, Runal John Steve

ABSTRACT

Acute respiratory infections (ARI) cause a major disease burden in developed and developing countries. Viruses are important etiological agents of upper and lower respiratory infections (LRI). LRI is among the leading causes of death in children under-5 in low and middle-income countries. Viruses transmitted by respiratory route, disseminate rapidly causing epidemics. Seasonal coronaviruses (CoVs): CoV-OC43, CoV-229E, CoV-NL63, and CoV-HKU1 are endemic viruses and known to circulate throughout the year. CoVs have also caused outbreaks (epidemics and a pandemic) in the past two decades. The abundance and wide range of animal hosts and ability to use cellular receptors present in humans are important factors in epidemic CoV emergence.

Severe acute respiratory syndrome (SARS) and Middle East respiratory syndrome (MERS) outbreaks were caused by SARS-CoV and MERS-CoV, respectively. These agents were zoonotic viruses and animal-to-human spillover presented as severe respiratory disease with high mortality. SARS-CoV emerged from bats with palm civets as intermediate hosts in 2002–2003. MERS-CoV emerged in 2012 by transmission from camels to humans. Currently, only supportive treatment is available. Stringent infection control measures like hand-washing, avoidance of over-crowding are measures to effectively reduce transmission of these epidemic CoVs.

"It's not what happens to you, but how you react to it that matters"

—Epictetus

INTRODUCTION

RESPIRATORY VIRAL INFECTIONS

Acute respiratory infections cause significant morbidity and mortality, globally. The ARI disease spectrum ranges from mild self-limiting URI like rhinitis and sinusitis to severe and potentially life-threatening LRI such as bronchiolitis and pneumonia. According to the Global Burden of Disease (GBD) study, 2016, LRI excluding tuberculosis, is the third leading cause of mortality worldwide, accounting for ~2,380,000 deaths among all age groups, with ~660,000 in children <5 years and ~1,081,000 in the elderly (>70 years). While the burden of LRI in developing countries is manyfold higher than the developed world, it is noteworthy that the former have a disproportionate burden of mortality (99%) compared to developed countries. Bacteria (*Streptococcus pneumoniae* and *Haemophilus influenzae*) and viruses (respiratory syncytial virus and influenza viruses) account for a large proportion of disease burden, hospitalization, and mortality seen in LRI.

Other viral etiologies including rhinovirus, adenovirus, parainfluenza virus 1-4, and Metapneumovirus are frequently codetected pathogens across all age groups and geographic locations. Monoinfections with single viral pathogens do occur frequently, but multiple pathogens are also codetected in ARI. The detection of coinfection in cases of ARI do not imply higher disease severity, but are primarily due to the use of highly sensitive molecular methods like polymerase chain reaction (PCR) for diagnosis. CoVs are the second frequently detected viruses in cases of "common cold" syndrome after rhinoviruses. Coronavirus (CoV) infection mainly presents as mild disease, but on occasion can cause severe disease necessitating hospitalization.

HISTORICAL PERSPECTIVE

Coronaviruses (CoVs) are single-stranded ribonucleic acid (RNA) viruses, belonging to the Family *Coronaviridae*. CoVs infect humans and diverse animals' hosts including rodents, pigs, cats, horses, birds, and bats. Over the span of the last two decades, three novel CoVs have emerged from animal reservoirs to cause epidemics with high case fatality as well as the recent pandemic [coronavirus disease-2019 (COVID-19)]. These viruses emerge from the animal reservoir (mainly bats) by transmission to intermediate hosts and resultant spillover occurring at the animal-human interface.

Prior to 2019, six CoVs have circulated in the human population causing seasonal or epidemic respiratory disease. The "seasonal" CoVs are commonly encountered viruses and are endemic in the population with periodic increases in activity. These CoVs, CoV-OC43, CoV-229E, CoV-NL63, and CoV-HKU1 cause mostly mild upper respiratory tract infection, and rarely, severe disease in infants, young children, and the elderly and individuals with preexisting illness. These viruses discovered between 1960 and 2006 are well-established agents of ARI. The epidemic CoVs, SARS-CoV, and MERS-CoV, caused clusters of severe lower respiratory tract disease with high mortality which have either been controlled or are currently restricted geographically with sporadic case detection. COVID-19 caused by SARS-CoV-2 is the first pandemic caused by a CoV.

TAXONOMY AND CLASSIFICATION

As the International Committee on Taxonomy of Viruses (ICTV), CoVs belong to Order *Nidovirales*, Family *Coronaviridae*, subfamily *Orthocoronaviridae* and comprise four genera—*Alphacoronavirus*, *Betacoronavirus*, *Gammacoronavirus*, and *Deltacoronavirus*. CoV of medical importance, belong to *Alphacoronavirus* and *Betacoronavirus*. Seven viruses are currently known to infect humans, namely, CoV-NL63 and CoV-229E (*Alphacoronavirus*), CoV-OC43, CoV-HKU1, SARS-CoV, MERS-CoV, and SARS-CoV-2 (*Betacoronavirus*). A notable feature of CoVs detected in animal hosts is their ability to jump the species barrier and cause infections in humans. CoVs have a very diverse animal reservoir and vary widely in specificity of receptors used to gain entry into host cells. Cross-species transmission is dependent on the intersection of human activities within ecological niches of animal hosts (reservoir and intermediate). The ability of a zoonotic virus to utilize receptors on human epithelial cells results in a productive viral infection in the spillover host. After an initial stage of adaptation in the host, onward transmission between humans occurs. In the recent past, members of *Betacoronavirus* exclusively have crossed over from the animals to humans resulting in epidemics or pandemics. The classification and known animal reservoirs of genus *Betacoronavirus* is represented in **Figure 1 A**. The SARS-CoV and SARS-CoV-2 belongs to a separate subgenus *Sarbecovirus* while MERS-CoV belongs to subgenus *Merbecovirus*. Genus *Betacoronavirus* also consists of diverse unrelated viruses that are found in bats that retain the potential to spillover into humans. The reservoirs and intermediate hosts for members of *Betacoronavirus* include bats, camels, rodents, civet cats, and racoons.

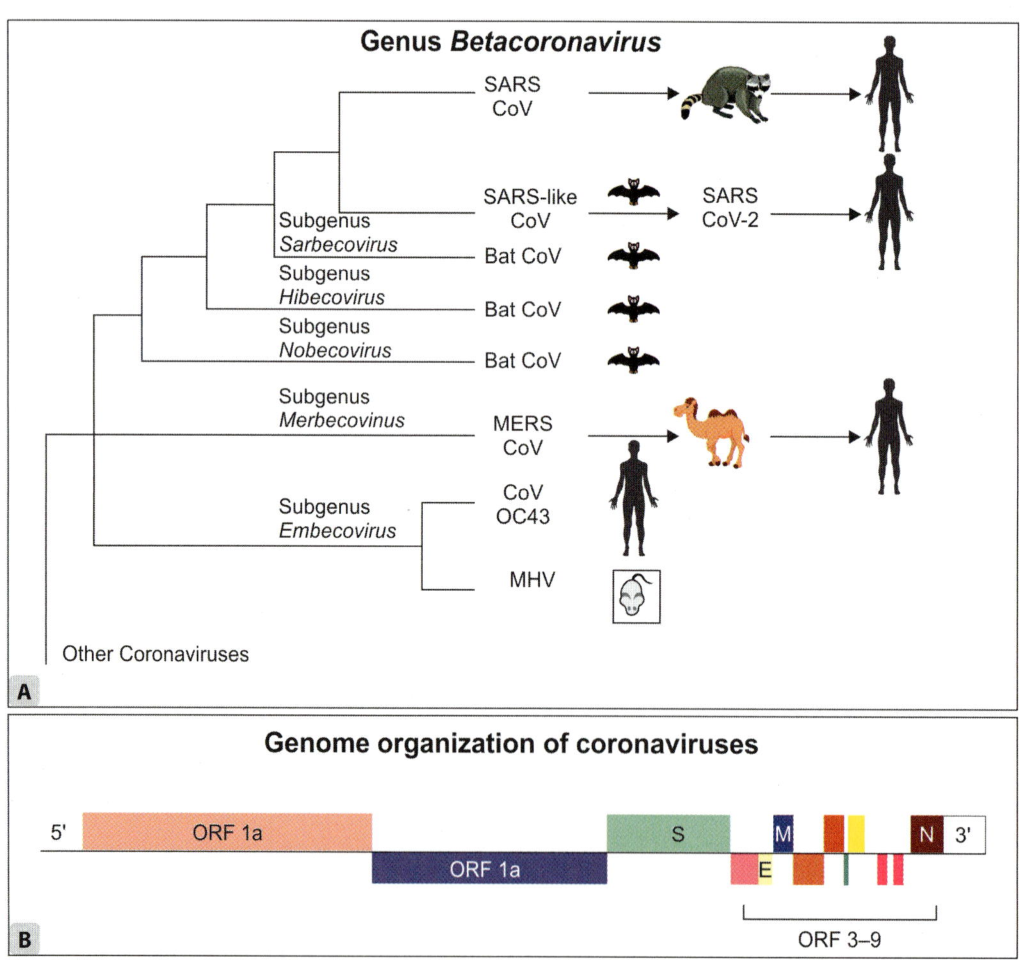

(CoV: coronavirus; MERS: Middle East respiratory syndrome; MHV: mouse hepatitis virus; ORF: open reading frame; SARS: severe acute respiratory syndrome)

FIGURES 1 A & B: **(A)** Classification and known animal reservoirs of genus *Betacoronavirus*; **(B)** Genome organization of CoVs.

VIRUS GENOME STRUCTURE

Coronaviruses are named based on the characteristic "crown-like" surface structures observed on electron microscopy. CoVs are enveloped spherical viruses, 50–200 nm in diameter and possess a nonsegmented, positive-sense, single-stranded RNA genome between 26 and 32 kilobases (kb) in length. SARS-CoV and MERS-CoV reference genomes are 29,751nt (NC_004718) and 30,119nt (NC_019843) in length, respectively.

Coronaviruses share a genome organization that includes structural and nonstructural genes which is broadly similar across genera. The genome organization of CoVs is depicted in **Figure 1 B**. The untranslated region (UTR) on the 5′ end of the genome is followed by the open reading frame (ORF) 1a and 1b that code nonstructural proteins (nsp) including proteases, RNA-dependent RNA polymerase (RdRp), helicase, and interspersed nsp. Following this are the structural genes S (spike), E (envelope), M (membrane), and N (nucleocapsid) and the genome termination at the three prime UTR (3′-UTR) with a polyadenylated end. The S protein has a role in host cell entry by binding the host receptor at the receptor-binding domain (RBD). The E and M proteins play a role in virus assembly and release. The N protein binds the viral genome and has a role in virus assembly. CoVs produce many subgenomic RNAs denoted as numbered ORFs that play a role in synthesis of structural proteins.

OUTBREAKS CAUSED BY CORONAVIRUSES

SEASONAL CORONAVIRUSES

Seasonal CoVs; CoV-OC43, CoV-229E, CoV-NL63, and CoV-HKU1 are endemic and have been demonstrated to circulate during winter in temperate regions and year-round in the tropics. The majority of cases occur in children and the elderly, but sporadic infections occur across all age-groups. These viruses cause outbreaks in special settings like long-term care facilities or bone marrow transplant units, but also have occasionally been associated with outbreaks in the general population. Many studies have been conducted on ARI in India, but to date only a single study has reported seasonal CoVs in severe acute respiratory infection (SARI) cases from Southwest India. The detection rate of CoVs in SARI cases was 1.04%, with detection of CoV-OC43, CoV-229E, CoV-NL63, but no CoV-HKU1.

CORONAVIRUSES CAUSING EPIDEMICS

Of the known CoVs causing human infections, SARS-CoV and MERS-CoV have caused outbreaks of variable severity in the last 2 decades.

Severe acute respiratory syndrome coronavirus: An outbreak of severe respiratory illness occurred in Guangdong Province of China in April 2002. This syndrome referred to as severe acute respiratory syndrome (SARS), was caused by SARS-CoV, that had not been previously encountered in humans. From its origin in Guangdong province in China, this virus spread initially within the province and onward to larger urban centers in China and also spread rapidly to countries in Southeast Asia and North America (Canada). One of the modes of dissemination outside China was through air travelers departing from China and Hong Kong. Between February and May, 2003, though there were 40 probable symptomatic SARS cases travelling by air, only 29 secondary cases could be linked to them. However, on one flight from Hong Kong to Beijing, 22 of 119 (18%) copassengers contracted the virus and became ill, after contact with a single symptomatic passenger. This is archetypal of "super-spreader" events that were first documented in this epidemic. The overall impact of this outbreak in 2002–2003 was low with ~8,098 cases occurring and 774 deaths recorded (mortality rate 9%). However, mortality approached ~50% in individuals over 60 years of age. No cases of SARS were detected in India. The SARS epidemic was controlled in a short-time frame due to implementation of rapid control measures and no further cases were reported.

Middle East respiratory syndrome coronavirus: In 2012, an epidemic cluster of cases clinically manifesting as severe respiratory disease with high mortality was described in humans in Saudi Arabia. The causative agent was identified to be a novel CoV named MERS-CoV. MERS-CoV causes a series of respiratory disease outbreaks in Saudi Arabia and other countries in the Middle East from 2012. Majority of epidemic clusters due to MERS-CoV occurred in the Middle East, with the notable exception of South Korea where an imported epidemic occurred in May, 2015. While the agent was found to be poorly transmissible, outbreaks were documented among healthcare workers in Saudi Arabia, United Arab Emirates, and Republic of Korea. Between April, 2012 and December 2019, 2,499 laboratory-confirmed cases of MERS-CoV infection were detected, and 858 deaths (34.3% mortality) were reported from 27 countries to World Health Organization (WHO), with the majority of cases reported by Saudi Arabia (2,106 cases, 780 deaths). The Korean outbreak in 2015 resulted in 186 cases and 38 recorded deaths. MERS-CoV continues to remain a priority pathogen, according to WHO, with potential to cause an outbreak of severe disease with high mortality. Sporadic cases continue to be reported with the last case being reported in January, 2020. No cases have been reported in India.

VIRAL ORIGINS AND DISCOVERY

Origin of severe acute respiratory syndrome coronavirus: Detailed epidemiological and virological investigations on the origins of the SARS outbreak, pointed to a history of animal exposure prior to manifesting symptoms of SARS, suggesting a zoonotic origin. CoVs related to human SARS-CoV were discovered in horseshoe bats (*Rhinolophus* species). These viruses, referred to a SARS-related coronaviruses (SARSr-CoVs), were closely related to the human SARS-CoV outbreak strain (Urbani strain) in sequencing studies. Serological reactivity to SARSr-CoV in bats, further supported the finding that the primary animal reservoir of SARS-CoV was in bats. Viruses related to SARS-CoV from the human outbreak were also independently identified in Himalayan palm civets and raccoon dogs in a live market in Shenzhen, China. These results indicate that bats were probably the natural reservoirs of SARS-CoV and palm civets were intermediate hosts. The currently accepted hypothesis for SARS-CoV emergence is that the most recent common ancestor originated by recombination within bats and further transmitted to palm civets (or other unknown intermediate reservoir hosts). Infected civets were transported to, housed and traded in the live animal markets resulting in further mutations before transmission to humans.

Origin of Middle East respiratory syndrome coronavirus: Extensive epidemiological and laboratory investigations (including genome sequencing of the novel virus) were undertaken into MERS clusters in an attempt to uncover the potential animal reservoir. Some cases of humans with disease and majority of cases with serological evidence of virus exposure reported close and prolonged contact with dromedary camels. The human MERS-CoV strain could be isolated in cell lines derived from camels. Animal inoculation experiments with the epidemic human strain caused infection of camels with recovery of virus from respiratory secretions 7 days postinoculation. Further, serological studies in camels from Middle East and Africa showed a high seroprevalence of antibodies to MERS-CoV providing supporting evidence that dromedary camels are the probable reservoir hosts of MERS-CoV.

The human epidemic viruses from the MERS outbreak closely clustered with bat viruses (CoV HKU4 and CoV HKU5) found in the bat species *Tylonycteris spp*. These bat viruses formed a distinct phylogenetic subgroup within *Betacoronavirus*, but divergent from SARS and SARSr-CoVs. Dipeptidyl peptidase-4 (DPP4) was found to be the receptor for viral entry for these bat viruses, similar to MERS-CoV. This suggests an ancestral linkage between MERS-CoV and circulating bat CoV, indicating that bats may be the reservoir of MERS-CoV.

CLINICAL PRESENTATION

Seasonal CoVs are generally thought of in the context of mild upper respiratory illness or "common cold". However, subclinical infections are also thought to occur frequently. These viruses are endemic in human populations, causing ~10% of respiratory tract infections annually. In general, incubation period of CoV infection is ~4–6 days with longer duration in certain special populations (e.g., immunosuppressed and transplant recipients). The spectrum of illness ranges from URI (common cold and rhinitis) to LRI (bronchiolitis, pneumonia, and croup). Severe disease is seen among neonates, the elderly, and individuals with underlying illness. In contrast to seasonal CoVs, epidemic CoV (SARS-CoV and MERS-CoV) generally present as a severe disease syndrome resulting in high mortality (10–50%).

Severe acute respiratory syndrome: The incubation period of SARS during the outbreak in 2003 ranged from 2 to 14 days. The disease presented as: (1) early phase with a history of fever, cough, sore throat, and symptoms of respiratory involvement of 3–7 days duration and (2) progressive phase between 7 and 14 days, where disease progressed from an uncomplicated respiratory illness to a rapid deterioration due to viral pneumonia resulting in respiratory failure and death in ~20% of cases. Noteworthy characteristics of SARS at presentation are: (1) absence of upper respiratory symptoms, (2) presence of dry cough, (3) minimal auscultatory findings, and (4) consolidation on chest radiographs. This constellation of features constituted the clinical case definition of SARS. Contact with a known case of SARS or visit to food market handling/involved with slaughter of animals was considered as high-risk individuals.

Middle East respiratory syndrome: Studies of human-to-human MERS-CoV transmission among case clusters in Saudi Arabia in 2012, estimated the incubation period to be 2–15 days. The most common manifestations of MERS-CoV infection was an influenza-like illness with fever, nonproductive cough, sore throat, chills or rigors, chest pain, and dyspnea, rapidly progressing to pneumonia. Gastrointestinal complaints such as abdominal pain, vomiting, and diarrhea were also reported. A prominent feature of MERS disease is the rapid clinical deterioration within days to a week after symptom onset. The median time to hospitalization post symptom onset was 4 days and to intensive care admission was 5 days. Acute kidney injury occurred in about 50% of MERS cases as a complication after 1 week of symptom onset. Notably, person with high intensity and/or frequent contact with camels (e.g., dromedary workers, veterinary, and slaughterhouse workers) often presented with severe infections.

The salient features of SARS and MERS are shown in **Table 1**.

CONTROL MEASURES

The incubation period of respiratory disease is the length of time elapsed between exposure to an infectious agent and first onset of symptoms. This time period is of particularly relevance as it informs the length of quarantine required. However, as the point of exposure may not always be apparent (e.g., in the case of asymptomatic infections), a reliable measure of infectivity in a transmission chain is the serial interval. The serial interval is the time period from onset of symptoms in a primary case to that in a secondary case. Estimating the serial interval and the period of "peak" infectiousness has implications for effective and early control of a respiratory virus epidemic.

Effective virus control measures in both community and nosocomial settings includes early detection of disease, strict isolation of patients, adherence to droplet, and contact precautions and compliance with appropriate personal protective equipment. Within the community,

TABLE 1 Salient features of SARS and MERS.

Characteristic	SARS	MERS
Causative agent	SARS-CoV	MERS-CoV
Taxonomy	Genus *Betacoronavirus*; Subgenus *Sarbecovirus*	Genus *Betacoronavirus*; Subgenus *Merbecovirus*
First reported in (year)	China (2002)	Saudi Arabia (2012)
Reservoir hosts	Bats (*Rhinolophus species*)	Bats (*Tylonycteris species*)
Intermediate hosts	Palm civets	Dromedary camels
Receptor for virus entry	Angiotensin-converting enzyme 2	Dipeptidyl peptidase-4
Incubation period	2–14 days	2–15 days
Clinical presentation	Acute febrile respiratory illness, cough, rapid progression to pneumonia, and death due to respiratory failure	Febrile respiratory illness, cough, breathlessness, progression to LRI requiring hospitalization, and death due to multiorgan failure
Total number of cases	8,098 (2002–2003)	2,499 (2012–2019)
Total number of deaths	774	858
Case fatality ratio	~15%	~35%
Treatment/prevention	Supportive treatment/no licensed vaccine	Supportive treatment/no licensed vaccine

(CoV: coronavirus; LRI: lower respiratory infection; MERS: Middle East respiratory syndrome; SARS: severe acute respiratory syndrome)

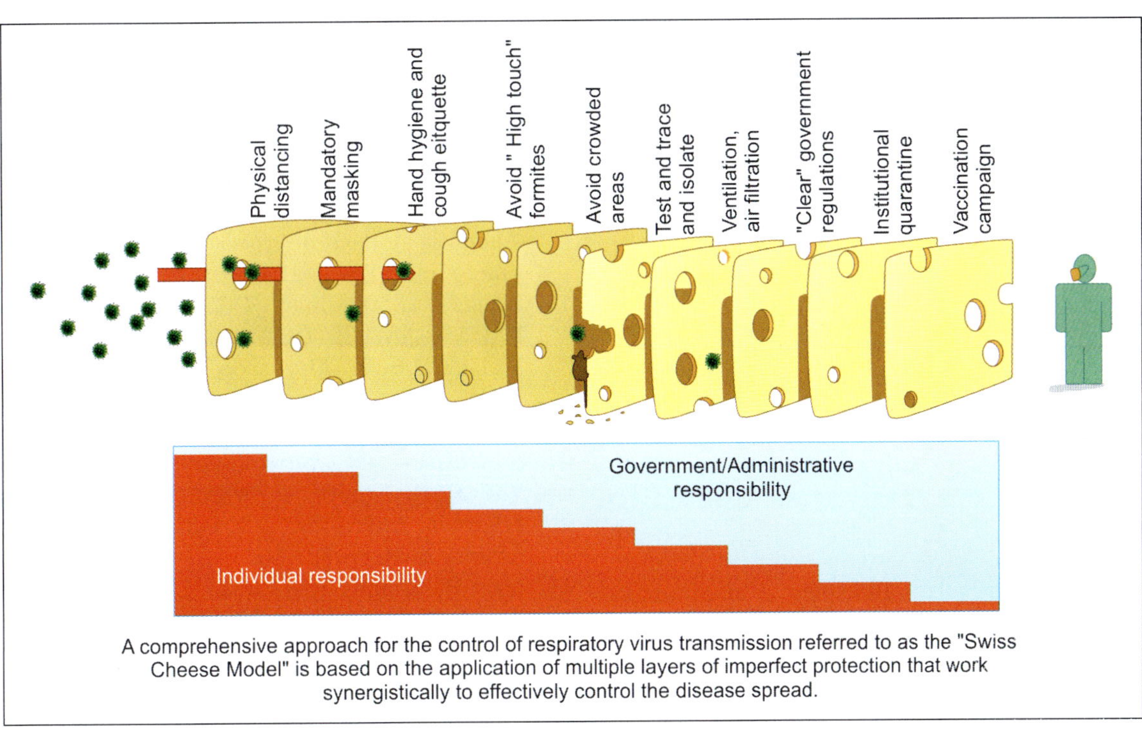

FIGURE 2: "Swiss Cheese Model" for respiratory virus control.

Source: Adapted from: https://virologydownunder.com/the-swiss-cheese-infographic-thatwent-viral/ (under a CC BY 4.0 open-access license)

disease control can be achieved primarily by tracing and quarantine of contacts. Early on in an outbreak, development of validated diagnostics to accurately detect and quarantine active cases from contact with the general public are crucial to the epidemic mitigation. Further measures include imposition of a strict lockdown of all social gatherings and enforcing mandatory public health measures such as social distancing and compulsory public mask usage. Lastly, an effective vaccine could rapidly control an ongoing epidemic and also potentially prevent further outbreaks. A comprehensive approach for the control of respiratory virus transmission referred to as the "Swiss Cheese Model" is based on the application of multiple layers of imperfect protection that work synergistically to effectively control pathogen spread, thus mitigating an epidemic (**Fig. 2**). This model of control consists of measures that require individual responsibility as well as governmental or administrative measures. The former are under the control of the individual while population level measures are under administrative control of public health authorities. The combined effect of these measures reduces transmission as seen in the case of SARS and MERS, where super-spreaders were responsible for large outbreaks and clusters among healthcare workers.

Measures implemented for severe acute respiratory syndrome: The SARS outbreak of 2002–2003 was controlled effectively with no further cases reported after 2004. No vaccine or treatment options were available to ameliorate the effects of this outbreak. No community measures were employed to control the outbreak except in restricted affected areas (Hong Kong, Singapore, and Canada). The overarching strategy employed in this outbreak involved early detection and quarantine of cases prior to the infectious period. The relatively prolonged incubation period allowed asymptomatic air travelers to spread the disease to other regions, hence contact tracing and airline screening were efficient measures for the early identification of suspected symptomatic cases to mitigate the outbreak.

Measures implemented for middle east respiratory syndrome: Preparedness measures for the influenza A (pH1N1) pandemic enabled a rapid and effective response to the primary outbreak in the Middle East in 2012. Adequate respiratory control measures employed were sufficient to restrict the spread of the epidemic. Widespread public health measures were not warranted as sustained human-to-human transmission was not demonstrable. The MERS outbreak resulted in many healthcare-associated clusters which were controlled by adequate isolation and respiratory control measures. The outbreak in Republic of Korea in 2015, which was an importation caused by an infected air traveler, was also effectively controlled in a short-time frame by appropriate infection control measures. No widespread public health measures were employed.

SUMMARY AND KEY LEARNING POINTS

- SARS and MERS are caused by SARS CoV and MERS CoV, respectively.
- Both viruses present as severe respiratory disease with high mortality rate. Both viruses emerged from an animal reservoir mostly bats and spillover into humans through an intermediate host (civet cat or dromedary camels).
- The SARS outbreak was effectively controlled by overarching public health measures, but MERS cases continue to smoulder, especially in the Middle East.

RECOMMENDED READING

1. Drosten C, Günther S, Preiser W, van der Werf S, Brodt HR, Becker S, et al. Identification of a novel coronavirus in patients with severe acute respiratory syndrome. N Engl J Med. 2003;348(20):1967-76.
2. Peiris JSM, Lai ST, Poon LLM, Guan Y, Yam LY, Lim W, et al. Coronavirus as a possible cause of severe acute respiratory syndrome. Lancet. 2003;361:1319-25.
3. Cherry JD, Krogstad P. SARS: The First Pandemic of the 21st Century. Pediatr Res. 2004;56(1):1-5.
4. Rota PA, Oberste MS, Monroe SS, Nix WA, Campagnoli R, Icenogle JP, et al, Characterization of a novel coronavirus associated with severe acute respiratory syndrome. Science. 2003;300(5624):1394-9.
5. Zaki AM, van Boheemen S, Bestebroer TM, Osterhaus AD, Fouchier RA. Isolation of a Novel Coronavirus from a Man with Pneumonia in Saudi Arabia. N Engl J Med. 2012;19:1814-20.
6. Cui J, Li F, Shi ZL. Origin and evolution of pathogenic coronaviruses. Nat Rev Microbiol. 2019;17:181-92.
7. de Wit E, van Doremalen N, Falzarano D, Munster VJ. SARS and MERS: recent insights into emerging coronaviruses. Nat Rev Microbiol. 2016;14(8):523-34.
8. Petrosillo N, Viceconte G, Ergonul O, Ippolito G, Petersen E. COVID-19, SARS and MERS: are they closely related? Clin Microbiol Infect. 2020;26(6):729-34.
9. Abdelrahman Z, Li M, Wang X. Comparative Review of SARS-CoV-2, SARS-CoV, MERS-CoV, and Influenza A Respiratory Viruses. Front Immunol. 2020;11:552909.
10. Ghai RR, Carpenter A, Liew AY, Martin KB, Herring MK, Gerber SI, et al. Animal reservoirs and hosts for emerging alphacoronaviruses and betacoronaviruses. Emerg Infect Dis. 2021;27:1015-22.
11. Masters PS, Perlman S. Coronaviridae. In: Knipe DM, Howley PM (Eds). Fields Virology, 6th edition. Philadelphia, PA: Lippincott Williams & Wilkins; 2013. pp. 825-58.
2. Siddell SG, Ziebuhr J, Snijder EJ. Coronaviruses, toroviruses, and arteriviruses. In: Mahy BWJ, Meulen VT (Eds). Topley & Wilson's Microbiology and Microbial Infections, 11th edition. London: Hodder Arnold; 2005. pp. 823-56.
13. Nair H, Simões EA, Rudan I, Gessner BD, Azziz-Baumgartner E, Zhang JS, et al. Severe Acute Lower Respiratory Infections Working Group. Global and regional burden of hospital admissions for severe acute lower respiratory infections in young children in 2010: a systematic analysis. Lancet. 2013;381(9875):1380-90.
14. Shi T, McLean K, Campbell H, Nair H. Aetiological role of common respiratory viruses in acute lower respiratory infections in children under five years: A systematic review and meta-analysis. J Glob Health. 2015;5(1):010408.

CHAPTER 54

COVID-19: Transmission, Pathophysiology, and Diagnosis

Navneet Arora, Ritin Mohindra, Vikas Suri

ABSTRACT

A novel coronavirus disease, designated as COVID-19, is responsible for the current ongoing pandemic. It has caused a significant mortality and morbidity and till date has no definitive cure. Early studies point to the zoonotic origin of the virus, and it belongs to family Coronaviridae (subfamily Orthocoronavirinae) and produces a broad spectrum of diseases ranging from the earlier smaller outbreaks of severe acute respiratory syndrome (SARS) and Middle East respiratory syndrome (MERS) to the recent pandemic of COVID-19. The main mode of transmission is via contact and droplet spread. It is highly transmissible and has a comparatively low mortality. Clinical features vary from a simple flu-like symptoms to acute severe respiratory syndrome. Preventive measures are the only effective known techniques to prevent this infection.

"Sometimes, the best thing we can do for our patients is to tell them what the best behavior is and then negotiate something they can live with"

—Nancy Dickey

INTRODUCTION

A new type of viral infection emerged in Wuhan city, Hubei province, China, on 12 December, 2019 and was officially designated as COVID-19 by the World Health Organization (WHO) on 11 February, 2020. SARS coronavirus 2 (SARS-CoV-2) is responsible for the ongoing pandemic causing life-threatening complications. Earlier known as 2019-nCov, the virus that causes coronavirus disease 2019 (COVID-19) is designated as SARS-CoV-2, and is a single-stranded, positive-sense RNA (ribonucleic acid) virus, and appears as "solar corona." Early studies point toward the zoonotic origin of coronavirus. Possibilities of other sources of origin are still under investigation. The codon usage studies suggest a probable origin of this novel coronavirus to bats.

Phylogenetic analysis shows an 88% similarity between SARS-CoV-2 and two SARS-like CoVs derived from bats (bat-SL-CoVC45 and bat-SL-CovZXC21). As compared to the previously known human CoV, COVID-19 has a higher transmission competence. SARS-CoV-2 belongs to the family Coronaviridae (subfamily Orthocoronavirinae) and produces a broad spectrum of diseases. The current COVID-19 outbreak is the third CoV outbreak in humans over the past two decades. The previous two outbreaks resulted in lesser deaths since they involved less number of cases, although the percentage mortality was higher. A comparison of the three outbreaks is shown in **Table 1**. The ability of coronavirus to infect multiple host species is due to high-frequency mutation, which is a result of the instability of the RNA-dependent RNA polymerase along with higher rates of homologous RNA recombination. Coronavirus mainly encodes for four major structural proteins—spike protein (S), membrane protein (M), an envelope protein (E), and nucleocapsid protein (N). Spike protein can induce host immune response and is the most immunodominant protein of coronavirus. The membrane protein provides a definitive shape to the virus. The envelop protein plays a role in the pathogenesis, assembly, and release of the virus (**Fig. 1**).

TABLE 1 Comparison of key features of SARS-CoV, MERS-CoV, and SARS-CoV-2.

	SARS-CoV	MERS-CoV	SARS-CoV-2
Year of outbreak	2003	2012	2019
Countries affected (no.)	29	27	220
Confirmed cases	8,096	2,538	>150 million (May 21)
Mortality	9.2%	34%	2.2%
Receptor for viral entry	ACE-2	DPP-4	ACE-2
Viral replication in URT	No	No	Yes
Viral replication in LRT	Yes	Yes	Yes
Peak viral load from symptom	~10 days	~10 days	3–5 days

(ACE-2: angiotensin-converting enzyme 2; DPP-4: dipeptidyl peptidase-4; LRT: lower respiratory tract; MERS: Middle East respiratory syndrome; SARS-CoV-2: severe acute respiratory syndrome coronavirus 2; URT: upper respiratory tract)

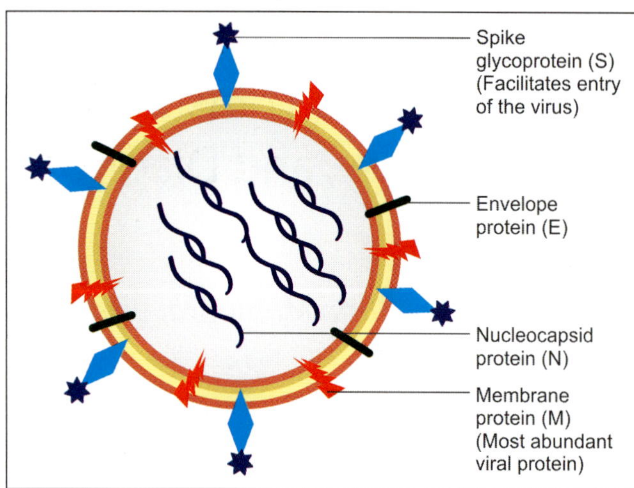

(SARS-CoV-2: severe acute respiratory syndrome coronavirus 2)

FIGURE 1: Structure of SARS-CoV-2 virus.

TRANSMISSION

Severe acute respiratory syndrome CoV2 has low pathogenicity and moderate transmissibility as compared to various other emerging infections. The infection fatality risk (IFR) ranges from 0.3 to 0.6%. A combination of viral, host, and environmental factors play a vital role in coronavirus transmission. A minimum yet unknown dose of replication-competent virus is required to be delivered to a vulnerable anatomical site in a susceptible host. The viral spike protein (S) binding to the host angiotensin-converting enzyme 2 (ACE-2) receptor is a critical step in viral entry into the cell. Coronavirus is predominantly spread by person-to-person transmission. The various modes proposed for coronavirus transmission include contact, droplet, airborne, fomite, fecal-oral, bloodborne, mother-to-child, and animal-to-human transmission. The dominant route of viral transmission is respiratory.

CONTACT AND DROPLET TRANSMISSION

Secretions, such as saliva or respiratory droplets, or nuclei from an infected person, lead to the transmission of coronavirus disease. Respiratory droplets are >5–10 μm in diameter, whereas respiratory nuclei (aerosols) are >5 μm in size. Respiratory droplet transmission mainly occurs when the person is in close contact (within 1 m) with an infected person with coronavirus disease symptoms.

AIRBORNE

Dissemination of infected aerosols in the air over long distances and time leads to the airborne spread of coronavirus. The majority of aerosol transmission occurs during aerosol-generating medical procedures. Outside of medical facilities, there is no reported airborne transmission of coronavirus. However, more studies are required to confirm the same.

FOMITE TRANSMISSION

Contaminated surface or objects (fomite) by a coronavirus, theoretically, may lead to the spread of infection. Despite consistent evidence of detection of SARS-CoV-2 on surfaces, there is not a single case reported to date with this mode of transmission.

OTHER POTENTIAL MODES OF TRANSMISSION

Severe acute respiratory syndrome CoV2 RNA has been detected in the urine or feces of various individuals, but there is no report to establish that transmission of SARS-CoV2 may occur by this route. The role of bloodborne transmission of SARS-CoV-2 remains uncertain, and the possibility of transmission via this route is very low, seeing the low viral titers in serum and plasma. Currently, there is no evidence for intrauterine transmission of SARS-CoV-2 from infected pregnant mothers to their fetuses. Breastfeeding does not seem to increase the risk of transmission, although the data is limited. Humans infected with SARS-CoV-2 can infect other mammals like dogs, cats, and farmed mink.

PATHOPHYSIOLOGY

Once transmitted, the virus binds to the host cell receptors via spike protein (S) and enters the host cell through endocytosis or membrane fusion. Spike protein has two components, namely S_1 and S_2. S_1 is responsible for binding the virus to the host cell receptor, whereas S_2 helps in the fusion of viral and host cell membrane. The functional receptor for SARS-CoV-2 is the ACE-2 receptor, which is highly expressed in the pulmonary epithelium. After entering the cell, the virus releases its contents into the cell, forms a negative strand of RNA through RNA polymerase activity, and synthesizes new proteins in the cytoplasm. The viral proteins bind to the new genomic RNA and form new viral particles. These viral particles invade other healthy cells and produce infection, which is transmitted via respiratory droplets. Infection by COVID-19 occurs in three phases: (1) the asymptomatic phase, (2) invasion of the upper respiratory tract, and (3) acute respiratory distress syndrome.

ASYMPTOMATIC PHASE

The infective aerosols bind to the nasal epithelial cells. They attach to the ACE-2 receptors and undergo local replication and propagation. There is a limited immune response generated in this phase, and this phase lasts for a couple of days. The asymptomatic phase is characterized by a low viral load but high infectivity. The virus can be detected via nasal swab testing in this phase.

INVASION OF THE UPPER RESPIRATORY TRACT

As the virus migrates via conducting airways to the upper respiratory tract, the patient develops symptoms such as fever, malaise, and dry cough. The immune response in this phase of the illness is high and is sufficient to contain the spread of the infection. In majority of the patients the disease does not progress beyond this phase.

ACUTE RESPIRATORY DISTRESS SYNDROME

In 20% of patients, the virus invades type 2 alveolar epithelial cells and undergoes replication. The viral-laden pneumocytes release various inflammatory markers [interleukin-1 (IL-1), IL-6, IL-8, IL-120, tumor necrosis factor-α (TNF-α), and interferon-λ (INF-λ)]. The IL-6 is a master cytokine since it has multiple effects in the body (**Fig. 2**). This results in a "cytokine storm" and leads to accumulation and sequestration of neutrophil, CD4 helper T cells, and CD8 cytotoxic T cells. Along with fighting off the virus, they result in injury to the lung tissue as well. New viral particles are released by the other infected pneumocytes, leading to a continuous immune response, resulting in subsequent loss of type 1 and type 2 pneumocytes, diffuse alveolar damage, eventually leading to acute respiratory distress syndrome.

The lung involvement in COVID-19 is complex and is due to multiple factors including endothelial damage, alveolitis, in situ thrombosis, consolidation, atelectasis, and angiogenesis (**Fig. 3**). Many patients are developing fibrosis which is prolonging hospital stay. It is known as post COVID lung and is responsible for late mortality and long-term morbidity in these patients.

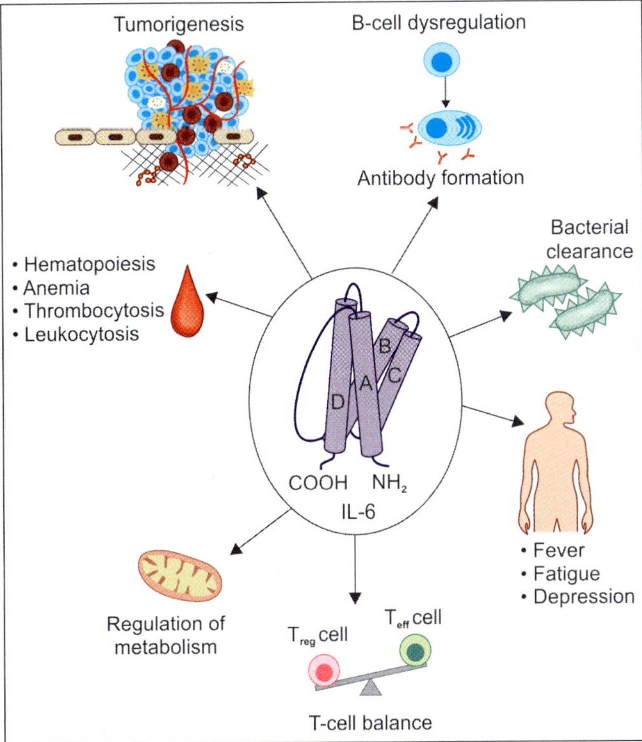

FIGURE 2: Multiple effects of interleukin-6 (IL-6), a master cytokine.

The hypercoagulable state in COVID-19 further complicates the clinical picture. The mechanisms suggested for this are antiphospholipid syndrome, disseminated intravascular coagulation (DIC), and complement cascade activation. Both pulmonary thromboembolism in larger pulmonary arteries and multiple small clots in distal branches have been described as shown in **Figure 4**.

The cytokine storm, hypercoagulable state, and the immune inflammatory state result in involvement of multiple organs in the body. The extrapulmonary clinical manifestations of COVID-19 are shown in **Box 1**.

DIAGNOSIS

Coronavirus disease 2019 cannot be reliably distinguished from other respiratory infections based on clinical features, so accurate molecular diagnostic tests are necessary for confirming the diagnosis. There are various diagnostic modalities available for the diagnosis of COVID-19.

NUCLEIC ACID AMPLIFICATION TESTS (INCLUDING RT-PCR)

Direct detection of SARS-CoV-2 RNA by nucleic acid amplification test (NAAT) confirms the diagnosis of coronavirus disease. The most commonly used NAAT is reverse-transcriptase polymerase chain reaction (RT-PCR). RT-PCR can be performed on various types of samples, and the sensitivity of the test depends on the type of sample used for the test. Different types of samples used for NAAT are nasopharyngeal, oropharyngeal, salvia, sputum, and lower respiratory samples like tracheal aspirate or bronchoalveolar lavage (BAL) fluid. The primary and preferred sampling method is from the upper respiratory tract, the nasopharyngeal swabs. The specificity of RT-PCR is very high. On the other hand, the sensitivity of

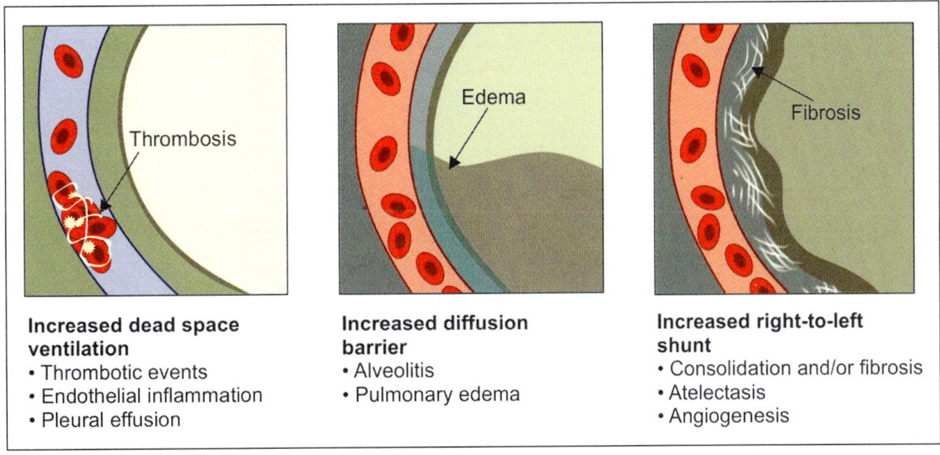

FIGURE 3: Mechanisms of lung involvement in COVID-19.

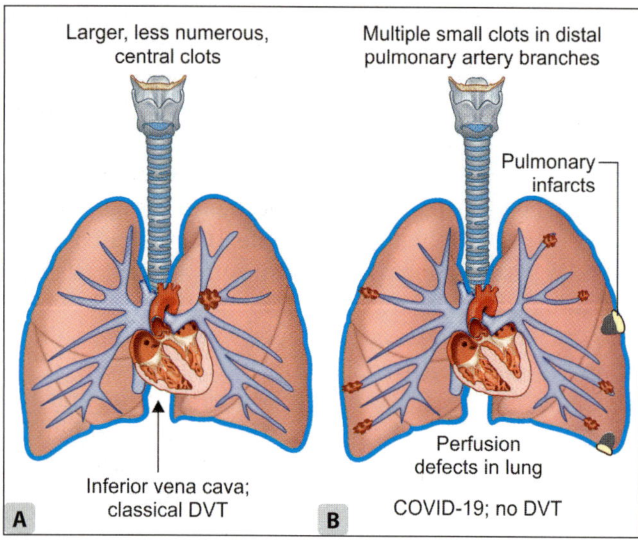

(DVT: deep vein thrombosis)

FIGURE 4: Pulmonary artery filling defects in severe COVID-19. **(A)** Typical pulmonary emboli; **(B)** Pulmonary intravascular coagulopathy.

BOX 1	Extrapulmonary clinical manifestations of COVID-19.
Nervous system:	
• Encephalitis	
• Headache	
• Ageusia and anosmia	
• Encephalopathy	
• Guillain–Barré syndrome	
• Stroke	
• Myalgia	
Kidney:	
• Acute kidney injury	
• Proteinuria	
• Hematuria	
• Metabolic acidosis	
• Electrolyte imbalances	
Liver and endocrine system:	
• Elevated aminotransferases	
• Elevated conjugated bilirubin	
• Low serum albumin	
• Hyperglycemia	
• Diabetic ketoacidosis	
Gastrointestinal tract:	
• Diarrhea	
• Nausea and vomiting	
• Abdominal pain	
• Mesenteric ischemia (rare)	
• Gastrointestinal bleeding (rare)	

Continued...

Continued...

Cardiovascular system:
• Myocardial injury, myocarditis
• Thromboembolism and endotheliitis
• Cardiac arrhythmias
• Cardiogenic shock
• Myocardial ischemia, acute coronary syndrome
• Cardiomyopathy (biventricular, left ventricular, or right ventricular)
Skin:
• Petechiae
• Pernio-like skin lesions
• Livedo reticularis
• Erythematous rash
• Urticaria
• Vesicles

RT-PCR is estimated to be around 66–80%. A single negative test does not exclude infection.

ANTIGEN TESTING

Antigen testing can be performed rapidly and gives quick results as compared to NAAT. It is less sensitive than NAAT but can be used as a screening tool in areas of a high prevalence of the disease. Antigen testing yields better results when used between the first 5–7 days of the disease onset. Negative antigen tests do not exclude the infection. In a low prevalence setting, a negative antigen test should be confirmed by a NAAT. The average sensitivity of antigen test for symptomatic individuals is 78%, and it reduces to 58% for asymptomatic individuals; however, the specificity of an antigen test is as high as 99.6%.

BLOOD INVESTIGATIONS

The most common laboratory abnormalities seen in a patient suffering from COVID-19 are leukopenia or leukocytosis, lymphopenia (63%), and elevated alanine aminotransferase and aspartate aminotransferase. Inflammatory markers such as C-reactive protein (CRP), IL-6, ferritin, fibrinogen, and D-dimer are usually elevated.

RADIOLOGICAL FINDINGS

A chest X-ray is the initial radiological investigation available for the COVID-19 patients. Though less sensitive (59%), it is a valuable investigation in a resource-constrained setting. It helps determine the severity, supports the diagnosis, and assesses the treatment response. Peripheral consolidation, with central sparing (reverse batwing appearance), is a characteristic finding in COVID-19-related pneumonia. The characteristic pattern of changes in chest X-ray in COVID-related lung involvement

BOX 2 Characteristics features in chest X-ray among patients with COVID-19.

Characteristic pattern

- Bilateral subpleural opacities that are relatively symmetrical, of large volume (>20% of lung) and predominantly affect the outer one-third of the lung
    - High confidence that the opacities are not artifactual and related to the chest wall

High suspicion pattern

- Unilateral subpleural opacity that are of large volume (>20% of lung)
- Bilateral large volume patchy or ill-defined opacities
    - Nonapical predominant
    - Nonperihilar distribution
    - Do not fit the characteristic pattern
    - High confidence that the opacities are not artifactual and related to the chest wall

is shown in **Box 2**. A high-resolution computed tomography of the chest (CT chest) exhibits ground-glass opacities, particularly on the peripheral and lower lobes. Multiple lobular and subsegmental areas of consolidation are seen in severe disease. The typical findings on CT chest in COVID-19 and those which are less likely are shown in **Table 2**. The CO-RADS (COVID-19 Reporting and Data System) scoring system from 1 to 6 indicates the probability of COVID-19 (**Table 3**). This is a common method of reporting which has been used in the pandemic. CT chest has at times been used indiscriminately for diagnosis of this condition due to the typical pattern of changes. It is recommended only when there is clinical evidence of lung involvement in the form of hypoxemia.

MANAGEMENT

The management of COVID-19 is primarily supportive, as there are no specific drugs yet. The primary purpose of treatment is to provide symptomatic relief and to prevent respiratory failure. Isolation of the infected patient to prevent disease transmission to close contacts and healthcare workers is important. There is no evidence for the use of antibiotics for the prevention of secondary bacterial superinfections. Anticoagulation with unfractionated heparin or low-molecular-weight heparin should be initiated in the hospitalized patients, especially when the D-dimer value is four times the normal.

STEROIDS

In patients who are suffering from severe or critical COVID-19 infection use of dexamethasone is recommended. Dexamethasone is given as a once-daily dose of 6 mg, for 10 days or until discharge, whichever is shorter. Other glucocorticoids (hydrocortisone, methylprednisolone, or prednisone) at equivalent doses may be considered if dexamethasone is unavailable. Dexamethasone should be avoided in mild to moderate disease and should only be reserved for severe COVID-19 infection. Patients on treatment with dexamethasone or equivalent glucocorticoids should be monitored for secondary infections (bacterial, fungal, and other opportunistic organisms) and hyperglycemia. Patients, who cannot receive steroids due to contraindications, should be started on baricitinib (4 mg daily for 14 days).

TABLE 2 Computed tomography: Chest findings COVID-19 lung.

Typical findings	Atypical findings
• Multifocal ground-glass opacities • Peripheral and basal distribution • Unsharp demarcation • Vascular thickening • Crazy paving • Ground glass and consolidations • Spider web	• Central or peribronchovascular • More apical distribution • Lymphadenopathy **Very atypical** • Cavitation-calcification • Tree-in-bud, bronchiolitis • Nodular pattern • Mass • Pleural thickening

TABLE 3 Scoring system used for reporting CT chest in patients with COVID-19.

Score	Level of suspicion	CT findings
CO-RADS 1	No	Normal or noninfectious abnormalities
CO-RADS 2	Low	Abnormalities consistent with infections other than COVID-19
CO-RADS 3	Indeterminate	Unclear whether COVID-19 is present
CO-RADS 4	High	Abnormalities suspicious for COVID-19
CO-RADS 5	Very high	Typical COVID-19
CO-RADS 6	PCR +	

(CO-RADS: COVID-19 Reporting and Data System; CT: computed tomography)

ANTIVIRAL DRUGS

Currently, there are no approved antiviral drugs for treating COVID-19 infection. Remdesivir, a nucleotide analog, is used in the off-label treatment of severe COVID-19 disease. According to various studies, there is no mortality benefit with this antiviral drug, but it reduces the duration of hospital stay. Remdesivir should be reserved only for hospitalized patients with severe COVID-19 infection and should not be used in mild disease. Severe illness is defined as patients with $SpO_2 \leq 94\%$ on room air, including patients on supplemental oxygen. It should be given for 5 days in patients who are on supplemental oxygen and not on mechanical ventilation. In patients on mechanical ventilation or extracorporeal membrane oxygenation (ECMO), the duration of remdesivir should be extended to 10 days.

MONOCLONAL ANTIBODIES

Markedly elevated inflammatory markers and elevated proinflammatory cytokines (IL-6) are associated with a critical and fatal disease. Tocilizumab is an IL-6 receptor blocker used in hospitalized patients with severe or critical COVID-19 infection and elevated markers of systemic inflammation. Critical illness is defined as patients on mechanical ventilation and/or ECMO. It also includes end-organ dysfunction. Tocilizumab is given along with standard care in this set of patients at a dose of 8 mg/kg as a single dose. Criteria for systemic inflammation were defined as CRP value of ≥75 mg/L.

RECOMMENDED READINGS

1. Zhu N, Zhang D, Wang W, Li X, Yang B, Song J, et al. China Novel Coronavirus Investigating and Research Team. A Novel Coronavirus from Patients with Pneumonia in China, 2019. N Engl J Med. 2020;382(8): 727-33.
2. Munster VJ, Koopmans M, van Doremalen N, van Riel D, de Wit E. A Novel Coronavirus Emerging in China - Key Questions for Impact Assessment. N Engl J Med. 2020;382(8):692-4.
3. Su S, Wong G, Shi W, Liu J, Lai ACK, Zhou J, et al. Epidemiology, Genetic Recombination, and Pathogenesis of Coronaviruses. Trends Microbiol. 2016;24(6): 490-502.
4. Ng OW, Tan YJ. Understanding bat SARS-like coronaviruses for the preparation of future coronavirus outbreaks - Implications for coronavirus vaccine development. Hum Vaccin Immunother. 2017;13(1): 186-9.
5. Meyerowitz EA, Richterman A, Gandhi RT, Sax PE. Transmission of SARS-CoV-2: A Review of Viral, Host, and Environmental Factors. Ann Intern Med. 2021;174(1):69-79.
6. WHO. (2020). Modes of transmission of virus causing COVID-19: implications for IPC precaution recommendations. [online] Available from https://www.who.int/news-room/commentaries/detail/modes-of-transmission-of-virus-causing-covid-19-implications-for-ipc-precaution-recommendations
7. Parasher A. COVID-19: Current understanding of its Pathophysiology, Clinical presentation and Treatment. Postgrad Med J. 2021;97(1147):312-20.
8. Pascarella G, Strumia A, Piliego C, Bruno F, Del Buono R, Costa F, et al. COVID-19 diagnosis and management: a comprehensive review. J Intern Med. 2020;288(2):192-206.
9. Arora N, Kumar HM. 'The photographic negative of pulmonary oedema' in COVID-19 pneumonia. Postgrad Med J. 2021;97(1148):401.
10. IDSA. (2021). COVID-19 Guideline, Part 1: Treatment and Management. [online] Available from https://www.idsociety.org/COVID19guidelines

CHAPTER 55

COVID-19: Clinical Presentation and Management

Ram Gopalakrishnan, Bikram Das, Haripriya Reddy Challa

ABSTRACT

Coronavirus disease-2019 (COVID-19) is the disease caused by severe acute respiratory syndrome coronavirus-2 (SARS-CoV-2). Disease is transmitted from one person to another through droplets; wearing a face mask and physical distancing are important in curtailing the pandemic. COVID-19 is predominantly a respiratory illness, but can involve many other organ systems. Molecular testing [reverse transcription-polymerase chain reaction (RT-PCR)] and imaging are the mainstays of diagnosis.

The management of COVID-19 is based on severity: Mild (category A, without hypoxia, usually managed as an outpatient), moderate [category B, with hypoxia oxygen saturation (SpO_2) 90–93% on room air], and severe (SpO_2 <90% at room air). Dexamethasone reduces mortality and is the therapy of choice for patients requiring oxygen supplementation. Tocilizumab reduces mortality if started early in severely ill patients. All hospitalized patients without contraindications should be treated with low-molecular-weight heparin (LMWH) for deep vein thrombosis (DVT) prophylaxis. Remdesivir is an antiviral for use in moderate ill patients requiring low-flow oxygen and should be started within 10 days from the onset of symptoms. Severe disease may progress to acute respiratory distress syndrome (ARDS) and respiratory failure. Complications such as hospital-acquired infection, COVID-associated pulmonary aspergillosis (CAPA), pulmonary embolism, and pneumothorax can occur.

"There are things known and there are things unknown, and in between are the doors of perception"
—**Aldous Huxley**

ETIOLOGY

Coronavirus disease-2019 is the name given to the disease caused by the new coronavirus, which was initially called novel coronavirus-2019 and later named as SARS-CoV-2 because of its resemblance with SARS-CoV viral genome. SARS-CoV, SARS-CoV-2, and Middle East respiratory syndrome coronavirus (MERS-CoV) are all closely related emerging coronaviruses that have caused epidemics in the last two decades.

VIRUS STRUCTURE

Coronaviruses have club-shaped trimeric surface spike glycoproteins that give the virions the appearance of a crown, hence their name (from the Latin corona meaning "crown") (**Fig. 1**).

TRANSMISSION

The transmission of COVID-19 is mainly through droplets spread and uncommonly via fomites. Airborne transmission of virus is also possible, especially in crowded poorly ventilated indoor areas. The S protein of SARS-CoV-2 binds to angiotensin-converting enzyme 2 (ACE-2) receptors which is the host receptor that is highly expressed on upper airway and pulmonary epithelial cells. The simplified CDC guidelines to prevent spread of infection are shown in **Figure 2**.

CLINICAL PRESENTATION

The incubation period of COVID-19 is 5–6 days on average, but can be up to 14 days. For up to 2 days before onset of symptoms, the infected individuals can shed virus (asymptomatic or presymptomatic shedding) and transmit the virus to contacts. The most common presenting symptoms are fever, sore throat, myalgia, malaise, rhinorrhea, dry cough, headache, loss of smell and taste is common, the former strongly suggestive of the disease. Dyspnea indicates worsening pneumonitis and is a sign of severe disease. Some patients may also present with gastrointestinal symptoms such as abdominal pain, vomiting, and loose stools. Extrapulmonary manifestations of COVID-19 include neurologic features [insomnia, headache, stroke, seizures, acute disseminated encephalomyelitis (ADEM), and meningoencephalitis], the heart [myocarditis, myocardial ischemia non-ST elevation myocardial infarction (NSTEMI) and ST-elevation myocardial infarction (STEMI), heart failure], thromboembolism (DVT pulmonary embolism and catheter-related thrombosis), and skin rash (petechiae, maculopapular rash, urticaria, and livedo reticularis) (**Table 1**).

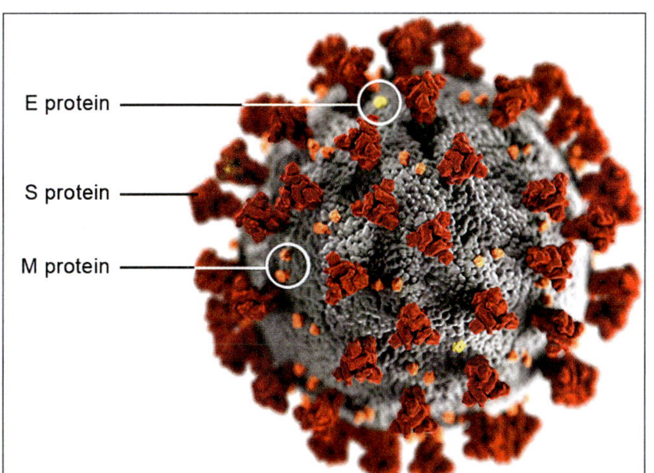

FIGURE 1: Illustration, created at the Centers for Disease Control and Prevention (CDC), revealing ultrastructural morphology exhibited by coronaviruses.

DIAGNOSIS AND IMAGING

MOLECULAR TESTS

Specimens are collected either from the upper respiratory tract and nasopharyngeal and oropharyngeal swabs or from the lower respiratory tract using expectorated sputum, bronchoalveolar lavage, or tracheal aspirate (only for mechanically ventilated patients). Sensitivity depends on the type of specimen with oral and nasal swabs having lower sensitivities of 50–65% and lower respiratory samples having higher sensitivities up to 93%.

False negative results are seen due to several reasons: Poor quality of specimen containing little patient material, specimen collection very early or late into infection, nonmaintenance of cold chain, and technical reasons inherent in the test, e.g., PCR inhibition and mutated virus targets.

SEROLOGY

There are two general types of antibodies; neutralizing antibodies (NAbs) and non-NAbs that start to develop a week after onset of symptoms. Commercially available anti-SARS-CoV-2 antibody tests use different technologies to qualitatively measure single immunoglobulin class or total antibody, but do not differentiate NAbs and binding antibodies. Currently guidelines recommend the use of serological tests only to detect evidence of SARS-CoV-2 infection 2 weeks after symptom onset.

BLOOD TESTS

Decreased total leukocyte count with lymphocytopenia and an elevated neutrophil-to-lymphocyte ratio seen in most patients. Levels of D-dimer, lactate dehydrogenase (LDH), C-reactive protein (CRP), and ferritin are elevated and serve as prognostic markers of inflammation. Red cell distribution width (RDW) >14.5% at diagnosis or a rise in RDW during hospitalization predicts increased mortality.

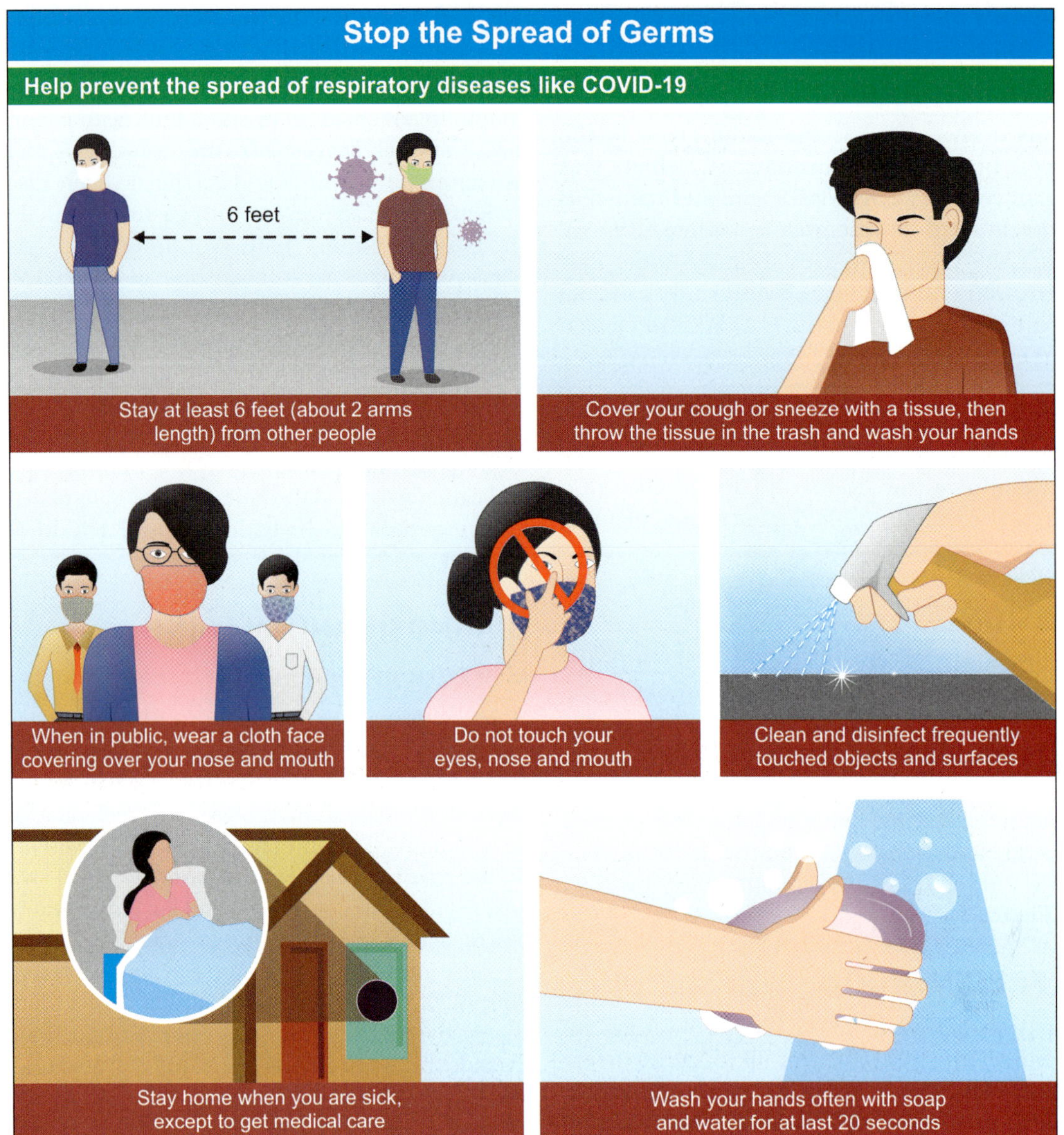

(COVID-19: coronavirus disease-2019)

FIGURE 2: Centers for Disease Control and Prevention (CDC) poster illustrating the effective interventions to prevent the spread of virus.

TABLE 1 Complications in patients with COVID-19.

Frequency	Complication
Commonly seen	• Acute respiratory distress syndrome • Acute respiratory failure • Sepsis • Disseminated intravascular coagulation • Acute liver and kidney injury • Pulmonary embolism
Rare	• Multisystem inflammatory syndrome • Coronavirus-associated pulmonary aspergillosis (CAPA) • Neurological complications

IMAGING

Chest-X ray is relatively insensitive in early pneumonia in comparison to high-resolution computed tomography (HRCT) chest, which is the preferred modality for diagnosing COVID-19 pneumonia, especially in PCR negative patients. The hallmark features on CT imaging include bilateral peripheral ground glass opacities and consolidations of the lung with peak of involvement between 6 and 11 days of symptom onset **Figures 3** to **5**.

MANAGEMENT

The clinical management of COVID-19 depends on the severity of illness as well as the duration of illness (**Table 2**).

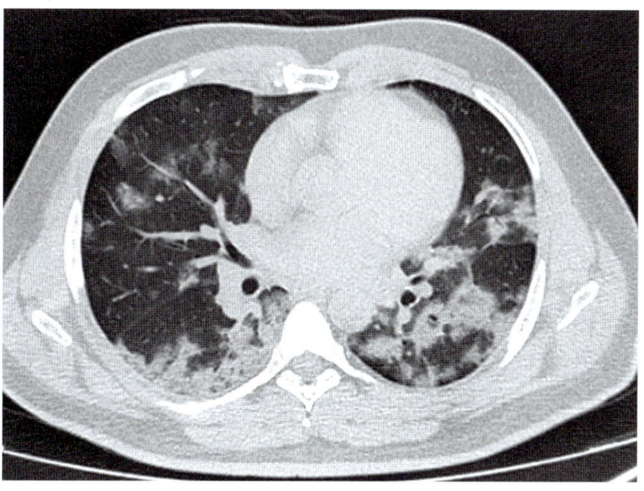

(COVID-19: coronavirus disease-2019; CT: computed tomography)

FIGURE 4: Plain CT scan of chest of a patient with moderate COVID-19.

RISK STRATIFICATION

Severe pneumonia can progress to ARDS or septic shock. ARDS can be categorized as follows:

- *Mild ARDS*: Partial pressure of oxygen/fractional inspired oxygen (PaO_2/FiO_2) of 200 to 300 mm Hg [with positive end-expiratory pressure (PEEP) or continuous positive airway pressure (CPAP) ≥5 cm H_2O]
- *Moderate ARDS*: PaO_2/FiO_2 of 100 to 200 mm Hg (with PEEP ≥5 cm H_20)
- *Severe ARDS*: PaO_2/FiO_2 ≤100 mm Hg (with PEEP ≥5 cm H_2O)

When PaO_2 is not available, SpO_2/FiO_2 ≤315 suggests ARDS (including in nonventilated patients).

Several risk factors what predispose to severe disease and increase mortality are presented in **Table 3**.

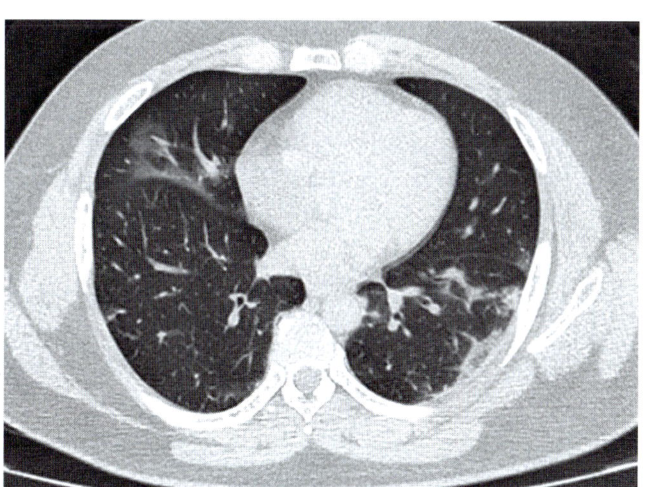

(COVID-19: coronavirus disease-2019; CT: computed tomography)

FIGURE 3: Plain CT scan of chest of a patient with mild COVID-19.

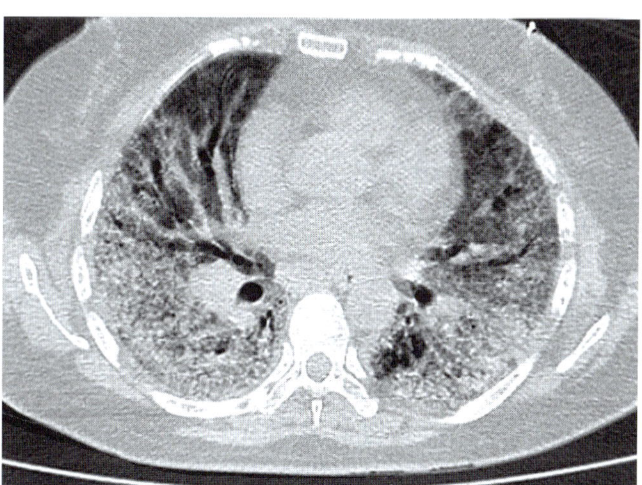

(COVID-19: coronavirus disease-2019; CT: computed tomography)

FIGURE 5: Plain CT scan of chest of a patient with severe COVID-19.

TABLE 2 Severity category.

Guidelines	Mild	Moderate	Severe
World Health Organization (WHO) (interim guidance, 27 May, 2020)	Symptomatic patients without evidence of viral pneumonia or hypoxia	Clinical signs of pneumonia*, no signs of severe pneumonia, and oxygen saturation (SpO_2) ≥ 90% on room air	Clinical signs of pneumonia* plus one of the following: • Respiratory rate >30 breaths/min • Severe respiratory distress • SpO_2 < 90% on room air
Government of India Ministry of Health and Family Welfare (version 3, June 2020)	Uncomplicated upper respiratory tract infection without evidence of breathlessness or hypoxia (normal saturation)	Clinical features of dyspnea and/or hypoxia, fever, cough, including SpO_2 < 94% (range 90–94%) on room air and respiratory rate ≥24 breaths/min	Clinical signs of pneumonia plus one of the following: • Respiratory rate >30 breaths/min • Severe respiratory distress • SpO_2 < 90% on room air**

*Fever, cough, dyspnea, and fast breathing.

**Individuals who have respiratory failure, septic shock, and multiple organ dysfunction should be considered in the critical illness group.

TABLE 3 Risk factors.

High risk	Possibly increased risk
• Age >60 years (risk increases with increasing age) • Type 2 diabetes mellitus • Chronic kidney disease • COPD • Pregnancy • Obesity (BMI > 30, risk increases further if >40) • Solid-organ transplant • Congestive heart failure, coronary artery disease, and cardiomyopathy • Sickle cell disease • Cancer and hematologic malignancy, especially with recent chemotherapy • Smoking	• Asthma (moderate to severe) • Cystic fibrosis • Hypertension • Type 1 diabetes mellitus • Solid-organ malignancy • Cerebrovascular accident • BMI > 25–30 • Chronic liver disease • Psychiatric illness and dementia • Immunocompromised state (HIV/immunosuppressed/immunodeficiency) • Obstructive sleep apnea • Thalassemia • Pulmonary fibrosis

(BMI: body mass index; COPD: chronic obstructive pulmonary disease; HIV: human immunodeficiency virus)

TREATMENT CHOICES

OXYGEN THERAPY

Different levels of oxygen therapy available as per the patient's level of consciousness, the severity of hypoxemia, and hemodynamic status.

- Nasal cannula
- Face mask
- Face mask with reservoir bag
- High-flow nasal oxygen (HFNO)
- NIV
- Invasive ventilation
- Extracorporeal membrane oxygenation (ECMO)

DEXAMETHASONE

- *Mechanism of action (MOA)*: Broad-spectrum immunomodulator.
- Dose is 8 mg once daily intravenous (IV)/orally for 7–10 days (or till discharge, if earlier).
- Dexamethasone reduces mortality in those who required therapy with supplemental oxygen or mechanical ventilation.
- May increase mortality in hospitalized patients who do not require oxygen.
- Alternatives are hydrocortisone 50 mg IV q8h or methylprednisolone 40 mg/day.
- *Adverse effects*: Hyperglycemia, hypertension, and opportunistic infection (hospital-acquired infection, strongyloides hyperinfection, CAPA, and invasive mucormycosis).

REMDESIVIR

- *MOA*: Inhibits ribonucleic acid (RNA)-dependent RNA polymerase activity.
- Dose is 200 mg IV on day 1, followed by 100 mg daily for 4 more days.
- Does not reduce mortality but reduces duration of hospital stay and improves oxygenation in patients requiring oxygen, but not on high-flow oxygen/noninvasive ventilation (NIV)/high-flow nasal cannula (HFNC)/mechanical ventilation.
- Benefit is more significant if started early in the disease (<10 days after symptom onset).
- *Adverse effects*: Abnormal liver function tests (LFTs) [measure at baseline, avoid if >5 upper limits of normal (ULN), monitor LFT while on the drug].

LOW MOLECULAR WEIGHT HEPARIN

- *MOA*: Anticoagulation and prevention of thrombosis [DVT and pulmonary thromboembolism (PE)].
- Start prophylactic dose LMWH [e.g., enoxaparin 1 mg/kg subcutaneously (SC) q24h] for all admitted patients.
- Start therapeutic anticoagulation for proven or strongly suspected DVT or PE till excluded on venous Doppler/CT pulmonary angiography.
- Repeat prothrombin time (PT), platelet count, and D-dimer every 2–3 days in patients who do not show improvement.
- *Contraindications*:
    - Active bleeding or a platelet count of $<25 \times 10^9$/L.
    - Decompensated liver disease with coagulopathy.
    - Prolonged activated partial thromboplastin time (aPTT) is not a contraindication to anticoagulation.

EXPERIMENTAL THERAPIES

Tocilizumab:

- *MOA*: Interleukin-6 receptor blocker.
- Administer single dose within 24 hours of worsening in patients on $FiO_2 > 0.4$ or higher levels of respiratory support with increasing hypoxemia/hypotension despite steroids/antivirals.
- Dose is 8 mg/kg or 400 mg IV, can repeat another dose after 12 hours (not to exceed 800 mg of total dose).
- Avoid if infection is present or suspected.

Convalescent plasma:

- *MOA*: Passive source of neutralizing antibody as antiviral and immunomodulator.
- Not associated with a reduction in mortality or progression to severe COVID-19.
- Consider for nonintubated severely ill patients presenting within 3 days of diagnosis.
- Dose is 200–250 mL, followed by a second dose, if needed 24 hours later.
- *Adverse effect*: Hypersensitivity reaction (rare)

Baricitinib:
- *MOA*: Selective inhibitor of Janus kinase (JAK) 1 and 2, which inhibits intracellular signaling pathway of cytokines.
- Accelerates recovery by a day but does not reduce mortality, when given in combination with remdesivir.
- Consider for patients in whom steroids are contra-indicated.
- Dose is 4 mg [either orally (two 2-mg tablets) or through a nasogastric tube] for 14 days or until hospital discharge.

LANDMARK TRIALS

RECOVERY

- Randomized controlled trial (RCT) in the UK comparing treatment outcome in standard of care arm versus five comparator arms, i.e., dexamethasone, hydroxychloroquine (HCQ), tocilizumab, convalescent plasma therapy (CPT), and lopinavir/ritonavir (LPV/r).
- Dexamethasone arm showed lower 28-day mortality among those receiving either invasive mechanical ventilation or oxygen, but not among those receiving no respiratory support. No mortality benefit with either LPV/r or HCQ.

SOLIDARITY

- RCT conducted by World Health Organization (WHO) involving 30 countries compared standard of care versus treatment with one of four arms with remdesivir, HCQ (or chloroquine), ritonavir/lopinavir, and interferon (IFN)-β combination.
- All four treatment arms showed no or little effect on overall mortality, initiation of ventilation, and duration of hospital stay in hospitalized patients.
- Showed reduction in mortality from 33 to 27% if tocilizumab given within 24 hours of worsening in patients on dexamethasone requiring $FiO_2 > 0.4$ or higher levels of respiratory support.

ADAPTIVE COVID-19 TREATMENT TRIAL-1

- Double-blind RCT of remdesivir versus standard of care was conducted by the National Institutes of Health (NIH), USA with a primary endpoint of time to recovery and improvement in ordinal scale of severity of pneumonia.
- Median time to recovery was 10 days for patients treated with remdesivir compared with 15 days for placebo.
- Benefit was statistically significant only in patients on minimal amounts of supplemental oxygen (ordinal scale 5), but not in patients not needing oxygen, those needing higher levels of oxygen or intubated patients.

PLACID

- Open level, parallel-arm (Phase II, Multicenter Randomized Controlled Trial) of convalescent plasma (CP) versus standard of care involving 39 public and private hospitals conducted in India.
- Showed that CP was not associated with a reduction in all-cause mortality at 28 days or progression to severe COVID-19.

SEVERITY AND MANAGEMENT

MILD CATEGORY

- Symptomatic management as outpatients is indicated in the majority.
- There is no role for antiviral agents, anticoagulation, or steroids.
- Home isolation is needed for 10 days from the date of onset of the first symptom.
- Patients aged >60 years or those with risk factors for worsening can use pulse oximetry monitoring every 4 hours. A walk test for 3–6 minutes might help to unmask impending hypoxia.
- However, patients must be admitted to the hospital if clinical condition worsens or SpO_2 falls to <94% on room air or persistence of fever for >7 days (**Flowchart 1**).

MODERATE CATEGORY

- This group of patients should be admitted to the COVID ward in airborne isolation.
- Dexamethasone should be started.
- Low-molecular-weight heparin should be started in all hospitalized patients except for those with contraindications.
- Remdesivir can be considered for those presenting early (within 10 days of onset of symptom) and requiring low flow oxygen <5 L/min to maintain SpO_2 >90%/ACTT-1 (Adaptive COVID-19 Treatment Trial-1) ordinal scale 5.
- Appropriate oxygen therapy, usually through a nasal cannula or Venturi device, along with awake proning, helps in better oxygenation.

SEVERE CATEGORY

- Patients should be admitted to a COVID intensive care unit (ICU).
- Dexamethasone should be started.
- Anticoagulation with LMWH should be given to patients without any contraindication.
- There is no effective antiviral of proven benefit in the severe category of COVID-19 patients.
- A single dose of ivermectin 12 mg can be considered as prophylaxis for strongyloides hyperinfection syndrome in patients on steroids.
- Management of ARDS and sepsis should be done as per standard protocol.
- Experimental drugs can be considered on a case-bycase basis (**Flowchart 1**).

MANAGEMENT OF COMPLICATIONS

ACUTE RESPIRATORY DISTRESS SYNDROME

- Low tidal volumes [4–8 mL/kg predicted body weight (PBW)] and lower inspiratory pressures (plateau pressure <30 cm H_2O).

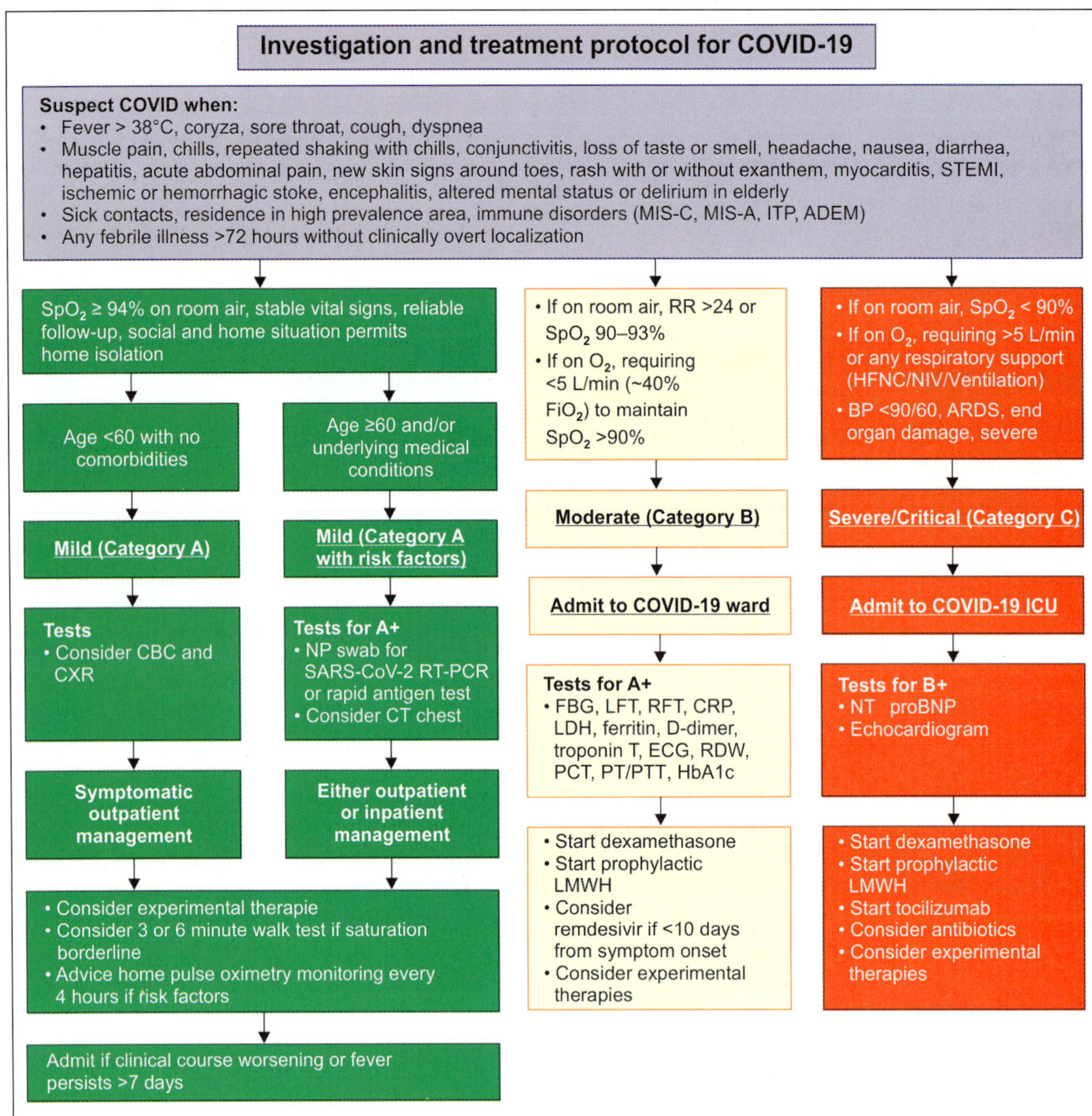

(ADEM: acute disseminated encephalomyelitis; FiO_2: fraction of inspired oxygen; HFNC: high-flow nasal cannula; ICU: intensive care unit; ITP: immune thrombocytopenic purpura; MAS: macrophage activation syndrome; MIS-A: multisystem inflammatory syndrome in adults; MIS-C: multisystem inflammatory syndrome in children; NP: nasopharyngeal; NT-proBNP: N-terminal pro-brain natriuretic peptide; RDW: red cell distribution width)

FLOWCHART 1: Algorithm for investigation and treatment.

- Hypercapnia is permitted if meeting the pH goal of 7.30–7.45.
- In patients with severe ARDS, prone ventilation for 16–18 hours per day is recommended.
- In patients with moderate or severe ARDS, higher PEEP is suggested instead of lower PEEP.

PULMONARY EMBOLISM

- Intermediate-low-risk or intermediate-high-risk PE should be managed initially with anticoagulation and close monitoring.
- Massive or high-risk PE with hypotension or sudden cardiac arrest thrombolytic therapy should be initiated urgently.
- In refractory shock or cardiac arrest, ECMO could be an option, combined with surgical embolectomy or catheter-directed treatment.

Anticoagulation after discharge:

- At discharge, consider starting patients at high risk [modified International Medical Prevention Registry on Venous Thromboembolism-Venous Thromboembolism (IMPROVE-VTE) score >4, D-dimer more than two times upper limit, age >75 years, and underlying malignancy] on DVT prophylaxis.

- Rivaroxaban 10 mg once PO daily (or equivalent agent) for 4 weeks.
- Patients with proven DVT/PE should be prescribed therapeutic anticoagulation for 3 months.

RECOMMENDED READINGS

1. Galbadage T, Peterson BM, Gunasekera RS. Does COVID-19 Spread through Droplets Alone? Front Public Health. 2020;8:163.
2. Parasher A. COVID-19: Current understanding of its pathophysiology, clinical presentation and treatment. Postgrad Med J. 2021;97(1147):312-20.
3. Government of India Ministry of Health and Family Welfare. (2020). Clinical Management Protocol: COVID-19. [online] Available from https://www.mohfw.gov.in/pdf/UpdatedClinical Management Protocolfor COVID19dated03072020.pdf.
4. Centers for Disease Control and Prevention. (2021). Interim Clinical Guidance for Management of Patients with Confirmed Coronavirus Disease (COVID-19) [online] Available from cdc.gov/coronavirus/2019ncov/hcp/clinical-guidance-management-patients. html.
5. National Institutes of Health. (2021). Coronavirus Disease 2019 (COVID-19) Treatment Guidelines. [online] Available from https://www.covid19treatment guidelines.nih.gov.
6. WHO. (2020). Clinical management of COVID-19: interim guidance. [online] Available from https://apps. who.int/iris/handle/10665/332196.
7. RECOVERY Collaborative Group; Horby P, Lim WS, Emberson JR, Mafham M, Bell JL, et al. Dexamethasone in Hospitalized Patients with Covid-19. N Engl J Med. 2021;384(8):693-704.
8. Beigel JH, Tomashek KM, Dodd LE, Mehta AK, Zingman BS, Kalil AC, et al. Remdesivir for the Treatment of Covid-19—Final Report. N Engl J Med. 2020;383:1813-26.
9. WHO Solidarity Trial Consortium, Pan H, Peto R, Henao-Restrepo AM, Preziosi MP, Sathiyamoorthy V, et al. Repurposed Antiviral Drugs for Covid-19—Interim WHO Solidarity Trial Results. N Engl J Med. 2021;384:497-511.
10. Moores LK, Tritschler T, Brosnahan S, Carrier M, Collen JF, Doerschug K, et al. Prevention, Diagnosis, and Treatment of VTE in Patients With Coronavirus Disease 2019: CHEST Guideline and Expert Panel Report. Chest. 2020;158(3):1143-63.
11. Aoyama H, Uchida K, Aoyama K, Pechlivanoglou P, Englesakis M, Yamada Y, et al. Assessment of therapeutic interventions and lung-protective ventilation in patients with moderate to severe acute respiratory distress syndrome: a systematic review and network meta-analysis. JAMA Netw Open. 2019;2:e198116.

CHAPTER 56

Mucormycosis in COVID-19 Pandemic: The New Challenge

Jagdish Chander

ABSTRACT

Mucormycosis is a rapidly destructive necrotizing fungal infection usually seen among diabetic patients and in those with other immunocompromised backgrounds. This occurs due to disruption of normal protective barrier hence local risk factors include trauma, burns, surgery, surgical splints, arterial lines, injection/biopsy sites, tattoos, and even insect or spider bites. The systemic risk factors are hyperglycemia, ketoacidosis, malignancy, leucopenia, and immunosuppressive therapy; however, infections in immunocompetent host are now well described. Mucormycetes are upcoming as emerging agents leading to fatal consequences, if not timely detected/treated. Coronavirus disease 2019 (COVID-19) pandemic has led to ~40,845 cases of rhino-orbito-cerebral mucormycosis in India during a very short span of time.

In the mainstream media, mucormycosis is being proposed as "black fungus" during this pandemic. It is rather a misnomer and should not be used because there is already a category of "black fungi" described in the medical literature. Ideally, it should be called as COVID-19-associated mucormycosis (CAM). Out of a total of six types of mucormycosis rhino-orbito-cerebral and pulmonary types are commonly encountered in this pandemic. Recently, it has been announced as a notifiable disease by various states of India. Eventually on May 20, 2021 the Indian Council of Medical Research/Government of India (ICMR/GOI) also declared this disease under Epidemic Diseases Act, 1897, wherein all government and private health facilities and medical colleges will follow guidelines for its screening, diagnosis, and management. Therefore, it has become an acute emergency being a life-threatening to the patients thereby a new challenge to the medical fraternity at large.

"Extreme hopes are born from extreme misery"

—Bertrand Russell

INTRODUCTION

The fungal infections are being increasingly reported during the last four decades. Some of them like candidiasis, cryptococcosis, pneumocystosis, talaromycosis, aspergillosis etc., were frequently encountered after the onset of acquired immunodeficiency syndrome (AIDS) pandemic during mid-1980s to the extent that they were coined as AIDS-defining illnesses. However, lately another disease was also added to this opportunistic list, not going parallel with other ones and that is mucormycosis. This has now posed a very grave challenge during this on-going pandemic of COVID-19.

The mainstream media has labeled it as a "black fungus," which is basically a misnomer because there is different category of "black fungi" already existing in the medical literature causing tinea nigra, chromoblastomycosis, phaeohyphomycosis etc. The deciding factor for any "black fungus" is presence of melanin in the fungal cell wall otherwise they are considered as hyaline (colorless) and the Mucorales are hyaline fungi. There is no end to such type of nomenclature as of now there is "white fungus" or "yellow fungus" and tomorrow there will be red, blue, or green fungi, which should be discouraged.

Ideally, it should be called as COVID-19-associated mucormycosis (CAM). The recent upsurge in cases is because of the on-going pandemic of COVID-19, contributed by various risk factors. During the first wave of pandemic such patients were not observed but in the second wave large number of cases, like a sort of tsunami, are being reported amounting ~40,845, majority of them being life-threatening.

PRE-COVID-19 PERIOD

Mucormycosis, the so-called "black fungus" disease, is an acute infection caused by several agents belonging to phylum Glomeromycota. These saprotrophic fungi are found ubiquitously in the soil and environment in our surrounding vicinity. In the past, these Mucoralean fungi used to be considered as nonpathogenic to man and animals. Not only that rather they used to be treated as fungal contaminants in any of the diagnostic microbiology laboratory. However, understanding about Mucormycetes has now entirely changed as these are emerging highly opportunistic pathogenic organisms invariably entailing fatal consequences, especially when an obvious underlying predisposing factor like diabetes mellitus already exists in a particular clinical setting. The cases are being increasingly reported among healthy individuals also where there is no apparent underlying risk factor present.

Moreover, unlike other fungal diseases, even the AIDS, pandemic could not significantly affect the incidence and prevalence of mucormycosis during last four decades, however, upsurge in number of diabetic patients has really changed the entire scenario more or less like an epidemic in the indian subcontinent posing a very serious health threat. In one of the Textbook of Medical Mycology in 2018, it was predicted that this disease is going to destroy India shortly, in a couple of years. This warning now has come true keeping in view of the magnitude of the disease being faced throughout the country.

MUCORMYCOSIS IN COVID-19

The basic question is why there is upsurge of cases of mucormycosis during this pandemic of COVID-19. This was not there during its first wave in 2020 and now all of a sudden, within a short span of time, so many cases are being reported all over the country. This began with a few case reports from Ganga Ram Hospital, New Delhi and almost simultaneously from Gujarat state. Subsequently cases started pouring in almost every state of the country. Most of the patients had recovered from COVID-19 thereby were actually discharged from the hospital but some of them came back again with this fulminant disease. The various risk factors are speculated and/or contemplated; however, evidence-based studies are yet to be carried out before reaching a definitive conclusion.

There is injudicious use of steroids in the course of treatment of COVID-19 and that too in high doses than the prescribed ones and for a prolonged duration. The other risk factors may be prolonged use of contaminated masks without changing *as per the prescribed guidelines.* There is strong possibility of the use of contaminated accessory while inhaling oxygen among patients. During the second wave of COVID-19 pandemic, there was acute shortage of medical oxygen in the country hence most of the hospitals had to shift on to the industrial oxygen. Although it is said that there is no basic difference between both these oxygen types except minor one of dispensing but public at large still suspect it to be one of the causes. The humidifiers used while delivering the oxygen, i.e., *distilled water versus sterile* or tap water, is also suspected to be a source. Moreover, frequent steam inhalation is also considered as one of the risk factors.

There is higher level of iron in the form of ferritin among the COVID-19 patients, which is also favorable for the growth of Mucormycetes. In addition all the patients of COVID-19 are taking zinc as a preventive and/or therapeutic agent, which is also *conducive ground for the fungal growth.* This fungal infection also affects people who are already on some medication like *prolonged use of antibiotics.* Some of the reports state that the delta strain of the SARS-CoV-2 (severe acute respiratory syndrome-Coronavirus-2) (B.1.617.2) is targeting the islets of Langerhans in pancreas through angiotensin-converting enzyme 2 (ACE2) receptors, affecting insulin production thereby leading to diabetic state among patients during their recovery period.

Recently, mucormycosis has been declared as a notifiable disease by various Indian states beginning with Rajasthan. Eventually Indian Council of Medical Research (ICMR)/Government of India (GOI) also on May 20, 2021 declared this disease under Epidemic Diseases Act, 1897, wherein all government and private health facilities and medical colleges will follow guidelines for its screening, diagnosis, and management. The advisory goes on to say that mucormycosis, if uncared for, may turn fatal. To prevent disease, blood glucose level should be monitored during post-COVID period. Now, all the cases reported, are to be conveyed to the World Bank-funded Integrated Disease Surveillance Project (IDSP) of the respective states and union territories.

In addition to the ICMR/GOI, Fungal Infection Study Forum (FISF), European Confederation of Medical Mycology (ECMM), and International Society for Human and Animal Mycology (ISHAM) have also released their respective guidelines on this acutely emerging disease during the COVID-19 pandemic. After mycetoma and chromoblastomycosis, which were declared as Neglected Tropical Disease (NTD) by World Health Organization (WHO), CAM got this much of importance. The International Forum on Zygomycosis held three meetings in Greece since 2008 under the leadership of Petrikkos, wherein most of the aspects of this emerging disease were discussed at length.

These fungi are seen as broad, nonseptate hyphae in tissue with a predilection to invade blood vessels due to their angioinvasive nature thereby leading to extensive necrosis of the surrounding area and formation of embolism. Since morphology of these organisms is indistinguishable in histopathological sections hence culture is essential for an exact identification of the causative fungal species. The course and outcome of disease differ according to anatomical site involved as well as nature of fungal species isolated in a particular patient.

CLASSIFICATION

The nomenclature, mucormycosis, is an umbrella term used for diseases caused by many nonseptate filamentous fungal species. Classified under orders Mucorales and Entomophthorales, they were previously considered members of phylum Zygomycota and now are elevated to the rank of subphylum Mucoromycotina and Entomophthoromycotina under phylum Glomeromycota. Some investigators prefer to call disease caused by members belonging to subphylum Mucoromycotina as mucormycosis and to subphylum Entomophthoromycotina as entomophthoromycosis or subcutaneous Mucormycosis, which is further subdivided into two types, i.e., conidiobolomycosis and basidiobolomycosis (**Box 1**).

As there are fungi in same class Mucormycetes, which produce syndromes quite different from those caused by members of subphylum Mucoromycotina thus some workers prefer a more restrictive designation, zygomycosis, as an appropriate term. However, due to changes in taxonomy and expanded range of etiological agents, term mucormycosis should be preferred over obsolete term, zygomycosis, or the present newly-coined one, “black fungus” during this ongoing COVID-19 pandemic. The older synonym, like phycomycosis, is also now an obsolete term, which denoted that infection was once caused by Phycomycetes.

The Mucormycete is a group of lower fungi and their hyphae are generally nonseptate or sparsely septate. However, when these septa occur they are solid cross-walls with no pores and there is no flow of cytoplasmic material between cells. These reproduce asexually by way of sporangiospores formed within a sac called as sporangium and/or by means of conidial development. These fungi also reproduce sexually by formation of a single, dark, thick-walled spore called zygospore. Based on zygospore formation, these fungi were classified under phylum Zygomycota. The various causative agents of mucormycosis and Entomophthoromycosis are shown in **Box 2**.

EPIDEMIOLOGICAL ASPECTS

The fungal species belonging to order Mucorales are ubiquitously found prevalent in the environment. They are found in food items, soil, air, and frequently encountered as laboratory contaminants. The clinical forms of mucormycosis occur following infection by Mucoralean fungi, which are found as saprotrophic in the environment and on a wide range of substrates including soil. However, during the pandemic of COVID-19, majority of the cases are

BOX 1	Broad categories of Mucormycetes and Entomophthoromycetes.
Phylum: Glomeromycota (former Zygomycota)	
Subphylum: Mucoromycotina (Mucormycetes)	
Mucoromycotina: Mucormycosis	
Acute angioinvasive infection in immunocompromised individuals	
Entomophthoromycotina: Entomophthoromycosis	
Chronic subcutaneous infections in immunocompetent individuals	

BOX 2 Causative Agents of Mucormycosis and Entomophthoromycosis.

Mucoromycotina: Mucormycosis

- *Rhizopus arrhizus (Rhizopus oryzae)*
- *Rhizopus microsporus* var. *rhizopodiformis*
- *Lichtheimia corymbifera (Mycocladus corymbiferus, Absidia corymbifera)*
- *Rhizomucor pusillus*
- *Mucor* species
- *Cunninghamella* species
- *Syncephalastrum* species
- *Apophysomyces elegans, A. variabilis, A. trapeziformis, A ossiformis*, and *A. mexicanus*
- *Saksenaea vasiformis, S. erythrospora, S. oblongispora, S. loutrophoriformis*
- *Cokeromyces recurvatus* and others species

Entomophthoromycotina: Entomophthoromycosis

- Conidiobolomycosis—*Conidiobolus coronatus*
- Basidiobolomycosis—*Basidiobolus ranarum*

rhino-orbital mucormycosis and a few belong to pulmonary type.

The spores of these fungi are widely distributed, growing on leaf litter and other decaying carbohydrate substrates. The spores are not as abundant in free air as *Alternaria* and *Cladosporium* species, but can be found in large number in damp interiors and around composing vegetation and even present as "bread molds" appearing as grayish, fluffy, and rapidly spreading growth. Because of their rapid growth and prolific spore-forming capacity, inhalation of conidia is a routine occurrence. It is now third most common invasive mycoses after candidiasis and aspergillosis.

The virulence of these fungi is clearly of low order and usually sporadic infections occur throughout world particularly in severely debilitated patients. Being an opportunistic infection, mucormycosis is produced by contaminant fungi in a host whose immunological defense mechanisms are weakened by endogenous causes like diabetes mellitus in Southeast Asia and malignancy, leukemia, or exogenous causes like immunosuppressive therapy in the Western world. The breakthrough mucormycosis cases have also been reported among patients with hematologic malignancies receiving hematopoietic stem cell transplants or intensive chemotherapy, who were given voriconazole for preventing aspergillosis.

IMMUNOLOGICAL ASPECTS

The neutrophils appear to play a major role in defense of host from infection caused by Mucormycetes. In normal hosts, macrophages prevent initiation of infection by phagocytosis and oxidative killing of spores. On the other hand in hosts with diabetes mellitus and other underlying factor, monocytes/macrophages are dysfunctional and fail to suppress spore germination process. The hosts with neutrophil defects, either qualitative or quantitative, are predisposed to infection by fungal agents of this class. The clinical entities include rhinocerebral mucormycosis in diabetic ketoacidosis and invasive infection with *Rhizopus, Lichtheimia,* and *Cunninghamella* species in case of treated malignancies and granulocytopenia. Like *Aspergillus* species, agents of mucormycosis have a predilection for vascular invasion causing thrombosis and infarction leading to necrosis of the affected tissue. In such type of clinical setting, infection with Mucormycetes carries very poor prognosis.

The other predisposing factors of mucormycosis are granulocytopenia, particularly in hematological malignancies, uncontrolled diabetes mellitus, and immunosuppressive conditions, in addition to long-term intake of corticosteroids. In human immunodeficiency virus (HIV) patients, however, mucormycosis cases have been reported but very rarely and frequency is not as much as candidiasis, cryptococcosis, and other opportunistic fungal infections, which is one of exceptional feature. It may be because HIV infection does not appear to increase risk of developing mucormycosis probably because neutrophils, as opposed to T-lymphocytes, play a major role in defense against Mucorales. If at all it is there, this occurs in context of intravenous drug abuse.

PATHOGENESIS AND PATHOLOGY

Similar to aspergillosis, phagocytes, polymorphonuclear neutrophils, and macrophages play a significant role among patients of mucormycosis. Infection can occur by inhalation, percutaneous inoculation, or ingestion. The spores are inhaled into lungs where they are ingested by alveolar macrophages. These cells are known to inhibit the germination of ingested spores to some extent but their activity to kill them is limited. Further, when they evade antifungal activity of macrophages and germinate into mycelial form, polymorphonuclear neutrophils and peripheral monocytes are expected to work against fungi. The former, which possess property of fungicidal activities against Mucormycetes, are known to play an important role in defense against mucormycosis, therefore, leukocytopenic patients are extremely susceptible. The increased risk of mucormycosis in patients with ketoacidosis may also be due to release of iron bound to proteins. Due to ketoacidosis, low serum pH diminishes the phagocytic effect of macrophages, chemotactic, and oxidative burst of neutrophils.

The most commonly encountered mucormycete, *Rhizopus arrhizus*, has several virulence factors like angioinvasive nature, growth at or above body temperature, production of destructive enzymes, dormant spores which are resistant to destruction at extremes of temperature along with active ketone reductase system, and hydroxamate siderophores. The diabetic patients with ketoacidosis are usually more affected by mucormycosis. *Rhizopus* species have an active ketone reductase system hence thrive in high glucose and acidotic conditions. These patients also have decreased phagocytic activity because of an impaired glutathione pathway. The exact mechanism of increased susceptibility among these patients remains somewhat unknown, probably a combination of metabolic abnormalities present in the patients with diabetes. Hyperglycemia or acidosis alone does not permit fungal growth *in vivo* although acidosis without hyperglycemia has been reported with invasive mucormycosis. The normal serum inhibits *Rhizopus* species whereas serum from patients of diabetic ketoacidosis stimulates its growth.

This has been observed that patients, on dialysis and iron overload, who are being treated with deferoxamine, an iron chelator, are more susceptible to mucormycosis. It is probably because Mucorales use this chelator as a siderophore to obtain more iron. The other risk factors include neutropenia, high-dose systemic steroids, protein-calorie malnutrition, solid organ and bone marrow transplants, immunodeficiency, leukemia, and intravenous drug abusers who may inject spores of Mucorales with the drugs and then present with space-occupying lesions of central nervous system.

The Mucormycetes have a predilection for elastic lamina of large and small arteries causing thrombosis, hemorrhage, and infarction. Hence angioinvasion, thrombosis, ischemia, and tissue necrosis are primary histopathological features of mucormycosis. In AIDS, neutrophil function remains relatively intact and this may be probable reason for less frequency of mucormycosis among these patients, therefore, as such it does not seem to be a significant risk factor.

CLINICAL MANIFESTATIONS

As such the nomenclature as mucormycosis comes from Mucorales and not from its genus *Mucor*. Irrespective of the genus or species, based on the sites involved by fungi, the disease is called mucormycosis, which presents as the following six clinical categories. Each category is associated with certain underlying disorders, relationship and existence of variable factor. However, recently the cases have been reported in immunocompetent individuals also without any underlying factor. The clinical manifestations are: (1) Rhino-orbito-cerebral, (2) Pulmonary, (3) Cutaneous, (4) Gastrointestinal, (5) Isolated renal, and (6) Disseminated mucormycosis.

RHINO-ORBITO-CEREBRAL TYPE

This is the most common and fulminating type of mucormycosis, which may lead to fatal consequences within a week of onset of disease if left untreated among the COVID-19 or otherwise in general patients. It is invariably associated either with acute onset of diabetes mellitus, hyperglycemia with ketoacidosis, or with debilitating diseases such as leukemia and lymphoma. The COVID-19 patients are usually given steroids in high doses and for prolonged duration to avert cytokine storm. Most commonly, it spreads from nasal mucosa to turbinate bones, paranasal sinuses, orbit and palate with eventual extension into brain where massive invasion of blood vessels cause major infarct. The destruction of bones is often revealed by imaging techniques like computed tomography (CT) or magnetic resonance imaging (MRI). Several species of Mucormycetes have been implicated as etiological agents but majority of cases are caused by *Rhizopus arrhizus*. The others are *R. microsporus*, *R. homothallicus*, *Syncephalastrum* etc. (See **Box 2**).

The presenting symptoms include facial pain, headache, lethargy, and in advanced cases, loss of vision. If there is no obvious reason for diplopia in diabetic patients, mucormycosis may be suspected. The physical examination reveal brownish, bloodstained nasal discharge on the affected side, black eschar on palate due to hemorrhage and tissue necrosis, with fixed and dilated pupil with global proptosis and ptosis with dysfunction of cranial nerves, especially fifth and seventh nerves. There is an extensive and rapid destruction of surrounding tissues. Sometimes, spread may also occur to lungs, gastrointestinal tract, skin, and occasionally to other organs. The rhinocerebral mucormycosis is usually fatal as patient dies within a week's time and is diagnosed on autopsy, if clinician could not reach tentative diagnosis during life.

The signs and symptoms of orbital mucormycosis include chemosis, periorbital cellulitis, ophthalmoplegia,

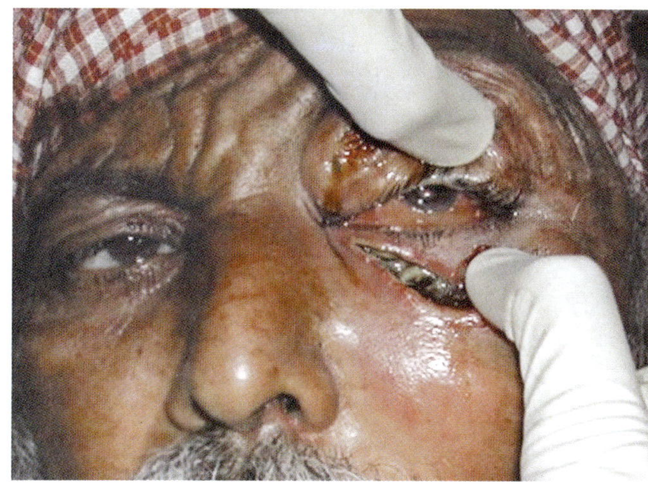

FIGURE 1: Swelling over left orbital area of a COVID-19 patient with proptosis, ophthalmoplegia, restricted eye movement, necrosis of lids with black eschar, and conjunctival chemosis.

proptosis, ptosis, abrupt visual loss, orbital pain, and facial hypoesthesia (**Fig. 1**). The infection may disseminate to lungs, other organ systems, and may spread from orbit into brain, leading to frontal lobe necrosis and abscesses formation. These features result from invasion of fungus through cribriform plate. The fungi invade blood vessels and cause necrotizing vasculitis, resulting in thrombosis of vessel lumen. Unless diagnosed and treated early, mucormycosis is often fatal due to cerebral involvement. An overall mortality among these patients is very high; however, chances of survival are ~50% if timely diagnosis and proper treatment is imparted.

PULMONARY TYPE

Among the patients of COVID-19, the pulmonary disease is the second most common presentation and is caused through inhalation of sporangiospores of Mucormycetes. They are usually immunocompromised by virtue of lack of circulating neutrophils, secondary to some underlying hematologic malignancy such as leukemia, lymphoma, profound immunosuppression, or even bone marrow transplantation. The lesions may be focal or diffuse and usually uncommon in patients having underlying diabetes mellitus in comparison to rhinocerebral type. The invasion of blood vessel may result in destruction of lung parenchyma. The usual course of disease takes about 1–4 weeks from onset till the terminal stages of illness. The clinical manifestations are nonspecific and may include chest pain, dyspnea, and hemoptysis.

The chest X-rays show evidence of infiltration, usually involving an anatomical segment but typically progressing to involve multiple adjoining areas. High-resolution chest CT scan is the best method of determining the extent of pulmonary mucormycosis. The disease can be suspected when patients have a reverse halo sign on CT of the chest, along with the associated clinical findings, which is in comparison to the halo sign of invasive pulmonary aspergillosis. The ground glass opacities due to COVID-19 and superimposed shadows caused by pulmonary

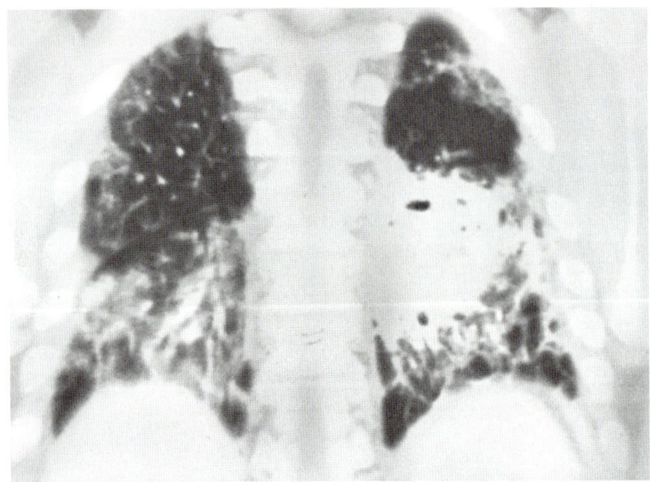

FIGURE 2: Coronal section of CT scan of COVID-19 patient shows homogeneous shadow with cavity formation in the left lung with surrounding halo. Also seen are ground glass opacities in the lower lobe of right lung.

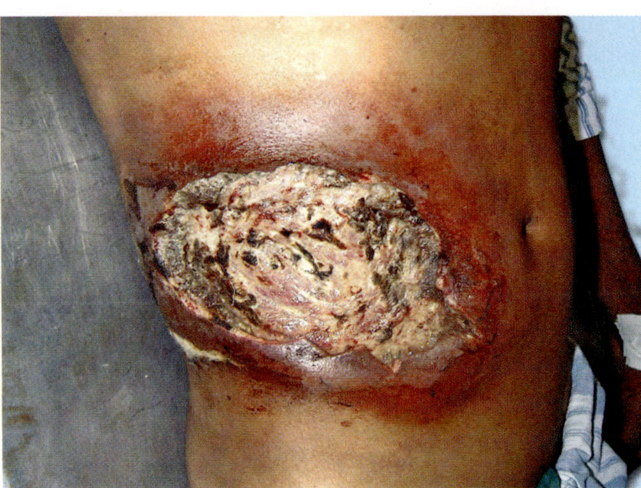

FIGURE 3: Extensive necrotizing cutaneous lesion over the right side of the abdominal wall of a patient.

mucormycosis really pose a very difficult and challenging situation (**Fig. 2**). Above all if the CT score of COVID-19 is on higher side like 16/25, then condition becomes grim. The overall prognosis is better in localized lesion as compared to the diffuse or bilateral involvement of the lungs. Very rarely members of order Mucorales are found to involve preformed cavities as fungus balls with their radiological picture present very similar to that of aspergilloma. Among COVID-19 patients cavities may otherwise be formed without pre-existing one and have a rapid and fulminant course.

CUTANEOUS TYPE

The cutaneous manifestations are not commonly found among the COVID-19 patients but otherwise these are varied and range from pustules or vesicles to wounds with wider areas of necrotic zones. In their early stages, lesions resemble ecthyma gangrenosum; cotton-like growth may be seen over surface of tissues, a clinical sign known as "hairy pus." The cutaneous type of mucormycosis can be either primary infection or secondary to the disseminated form. It is relatively benign form of disease in comparison to the other clinical types. The primary cutaneous lesions have rarely been reported which is due to direct inoculation of fungus into skin. It usually occurs among patients with severe burns, superficial ulcers in diabetic patients, gangrenous cellulitis in trauma patients, and infections associated with contaminated elasticized wound dressings. The lesions are painful; progressively enlarge with nodular ecchymotic areas of cutaneous infarction. Necrotizing fasciitis may be secondary to cutaneous or subcutaneous mucormycosis and has a very high mortality (**Fig. 3**).

The histopathological examination shows focal necrosis of parenchyma and adipose tissue. The biopsy and culture of skin lesions should be performed as early as possible, which is the diagnostic procedure of choice in this disease. *Lichtheimia corymbifera* and *Saksenaea vasiformis* have also been reported in cutaneous mucormycosis particularly among diabetic patients. The primary cutaneous mucormycosis caused by *S. vasiformis* and *Apophysomyces variabilis* should be suspected when blistering, necrotic lesions develop within a few days of traumatic injury due to potential contamination of wound with dust or soil. Cutaneous mucormycosis has a much more favorable prognosis than more deeply invasive forms but it is still associated with significant fatality and long-term morbidity. This may also be observed as a manifestation of disseminated disease in patients with leukemia.

GASTROINTESTINAL TYPE

Very rarely gangrenous lesions of intestine are reported among the COVID-19 patients due to mucormycosis. Some of the cases have recently been encountered from Rajkot in Gujarat. As such this type occurs in general accounting for about 7% of all cases of mucormycosis, most often involving stomach. It is primarily found among patients suffering from extreme malnutrition and is acquired by ingesting food contaminated with fungal spores. Ingestion of fermented milk, porridge and alcohol made from corn, and herbal products have been implicated in gastrointestinal mucormycosis. The lesions in stomach are followed by colon, ileum, and esophagus. This may follow surgery from filthy trauma to abdomen or contaminated ileostomy. Ulceration of gastric mucosa with thrombosis of associated vessels has been observed. The disease is usually found in adult patients but has also been reported in children.

In this type, Mucormycetes fungi either colonize or invade gastric mucosa. In invasive variant, there is involvement of vessel walls producing thrombosis, hemorrhage, necrosis, and ulceration of local tissue and usually has a fatal outcome. Intestinal tract involvement is rare with terminal ileum, cecum, and colon being the primarily affected sites.

The signs and symptoms of abdominal mucormycosis vary considerably and depend on site as well as extent of involvement. These are nonspecific such as abdominal pain, diarrhea, hematemesis, and melena. The patients on dialysis are reported to develop mucormycosis as most of them are treated with desferrioxamine (deferoxamine and desferal) used as chelator for either iron or aluminum and may be for both.

Earlier, diagnosis of gastric mucormycosis used to be made on the basis of postmortem examination and was rarely feasible during life. More recently, endoscopic biopsies have established diagnosis at an earlier stage, allowing attempt to a successful treatment. Gastric brushing is less invasive than biopsy and allows early identification of organisms as compared to histopathological processing. A very similar type of disease is caused by *Basidiobolus ranarum*, members of order Entomophthorales, which is very rare clinical entity and > 80 cases have been reported.

ISOLATED RENAL TYPE

The isolated renal mucormycosis is also not commonly seen with COVID-19 and is one of the emerging clinical entities, which is an unusual cause of renal infarction and may be fatal if not timely detected. Any of the species of Mucorales may infect the kidneys. The patients usually present with flank pain, fever, and pyuria. In due course of time, there is infarct of renal tissue leading to hematuria. Most of these patients are presumed to be suffering from bacterial pyelonephritis hence do not respond to routinely prescribed antibacterial antibiotics. In the immunocompromised patients, there are clinical features of acute pyelonephritis. There is renal enlargement with or without perinephric collection on ultrasonography. In such a situation, contrast-enhanced CT or MRI is indicated to have more clearer view. In case of infarction or multiple abscesses in parenchyma, renal biopsy is indicated to establish tissue diagnosis. A combination of aggressive surgical and medical treatment may improve the outcome of patients. The overall survival of isolated renal mucormycosis is around 65% and mortality is almost cent percent for those who have not undergone nephrectomy. Therefore, a high index of suspicion and awareness among clinicians about the protean manifestations of mucormycosis is significant to establish timely and proper diagnosis of such a fatal condition.

DISSEMINATED TYPE

If the COVID-19 advances, Mucormycetes may become widely disseminated affecting lungs, kidney, gastrointestinal tract, heart, and brain, however, lungs being the most commonly involved site. The clinical syndromes most frequently reported include pneumonia, stroke, subarachnoid hemorrhage, brain abscess, cellulitis, or gangrene of a skin structure. In addition, gastrointestinal bleeding, peritonitis, acute myocardial infarction, hepatitis, and superior vena cava syndrome have been related to mucormycosis. The vessel invasion with infarction of surrounding parenchyma is seen with a striking absence of inflammatory cells; however, antemortem diagnosis is very rare. In cardiac patients, ultrastructural studies have revealed presence of a thick-walled fungus that participates in formation of thrombus, which crosses coronary arteries in a "corkscrew" pattern. Thin-walled branching structures are also observed occluding microcirculation of preserved cardiac areas. These structures could be plasma membranes left after fungus loses its thick wall.

The portal of entry into human body is probably through traumatized skin followed by invasion of blood vessels and dissemination to body organs. This has been reported with infections caused by *A. elegans*, *S. vasiformis*, and *Rhizopus* species. Cerebral dissemination is caused by hematogenous and lymphogenous seeding by abscess formation, particularly in intravenous drug abusers. In mucormycotic aneurysms (cerebral), numerous nonseptate hyphae are seen obstructing cerebral arteries. There is formation of perinephric abscess also that can be visualized on ultrasonography, CT, or MRI. Other infections without rhinocerebral involvement may occur in severely immunocompromised patients.

DIFFERENTIAL DIAGNOSIS

Rhinocerebral mucormycosis is an acute and distinctive condition, but it can be confused with cavernous sinus thrombosis, bacterial orbital cellulitis or rhinocerebral aspergillosis or scedosporiosis. Clinically, pulmonary mucormycosis cannot be distinguished from gram-negative bacterial pneumonia, aspergillosis, or scedosporiosis. The histopathological examination is useful in establishing the correct diagnosis.

The cutaneous and subcutaneous lesions caused by oomycetes like *Pythium insidiosum* are invariably confused with mucormycosis. However, hyphae are intensely stained with periodic acid-Schiff (PAS) than hematoxylin and eosin (H&E) in case of pythiosis insidiosi, which is other way round in mucormycosis and is helpful in differentiation of the similar looking pseudofungal clinical entity.

DIAGNOSIS

RADIOLOGICAL FINDINGS

It has recently been established that CT and particularly MRI are most helpful in enabling an early detection of orbital, sinus, meningeal, intraparenchymal, and cerebral lesions as well as intracranial vascular occlusion, even before clinical signs develop. T1- and T2-weighted images are taken to know the extent of lesions. These imaging techniques are helpful in defining extent of soft tissue and bone destruction and are more useful in planning surgical intervention in addition to establishing the diagnosis.

LABORATORY FINDINGS

A thorough knowledge of mucormycosis with high index of suspicion is of paramount importance to establish an early diagnosis thereby appropriate treatment. The diagnosis of rhinocerebral mucormycosis is challenging and that too in COVID-19 times because of rapid fulminating course of disease and doubtful significance of isolates, which are commonly encountered as laboratory contaminants also. One has to compete with the race of time. Therefore, detection of fungus in tissues is supplemented to establish significance of cultural isolate. The clinical materials from infected site, nasal discharge, or sputum may contain fungal elements; however, deeper tissue section may also be required. Detection of galactomannan or β-glucans in patients' serum, which is often helpful in diagnosis of other systemic fungal infection, is of little value because Mucormycetes produce very minute GM or β-glucan.

Direct fungal examination: The microscopic examination of nasal discharge or biopsy material in potassium hydroxide/calcofluor-white (KOH/CFW) wet mount shows characteristic broad, nonseptate, ribbon-like hyphae with wide-angle or right-angle branching at irregular intervals (**Figs. 4** and **5**). These hyphae usually are very sparsely distributed in infected tissue and therefore special fungal stains are mandatory like H&E, PAS (**Figs. 6** and **7**), and Gomori's methenamine silver (GMS). These Mucormycetes are poorly stained with PAS, Gridley, and Gram stains but very well seen in H&E and GMS stain. The inflammatory response is of neutrophilic nature and is associated with infarct, vascular, and perineural invasion. Sometimes, distorted hyphae are also seen in the tissues. The disease has also been established on the basis of fine-needle aspiration cytology from the affected site like in case of isolated renal mucormycosis.

The hyphal elements of Mucormycetes can be recognized as nonseptate thick-walled (10–20 μm across) hyphae, with wide-angle branching. Due to absence of cross-walls, fluids from hyphae are free to escape during handling of tissues, hyphae collapse, and crinkle giving characteristic ribbon-like appearance. They do not radiate from a single point in tissue. These features distinguish them from slender hyphae of *Aspergillus* species, which have regular dichotomous branching with frequent septation. Therefore, it is recommended not to homogenize tissue material and specimens must be directly inoculated on to culture media to keep viability of fungal cells.

Culture of fungi: As stated above, the hyphal elements of Mucormycetes are prone to physical damage; therefore, specimens must be directly inoculated onto fungal culture media avoiding undue grinding. The relevance of isolates in clinical material may be difficult to establish if coenocytic hyphal elements are not seen in direct examination of KOH/CFW wet mount or histopathological section. Hence, repeated trial to isolate organism from consecutive specimens provides strong evidence that isolate may be clinically significant.

The Mucormycetes can be easily grown on conventional media like Sabouraud dextrose agar (SDA) with antibiotics at both temperatures, i.e., 25°C and 37°C. The Mucorales grow on standard fungal culture media without cycloheximide, as it is inhibitory to most of them except *Apophysomyces* species. Although the Mucormycetes are not fastidious fungi still sometimes they fail to grow during primary isolation. Therefore, to avoid growth failure, some portion of tissue may be kept in water added with a few drops of Malt Yeast Broth. In about 50% of cases there is no growth despite direct demonstration of the fungi. In such circumstance, it is better to do molecular technique directly from the sample and the diagnosis can be established.

The rapidly growing mycelial colonies are floccose, dense, and have hairy appearance. The mycelia are described as fibrous or cotton-candy growth, which is very vigorous hence some of Mucormycetes of order Mucorales are called as "lid-lifters" as they press upon lid of Petri dish from below (**Fig. 8**). The isolate is identified on the basis of morphological features observed in lactophenol cotton blue (LCB) mount followed by molecular sequencing for confirmation (**Fig. 9**). The antifungal susceptibility testing is also done to establish

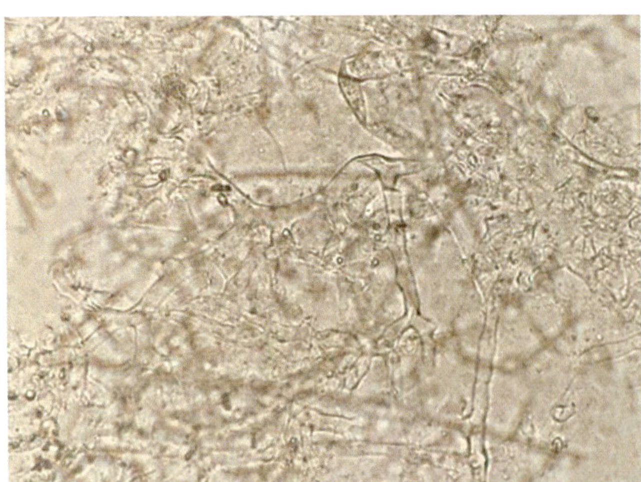

(KOH: Potassium hydroxide)

FIGURE 4: Broad, ribbon-like, nonseptate hyphae with wide angle branching seen in wet mount (KOH × 400).

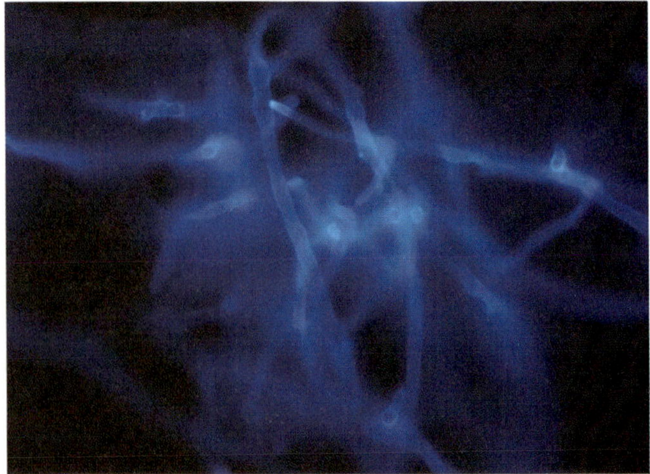

(CFW: Calcofluor-white)

FIGURE 5: Broad, ribbon-like, nonseptate hyphae with wide angle branching seen in wet mount (CFW × 400).

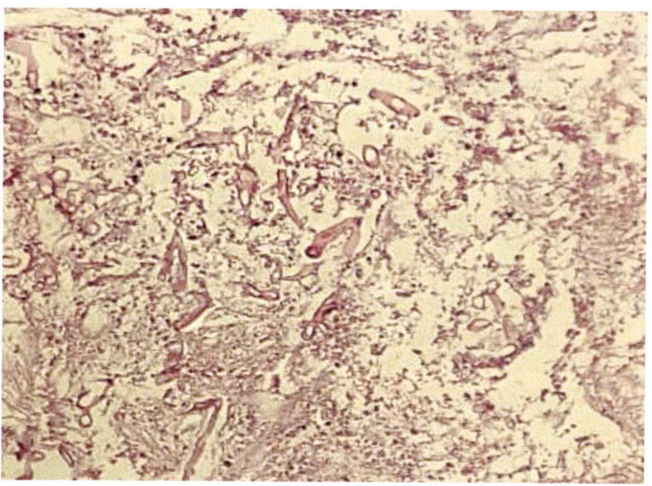

(H&E: Hematoxylin and Eosin)

FIGURE 6: Nonseptate hyphae of Mucormycetes with wide-angle branching in a tissue sections (H&E × 400).

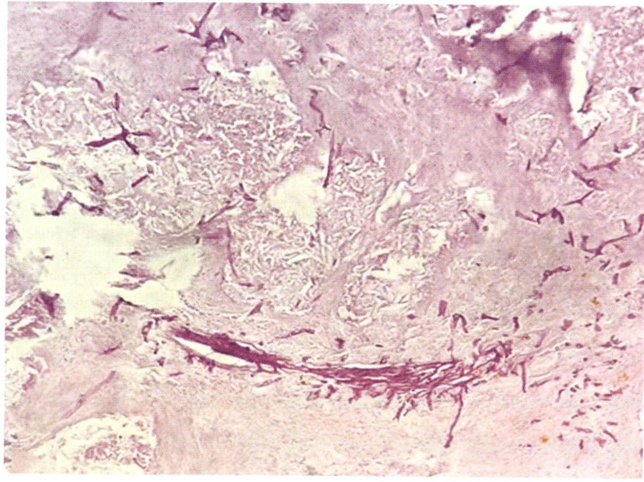

(PAS: Periodic acid–Schiff)

FIGURE 7: Nonseptate hyphae of Mucormycetes with wide-angle branching in a tissue sections (PAS × 200).

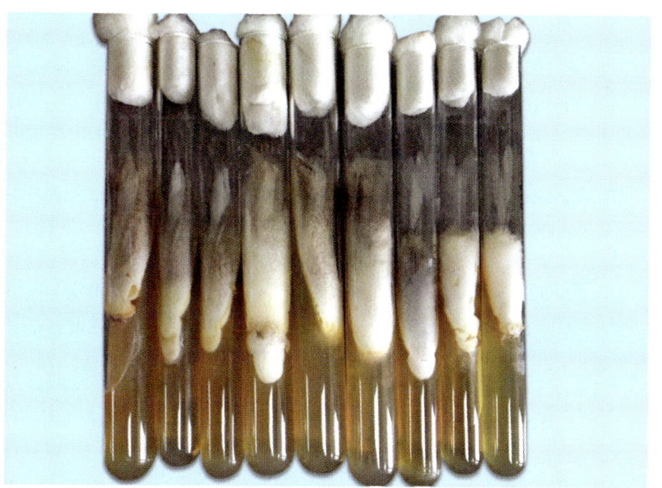

FIGURE 8: Grayish mycelial growth of *Rhizopus arrhizus* in multiple tubes after 3 days of incubation on Sabouraud dextrose agar (SDA).

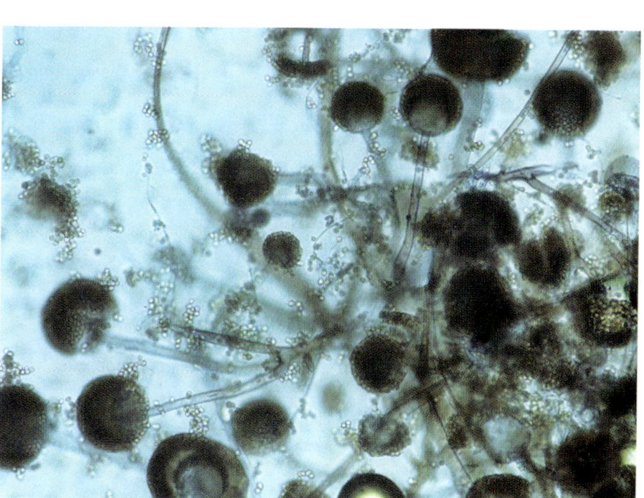

(LCB: Lactophenol cotton blue)

FIGURE 9: Nonseptate hyphae of *Rhizopus* species with rhizoids, sporangia, and sporangiospores (LCB × 400).

whether the isolate is sensitive to a particular drug or not using CLSI or EUCAST methods.

As such there is no satisfactory serological procedure, which can be relied upon to establish final diagnosis of any of clinical forms of mucormycosis or their causative fungal agents. In a study serological diagnosis of antibody production is 73% sensitive and 100% specific when using homogenate antigens. The serological cross-reactions have been reported among other potentially pathogenic species. Ouchterlony technique of patients' serum demonstrates multiple precipitation bands against cytoplasmic antigen prepared from *B. ranarum* isolate. The enzyme-linked immunosorbent assay (ELISA) may also be performed to detect antibodies produced in invasive types of infections. However, serodiagnosis of mucormycosis still remains investigational and cannot yet be recommended for the routine use in a diagnostic microbiology laboratory.

TREATMENT OF MUCORMYCOSIS

Proper management of COVID-19 infection is to be instituted, *depending on the stage and severity* of the disease, with all prescribed precautions. Try to avoid steroids therapy as far as possible. However, if indicated then regulated dose to be given for a minimum time period. Immediately remove all the risk factors like diabetes mellitus by starting insulin or other antidiabetic regimens. Mucormycosis is an increasingly emerging fungal infection with a formidable mortality in otherwise normal circumstances and particularly during COVID-19. Physicians/surgeons do not normally contemplate fungi with necrotizing infections entailing delay in diagnosis thereby rapid progression of the undergoing infection, may go to the irreversible level. Hence, there is a need for creating awareness among the clinicians to have high index of suspicion to establish appropriate diagnosis at an early stage of the fungal disease so that specific treatment can be instituted well in time.

During this pandemic of COVID-19, WHO, ISHAM, ECMM, and ICMR/GOI have issued clinical guidelines for the diagnosis and management of mucormycosis. The consensus has been derived from experiences of clinicians treating such cases. As mucormycosis is a life-threatening condition, hence invariably it proves to be fatal within a very short span, particularly when specific diagnosis is not established well in time thereby leading to a delay in surgery as well as institution of proper antifungal regimen.

The therapy can be divided in *four concurrent approaches*. These are: (1) Rapid correction of underlying predisposing condition of the host like diabetic ketoacidosis using insulin; (2) Surgical debridement of necrotizing tissue for better circulation and penetration of drugs; (3) Antifungal therapy; and (4) Consideration of adjunctive treatment such as hyperbaric oxygen. A combination of surgical debridement and antifungal drugs is required for an ideal treatment of mucormycosis. The temptation for small daily piecemeal type bedside debridement should be avoided, which further aggravates morbidity and mortality among the patients. It should be preferably done under general anesthesia taking adequate surrounding healthy tissue for debridement.

There are *only three drugs*, which are available for treating mucormycosis, i.e., intravenous amphotericin B (conventional/liposomal), posaconazole, and isavuconazole. It is observed to start with higher doses of antifungal drugs instead of stepwise increment. Drug resistance may be another hurdle but in case of majority of mucormycetes strains, these are found to be sensitive. Surgical debridement is the mainstay of therapy for mucormycosis. Topical amphotericin B gel is a useful adjunct, which is applied locally after surgery, with a gauge. Skin grafting or denture application to repair defects remaining after surgical debridement is usually successful.

The azole derivatives are not useful in treating mucormycosis due to lack of both *in vivo* and *in vitro* antifungal activity. However, posaconazole and isavuconazole are found useful, which are available for oral as well as intravenous use. Some of the azole, like voriconazole, is otherwise counterproductive which enhances the disease process in a mucormycosis patient. Similarly, echinocandins have no role in the treatment and there is no oral chemoprophylactic agent available for this fungal disease. Cytokines such as gamma interferon and granulocyte-macrophage colony-stimulating factors have also been used to treat mucormycosis.

Most of the times, the guidelines prove to be toothless because there is nothing mandatory. Hence, keeping in view of the rapid and devastating course of mucormycosis, every institution should resort to its local mandatory protocol, wherein KOH/CFW wet mount should be performed within half an hour of the arrival of suspected patient followed by surgical debridement within 2 hours. If this promptness is adopted, the patients may not require antifungal drugs also, which are now in scarcity due to increased demand. However, antifungal regimen is to be instituted as per the clinical and financial condition of the patient. If such measures are not followed in letter and spirit one is bound to lose the patient of a simply treatable disease. All the COVID-19 patients should be made cautious at the time of discharge that they should check and regulate their sugar level at least for a period of 4–6 weeks.

RECOMMENDED READINGS

1. Alvarez E, Stchigel AM, Cano J, Sutton DA, Fothergill AW, Chander J, et al. Molecular phylogenetic diversity of the emerging mucoralean fungus *Apophysomyces*: Proposal of three new species. Rev Iberoam Micol. 2010;27:80-9.
2. Chander J, Singla N, Kaur M, Punia RS, Attri A, Alastruey-Izquierdo A, et al. *Saksenaea erythrospora*, an emerging mucoralean fungus causing severe necrotizing skin and soft tissue infections—A study from a tertiary care hospital in north India. Infect Dis (Lond). 2017;49:170-7.
3. Chander J. Textbook of Medical Mycology, 4th edition. New Delhi: Jaypee Brothers Medical Publishers (P) Ltd.; 2018.
4. Garg D, Muthu V, Sehgal IS, Ramachandran R, Kaur H, Bhalla A, et al. Coronavirus Disease (COVID-19) Associated Mucormycosis (CAM): Case report and systematic review of literature. Mycopathologia. 2021;186:289-98.
5. Mehta S, Pandey A. Rhino-orbital mucormycosis associated with COVID-19. Cureus. 2020;12:e10726.
6. Monte Junior ESD, Santos MELD, Ribeiro IB, Luz GO, Baba ER, Hirsch BS, et al. Rare and fatal gastrointestinal mucormycosis (zygomycosis) in a COVID-19 patient: A case report. Clin Endosc. 2020;53:746-9.
7. Revannavar SM, Supriya PS, Samaga L, Vineeth VK. COVID-19 triggering mucormycosis in a susceptible patient: A new phenomenon in the developing world? BMJ Case Rep. 2021;14:e241663.
8. Saldanha M, Reddy R, Vincent MJ. Paranasal mucormycosis in COVID-19 patient. Indian J Otolaryngol Head Neck Surg. 2021;22:1-4.
9. Sarkar S, Gokhale T, Choudhury SS, Deb AK. COVID-19 and orbital mucormycosis. Indian J Ophthalmol. 2021;69:1002-4.
10. Sen M, Honavar SG, Sharma N, Sachdev MS. COVID-19 and Eye: A review of ophthalmic manifestations of COVID-19. Indian J Ophthalmol. 2021;69:488-509.
11. Sen M, Lahane S, Lahane TP, Parekh R, Honavar SG. Mucor in a viral land: A tale of two pathogens. Indian J Ophthalmol. 2021;69:244-52.
12. Sharma S, Grover M, Bhargava S, Samdani S, Kataria T. Post coronavirus disease mucormycosis: A deadly addition to the pandemic spectrum. J Laryngol Otol. 2021;8:1-6.
13. Sutton DA, Stchigel AM, Chander J, Guarro J, Cano-Lira JF. *Saksenaea loutrophoriformis*. Fungal Planet. 2017;38:558-624.
14. Szarpak L, Chirico F, Pruc M, Szarpak L, Dzieciatkowski T, Rafique Z. Mucormycosis—A serious threat in the COVID-19 pandemic? J Infect. 2021 May 21:S0163-4453(21)00257-7.

CHAPTER

57

COVID-19 Vaccines

Savita Verma, Jyoti Sharma

ABSTRACT

The severe acute respiratory syndrome coronavirus 2 (SARS-CoV-2) pandemic has severely ravaged health systems and economic and social progress globally. While the most serious threat from infection includes acute respiratory distress syndrome, multiorgan failure, and death, the long-term sequelae from mild disease have also caused devastation. Vaccination constitutes the most promising path to protect against severe disease and preferably drive herd immunity to halt transmission of the virus. In response to the pandemic, the vaccine development process has been fast-tracked. Many SARS-CoV-2 vaccines have been authorized or approved for emergency use within last 1 year and more are expected to be licensed in 2021.

Coronavirus disease 2019 (COVID-19) vaccines are novel in terms of specificity, their manufacturing platforms like messenger ribonucleic acid (mRNA) and rapid and widespread use across the global population. But having licensed vaccines is not enough to achieve global control of COVID-19; they also need to be produced at a large scale, at affordable price, and allocated globally for equitable distribution of the vaccines. This chapter discusses regarding COVID-19 vaccine candidates authorized/approved or in development, technology behind them, triggering of innate immunity for durable immunological memory and the future implications of protecting populations with these vaccines.

"The art of progress is to preserve order amid change and to preserve change amid order"

—Alfred N Whitehead

INTRODUCTION

Coronavirus disease 2019 is an infectious disease caused by newly discovered coronavirus (CoV) now named as the SARS-CoV-2, which has spread rapidly throughout the world. In March 2020, COVID-19 outbreak was declared as a pandemic by the World Health Organization (WHO). This pandemic has severely ravaged health systems and economic and social progress globally. There are about 113,820,168 million confirmed COVID-19 cases and 2,527,891 deaths reported worldwide (WHO).

The COVID-19 pandemic is unlikely to end until there is a global rollout of vaccines that protect against severe disease and preferably drive herd immunity to halt transmission of the virus. Although strong measures such as social distancing, better diagnostics, and treatment facilities have been adopted to contain the spread of COVID-19 by many countries including India, but the spread of the disease can only be prevented by enhancing a lasting immunity through vaccines. The process of development of COVID-19 vaccines has been fast-tracked in response to pandemic. Globally, over 300 candidate vaccines are in different stages of development. Drug Controller General of India (DCGI) has given permission for restricted use of two COVID-19 vaccines in the first week of January 2021; Covishield, a recombinant vaccine in collaboration of Serum Institute of India and AstraZeneca and Covaxin, a killed vaccine indigenously produced by Bharat Biotech Ltd. On 16th January, 2021 the COVID-19 vaccine drive was launched in India.

Coronavirus disease 2019 vaccines are novel in terms of specificity, their manufacturing platforms like mRNA and rapid and widespread use across the global population. But having licensed vaccines is not enough to achieve global control of COVID-19; they also need to be produced at a large scale, at affordable price, and allocated globally for equitable distribution of the vaccines. This chapter discusses regarding COVID-19 vaccine candidates authorized/approved or in development, technology behind them, triggering of innate immunity to promote durable immunological memory, and the future implications of protecting populations with these vaccines.

STRUCTURE OF CORONAVIRUS

Coronavirus is a spherical or pleomorphic enveloped particle containing single-stranded (positive-sense) RNA associated with a nucleoprotein within a capsid comprised of matrix protein. The envelope bears club-shaped glycoprotein projections. Some coronaviruses also contain a hemagglutinin esterase (HE) protein. The structure of SARS-CoV-2 consists of the following: A spike protein (S), HE dimer, a membrane glycoprotein (M), an envelope protein (E) a nucleocapsid protein (N), and RNA as seen in the **Figure 1 in chapter 54**.

Coronaviruses are zoonotic and are transmitted between animals and humans. Coronaviruses cause diseases such as the Middle East respiratory syndrome (MERS) and severe acute respiratory syndrome (SARS) and more mild illnesses including the common cold. The most common signs of infection with COVID-19 include fever, dry cough, shortness of breath or difficulty in breathing, and tiredness or fatigue. Most people have mild disease and recover without requiring hospitalization. However, globally, around 20% of people who contract COVID-19 become more seriously ill and require hospitalization and intensive care facilities. In more severe cases, the infection can cause pneumonia, SARS, kidney failure, and even lead to death.

COVID-19 VACCINE DEVELOPMENT

CHALLENGES

New vaccine development for COVID-19 was challenging as the reference reagents such as antibodies, reference vaccine for testing, and virus strain suitable for vaccine development were not available. Hence fundamental work was required to qualify, any virus strain to be used as a vaccine strain. Extensive validation was required to qualify primary in-house reference reagents. However, the most challenging aspect of a new vaccine development is the derivation and rationalization of vaccine doses for clinical testing. The use of different platform technologies rendered comparison of protective correlates induced by the different candidate vaccines difficult to assess.

Multiple platforms are being used and many more are under development for COVID-19 vaccines. Among those with the greatest potential for speed are DNA (deoxyribonucleic acid) and RNA-based platforms, followed by those for developing recombinant-subunit vaccines. Both DNA and messenger RNA (mRNA) encode production of the SARS-CoV-2 spike (S) protein, which is the primary target for neutralizing antibodies generated from natural infection. RNA and DNA vaccines can be made quickly because they require no culture or fermentation, instead use synthetic processes.

PACE OF DEVELOPMENT

Several factors have enabled the rapid development of COVID-19 vaccines:

- The role of the spike protein in causing pathogenesis of CoV was established;
- The knowledge that neutralizing antibodies against these spike proteins play an important role in providing immunity;
- Nucleic acid vaccine technology platforms were already in place which can create vaccines and manufacture thousands of doses quickly once a genetic sequence of virus is known;
- Information that the development activities can be conducted in parallel, rather than sequentially, without increasing risks for study participants.

IMMUNE ACTIVATION

A vaccine exposes the body to an antigen that does not cause disease but provides an adaptive immune response that can block or kill the virus if a person becomes infected similar to the actual infection (**Fig. 1**). For generation of adaptive immunity, a vaccine requires an antigen which is pathogen-specific and an adjuvant which stimulates the innate immune system and provides the necessary second signal for T cell activation without inducing systemic inflammation that can lead to severe side effects. For example, in mRNA vaccines, the mRNA can serve as both antigen (encoding the viral protein) and adjuvant. Early trials results show that COVID-19 vaccines generate virus-specific neutralizing antibody titers for several months postvaccination, while virus-specific T cell responses remain to be fully elucidated.

PROCESS OF DEVELOPMENT

The development of a vaccine is a time-consuming process that traditionally takes 10–15 years from project start and initial discovery until the final approval of a new product and includes various phases done in sequential manner as shown in **Figure 2**. However, due to urgent demand of COVID-19 vaccines, the development process has been fast-tracked; intense global efforts in research and development activity around the world have been triggered to accelerate the development of these vaccines. There has been more international scientific and development cooperation, early sharing of vaccine protocols and data results, intensive planning activities for clinical trials (like rapid enrollment of participants), fast-track regulatory programs (like special committees for COVID-19), Public-Private-partnerships (increased financial support), frequent discussions and alignment with regulatory agencies and simultaneous manufacturing which has helped in rapid COVID-19 vaccine development and ensured that various phases of the trials are going on simultaneously in parallel (**Fig. 2**).

VACCINES FOR COVID-19

Different types of vaccines work by different mechanisms but the underlying process with all vaccines is to produce "memory" T-lymphocytes and B-lymphocytes that help the body to fight against the virus whenever it attacks in the future. The potential COVID-19 vaccine targets could be whole cell antigen (WCA), spike protein (S protein) (the full-length S protein, RBD, NTD, S1 subunit, FP), nucleocapsid protein (N protein), membrane protein (M protein), or envelope protein (E protein). The COVID-19 vaccines under development are using various scientific techniques which have been categorized into four groups (**Figs. 3 A and B**).

Virus vaccines: These vaccines use the virus itself in a weakened or inactivated form. Vaccines against measles and polio (oral) are made in this manner. Weakened virus and inactivated virus vaccines are the two types of vaccines under development in this category.

Viral vector vaccines: In the development of these vaccines, a virus (such as AdV or measles), is genetically engineered to produce CoV proteins in the body, but the virus is weakened (can replicate within cells) and nonreplicating viral vector (cannot replicate within cells).

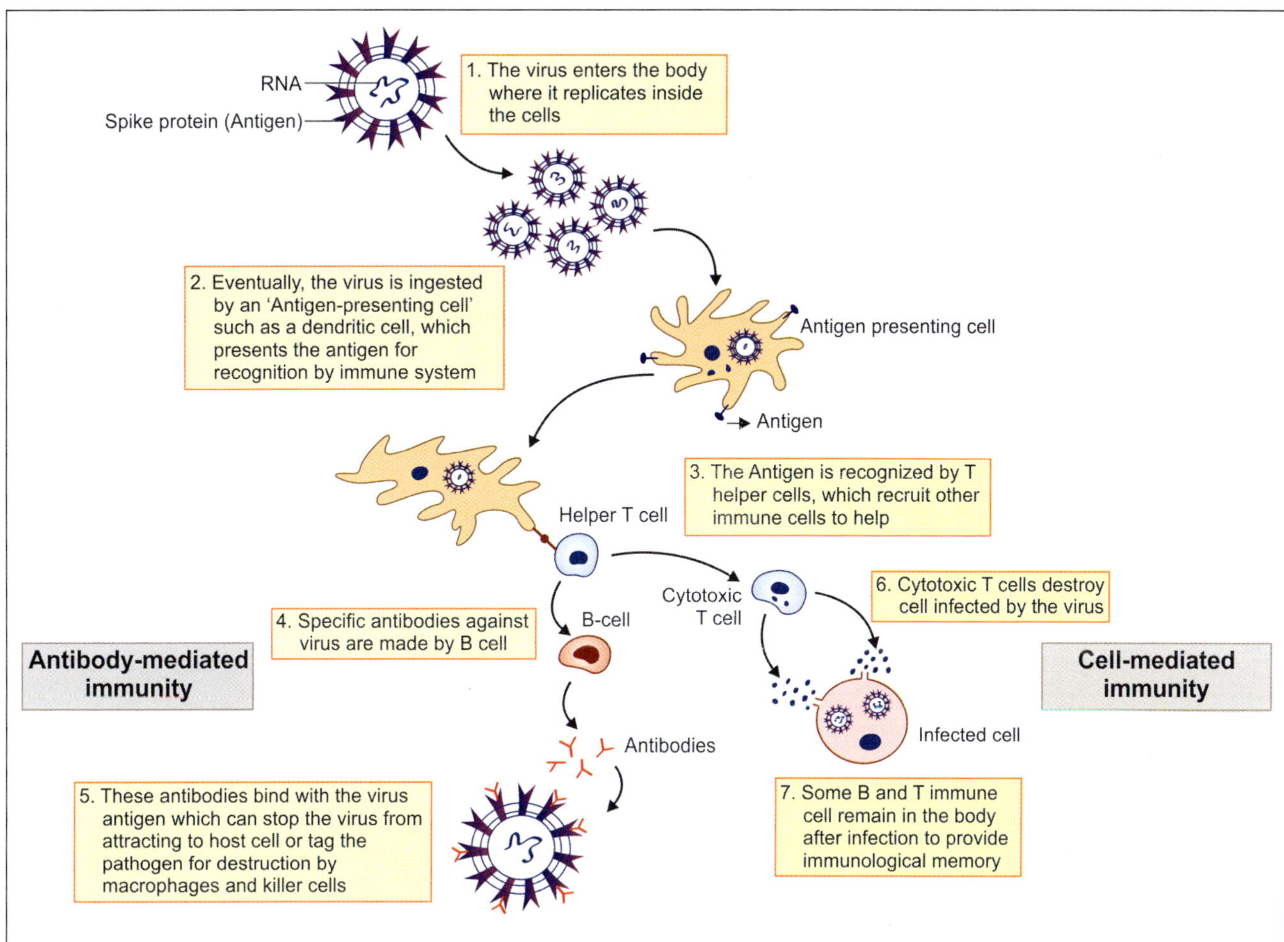

FIGURE 1: Immune activation with coronavirus disease 2019 vaccine.

Nucleic acid vaccines: In these vaccines, nucleic acid (DNA or RNA) is inserted into human cells. These human cells then produce copies of the virus protein which produces an immune response. DNA vaccine and RNA vaccine are the two types of vaccines under development in this category.

Protein-based vaccines: These vaccines use virus protein fragments or protein shells which are injected directly into the body. The two types of protein-based vaccines being developed against the CoV are the protein subunit vaccines and virus-like particle vaccines.

Vaccines which have been developed for COVID-19 have certain common characteristics which are as follows:

- Most are liquid products (few are freeze-dried)
- Majority are given as intramuscular injection
- Majority have two-dose schedule; 21–28 days apart
- Most vaccines are provided in a multidose vial
- Most vaccines have a targeted temperature range of 2–8°C; however some have temperature requirements of –60°C and a shorter life.

APPROVED/AUTHORIZED VACCINES

As of 1st March 2021, at least 11 different vaccines across the four platforms have been authorized/approved for emergency/restricted use in different countries (**Table 1**). More than a dozen countries have already initiated mass vaccination against COVID-19. Vulnerable populations in all countries are the highest priority for vaccination. There are more than 300 additional vaccine candidates under development—including many with new mechanisms of action—that could prove to be effective and cheaper and easier to distribute, of which more than 60 are in clinical trials.

A brief note of the two vaccines available in India with contraindications, possible side effects and experience so far is desirable.

VACCINES AVAILABLE IN INDIA

Two vaccines produced in India, "COVISHIELD" and "COVAXIN," have been authorized for restricted use in India in the first week of January 2021. India launched its vaccine drive, the world's largest inoculation effort, in early January across 3,006 vaccination centers. It has vaccinated nearly 30 million people so far—healthcare and frontline workers were given priority in the first phase. According to health officials, India has administered 3,71,43,255 vaccine doses across the country as of 16 March, 2021. People over 60 years and those who are between 45 and 59 years but have other illnesses are now getting vaccinated. The government

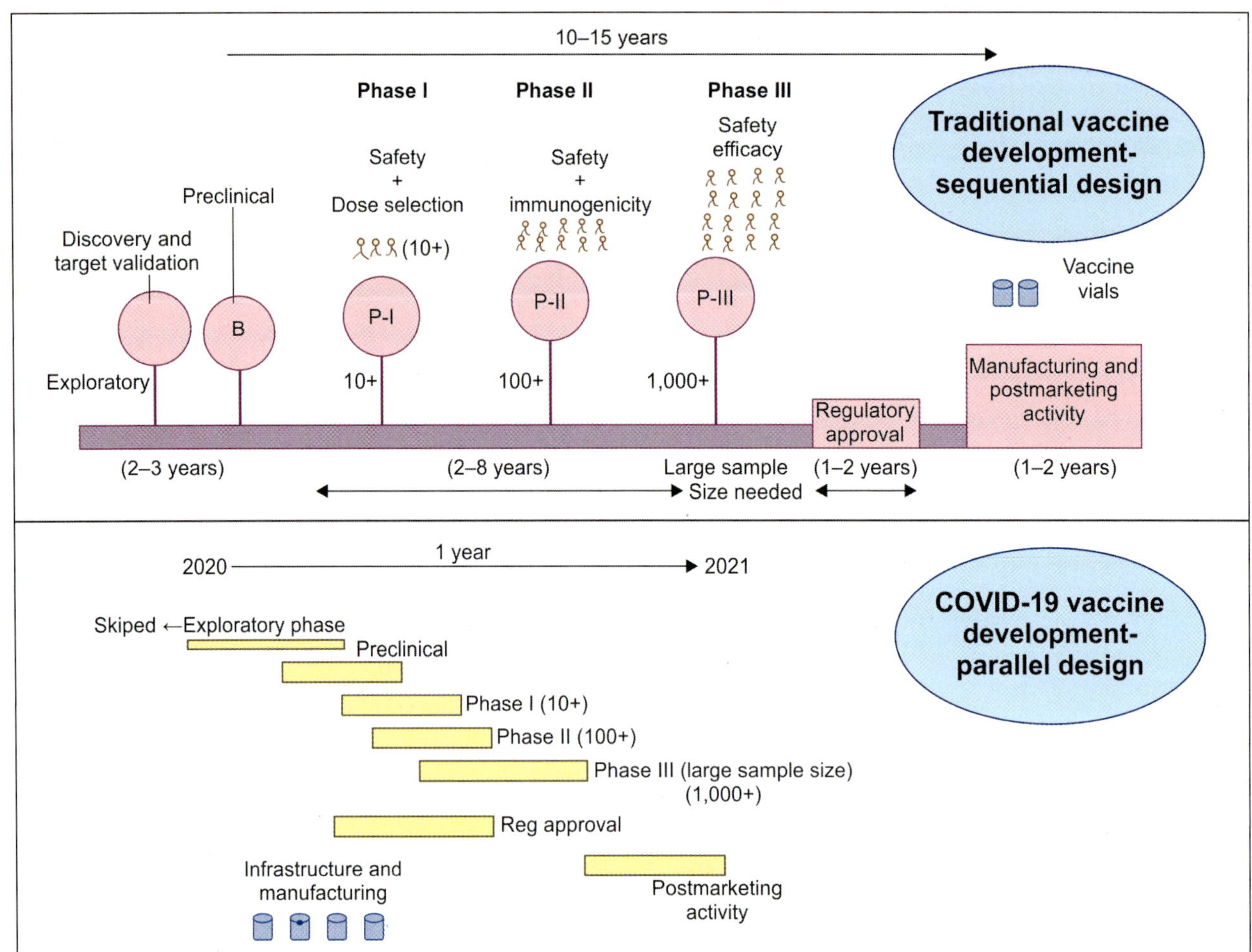

FIGURE 2: Traditional versus coronavirus disease 2019 (COVID-19) vaccine development.

aims to cover 250 million "priority people" by the end of July 2021. The country is a vaccine powerhouse; it makes 60% of the world's vaccines and is home to half a dozen major manufacturers.

The characteristics of the two vaccines have been depicted in **Table 2.**

COVAXIN is an indigenous COVID-19 vaccine made in India. This is an inactivated vaccine which is developed and manufactured in Bharat Biotech's BSL-3 (Bio-Safety Level 3) high containment facility and uses a tried and tested technology platform used by other vaccines like polio vaccine. It can produce antibodies against many regions of the complete virus. Since this vaccine contains a full inactivated virus with all its 29 proteins intact, the immunity provoked by it is expected to be more comprehensive and closer to natural immunity arising out of an infection. However, these vaccines require an adjuvant to provoke immunity. For this purpose, alum is commonly used which mainly provokes Th-2 type immunity which also leads to more side effects. Hence, Bharat Biotech has used an alternative adjuvant "Algel-IMDG (imidazoquinolinone)" which stimulates Th-1 type immunity that is also generated by mRNA/DNA vaccines. On 3 March, 2021, interim results of Phase III trial of COVAXIN which is being conducted on 25,600 participants in India has shown an efficacy of 81%.

COVISHIELD, the Oxford-AstraZeneca vaccine, is being manufactured locally by the Serum Institute of India (SII), the world's largest vaccine manufacturer. The vaccine is made from a weakened version of a common cold virus (known as an adenovirus) from chimpanzees. It has been modified to look more like coronavirus—although it cannot cause illness. This vaccine produces antibodies against only a specific region of the virus. It contains a portion of the DNA that codes for the spike protein (S-protein). Once inside the cells, the DNA part first needs to enter the nucleus to create its mirror image (complementary RNA). Then this RNA comes out in the cytoplasm as a messenger and starts making S-protein through a machine available for this purpose called ribosome. Since it is S-protein that provokes immunity it may not be as close to natural immunity as created by COVAXIN. Any long-term side effects of the DNA material remaining inside the nucleus (e.g., integration in human DNA) are not known yet. So far, DNA vaccines were only being tried out for treating cancer patients and never used for preventing infections in normal subjects.

Sputnik V is the first foreign vaccine to be granted restricted use authorization based on the results of the clinical trials in Russia as well as local Phase III clinical trial in India; while COVID-19 vaccines like Moderna and Pfizer have been granted restricted emergency use authorization

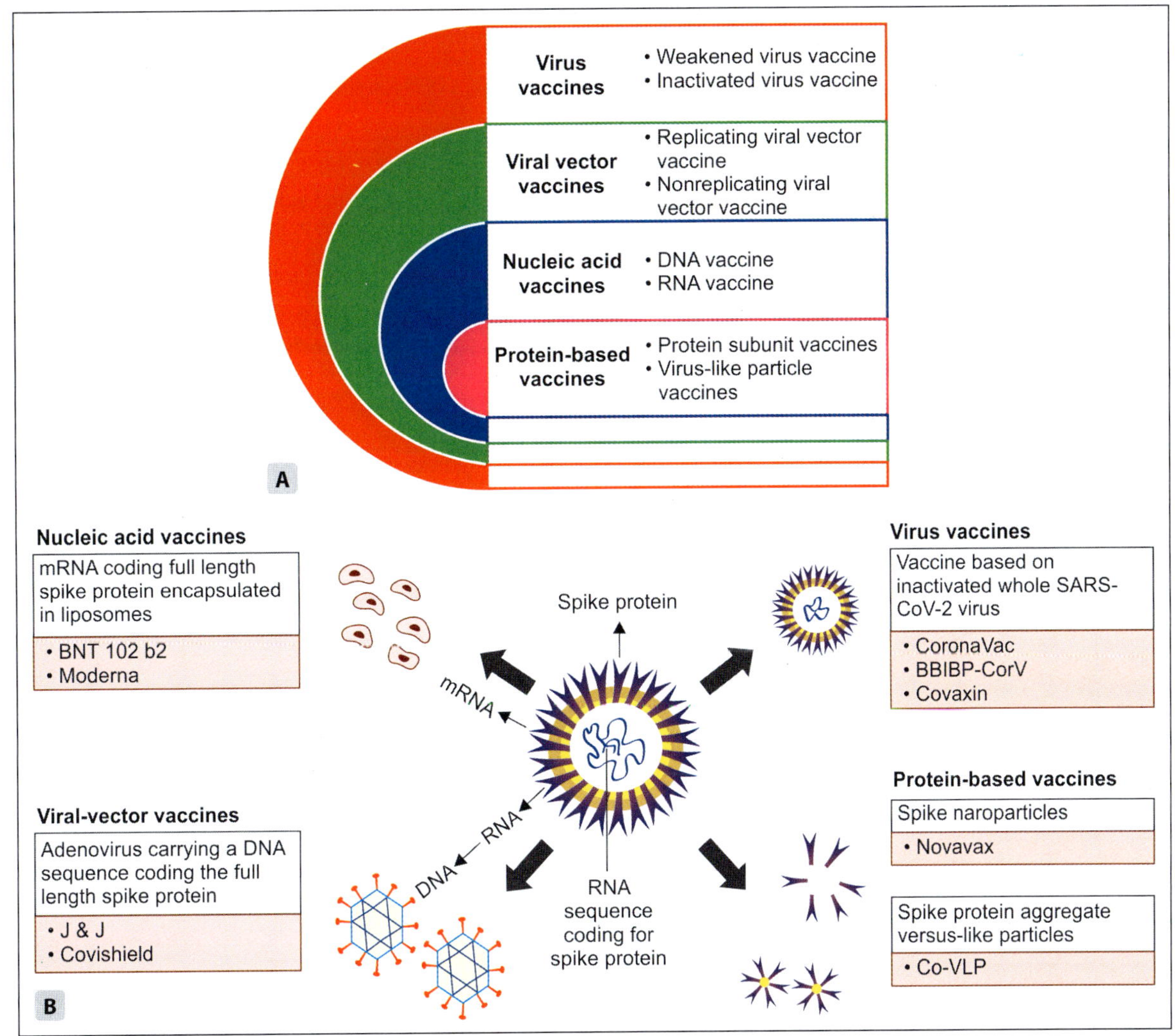

(COVID-19: coronavirus disease 2019; DNA: deoxyribonucleic acid; mRNA: messenger ribonucleic acid; RNA: ribonucleic acid; SARS-CoV-2: severe acute respiratory syndrome coronavirus 2)

FIGURES 3 A & B: Platforms for COVID-19 vaccines.

TABLE 1 Authorized/approved COVID-19 vaccines.

Vaccine	Type	Developer	Country of origin	Doses
Comirnaty (BNT162b2)	mRNA-based vaccine	Pfizer, BioNTech	Multinational	2, IM
Moderna Covid-19 vaccine (mRNA 1273)	mRNA-based vaccine	Moderna	US	2, IM
AZD1222/Covishield	Adenovirus vaccine	Oxford-AstraZeneca	UK	2, IM
Sputnik V	Nonreplicating viral vector	Gamaleya research institute	Russia	2, IM
CoronaVac	Inactivated vaccine (formalin with alum adjuvant)	Sinovac	China	2, IM
BBIBP-CorV	Inactivated vaccine	Sinopharm-Beijing Institute of Biological Products	China	2, IM
EpiVacCorona	Peptide vaccine	VECTOR Institute	Russia	2, IM
Convidicea (Ad5-nCoV)	Recombinant vaccine (adenovirus type 5 vector)	CanSino Biologics	China	1, IM
Covaxin	Inactivated vaccine	Bharat Biotech; ICMR	India	2, IM
No name announced	Inactivated vaccine	Sinopharm-Wuhan institute of biological products	China	2, IM
JNJ-78436735	Nonreplicating viral vector	Janssen vaccines (Johnson & Johnson)	Netherlands, US	1, IM

(COVID-19: coronavirus disease 2019; ICMR: Indian Council of Medical Research; IM: intramuscular; mRNA: messenger ribonucleic acid)

TABLE 2 Characteristics of the two Indian vaccines.

Features	COVISHIELD	COVAXIN
Type	**Viral vector vaccine**	**Inactivated vaccine**
Chemical ingredients	L-histidine ethanol, L-histidine hydrochloride monohydrate, magnesium chloride hexahydrate, polysorbate 80, sucrose, sodium chloride, disodium edetate dihydrate (EDTA), water for injection	Aluminum hydroxide gel, Imidazoquinolinone, 2-phenoxyethanol, phosphate buffer saline
Storage	2–8°C	2–8°C
Developed by	AstraZeneca along with Oxford university and manufactured by SII	Bharat Biotech along with the Indian Council of Medical Research (ICMR) and National Institute of Virology (NIV)
Dosage regimen	2 doses 4–8 weeks apart	2 doses 4 weeks apart
Efficacy	70% when 2 doses are administered 4 weeks apart, efficacy improves to 82.4% with a 12-week gap	Phase-3 interim results show an efficacy of 81%
Protection against mutations	Effective against UK variant No data on efficacy against the mutants found in South Africa and Brazil	Effective against UK, South Africa, and Brazil variant
Side effects:		
• Tenderness, pain, itching, swelling at the injection site	Yes	Yes
• Fever	Yes	Yes
• Fatigue/Malaise/Weakness	Yes	Yes
• Headache	Yes	Yes
• Nausea/Vomiting	Yes	Yes
• Rashes	Yes	Yes
• Stiffness in upper arm	No	Yes
• Bodyache	No	Yes
• Anaphylaxis	Yes	No
• Joint pain/Muscle ache	Yes	No
• Enlarged lymph nodes	Yes	No
• Excessive sweating, itchy skin	Yes	No
• Feeling dizzy, decreased appetite, abdominal pain	Yes	No
Contraindications	• Any history of allergies • Fever • Bleeding disorder or if on a blood thinner • Immunocompromised • Pregnant/ breastfeeding • Received another COVID-19 vaccine	• Any history of allergies • Fever • Bleeding disorder or if on a blood thinner • Immunocompromised • Pregnant/breastfeeding • Received another COVID-19 vaccine

in light of the huge vaccination requirements due to the recent surge of COVID-19 cases in India without the need to conduct postapproval bridging trials. The details of these vaccines have been summarized in **Table 3**.

NONINJECTABLE VACCINES

Most of the COVID-19 vaccines developed or under development are injectables. However, some vaccine candidates are being developed as noninjectables for ease of administration (**Table 4**).

VARIANTS AND VACCINES

Under the pressure of rising immunity in the population through natural infections or vaccination, the SARS-CoV-2 virus is adapting, leading to rise of new variants. These mutations in the SARS-CoV-2 genome can occur at any site. RNA viruses mutate frequently unlike the human DNA genome, which is slow to mutate. A mutation may alter the viral function (e.g., enhance receptor binding), or may have no discernible function. A new virus variant emerges when the virus develops one or more mutations that differentiate

TABLE 3 Foreign-approved coronavirus disease 2019 vaccines available in India.

Features	Sputnik V	Moderna	Comirnaty (Pfizer)
Type	Non replicating viral vector	mRNA-based vaccine	mRNA-based vaccine
Chemical features	• Component I: Recombinant adenovirus serotype 26 particles containing the SARS-CoV-2 protein S gene, in the amount of (1.0 ± 0.5) × 1011 particles per dose of 0.5 mL • Component II: Recombinant adenovirus serotype 5 particles-containing SARS-CoV-2 protein S gene, in the amount of (1.0 ± 0.5) × 1011 particles per dose of 0.5 mL	Nucleoside-modified mRNA encoding spike (S) protein, lipids-SM-102, polyethylene glycol, cholesterol, 1,2-distearoyl-sn-glycero-3-phosphocholine, tromethamine, acetic acid, sodium acetate, sucrose	mRNA molecule, PEGylated lipids, 1,2-distearoyl-sn-glycero-3-phosphocholine,monobasic potassium phosphate, potassium chloride, sodium chloride, sucrose
Storage	2–8°C	• 2–8°C for upto 30 days • –20°C for upto 4 months	Between –80°C and –60°C
Developed by	Gamaleya Research Institute of Epidemiology and Microbiology, Moscow, Russia	Moderna	Pfizer, BioNTech
Dosage regimen	2 doses 21 days apart	2 doses 4-6 weeks apart	2 doses 21 days apart
Efficacy	Interim Phase-III results show an efficacy of 91.6%	94.1%	95%
Protection against mutations	Effective against UK, South Africa, Brazil, and Indian variants	Effective against UK, South Africa, Brazil, and Indian variants	Effective against UK, South Africa, Brazil, and Indian variants
Side effects	Tenderness, pain, itching, swelling at the injection site, stiffness in upper arm, fever, malaise, headache, nausea, vomiting, bodyache, rashes	Tenderness, pain, itching, swelling at the injection site, fatigue, headache, muscle pain, joint pain, nausea and vomiting. Rarely can cause anaphylaxis, Bell's palsy	Tenderness, pain, itching, swelling at the injection site, fatigue, headache, muscle pain, joint pain, nausea. Rarely can cause anaphylaxis, myocarditis, pericarditis

TABLE 4 Noninjectable investigational vaccines.

Vaccine	Comments
VXA-CoV2-1 oral vaccine (Vaxart)	Recombinant adenovirus vector type 5 (Ad5) expressing coronavirus antigen and a toll-like receptor 3 (TLR3) agonist as an adjuvant. Preliminary phase 1 trial ($n = 495$) showed induced CD8 T-cell responses to the viral spike protein. Neutralizing antibodies not detected in most subjects
hAd5 T-cell (ImmunityBio and NantKwest)	• Vaccine targets inner nucleocapsid (N) and outer spike (S) protein, which have been engineered to activate T cells and antibodies against SARS-CoV-2, respectively • Phase 1 trial expanded to include the initial subcutaneous (SC) prime vaccine with a room-temperature oral or sublingual booster to induce comprehensive immune protection and generate both systemic and mucosal antibodies
Intranasal COVID-19 vaccine (AdCOVID; Altimmune, Inc	Phase 1 dose-ranging study of 1 or 2 intranasal doses initiated in February 2021. The trial will evaluate safety and immunogenicity in up to 180 participants aged 18–55 years
ChAdOx1 nCov-19 inhaled (University of Oxford)	Dose-ranging trial for orally inhaled vaccine beginning phases 1 trial in 30 volunteers in Fall 2020
saRNA inhaled (Imperial College of London)	Dose-ranging trial for orally inhaled vaccine beginning phases 1 trial in 30 volunteers in Fall 2020
PittCoVacc (University of Pittsburgh School of Medicine)	Vaccine candidate using transdermal microneedle for coronavirus disease 2019 (COVID-19); testing in mice produced antibodies over a 2-week period; microneedles are made of sugar, making it easy to mass-produce and store without refrigeration

TABLE 5 Coronavirus disease 2019 (COVID-19) variants.

Variant	Name	WHO label	First detected	Comments
UK	B.1.1.7	Alpha	December 2020	Spreads more easily and rapidly and potentially 30% more lethal than wild type version
South Africa	B.1.351	Beta	Early October 2020	Less responsive to existing vaccines and antibody therapies
Brazil	P.1	Gamma	Early January 2021	Have a group of additional mutations that affects its ability to be recognized by antibodies
New York	B.1.526	–	January–February 2021	Mutation of concern is called E484K, which has been observed in at least 59 different lineages of coronavirus. Evolving independently around the world
California	B.1.427/B.1.429	–	January–February 2021	L452R mutation affects the virus's spike protein, which may allow it to attack itself more efficiently to cells, making it more infectious
India	B.1.617.1 B.1.617.2	Kappa Delta	October 2020	More commonly known as the double mutant strain. Found to have E484Q mutation which has characteristics of previously detected mutations; E484K and L452R mutation making it highly transmissible and helps the virus to evade the body's immune response.
Vietnam	Hybrid variant	–	May 2021	It has combined mutations first found in India and UK and is highly transmissible due to rapid replication

TABLE 6 Next-generation vaccines.

Sponsor/Institution	Mechanism	Trial phase
University of Washington	Designed protein nanoparticle	Preclinical
Pfizer	mRNA-based vaccine (after modification)	Not declared yet
Moderna	mRNA-based vaccine (after modification)	Not declared yet
Novavax	Protein subunit	Phase 3

(mRNA: messenger ribonucleic acid)

it from the predominant virus variants circulating in a population. SARS-CoV-2 has already evolved several new variants (**Table 5**). There is a growing concern over future waves of COVID-19 infection and variants of the SARS-CoV-2 virus. With emergency authorizations for several COVID-19 vaccines under our belt, the question remains if these vaccines will be enough to carry us through the end of the pandemic.

NEXT GENERATION VACCINES

For a new vaccine to be next-generation, it must take a different approach than using the SARS-CoV-2 virus's mRNA to tell the body's cells to produce the virus's distinctive spike protein. Next-generation vaccines will be those which will be able to take care of spike mutations as well as provide a potent T cellular response. Another target to consider is the nucleocapsid which might add to the T cell immune response. "Next-generation" COVID-19 vaccines are being developed, many of whom are working with novel techniques. mRNA technology has emerged as a key technology to rapidly provide potent, flexible, and easy to manufacture vaccines. This platform can be used to update first-generation vaccines based on the new strains of the SARS-CoV-2 virus which pose biggest concern allowing for reformulation more quickly than traditional vaccine technology. Some of the next-generation vaccines under development are shown in **Table 6**.

OPEN QUESTIONS

- Will the new vaccines be able to control the COVID-19 pandemic?
- What will be the long-term efficacy and possible side effects?
- Will it be possible to overcome financial and political problems and allow COVID-19 vaccines to be available with equity for the entire population?

RECOMMENDED READINGS

1. WHO. (2021). WHO Coronavirus (COVID-19) Dashboard. [online] Available from https://covid19.who.int/.
2. WHO. (2021). Draft landscape and tracker of COVID-19 candidate vaccines. [online] Available from https://

www.who.int/publications/m/item/draft-landscape-of-covid-19-candidate-vaccines.
3. Mousavizadeh L, Ghasem S. Genotype and phenotype of COVID-19: Their roles in pathogenesis. J Microbiol Immunol Infect. 2021;54(2):159-63.
4. CDC. (2021). Symptoms of COVID-19. [online] Available from https://www.cdc.gov/coronavirus/2019-ncov/symptoms-testing/symptoms.html.
5. Heaton PM. The Covid-19 Vaccine-Development Multiverse. N Engl J Med. 2020;383:1986-8.
6. London School of Hygiene & Tropical Medicine. (2021). COVID-19 vaccine tracker. [online] Available from https://vac-lshtm.shinyapps.io/ncov_vaccine_landscape.
7. MOHFW. [2021]. [online] Available from https://www.mohfw.gov.in/covid_vaccination/vaccination/index.html.
8. Bharat Biotech. (20121). Covaxin. [online] Available from https://www.bharatbiotech.com/covaxin.html
9. SII. (2021). [online] Available from https://www.seruminstitute.com/product_covishield.php
10. David J Cennimo. (2021). COVID-19 Vaccines. [online] Available from https://emedicine.medscape.com/article/2500139-overview#a4.

Other Infections

CHAPTER 58

Tropical Fever: Diagnosis and Management

Vikas Suri, Ashish Bhalla

ABSTRACT

Acute tropical fever refers to a febrile illness occurring in tropics of ≤2 weeks duration with no indication of an organ-specific disease or a focal site of infection. The differential diagnosis for tropical fevers includes variety of parasitic, viral, and bacterial infections. Clinically it may be very difficult to differentiate between these infections as classic pattern described in the books may be missing due to early presentation and consumption of drugs available over-the-counter, which may modify the course of the illness. A high index of clinical suspicion and appropriate and timely laboratory investigation are important steps in the management. Etiology of tropical fevers varies according to geographic region and season. A syndromic approach in diagnosing of tropical fevers is recommended to help better management.

"Silence is a profound melody, for those who can hear it above all the noise"

—Socrates

INTRODUCTION

Fever is the most common chief complaint of the patients presenting to the emergency department. Acute tropical fevers refer to a febrile illness occurring in tropics of ≤2 weeks duration with no indication of an organ-specific disease or a focal site of infection. The differential diagnosis for tropical fevers includes infections such as malaria, dengue fever, enteric fever, leptospirosis, rickettsiosis, hantavirus, and Japanese encephalitis (**Table 1**).

ETIOLOGIES

Common etiologies observed are shown in **Table 1**.

APPROACH IN EMERGENCY AND CONCEPT OF "TROPICODROMES"

In a busy emergency clinical judgment is more important as only laboratory tests alone cannot diagnose/exclude a particular diagnosis. We should always look for "alarming features" which help the clinician in deciding for intensive care unit (ICU)/critical area monitoring. These alarming signs and symptoms include pulse rate of >120/min, a systolic blood pressure (SBP) <100 mm Hg, respiratory rate (RR) >22/min; oxygen saturation (SpO_2) <92%, temperature >104°F or >41.5°C, altered sensorium/seizures/severe headache, cold

TABLE 1 Etiologies of acute febrile tropical fever.

Malaria	
Bacterial infections	Enteric fever
	Rickettsial disease—scrub typhus, murine typhus, and spotted fever
	Leptospirosis
	Q fever
	Melioidosis
Viral infections	Dengue fever
	Influenza (A or B)
	Measles and rubella
	Chikungunya and other viral hemorrhagic fevers
	Acute viral hepatitis (Hepatitis A/B/E and others)
	Yellow fever
	Japanese encephalitis
	Human immunodeficiency virus
	Epstein–Barr virus, adenovirus, and mumps
Noninfectious etiology	Connective tissue disorders like systemic lupus erythematosus etc.
A significant number of patients remain with unknown diagnosis. Coinfections with two different organisms have also been reported.	

extremities/hypotension/inability to stand/postural dizziness, breathlessness/tachypnea/cyanosis, recurrent vomiting, profuse diarrhea/severe abdominal pain/dehydration, decreased urine output, bleeding manifestations, and muscle paralysis.

Tropical fevers vary according to region and season. A syndromic approach in diagnosing and managing these tropical fevers is of utmost importance. Common "Tropicodromes" are shown in **Table 2**.

Early initiation of definitive and supportive management, especially in an emergency setting, can improve the outcome of the patient. Upfront recommended investigations include rapid diagnostic tests (RDTs)/thick smear for malaria, hemogram, dengue NS1 antigen during the first 5 days of fever, and dengue/scrub/*Leptospira* immunoglobulin M (IgM) enzyme-linked immunosorbent assay (ELISA) after day 5 of fever. It is important to withdraw blood and urine cultures before antibiotic initiation as prior antimicrobial use may decrease the chances of a definite organism. Optional investigations to be considered are throat swab for influenza, chest X-ray, ultrasonography (USG) abdomen. The widespread use of RDTs in the diagnosis of malaria has helped in deciding specific artemisinin based at bedside. Points of care tests are being developed to expedite the early diagnosis of common tropical infections like scrub typhus/dengue and leptospirosis. More work is needed to increase the sensitivity and specificity of these tests. Approach to acute febrile tropical fever is presented in **Flowchart 1**.

TABLE 2 Tropicodromes.

Tropicodromes	Possible etiology
Fever with renal failure	Scrub typhus, leptospirosis, melioidosis, dengue fever (DHSS), acute viral hepatitis (hepatitis A/B/E and others), and yellow fever
Fever with liver failure	Acute viral hepatitis (hepatitis A/B/E and others), scrub typhus, leptospirosis, dengue fever, and yellow fever
Fever with altered sensorium	Malaria, tubercular meningitis, encephalitis (HSV/JE), scrub typhus, and leptospirosis
Fever with rash	Scrub typhus, leptospirosis, dengue fever (DHSS), and viral exanthems
Fever with ARDS	Malaria, scrub typhus, leptospirosis, melioidosis, and dengue fever (DHSS)

(ARDS: acute respiratory distress syndrome; DHSS: dengue hemorrhagic shock syndrome; HSV: herpes simplex virus; JE: Japanese encephalitis)

Empirical treatment with ceftriaxone and either doxycycline or azithromycin covers most of the tropical fevers (**Table 3**). In medical centers with limited diagnostic work up, this empirical treatment can help to reduce the mortality till better and suitable diagnostics for limited resource settings are made available (**Flowchart 2**).

SPECIFIC TROPICAL FEVERS

MALARIA

It is caused by protozoa of the genus *Plasmodium.* The five species known to infect humans are: (1) *P. falciparum,* (2) *P. vivax,* (3) *P. malariae,* (4) *P. ovale,* and sometimes (5) *P. knowlesi* (not seen in India). Mosquito is the vector and the definitive host in which sexual development occurs while human is its intermediate host.

In India, out of nine species of malaria vectors, the major vectors are *Anopheles culicifacies* in rural areas, breeds in clean ground water collections, and *Anopheles stephensi* in urban areas, breeds in man-made water containers in domestic and peridomestic situations such as tanks, wells, and cisterns. Female *Anopheles* as they feed on vertebrates inject sporozoites into blood, which starts the asexual development.

The incubation period is usually 12–35 days depending on the species. Presentation can be classified as uncomplicated and complicated or severe malaria to decide the line of management. In uncomplicated malaria, symptoms are nonspecific such as fever, chills, malaise, fatigue, diaphoresis (sweating), headache, cough, anorexia, nausea, vomiting, abdominal pain, diarrhea, arthralgias, and myalgias. Physical findings include mild anemia, mild jaundice, and splenomegaly which more often represent repeated infections in endemic region.

The standard tool of diagnosis is microscopy. Thick and thin films are made usually with Giemsa stain. Thick film increase sensitivity and thin film helps in species identification. The sensitivity of microscopy is excellent and can detect as low as 4–20 parasites/μL of blood. RDTs are simple, sensitive, and specific and can be used at field level with minimal training. Both microscopy and RDTs have similar levels of detection at around 50 parasites/μL. In endemic areas, the sensitivity and specificity of RDTs targeting histidine-rich protein 2 (HRP2) and *Plasmodium* lactate dehydrogenase (pLDH) appears to be 93–98% compared to microscopy.

Definitive treatment includes chloroquine for uncomplicated *P. vivax* and artemisinin-based therapies for *P. falciparum* or severe malaria. Drugs usually used in chemoprophylaxis are doxycycline, atovaquone-proguanil and primaquine. Malaria prevention measures include usage of insecticide-treated nets, indoor residual spraying with insecticides and prompt and effective case management of malaria illness to reduce transmission.

SCRUB TYPHUS

It Scrub typhus is widely prevalent with significant morbidity and mortality in India. Scrub typhus is seen in the countries that form the "tsutsugamushi triangle", which extends from Pakistan and Afghanistan in the West, to Eastern Russia in the North, to Northern Australia in the South, and Pacific island countries in the East. The endemic countries are India and its neighboring countries Myanmar, Sri Lanka, Nepal, and also Malaysia, Indonesia, Papua New Guinea, Korea, Japan, China, Thailand, Laos, Cambodia, Vietnam, and the other Pacific and Indian Ocean islands.

The causative organism, *Orientia tsutsugamushi*, is an obligate intracellular gram-negative bacterium, which grows freely in the cytoplasm of infected cells. Five major serotypes seen are: Boryon, Gilliam, Karp, Kato, and Kawazaki. In India, serotypes observed are predominantly Kato-like strains, especially in the South and Northeast, followed by Karp-like strains and Gilliam and Ikeda strains. It is transmitted to humans by larvae of trombiculid mites—chiggers (*Leptotrombidium*) during feeding, which are also the reservoirs of the agent. Rodents play a key role in maintenance of chigger population, though they are not reservoir of *Orientia tsutsugamushi.* Environmental risk factors for scrub typhus include exposure to bushes, piles of wood, domestic animals and rodents, living at the edge of the village, living in the houses near grassland, vegetable field or ditch, house yard without cement floor, and piling weeds in the house or yard. Most cases occur between August and February.

The incubation period is 5–20 days. The early clinical manifestations are fever, myalgia, headache, generalized

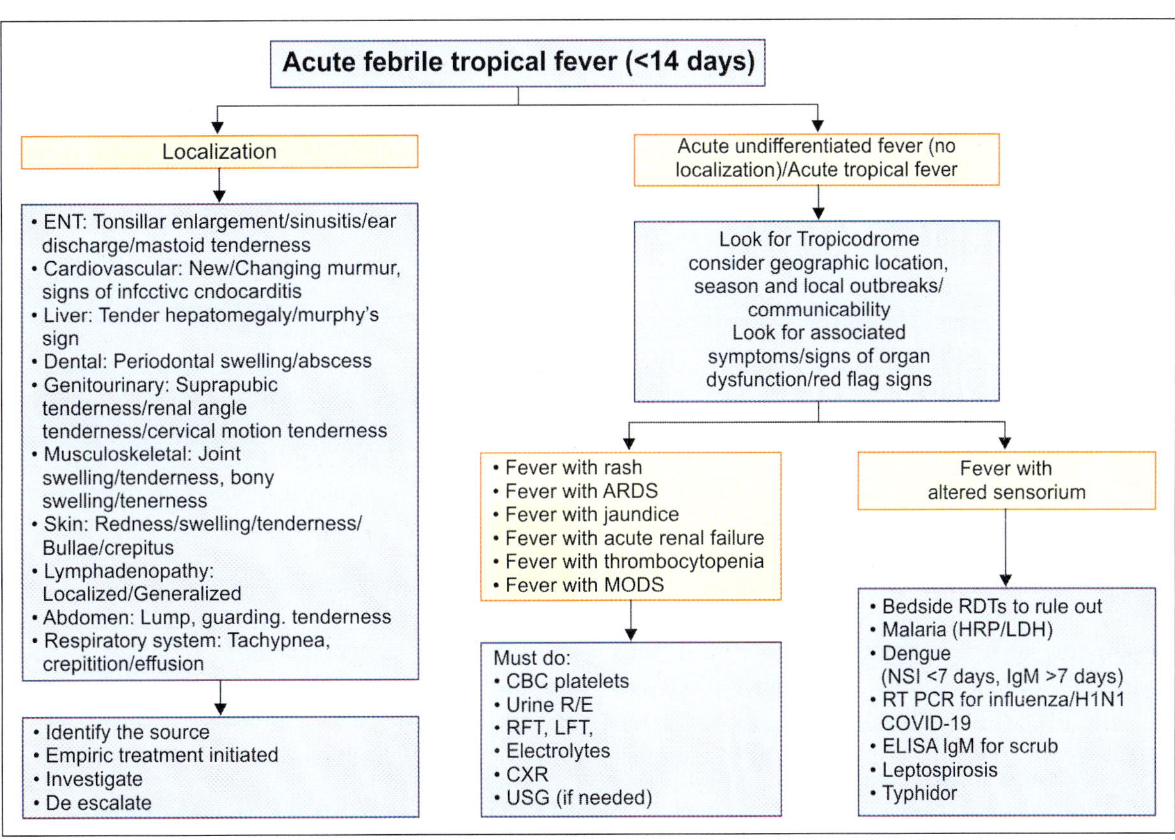

(ELISA: enzyme-linked immunosorbent assay; HRP: histidine-rich protein; IgM: immunoglobulin M; MODS: multiple organ dysfunction syndrome; RDTs: rapid diagnostic tests)

FLOWCHART 1: Approach to acute febrile tropical fever.

Source: Adapted from Singhi S, Chaudhary D, Varghese GM, Bhalla A, Karthi N, Kalantri S, et al. Tropical fevers: Management guidelines. Indian J CritCare Med. 2014;18:62-9.

TABLE 3 Syndromic management of acute tropical fever.

Fever with thrombocytopenia	**Fever with jaundice**
• Antipyretics for control of fever • IV fluids • Avoid aspirin/NSAIDs/anticoagulants • Watch for complications: bleeding, dyspnea, and shock • Platelet transfusion if the platelet count <10,000 or clinically overt bleeding • No role of steroids • Specific therapy once the diagnosis is established	• Antipyretics for control of fever IV fluids • Injection ceftriaxone 2 g IV BD Tablet doxycycline 100 mg BD • Watch for urine output, seizures, encephalopathy, bleeding, FFP/cryoprecipitate for bleeding • Specific therapy once the diagnosis is established
Fever with encephalopathy (Flowchart 3) • IV fluids • Antipyretics for control of fever • Injection ceftriaxone 2 g IV BD • IV acyclovir 10 mg/kg in adults (up to 20 mg/kg in children) intravenously every 8 hours • Injection doxycycline 200 mg stat and 100 mg OD (if scrub typhus is a strong possibility) • IV mannitol for raised ICP • Dexamethasone 8 mg BD (in pyogenic meningitis, before antibiotics) • Watch for seizures, dip in sensorium • Specific therapy once the diagnosis is established	**Fever with respiratory distress** • Antipyretics for control of fever IV fluids • Oxygen by venturi mask • Injection ceftriaxone 2 g IV BD • Injection azithromycin 500 mg IV OD or injection doxycyclin (if hepatitis) • Tablet oseltamivir 150 mg BD, if H1N1 suspected • Watch for impending respiratory failure, shock, renal failure, and alveolar hemorrhage • Specific therapy once diagnosis is established
Fever with renal failure • Antipyretics for control of fever • Injection ceftriaxone 2 g IV BD* • Tablet doxycycline 100 mg BD* • IV fluids according to CVP • Watch for encephalopathy, bleeding, seizures, and ARDS • Renal replacement therapy (intermittent HD/CRRT) • Specific therapy once the diagnosis is established	**Fever with MODS** • IV fluids • Antipyretics for control of fever • Injection ceftriaxone 2 g IV BD • Tablet doxycycline 100 mg BD/injection azithromycin • Watch for complications: Encephalopathy, bleeding, seizures, and ARDS • Supportive therapy as and when indicated

Ceftriaxone 2 g IV BD* (twice a day × 7 days), doxycycline 100 mg BD* (twice a day × 1 day, once a day × 5 days)

(CRRT: continuous renal replacement therapy; FPP: fresh frozen plasma; ICP: intracranial pressure; MODS: multiple organ dysfunction syndrome)

Source: Adapted from Singhi S, Chaudhary D, Varghese GM, Bhalla A, Karthi N, Kalantri S, et al. Tropical fevers: Management guidelines. Indian J Crit Care Med. 2014;18:62-9.

lymphadenopathy, gastrointestinal symptoms, cough, transient hearing loss, eschar, and rash. Eschar is a pathognomonic sign of scrub typhus and usually found on the neck, axillae, chest, abdomen, and groin and its detection rate varies greatly from 7 to 97%. Other associated complications are acute respiratory distress syndrome, interstitial pneumonitis, meningoencephalitis, acute renal failure, shock, gastrointestinal bleeding, and coagulopathy.

Abnormal laboratory findings seen are thrombocytopenia, leukopenia or leukocytosis, elevations in hepatic enzymes, bilirubin, and creatinine. Weil-Felix test is useful in establishing presumptive diagnosis of typhus fever at primary healthcare level, but lacks high sensitivity and specificity. It is based on the detection of antibodies to various *Proteus* species which contain antigens with cross-reacting epitomes to antigens from members of the genus *Rickettsia* with the exception of *R. akari*. The criterion for a positive result is either one determination of a titer of 1:320 or greater or a fourfold rise in titer starting from 1:20. False positive results can occur with malaria, undulant fever, infectious mononucleosis, tuberculosis, liver disease, and urinary tract infections by *Proteus*. Though indirect immunofluorescent antibody assay (IFA) and immunoperoxidase assay (IPA) are recommended by the World Health Organization as the gold standard methods for the serodiagnosis, IgM ELISA against a recombinant 56 kDa protein is a reliable method for the early detection of scrub typhus. The sensitivity observed with IgM ELISA was 86.5%.

Doxycycline is the drug of choice for the treatment. Alternative drugs are azithromycin, rifampicin, and chloramphenicol. Treatment of scrub typhus with antibiotics must be initiated early in the course of the disease, based on a presumptive diagnosis, to decrease morbidity and mortality.

TYPHOID AND PARATYPHOID FEVER

They are endemic in many areas of the underdeveloped and developing world, while rare in developed nations. The organism that usually causes the enteric fever syndrome is *S. enterica serotype typhi*. Other *Salmonellae* species that can cause a similar syndrome are *Salmonella paratyphi A, Salmonella paratyphi B, Salmonella paratyphi C,* and *Salmonella choleraesuis*. Enteric infection is acquired by

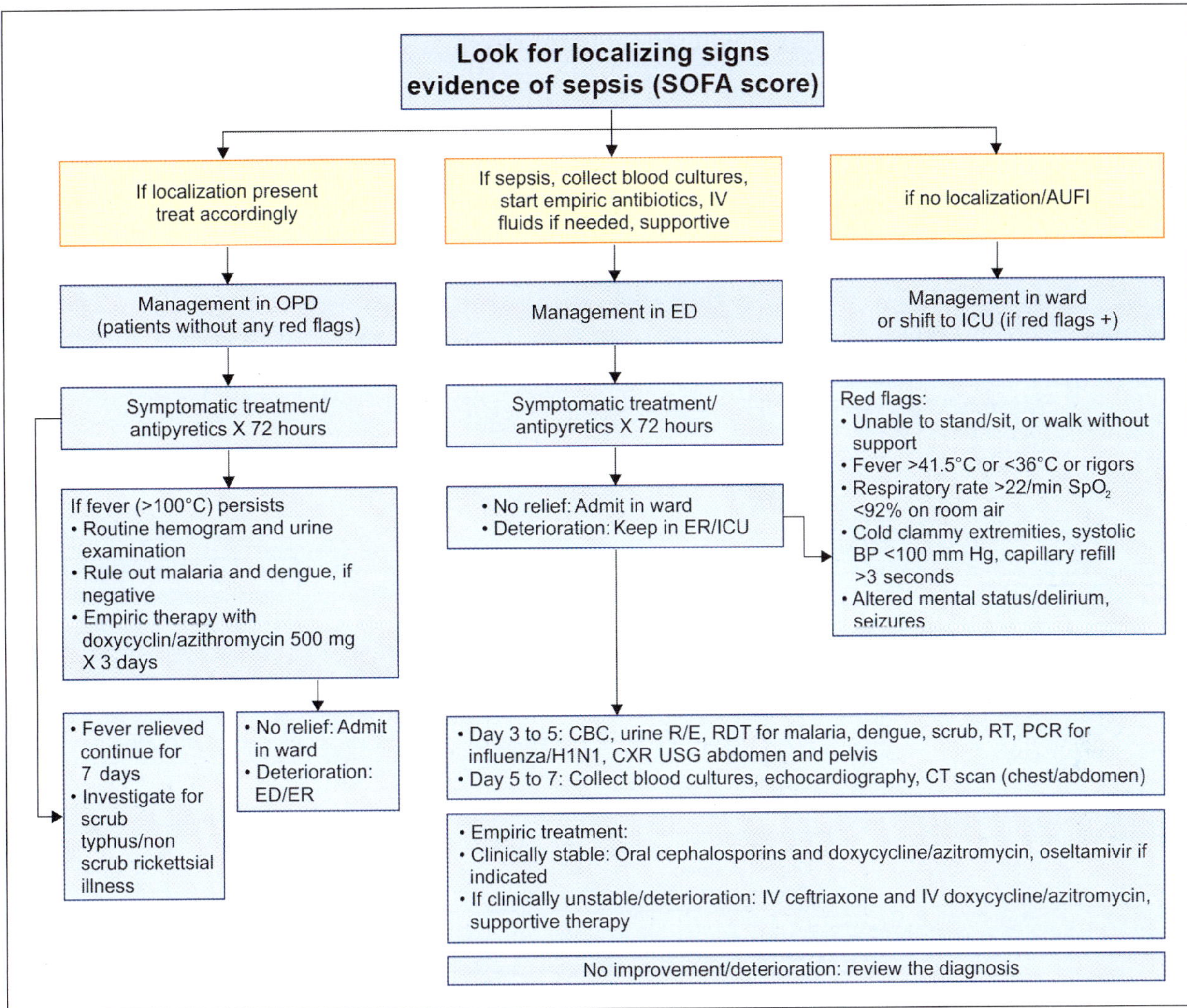

(AUFI: acute undifferentiated febrile illnesses; ED: emergency department; RDT: rapid diagnostic test; SOFA: sequential organ failure assessment)

FLOWCHART 2: Management of acute febrile illness/acute tropical fever.

Source: Adapted from Thangarasu S, Natrajan P, Rajavelu P, Rajagopalan A, Devey JSS. A protocol for the emergency department management of acute undifferentiated febrile illness in India. Int J Emerg Med. 2011;4:57.

Bhargava A, Ralph R, Chaterjee B, Bottieu E. Assessment and initial management of acute undifferentiated fever in tropical and sub tropical regions. BMJ. 2018;363(4766):145-53.

ingestion of food or water contaminated by human excreta that contain the pathogenic agents. Chronic gallbladder carriers form the long-term reservoirs. Persons with subclinical and clinical infection (short-term excreters) also act as reservoirs, especially in endemic regions.

Incubation period is about 5–21 days. In untreated individuals, the natural course of the disease in the first week, rising ("stepwise") fever develops corresponding to bacteremia and relative bradycardia may be seen. In the second week, abdominal pain develops and rose spots, which are faint salmon-colored macules on the trunk and abdomen, may be seen. During the third week, hepatosplenomegaly, intestinal perforation or bleeding may occur leading to secondary bacteremia and peritonitis. Introduction of antibiotics had altered the course of the disease and the mortality rate decreased to <1%.

Physical findings seen are relative bradycardia, rash (rose spots), coated tongue, hepatosplenomegaly, and sometimes abdominal tenderness. Gastrointestinal complications (seen in 10–15% cases) include gastrointestinal bleeding and intestinal perforation which most commonly occur in the third to fourth week of illness.

The definitive diagnosis requires the isolation of *S. typhi* or *S. paratyphi* from blood, bone marrow, or other sterile sites such as rose spots, stool, or intestinal secretions. Blood culture sensitivity varies between 40% and 80% depending on technique used. Bone marrow culture is 55–90% sensitive and yield is not reduced at least till 5 days of antibiotic usage. Stool cultures sensitivity increases by third week of illness. Serological tests include Widal and Typhidot IgM. Widal agglutination test is considered to be positive if a four-fold or greater increase

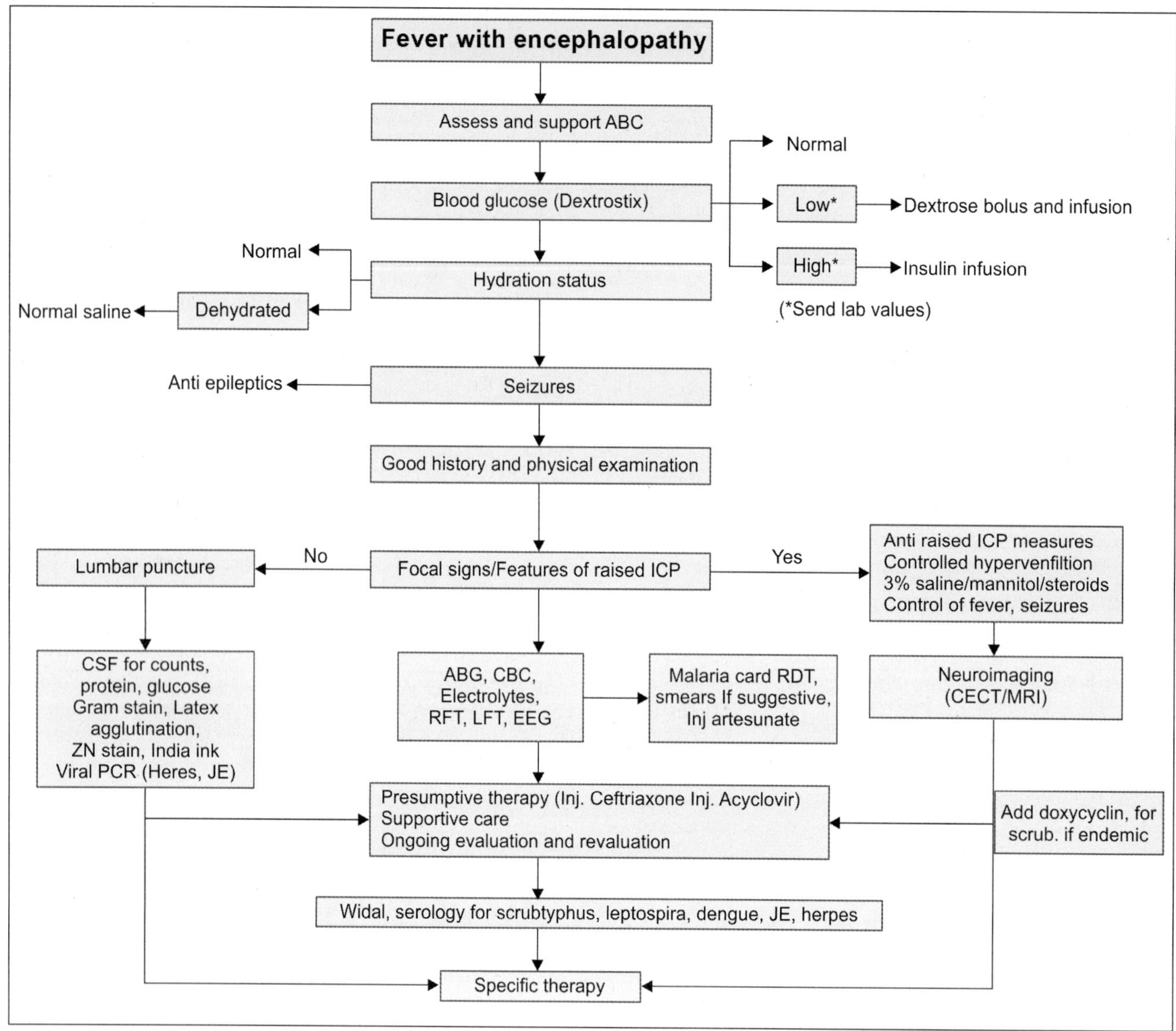

(ABC: airway, breathing, and circulation; CECT: contrast-enhanced computed tomography; ICP: intracranial pressure; JE: Japanese encephalitis; RDT: rapid diagnostic test; ZN: Ziehl–Neelsen)

FLOWCHART 3: Approach to fever with encephalopathy.

Source: Adapted from Singhi S, Chaudhary D, Varghese GM, Bhalla A, Karthi N, Kalantri S, et al. Tropical fevers: Management guidelines. Indian J Crit Care Med. 2014;18:62-9.

in titer in paired samples of acute and convalescent sera is documented. Sensitivity of Widal test varies between 46% and 94% and is of limited clinical utility in endemic areas because of false positive results. Typhidot IgM is an indirect solid phase immunochromatographic assay designed for the qualitative detection of antibodies against specific *Salmonella typhi* antigen in blood. Typhidot IgM, though easy and affordable has varied sensitivity and specificity.

Ceftriaxone, high dose azithromycin remain the main drugs for treatment of enteric fever. Around 1–5% of patients develop chronic carriage of *Salmonella* and these can be treated with oral amoxicillin, ciprofloxacin, norfloxacin, or trimethoprim/sulfamethoxazole for 4–6 weeks. Effective vaccines against *S. typhi* are available and include Ty21a, an oral live attenuated vaccine (doses given on days 1, 3, 5, and 7, with a booster every 5 years); and Vi polysaccharide parenteral vaccine (given in a single dose, with a booster every 2 years).

LEPTOSPIROSIS

It is a global public health problem and endemic in many areas of both tropical and temperate regions apart from being diagnosed in travelers to endemic regions. It has a peak incidence in summer and epidemics have been reported after periods of unusually heavy rainfall and monsoons.

The causative organism belongs to genus *Leptospira*, which was classified into 16 species of which at least seven are pathogenic. It is an important zoonosis affecting many wild and domestic animals, such as rodents, dogs, cats, livestock, and wild mammals. Humans commonly get infected through indirect contact with water or soil contaminated by the urine of infected animals or sometimes by direct contact with infected animals.

The incubation period of leptospirosis ranges from 2 to 26 days. Most cases are relatively mild and present as a febrile illness while some are severe and potentially fatal. Patients with mild leptospirosis present as a flu-like illness with fever, chills, headache, myalgia, nausea, vomiting, abdominal pain, and conjunctival suffusion. Myalgia and headache are usually severe. The natural course is usually a spontaneous resolution in 7–10 days. Severe leptospirosis is usually associated with renal insufficiency, hepatic dysfunction, hemorrhage, myocarditis, and a high mortality. The triad of hemorrhage, jaundice, and acute kidney injury in leptospirosis constitutes "Weil's syndrome".

The diagnosis can be confirmed by direct detection of the organisms [microscopy, antigen detection, deoxyribonucleic acid (DNA) detection, and culture] or by serologic methods. Serological tests are used most frequently for diagnosis. Assays include the microscopic agglutination test, macroscopic agglutination test, indirect hemagglutination, and ELISA. Microscopic agglutination test (MAT) is considered a reference standard assay. A definitive diagnosis of leptospirosis is based on isolation of the organism from the patient, on a positive result in the polymerase chain reaction (PCR), or on seroconversion or a rise in antibody titer (a four-fold or greater rise). In case of strong clinical suspicion, a single antibody titer of 1:200–1:800 in the MAT is evidence of recent or current infection.

Severe leptospirosis should be treated with intravenous (IV) penicillin or ceftriaxone or doxycycline. In mild cases, oral treatment with doxycycline, azithromycin, ampicillin, or amoxicillin is recommended. Preventive measures include avoidance of exposure to urine and tissues from infected animals through protective equipment such as proper eyewear and footwear. Rodent control strategies need to be taken. Chemoprophylaxis with doxycycline or azithromycin indicated in short-term exposure in high-risk areas.

DENGUE

It is caused by dengue viruses (family *Flaviviridae*, genus *Flavivirus*). The dengue virus complex has four antigenically related but distinct serotypes named one through four. Dengue is transmitted by *Aedes* mosquitoes. *Aedes aegypti* mosquitoes prefer to breed in man-made containers such as cement tanks, overhead tanks, underground tanks, tires, desert coolers, and discarded containers, where there is a possibility for water stagnation. *Aedes albopictus* mosquitoes prefer to breed in natural habitats such as tree holes and plantation. The incubation period is 3–14 days.

The disease presentation can be classified into two groups, which helps in better patient management and epidemiological surveillance. The WHO proposed classification includes two major categories, dengue with or without warning signs and severe dengue; the former includes dengue fever, and the latter includes dengue hemorrhagic fever/dengue shock syndrome (DHF/DSS) and other severe forms of infections previously referred to as atypical dengue. Laboratory diagnosis of dengue is made by detection of the virus or its components or by detection of the serological responses after infection (IgM and IgG levels).

During febrile phase (day 1 to days 4–5 of fever), NS1 Ag can be used. Both ELISA and rapid commercial tests are available for NS1 Ag detection. The sensitivity and specificity of NS1 antigen-capture ELISA ranges from 81 to 93% and 100%, respectively. A single serum sample collected after day 5 of fever onset is useful for IgM determination. Antidengue IgM kits evaluated showed test sensitivities of 21–99% and specificities of 77–98% compared with reference ELISAs. Serological cross reaction within *Flaviviruses* (such as Japanese encephalitis virus and West Nile virus) can occur. Other false-positive results are found in patients with malaria or past dengue infections.

Dengue fever is usually a self-limited illness, and only supportive care is required. Early and effective fluid replacement of lost plasma with Ringers lactate solution or with plasma expanders like starch or albumin 5% results in a good outcome. Prognosis depends on early recognition of shock, based on careful monitoring. Other supportive treatment includes transfusion of platelets, packed cells, or fresh frozen plasma depending on the requirement. A fall in the platelet count, (precedes the rise in hematocrit) is of great diagnostic and prognostic value. Preventive measures include vector control by proper disposal of solid waste, usage of insecticides, personal household protection like window screens, long-sleeved clothes, insecticide treated materials, coils and vaporizers, and active monitoring and surveillance to evaluate the effectiveness of interventions.

TAKE HOME POINTS

- In a country with endemic tropical infections, a possibility of acute tropical fever/infection should always be kept in mind in a febrile patient.
- A clinician should be aware of the epidemiology of tropical infections in the area where he/she is practicing.
- It is important to obtain travel history always as travel to an endemic area may result in tropical infections and may be difficult to diagnose if not suspected.
- A clinician should be aware of the outbreaks/epidemics of tropical infections in the area so as to suspect/manage tropical infections in people living or traveling to those areas.
- Syndromic approach to any fever would help narrow down the clinical possibilities and improve clinical management of acute tropical fevers.

RECOMMENDED READINGS

1. Joshi R, Colford JM Jr, Reingold AL, Kalantri S. Nonmalarial acute undifferentiated fever in a rural hospital in central India: diagnostic uncertainty and overtreatment with antimalarial agents. Am J Trop Med Hyg. 2008;78:393-9.

2. NVBDCP. National Vector Borne Disease Control Programme. [online] Available from http://www.nvbdcp.gov.in/malaria3.html.
3. Peter JV, Sudarsan TI, Prakash JA, Varghese GM. Severe scrub typhus infection: Clinical features, diagnostic challenges and management. World J Crit Care Med. 2015;4(3):244-50.
4. Prakash JA, Abraham OC, Mathai E. Evaluation of tests for serological diagnosis of scrub typhus. Trop Doct. 2006;36:212-3.
5. Guerrant RL, Walker DH, Weller PF. Tropical Infectious Diseases: Principles, Pathogens, and Practice, 3rd edition. Amsterdam, Netherlands: Elsevier Inc.; 2011.
6. Gupta SP, Gupta MS, Bhardwaj S, Chugh TD. Current clinical patterns of typhoid fever: a prospective study. J Trop Med Hyg. 1985;88:377-81.
7. World Health Organization. (2012). Handbook for Clinical Management of Dengue [online] Available from http://apps.who.int/iris/bitstream/10665/76887/1/9789241504713_eng.pdf.
8. Singhi S, Chaudhary D, Varghese GM, Bhalla A, Karthi N, Kalantri S, et al. Tropical fevers: Management guidelines. Indian J Crit Care Med. 2014;18:62-9.
9. Thangarasu S, Natrajan P, Rajavelu P, Rajagopalan A, Seelinger Devey JS. A protocol for the emergency department management of acute undifferentiated febrile illness in India. Int J Emerg Med. 2011 4:57.
10. Bhargava A, Ralph R, Chaterjee B, Bottieu E. Assessment and initial management of acute undifferentiated fever in tropical and sub tropical regions. BMJ 2018;363:k4766.

CHAPTER

59

Malaria

Manoj Kumar Mohapatra, Abhipsa Mohapatra

ABSTRACT

Malaria is a major public health problem in India with high morbidity and mortality. *Plasmodium falciparum* and *P. vivax* are two common parasites causing malaria. The former progresses to severe malaria and is responsible for almost all deaths due to malaria. However, recently severe malaria due to *P. vivax* has been encountered from different parts of the country. *P. falciparum* has developed resistance to frontline drugs except artemisinin compounds and quinine, whereas *P. vivax* still retains its sensitivity to chloroquine. Therefore, treatment of falciparum malaria is based on artemisinin-based combination therapy and quinine. Uncomplicated vivax malaria is treated with chloroquine and severe vivax malaria is treated like severe falciparum malaria.

"Inevitably, malaria parasites developed resistance to commonly used drugs, and the mosquito vectors became insecticide resistant"

—Anthony Fauci

INTRODUCTION

Malaria is an ancient parasitic disease which is very strongly associated with human beings since evolution. Still in 21st century it is a major global health problem.

EPIDEMIOLOGY

Malaria is a geographical disease with local and global impact. The incidence, clinical spectrum, and species causing malaria are different from one country to another and in a same country from one geographical area to another.

It affects about 97 countries of tropical and subtropical regions of the world and ranks among the top 10 killer diseases of the world. Even though malarial mortality has reduced by 47% globally, it afflicts >198 million people and causes about 584,000 deaths each year with 75% of the victims being from Africa.

In Southeast region of the World Health Organization (WHO), India alone contributes 80% of malaria cases. In India, currently around 880,000 cases of malaria are reported annually, of which 460,000 (about 50%) are due to falciparum malaria with 440 deaths. Malaria found in all states and Union territories but contributed the most (25.9%; in 2013, 37.1% in 2014) by Odisha state. Out of all deaths, Odisha state is second in the country where as Maharashtra is first in the year 2013 and Tripura in 2014.

SPECIES

Malaria is caused by one or more of the following *Plasmodium* species, i.e., *P. falciparum, P. vivax, P. malariae, P. ovale,* and *P. knowlesi* being transmitted by infected *Anopheles* mosquitoes. In Southeast Asia, the monkey parasite *P. knowlesi* causes malaria. In India, *P. falciparum and P. vivax* are common causes of malaria. Worldwide *P. falciparum* is responsible for most cases of severe malaria and death. However, malaria caused by *P. vivax, P. knowlesi,* and mixed species (*P. falciparum* and *P. vivax*) can progress to severe malaria.

Apart from individual species, infection due to both *P. falciparum* and *P. vivax* is also common in India. It is due to mosquito harboring multiple species of parasites and inoculation of a species to a patient with an existing infection with another.

LIFE CYCLE OF PARASITE

The parasite has a complex life cycle and to treat the patent and eradicate the disease, every stage is important.

LIVER STAGE

During bite, the mosquito inoculates the parasite (sporozoite) into the blood stream of human beings. The parasite invades the liver within minutes and start replicating (schizonts). *P. vivax* and *P. ovale* can remain dormant in the liver as hypnozoites and cause relapse. Drugs that target hypnozoites (primaquine) cause radical cure and prevents relapse.

BLOOD STAGE

After approximately 5–10 days, the liver cells rupture to release merozoites which invade the red blood cells (RBC). Inside RBC the merozoites go through various forms (rings, trophozoites, and schizonts) to form an average 20 merozoites/RBC that are released to blood stream to infect new RBC. During the release symptoms of high fever and other pathology of malaria develop. Drugs that target the blood stages are crucial for malaria case management. They cure malaria and prevent associated mortality.

TRANSMISSION STAGE

After several cycles of asexual reproduction, some parasites differentiate into male and female gametocytes in five stages. They contain half of chromosomes. Gametocidal drugs act at this stage.

MOSQUITO STAGE

After ingestion of male and female gametocytes by mosquito, they fuse in the midgut to form a zygote that further develops to sporozoites. Drugs at this stage are meant for prevention of transmission.

CLINICAL FEATURES

Plasmodia are intraerythrocytic parasites and they invade erythrocytes for their multiplication and further development. The erythrocytic stage of the parasite that includes parasite invasion, growth, replication, and rupture of RBC to release merozoites along with toxins that cause symptoms of malaria.

The clinical features of malaria depend on the species and whether it is uncomplicated or complicated malaria.

UNCOMPLICATED MALARIA

Fever: Fever is the most important symptoms of malaria. The fever is intermittent with chills and rigor. Periodicity is another feature of malarial fever.

Mechanism of fever in malaria: Fever in malaria coincides with the rupture of RBC releasing merozoites. Various parasite-derived toxins and cytokines are released that cause fever.

- *Hemozoin (Hz), toll-like receptors (TLRs), and fever*: Hz is released along with merozoites after rupture of RBC. Hz induces inflammation by activating TLR-9 through activation of nuclear factor-κβ that stimulates proinflammatory cytokines causing fever.
- *Pyrogenic cytokines*: Pyrogenic cytokines are formerly described as endogenous pyrogens. They are interleukin-1 and 6 and tumor necrosis factor. All these are released in malaria-causing fever.
- *Other pyrogens*: In malaria some other unidentified pyrogens play role in causation of fever.

Periodicity of fever: Malarial fever is intermittent with periodicity. *P. falciparum, P. vivax,* and *P. ovale* have tertian periodicity, i.e., the fever has a 2-day cycle. However, the typical tertian pattern is not found always in falciparum malaria. Due to benign nature of the disease *P. vivax* is described as benign tertian and *P. falciparum* malignant tertian malaria. *P. malariae* occurs every 3 days (quartan pattern). Malaria fever may occur daily (quotidian) in mixed species infection due to different erythrocytic cycle.

Paroxysm in malaria: The paroxysm of fever is associated with chill and rigor and typically consists of three stages, e.g., cold stage, hot stage, and diaphoresis. Cold stage is associated with chill. Patient clutches at blanket, curls up shivering. There is peripheral vasoconstriction and often goose pimples. Within minutes limbs shake and the teeth chatter, and temperature starts rising giving rise to hot stage. It is followed by vasodilatation and sweating known as "diaphoresis." Then fever subsides automatically. The cold stage lasts for 10–30 minutes, hot stage for about 10 minutes, and diaphoresis with defervescence within 4–8 hours. The typical paroxysm is observed in vivax malaria and after the paroxysm patient feels normal while in falciparum malaria the typical paroxysm is not observed and after paroxysm the patient has severe prostration.

Pyrogenic density (PD) of fever: Fever in malaria is causally related to rupture of RBC and parasitemia. The parasitemia at which fever occurs is known as PD. It is <500/μL for *P. vivax* and about 10,000/μL for *P. falciparum*. Hence, fever occurs early in vivax malaria seeking treatment and in falciparum malaria by the time fever starts there is already high parasitemia. However, *P. vivax* can give rise to fever as low as 100 parasites/μL whereas there may not be any fever in falciparum malaria with parasite count up to 100,000/ μL.

Nonfebrile clinical features: Apart from fever other clinical symptoms like headache, reeling of head, muscle pain, abdominal pain, nausea, vomiting, and dry cough may occur. The clinical features are very often indistinguishable from other viral and bacterial infections.

Hyperpyrexia in malaria: Hyperpyrexia is defined as fever >41.5°C or 106.7°F. Malaria is a cause of hyperpyrexia and is a medical emergency.

COMPLICATED MALARIA

The natural history of falciparum malaria showed that severe malaria represents a hierarchical continuum of abnormalities that start with asymptomatic infection, symptomatic uncomplicated malaria that progresses to complicated malaria with variable severity. It is notable that only about <1% of cases falciparum malaria may progress to severe disease.

The clinical picture of severe malaria is according to the organ affected in malaria that includes coma, convulsion, jaundice, anemia, oliguria etc. Intravascular hemolysis can also give rise to Blackwater fever.

Out of all species of malaria *P. falciparum* has the potentiality to cause severe malaria and is the cause of almost all deaths due to malaria. However, recently severe malaria due to *P. vivax,* mixed infection (due to *P. falciparum* and *P. vivax),* and *P. knowlesi* have also been reported.

Definition of severe malaria: "Complicated" and "severe" are the two terms frequently used in relation to falciparum malaria to describe the increasing severity of the disease. The diagnostic features of severe malaria have been set out by WHO in 2000 and revised in 2015.

Pathogenesis of severe malaria: There is no consensus on the pathogenesis of severe malaria including cerebral malaria. However, there are many hypotheses that describe the pathogenesis of severe malaria. But not a single scheme (hypothesis) could describe all the findings hence, multiple schemes hypothesis for pathogenesis has been proposed.

- *Sequestration hypothesis*: Sequestration of parasitized RBCs in the cerebral microvasculature has emerged as the primary pathophysiological event in cerebral malaria and other forms of severe malaria. After invasion by the parasite, knobs are formed on the RBC wall and *P. falciparum* erythrocyte membrane protein 1 (PfEMP1) is its main component. It causes cytoadherence to endothelial cells, described as "cytoadherence" or "cytoadhesion." Further, clumping of uninfected RBC occurs which is known as "rosetting." Platelets interact leading to further clumping. Sequestration causes cerebral occlusion of brain capillaries, reduction of microvascular flow, decreased nutrient supply to the brain, and damage to the vessel wall, leading to coma.
- *Inflammatory hypothesis*: This hypothesis proposes that increased levels of proinflammatory cytokines in *P. falciparum*-infected patients induces the expression of adhesion molecules in the brain endothelium, i.e., intercellular adhesion molecule-1 (ICAM-1), vascular cell adhesion molecule-1 (VCAM-1), and E-selectin. Systemic inflammation along with sequestration of parasitized RBCs leads to excessive endothelial activation with local secretion of proinflammatory mediators and impairment of blood–brain barrier (BBB).
- *Endothelial activation and coagulation dysfunction hypothesis*: Increased serum levels of the procoagulant von Willebrand factor and tissue factor support for a "coagulation dysfunction hypothesis" in development of cerebral malaria. It enhances cytoadherence and amplification of the coagulation cascade causing vascular leakage to the brain parenchyma and coma.
- *Innate immune hypothesis*: Innate immune system recognizes pathogens through pattern recognition receptors of which TLRs are important to detect pathogens and induce inflammation. TLRs present on endothelium play a role in the pathogenesis.
- *The BBB hypothesis*: The role of BBB in human cerebral malaria was postulated 40 years ago and the hypothesis was less favored for many years. Recently, many studies have been performed to uncover the extent of BBB alterations in cerebral malaria and it has been considered as final step of pathogenesis.

The BBB is a protective barrier for the human host during malaria infections. Unlike viruses and bacteria, the malaria parasites do not penetrate the brain parenchyma. After sequestration there is a constant and dynamic interplay between parasitized RBC, parasite-derived materials, host leukocytes, and the endothelial cells causing damage to BBB. Further, plugging of microvessels creates local hypertension which increases pressure on tight junctions leading to rupture of the BBB, causing hemorrhages and coma.

Definition of severe falciparum malaria (WHO guidelines 2015): Severe falciparum malaria is said to be present if one or more of the following are present in absence of identified alternative cause and in the presence of *P. falciparum* asexual parasitemia.

- *Impaired consciousness*: Glasgow Coma Scale score <11 in adult or Blantyre Coma Score <3 in children.
- *Prostration*: Generalized weakness, so that the person is unable to sit, stand, or walk without assistance.
- *Multiple convulsions*: More than two episodes within 24 hours.
- *Acidosis*: A base deficit of >8 mEq/L or if not available a plasma bicarbonate level of <15 mmol/L or venous plasma lactate ≥5 mmol/L. Severe acidosis manifests clinically as respiratory distress (rapid, deep, and labored breathing).
- *Hypoglycemia*: Blood or plasma glucose < 2.2 mmol/L (<40 mg/dL).

- *Severe malarial anemia*: Hemoglobin ≤ 5 g/dL or hematocrit ≤ 15% in children <12 years of age (<7 g/dL and <20%, respectively in adults) with a parasite count > 10,000/µL.
- *Renal impairment*: Plasma or serum creatinine >265 µmol/L (>3 mg/dL) or blood urea > 20 mmol/L.
- *Jaundice*: Plasma or serum bilirubin > 50 µmol/L (>3 mg/dL) with a parasite count of >100,000/µL.
- *Pulmonary edema*: Radiologically confirmed or oxygen saturation < 92% on room air with a respiratory rate > 30 breaths/min often with chest in drawing and crepitations.
- *Significant bleeding*: Recurrent or prolonged bleeding from nose, gums, or venipuncture sites, hematemesis, or melena.
- *Shock*:
  - Compensated shock: Capillary refill ≥ 3 seconds or temperature gradient on leg (mid to proximal limb), but no hypotension.
  - Decompensated shock: A systolic blood pressure of <70 mm Hg in children or <80 mm Hg in adults with evidence of impaired perfusion (cool peripheries, prolonged capillary refill).
- Hyperparasitemia: *P. falciparum* parasitemia > 10%.

Why *P. falciparum* causes severe malaria? *Plasmodium falciparum* has the potentiality to progress to severe disease causing death and almost all deaths of malaria are due to falciparum malaria. It causes severe disease due to:

- It invades RBC of all ages, i.e., reticulocytes, young, and senescent RBCs.
- A single RBC can be infected by multiple parasites.
- The number of merozoites released from a single RBC is about 25,000–30,000 that is 2–5 times higher than other species.
- The infected RBCs form rosette that binds to endothelial cells causing sequestration of microcirculation of brain, kidney, and other organs causing hypoxia and severe disease.
- The PD of falciparum malaria is high, i.e., 10,000/µL, which is more than vivax malaria (500/µL). Hence, the patient seeks medical advice later. Delay in treatment is a cause for development of severe malaria.
- Development of resistance of *P. falciparum* to various antimalarial drugs.

Severe malaria due to *P. vivax* malaria: Vivax malaria is the second most common cause of malaria. Though it is benign in nature, it may present with various complications. It has been reported from various parts of India and other countries.

Severe malaria due to mixed species infection: The mixed infection with *P. vivax* and *falciparum* reduces the risk of severe malaria by 4-fold, still then it is found in 17.0% cases of mixed infection.

In mixed species infection of *P. falciparum* with *P. malariae,* the later protects the severity of falciparum malaria.

The clinical features of severe malaria depend on the organ or organs involved. Mortality is high in multiorgan failure.

Organ dysfunction and assessment of severity: Though it is convenient and conventional to describe various complications of falciparum malaria in isolation, clinical reality, however, is that majority of patients present with a wide variety of combined complications leading to multi-organ failure. The important limitations of WHO criteria are lack of defining organ dysfunction and assessment of severity of organ dysfunction, which is required for risk stratification, prognostication, and planning of treatment. Organ dysfunctions can be defined and the severity can be assessed by Malaria Severity Score (MSS) and it has been given in **Tables 1** to **3**.

DIAGNOSIS OF MALARIA

CLINICAL

Fever is an important symptom of malaria. But the typical periodicity is absent in many cases. It can be intermittent with or without periodicity or continuous. Many cases have chills and rigors. Fever is often accompanied by headache, myalgia, arthralgia, anorexia, abdominal pain, nausea, and vomiting. At this stage, if treated, patient will be cured completely.

Therefore, all clinically suspected malaria cases should be investigated immediately by microscopy and/or rapid diagnostic test (RDT).

TABLE 1 Criteria for severity of malaria.

Criteria	Parameters	
General	• Fever ≥ 101°F • Presence of asexual form of *Plasmodium falciparum*	
Organ specific	**Organ system**	**Parameters for defining dysfunction**
	Neurologic	• Glasgow Coma Scale ≤ 13
	Renal (one or more)	• Urine output < 750 mL/24 h • Serum creatinine ≥ 1.2 mg/dL • Blood urea ≥ 36.0 mg/dL
	Hepatic	• Serum bilirubin ≥ 2.0 mg/dL
	Respiratory	• Respiratory rate ≥ 30 breaths/min
	Cardiac (one or more)	• Systolic blood pressure ≤ 90 mm Hg • Heart rate ≥ 120 beats/min or < 51 beats/min
	Metabolic	• Blood glucose ≤ 60 mg/dL
	Hematological (one or more)	• Hemoglobin < 10.0 g/dL • Platelet count < 80,000/µL • Total leukocyte count < 4,000/µL or > 12,000/µL

TABLE 2 Range of variables to assess the level of severity of organ dysfunction in malaria.

Parameters of organ dysfunction	Range of variables for different level of severity			
	Level 0	Level I	Level II	Level III
Neurologic:				
GCS score	14–15	10–13	7–9	0–6
Renal:				
Blood urea (mg/dL)	10.0–36.0	37.0–59.0	60.0–119.0	>120.0
Serum creatinine (mg/dL)	0.6–1.2	1.3–1.9	2.0–4.9	>5.0
Urine output (L/day)	0.75–3.9	0.5–0.75	0.4–0.5	<0.5
Cardiovascular:				
Heart rate/min	51–119	120–139	>140 or <51	
Systolic blood pressure (mm Hg)	90–160	70–89	41–69	
Respiratory:				
Respiration rate/min	20–30	31–40	>41	
Hematologic:				
Hemoglobin (g/dL)	10.0–13.9	7.0–9.9	<7.0	
TLC/cmm	4,001–16,000	2,001–4,000 or 10–20,000	<2,000	
Platelet/cmm	80,000–250,000	<80,000		
Hepatic:				
Serum bilirubin (mg/dL)	<2.0	≥2.0		
Metabolic:				
Blood glucose (mg/dL)	60.0–110.0	<60.0		

TABLE 3 Malaria Severity Score (MSS) of each organ dysfunction with different level of severity.

Organ dysfunction and score	Level of severity				
	Level 0	Level I	Level II	Level III	
Neurologic	Score 0	Score 1	Score 3	Score 5	
Renal	Score 0	Score 1	Score 3	Score 5	S
Cardiovascular	Score 0	Score 1	Score 3	x	C
Respiratory	Score 0	Score 1	Score 3	x	O
Hematologic	Score 0	Score 1	Score 3	x	R
Hepatic	Score 0	Score 1	x	x	E
Metabolic	Score 0	Score 1	x	x	

PARASITOLOGICAL

Microscopy: Microscopy of stained thick and thin blood smears is the gold standard for diagnosis of malaria. The advantages of microscopy are: (1) its high sensitivity, (2) to distinguish various species of parasites, (3) detection of low density of parasites, and (4) purpose of parasite load.

Rapid diagnostic test: Rapid diagnostic tests are based on the detection of circulating parasites antigens. Several types of RDTs are available. Some of them can only detect *P. falciparum*, while others can detect other parasites species also. Presently, a single kit detecting both *P. falciparum* and *vivax* is also available.

OTHER INVESTIGATIONS

Patient is investigated to diagnose the type of severe malaria, involvement of different organs, and to assess the severity. Hemoglobin (Hb), total leukocyte count, differential count, platelet count, blood glucose, urea, creatinine, liver function tests, and urine analysis are done. Recently, different biomarkers like procalcitonin, angiopoietin, and uric acids are also estimated to assess the prognosis.

TREATMENT

OBJECTIVES OF TREATMENT

- Early diagnosis and prompt effective treatment of malaria within 24–48 hours of symptoms to prevent progression to severe malaria.
- Rational use of antimalarials to limit misuse and promote full treatment for cases of true malaria.
- In cases of vivax malaria prevention of relapse is also another objective.

- The objective of treatment in severe malaria is to *prevent death*. During pregnancy, *saving life of the mother* is the primary objective.

ANTIMALARIAL DRUGS IN INDIA

Out of all the antimalarial drugs the following drugs are available for treatment under national drug policy.

- Chloroquine (oral)
- Oral artemisinin-based combination therapy (ACT).
  - ACT-SP—Artesunate + Sulfadoxine-pyrimethamine
  - ACT-AL—Artesunate + Lumefantrine
- Quinine dihydrochloride [oral and intravenous (IV)]
- Parenteral artesunate, artemether [intramuscular (IM)], and arteether (IM)
- Doxycycline (oral)
- Clindamycin (oral)
- Primaquine (oral)

UNCOMPLICATED FALCIPARUM MALARIA

One of the ACTs for 3 days followed by single dose of primaquine (0.25 mg/kg) as gametocidal drug has been recommended. ACTs are contraindicated in first trimester of pregnancy. Primaquin is contraindicated during pregnancy, lactation, and in infants (<6 months). Testing for glucose-6-phosphate dehydrogenase (G6PD) deficiency is not required.

In North-Eastern states of India: *ACT-AL (Artemether + Lumefantrine)*: The dose as per weight and age for 3 days. ACT-SP has not been recommended because of resistance to SP. ACT-AL is not recommended during first trimester of pregnancy and children <5 kg weight.

Uncomplicated falciparum malaria in special risk groups:

- *First trimester pregnancy*: 7 days quinine + clindamycin
- *Infants <5 kg body weight*: ACT at same mg/kg body weight as for children weighing 5 kg
- *HIV coinfected*: Avoid ACT-SP if treated with cotrimoxazole and avoid artesunate + amodiaquine if being treated with efavirenz or zidovudine.
- *Nonimmune travelers*: ACT

UNCOMPLICATED *P. VIVAX, P. OVALE, P. MALARIAE* OR *P. KNOWLESI* MALARIA

- *Chloroquine susceptible*: ACT or chloroquine (except first trimester pregnancy)
- *Chloroquine resistant*: ACT (except in first trimester pregnancy). Quinine in first trimester pregnancy

Prevention of relapse in *P. vivax* or *P. ovale:*

Primaquine:

- 0.25–0.5 mg/kg for 14 days except pregnant women, infants <6 months, women breastfeeding infants <6 months, and those with G6PD deficiency.
- 0.75 mg/kg once a week for 8 weeks in those with G6PD deficiency with close medical supervision for hemolysis.
- Chloroquine weekly in pregnant and breastfeeding women.

TREATMENT OF SEVERE MALARIA

Severe malaria is a medical emergency and preferably be treated in a health facility with experience and expertise in treating such cases. Before administering antimalarials, one should collect blood for RDT and/or smear. The recommended antimalarials are artemisinin derivatives or quinine irrespective of chloroquine resistance status.

- *Artesunate*: 2.4 mg/kg IV or IM given on admission (0 h), then at 12 hour and 24 hour, then once a day
  Or
- *Artemether*: 3.2 mg/kg given on admission, then 1.6 mg/kg/day IM
  Or
- *Arteether*: 150 mg daily IM for 3 days in adults only

After the patient become conscious or able to take orally then full course of area-specific oral ACT should be given.

In North-Eastern states of India: Age-specific *ACT-AL* for 3 days + *Primaquine* single dose on 2nd day

In other states of India:

- *ACT-SP* for 3 days + primaquine single dose on 2nd day
- Quinine is the second drug of choice given at the dose of 20 mg quinine salt/kg body weight on admission (IV infusion or divided IM injection) followed by maintenance dose of 10 mg/kg 8 hourly with infusion rate not exceeding 5 mg/kg/hours. Loading dose should not be given, if the patient has already received quinine. Once the patient is able to take orally, *Quinine* 10 mg/kg three times a day with *doxycycline* 100 mg once a day is administered to complete 7 days of treatment in total. For pregnant women and children under 8 years of age, *Clindamycin* 10 mg/kg 12 hourly (instead of doxycycline) is administered to complete 7 days of treatment including the days on parenteral quinine. Area specific ACTs can also be administered instead of oral quinine.
- Or *Clindamycin* 10 mg/kg 12 hourly for pregnant women and children under 8 hours of age to complete 7 days of treatment (including the days on parenteral therapy).
- Or area specific ACT is administered.

Notes:

- Pregnant women with severe malaria in any trimester can be treated with artemisinin derivatives. This reduces risk of hypoglycemia due to quinine.
- Parenteral treatment for a minimum of 48 hours.
- Quinine or ACT orally should be given once the patient is able to take orally.
- Mefloquine should be avoided in cerebral malaria due to neuropsychiatric complications associated with it.
- Corticosteroid, IV mannitol, heparin, and adrenaline are not recommended for use.

MANAGEMENT OF COMPLICATIONS

- *Cerebral malaria*: Maintain airway, place patient on his side, and exclude other causes of coma.
- *Hyperpyrexia*: Tepid sponging, fanning, cooling blanket, and paracetamol
- *Convulsions*: IV or rectal diazepam, lorazepam, and intramuscular paraldehyde
- *Hypoglycemia*: Glucose infusion
- *Severe anemia*: Fresh screened whole blood
- *Acute pulmonary edema*: Oxygen, diuretic, no IV fluid, intubate, and ventilate with positive end-expiratory pressure
- *Acute kidney injury*: Fluid balance, hemodialysis or/if not available peritoneal dialysis.
- *Spontaneous bleeding and coagulopathy*: Fresh blood, fresh frozen plasma (FFP), platelets, and vitamin K injection.
- *Metabolic acidosis*: Exclude or treat hypoglycemia, fluid balance, sepsis, if severe hemofiltration or hemodialysis.
- *Shock*: Blood culture, broad-spectrum antibiotics, and correction of hemodynamics
- *Other aspects*: Cautious fluid administration is recommended. General recommendation is not possible, and treatment must be individualized. Antibiotics should be given as sepsis is common.

CHEMOPROPHYLAXIS

- *Short term (up to 6 weeks)*: It should be started 2 days before and continued for 4 weeks after leaving the malaria area.

  Doxycycline 100 mg daily for adults and 1.5 mg/kg for children. (Contraindicated in children <8 years and pregnant women)
- *For longer stay (>6 weeks)*: Mefloquine (250 mg) weekly for adults 2 weeks before, during, and 4 weeks after exposure.

It is contraindicated in persons with history of convulsion, neuropsychiatric, and cardiac problems.

RECOMMENDED READINGS

1. Guidelines for the treatment of Malaria, 3rd edition. World Health Organization, 2015; pp. 1-62. [online] Available from www.who.int.
2. Mohapatra MK, Das SP. The malaria severity score: a method for severity assessment and risk prediction of hospital mortality for falciparum malaria in adults. J Asso Phys Ind. 2009;57:119-26.
3. Severe falciparum malaria. World Health Organization, Communicable Diseases Cluster. Trans R Soc Trop Med Hyg. 2000;94:S1-90.

CHAPTER 60

Other Protozoal Infections: Leishmaniasis, Toxoplasmosis, Trypanosomiasis, Trichomoniasis, Amoebiasis and Giardiasis

Agnibho Mondal, Mehebubar Rahman, Rama Prosad Goswami

ABSTRACT

In India, visceral leishmaniasis (VL) is primarily caused by *Leishmania donovani* and transmitted by *Phlebotomus argentipes*. Classical pentad includes fever, progressive weight loss, hepatosplenomegaly, pancytopenia, and hypergammaglobulinemia in endemic areas. The diagnosis is confirmed by demonstration of parasites and immunochromatographic rK39 test. Preferred treatment is liposomal amphotericin B in India. Immunocompromised patients may need secondary prophylaxis to prevent relapse.

Post-kala-azar dermal leishmaniasis (PKDL) may follow later after treatment of VL. Diagnosis requires demonstration of parasites from the skin lesions or polymerase chain reaction (PCR). It is usually treated by liposomal amphotericin B or miltefosine in India.

Toxoplasmosis is caused by *Toxoplasma gondii* and may involve many different sites including lymph nodes, lung, eye, and brain. Acquired toxoplasmosis in mother during pregnancy may result in congenital toxoplasmosis in the child. Diagnosis requires a battery of tests including serology, PCR, histopathology, parasite isolation, and radiology. The preferred regimen for toxoplasmosis is pyrimethamine plus sulfadiazine plus folinic acid.

American trypanosomiasis can be both acute and chronic. Heart is commonly involved. Treatment of choice is benznidazole. African trypanosomiasis has a hemolymphatic phase and a meningoencephalitic phase. Cerebrospinal fluid (CSF) examination is often helpful in diagnosis. Treatment options include fexinidazole, pentamidine, nifurtimox, eflornithine, suramin, and melarsoprol.

Trichomonas vaginalis causes vaginitis in women and urethritis in men. It is treated with metronidazole or tinidazole.

Amoebiasis may manifest as diarrhea, dysentery, liver abscess, or metastatic amoebiasis. Antigen detection is better than microscopy and PCR is the gold standard of diagnosis. Treatment involves metronidazole or tinidazole followed by a luminal agent.

Giardiasis should be suspected in all patients with prolonged diarrhea particularly associated with malabsorption and weight loss, travel to endemic area, or sexual risk behavior. The drug of choice is tinidazole or metronidazole.

"It's humbling to think that all animals, including human beings, are parasites of the plant world"

—Isaac Asimov

LEISHMANIASIS

Leishmaniasis is caused by the protozoan parasites in the genus *Leishmania* (**Table 1**). Three types of leishmaniasis are seen in human hosts (**Table 2**):

1. Visceral leishmaniasis
2. Cutaneous leishmaniasis
3. Mucosal leishmaniasis

VISCERAL LEISHMANIASIS

Visceral leishmaniasis or kala-azar is endemic in 75 tropical and subtropical countries. India, Bangladesh, Brazil, Ethiopia, Sudan, and South Sudan together are responsible for more than 90% cases worldwide.

In the Indian subcontinent the disease is caused by *L. donovani* which is transmitted by the vector *P. argentipes* and humans are the reservoirs. The ratio of latent VL to active VL may be in the range of 4:1 to 50:1 in an endemic region (**Table 3**).

The incubation period can vary between 2 and 8 months. The disease may remain latent in most infected persons. However, such persons may develop active VL after many years of latent infection (2–29% within 3 years).

Clinical features: The classic pentad of VL includes:

- Fever
- Progressive weight loss
- Hepatosplenomegaly
- Pancytopenia
- Hypergammaglobulinemia

In endemic areas low-grade symptoms may be present for weeks to months before the patient seeks medical attention. The spleen can be massively enlarged and it is soft to firm and nontender (a hard spleen points toward other diagnoses). Lymphadenopathy is common in Sudan but it is not seen in other geographic areas.

Visceral leishmaniasis may also present acutely in nonimmune persons which is characterized by abrupt onset high fever and chills, sometimes with a periodicity mimicking malaria.

Typical laboratory findings include:

- Anemia (normocytic and normochromic)

TABLE 1 Host-vector-organism.

Organism	*Leishmania*
Vector	Sand fly (*Lutzomyia* and *Phlebotomus*)
Host	Mammalian species
Infective form to vector	Amastigotes
Infective form to host	Promastigotes

TABLE 2 Organisms causing leishmaniasis.

Disease	Region/character	Organism
Visceral leishmaniasis	South Asia East Africa	*Leishmania donovani*
	Americas Mediterranean	*Leishmania infantum*
	Rare and atypical	• *Leishmania amazonensis* • *Leishmania martiniquensis* • *Leishmania tropica*
Post-kala-azar dermal leishmaniasis	South Asia (macular) East Africa (nodular)	*Leishmania donovani*
	Rare and immuno-compromization related	*Leishmania infantum*
Old world cutaneous leishmaniasis	Africa Mediterranean Southwest and Central Asia	• *Leishmania major (wet, rural oriental sore)* • *Leishmania tropica (dry urban oriental sore)*
	Ethiopia	*Leishmania aethiopica*
	Less common	• *Leishmania donovani* • *Leishmania infantum*
New world cataneous leishmaniasis	Texas to South America	*Leishmania Mexicana*
	Central to South America	*Leishmania braziliensis*
	Northern Amazon Basin	*Leishmania guyanensis*
	Panama Costa rica Colombia	*Leishmania panamensis*
	Peru	*Leishmania peruviana*
	Central and South America	*Leishmania infantum* (Other include amazonensis, colombiensis, venezuelensis, naiffi, pifanoi, garnhami etc.)

- Leukopenia (severe eosinopenia is common)
- Thrombocytopenia
- Hypergammaglobulinemia (can be as high as 9 g/dL)
- High erythrocyte sedimentation rate (ESR)

Diagnosis: The classical pentad has high positive predictive value in endemic region. Parasitological diagnosis is the gold standard.

Splenic aspiration has high sensitivity (93–99%) and can also be used for quantification of parasite burden and monitoring of treatment response. However, it has the risk of life-threatening hemorrhage.

Bone marrow aspiration is a safer alternative but it is less sensitive (60–85%). Liver biopsy is even less sensitive.

Molecular approaches can reach up to 93% sensitivity and 96% specificity. Quantitative PCR assay can assess parasite burden and is also useful for monitoring treatment response.

Immunologic tests include rK39 immunochromatography and direct agglutination test (DAT) using blood sample. Both have high specificity (>90%). The rK39 strip test can also be performed using urine sample (Goswami RP et al.).

A new enzyme-linked immunosorbent assay (ELISA)-based *L. donovani* promastigote membrane antigen (LAg) shows promise as an easily applicable diagnostic tool (Saha S et al.). A 2016 study from India (Ejazi SA et al.) found the sensitivity and specificity of the dipstick test to be 100%.

TABLE 3 Immune response to leishmaniasis.

Protective immune response	Ineffective immune response
• IL-12 • IFN-γ • TNF-α • Macrophages • Th1 CD4 cells	• IL-10 • TGF-β • Nonspecific B-cell proliferation and antibody production

(IFN: interferon; IL: interleukin; TGF: transforming growth factor; TNF: tumor necrosis factor)

A meta-analysis in 2018 found that kala-azar latex agglutination test (KAtex) had good specificity (97%) but suffered from poor sensitivity (77%).

Immunocompromised hosts: Immunocompromised patients with *Leishmania* infection have higher risk of progressing to clinical VL (4-fold in transplant patients and 100–2,300-fold in HIV patients). The impaired cell-mediated immunity causes higher parasite burden. VL coinfection also causes progression of HIV infection.

Atypical presentations are much more common in patients with CD4 count <50 cells/mm^3 and include:
- Atypical skin lesions
- Gastrointestinal tract involvement (chronic diarrhea, malabsorption etc.)
- Airway, pleural, or pericardial involvement
- Eye involvement like anterior uveitis

Parasitological diagnosis is easier with the usual samples. PCR remains highly sensitive but serology may be less sensitive in these patients.

Treatment: The treatment options for VL include liposomal amphotericin B, pentavalent antimony, miltefosine, and paromomycin.

The treatment regimens as proposed by the National Vector Borne Disease Control and Prevention, India are summarized in **Table 4**.

Liposomal amphotericin B: In India and in other regions outside East Africa, the preferred treatment for VL is liposomal amphotericin B which can be used in all age groups and even in pregnancy. It is generally less toxic but adverse reactions may include fever, rigor, nausea, vomiting, hypokalemia, and nephrotoxicity.

Liposomal amphotericin B, branded as AmBisome (Gilead Pharmaceuticals, Foster City, CA), is recommended by World Health Organization (WHO) for management of VL and it is available in India with preferential pricing for developing countries. Authors used a liposomal amphotericin B preparation, developed in India and commercially available as Fungisome™ (Lifecare Innovations Ltd., Gurgaon, Haryana, India), for the treatment of VL.

TABLE 4 Treatment options for visceral leishmaniasis in India.

Drug	Dose		Duration
Liposomal amphotericin B	10 mg/kg		Single dose infusion
Miltefosine + Paromomycin	Miltefosine daily dose as below		10 days
	Paromomycin 11 mg/kg IM		
Amphotericin B deoxycholate	0.75–1 mg/kg/day indusion daily or on alternate days		15–20 doses
Miltefosine	2–11 years	2.5 mg/kg/day	28 days
	>12 years and <25 kg body weight	50 mg/day	
	25–50 kg body weight	100 mg/day	
	>50 kg body weight	150 mg/day	
Pentavalent antimonials	Sb5 + 20 mg/kg/day IV or IM		30 days

Note: Pentavalent antimonials can only be used in regions where they are still effective (Indian states of Jharkhand, West Bengal, and Uttar Pradesh)

(IM: intramuscular; IV: intravenous)

Fungisome requires sonication for 45 minutes before administration. Like AmBisome, Fungisome is also an intravenous infusion (normal saline in contrast to 5% dextrose for AmBisome). Authors observed a short course 2-day regimen of 15 mg/kg Fungisome yielded 100% cure rate at 6 months after completion of treatment.

Miltefosine: Miltefosine is the only oral agent available for the treatment of VL. Miltefosine can be used in VL patients in the age range of 2–65 years. Adverse reactions of miltefosine include nausea, vomiting, dizziness, scrotal pain, nephrotoxicity, and hepatotoxicity. Miltefosine is teratogenic and is contraindicated in pregnancy.

Paromomycin: Paromomycin is used in combination with miltefosine in India. The adverse effects of paromomycin include injection site pain, raised aspartate aminotransferase, reversible ototoxicity, and nephrotoxicity.

Amphotericin B deoxycholate: Amphotericin B deoxycholate generally has poorer tolerability than liposomal amphotericin B. However, it has been used as a second-line agent when other agents like miltefosine cannot be used.

Combination therapies: Combination therapies for VL may include liposomal amphotericin B followed by miltefosine or paromomycin or both.

In a study from India, one dose of liposomal amphotericin B (5 mg/kg) followed by miltefosine for 7 days, paromomycin for 10 days, or both miltefosine and paromomycin simultaneously for 10 days produced a cure rate of >97% (Sundar S et al.).

In another Indian study on combination therapy for VL (Goswami RP et al.), single dose 7.5 mg/kg Fungisome followed by miltefosine (2.5 mg/kg/day for 14 days) achieved 100% cure rate. There was no relapse and no incidence of PKDL over a follow-up period of 5 years.

Treatment of HIV and VL coinfection: Presence of VL coinfection is a criteria of stage 4 HIV disease. HIV patients have a higher relapse rate of VL. Moreover, VL can also present as immune reconstitution inflammatory syndrome in patients with HIV infection.

A higher dose of liposomal amphotericin B is needed in these patients. The recommended regimen in India is a total dose of 40 mg/kg divided over 10 doses, i.e., 3–5 mg/kg on days 1–5, 10, 17, 24, 31, and 38.

Secondary prophylaxis: Secondary prophylaxis is beneficial in immunocompromised patients due to high relapse rate (**Table 5**).

In a study conducted in Eastern India (Goswami RP et al.), the secondary prophylaxis with liposomal amphotericin B or amphotericin B deoxycholate (1 mg/kg monthly) in HIV-VL coinfected patients significantly reduced relapse as well as mortality (100% in 6 months follow-up).

POST-KALA-AZAR DERMAL LEISHMANIASIS

Post-kala-azar dermal leishmaniasis manifests as macular, papular, nodular, or verrucous skin lesions after treatment of VL (**Table 6**).

The diagnosis can be done clinically. However, it is also possible to demonstrate amastigotes in the slit skin smear or by PCR.

Post-kala-azar dermal leishmaniasis patients are infectious to sand flies and hence may act as a reservoir of *Leishmania* in a community. Effective treatment of PKDL patients may be helpful in eliminating VL.

Treatment: The treatment of PKDL typically requires longer duration and outcome is frequently unsatisfactory. The approved regimens in India are summarized in **Table 7**.

Prevention:

Elimination of human reservoir:
- Improved basic health system
- Improved testing and treatment of cases
- Effective treatment of PKDL patients

Vector control:
- Insect repellents (e.g., N, N-diethyl-meta-toluamide)
- Insecticides (e.g., permethrin)
- Insecticide treated bed nets
- Indoor residual spray (e.g., dichlorodiethyltrichloroethane)

TABLE 5 Secondary prophylaxis for leishmaniasis.

Regimen	Dose
Amphotericin B lipid complex	3 mg/kg IV every 3 weeks
Pentamidine	4 mg/kg IV every 2–4 weeks
Liposomal amphotericin B	3–5 mg/kg IV every 3–4 weeks
SbV	20 mg/kg IM or IV every 3–4 weeks

(IM: intramuscular; IV: intravenous)

TABLE 6 Characteristics of PKDL according to geographic regions.

	India	Sudan
Percentage of VL developing PKDL	5–10%	50%
Onset after VL treatment	2–4 years	0–6 months
Character of lesion	Macular	Papulonodular
Time to resolve	Chronic	Within 12 months

(PKDL: post-kala-azar dermal leishmaniasis; VL: visceral leishmaniasis)

TABLE 7 Treatment regimen for PKDL in India.

Drug	Dose	Duration
Miltefosine	Daily dose same as VL	12 weeks
Amphotericin B deoxycholate	1 mg/kg/day infusion	60–80 doses over 4 months
Liposomal amphotericin B	5 mg/kg twice weekly	3 weeks

(PKDL: post-kala-azar dermal leishmaniasis; VL: visceral leishmaniasis)

Animal reservoir control (L. infantum):
- Immunizing dogs
- Insecticide-treated dog collars
- Culling feral dogs
- Serological identification of infected dogs

No form of chemoprophylaxis is available for preventing leishmaniasis.

Several vaccines for canine species are available with variable efficacy, but till now no vaccine is available for humans. However, several vaccines are in development.

TOXOPLASMOSIS

Toxoplasmosis in humans is caused by the organism *T. gondii* which belongs to the subphylum Apicomplexa, class Sporozoa.

The sexual stage of toxoplasma life cycle occurs in the small bowel of cats; hence they act as disease amplifier in the nature.

Transmission to human can occur via:
- Ingestion of undercooked meat containing tissue cysts
- Ingestion water or food contaminated with oocysts
- Transmission from mother to child

Clinical manifestations:

Immunocompetent patient: Often asymptomatic. In symptomatic cases the most common manifestation is painless cervical lymphadenopathy.

Immunocompromised patient: In the organ transplant recipients, toxoplasmosis may develop either through the transplanted organ or as a reactivation due to the immunosuppression.

In HIV patients *T. gondii* usually causes encephalitis, pneumonitis, and chorioretinitis. The most common manifestation is focal central nervous system (CNS) lesions.

Immune reconstitution inflammatory syndrome (IRIS) associated with toxoplasmosis is a rare entity.

Ocular toxoplasmosis: Features of ocular toxoplasmosis are summarized in **Table 8**.

Toxoplasmosis in pregnancy: Vast majority of pregnant women with toxoplasmosis are asymptomatic. Hence, all pregnant women should be screened for toxoplasmosis due to the risk of mother to child transmission.

TABLE 8 Toxoplasma chorioretinitis.

Ocular toxoplasmosis as reactivation of congenital infection	Ocular toxoplasmosis due to acquired infection
More severe disease	Less severe disease
2nd and 3rd decade of life	Between 4th and 6th decades of life
Bilateral disease	Unilateral disease
Old retinal scars	No old scars in retina
Macular involvement	Macular spring

Congenital toxoplasmosis: Infection acquired in first or second trimester are more severe, whereas infection acquired in the third trimester is often subclinical.

The classical Sabin's tetrad: Hydrocephalus, chorioretinitis, cerebral calcification, convulsions. *Pentad* includes mental retardation.

Diagnosis:

Serology: No single serological test can confirm the diagnosis and a battery of tests are often required.

Immunoglobulin G (IgG) antibody test: IgG usually appears within 1–2 weeks of acquisition of infection, peaks within 1–2 months and falls at variable rates. IgG usually persists for life at relatively low titers.

Immunoglobulin G avidity test: During acute infection, IgG binds antigen weakly (low avidity) whereas in chronic infection, patients have more strongly binding antibodies (high avidity).

A high avidity test indicates that the patient was infected at least 3–5 months earlier.

Immunoglobulin M antibody test: IgM appears earlier and declines faster in comparison to IgG. IgM is often used to determine whether an infection is new or old. However, the reliability of this method is not without doubt as IgM may persist for long duration in some pregnant women.

Other immunoglobulins: IgA antibodies may be detected in acute toxoplasmosis in adults and congenital toxoplasmosis in neonates.

Similarly, IgE antibodies can be detected in acute toxoplasmosis in adults, congenital toxoplasmosis in neonates and toxoplasmic chorioretinitis in children. IgE persists for even shorter duration compared to both IgM and IgA (**Table 9**).

Polymerase chain reaction: Cerebrospinal fluid PCR in toxoplasmic encephalitis (TE) has a sensitivity of 11–77% but a specificity of 100%.

Histology: Demonstration of tachyzoites in tissue sections/ aspirations or body fluids.

TABLE 9 Interpretation of *Toxoplasma* antibody tests.

IgG result	IgM result	Interpretation
Negative	Negative	No serologic evidence of infection with *Toxoplasma*
Negative	Positive	• Possible acute infection/false-positive IgM result • Repeat test
Positive	Negative	Chronic *Toxoplasma* infection
Positive	Positive	• Possible recent infection/false positive IgM reaction • Send sample to reference laboratory

(Ig: immunoglobulin)

Radiologic method: In HIV patients with TE, multiple ring-enhancing lesions may be seen on computed tomography CT scan. If the patient is not on anti-*Toxoplasma* prophylaxis and *Toxoplasma* IgG is detectable, then multiple ring-enhancing lesion on CT or MRI has 80% positive predictive value for TE.

Diagnosis of CNS toxoplasmosis in HIV patient: Treat on the basis of empirical diagnosis:

1. Clinical—focal CNS sign
2. Serological—Toxoplasma IgG
3. Radiological—CT/MRI with contrast showing ring-enhancing lesions

If no improvement by 10–14 days or clinical deterioration within 1 week, consider lumber puncture and PCR for *Toxoplasma* to exclude or confirm diagnosis along with acid-fast bacillus (AFB), Giemsa, and Gram stain.

Treatment: Current treatment regimens are summarized in **Table 10**.

Other treatment options include:

- Pyrimethamine-folinic acid *plus* clarithromycin *or* dapsone *or* azithromycin
- Sulfadiazine *plus* atovaquone

The treatment is recommended for 4–6 weeks after resolution of all the signs and symptoms—often for 6 months or longer. Therapy for toxoplasmosis in acquired immunodeficiency syndrome (AIDS) includes induction, maintenance (secondary prophylaxis), and primary prophylaxis. Maintenance therapy (pyrimethamine 25 mg once + SDZ 500 mg four times/day) is recommended for all patients until CD4 count rises above 200/mm^3 for at least 6 months.

The current standard treatment often encounters problems of poor tolerability, adverse effects, frequent dropouts, and nonavailability of pyrimethamine/sulfadiazine in some parts of India. The author (Goswami et al., 2015) had to use the combination of two effective alternative agents for toxoplasmosis, cotrimoxazole and clindamycin, on compassionate grounds. Complete response occurred more commonly with this regimen (80% vs. 31.25%) with lower mortality (12% vs. 37.5%) and toxicity (24% vs. 62.5%).

Maternal treatment to prevent transmission to the fetus has been with spiramycin (3 g/day). Spiramycin is indicated for treatment in pregnancy before 14 weeks of gestation after which pyrimethamine + SDZ + folinic acid regimen is recommended as spiramycin does not reliably cross the placenta.

Prevention:

- Avoid direct contact with cat feces and disinfect cat litter before handling.
- Avoid mucous membrane contact with raw meat and wash hands after handling it.
- Freeze meat to -20°C for 48 hours and cook meat to 67°C.
- Wash fruits or vegetable before consumption.
- Avoid drinking untreated water and unpasteurized milk.

In HIV patients trimethoprim-sulfamethoxazole (TMP-SMX) prophylaxis for pneumocystis pneumonia (PCP) is also effective against toxoplasmosis. Another option in transplant recipients is prophylactic treatment with pyrimethamine (25 mg OD for 6 weeks after transplantation).

TRYPANOSOMIASIS

CHAGAS DISEASE (AMERICAN TRYPANOSOMIASIS)

Chagas disease is caused by *Trypanosoma cruzi* which is found in central and south America (**Table 11**).

TABLE 10 Treatment regimens for toxoplasmosis.

	Immunocompetent	Immunocompromised
Preferred regimen		
Pyrimethamine (PO)	50 mg BD for 2 days; then 25–50 mg daily	200 mg loading dose; then 50 mg (<60 kg body weight) or 75 mg (<60 kg body weight) daily
Plus		
Sulfadiazine (PO)	1 g QDS	1 g (<60 kg body weight) or 1.5 g (<60 kg body weight) daily
Plus		
Folinic acid (PO)	10–20 mg daily (till 1 week after pyrimethamine therapy)	
Alternate regimen		
Pyrimethamine (PO)	Same as above	
Plus		
Folinic acid (PO)	Same as above	
Plus		
Clindamycin (PO/IV)	300 mg QDS	600–1,200 mg QDS
Plus		
Atovaquone (PO)	1,500 mg BD	

TABLE 11	Organism, host, and vector of Chagas disease.
Organism	*Trypanosoma cruzi*
Host	Various mammalian species (Humans are accidental host)
Vector	Triatomines (type of reduviid bugs)
Infective form to vector	Circulating trypomastigotes (while taking blood meal)
Infective form to host	Metacyclic trypomastigotes (feces of insects)

Epidemiology: The disease can be found in the region extending from southern half of United States to southern Argentina.

The disease can be transmitted by—contamination of mucus membrane, conjunctiva or skin-breaks with infected feces of vectors, ingestion of the infected insects or excreta, blood transfusion, and vertical transmission.

Clinical features:

Acute Chagas disease:

- *Chagoma* at the site of entry, which involves swelling, erythema, induration, and local lymph node involvement. (when portal of entry is skin)
- Classic *Romana sign* which involves painless edema of palpebrae and periocular tissue. (when portal of entry is conjunctiva)
- Fever, malaise, anorexia, facial, and pedal edema
- Generalized lymphadenopathy and hepatosplenomegaly
- Meningoencephalitis and myocarditis

Chronic Chagas disease: Most common involved organ is the heart:

- Arrhythmias
- Cardiomyopathy primarily involving right ventricle with features of right heart failure
- Thromboembolism to brain or other areas

Patients with megaesophagus may have dysphagia, odynophagia, chest pain, cough, and regurgitation.

On the other hand, patients with megacolon may have chronic constipation and abdominal pain.

Reactivation of Chagas disease: Chagas disease may be reactivated in immunocompromised patients including transplant recipients and HIV-infected individuals. Such reactivation often produces skin lesions and cerebral mass lesions.

Diagnosis:

Acute Chagas disease: *Consistent history*:

- Residence in an endemic area with known vector-borne transmission
- Blood transfusion in an endemic area without effective screening programs

Detection of parasite:

- Motile parasites in anticoagulated blood or buffy coat
- Giemsa-stained smears

TABLE 12	Drugs used in Chagas disease.		
	Benzidazole	**Nifurtimox**	
Dose	5 mg/kg/day	Adults	8–10 mg/kg/day
		Adolescents	12.5–1.5 mg/kg/day
		Children (1–10 years)	15–20 mg/kg/day
Duration	60 days	90–120 day	
Adverse reactions	Peripheral neuropathy, rash, granulocytopenia	Gastrointestinal and neurological symptoms	

Polymerase chain reaction assays are a better alternative to the culture due to the higher sensitivity and shorter duration.

Serologic diagnosis using serum IgM is not useful in Chagas disease.

Chronic Chagas disease: The diagnosis of chronic Chagas disease is done by detection of specific IgG in serum. Demonstration of parasites is not needed. Common methods of IgG detection involve ELISA, indirect hemagglutination, chemiluminescence, and indirect immunofluorescence.

Treatment: Treatment options are benznidazole and nifurtimox. Both drugs are oral and none of them can be used in pregnancy (**Table 12**).

According to 2018 WHO recommendation both children and adults with chronic Chagas disease should be treated with trypanocidal drugs if no specific organ damage is present. However, adults with specific organ damage should not be treated with trypanocidal drugs.

Management of cardiac involvement is supportive. Megaesophagus in Chagas disease is treated as idiopathic achalasia which involves balloon dilatation of lower esophageal sphincter.

Prevention:

- Immigrants from endemic regions should be screened.
- Treatment of chronically infected women of childbearing age group may reduce congenital Chagas disease.

SLEEPING SICKNESS (AFRICAN TRYPANOSOMIASIS)

Two organisms are responsible for African trypanosomiasis:

1. West Africa: *T. brucei* gambiense
2. East Africa: *T. brucei* rhodesiensi

The disease is transmitted by tsetse flies (genus *Glossina*) while taking blood meals from mammalian hosts. The disease is limited to the sub-Saharan Africa.

Clinical features: Painful, indurated trypanosomal chancre may develop at the site of inoculation 1–2 weeks after the insect bite. However, in reality they are rarely seen.

West African: *Stage 1 (hemolymphatic)*:

- Fever may appear 1–2 weeks after infection and is characterized by intermittent bouts of high temperature lasting several days with extended afebrile periods.
- Lymphadenopathy is common. Posterior cervical lymph nodes are enlarged in as many as 85% hospitalized patients (classic Winterbottom's sign).
- Transient edema of face, hands, and periarticular area
- Pruritus and erythematous rash

Stage 2 (meningoencephalitic):

- Appears months or years after infection
- Irritability, personality change, and loss of concentration
- Progressive daytime somnolence
- Severe headache
- Extrapyramidal symptoms

East African: Although similar, the east African trypanosomiasis follows a more acute course. If left untreated, death may happen within weeks to months, sometimes without a clear distinction between the hemolymphatic and the meningoencephalitic stage.

Diagnosis:

- High index of suspicion is required in people returning from endemic areas.
- Microscopic examination of the fluid from chancre, lymph node aspiration, blood smear, and buffy coat
- PCR and loop-mediated amplification of DNA (LAMP)-based assays are newer alternatives for diagnosis
- CSF examination is mandatory. It may show high cell count, increased opening pressure and even trypanosomes may be present.
- Bone marrow examination
- Culture in liquid medium
- CATT (card agglutination trypanosomiasis test) and RDTs (rapid diagnostic test) are also available commercially.

Treatment:

African trypanosomiasis caused by:

- *Rhodesiense* is treated with suramin in stage 1 and melarsoprol in stage 2.
- *Gambiense* is treated with pentamidine in stage 1 and eflornithine in stage 2 (**Flowchart 1**).

Prevention:

Prevention strategies include avoiding infected insects (clothing and insect repellent). Chemoprophylaxis is not recommended due to high toxicity and no vaccine is available.

TRICHOMONIASIS

Organism: *Trichomonas vaginalis.* They cause vaginitis in women, urethritis in men but often remain asymptomatic.

Trichomonas is often associated with other sexually transmitted diseases (STDs) and its presence indicates high risk sexual behavior.

Clinical manifestation: Clinical features are summarized in **Table 13**.

Diagnosis:

- Direct microscopic examination of vaginal fluid for motile trichomonads
- Nucleic acid amplification tests (gold standard)
- Culture (may take up to 7 days but can determine drug susceptibility)
- Affirm VPIII—nucleic acid probe hybridization semiautomatic system
- OSOM trichomonas rapid test—immunochromatographic capillary flow dipstick technology

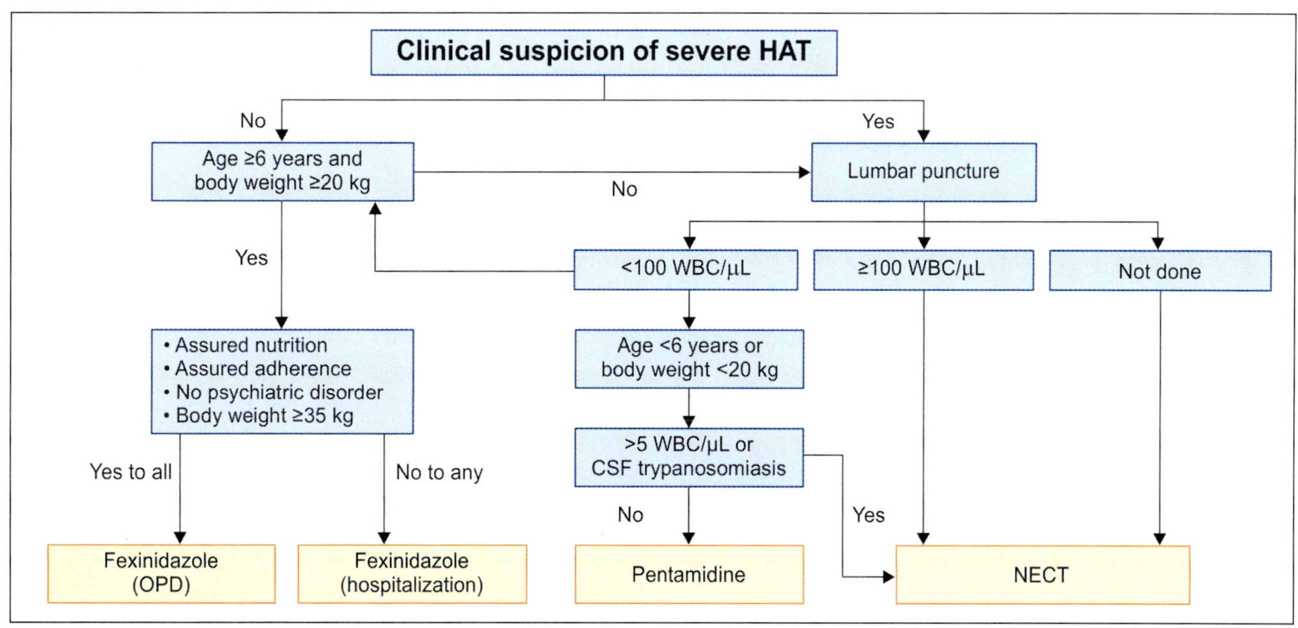

(CSF: cerebrospinal fluid; HAT: human African trypanosomiasis: NECT: nifurtimox–eflornithine combination therapy; WBC: white blood cell)

FLOWCHART 1: WHO guideline for treatment of *gambiense* African trypanosomiasis.

TABLE 13 Clinical manifestations and laboratory findings of trichomoniasis.

Clinical manifestations of trichomoniasis	
Symptoms	• Asymptomatic • Pruritus • Malodorous discharge • Dysuria • Dyspareunia
Signs	• Excessive frothy discharge • Vulval and/or vaginal inflammation • Colpitis macularis • Strawberry cervix
Investigation	• pH >4.5 • Positive whiff test • Excess polymorphonuclear neutrophils

Treatment: Trichomoniasis can be easily treated by metronidazole or tinidazole (single 2 g oral dose). However, the sexual partner must also be treated.

Resistance to metronidazole and tinidazole may be seen in 2.5–10% cases and <1% cases, respectively. In patients not responding to the usual metronidazole therapy the recommended regimen is metronidazole 500 mg twice daily for 7 days or tinidazole 2 g immediately. If even this regimen fails, metronidazole or tinidazole 2 g once daily for 5 days is recommended.

Complications: Trichomoniasis may be associated with:

- Preterm delivery
- Low birth weight
- Premature rupture of membranes

Trichomoniasis may also facilitate infection by HIV.

AMOEBIASIS

Amoebiasis is a human infection by *Entamoeba* species. *E. histolytica* causes amoebic colitis and liver abscess while *E. moshkovskii* causes diarrhea. *E. Bangladeshi* and *E. dispar* are nonpathogenic.

Pathogenesis: *Entamoeba histolytica* causes tissue destruction by a contact-dependent process called "trogocytosis-like":

- Adherence
- Cytolysis
- Phagocytosis

Clinical manifestations: The clinical manifestations of amoebiasis include following as described here.

Asymptomatic intraluminal amoebiasis: Intraluminal amoebiasis may persist without any clinical manifestation.

Amoebic diarrhea: This is the most common disease manifestation of amoebiasis. Mean duration is 3 days.

Amoebic dysentery or colitis: Amoebic dysentery is defined as diarrhea with mucus and visible or microscopic blood in a patient with *E. histolytica* infection. The most common clinical features are increasingly severe diarrhea with general abdominal tenderness and pain.

Amoebic liver abscess: Amoebic liver abscess is 10 times more common in men than women.

The symptoms may include:

- Fever
- Constant dull aching abdominal pain in the right upper quadrant or epigastrium
- Right-sided pleural effusion, pain, and cough
- Presentation can be both acute and subacute. In 80% cases the abscess is single and located in the right lobe of liver. There is usually leukocytosis and elevated alkaline phosphatase level.

Metastatic amoebiasis: Metastatic amoebiasis extends from liver abscesses to extrahepatic sites, such as:

- Thoracic amoebiasis (empyema, bronchohepatic fistula, and pleuropulmonary abscess)
- Pericardial involvement (acute pericarditis, tamponade, and pneumopericardium)
- Cerebral amoebic abscess

Diagnosis:

Stool ova and parasite examination: Although used traditionally, this method is inadequate for diagnosing amoebiasis.

Culture: This also suffers from poor sensitivity and specificity.

Antigen detection: Fecal antigen detection can be done by Gal/GalNAc adherence lectin detection by TechLab *E. HISTOLYTICA II* ELISA. It can differentiate *E. histolytica* from *E. dispar* and *E. moshkovskii* and *it is rapid (<2 h).*

Polymerase chain reaction: This is the gold standard for the diagnosis of amoebiasis.

Serologic tests: RIDASCREEN *E. histolytica* IgG enzyme immunoassay (sensitivity 97%), Microtiter ELISA, and indirect hemagglutinin assay (98–99%), can be used for serologic diagnosis of amoebic liver abscess and as an adjunct in intestinal amoebiasis. However, serologic tests are best used in conjunction with antigen detection or PCR.

Colonoscopy and biopsy: Colonoscopy and biopsy may be useful for diagnosing intestinal amoebiasis.

Imaging: Useful imaging modalities include ultrasound, CT, and magnetic resonance imaging. They are especially helpful in diagnosing amoebic liver abscess.

Treatment: All infections with *E. histolytica*, including asymptomatic infections, should be treated. Therapeutic aspiration of amoebic liver abscess may be considered if there is no clinical response to medical therapy within 5–7 days, high risk of abscess rupture (cavity diameter >5–10 cm) or lesion in left lobe (**Table 14**).

Prevention:

- Prevention of fecal contamination of food
- Safe sexual practices
- Proper maintenance of municipal water supply

No vaccine is yet available for prevention of amoebiasis.

TABLE 14 Medical management of amoebiasis in India.

Drug	Dose	Adverse effects
Amoebic liver abscess		
Metronidazole	800 mg PO TDS for 10 days	• GI side effects • Disulfiram-like reaction • Neurotoxicity
Or		
Tinidazole	2 g PO OD for 5 days	• GI side effects • Disulfiram like reaction
Followed by luminal agent		
Paromomycin		GI side effects
Or		
Diloxanide furoate	500 mg PO TDS for 10 days	• GI side effects • Pruritus • Urticaria
Amoebic colitis		
Metronidazole	800 mg PO TDS for 10 days	
Tinidazole	2 g PO OD for 5 days	
Luminal agent		
Asymptomatic intestinal colonization		
Luminal agent		

(GI: gastrointestinal)

GIARDIASIS

Giardiasis is caused by *Giardia lamblia,* an intestinal flagellate, transmitted via feco-oral route and inadequately treated water supply.

Clinical manifestations: The incubation period is 1–2 weeks. The clinical manifestations are varied and can be asymptomatic to severe diarrhea requiring hospitalization. The symptoms of giardiasis include diarrhea, malaise, flatulence, foul smelling greasy stool, abdominal cramps, bloating, nausea, anorexia, vomiting, weight loss, fever, urticaria etc. One of the most important distinguishing features is the prolonged duration of diarrhea with waxing and waning usually accompanied by weight loss.

In nonendemic areas post-*Giardia* irritable bowel syndrome is being increasingly recognized.

For traveler's diarrhea, giardiasis is common in long-term travelers whereas bacteria are common in short-term traveler.

Diagnosis: Giardiasis should be suspected in all patients with prolonged diarrhea particularly associated with malabsorption and weight loss, travel to endemic area or sexual risk behavior.

Traditional method of diagnosis is by microscopic examination of stool for ova, parasites, and cyst. At least three stool samples should be examined over multiple days for a 90% sensitivity.

Other methods include assays for detection of *Giardia*-soluble specific cyst wall antigen, cyst detection with immunofluorescence, and PCR.

Treatment: Treatment options are summarized in **Table 15**.

Prevention:
- Proper treatment of drinking water supply including halogenation, coagulation-flocculation, sedimentation, and filtration
- Boiling water and halogenation while visiting endemic areas
- Treatment of all children, regardless of symptoms, in case of giardiasis breakout in day-care centers.

TABLE 15 Treatment options for giardiasis in India.

Drug	Dose	
	Adult	Pediatric
Tinidazole	2 g single dose	50 mg/kg single dose
Metronidazole	200 mg TDS for 5–7 days	5 mg/kg for 7 days
Nitazoxanide	500 mg BD for 3 days	12–47 months: 100 mg BD for 3 days 4–11 years: 200 mg BD for 3 days
Albendazole	400 mg QDS for 5 days	15 mg/kg/day for 5–7 days (400 mg maximum)
Paromomycin	500 mg TDS for 5–10 days	30 mg/kg/day (in 3 doses) for 5–10 days
Quinacrine	100 mg TDS for 5–7 days	2 mg/kg TDS for 7 days
Furazolidone	100 mg QDS for 7–10 days	1.25–2 mg/kg QDS for 10 days

RECOMMENDED READINGS

1. Bennet J, Dolin R, Blaser M (Eds). Mandell, Douglas, and Bennet's Principles and Practice of Infectious Diseases, 9th edition. Philadelphia: Elsevier; 2019.
2. Farrar J, Hotez PJ, Junghanss T, Kang G, Lalloo D, White NJ, (Eds). Manson's Tropical Diseases, 23rd edition. Edinburgh: Elsevier Saunders; 2014.

3. Jameson J, Fauci A, Kasper D, Hauser S, Longo D, Loscalzo J (Eds). Harrison's Principles of Internal Medicine, 20th edition. McGraw-Hill Education; 2018.
4. National Vector Borne Disease Control Programme. Accelerated Plan for Kala-azar Elimination. National Vector Borne Disease Control Programme; 2017.
5. Goswami RP, Bairagi B, Kundu PK. K39 strip test--easy, reliable and cost-effective field diagnosis for visceral leishmaniasis in India. J Assoc Physicians India. 2003;51:759-61.
6. Goswami RP, Goswami RP, Das S, Ray Y, Rahman M. Testing urine samples with rK39 strip as the simplest non-invasive field diagnosis for visceral leishmaniasis: an early report from eastern India. J Postgrad Med. 2012;58(3):180-4.
7. Goswami RP, Rahman M, Guha SK. Utility of K39 strip test in visceral leishmaniasis (VL) and HIV co-infected patients: an early report from Eastern India. J Assoc Physicians India. 2007;55:154-5.
8. Goswami RP, Goswami RP, Das S, Satpati A, Rahman M. Short-Course Treatment Regimen of Indian Visceral Leishmaniasis with an Indian Liposomal Amphotericin B Preparation (Fungisome™). Am J Trop Med Hyg. 2016;94(1):93-8.
9. Goswami RP, Rahman M, Das S, Tripathi SK, Goswami RP. Combination Therapy Against Indian Visceral Leishmaniasis with Liposomal Amphotericin B (Fungisome™) and Short-Course Miltefosine in Comparison to Miltefosine Monotherapy. Am J Trop Med Hyg. 2020;103(1):308-14.
10. Goswami RP, Goswami RP, Basu A, Ray Y, Rahman M, Tripathi SK. Protective Efficacy of Secondary Prophylaxis Against Visceral Leishmaniasis in Human Immunodeficiency Virus Coinfected Patients Over the Past 10 Years in Eastern India. Am J Trop Med Hyg. 2017;96(2):285-91.
11. Sundar S, Sinha PK, Rai M, Verma DK, Nawin K, Alam S, et al. Comparison of short-course multidrug treatment with standard therapy for visceral leishmaniasis in India: an open-label, non-inferiority, randomised controlled trial. The Lancet. 2011;377(9764):477-86.
12. Ejazi SA, Bhattacharya P, Bakhteyar MAK, Mumtaz AA, Pandey K, Das VNR, et al. Noninvasive Diagnosis of Visceral Leishmaniasis: Development and Evaluation of Two Urine-Based Immunoassays for Detection of Leishmania donovani Infection in India. PLoS Negl Trop Dis. 2016;10(10):e0005035.
13. Saha S. Goswami R, Pramanik N, Guha SK, Saha B, Rahman M, et al. Easy Test for Visceral Leishmaniasis and Post-Kala-azar Dermal Leishmaniasis. Emerg Infect Dis. 2011;17(7):1304-6.
14. Goswami RP, Goswami RP, Rahman M, Ray Y, Tripathi SK. Alternative treatment approach to cerebral toxoplasmosis in HIV/AIDS: experience from a resource-poor setting. Int J STD AIDS. 2015;26(12):864-9.
15. World Health Organization. Guidelines for the Diagnosis and Treatment of Chagas Disease. Washington D.C.: World Health Organization; 2019.
16. World Health Organization. WHO interim guidelines for the treatment of gambiense human African trypanosomiasis. [online] Available from https://www.ncbi.nlm.nih.gov/books/NBK545514/

CHAPTER 61

Diseases of Rickettsiae, *Mycoplasma*, and Chlamydiae

Sanjay K Mahajan, Sanyam K Mahajan

ABSTRACT

Rickettsiae are a rather diverse collection of organisms with several differences; this prohibits their description as a single homogenous group. Rickettsiae are maintained in nature through a cycle involving reservoir in mammals and arthropod vectors. The public health impact of these on lives or productivity lost is largely unmeasured, but suspected to be quite high worldwide. The diseases caused by *Rickettsia* and *Orientia* species are often collectively referred to as rickettsioses.

Mycoplasma is the smallest and simplest self-limiting bacteria and lacks cell wall structure. *Mycoplasma pneumoniae* causes "atypical pneumonia" whereas *Mycoplasma hominis* and *Mycoplasma genitalium* are classified as genital mycoplasmas.

Chlamydia trachomatis is an obligate intracellular parasite as it grows only inside a host cell and cannot synthesize its own adenosine triphosphate (ATP) or grow on any artificial medium, it was believed for a long period of time to be a virus. The infection affects eyes and sexually transmitted infections, predominantly affects women, especially adolescent females. The clinical course of *C. trachomatis* is varies considerably and majority of infections remain asymptomatic; however, in few females can lead to pelvic inflammatory disease and tubal pregnancy.

"A body is a cell state in which every cell is a citizen. Disease is merely the conflict of the citizens of the state brought about by action of external forces"

—Rudolf Virchow

RICKETTSIAE

Rickettsiae comprise a group of microorganisms that phylogenetically occupy a position between bacteria and viruses. The genus *Rickettsia* is included in the bacterial tribe rickettsiae, family Rickettsiaceae, and order Rickettsiales. The taxonomy of Rickettsiales is complex and continues to be updated. Rickettsiae are a rather diverse collection of organisms with several differences; this prohibits their description as a single homogenous group. A general characteristic of rickettsiae is that mammals and arthropods are natural hosts. Rickettsioses usually are transmitted to humans by arthropods. The Rickettsiaceae family is maintained in nature through a cycle involving reservoir in mammals and arthropod vectors. They are obligate intracellular gram-negative coccobacillary forms that multiply within eukaryotic cells. Eighteen rickettsioses, caused by organisms within the genus of rickettsiae, are recognized and can be divided into the following three biogroups:

1. *Typhus group*: Causing classical epidemic typhus caused by *Rickettsia prowazekii* and *Rickettsia typhi* transmitted by human body louse and rat flea, respectively.
2. *Spotted fever group (SFG)*: Containing a large number of species *Rickettsia rickettsii, Rickettsia conorii* etc., transmitted from rodents and other animals by ticks (except *Rickettsia akari*) Rocky Mountain spotted fever (RMSF) is prototype.
3. *Scrub typhus*: Caused by *Orientia tsutsugamushi* and transmitted by larval trombiculid mites.

The diseases caused by *Rickettsia* and *Orientia* species are often collectively referred to as rickettsioses.

Tick-borne lymphadenopathy (TIBOLA) and *Dermacentor*-borne-necrosis-eschar-lymphadenopathy (DEBONEL) related to *Rickettsia slovaca* infection, as well as lymphangitis-associated rickettsiosis attributed to *Rickettsia sibirica* infection are new or emerging rickettsioses.

SPOTTED FEVER GROUP RICKETTSIAE

The spotted fevers compose a large group (15 rickettsioses) of tick- and mite-borne zoonotic infections that are caused by closely related rickettsiae. They include RMSF, boutonneuse fever, African tick bite fever, North Asian tick typhus, Queensland tick typhus, Finders Island spotted fever, Japanese spotted fever, and rickettsial pox. These diseases have a broad spectrum of severity and RMSF is most virulent.

Rocky Mountain spotted fever: The etiological agent *Rickettsia rickettsii*, belong to the SFG rickettsiae and are obligate intracellular bacteria. The spotted fever rickettsiae have been found in every continent except Antarctica. The tick of *Dermacentor* species, *Rhipicephalus sanguineus,* and *Amblyomma cajennense* are both vector and main reservoir. *Rickettsia rickettsii*, is transmitted trans-stadially (stage to stage) and transovarially in tick and thus maintains infection in nature. The tick transmits the disease to human during feeding. Rickettsiae are injected from salivary glands of attached tick or by exposure to infected tick hemolymph while removing tick from person or animal, especially if tick is crushed between fingers.

Pathophysiology: Rickettsiae microorganisms appear to exert their pathologic effects by invading the endothelial lining of the vasculature within the various organs affected. The most important pathophysiologic effect is increased vascular permeability with consequent edema, loss of blood volume, hypoalbuminemia, decreased osmotic pressure, and hypotension. The consequent of cell-to-cell spread of rickettsiae in body in a focal network of hundreds of contiguous infected endothelial cells corresponding to the lesion and manifest as maculopapular rash. The vascular injury and subsequent host lymphohistiocytic response correspond to distribution of rickettsiae and include interstitial pneumonia, interstitial myocarditis, perivascular glial nodules of central nervous system, and similar vascular lesions in skin, gastrointestinal tract, pancreas, liver, skeletal muscles and kidneys. Platelets are consumed locally.

Clinical manifestations: The incubation period ranges from 2 to 14 days. The disease begins with fever, myalgia, and headache. Headache is usually quite severe, onset of nausea, vomiting, pain abdomen, diarrhea, and abdominal tenderness occur in substantial number of patients. The rash, the major diagnostic sign, appear in a small number of cases on first day and in about 50% cases by third day of onset of fever. RMSF occurs more often in older patients and in black patients. Focal neurological deficits, transient deafness, meningismus, and photophobia may suggest meningitis or meningoencephalitis. The cerebrospinal fluid contains increase leukocytes (either lymphocyte of polymorphs). Fulminant RMSE is more often observed in black males with glucose-6-phosphatase dehydrogenase deficiency. Older age, male gender, and possibly alcoholism are other risk factors associated with fatal outcome. In classic RMSF, death occurs 8–15 days after onset of symptoms when appropriate is not given in a timely manner. In fulminant RMSF, death occurs within first 5 days.

Other spotted fever group rickettsiae: Among eight other SFG rickettsial species known to be pathogenic for human, *R. conorii, R. sibirica, R. japonica, R. australis, R. honei, R. africae,* and *R. slovaca* are considered to be transmitted by tick bite. *R. conorii* infection has been designated by many geographic names: Marseilles fever, Mediterranean spotted fever, Kenya tick typhus, and Indian tick typhus. Flea-borne spotted fever is caused by *R. felis*, suspected to be endemic globally and is an incompletely defined emerging disease which causes a murine typhus-like illness.

Boutonneuse fever occurs in Mediterranean locations mainly in warm months with peak incidence from July to September, and causes death up to 5% in hospitalized patients.

Rickettsia akari causes a nonfatal febrile illness called rickettsial pox and presents with fever with chills, headache, myalgia, especially backache, photophobia, generalized maculopapular rash, and eschar with painless regional lymphadenopathy.

Indian tick typhus is a SFG *Rickettsia* (*Rickettsia conorii*) and was isolated in 1950 from a brown dog tick (*Rhipicephalus sanguineus*). The rash is frequently purpuric, and an inoculation eschar at the bite site is rarely found and the disease as known in India is mild to moderately severe.

TYPHUS GROUP RICKETTSIAE

Epidemic or louse-borne typhus: Louse-borne typhus is the prototype of the typhus group rickettsial diseases. It is known as epidemic typhus, classic typhus, typhus exanthematicus, tabardillo, fleckfieber, and jail fever. The occurrence of typhus parallels the history of war and famine. An astonishing 30 million cases occurred in Soviet Union and Eastern Europe during 1918–1922 with an estimated 3 million deaths. The etiological agent *Rickettsia prowazekii* is an intracellular coccobacillary bacteria and is transmitted from person to person by body louse.

The cycle is thought to be initiated by a human case of recrudescence typhus or by a recently introduced case of primary louse-borne typhus. The louse is infected by feeding on a rickettsemic person. When the louse takes a blood meal, it defecates. The irritation causes the host to scratch the site, thereby contaminating the bite wound with louse feces. Chronic human carriage of *R. prowazekii* may result in later relapse of typhus fever called Brill–Zinsser disease who are thought to form a source of potential infection when louse infestation becomes common in prisons and refugee camps or unsanitary conditions.

Pathophysiology: The pathology is similar to that described for the SFG of rickettsial diseases. However, typhus group rickettsiae extensively multiply and accumulate intracellularly until they burst the endothelial cell and disseminate into the bloodstream. The angiitis is most marked in the skin, heart, nervous system, skeletal muscle, and kidneys. If local thrombosis is extensive, it can cause gangrene of skin and distal part of extremities.

Clinical manifestations: After an incubation period of 7–12 days, an abrupt onset with intense headache, chills, fever, and myalgia are characteristic. The fever worsens quickly and become unremitting and remains high until death or if untreated, resolution by crisis toward the end of the second week. The conjunctivae are suffused and face congested. There may be epistaxis, dry cough, delirium, and splenomegaly is common. The typhus rash appears on the second to fourth day of fever. It begins in axillary folds and upper part of trunk and spreads centrifugally to limbs. There is no eschar, meningoencephalitis may occur in 50% with meningism, tinnitus, hyperacusis followed by deafness, dysphagia, dysphoria, agitated delirium, and coma. Some survivors may suffer transverse myelitis, hemiparesis, peripheral neuropathy with hyperesthesia, and prolonged psychiatric disturbances. Secondary infection leading to bronchopneumonia, suppurative parotitis, otitis media, and peripheral blood vessels occlusion may occur. During recovery, myocarditis may occur with or without specific treatment. In untreated uncomplicated louse-borne typhus, fever lyses after 2 weeks of illness; recovery of normal mentation is rapid. In population at risk of epidemic typhus fever, nutrition and general immunity to infection are inadequate and illness is often severe with overall mortality rate up to 20% and >50% in the weak and aged. Louse-borne typhus is a mild disease in children.

Brill–Zinsser disease (i.e., relapsing louse-borne typhus): Brill–Zinsser disease occurs as recrudescence of previous infection with *Rickettsia prowazekii*. Its pathogen is unknown but recrudescence is presumed to be precipitated by stress or a waning immune system. The pathology is similar to that described for the other rickettsial diseases. However, the organisms appear to lie dormant, most likely in the cells of the reticuloendothelial system, until they are reactivated by an unknown stressor, multiply, and cause another acute but milder infection. The illness is similar to louse-borne typhus but it is usually milder.

Murine typhus: Murine typhus (endemic and shop typhus) is caused by *Rickettsia typhi (Rickettsia mooseri)* transmitted by rat flea *(Xenopsylla cheopis)*. It is believed to be mild but illness may be severe and can cause death. It may occur in epidemics or with high prevalence in certain regions. Human are infected by close contact with rodents and fleas in granaries, breweries, shops and food stores, and domestically in developing countries. Flea feces infected with rickettsiae contaminate the flea bite, which is then scratched, so inoculating the infection or may be inhaled when dried or rubbed into the conjunctiva.

Clinical manifestations: After an incubation period of 1–2 weeks there is an abrupt onset of illness and the initial presentation if often nonspecific. Fever, severe headache, chills, myalgia, rash, nausea and vomiting, rash, and hepatosplenomegaly are reported. The clinical course of murine typhus is usually uncomplicated. However, about 10% patients may develop central nervous system abnormalities, renal insufficiency, hepatic insufficiency, reparatory failure, and hematemesis requiring intensive care. About 4% of hospitalized patients will die of infection.

SCRUB TYPHUS

Scrub typhus, a zoonosis, was known in Japanese folklore to be associated with the jungle mite or chigger which was named "dangerous bug" (*tsutsugamushi*). The illness was described by Hashimoto in 1810. Ogata in 1931 isolated the organism and named it *Rickettsia tsutsugamushi*. Now it has been reclassified as *Orientia tsutsugamushi*. An estimated one billion people are at risk for scrub typhus and one million cases occur annually. Interest in this infection is reemerging because of descriptions of strains of

O. tsutsugamushi with reduced susceptibility to antibiotics and because of the surprising interactions between scrub typhus and the human immunodeficiency virus. Increasing prevalence of the scrub typhus has been reported from some Asian countries and may coincide with the widespread use of beta-lactam antibiotics or to urbanization into rural areas. Scrub typhus is a zoonosis and is a widespread disease in Asia and Pacific Islands. It also occurs in Japan, South Korea, Nepal, Northern Pakistan, South China, Papua New Guinea, Queensland, and Northern New South Wales. Scrub typhus is known to occur all over India.

Clinical manifestations: The clinical manifestations of this disease range from subclinical disease to organ failure to fatal disease. The clinical picture of scrub typhus is typically associated with fever, rash, myalgia, and diffuses lymphadenopathy. A necrotic eschar at the inoculating site of the mite is pathognomic of scrub typhus (**Figs. 1** and **2**). Cough sometimes accompanied by infiltrates on the chest radiograph is one of the most common presentations of scrub typhus infection. In severe cases, tachypnea progresses to dyspnea, the patient becomes cyanotic, and full-blown adult respiratory distress syndrome may develop.

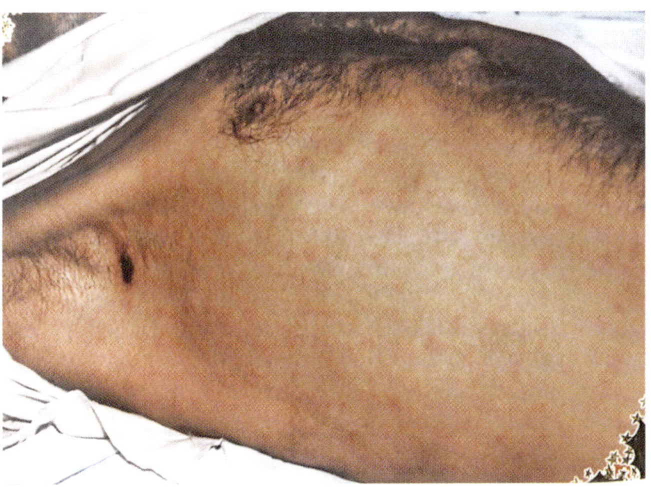

FIGURE 1: Photograph of a patient of scrub typhus showing rash and eschar in axilla.

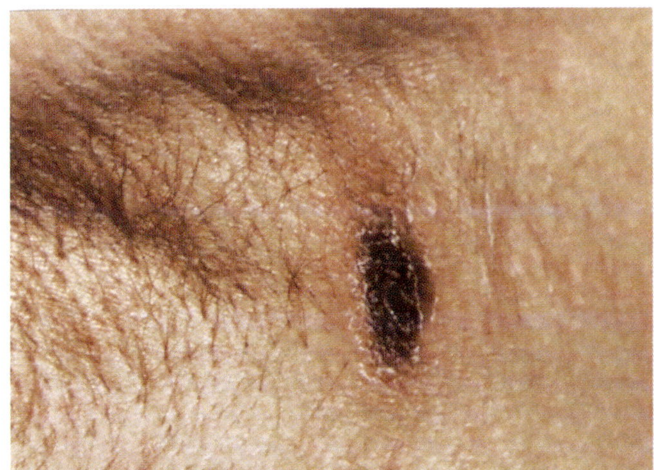

FIGURE 2: Photograph of a patient of scrub typhus showing details of eschar.

Rickettsioses in India: The rickettsial diseases once thought to have been eradicated from India are reemerging in many parts of our country. The presence of rickettsial diseases in India has been documented in Jammu and Kashmir, Himachal Pradesh, Uttaranchal, Rajasthan, Assam, West Bengal, Maharashtra, Pondicherry, Kerala, and Tamil Nadu. There are many reports of occurrence of rickettsial diseases from hills of North and Eastern parts of India as well from Southern plateau in last few years. Recently both scrub typhus and SFG rickettsioses have been reported from Haryana, which is situated in plains of North India.

TIBOLA AND DEBONEL

Patients may develop persistent asthenia and alopecia at the site of the eschar. The tick (*Dermacentor* species) bite is commonly located on the scalp region with a characteristic local reaction (eschar) and painful lymph nodes in the occipital region and/or behind the sternocleidomastoid muscle. The most frequent general symptoms were low-grade fever, fatigue, dizziness, headache, sweat, myalgia, arthralgia, and loss of appetite. Without treatment, the symptoms were seen to persist for as long as 18 months. Doxycycline treatment can shorten the usually benign illness.

DIAGNOSIS OF RICKETTSIAL DISEASES

In *Weil-Felix test*, cells of *Proteus vulgaris* OX-2 react strongly with sera from persons infected with *SFG rickettsiae* with the exception of those with *RMSF*, and whole cells of *P. vulgaris* OX-19 react with sera from persons infected with typhus group rickettsiae as well as with *RMSF*. However, *Proteus vulgaris* OXK will react in patients suffering from scrub typhus. The value of testing two sequential serum or plasma samples together to show a rising antibody level is considerably more important in confirming acute infection with rickettsial agents because antibody titers may persist in some patients for years after the original exposure.

The detection of immunoglobulin M (IgM) antibodies by *enzyme-linked immunosorbent assay (ELISA)* has got high sensitivity and specificity. *Immunofluorescence assay (IFA)* is currently considered to be the reference serological method. However, it cannot determine the causative agent to the species level. *Polymerase chain reaction (PCR)* to detect rickettsiae in blood or tissue provides promise for early diagnosis. However, serology remains the mainstay of diagnosis because these other tests are expensive.

TREATMENT

Adequate antibiotic therapy initiated early in the first week of illness is highly effective. Fever usually subsides within 24–72 hours after starting antibiotic therapy. If fever fails to subside with the use of a suitable antibiotic, the diagnosis of rickettsial disease should be reconsidered. Doxycycline, 200 mg/day PO/IV divided bid, is the drug of choice. In louse-borne (epidemic) typhus, single oral dose of 200 mg, and repeat once later if necessary or in a short course of 100–200 mg daily for 3 days. Chloramphenicol, 500 mg 6 hourly orally or intravenously for 7 days, may be used as an alternative but may not be as effective against rickettsiae as doxycycline. Tetracycline can also be used in dosage of 500 mg 6 hourly orally or intravenously for 7 day. The treatment with macrolide compounds clarithromycin and azithromycin can be considered a valid alternative therapy for children aged < 8 years and pregnant females. Rickettsiae are also sensitive to rifampicin and quinolones. Recent data from Europe suggest that fluoroquinolones may be effective in the treatment of certain rickettsioses. However, quinolones have been associated with clinical failures despite good in vitro activity. Sulfonamides were found to have a harmful effect either by delaying the institution of proper antimicrobial therapy or by directly stimulating growth of the organisms and are contraindicated in rickettsial infections.

As per recommendations of *Tick-borne Rickettsial Diseases Working Group* of Centre for Disease Control (CDC), Atlanta for management of rickettsial infections:

- The patients suspected to be suffering from rickettsial infection with evidence of organ dysfunction and severe thrombocytopenia, mental status changes, and the need for supportive therapy should be hospitalized.
- If laboratory testing of a patient with a history compatible with rickettsial diseases reveals leukopenia or thrombocytopenia, or metabolic abnormalities, the clinician should consider obtaining blood cultures for other likely pathogens and specific laboratory tests and initiating empiric oral antimicrobial therapy that will effectively treat rickettsial diseases.
- Delay in treatment can lead to severe disease and fatal outcome for rickettsial infection; doxycycline is therapy of choice in nearly all clinical situations. Typically when started early, fever tend to subsides within 24–48 hours after treatment.
- If a patient fails to respond to early treatment with a tetracycline antibiotic (i.e., within 48 hours), this response might be an indication that their condition is not a rickettsial diseases. Severely ill patients might require longer periods before clinical improvement is noted, especially if they have multiple organ dysfunction.

MYCOPLASMA

Mycoplasma is the smallest and simplest self-limiting bacteria and distinguished from bacteria by the lack of cell wall structure. *Mycoplasma pneumoniae* causes "atypical pneumonia" whereas *Mycoplasma hominis, Mycoplasma genitalium, Ureaplasma urealyticum*, and *Ureaplasma parvum* are classified as genital mycoplasmas. *Ureaplasma urealyticum*, and *Ureaplasma parvum* have been classified separately recently.

MYCOPLASMA PNEUMONIAE

This organism is thought to be responsible for about 40% community-acquired pneumonia. *M. pneumoniae* affects the upper or lower respiratory tracts or both and symptoms commonly appear gradually, and can persist for weeks or months. The *M. pneumoniae* is milder, associated with slower onset and lack lobar consolidation and resolution by crisis.

On auscultation of chest, the classic features of consolidation are lacking due to the fact that alveoli are not involved and localized or scattered rhonchi are audible. About 25% patients can experience extrapulmonary complications which can overshadow pulmonary involvement.

Encephalitis and meningoencephalitis, vomiting, abdominal pain, diarrhea, Stevens-Johnson syndrome, erythema multiforme and toxic epidermal necrolysis, autoimmune hemolytic anemia, autoimmune thrombocytopenia and disseminated intravascular coagulation, nonspecific myalgias, arthralgias and polyarthropathies, progressive glomerulonephritis, nephrotic syndrome, transient massive proteinuria, chronic renal failure due to cold agglutinin, acute interstitial nephritis, acute renal failure due to acute nephritis, hemoglobinuria or hemolytic uremic syndrome, isolated hematuria, and cystitis or urethritis are some of extrapulmonary manifestations of *M. pneumoniae*.

Mycoplasma pneumoniae is primarily considered as a causative agent of community-acquired pneumonia, but preceding infection with this organism has been associated with exacerbation of bronchial asthma which if difficult to control. The presence of interstitial infiltrate, alveolar infiltrates on chest X-ray, and bronchial wall thickening on chest computed tomography (CT) are common findings on imaging. The culture of *M. pneumoniae*, need specialized techniques, take many days for growth detection, and is successful in only 30–60% of the serologically diagnosed. The four-fold rise in titer between acute and convalescent sera, detection of *M. pneumoniae-specific antigen or M. pneumoniae-specific genetic components* are considered diagnostic.

The treatment consists of azithromycin, 500 mg on day 1, followed by 250 mg once a day from day 2 to day 4, or doxycycline 100 mg twice a day for 14 days or moxifloxacin 400 mg once a day for 14 days.

GENITAL MYCOPLASMAS

The genital mycoplasmas are primarily sexually transmitted but can be transmitted to infant at the time of birth which may persist in children in to adulthood. *U. urealyticum* causes urethritis in sexually inexperienced men; however, after multiple exposures to this organism leads to development of immunity. *M. hominis* has been implicated for causing postpartum fever, bacteremia, and postoperative mediastinal and wound infections. *M. genitalium* is associated with urethritis in men and endocervicitis in women.

Tetracycline classes of drugs are effective against ureaplasmas and *M. hominis,* macrolides are effective against ureaplasmas but partially effective against *M. genitalium.* Quinolones, especially moxifloxacin, are active against all of the genital mycoplasmas.

TABLE 1 The clinical spectrum of *Chlamydia trachomatis*.

Females		Males	Infants
Lower genital tract	**Upper genital tract**		
• Asymptomatic (up to 70%) • Cervicitis • Urethritis	Pelvic pain, menstrual abnormalities, pelvic inflammatory disease, endometritis, salpingitis, and pelvic peritonitis	• Asymptomatic (up to 50%) • Nongonococcal urethritis, epididymitis, lymphogranuloma venereum, and Reiter's syndrome	Conjunctivitis and pneumonia
Ocular	**Sequelae**	**Sequelae**	**In men who have sex with men**
Chronic conjunctivitis	• Infertility • Chronic pelvic pain • Ectopic pregnancy • Perihepatitis (Fitz–Hugh–Curtis syndrome) • Reiter's syndrome (reactive arthritis)	Abnormal pulmonary function tests	• Proctitis • Proctocolitis

CHLAMYDIA

Chlamydia trachomatis is an obligate intracellular bacterium and it mainly infects ocular and genitourinary epithelium. The ocular disease is one of the leading causes of blindness worldwide. The genital infections caused by *Chlamydia* are also very common bacterial sexually transmitted infection. Lymphogranuloma venereum (LGV) is also a chlamydia sexually transmitted infection leading to enlarged lymph nodes of severe proctitis. The clinical spectrum of *Chlamydia trachomatis* is given in **Table 1**.

Lymphogranuloma venereum is sexually transmitted, caused by different strain types of *C. Trachomatis*. It is a chronic infection of the lymphatic system that if untreated can result in complications involving the genital organs, joints, heart, liver, eyes or, rarely, the brain.

The majorities of genital infections remain asymptomatic and act as source of infection. The diagnosis of trachoma in endemic areas is by physical examination as per criteria established by the World Health Organization. The diagnosis of genital infections require microbiologic testing, ideally by nucleic acid amplification tests (NAATs) of first-catch urine in men and vaginal swabs in women.

The single dose azithromycin is treatment for trachoma usually provided as mass treatment. The treatment of uncomplicated urogenital infection is azithromycin 1 g as single dose or doxycycline 100 mg twice a day for 7 days. The treatment of sexual partner is important to prevent reinfection.

Trachoma can be prevented by frequent washing of face, practice of hygiene practices, and access to clean water.

The screening of females in sexually active age group annually and screening of all pregnant females is recommended. One-time screening and treatment in women decreases risk of symptomatic pelvic inflammatory disease in the following year.

CHLAMYDIA PSITTACI (PSITTACOSIS)

It causes pneumonia after exposure to infected birds. The diagnosis is commonly made by serology and if available by PCR. The treatment should not be delayed as diagnosis may not be available early. Doxycyclines or tetracyclines are drugs of choice; however, macrolides and fluoroquinolones are also effective.

CHLAMYDIA PNEUMONIAE

It is primarily a respiratory pathogen causing community-acquired atypical pneumonia and is known to cause epidemics in schools, nursing homes, and military bases. It can cause persistent subclinical infection. *Chlamydia pneumoniae* can lead to a spectrum of respiratory and nonrespiratory clinical syndromes. Severe infection has the potential to cause multiple organ dysfunction syndrome.

The diagnosis is established by the microimmunofluorescence technique by demonstrating either a four-fold rise in antibody titers, IgM antibody titer of 1: >16 or an IgG antibody titer of 1: >512. The diagnosis using PCR or cultures is only performed in a few laboratories. The treatment with erythromycin, clarithromycin, doxycycline, levofloxacin, or moxifloxacin for 10 days or 5 days course with azithromycin is effective.

RECOMMENDED READINGS

1. Bennet JE, Doalin R, Blaser MJ. Principles and Practice of Infectious Diseases. Philadelphia: Elsevier; 2017.
2. Cook GC, Zumla A. Manson's Tropical Diseases, 22nd edition. London: Saunders Elsevier Science, Health Sciences Division; 2009.
3. Walker DH. Rickettsial diseases including ehrlichioses. In: Warrel DA, Cox TM, Firth JD (Eds). Oxford Textbook of Medicine, 4th edition. Oxford: Oxford University Press; 2003. pp. 623-31.
4. Mahajan SK. Rickettsial diseases. J Assoc Physicians India. 2012;60:37-44.
5. La Scola B, Raoult D. Laboratory Diagnosis of Rickettsioses: Current Approaches to Diagnosis of Old and New Rickettsial Diseases. J Cli Micro. 1997;35(11):2715-27.

6. Cowan G. Rickettsial diseases: the typhus group of fevers—a review. Postgrad Med J. 2000;76:269-72.
7. Alvarez-Eicoro S, Enzler MJ. The macrolide: erythromycin, clarithromycin and azithromycin. Mayo Clin Proc. 1999;74:613-34.
8. Chapman AS, Bakken JS, Folk SM, Paddock CD, Bloch KC, Krusell A, et al. Diagnosis and management of tickborne rickettsial diseases: Rocky Mountain spotted fever, ehrlichioses, and anaplasmosis—United States: a practical guide for physicians and other health-care workers and public health professionals. MMWR Recomm Rep. 2006;55(RR-4):1-27.
9. Kashyap S, Sarkar M. *Mycoplasma pneumonia*: Clinical features and management. Lung India. 2010;27(2):75-85.
10. Black CM. Chlamydial Infection: A Clinical and Public Health Perspective. Basel: Karger; 2013. pp. 1-8.

CHAPTER 62

Other Mycobacterial Infections: Leprosy and Nontuberculous Mycobacteria

SK Baruah, Bhaskar Thakuria, Hitakalpa Baishya

ABSTRACT

Leprosy is a chronic infectious disease caused by *Mycobacterium leprae*. India has the highest burden of the disease. *M. leprae* is acid fast when stained by Ziehl–Neelsen (ZN) stain or a modified Fite stain. Humans are major host and reservoir. The major features are skin lesions, thickened peripheral nerves, and acid fast bacilli (AFB) on slit skin smears or biopsy. It is divided into five groups: Tuberculoid (TT), borderline tuberculoid (BT), mid borderline (BB), borderline lepromatous (BL), and lepromatous leprosy (LL). The World Health Organization (WHO) has classified it to paucibacillary (PB) and multibacillary (MB). Lepra reaction and Lucio's phenomenon may occur. Rifampicin, clofazimine, and dapsone are used for treating leprosy. Lepra reactions may require glucocorticoids. The National Leprosy Control Programme strategies and plans, though formulated centrally are implemented by states and union territories (UTs) with support from WHO, International Federation of Anti-Leprosy Association (ILEP), and nongovernment organizations (NGOs).

Nontuberculous mycobacteria (NTM) are environmental organisms capable of causing infection in immunocompromised and immunocompetent hosts. Disease is acquired by human from environment exposure. NTM are classified according to the rate of growth and pigment production at cultures. They are acid fast and produce positive Mantoux test but CBNAAT negative. NTM can produce pulmonary disease, lymphadenitis, skin and soft tissue infections, and disseminated disease. Treatment should contain at two drugs of proven efficacy. Macrolides and some antitubercular drugs are effective against NTM.

"Neglect starts out as an infection then becomes a disease"

—Jim Rohn

LEPROSY

INTRODUCTION

Leprosy (Hansen's disease) is a chronic infectious granulomatous disease caused by *M. leprae. M. leprae* was discovered by Hansen in Norway in 1873. The WHO has listed it as one of the neglected tropical diseases.

There were 208,619 new leprosy cases registered worldwide in 2018 as per official figures from 159 countries from the six WHO regions. The global prevalence rate of leprosy at the end of 2018 was 0.2/10,000.

India, which has the highest burden of disease accounted for 120,334 new cases in 2017–2018.

EPIDEMIOLOGY

Mycobacterium leprae is an obligate intracellular bacillus that is gram positive and acid fast when stained by ZN or a modified Fite stain. It has a generation time of 12–14 days.

Mycobacterium leprae can remain viable outside the human body for up to 9 days and its survival is optimal at high humidity.

Humans are considered to be the major host and reservoir of *M. leprae*. Other animals such as armadillos, chimpanzee, mangabey, and macaque monkeys have also been incriminated as a reservoir of infection.

There may be multiple routes of transmission, of which nasal droplet infection and contact with infected soil have been considered important.

CLASSIFICATION AND CLINICAL SPECTRUM

The clinical manifestations of leprosy are largely confined to skin, peripheral nervous system, upper respiratory tract, eyes, and testes. Leprosy has varied manifestations which

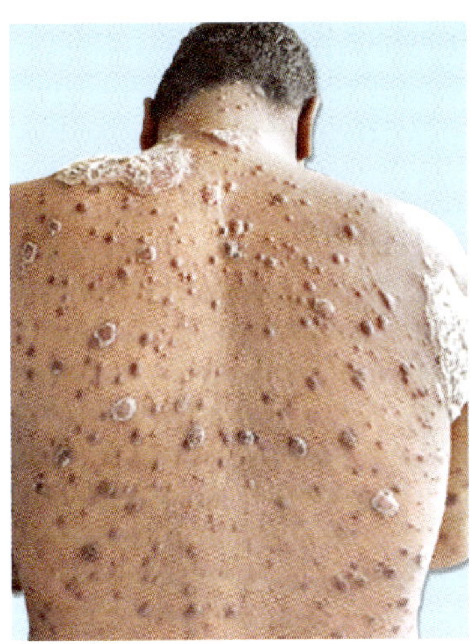

FIGURE 1: Lepromatous leprosy: Nodular lesions on trunk.

Source: Gauhati Medical College.

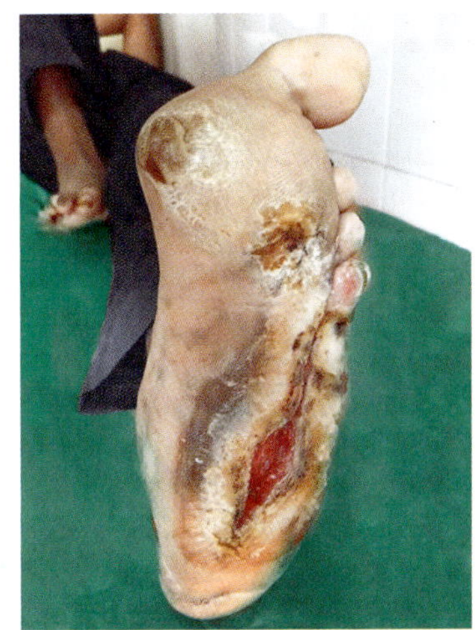

FIGURE 2: Complication of lepromatous leprosy: Foot ulcer.

Source: Gauhati Medical College.

may include hypoesthetic, hypopigmented or erythematous macules, localized paresthesias painless nodules over face, ears, elbows and knees, blistering on hands and feet, nasal stuffiness, facial deformity etc. (**Fig. 1**). The three cardinal features of leprosy are:

1. Skin lesions, typically anesthetic at TT end of the spectrum
2. Thickened peripheral nerves
3. AFB on slit skin smears or biopsy

As per the Ridley–Jopling classification, leprosy is divided into five groups: TT, BT, BB, BL, and LL.

The WHO has classified leprosy as PB (≤5 lesions or skin smear negative for AFB) and MB (>5 lesions or skin smear positive for AFB) for the ease of treatment.

COMPLICATIONS

- As a consequence of neuropathy leading to insensitivity and myopathy, the extremities are affected in the form of wrist drop, foot drop, plantar ulceration, Charcot's joint, and loss of distal digits in few cases with LL disease (**Fig. 2**).
- Chronic nasal congestion and epistaxis may be seen in cases of LL due to bacillary invasion of nasal mucosa. Long untreated cases may present with saddle nose deformity and anosmia.
- Leprosy is a major cause of blindness in the developing world. Lagophthalmos, corneal ulceration, and opacities are seen owing to cranial nerve palsies. In LL due to bacillary invasion of the anterior chamber and in cases of erythema nodosum leprosum (ENL), uveitis with consequent glaucoma, and cataract may be seen.
- Male patients with LL may become impotent and infertile owing to testicular dysfunction associated with decreased testosterone levels, elevated luteinizing hormone (LH) and follicle-stimulating hormone (FSH) levels, aspermia, or hypospermia.
- Secondary amyloidosis resulting in hepatic and renal abnormalities is a complication of LL and ENL which has become infrequent in the postmultidrug therapy (MDT) era.
- Mostly the patient with BT leprosy may present with nerve abscess, usually the ulnar nerve. Rapid surgical decompression is necessary to prevent irreversible sequelae, though glucocorticoids may reduce signs of inflammation.

LEPRA REACTIONS

These reactions may occur spontaneously superimposed on the cardinal features of leprosy or after initiation of MDT.

Type 1 lepra reaction (reversal reaction) is a cell-mediated hypersensitivity reaction that manifest as appearance of new skin lesions, swelling of existing lesions, painful and tender peripheral nerves, and sudden loss of nerve function.

Type 2 lepra reaction (ENL) is immune complex-mediated hypersensitivity reaction which presents as fever, edema, tender papules and nodules, iritis, orchitis, myositis, and lymphadenitis.

Lucio's phenomenon is an unusual reaction probably mediated by immune complexes. It is seen exclusively in patients with diffuse lepromatosis form of LL, mostly untreated cases. Patients with this reaction develop recurrent crops of large, sharply marginated, and ulcerative lesions particularly on the lower extremities that may be generalized. Histologically, the lesions are characterized by ischemic necrosis of the epidermis and superficial dermis, heavy parasitism of endothelial cells with AFB, and endothelial proliferation and thrombus formation in the larger vessels of the deeper dermis.

TREATMENT

The standard adult treatment regimen for MB leprosy (12 months) is:

- Rifampicin 600 mg once a month
- Clofazimine 300 mg once a month and 50 mg daily

- Dapsone 100 mg daily
- The standard adult treatment regimen for PB leprosy (6 months) is:
  - Rifampicin 600 mg once a month
  - Dapsone 100 mg daily

Type 1 lepra reaction is treated with anti-inflammatory agents and severe cases with glucocorticoids with gradual dose tapering over 3–6 months.

Treatment of ENL is individualized. Mild cases are treated with antipyretics alone. Glucocorticoids are effective in controlling the reaction. In case of recurrence, thalidomide or high-dose clofazimine is used judiciously.

Leprosy patients with rifampicin resistance may be treated using at least two of the following second-line drugs: Clarithromycin, minocycline or a quinolone (ofloxacin, levofloxacin, or moxifloxacin), plus clofazimine daily for 6 months followed by clofazimine plus one of the second-line drugs daily for additional 18 months.

Patients with both rifampicin and ofloxacin resistance may be treated with the following drugs: Clarithromycin, minocycline, and clofazimine for 6 months followed by clarithromycin or minocycline plus clofazimine for another 18 months.

IMMUNOPROPHYLAXIS

Vaccination at birth with Bacillus Calmette-Guérin (BCG) has shown variable efficacy ranging from 0% to 80%. A small-sized clinical trial in India studied a combination of MDT and immunotherapy with BCG in newly diagnosed leprosy patients and found a significant reduction in duration of reactions, incidence of ENL, and time to achieve bacterial clearance.

LepVax and *Mycobacterium indicus pranii* (MIP) are two candidate vaccines which has shown efficacy in prevention of leprosy. MIP is currently being evaluated as a prophylactic and therapeutic vaccine in two high endemic districts of India in combination with a single-dose rifampicin (SDR).

CHEMOPROPHYLAXIS

Chemoprophylaxis with SDR is recommended for contacts of leprosy patients (adults and children >2 years) after excluding leprosy and tuberculosis (TB). The recommended dose is given in **Table 1**.

TABLE 1 Chemoprophylaxis for leprosy.

Age	Rifampicin single dose
≥15 years	600 mg
10–14 years	450 mg
6–9 years (≥20 kg)	300 mg
>2 years (<20 kg)	10–15 mg/kg

PRESENT INDIAN SCENARIO

- India is among the 22 "global priority countries" that contribute to 95% of the world numbers of leprosy and 60% of new cases reported globally warranting a sustained effort to bring the numbers down.
- As per the WHO latest update, despite of significant reduction in prevalence of leprosy worldwide, new cases continue to arise indicating continued transmission.
- The National Leprosy Eradication Programme (NLEP) strategies and plans though formulated centrally are implemented by states and UTs with support from WHO, ILEP, and NGOs. In addition to achieving the national elimination target by end of 2005, India succeeded in achieving elimination at the state level in 34 states/UTs out of 36 by the end of 2011–2012. Only Chhattisgarh and Dadra and Nagar Haveli were yet to achieve elimination.
- Four alarming trends were brought to the notice in August 2016, by the deputy director general for leprosy:
  1. There are pockets of high endemicity with ongoing transmission.
  2. There are many hidden cases in the community as revealed by the Indian Council of Medical Research (ICMR) sample survey.
  3. New case detection rate has remained almost same since 2005.
  4. Disability rates have been rising due to delay in diagnosis.
- NLEP has advocated a pronged approach in order to address these challenges:
  - Leprosy Case Detection Campaign (LCDC) in endemic districts.
  - Focused leprosy awareness campaign using Accredited Social Health Activist (ASHA) and Multipurpose Worker (MPW) in hotspots where new cases with grade 2 disability are detected.
  - Area specific plans for case detection in hard-to-reach areas.
- The SPARSH leprosy awareness campaign was launched on 30 January, 2017 with the aim of promoting awareness and addressing the issues of stigma and discrimination.
- NLEP has also launched *Nikusth* a web-based reporting system for leprosy. It will also be helpful in keeping track of all the activities being implemented under NLEP.

AREAS OF CONCERN

Few challenges like delay in detecting new patients, discrimination against those affected, lack of effective monitoring of treatment adherence by healthcare workers, and prevention of disability and need of medical rehabilitation need to be addressed.

Community education regarding early signs and symptoms of leprosy and its curability by MDT is needed to encourage people for self-reporting and reduce social stigma.

The WHO has identified research areas for diagnosis [polymerase chain reaction (PCR) on tissue samples, ultrasound and other imaging tests, new biomarkers etc.], treatment (shorter MDT for MB leprosy with study on effects in terms of bacteriological outcomes and drug-resistant leprosy), chemoprophylaxis, and immunoprophylaxis (existing and new vaccines).

NONTUBERCULOUS MYCOBACTERIA

Nontuberculous mycobacteria are environmental organisms capable of causing infection in immunocompromised and immunocompetent hosts. There are more than 125 different types, of which around 40 species are involved in human disease. NTM are mycobacteria other than *Mycobacterium tuberculosis*, its close relatives (*M. bovis, M. caprae, M. africanum, M. canetti, and M. pinnipedii*) and *M. leprae*. They are also often referred to by various other names such as atypical mycobacteria, mycobacteria other than tuberculosis (MOTT), environmental mycobacteria, and opportunistic mycobacteria.

Nontuberculous mycobacteria are found throughout the environment viz. natural water sources, drinking water distribution systems (biofilm formation), hot tubs and spas, acidic brown water swamps, potting soils, boreal forest soils and pits, metal removal fluid systems etc. Thus, their habitat is intimately shared with those of humans.

EPIDEMIOLOGY

Nontuberculous mycobacteria are widely distributed in the environment. Organisms found in soil and water, both natural and treated water sources. *M. kansasii, M. xenopi,* and *M. simiae* are almost exclusively isolated from municipal water sources. There is no evidence of animal-to-human or human-to-human transmission of NTM, except in patients of cystic fibrosis. Human disease is acquired from environment exposures. They are relatively resistant to chlorination and ozonization. Key distinguishing features between *M. tuberculosis* and NTM are tabulated in **Table 2**.

They basically differ in terms of pathogenicity, infection rates, and transmission routes.

CLASSIFICATION

Nontuberculous mycobacteria are classified based on their rate of growth and pigment production at culture as above (**Box 1**). It is important to note that atypical mycobacteria are acid-fast and also produce positive Mantoux skin test mimicking *M. tuberculosis*. Atypical mycobacteria give sputum cartridge based nucleic acid amplification test (CBNAAT) negative results.

Mycobacterium kansasii forms visible niacin-negative, photochromogenic colonies on Löwenstein-Jensen (LJ) media at 2–3 weeks. After 2 weeks in ambient light, the colonies turn bright yellow or orange (**Fig. 3**).

Smooth and buff colored colonies on LJ media are suggestive of *M. avium* complex (MAC). *M. scrofulaceum*

BOX 1 Runyon classification basis–pigment production and rate of growth.

- **Group I: Photochromogens**
  - Form pigment after exposure to light
  - Example: *Mycobacterium kansasii*
  - Habitat: Water and animals
  - Causes: Pulmonary, skin, systemic, LN infections
- **Group II: Scotochromogens**
  - Pigment produced in dark
  - Example: *M. scrofulaceum*
  - Habitat: Water, soil, fomites
  - Causes: Cervical lymphadenitis in children
- **Group III: Nonphotochromogens**
  - No pigment production
  - Examples: *M. intracellulare, M. avium* and *M. xenopi*
  - Habitat: Soil, seawater, animals
  - Causes: Pulmonary, gastrointestinal, renal, systemic, LN infections, pulmonary epididymis
- **Group IV: Rapid growers**
  - Colonies appear within 7 days
  - Example: *M. fortuitum*
  - Habitat: Water, soil and animals
  - Causes: Pulmonary, gastrointestinal, renal, systemic, LN infections

(LN: lymph node)

TABLE 2 Comparison of *Mycobacterium tuberculosis* and nontuberculous mycobacteria.

Nontuberculous	*Mycobacterium tuberculosis*
Not obligate pathogens – normally live free in the enviroment	Obligate pathogens: Require host
Low virulence: Not usually pathogenic in the absence of predisposing conditions	Human-to-human transmission
Infection rates increasing, especially in developed countries	Infection rates decreasing, especially in developed countries
Large heterogeneous group of species	*Mycobacterium tuberculosis* complex contains small group of closely ralated subspecies

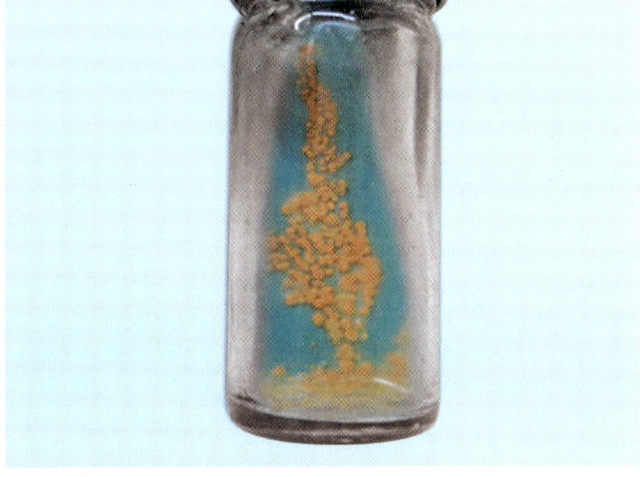

FIGURE 3: Growth of *Mycobacterium kansasii* in Löwenstein–Jensen (LJ) media.

produced yellow pigment when incubated in the darkness on LJ media. Whereas, *M. tuberculosis* colonies appears on LJ media as buff colored, dry, irregular colonies with wrinkled surface, and not easily emulsifiable (buff, rough, and tough colonies).

Important members of the photochromogens are *M. kansasii, M. marinum,* and *M. simiae. M. kansasii* causes chronic pulmonary disease resembling TB. It may also occasionally cause infections of the cervical nodes, penetrating wound infections and granulomatous synovitis. It can also produce generalized infection in human immunodeficiency virus (HIV) patients. *M. marinum* causes a warty skin lesion known as swimming pool or fish tank granuloma. It closely resembles *M. kansasii* but can be differentiated by its poor growth at 37°C, negative nitrate, and positive pyrazinamide hydrolase.

Scotochromogens form pigmented colonies even in dark. They are widely distributed in environment and sometime contaminate cultures of *tubercle bacilli*. Under this group, *M. scrofulaceum* cause cervical adenitis (scrofula) in children. *M. gordonae* is often found in tap water. It is a common contaminant of clinical specimens and is a rare cause of pulmonary disease. *M. szulgai* is an uncommon cause of pulmonary disease and bursitis.

Medically important nonphotochromogens are *M. avium, M. intracellulare, M. xenopi,* and *M. ulcerans. M. avium,* which causes natural TB in birds and lymphadenopathy in pigs, is one of the most common opportunistic human pathogens. *M. intracellulare* is commonly known as *Battey bacillus*. Both *M. avium* and *M. intracellulare* are so similar that they are commonly considered as one group, the MAC. MAC cause lymphadenopathy, pulmonary lesions or disseminated disease, particularly in acquired immunodeficiency syndrome (AIDS) patients. *M. xenopi,* originally isolated from toads, may occasionally cause chronic lung disease in human beings. *M. ulcerans* is the etiologic agent of buruli ulcer.

Rapid growers are a heterogenous group of mycobacteria capable of rapid growth, colonies appearing within 7 days of incubation. Within the group photochromogenic, scotochromogenic, and nonchromogenic species occur. Most of these are purely environmental saprophytes. Medically important species are *M. fortuitum* and *M. chelonae*. Both occasionally cause pulmonary or disseminated disease, but are principally responsible for postinjection abscess and wound infections (**Fig. 4**).

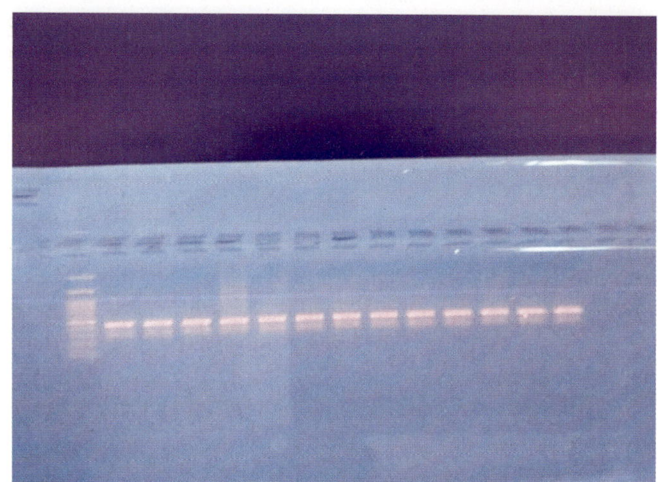

FIGURE 4: Polymerase chain reaction (PCR) for hsp65, rpoB, and 16S rRNA.

PATHOGENESIS

In HIV infected patients disseminated NTM infection typically occurred only after CD4 T-lymphocyte is <50/μL. In those without preexisting HIV infection disseminated NTM infection is associated with specific mutation in interferon (INF) gamma, interleukin 12 (IL-12) synthesis and response path, IFN-γ receptor 1, IFN-γ receptor 2, IL-12 receptor beta-1 subunit, IL-12 subunit p40 (the signal transducer and activator of transcription), and the nuclear factor-kappa beta essential modulator. The constellation of pulmonary disease due to NTM in a tall and thin woman who may have chest wall abnormalities is often referred to as Lady Windermere syndrome. Sometimes pulmonary hypersensitivity occurs to NTM (most commonly MAC organisms) which is often referred to as hot tub lung.

Risk factors for NTM infection are immunosuppression (HIV and medications), aging, cystic fibrosis, fibronodular bronchiectasis, predisposing lung diseases, chronic obstructive pulmonary disease (COPD), pneumoconiosis, prior TB, pulmonary alveolar proteinosis, esophageal motility disorders etc.

CLINICAL FEATURES

Various lesions produced by NTM are pulmonary lesions, localized lymphadenitis, skin and soft tissue infections, and disseminated disease.

Pulmonary disease: Common etiologic agents for pulmonary disease are MAC, *M. kansasii, M. abscessus,* and *M. xenopi*. The clinical, radiological, and microbiological factors or diagnosis of NTM pulmonary disease are given in **Box 2**.

Lymph node disease: Common etiologic agents are *MAC; M. scrofulaceum, M. kansasii, M. malmoense,* and *M. haemophilum*. Lymph node disease usually occurs in children below 5 years of age. MAC is the most common organism followed by *M. scrofulaceum*. Unilateral, submandibular lymph node most commonly involved. Onset of symptoms is usually subacute. Skin induration and sinus tract formation may occur. For diagnosis fine needle or excisional biopsy is needed and TB must be ruled out.

Skin and soft tissue infection: Common etiological agents are *M. marinum* which causes fish tank granuloma/swimming pool granuloma, *M. ulcerans* (which causes Buruli ulcer), *M. fortuitum,* and *M. abscessus/chelonae.*

- *Swimming pool granuloma*: It is caused by *M. marinum* and is also known as fish tank granuloma. *M marinum* occurs as saprophyte in fresh or salt water. Human infection originates from contaminated swimming pools or fish tanks. The bacilli enter through scratches

BOX 2 Diagnostic Criteria of NTM pulmonary disease.

Clinical, radiological, and microbiological all required

Clinical:

- Pulmonary symptoms (Cough, fatigue, weight loss. Fever and hemoptysis are less common and suggest advance/extensive disease)

and

- Exclusion of other disease (Such as TB, malignancy)

Chest imaging:

- Radiograph: Nodular or cavitary lesion on chest radiograph

or

- High-resolution computed tomography (HRCT): Multifocal bronchiectasis with multiple small nodules

Microbiologic:

- Positive cultures from two separate sputum specimens

or

- Positive culture from >1 bronchial wash or bronchoalveolar lavage (BAL)

or

- Lung biopsy with histopathologic changes of granulomatous inflammation or AFB *plus* positive NTM culture

and abrasions and cause warty lesion similar to those seen in skin TB. The lesion begin as a papule and breaks down to form an indolent ulcer. The disease is usually self-limiting, although chemotherapy with minocycline, cotrimoxazole, or rifampicin with ethambutol hatens its resolution.

- *Buruli ulcer*: The disease is caused by *M. ulcerans*. The name is derived from Buruli district of Uganda where a large outbreak was extensively investigated. Ulcers are usually seen on legs or arms and are believed to follow infection through minor injuries. After an incubation period of few weeks, indurated nodules appear, which breaks down forming indolent ulcers which slowly extend under the skin. When the immunoreactive phase sets in, ulcers heal with disfiguring scars.

Disseminated disease: Common etiological agents are *MAC, M. genavense, M. abscessus/chelonae,* and *M. haemophilum*. Any mycobacterium may cause disease in association with significant immunosuppression viz. HIV (CD4 <50), and any localized lesion may disseminate. Symptoms are fever, weight loss, and diarrhea. Disease can occur at any site and no prior trauma is necessary for initiation.

TREATMENT

- Patients should be carefully evaluated to determine the significance of a NTM isolate. The presence of the organism in a sterile site or repeatedly from airway secretions in association with a compatible clinical and radiologic picture confirms the diagnosis.
- Treatment of rapidly growing mycobacteria should be guided by in vitro susceptibilities. Other drug susceptibility testing is not standardized.
- Treatment should usually combine at least two drugs of proven efficacy.
- Contact follow-up is not necessary since NTM are not transmitted from person to person.
- Duration of therapy has not been determined; in general, 6–12 months is required following negative cultures.
- In soft tissue infections, because of rapidly growing mycobacteria, a combination of debridement and treatment with antimicrobials is recommended. For selection of antimicrobial agents, consultation with the laboratory should be undertaken regarding the reliability of in vitro testing.

***Mycobacterium avium* complex pulmonary disease:**

- *For Nodular/bronchiectatic MAC lung disease*: Initial three time weekly regimen consisting of clarithromycin 1,000 mg or azithromycin 500 mg, rifampin 600 mg, and ethambutol 25 mg/kg body weight (BW). Patients to be followed with sputum culture monthly. Treatment to be continued until culture negative for 1 year.
- *Fibrocavitary or severe nodular/bronchiectasis*: Initially daily treatment consisting of clarithromycin 500–1,000 mg or azithromycin 250 mg/day, rifampin 600 mg, or rifabutin 150–300 mg, ethambutol 15 mg/kg BW, ± 3 times weekly amikacin or streptomycin for 3 months. Treatment continued until culture negative for 1 year.

Macrolide-resistant *Mycobacterium avium* complex lung disease: It is analogous to treatment for drug-resistant TB. Risk factor for development of macrolide-resistant MAC lung disease is macrolide monotherapy or inadequate companion drug use. Management principles include use of parenteral aminoglycosides: Parenteral streptomycin or amikacin or surgical resection (debulking). The four drug regimen that is often used includes isoniazid (INH), rifampin, ethambutol, and streptomycin for 3–6 months.

Disseminated *Mycobacterium avium* complex infections: Clarithromycin 500 mg BID or azithromycin 500 mg/day and ethambutol 15 mg/kg/day ± rifabutin 300 mg/day (interferes with metabolism of protease inhibitors and non-nucleoside reverse transcriptase inhibitors). Therapy discontinued with resolution of symptoms and reconstitution of cell-mediated immune function (CD4 count >100/μL for 12 months). Otherwise, treatment should be lifelong.

Prophylaxis of disseminated Mycobacterium avium complex disease: It is indicated when CD4 T-lymphocyte count is <50 cells/μL. Antimicrobial agents used are azithromycin 1,200 mg/week or clarithromycin 1,000 mg/day, or rifabutin 300 mg/day.

***Mycobacterium kansasii* pulmonary disease:** Treatment is similar to TB. Regimen usually includes: INH 300 mg/day, rifampin 600 mg/day, ethambutol 15 mg/kg/day, until culture negative for 1 year. Pyrazinamide is not effective against *M. Kansasii*. Other drugs with activity against *M. Kansasii* include macrolide, fluoroquinolone, and cotrimoxazole.

***Mycobacterium marinum* infection:** This infection can be treated with variety of antibiotics including doxycycline 200 mg/day or clarithromycin 500 mg/day or rifampin 600 mg/day or minocycline 200 mg/day or ciprofloxacin 1,000 mg/day or trimethoprim-sulfamethoxazole 160/800 mg/day. Total duration of therapy is for 2–12 months.

***Mycobacterium abscessus* pulmonary disease:** There is no drug regimen. Clarithromycin 1,000 mg/day and multidrug regimen is usually used. Surgical resection of localized disease is another viable alternative.

Nontuberculous mycobacteria cervical adenitis: It is mostly due to MAC. Surgical resection is associated with >90% cure rate. A macrolide-based regimen is frequently used for extensive MAC lymphadenitis.

RECOMMENDED READINGS

1. WHO. Leprosy elimination. [online] Available from www.who.int/lep/resources.
2. WHO. (2018). Guidelines for the diagnosis, treatment and prevention of leprosy. [online] Available from https://apps.who.int/iris/bitstream/handle/10665/274127/9789290226383-eng.pdf?ua=1.
3. Katoch K, Katoch VM, Natarajan M, Gupta UD, Sharma VD, Shivanavar CT. 10-12 years follow up of highly bacillated BL/LL leprosy patients on combined chemotherapy and immunotherapy. Vaccine. 2004;22(27-28):3649-57.
4. Kumar S. India resurrects forgotten leprosy vaccine. Science. 2017;356(6342):999.
5. National Leprosy Eradication Programme. Revised operational guidelines for leprosy case detection campaign. Central Leprosy Division. Directorate General of Health Services. Government of India: Ministry of Health and Family Welfare; 2016.
6. Falkinham JO 3rd. Epidemiology of infection by nontuberculous mycobacteria. Clin Microbiol Rev. 1996;9:177-215.
7. Primm TP, Lucero CA, Falkinham JO 3rd. Health impacts of environmental mycobacteria. Clin Microbiol Rev. 2004;17:98-106.
8. Tortoli E. Clinical manifestations of nontuberculous mycobacteria infections. Clin Microbiol Infect. 2009;15:906-10.
9. McShane PJ, Glassroth J. Pulmonary Disease Due to Nontuberculous Mycobacteria: Current State and New Insights. Chest. 2015;148:1517-27.
10. Johnson MM, Odell JA. Nontuberculous mycobacterial pulmonary infections. J Thorac Dis. 2014;6:210-20.
11. Griffith DE, Aksamit T, Brown-Elliott BA, Catanzaro A, Daley C, Gordin F, et al. An official ATS/IDSA statement: diagnosis, treatment, and prevention of nontuberculous mycobacterial diseases. Am J Respir Crit Care Med. 2007;175:367-416.
12. Singh K, Kumari R, Tripathy R, Gupta S, Anupurba S. Detection of clinically important non tuberculous mycobacteria (NTM) from pulmonary samples through one-step multiplex PCR assay. BMC Microbiol. 2020;20:267.

CHAPTER

63

Spirochetal Infections: Syphilis, Leptospirosis, and Others

Gurinder Mohan, Akanksha, Jaspreet Kaur

ABSTRACT

Spirochetales include four genera that are pathogenic organisms for humans and other animals: *Leptospira* species (leptospirosis); *Borrelia* species (relapsing fever and Lyme disease); *Brachyspira* species [gastrointestinal (GI) infections] and *Treponema* species (syphilis and endemic treponematosis). The *Treponema* subspecies include *T. pallidum* subspecies pallidum (venereal syphilis); *T. pallidum* subspecies pertenue (yaws); *T. pallidum* subspecies endemicum (endemic syphilis or bejel); and *T. carateum* (pinta). *Treponema pallidum* causes venereal syphilis which is staged into early and late syphilis. Early syphilis includes primary, secondary, and early latent syphilis. Late syphilis further includes tertiary and late latent syphilis. Every patient with high-risk behavior, human immunodeficiency virus (HIV) infection, and pregnancy should be screened for syphilis with nontreponemal serologic tests whereas for confirmation treponemal serologic tests are performed. Yaws, bejel, and pinta are nonsexually transmitted and are largely limited to tropical regions. These are usually transmitted during childhood and cause late severe clinical manifestations after initial infection.

Further, leptospirosis which is a zoonotic infection, is caused after exposure to rodents, it is staged as mild or severe infection depending upon the immune reaction involved. Severe manifestation includes Weil's disease, an icterohemorrhagic disease, which includes hemorrhage, jaundice, and acute kidney injury. For the diagnosis of leptospirosis serologic testing should be performed in immune phase of the disease, and in early phase isolation of organism should be the preferred diagnostic test. *Borrelia* species cause relapsing fever and Lyme disease. Relapsing fever is further of two types: Tick-borne relapsing fever (TBRF) and louse-borne relapsing fever (LBRF).

"Infectious diseases are impossible to cover up. You may be able to cover up figures but you cannot cover up the viruses"

—Gao Qiang

SYPHILIS

It is a venereal disease.

CAUSATIVE AGENT

Treponema pallidum subspecies *pallidum* is the causative agent. Human are the natural host.

TRANSMISSION

- Sexual contact
- Blood transfusion
- Infection in utero
- Organ transplantation

Individuals who are sexual contact of infected person if remain asymptomatic and untreated, will develop infectious syphilis. Hence, it is essential to identify and treat all recently exposed sexual contacts.

Regions most affected by syphilis are Sub-Saharan Africa, South America, China, and Southeast Asia.

PATHOGENESIS

Treponema pallidum penetrates intact mucous membrane or abrasion in skin

↓

Enters lymphatics and blood within hours

↓

Disseminates to tissues

↓

Primary lesion appears at inoculation site (histopathology shows perivascular infiltration of CD4 and CD8 T lymphocytes, plasma cell, and macrophages)

↓

Primary lesion heals spontaneously due to phagocytosis by macrophages

↓

After 6–12 weeks, secondary syphilis appears (due to variation of surface antigen, immune evasion occurs)

↓

Within 2–6 weeks, it generally subsides

↓

Patient enters latent syphilis

Coexpression of HIV receptors (CCR5 and DC-SIGN) on dendritic cells explains the link between syphilis and HIV.

CLINICAL MANIFESTATIONS

Syphilis is staged as:
- Early syphilis includes primary, secondary, and early latent syphilis.
- Late syphilis includes tertiary and late latent syphilis.

Primary syphilis: Typical primary chancre (**Fig. 1**) is single painless papule which erodes to have an indurated edge accompanied by bilateral, nontender, nonsuppurative, and firm lymphadenopathy.

Site: Penis in heterosexual, anal/rectum in homosexual men, cervix or labia in female.

Primary syphilis usually not recognized in females and homosexual men.

Secondary syphilis:
- *Generalized symptoms*: Constitutional symptoms (fever, malaise, anorexia, weight loss, and sore throat) and generalized nontender lymphadenopathy
- *Dermatological findings*: Rash consists of macular, papular, papulosquamous, pustule (**Figs. 2 A** and **B**), lues maligna (**Fig. 3**), and moth-eaten alopecia (**Fig. 4**)

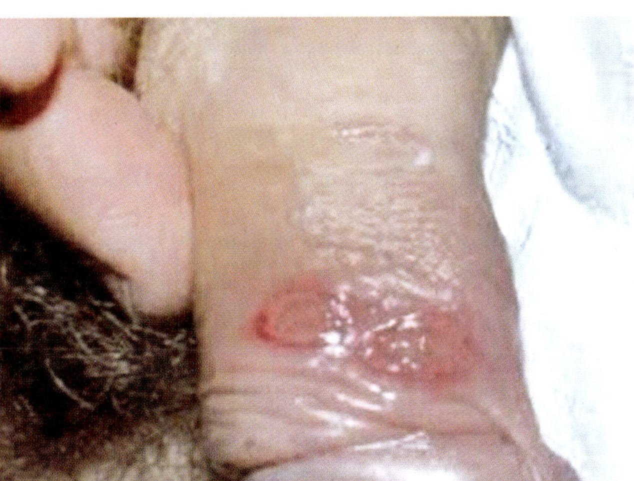

FIGURE 1: Primary chancre on penis in syphilis.

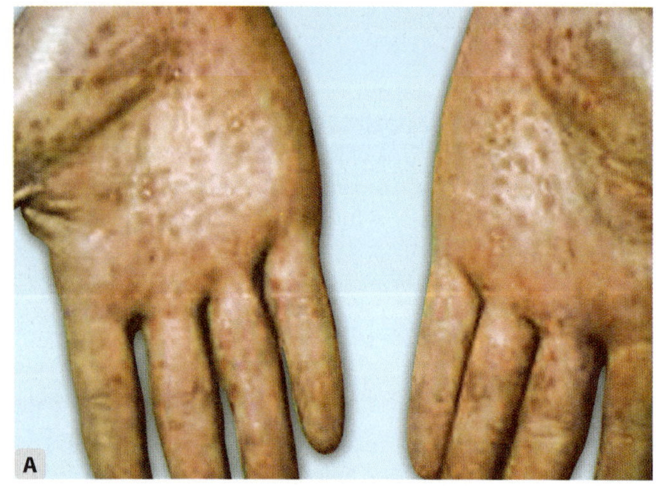

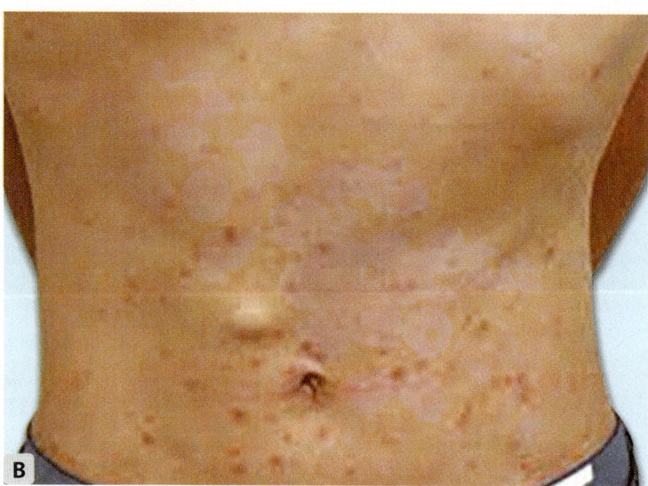

FIGURES 2 A & B: Cutaneous lesions in secondary syphilis.

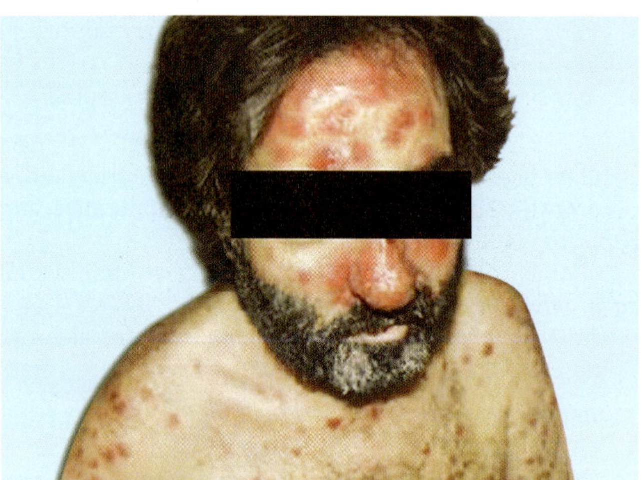

FIGURE 3: Lues maligna cutaneous lesions in secondary syphilis in human immunodeficiency virus (HIV).

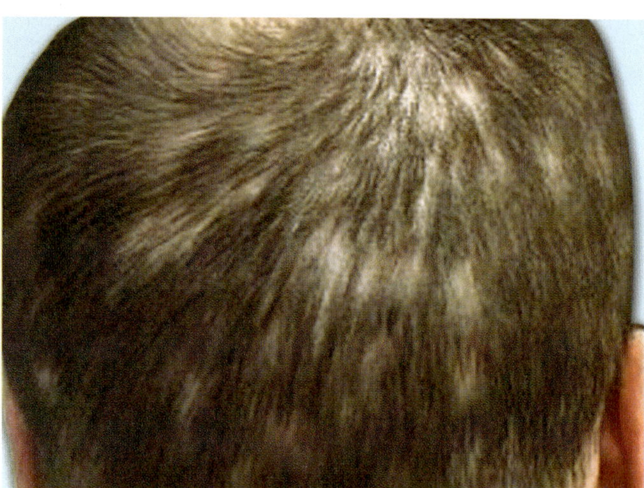

FIGURE 4: Moth-eaten alopecia seen in secondary syphilis.

Initially lesions are pink, nonpruritic, discrete macules over trunk, and extremities which progress to papular lesions, even involving palms and soles.

Severe necrotic lesion (lues maligna) (**Fig. 3**) may appear in HIV infection where primary and secondary manifestations may coexist.

Moist, intertriginous papules enlarge to produce pink or gray white infectious painless erosion with red periphery called as *condylomata lata* (**Fig. 5**) commonly involving oral or genital mucosa.

Gastrointestinal findings: Hepatitis (cholestatic pattern) and GI ulcerations

Musculoskeletal findings: Synovitis, osteitis, and periostitis

Renal abnormalities: Albuminuria, nephrotic syndrome (membranous glomerulopathy) or acute nephritis with hypertension, and acute renal failure

Neurological findings: Headache, meningitis, cranial neuritis, meningovascular disease, or stroke

Ocular findings: Anterior, posterior, or panuveitis. Retinal necrosis and optic neuritis may also occur and indicate emergent therapy

Tertiary syphilis:

Cardiovascular syphilis: Dilated aorta and aortic valve regurgitation, syphilitic aneurysms (**Fig. 6**) rarely leading to dissection, and coronary artery stenosis.

Gummatous syphilis: Gumma may present as ulcer, granulomatous lesion with round irregular or serpiginous shape (**Fig. 7**).

Neurosyphilis: May be asymptomatic or symptomatic syphilis.

Asymptomatic neurosyphilis: No neurological symptom or sign with cerebrospinal fluid (CSF) abnormality, associated with HIV infection, hence should be treated.

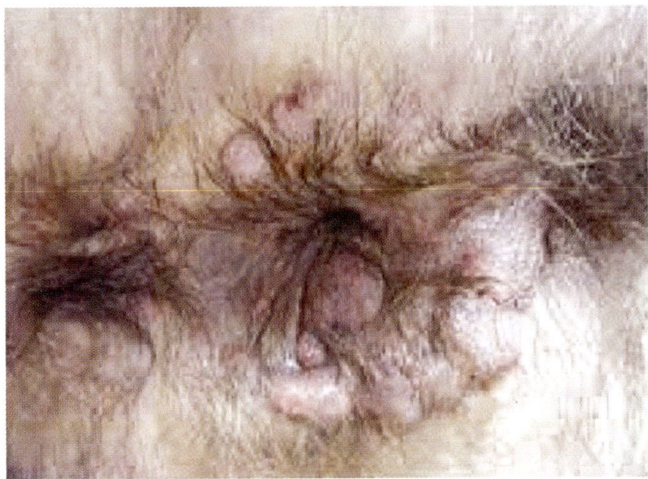

FIGURE 5: Condylomata lata seen in secondary syphilis.

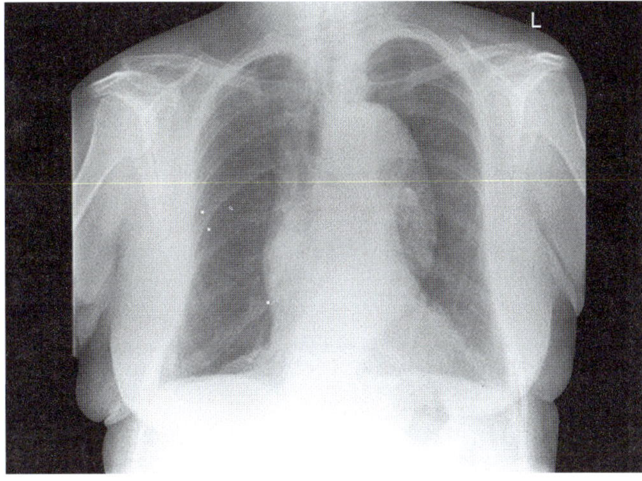

FIGURE 6: Chest X-ray showing saccular aneurysm of the ascending aorta.

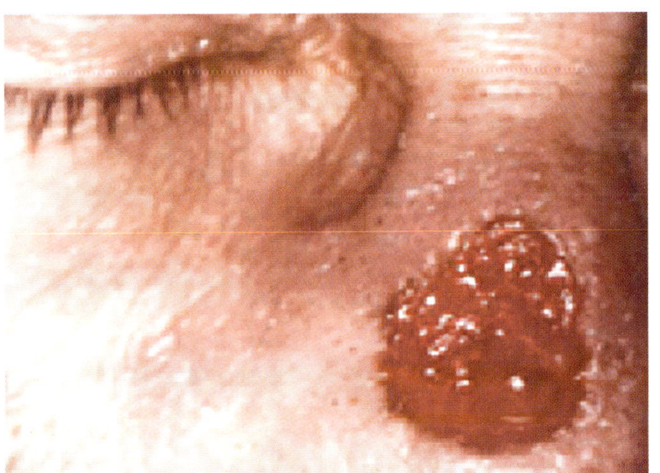

FIGURE 7: Gummatous lesion over the nose.

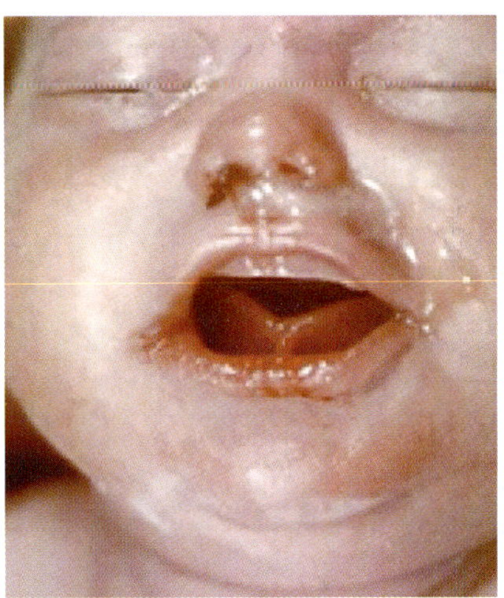

FIGURE 8: Snuffles in congenital syphilis.

Symptomatic neurosyphilis:

- *Meningeal*: Consists of meningism, seizures, cranial nerve involvement, and altered sensorium
- *Meningovascular*: Manifests after subacute encephalitic syndrome followed by gradual progressive vascular syndrome (middle cerebral artery stroke syndrome)
- *Parenchymatous syphilis*: General paresis: P (personality change), A (affect), R (reflex), E (eye Argyll Robertson Pupil), S (sensorium), I (intellect), and S (speech)
- *Tabes dorsalis*: Demyelination of posterior column, dorsal root ganglion (ataxia, foot drop, bladder disturbance, paresthesia, impotence, areflexia, loss of pain, temperature, and position sense), and optic atrophy can also be seen.

Latent syphilis: It is labelled when serological tests for syphilis are positive with normal CSF examination in the absence of clinical features of syphilis. Pregnant female with latent syphilis transmit *T. pallidum* to fetus till 4 years of acquisition. It is diagnosed on the basis of history of primary or secondary syphilis, history of syphilis exposure, and delivery of newborn from infected mother.

Early latent syphilis: Limited to first year after infection.

Late latent syphilis: Limited to duration ≥1 year or unknown period (noninfectious).

Syphilis may be transmitted during this phase. Possible future outcomes are lifelong infection, late syphilis, and spontaneous cure.

Congenital syphilis: It can transmit through placenta from syphilitic mother to fetus at any stage of pregnancy. Fetal damage does not occur after fourth month of gestation, so adequate treatment of mother before sixteenth weeks of gestation is needed.

Risk of transmission of syphilis to fetus during early syphilis is 75–95%, 35% in maternal syphilis of duration >2 years.

Clinical feature of syphilis appears early (within 2 years of life, usually 2–10 weeks of age) or late (after 2 years).

Early features include snuffles (**Fig. 8**), mucocutaneous lesion, bony changes (periostitis), rhinitis, hepatosplenomegaly, lymphadenopathy, anemia, thrombocytopenia, leukocytosis, and jaundice.

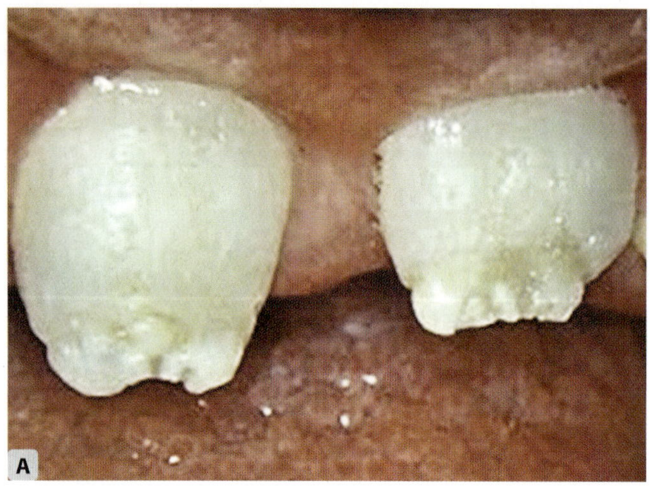
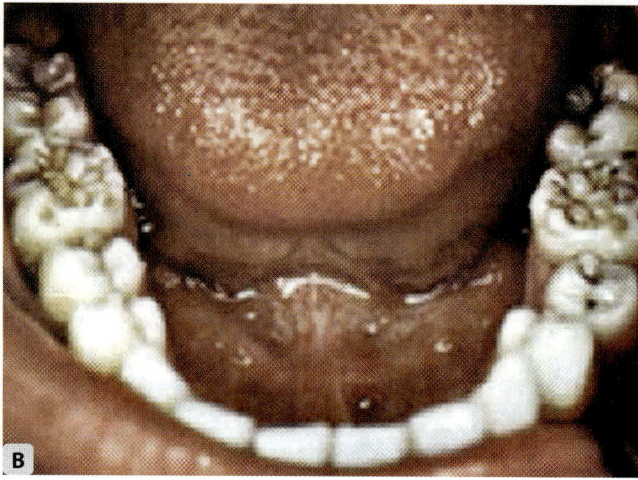

FIGURES 9 A & B: **(A)** Hutchinson teeth and **(B)** mulberry molars in congenital syphilis.

Late features are subclinical, include interstitial keratitis, 8th nerve deafness, recurrent arthropathy, neurosyphilis, Hutchinson teeth (centrally notched, wide spaced, and peg-shaped upper central incisors), mulberry molars (multiple poorly developed cusps), saddle nose, and saber shins (**Figs. 9 A** and **B**).

LABORATORY DIAGNOSIS

Whom to test:

- Asymptomatic high-risk patients [men who have sex with men (MSM), sexual partners with early syphilis, and pregnancy]
- Symptomatic patients
- HIV infected

Serologic testing: Various serologic tests are shown in **Table 1**.

Direct methods for diagnosis: Dark-field microscopy and direct fluorescent antibody testing detect organism. Polymerase chain reaction (PCR) for *T. pallidum*.

Diagnosis of neurosyphilis: Firstly perform nontreponemal test, i.e., CSF venereal disease research laboratory (VDRL). If CSF VDRL is negative and neurosyphilis is strongly suspected, perform CSF fluorescent treponemal antibody absorption (FTA-ABS).

Nonspecific CSF findings include increased cells and CSF proteins.

Table 2 shows interpretation of the serologic tests in syphilis.

Causes of false positive states:

- Pregnancy, acute febrile illness (endocarditis and rickettsial disease), and recent immunization
- Chronic conditions such as systemic lupus erythematosus (SLE), intravenous (IV) drug abuse, chronic lung disease (CLD), and HIV

Usually transitory and last for ≤6 months.

TABLE 1 Various serologic tests available for syphilis.

Nontreponemal tests	Treponemal tests
Detect serum reactivity to cardiolipin cholesterol lecithin antigen	Detect antibodies to treponemal specific antigen
Includes RPR, VDRL, and TRUST	Includes FTA-ABS, MHA-TP, TPPA, TP-EIA, and CIA
Used as initial screening test	Used as confirmatory tests
Semiquantitative	Qualitative
Used to assess the response to therapy	Remain positive throughout life
Less specific	More specific

(CIA: chemiluminescence immunoassay; FTA-ABS: fluorescent treponemal antibody absorption; MHA-TP: microhemagglutination assay for antibody to *Treponema pallidum*; RPR: rapid plasma regain; TP-EIA: *Treponema pallidum* enzyme immunoassay; TPPA: *Treponema pallidum* particle agglutination assay; TRUST: toluidine red unheated serum test; VDRL: venereal disease research laboratory)

Causes of false negative tests:

- Testing prior to antibody formation.
- Prozone reaction—inability to visualize agglutination due to overabundance of antibodies, they interfere with clumping of antigen—antibody complexes. Usually associated with pregnancy, HIV coinfection, and neurosyphilis.
- Early treatment—seroreversion of both nontreponemal and treponemal tests is uncommon.
- Seronegative late syphilis—seen with advanced immunosuppression, as in B cell failure during late stages of HIV.

TREATMENT

Table 3 shows treatment of syphilis. A common complications of treatment is the Jarisch-Herxheimer reaction.

Jarisch-Herxheimer reaction: An acute febrile reaction accompanied by headache, myalgia, rash, and hypotension

TABLE 2 Interpretation of the serologic tests in syphilis.

History	Nontreponemal test	Treponemal test	Interpretation
Symptomatic	Reactive	Reactive	Syphilis
Asymptomatic	Reactive	Reactive	New infection
Symptomatic	Nonreactive	Reactive	Very early syphilis
Without history of previous treatment	Nonreactive	Reactive	Early/late syphilis
Previously treated syphilis	Declining titer/nonreactive	Reactive	Treated syphilis
Previously treated	Fourfold or greater increase in titer	Reactive	New infection
On adequate treatment	Persistently reactive low titer (1:8)	Reactive	Serofast state
Asymptomatic	Reactive	Nonreactive	False positive
Symptoms of early syphilis	Nonreactive	Reactive	False negative
Without past diagnosis of syphilis	Reactive	Reactive	Early latent syphilis
On treatment	Less than fourfold titer fall	Reactive	Treatment failure

TABLE 3 Treatment of syphilis.

Stage of syphilis	Patient without penicillin allergy	Patient with confirmed penicillin allergy
Primary, secondary, or early latent	• CSF normal or not examined: Penicillin G benzathine (single dose of 2.4 MU IM) • CSF abnormal: Treat as neurosyphilis	• CSF normal or not examined: Tetracycline HCl (500 mg PO qid) or doxycycline (100 mg PO bid) for 2 weeks • CSF abnormal: Treat as neurosyphilis
Late latent, cardiovascular, or benign tertiary	• CSF normal or not examined: Penicillin G benzathine (single dose of 2.4 MU IM weekly for 3 weeks) • CSF abnormal: Treat as neurosyphilis	• CSF normal or not examined: Tetracycline HCl (500 mg PO qid) or doxycycline (100 mg PO bid) for 4 weeks • CSF normal and patient infected with HIV: Desensitize* and treat with penicillin, if compliance cannot assured • CSF abnormal: Treat as neurosyphilis
Neurosyphilis (asymptomatic or symptomatic)	Aqueous crystalline penicillin G (18–24 mU/day IV, given as 3–4 mUq4h or continuous infusion) for 10–14 days Or Aqueous procaine penicillin G (2.4 mU/day IM plus oral probenecid (500 mg qid) both for 10–14 days	Desensitize and treat with penicillin
Syphilis in pregnancy	According to stage	• Desensitize and treat with penicillin • If desensitization not possible alternate regimen • Primary, secondary, or latent <2 years • Erythromycin 500 mg PO qid for 2 weeks • Ceftriaxone 1 g IM OD for 2 weeks • Azithromycin 2 g PO once • Late syphilis: Erythromycin 500 mg qid for 1 month
Treatment failure	• Evidence of new infection, HIV testing • Perform LP and treat as neurosyphilis	Desensitization with penicillin

* Desensitization involves exposure of patient to small amount of penicillin and gradual increase till effective level. Oral desensitization is safe and simpler.

(CSF: cerebrospinal fluid; HIV: human immunodeficiency virus; IM: intramuscular; IV: intravenous; LP: lumbar puncture)

resulting from the release of large amounts of treponemal lipopolysaccharides from dying spirochetes and increased circulating cytokine levels [tumor necrosis factor alpha (TNFα), interleukin 6, and interleukin 8].

ENDEMIC TREPONEMATOSIS

Table 4 shows the comparison of venereal syphilis and nonsexually transmitted endemic treponematosis.

Diagnosis:

- Reactive syphilis serology in any person migrated from endemic area
- PCR to confirm infection

Treatment:

- Azithromycin (30 mg/kg) maximum up to 2 g
- Benzathine penicillin G (1.2 million units IM for adults or 60,000 units for children ≤10 years)

TABLE 4 **Comparison of venereal syphilis and nonsexually transmitted endemic treponematosis.**

Features	Venereal syphilis	Yaws	Endemic syphilis	Pinta
Organism	*Treponema pallidum* subspecies *pallidum*	*Treponema pallidum* subspecies *pertenue*	*Treponema pallidum* subspecies *endemicum*	*Treponema carateum*
Transmission mode	Sexual and transplacental	Skin-to-skin	Mouth-to-mouth	Skin-to-skin
Usual age of acquisition	Sexual and in utero	Early childhood	Early childhood	Late childhood
Primary lesion	Chancre	Papilloma (**Figs. 10 A** and **B**) (ulcerative)	Mucosal papule	Mucosal papule with pruritus
Location	Genital, oral, and anal	Extremities	Oral	• Extremities • Face
Secondary lesions	Skin rash, mucocutaneous lesion, and condylomata lata	• Condylomata lata, cutaneous papillomatous lesion • Ulcerative lesion • Osteoperiostitis (**Fig. 11**)	Mucocutaneous lesion, condylomata lata, and osteoperiostitis	Pintides and pruritic
Infectious relapses	25%	Common	unknown	Unknown
Late complication	Gumma, CVS, and CNS involvement	Destructive lesion (nose, bone, and cartilage)	Destructive lesion (nose, bone, and cartilage)	Nondestructive and achromic macules
Regions		Tropical	Arid climate	Temperate

(CNS: central nervous system; CVS: cardiovascular system)

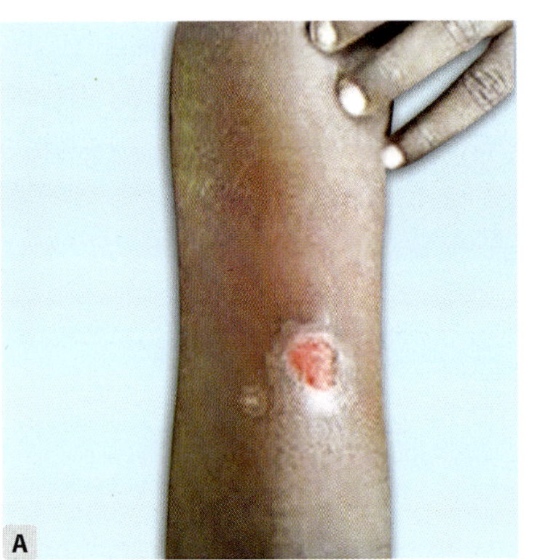

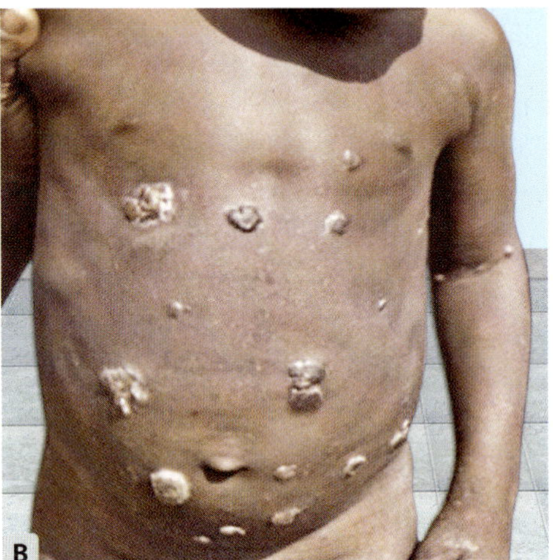

FIGURES 10 A & B: Cutaneous lesions (papillomatosis) in yaws.

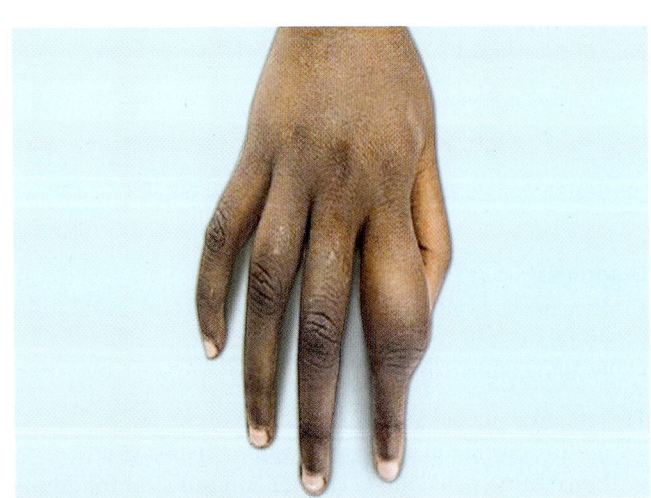

FIGURE 11: Periostitis seen in yaws.

LEPTOSPIROSIS

- It is a zoonotic disease.
- *Leptospira* species are the causative agent.
- Water serves as the vehicle for leptospirosis.
- Rodents, especially rats are the reservoir.
- Humans are the host for leptospirosis.
- The genus *Leptospira* comprised two species: The pathogenic *L. interrogans* and free-living *L. biflexa*.

TRANSMISSION

It commonly occurs in tropics (rainy season) and subtropics (summer and winter season). Transmission of *Leptospira* occurs with direct contact with urine, blood, tissue, or bite from infected animal. It can present as an endemic or an epidemic disease.

High-risk groups for leptospirosis:

- Occupational groups include veterinarians, agricultural workers, slaughterhouse employee, and workers in fish industry
- Recreational activities such as swimming, trekking, caving, and rafting
- Domestic animal contact is prominent source of leptospirosis

PATHOGENESIS

Life cycle of *Leptospira* is shown in **Figure 12**.

- *Incubation period*: 1–2 weeks (1–30 days). It is described as biphasic.
- *Acute leptospiremic phase*: Fever of 3–10 days duration during which organism can be cultured from blood and detected by PCR.
- *Immune phase*: Appearance of antibodies coincides with disappearance of *Leptospira* from blood.
- *Leptospira* can be cultured from urine.
- Mild disease does not include second phase, severe disease may be monophasic and fulminant.

CLINICAL FEATURES

Vary from asymptomatic infection to fatal disease.

Mild leptospirosis:

- These patients are asymptomatic or present as flu-like illness, muscle pain is intense, and affects calves, back, and abdomen.
- Headache is localized to retro-orbital region resembling dengue fever.
- *Rash*: Macular, maculopapular, erythematous, or hemorrhagic
- Aseptic meningitis may be present
- On examination patient has:
    - Fever
    - Conjunctival suffusion
    - Pharyngeal injection
    - Lymphadenopathy
    - Mild jaundice
    - Hepatosplenomegaly
    - Crackles on lung auscultation
- Mild leptospirosis resolves within 7–10 days.

Severe leptospirosis: Severe leptospirosis is rapidly progressive, case fatality ranging from 1 to 50%.

Patients with increased mortality:

- Age >40 years
- Altered mental status
- Acute renal failure

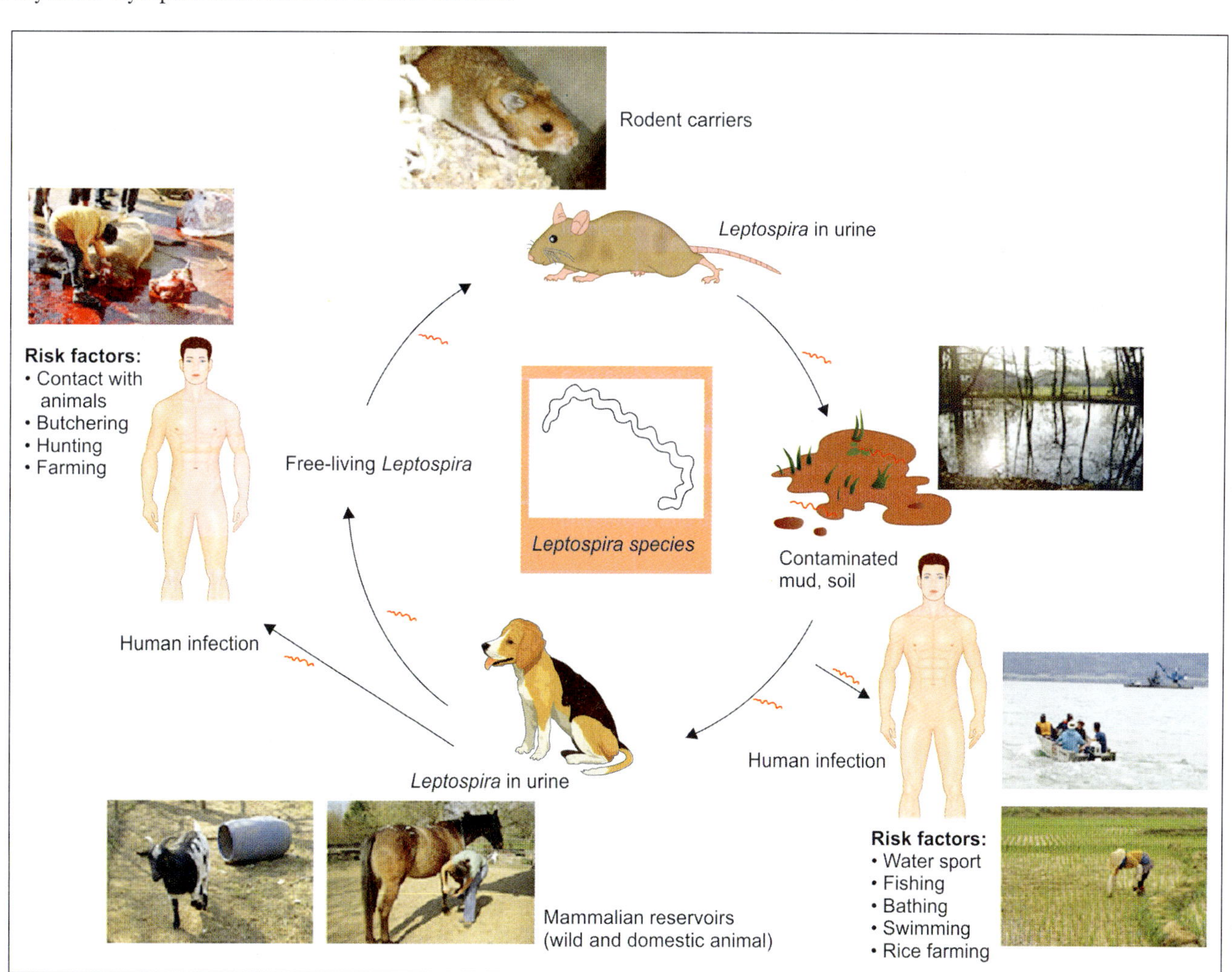

FIGURE 12: Life cycle of *Leptospira*.

- Respiratory insufficiency
- Hypotension
- Arrhythmia

Weil's syndrome:

- Triad of hemorrhage, jaundice, and acute kidney injury
- *Skin*: Petechiae, ecchymosis, and bleeding from venepuncture
- *Acute kidney injury*: Oliguric or nonoliguric and magnesiuria
- *Gastrointestinal tract (GIT)*: Melena, hematemesis, necrotizing pancreatitis, and cholecystitis
- *Pulmonary*: Hemorrhage, cough, chest pain, respiratory distress, and hemoptysis
- *Liver*: Profound jaundice and orange cast skin
- *CNS*: Meningitis
- *CVS*: Myocarditis and arrythmias
- Death due to septic shock with multiorgan failure
- *Sequelae*: Headache, myalgia, fever, and autoimmune uveitis

DIAGNOSIS

Table 5 shows the modified Faine's criteria for diagnosis of leptospirosis.

TABLE 5 Modified Faine's criteria for diagnosis of leptospirosis.

Criteria	Score
Part A: Clinical data	
Headache	2
Fever	2
If fever temperature >39°C	2
Conjunctival suffusion	4
Meningism	4
Muscle pain (especially calf muscles)	4
Conjunctival suffusion + meningism + muscle pain	10
Jaundice	1
Albuminuria or nitrogen retention	2
Part B: Epidemiological factors	
Rainfall	5
Contact with contaminated environment	4
Animal contact	1
Part C: Bacteriological and laboratory findings	
Isolation of *Leptospira* on culture	Diagnosis certain
Positive serology (any one of the three tests should be scored)	15
ELISA IgM positive	
SAT (slide agglutination test) positive	
MAT single high titer	
MAT rising titer (paired sera)	25
Total score	

By modified Faine's criteria score of ≥26 when using part A, part A + B or ≥ 25 using part A + B + C can be considered as current leptospirosis.

(ELISA: enzyme-linked immunosorbent assay; IgM: immunoglobulin M; MAT: microscopic agglutination test)

INVESTIGATIONS

- *Peripheral blood film (PBF)*: Leukocytosis (shift to left) and thrombocytopenia
- *Acute phase reactants (APR)*: Elevated erythrocyte sedimentation rate (ESR), C-reactive protein (CRP), and procalcitonin
- *Urinalysis*: Leukocytes, red blood cells (RBCs), hyaline or granular casts, mild proteinuria, magnesuria (hallmark of *Leptospira* nephropathy)
- *Renal function test (RFT)*: Azotemia
- *Electrolytes*: Hypokalemia, hyponatremia, and hypomagnesemia
- *Liver function test (LFT)*: Hyperbilirubinemia and transaminitis
- *Electrocardiogram (ECG)*: Nonspecific ST-T changes and arrhythmias.
- *CSF*: Pleocytosis (few cells to >1,000 cells/mcL predominant lymphocytes, early in disease course polymorphonuclear cells, later lymphocytes, protein elevated slightly, sugar normal
- Amylasemia, elevated creatine kinase (CK) levels
- *Chest X-ray* (**Fig. 13**): Patchy bilateral alveolar pattern (due to scattered alveolar hemorrhage), pleural based densities, diffuse ground glass attenuation typical of ARDS
- Affect lower lobes, pleural based densities, diffuse ground glass attenuation typical of ARDS

Definite diagnosis is made after isolation of organisms from the patient by PCR testing in the first week of illness (**Fig. 14**) and during the second week of illness, antibody detection can be done by MAC and ELISA.

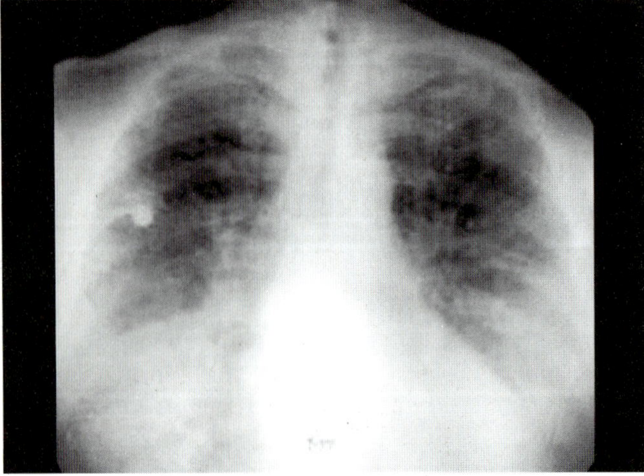

FIGURE 13: Severe pulmonary hemorrhages in leptospirosis.

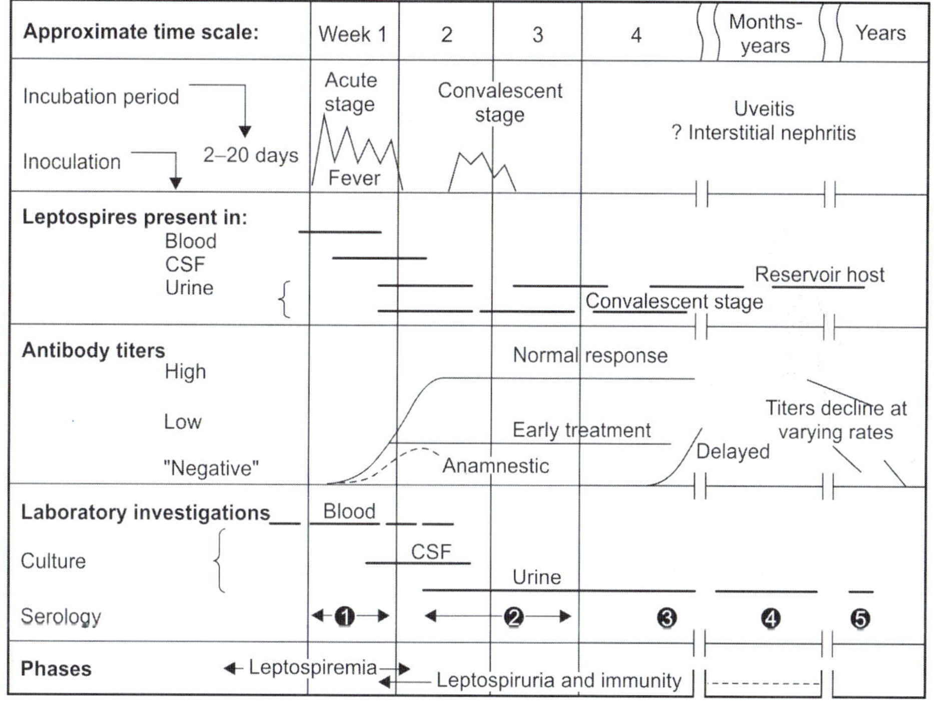

(CSF: cerebrospinal fluid)

FIGURE 14: Timing of the diagnostic tests for leptospirosis.

TABLE 6 Treatment of leptospirosis.

Indication	Treatment regimen
Mild leptospirosis	• Doxycycline (100 mg BD) Or amoxicillin (500 mg TDS) Or ampicillin (500 mg TDS)
Moderate/Severe leptospirosis	• Penicillin (1.5 MU IV or IM 6 hourly) Or ceftriaxone (2 g/day IV) Or cefotaxime 1 g IV 6 hourly Or doxycycline (loading dose of 200 mg IV, then 100 mg IV 12 hourly)
Chemoprophylaxis	• Doxycycline (200 mg once a week) Or azithromycin (250 mg once or twice a week)

(IM: intramuscular; IV: intravascular)

DIFFERENTIAL DIAGNOSIS

- Dengue
- Chikungunya
- Malaria
- Typhoid fever
- Rickettsial diseases

TREATMENT

Table 6 shows treatment of leptospirosis. All regimens are given for 7 days.

Supportive treatment:

- IV fluids
- Electrolyte resuscitation
- Peritoneal dialysis or hemodialysis
- Low tidal volume mechanical ventilation
- No steroids or desmopressin

PROGNOSIS

- Most patients recover
- *Post Leptospiral symptoms*: Depression like nature may persist for years
- Mortality is high during pregnancy

LYME BORRELIOSIS

- It is a zoonotic infection.
- It is caused by:
  - *Borrelia burgdorferi* sensu lato
  - *Borrelia garinii*
  - *Borrelia afzelii*
- The vector is ticks of the *Ixodes ricinus* complex (**Fig. 15**).
- The white-footed mouse and other rodents are the host.
- After several weeks, *B. burgdorferi* migrate into skin producing erythema migrans (EM), may spread via blood or lymph to other organs (**Fig. 16**).
- *Infection of humans*: Dead-end event for spirochete.

CLINICAL MANIFESTATIONS

Table 7 shows the stages and clinical manifestations of Lyme borreliosis.

Erythema migrans begins as red macule or papule at site of tick bite and slowly expand to form large annular lesion, develop bright red outer border and partial central clearing, and nontender. It can be located anywhere, especially thigh, groin, and axilla (**Fig. 17**).

DIAGNOSIS

- Recognition of specific clinical features accompanied by serological confirmation
- Isolation of spirochete from the culture [Barbour-Stoenner-Kelly (BSK) medium] in early infection
- PCR is more superior in late infection
- According to algorithm published by the American College of Physician, serological testing of Lyme disease is recommended only for patient with at least intermediate probability of Lyme disease
- The Centers for Disease Control and Prevention (CDC) recommends two-step approach in which sample is first tested by ELISA and positive results are then subjected to western blot.

DIFFERENTIAL DIAGNOSIS

- *Cellulitis or allergic reaction*: Lesion expands rapidly
- Relapsing fever
- Babesiosis

TREATMENT

Algorithm for testing and treatment of Lyme disease, treatment regimen, and duration of treatment for Lyme disease have been presented in **Tables 8** to **10**.

Immunoglobulin M positive response cannot be interpreted as confirmation of recent infection or reinfection unless clinical picture is appropriate.

Usually Lyme disease can be treated with oral antibiotic except:

- Severe objective neurological abnormality
- Third-degree atrioventricular (AV) block
- Arthritis not responding to oral therapy

Intravenous antibiotic is to be used, especially for 28 days:

- Ceftriaxone IV 2 g qd
- Cefotaxime IV 2 g tds
- Penicillin G, IV 5 million Uq6h

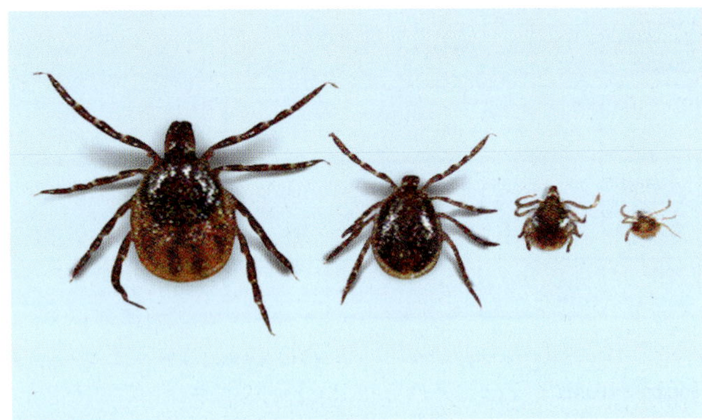

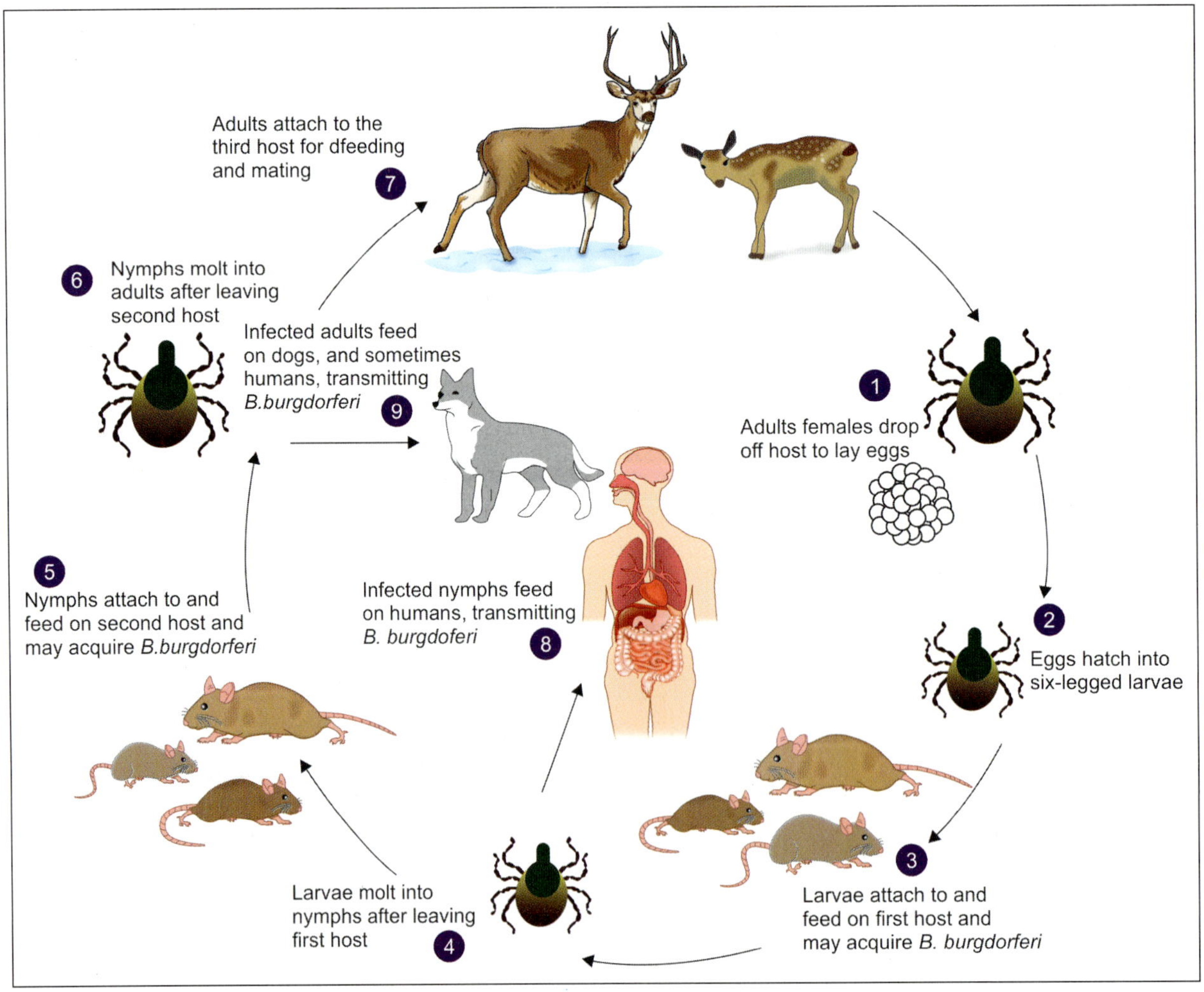

FIGURE 15: Hard ticks responsible for transmission of borreliosis.

FIGURE 16: Life cycle of the *Borrelia burgdorferi*.

TABLE 7 Stages and clinical manifestations of Lyme borreliosis.

Early infection	Stage 1 (localized infection)	• Erythema migrans (**Fig. 17**) • Borrelia lymphocytoma (**Fig. 18**)	
	Stage 2 (disseminated infection)	Skin: Secondary annular lesion Constitutional: Headache, fever, diffuse pain, and fatigue CNS manifestations: • Meningitis • Encephalopathy • Peripheral neuropathy • Cerebellar ataxia • Optic neuritis • Cranial neuritis • Radiculopathy • Myelitis • Radicular pain ↓ CSF pleocytosis (meningopolyneuritis or Bannwarth's syndrome) Cardiac abnormality: • Fluctuating degree of atrioventricular block • Myopericarditis • Cardiomyopathy Joint: Typical migratory pain	
Late infection	Stage 3 (persistent infection)	• Joint: Intermittent attacks of oligoarthritis (large joint) • Postinfectious antibiotic refractory arthritis • CNS: Subtle encephalopathy peripheral neuropathy encephalomyelitis • Skin: Acrodermatitis chronic atrophicans (reddish violaceous discolouration on acral surface of arm and leg) (**Fig. 19**)	Months after the onset of infection
Post Lyme syndrome (chronic Lyme disease)		• Fatigue • Subjective pain neurocognitive manifestation	Resolve within few months

(CNS: central nervous system; CSF: cerebrospinal fluid)

TABLE 8 Algorithm for testing and treatment of Lyme disease.

Pretest probability	Symptoms	Recommendation
High	Patient with erythema migrans	Empirical antibiotic treatment without serological testing
Intermediate	Patient with oligoarticular arthritis	Serological testing, antibiotic treatment if test positive
Low	Patient with nonspecific symptoms (arthralgia, myalgia, and fatigue)	Neither testing nor treatment

TABLE 9 Treatment regimen for Lyme disease.

Oral therapy	
First choice	Age ≥9 years, not pregnant → doxycycline 100 mg bid
	Age <9 years: amoxicillin, 50 mg/kg/day
Second choice (adults)	Amoxicillin, 500 mg tid
Third choice for all ages	Cefuroxime axetil, 500 mg bid
Fourth choice for all ages	Erythromycin 250 mg qid

TABLE 10 Duration of treatment for Lyme disease.

Localized skin infections	14 days
Early disseminated infection	21 days
Acrodermatitis	30 days
Arthritis	30–60 days

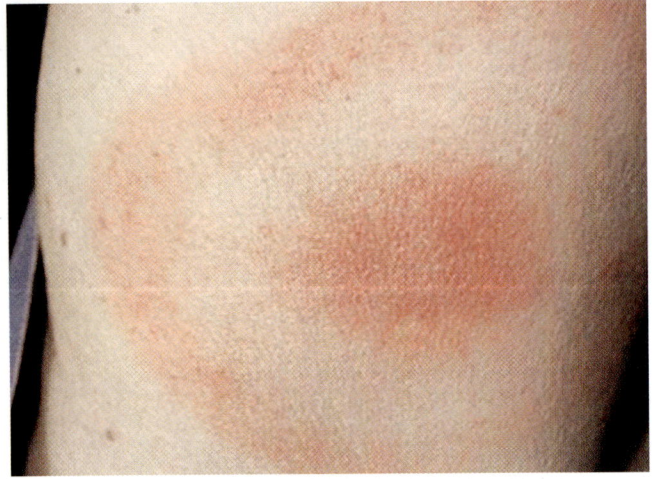

FIGURE 17: Erythema migrans seen in borreliosis.

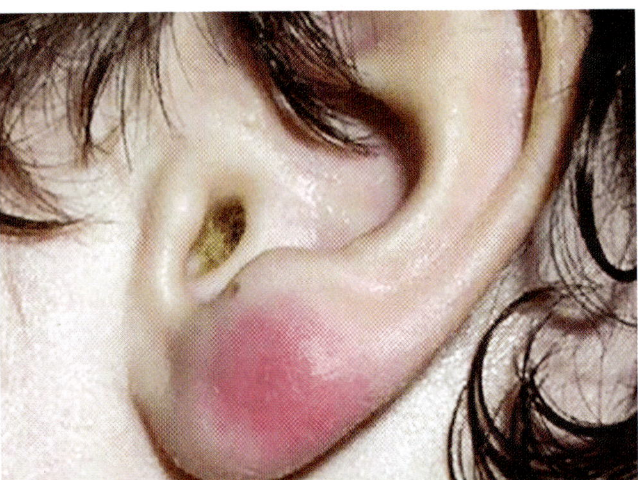

FIGURE 18: Borrelia lymphocytoma (bluish red swelling at the site of tick bite) on ear lobule.

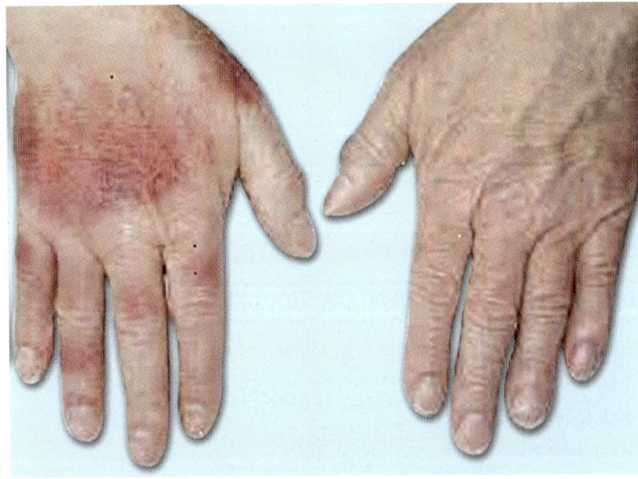

FIGURE 19: Acrodermatitis chronicum atrophicum in borreliosis.

Postinfectious antibiotic refractory arthritis responds to nonsteroidal anti-inflammatory drugs (NSAIDs) or disease-modifying antirheumatic drug (DMARD) and synovectomy.

PROPHYLAXIS AFTER TICK BITE

Single dose of 200 mg doxycycline given within 72 hours of tick bite. The response to treatment is best in early disease.

RELAPSING FEVER

CAUSATIVE AGENT

- The causative agent is *Borrelia* species
- Arthropod-borne infection
- Zoonotic infection
- Two major forms:
  i. Tick-borne relapsing fever (*Borrelia hermsii* and *Borrelia turicatae*) (due to soft tick bite)
  ii. Louse-borne relapsing fever (*Borrelia recurrentis*) (due to louse infestation)
- Extracellular organism, but presence inside cells denotes dead organism.

MODE OF TRANSMISSION

- Contact with louse or tick bearing spirochetes
- *Animal reservoir*: Rodents like rat
- Transplacental, transfusion spread, and contact through abraded skin have been reported
- Incubation period is 3–12 days

PATHOGENESIS

- Infection begins at louse or tick bite, followed by dissemination of spirochetes in blood
- Spirochete burden correlate with severity of symptoms
- Various antigenic phases occur during infection, so no standard serodiagnosis of *Borrelia*
- They have lipoprotein which binds to host cell

CLINICAL FEATURES

- Recurrent bouts of fever with spirochetemia separated by short free time due to antigenic variation by the spirochetes
- *Constitutional*: Fever, myalgia, chills, headache, and neck stiffness
- Fever (may be as high as 43°C)
- Tachycardia
- Lethargy
- Conjunctival injection
- Hepatosplenomegaly, jaundice, truncal petechial rash (louse borne)
- *CNS*: Meningitis, meningoencephalitis, and facial palsy (tick borne)

TABLE 11 Management of relapsing fever.

Tick-borne relapsing fever	Louse-borne relapsing fever
First choice	
• Age ≥9 years, not pregnant: Doxycycline 100 mg bid • Age <9 years: Erythromycin 12.5 mg/kg/day PO qid	• Age ≥9 years, not pregnant: Doxycycline 200 mg PO or: Tetracycline 500 mg PO qid/250–500 mg IV • Age <9 years: Erythromycin 12.5 mg/kg/day PO
Second choice	
Age ≥9 years, not pregnant: Tetracycline 500 mg qid	Penicillin G procaine IM 800,000 U adults 200,000 U children
Third choice	
Age ≥9 years: Erythromycin 500 mg qid	Age ≥9 years: Erythromycin 500 mg PO
Duration: 10 days	

Duration of disease:

- *Louse-borne relapsing fever*: Fever lasts for 6 days→ afebrile period of 9 days → relapse once
- *Tick-borne relapsing fever*: Fever lasts for 4 days → afebrile period of 10 days → relapse twice

In pregnancy:

- Placental damage
- Intrauterine growth retardation
- Miscarriage
- *Neonate*: Jaundice, sepsis, hemorrhage, and hepatosplenomegaly

DIAGNOSIS

- History of stay at mountains and high elevation areas, history of tick bite, and body's louse
- Direct visualization in Wright-stained blood smear (febrile period)
- Hemogram shows normocytic anemia, normal white blood cells (WBCs), and decreased platelets
- Prothrombin time (PT) and activated partial thromboplastin time (APTT) prolonged
- LFT and RFT abnormal
- *Urine*: Proteinuria and hematuria
- *CSF examination*: Lymphocytic pleocytosis and direct spirochetes visualized
- *Promising analysis*: Detection of glycerophosphodiester phosphodiesterase (GlpQ) and protein antigen of all relapsing fever

DIFFERENTIAL DIAGNOSIS

- Dengue
- Rocky mountain spotted fever
- Rickettsial infection

MANAGEMENT

Table 11 shows management of relapsing fever.

Meningitis/Encephalitis/Stuporous: Ceftriaxone 2 g IV qd or Na penicillin G 5 million U qid for 14 days.

A single dose antibiotic required for treatment of LBRF.

Multiple dosing of antibiotic required for treatment of TBRF.

RECOMMENDED READINGS

1. Leukehart SA. Spirochetal diseases. In: Jameson JL, Fauci AS, Kasper DL, Hauser SL, Longo DL, Loscalzo J (Eds). Harrison's Principles of Internal Medicine, 20th edition. California: McGraw Hill; 2018. pp. 1279-303.
2. Philip SS. Spirochetal infections. In: Papadakis MA, Mcphee SJ (Eds). Current Medical Diagnosis and Treatment, 59th edition. California: McGraw Hill; 2020. pp. 1510-26.
3. Butler T. The Jarisch–Herxheimer Reaction After Antibiotic Treatment of Spirochetal Infections: A Review of Recent Cases and Our Understanding of Pathogenesis. Am J Trop Med Hyg. 2017;96(1):46-52.
4. Goarant C. Leptospirosis: risk factors and management challenges in developing countries. Res Rep Trop Med. 2016;7:49-62.
5. Bandara K, Weerasekar MM, Gurasekara C, Ranasinghe N, Marasinghe C, Fernando N. Utility of modified Faine's criteria in diagnosis of leptospirosis. BMC Infect Dis. 2016;16(1):446.
6. Jerajani HR. Syphilis. In: Milind NY (Ed). API Textbook of Medicine, 11th edition. India: The Association of Physicians of India; 2019. pp. 182-6.
7. Gary WP. Lyme disease. In: Goldman L (Ed). Goldman-Cecil Medicine, 25th edition. New York: Elsevier; 2012. pp. 2021-7.
8. Sherif ZR, Muehlenbachs A. Relapsing fever and other Borrelia infections. In: Goldman L (Ed). Goldman-Cecil Medicine, 25th edition. New York: Elsevier; 2012. pp. 2027-8.

CHAPTER 64

Common Fungal Infections: Aspergillosis, Candidiasis

J Rajkumar, S Subramanian, G Balajee

ABSTRACT

Aspergillus species are found in the environment in water, food, air, and soil and affect patients with altered host immunity, particularly those with reduced pulmonary host defenses. Patients undergoing hematopoietic stem cell transplant (HSCT) are at the greatest risk of invasive aspergillosis (IA). The spectrum of aspergillosis encompasses noninvasive forms such as allergic bronchopulmonary aspergillosis (ABPA) and invasive forms like invasive pulmonary aspergillosis (IPA), disseminated disease. Diagnosis of IA requires microbiologic and/or histopathologic criteria to define proven infection. *Aspergillus* grow well on routine culture, although a fungal-specific media may improve yield. Voriconazole, a triazole, is considered as the drug of choice for primary therapy and is effective both in pulmonary aspergillosis and extrapulmonary aspergillosis.

Candida species are normal human flora and are typically found in the gastrointestinal (GI) tract and are common colonizers of the genitourinary tract and skin. The incidence of candidiasis due to nonalbicans *Candida* (NAC) species is increasing and *Candida auris* is a multidrug-resistant pathogen causing serious threat to global health. *Candida* organisms are with small, thin-walled, ovoid cells (blastospores) and form smooth, creamy white, glistening colonies. Risk factors include exposure to broad-spectrum antibiotics, indwelling intravenous (IV) catheters, hyperalimentation fluids, GI and thoracic surgery, neutropenia, and burns patients; gold standard of diagnosis in invasive candidiasis (IC) is culture, in particular culture from sterile sites, such as blood, peritoneal fluid, and pleural fluid. An echinocandin is appropriate in hemodynamically unstable patients, those previously exposed to an azole, and in those colonized with azole-resistant *Candida* species.

"I'm like a fungus; you can't get rid of me"

—Adam Baldwin

ASPERGILLOSIS

INTRODUCTION

Aspergillus species are found in the environment in water, food, air, and soil and thus have a clear environmental niche. Regional differences in precipitation, humidity, and temperature play a role in its environmental burden.

Patients with altered host immunity, particularly those with reduced pulmonary host defenses (e.g., those who use corticosteroids) that inhibit the activity of pulmonary macrophages or those who are neutropenic, have increased susceptibility to the organism. Outbreaks of IA do occur when patients are exposed to aerosols of *Aspergillus* conidia in association with construction and other environmental risks. The disease can also occur due to endogenous reactivation of prior infection.

MICROBIOLOGY

Aspergillus includes 250 species with several subgenera and multiple sections. The most common species causing invasive disease are *A. fumigatus*, followed by *A. flavus*, *A. terreus*, *A. niger* and *A. nidulans*. In recent times, cryptic *Aspergillus* species that are morphologically indistinguishable from the main *Aspergillus* sections have been detected. These organisms possess elevated triazole minimum inhibitory concentrations (MICs) and identification requires molecular methods like gene sequencing. The organisms include *A. lentulus*, *Neosartorya pseudofischeri*, *A. udagawae*, *A. viridinutans*, *A. fumigatiaffinis*, and *A. novofumigatus* and many others.

PREDISPOSING FACTORS

Patients undergoing HSCT are at the greatest risk of IA, in particular IPA and sinus disease. Prolonged neutropenia, defects in cell-mediated immunity, and prolonged immunosuppressive therapy for graft-versus-host disease (GVHD) are the risk factors in this population. The incidence is more in allogenic transplant recipients as compared to autologous transplant recipients. IA has a bimodal temporal distribution, i.e., early transplantation period (<20 days) and a second peak at >100 days after transplant (corticosteroid use and treatment of GVHD). Conditions like myeloproliferative syndromes requiring repeated courses of chemotherapy, solid organ transplantation (SOT), in particular, lung transplant recipients are other risk factors.

Chronic obstructive pulmonary disease, decompensated liver disease or cirrhosis, acquired immunodeficiency syndrome (AIDS), corticosteroid therapy for management

TABLE 1 **Risk factors for invasive aspergillosis.**

Low risk	Intermediate risk	High risk
• Autoimmune	• Myelodysplastic syndrome	• AML/MDS
• Solid tumor	• Chronic lymphocytic leukemia	• Lung transplantation
• Kidney transplantation	• Acute myeloblastic leukemia (consolidation phase)	• Allogenic HSCT with GVHD
• Autologous HSCT	• Heart transplantation	• Chronic granulomatous disease
• AIDS	• Liver transplantation	
• COPD with acute exacerbation	• Small bowel transplantation	
• Multiple myeloma	• Allogenic HSCT without GVHD	

(GVHD: graft-versus-host disease; HSCT: hematopoietic stem cell transplant; MDS: myelodysplastic syndrome)

of acute respiratory distress syndrome, impaired mucociliary clearance after resolution of pneumonia (viral or bacterial), immune deficiency following prolonged illness, patients with primary immunodeficiency, or those receiving immunosuppressive medications such as tumor necrosis factor-α blockers and autoimmune disease have also been identified as significant risk factors (**Table 1**).

PATHOGENESIS

The usual route of infection for IA is through inhalation of *Aspergillus* conidia into the lungs or paranasal sinuses. In the absence of effective host defenses after pulmonary exposure, the inhaled small resting conidia enlarge and germinate, resulting in transformation into hyphae. The process of hyphal growth and tissue invasion results in a hallmark feature of IA—vascular invasion and pulmonary infarction. The polymorphonuclear leukocytes, T-helper (Th) cytokines, have vital roles in innate and adaptive defense against *Aspergillus* and any defect in these mechanisms leads to invasive disease.

The immune response to *Aspergillus* antigens in ABPA as in both asthmatic patients and those with cystic fibrosis is a Th2 response. The formed hyphae release allergens that are processed by antigen-presenting cells bearing human leukocyte antigen (HLA)-DR2 or HLA-DR5 and presented to the T cells. The T cells respond by a Th2 response, with release of cytokines interleukin (IL)-4, IL-5, and IL-13 and thereby inflammatory response.

CLINICAL MANIFESTATIONS

The spectrum of aspergillosis encompasses a broad variety of clinical entities, from noninvasive forms, such as ABPA and chronic pulmonary aspergillosis syndromes, to IPA with possible widespread dissemination. Although most frequently affecting the lungs, aspergillosis can develop within virtually any organ system and disseminated disease is particularly common among patients with prolonged granulocytopenia following chemotherapy.

NONINVASIVE FORMS

Aspergilloma: An aspergilloma, or *Aspergillus* fungus ball, forms inside a pre-existing pulmonary cavity caused by emphysema, malignancy, or pulmonary tuberculosis and is seen on imaging as a freely moveable solid mass within a cavity. Clinical presentation may vary from asymptomatic, incidentally detected lesion to life-threatening hemoptysis requiring emergent intervention.

Allergic bronchopulmonary aspergillosis: Allergic bronchopulmonary aspergillosis is a clinical syndrome caused by hypersensitivity to *Aspergillus* species and is characterized by the presence of chronic immune activation, pulmonary infiltrates, and asthma. Bronchiectasis may also develop in time. Criteria for diagnosis include the presence of bronchial asthma, immediate skin reactivity to *A. fumigatus*, elevated serum immunoglobulin (Ig)-E titers, pulmonary infiltrates, central bronchiectasis, eosinophilia, and anti-IgG precipitins against *Aspergillus*.

INVASIVE DISEASE

Invasive pulmonary aspergillosis: Invasive pulmonary aspergillosis occurs 10–21 days following HSCT in the setting of profound granulocytopenia. Clinical manifestations of IPA include cough, fever, chest pain or pleuritic pain, dyspnea, and hemoptysis. The symptoms may be more subtle given their relative inability to mount an appropriate inflammatory response and patients may not have fever but present with hemoptysis and pleuritic chest pain, secondary to angioinvasion. The classic radiological finding associated with IPA in HRCT is the halo sign, which is an area of low attenuation surrounding a pulmonary nodule.

Central nervous system aspergillosis: Central nervous system (CNS) aspergillosis usually occurs in patients with neutropenia. Patients usually have previous or concurrent IPA or invasive sinus infection. The clinical presentation usually includes fever, neurologic deficits, seizures, mental status changes, and headache.

OTHER FORMS

Other forms of aspergillosis include tracheobronchial aspergillosis (TBA), sinus aspergillosis, and ocular aspergillosis.

DIAGNOSIS

Diagnosis of IA, requires microbiologic and/or histopathologic criteria to define proven infection. Obtaining appropriate specimens is crucial for early diagnosis;

bronchoscopy with bronchoalveolar lavage (BAL) is recommended for patients with suspected IPA with consideration of transbronchial biopsy or percutaneous needle biopsy depending on radiographic site of lesion.

Chest computed tomography (CT): It is the recommended imaging modality for suspected IPA. Typical CT findings include nodules, consolidative lesions, or wedge-shaped infarcts. The classic halo sign, a nodule surrounded by a perimeter of ground glass opacity reflecting hemorrhage, may be seen particularly in neutropenic patients. An air crescent, or cavity in a mass or nodule, is usually a late CT finding.

Routine culture: *Aspergillus* species grow well on routine culture, although a fungal-specific media may improve yield. Most species appear initially as small, fluffy white colonies on culture plates within 48 hours. Presumptive identification of the *Aspergillus* species complex is based on the gross and microscopic inspection of the colony along with molecular confirmation. Staining shows narrow septate hyphae with acute angle branching. Species identification and antifungal susceptibility testing (AFST) is recommended due to variable azole resistance among various species. Blood cultures with *Aspergillus* species usually are consistent with contamination and are rarely associated with IA even in high-risk patients.

Antigen detection of galactomannan (GM): Given the various challenges associated with obtaining cultures, nonculture-based diagnostics have been developed. Antigen detection of GM, a component of the *Aspergillus* cell wall, is the most frequently used methodology. It has a sensitivity of 44–90%, more so in hematological malignancy. False negative GM results may occur while on antifungal therapy and false positive results may occur with histoplasmosis, blastomycosis, and antibiotic use (piperacillin-tazobactam and amoxicillin-clavulanate).

Enzyme immunoassay (EIA): The use of serial EIA testing for screening high-risk patients has been found to be useful. Platelia EIA (BioRad, Hercules, CA) is recommended in symptomatic patients suspected of having IPA; it can also be used on BAL fluid, even for patients receiving antimold therapy.

Serum GM determination also provides prognostic information with declining values following appropriate therapy. BAL testing exhibits increased sensitivity compared with serum testing. Serum (1/3)-β-D-glucan (another component of the fungal cell wall) determination, though not specific for *Aspergillus*, has a good negative predictive value.

Lateral-flow device (LFD): An *Aspergillus*-specific lateral-flow device (LFD) has recently been developed as a point-of-care test for the diagnosis of IA and poses an upcoming alternative to GM determination.

Polymerase chain reaction (PCR): This testing has not been widely adopted due to a lack of standardization. However, BAL PCR seems to have a higher specificity (93%). The emergence of antifungal resistance in *Aspergillus* species has also led to the development of additional nucleic acid-based assays (AsperGenius, PathoNostics B.V., Netherlands) capable of identifying resistance mutations known to confer antifungal resistance. Sensitivity has been reported as 78% and specificity 100%.

TREATMENT

In suspected cases of IA, early initiation of antifungal treatment is strongly recommended while conducting diagnostic testing, mainly to limit progression of disease (**Table 2**).

Voriconazole: A triazole, is considered as the drug of choice for primary therapy in all patient populations. It is effective both in pulmonary aspergillosis and also for extrapulmonary aspergillosis such as CNS, ophthalmic, and disseminated disease. Adverse effects include liver function test abnormalities, gastrointestinal disturbances, skin rashes, hallucinations, and visual abnormalities. Posaconazole is another triazole that is highly active in vitro against *Aspergillus* species. Posaconazole prophylaxis

TABLE 2 Therapies for invasive aspergillosis.

Agent	Class	Route of administration	Dose
Primary therapy			
Voriconazole	Azole	IV/Oral	6 mg/kg (IV) q12h × 2 doses, followed by 4 mg/kg (IV) q12h or 200 mg (PO) q12h
Alternative primary therapy			
Amphotericin B	Polyene	IV	1–1.5 mg/kg/day
Liposomal amphotericin B	Polyene	IV	3 mg/kg/day
Posaconazole	Azole	IV	300 mg IV BID on day 1, then 300 mg IV OD
		Oral	• Suspension: 400 mg BID with food • Capsule: 300 mg BID on day 1 then OD
Itraconazole	Azole	Oral	200–600 mg/day

(BID: twice daily; IV: intravenous; OD: once daily; PO: oral)

has been used in high-risk patients undergoing bone marrow transplant with GVHD and in patients with acute myelogenous leukemia and myelodysplastic syndrome. Therapeutic drug monitoring (TDM) is recommended for all these agents. Isavuconazole has potent activity against *Aspergillus* species in vitro, including some isolates with decreased susceptibility to other triazoles. It has excellent bioavailability and has a prolonged half-life of 100–130 hours. Common side effects include nausea, vomiting, and diarrhea and hepatotoxicity.

Amphotericin B (AmB): Deoxycholate was the first-line therapeutic agent for IA for decades, with the exception of *A. terreus*, which is inherently resistant. Its use is limited with toxicity and poor outcomes and is recommended as alternative agent. Lipid formulations of AmB are less nephrotoxic, and are preferred to AmB deoxycholate. Echinocandins like caspofungin, micafungin, and anidulafungin inhibit the growth of *Aspergillus* species but they are fungistatic, rather than fungicidal. They are reserved for salvage therapy or in combination with another antifungal class.

Duration of therapy is usually 6–12 weeks for IPA depending on disease response to treatment and degree of immune suppression, at least 3 months for TBA or until resolution of infection. Adjunctive therapies for IA include reduction in immune suppression, surgery for localized disease, and colony-stimulating factors or granulocyte infusions for neutropenic patients.

CANDIDIASIS

"Your willpower behaves like an antibiotic, which protects you from the harmful virus; like failure"
—Anonymous

INTRODUCTION

Candida species are normal human flora and are typically found in the GI tract and are common colonizers of the genitourinary tract and skin. Candidemia ranks as the third or fourth most common cause of healthcare-associated bloodstream infection (BSI) particularly in intensive care settings. The advanced medical care, in terms of complex surgical procedures and comprehensive cancer treatments, has led to a steady rise in these infection in recent times.

EPIDEMIOLOGY

There are at least 15 distinct *Candida* species that cause human disease, but >95% of invasive disease are caused by the five most common pathogens: *C. albicans*, *C. glabrata*, *C. tropicalis*, *C. parapsilosis*, and *C. krusei*. There are more than 150 species of *Candida*. Some of them are *C. albicans*, *C. guilliermondii*, *C. krusei*, *C. parapsilosis*, *C. tropicalis*, *C. pseudotropicalis*, *C. lusitaniae*, *C. dubliniensis*, and *C. glabrata*. Although *Candida albicans* is the most prevalent species involved in both mucocutaneous and disseminated infections, the incidence of candidiasis due to NAC species is increasing and *C. auris* has emerged as a serious threat to global health—a multidrug-resistant pathogen.

MICROBIOLOGY

Candida organisms are with small, thin-walled, ovoid cells (blastospores) that reproduce by budding. They grow well in routine agar plates, blood culture bottles, and do not require special fungal media for growth. The organism stains gram positive and yeast forms, pseudohyphae and hyphae may be found on microscopic examination. Identification of the hyphae and pseudohyphae is facilitated with 10% potassium hydroxide, which clears the epithelial cells, and with fluorescent microscopic examination of calcofluor white-stained smears. *Candida* organisms form smooth, creamy white, glistening colonies and a rapid, presumptive identification of *C. albicans* can be made by placing the organism in serum and observing germ tube formation—small projections from the cell surface that appear within 90 minutes. Further identification and speciation procedures are based primarily on physiologic parameters and biochemical tests. *C. auris* is many times misidentified as *C. haemulonii* and needs molecular gene sequencing or matrix-assisted laser desorption/ionization time of flight (MALDI-TOF) MS for proper identification.

PATHOGENESIS

Invasive candidiasis results from a combination of increased fungal burden with an alteration of the skin and mucous membranes. *Candida* has a tendency for surface adherence and the formation of biofilms both on body surfaces as well as prosthetic devices, including urinary catheters and intravascular devices leading on to azole resistance and persistence. The capability of the organism to switch from yeast to hyphal phase appears to be the most virulent factor leading on to host damage.

All arms of the immune system are involved in the response to candidal infections. Lymphocytes are essential for cell-mediated immunity and prevention of mucosal disease. Monocytes and neutrophils damage and destroy pseudohyphae and blastospores. Complement and immunoglobulins are for optimal opsonization and intracellular killing. Any deficiency of these components can be associated with complicated or refractory disease.

Candida species has a tendency for biofilm formation. Biofilms are structured microbial communities that form on abiotic and biotic surfaces and are embedded in an extracellular matrix. In a clinical setting, a biofilm formed on human tissue (e.g., on a mucosal layer) or on an implanted medical device [e.g., a central venous catheter (CVC)] can serve as a source of infection that can spread to other parts of the body and also leads to difficulty in eradication due to poor drug penetration.

TABLE 3 Risk factors for invasive candidiasis.

Immunocompromised	Nonimmunocompromised
• Granulocytopenia • Stem cell transplant • Mucositis • Graft-versus-host disease • Type of chemotherapy • Organ transplants	• Broad-spectrum antibiotics • Any type of renal dialysis • Central venous catheter • IV drug use • Severity of illness • Total parenteral nutrition • GI perforation or surgery • Diabetes • Length of stay in ICU • Pancreatitis • Sepsis • Burns patients • Neonates

(GI: gastrointestinal; ICU: intensive care unit; IV: intravenous)

RISK FACTORS

The risk factors for IC include exposure to broad-spectrum antibiotics, indwelling IV catheters, hyper-alimentation fluids, GI and thoracic surgery, neutropenia, burns patients, IV heroin use, low-birth-weight neonates, and solid organ transplant patients on immunosuppressives (**Table 3**).

CLINICAL MANIFESTATIONS

Invasive candidiasis is most commonly manifest as candidemia, but it can occur at virtually any anatomic site. A few syndromes compose most cases and the classic manifestations are as discussed here.

Candidemia: Bloodstream infection with *Candida* is the most commonly recognized form of IC, accounting for more than half of all IC cases. CVCs and other intravascular devices are commonly implicated in candidemia; but other sources must be considered, especially among neutropenic patients in whom the GI tract is a common source. A positive blood culture result for *Candida* should be thoroughly investigated because of the high risk of morbidity and mortality (15–20%).

Acute disseminated candidiasis: Acute disseminated candidiasis is a life-threatening manifestation and occurs exclusively among patients with neutropenia secondary to cytotoxic chemotherapy for a hematologic malignancy. These patients are acutely ill, have positive blood cultures, and a characteristic diffuse, discrete hemorrhagic and papular rash consistent with small vessel vasculitis and multiple organs like the kidney, liver, spleen, and GI tract may be involved.

Endovascular infection: Endovascular *Candida* infection manifests as infective endocarditis (IE) and infection involving implantable intracardiac devices. Endocarditis should be suspected when blood cultures are persistently positive, when a patient with candidemia has persistent fever despite appropriate treatment, or when a new heart murmur, heart failure, or embolic phenomena occurs in the setting of candidemia. Most cases occur following cardiac valvular surgery; but other risk factors include injection drug use, cancer chemotherapy, prolonged presence of CVCs, and prior bacterial endocarditis.

Mucocutaneous candidiasis: Oral *Candida* infections are common and are characterized by creamy white, curd-like patches on the tongue and other mucous membranes; the patches are removable by scraping and leave a raw, bleeding, and painful surface. Other manifestations include: (1) Acute atrophic candidiasis, a nonspecific atrophy of the tongue that is thought to be a sequela of acute pseudo-membranous candidiasis; (2) Chronic atrophic candidiasis or "denture sore mouth," which is a chronic inflammatory reaction and epithelial thinning under the dental plates; (3) Angular cheilitis, an inflammatory reaction at the corners of the mouth (not exclusively due to *Candida*); (4) *Candida* leukoplakia, firm, white plaques affecting the cheek, lips, and tongue that have a protracted course.

Chronic disseminated candidiasis: Chronic disseminated candidiasis is seen almost exclusively among patients who undergone myeloablative chemotherapy associated with neutropenia. On recovery from neutropenia, patients with this disorder develop low-grade fever; right upper quadrant pain, often associated with a palpable and tender liver; splenomegaly; and an elevated serum alkaline phosphatase. Parenchymal lesions develop following neutrophil recovery, suggesting that an adequate host inflammatory response is a prerequisite to the development of radiographically visible lesions, which are rarely seen during the period of neutropenia. Imaging studies [magnetic resonance imaging (MRI), computed tomography (CT), or abdominal ultrasound] reveal multiple focal abnormalities in the liver, spleen, kidneys, and, rarely, the lungs.

Others: Endogenous infections of the eye can be manifested as isolated chorioretinitis or as chorioretinitis with extension into the vitreous, leading to vitritis. The source is mainly endogenous, as a consequence of candidemia. Vertebral osteomyelitis, with or without discitis, is an increasingly common disorder that is usually associated with unrecognized or untreated candidemia and manifests several weeks to months after the episode. *Candida* species may cause meningitis, septic arthritis, tenosynovitis, isolated involvement of the kidney, the intra-abdominal cavity, and, rarely, pneumonia.

DIAGNOSIS

The gold standard of diagnosis in IC is culture, in particular culture from sterile sites, such as blood, peritoneal fluid, and pleural fluid.

Blood cultures: It is identify only approximately 50% of all patients and are usually positive within 96 hours, though time to positivity is species-dependent, e.g., *C. glabrata* grows much more slowly than *C. albicans*. The volume of blood, antifungal drug exposure, and the specific blood culture technique also influence sensitivity.

Several reliable nonculture assays have been developed for providing the opportunity for earlier intervention with more targeted antifungal therapy. They include MALDI-TOF, peptide nucleic acid fluorescent in situ hybridization (PNA-FISH), the beta-D-glucan (BDG) (Fungitell, Associates of Cape Cod, Inc., East Falmouth, MA) assay, and the T2Candida assay (T2 Biosystems, Lexington, MA).

Matrix-assisted laser desorption/ionization time of flight is a postculture technique that uses mass spectroscopy and can provide species identification within 10–15 minutes once an organism is isolated. However, it requires pure growth of an organism on artificial media. PNA-FISH can be performed directly on a positive blood culture result rather than waiting for the growth of pure colonies.

Beta-D-glucan: It is a cell wall constituent of *Candida* species, *Aspergillus* species, *Pneumocystis jirovecii*, selected dematiaceous fungi, and several other fungi. Using a cut-off value of 80 pg/mL in patients with proven IC, in meta-analyses of BDG studies, the pooled sensitivity and specificity for diagnosing IC were 75–80% and 80%, respectively. Its performance is further optimized by requiring two successive positive assays to define a true positive result. The T2Candida assay is a polymerase chain reaction (PCR)-based assay that uses magnetic resonance detection to identify the presence of *Candida* organisms in whole blood. The assay provides the same paired species level result as does PNA-FISH. The advantage is that the assay is performed on whole blood, ideally collected in parallel with routine or fungal blood cultures, allowing the rapid diagnosis of candidemia with additional species level information.

TREATMENT

In the treatment of proven or suspected IC, several factors need to be considered. Severity of illness, associated comorbidities, possible source, prior antifungal exposure, clinical evidence of disseminated disease, the predominant species in the settings along with the susceptibility pattern. An echinocandin is appropriate in hemodynamically unstable patients, those previously exposed to an azole, and in those colonized with azole-resistant *Candida* species. For patients with documented candidemia, 14 days of effective antifungal therapy following the first negative blood culture is recommended. A dilated funduscopic examination during the 1st week of antifungal therapy in non-neutropenic patients is recommended for all patients with documented candidemia to exclude occult ocular involvement. For neutropenic patients, this procedure should be delayed until neutrophil recovery, as the characteristic findings of ocular candidiasis are often delayed.

Echinocandins: The echinocandins (caspofungin, anidulafungin, and micafungin) demonstrate significant fungicidal activity against most *Candida* species and is recommended as the initial therapy for most adult patients with candidemia. However, *C. parapsilosis* demonstrates innately higher minimum inhibitory concentrations (MICs) to the echinocandins compared with other *Candida* species. All echinocandins have minimal adverse effects. Echinocandins achieve therapeutic concentrations in all infection sites with the exception of the eye, central nervous system (CNS), and urine. They do not require dosage adjustment for renal insufficiency or dialysis.

Triazoles: Fluconazole, itraconazole, voriconazole, posaconazole, and a new expanded spectrum triazole, isavuconazole, demonstrate similar in vitro activity against most *Candida* species. Fluconazole is readily absorbed, with oral bioavailability resulting in concentrations equal to approximately 90% of those achieved by IV administration. Fluconazole has the greatest penetration into the CSF and vitreous, achieving concentrations of >70% of those in serum and is useful in treatment of CNS and intraocular *Candida* infections. It also achieves urine concentrations that are 10–20 times the concentrations in serum, thus, is the preferred treatment option for symptomatic cystitis. Voriconazole role is limited for infections due to *C. krusei* and fluconazole-resistant, voriconazole-susceptible *C. glabrata*. Itraconazole and posaconazole offer little benefit. Isavuconazole is a recently approved expanded spectrum triazole antifungal with excellent in vitro activity versus *Candida* species.

Amphotericin B: Amphotericin B (AmB) deoxycholate preparations have been extensively studied in IC. However, their usage has been limited by the toxicity and resistance patterns. Two lipid formulations of AmB (LFAmB) have been developed with relatively fewer toxic profiles.

RECOMMENDED READINGS

1. Segal BH. Aspergillosis. N Engl J Med. 2009;360:1870.
2. Meersseman W, Lagrou K, Maertens J, Van Wijngaerden E. Invasive aspergillosis in the intensive care unit. Clin Infect Dis. 2007;45:205.
3. Patterson TF, Thompson GR 3rd, Denning DW, et al. Practice Guidelines for the Diagnosis and Management of Aspergillosis: 2016 Update by the Infectious Diseases Society of America. Clin Infect Dis. 2016;63:e1.
4. Maertens JA, Raad II, Marr KA, et al. Isavuconazole versus voriconazole for primary treatment of invasive mould disease caused by *Aspergillus* and other filamentous fungi (SECURE): a phase 3, randomised-controlled, non-inferiority trial. Lancet. 2016;387:760.
5. Pappas PG, Kauffman CA, Andes DR, et al. Clinical Practice Guideline for the Management of Candidiasis: 2016 Update by the Infectious Diseases Society of America. Clin Infect Dis. 2016;62:e1.
6. Rex JH, Walsh TJ, Sobel JD, et al. Practice guidelines for the treatment of candidiasis. Infectious Diseases Society of America. Clin Infect Dis. 2000;30:662.
7. Morelli MK, Veve MP, Lorson W, Shorman MA. *Candida* spp. infective endocarditis: Characteristics and outcomes of twenty patients with a focus on injection drug use as a predisposing risk factor. Mycoses. 2021;64:181.

CHAPTER 65

Fungal Infections: Histoplasmosis, Blastomycosis, *Pneumocystis* Pneumonia, and Others

Immaculata Xess, Gagandeep Singh, Renu Yadav

ABSTRACT

Histoplasmosis is a systemic granulomatous disease caused by a dimorphic fungus known as *Histoplasma capsulatum*. The endemicity of *H. capsulatum* infection is mostly reported from Ohio and Mississippi river of North America. In India, most cases are reported from Northern and North Eastern states. Most of the immunocompetent individuals with low-level exposure are either asymptomatic and some may show mild or self-limited illness. Progressive disseminated histoplasmosis (PDH) is typically seen in immunocompromised host. PDH can cause respiratory failure, shock.

Blastomycosis is a systemic granulomatous disease caused by a dimorphic fungus *Blastomyces dermatitidis*. Blastomycosis is found in warm and moist soil of wooded areas, mostly reported from North America. Blastomycosis is not very uncommon in India. Sporadic cases have been reported from Uttar Pradesh, Madhya Pradesh, and Maharashtra. Pneumonia is the most common presentation of blastomycosis.

Pneumocystis jiroveci pneumonia (PJP), formerly known as *Pneumocystis carinii* pneumonia (PCP), is the most common opportunistic infection in persons with HIV infectoin. *Pneumocystis* is a genus of unicellular fungi found in the respiratory tracts of many mammals and humans. Disease occurs when both cellular and humoral immunity are defective. Currently the mortality in patients with PJP is 10–20% in HIV patients. The treatment of choices is trimethoprim-sulphamethoxazole. Second line agents include pentamidene, dapsone or atovaquone.

"There is no need for fiction in medicine, for the facts will beat anything you fancy"

—Sir Arthur C Doyle

HISTOPLASMOSIS

INTRODUCTION

Histoplasmosis is a systemic granulomatous disease caused by a dimorphic fungus known as *Histoplasma capsulatum*. The genus *Histoplasma* consists of only one species that is *H. capsulatum* and it has two varieties: *H. capsulatum* variety *capsulatum* and *H. capsulatum* variety *duboisii*. By using molecular analysis, eight clades of this fungus have been identified—two North American, two Latin American, and one each of Australian, Indonesian, Eurasian, and African clades.

EPIDEMIOLOGY

The endemicity of *H. capsulatum* infection is mostly reported from Ohio and Mississippi river of North America. It is also reported from some parts of Central America, South America, Africa, and Asia. In India, most cases are reported from Northern and North Eastern states; namely Uttar Pradesh (UP), New Delhi, Haryana, Punjab, West Bengal, Assam, and Bihar which form the plains of three major rivers in North India, namely Ganges, Yamuna, and Brahmaputra and it is also seen in people associated with agricultural activity (**Fig. 1**). Various attempts to isolate *H. capsulatum* from soil in India and bat habitats are failed because major soil type in India is alluvial soil. This soil is highly fertile but poor in organic and nitrogenous contents, which is necessary for the growth of *H. capsulatum*. However, because of the increase in histoplasmosis cases in India, the ecological niche for the organism should be further looked. In India, majority of people are related to the farming, poultry, or exposure to birds, and these can act as a major ecological niche for histoplasmosis. The epidemiology of *Histoplasma* is changing nowadays due to the acceleration in the international travels that lead to the occurrence of cases in the area where it was not reported previously. Recently cases have been reported from Western and Northwestern region, i.e., Gujarat and Rajasthan. According to a review study, the mean age of histoplasmosis is 45.1 ± 15.4 years, and male-to-female ratio was 6:1.

The transmission of *Histoplasma* is related to the disruption of the soil contaminated with bird or bat droppings that promotes the growth and sporulation of *Histoplasma*. The conditions which favor growth of *Histoplasma* in the soil are 22–29°C temperature and 67–87% humidity. The organism is mostly found within 20 cm of surface of soil that is acidic, moist, and contains high nitrogen content. Disruption of this soil leads to aerosolization of the microconidia of *Histoplasma* and exposure of humans nearby. Activities that are associated with *Histoplasma* transmission are demolition, remodeling of old buildings, excavation, and cutting of dead trees.

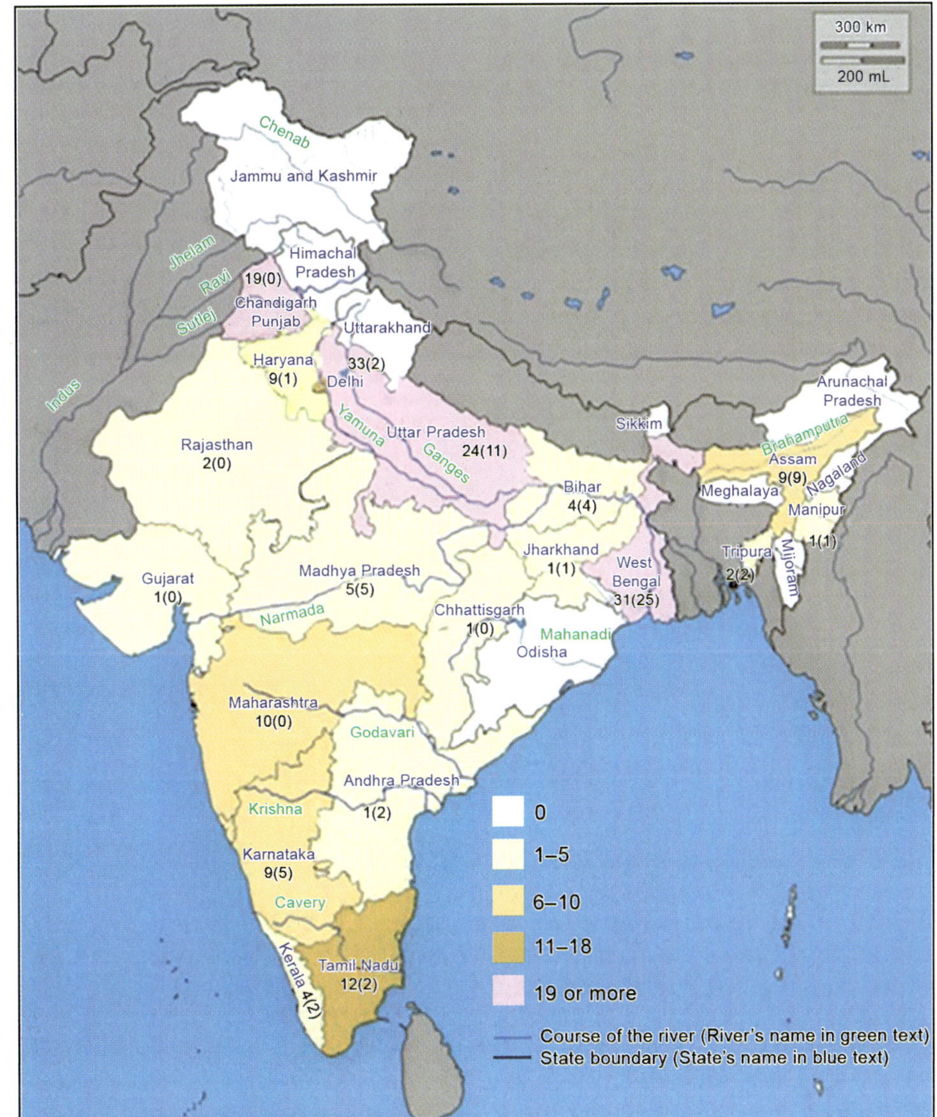

FIGURE 1: Map of India showing total cases reported from each state and cases with definite history of residence in parenthesis.

Source: Taken with permission from Gupta A, Ghosh A, Singh G, Xess I. A twenty-first-century perspective of disseminated histoplasmosis in India: literature review and retrospective analysis of published and unpublished cases at a tertiary care hospital in North India. Mycopathologia. 2017;182(11-12):1077-93.

Human-to-human transmission via the pulmonary route has not been reported.

PATHOGENESIS

Infection occurs due to the inhalation of microconidia from the contaminated soil. After inhalation, microconidia are engulfed by the alveolar macrophages where they transform into the budding yeast form which is an actively multiplying stage. This process depends on the availability of calcium and iron inside the phagocytes. Neutrophils and lymphocytes are also activated and recruited to the site of infection. These *Histoplasma* containing phagocytes are then translocated to the lymph nodes and then disseminate hematogenously throughout the reticuloendothelial system. Then after 2 weeks of infection, cellular immunity develops and T cells produce interferon γ which assist the macrophages in killing of *Histoplasma* and controlling the progression of disease. Interleukin 12 and tumor necrosis factor-α (TNF-α) also play an important role in cellular immunity to *H. capsulatum*. In the immunocompetent host, to contain the organism, macrophages, lymphocytes, and epithelial cells organize and lead to the formation of granulomas. These granulomas then fibrosed and become calcified hence calcified lung nodules, mediastinal lymph nodes, and hepatosplenic calcifications can be seen in healthy individuals from endemic areas. In immunocompromised patients, the infection is not properly contained and can disseminate throughout the reticuloendothelial system. Progressive disseminated histoplasmosis (PDH) can involve multiple organs, most commonly the lungs, bone marrow, spleen, liver, adrenal glands, and mucocutaneous membranes. Reactivation of latent histoplasmosis is rarely seen.

CLINICAL FEATURES

Most of the immunocompetent individuals with low-level exposure are either asymptomatic and some may show mild or self-limited illness. After 1–4 weeks of exposure, acute histoplasmosis leads to a flulike illness with fever, chills, sweats, headache, myalgia, anorexia, cough, dyspnea, and chest pain. In chest radiography, there is prominent hilar or mediastinal adenopathy and pulmonary infiltrates can be seen. Depending on the exposure these infiltrates may be focal with light exposure or diffuse with heavy exposure. In 5–10% patients of acute histoplasmosis rheumatologic symptoms, often associated with erythema nodosum can be seen. Pericarditis may also develop. All these manifestations represent inflammatory responses to the acute histoplasmosis rather than extrapulmonary spread. PDH is typically seen in immunocompromised host. PDH can cause respiratory failure, shock, coagulopathy, and multiorgan failure, meningitis or focal brain lesions, ulcerations of the oral mucosa, gastrointestinal ulcerations and bleeding, and adrenal insufficiency. Chronic cavitary histoplasmosis resembles with tuberculosis and mostly seen in smokers who have structural lung disease. Chronic cases are characterized by productive cough, dyspnea, low-grade fever, night sweats, and weight loss. An uncommon and serious complication of histoplasmosis is fibrosing mediastinitis that is progressive fibrosis around the hilar and mediastinal lymph nodes. It leads to the manifestations such as superior vena cava syndrome, obstruction of pulmonary vessels, and airway obstruction. The prognosis is worse if the mediastinal involvement is bilateral. In India, histoplasmosis is mainly extrapulmonary and patient mostly presents with hard palate or oral mucosa ulceration umblicated cutaneous lesions (**Fig. 2**), lymph node involvement, adrenal hyperplasia or they present with pyrexia of unknown origin. It can be a possibility that a large number of pulmonary histoplasmosis may be getting missed due to asymptomatic or milder symptomatology or getting misdiagnosed with tuberculosis due to lack of available diagnostic facilities.

LABORATORY DIAGNOSIS

The sample should be collected depending on the site of lesion; such as biopsy from lymph node, mucosal surfaces, lung nodule, adrenal gland, and bone marrow or scraping from skin (**Table 1**).

- *Direct microscopy*: Sample is processed and examined in 10% KOH-calcofluor-white mount and stained with Gram stain and Giemsa stain. Tissue section should be stained with periodic acid–Schiff (PAS), Grocott-Gomori's methenamine silver (GMS), Wright-Giemsa stain etc. However, all these diagnostic methods lack the sensitivity since they facilitate the diagnosis primarily in patients with chronic acute disseminated or sever pulmonary infections. The structure of *H. capsulatum* yeast is very similar to other pathogens. Presence of narrow-based budding intracellular yeast around 2–4 µm size is only suggestive of histoplasmosis (**Fig. 3**). The misidentifications occur principally with *Emergomyces* species, *Talaromyces marneffei, Candida glabrata, Blastomyces dermatitidis* (small form), *Cryptococcus neoformans, Leishmania donovani,* and *Toxoplasma gondii.*
- *Culture*: For the diagnosis of histoplasmosis, fungal culture is the gold standard test; however, it takes minimum 6–12 weeks depending on the inoculum size of the organism. It has significant limitations in patients with an asymptomatic or mild form. It requires special media blood or brain heart infusion agar with cysteine and incubated at 35–37°C. Very rarely it can be recovered from blood in disseminated histoplasmosis. On culture, initially the colonies are smooth, later become filamentous cottony and brownish with the

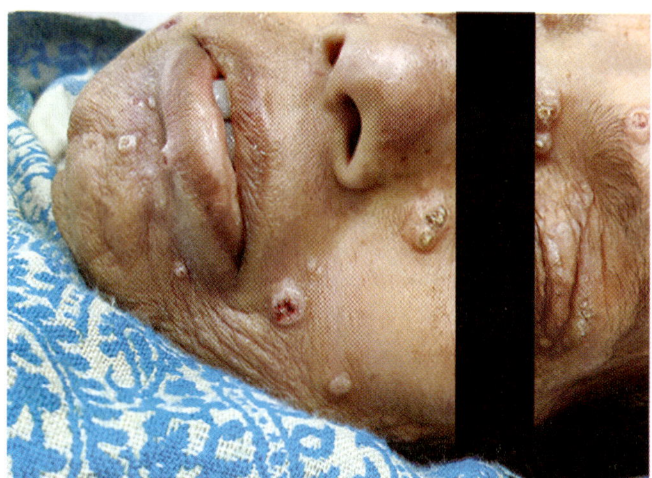

FIGURE 2: Cutaneous histoplasmosis with typical molluscum contagiosum-like lesions.

TABLE 1 Diagnosis of *Histoplasma capsulatum* according to disease type.

Type of histoplasmosis	Test	Sample
Acute pulmonary histoplasmosis	*Histoplasma* antigen test, cytopathology, and fungal culture	BAL fluid, serum, and urine
Chronic cavitary histoplasmosis	Immunodiffusion test, complement fixation test, and fungal culture	Sputum or BAL fluid
Progressive disseminated histoplasmosis	*Histoplasma* antigen test, fungal culture, and cytopathology	Serum, urine, blood or bone marrow aspirate, biopsy of affected organ
Histoplasmosis affecting central nervous system	*Histoplasma* antigen test, serology, and fungal culture	CSF

(BAL: bronchoalveolar lavage; CSF: cerebrospinal fluid)

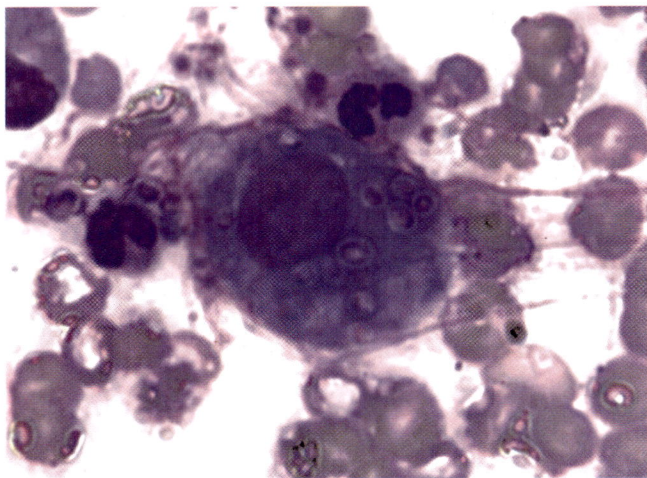

FIGURE 3: Giemsa stain showing intracellular yeasts approximately 2–4 µm size with morphology suggestive of *Histoplasma* (100X).

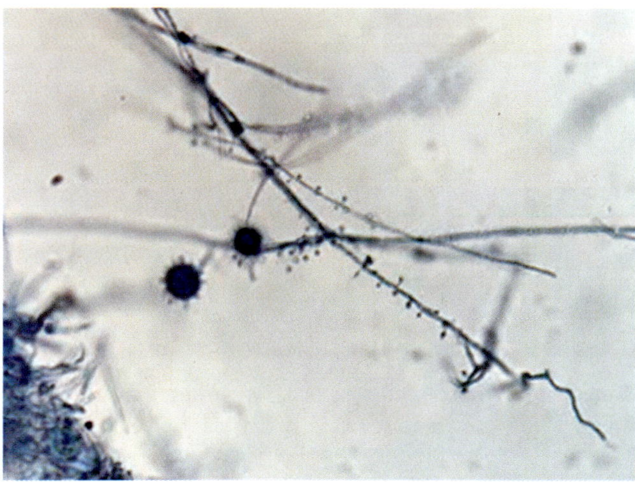

FIGURE 4: Lactophenol cotton blue (LPCB) mount of *Histoplasma* culture showing macroconidia and microconidia (40X).

age. Microscopically on lactophenol cotton blue preparation, it shows thin septate hyphae with micro- or macroconidia in various developmental stages (**Fig. 4**). The conversion from mold to yeast phase is necessary for accurate diagnosis of *Histoplasma*.

- *Antibody detection*: It is detected after 4–6 weeks of the infections. There are two methods routinely used; immunodiffusion (ID) test and compliment fixation test (CFT). These serological tests cross-reacts with *Blastomyces dermatitidis, Coccidioides immitis, Paracoccidioides brasiliensis, Aspergillus, and* also *Candida* and cryptococcal infections. In ID, presence of H and M precipitating band is considered to be conclusive of diagnosis of histoplasmosis. H band appears after M band in acute/progressive disease. It is only in 7% serum with patients in acute infections. It disappears more quickly than M antibodies; it is rarely detected after skin test. Antibodies to H antigen may be detected in 1–2 years after resolution of the diseases. M band is more frequently detected than H; it appears soon after infections. It is positive in past infections, acute, and chronic progressive diseases. It persists up to 3 years after the resolution of the diseases can be stimulated after skin infections.
- *Antigen detection assay*: This assay detects polysaccharide antigen in serum or urine by enzyme-linked immunosorbent assay (ELISA). Sensitivity of antigen detection in disseminated histoplasmosis is higher in immunocompromised patients than immunocompetent patients and in patients with more severe illness. That is why it is the mainstay of diagnosis, especially in the progressive histoplasmosis. It has got prognostic value for management of the patients.
- *Molecular diagnosis*: Main difficulty with molecular diagnosis in invasive fungal infection is extraction of deoxyribonucleic acid (DNA) from clinical samples. Recently, real-time polymerase chain reaction (PCR) has been evaluated for histidine kinase and glyceraldehyde-3 phosphate dehydrogenase gene; detected by florescence resonance energy transfer and hybridization assay. Analytical sensitivity of assay was 94% with 100% specificity and in clinical sample it was 73% and 100%.
- *Other tests*: Skin sensitivity test to histoplasmin antigen is used as an epidemiologic tool for determining *Histoplasma* cases.

According to the European Organization for Research and Treatment of Cancer/Mycoses Study Group Education and Research Consortium (EORTC/MSGERC) Criteria 2020, *Probable endemic mycoses* are defined by evidence of environmental exposure to the fungus, a compatible clinical illness, and the presence of antigen in any body fluid and histopathologic evidence of infection is generally lacking.

Proven endemic mycosis are defined as histopathology or direct microscopy of specimens obtained from an affected site showing intracellular yeast cells, recovery of the fungus by culture from an affected site, and blood culture yields the fungus.

TREATMENT

The treatment of acute pulmonary histoplasmosis is not required in immunocompetent patient with low degree of exposure, in asymptomatic or mild symptomatic patients, and when the illness resolves without therapy. The preferred treatment for histoplasmosis (**Table 2**) is liposomal amphotericin B in more severe cases followed by itraconazole.

Deoxycholate formulation can also be used but liposomal amphotericin B is more effective and better tolerated and dose can be manipulated for the treatment of PDH in patients with acquired immunodeficiency syndrome (AIDS). For the patients who cannot take itraconazole can use voriconazole, posaconazole, and isavuconazole as alternative.

TABLE 2 Recommended treatment for histoplasmosis.

Type of histoplasmosis	Treatment
Acute pulmonary histoplasmosis	Liposomal amphotericin B (3–5 mg/kg/day) ± glucocorticoids for 1–2 weeks; then itraconazole (200 mg bid) for 12 weeks. Monitor renal and hepatic function
Chronic cavitary histoplasmosis	Itraconazole (200 mg qd or bid) for at least 12 months. Monitor hepatic function
Progressive disseminated histoplasmosis	Lipid amphotericin B (3–5 mg/kg/day) for 1–2 weeks; then itraconazole (200 mg bid) for at least 12 months. Monitor renal and hepatic function
Histoplasmosis affecting central nervous system	Liposomal amphotericin B (5 mg/kg/day) for 4–6 weeks; then itraconazole (200 mg bid or tid) for at least 12 months. Monitor renal and hepatic function
Mediastinal lymphadenitis	No treatment. If symptomatic (e.g., dysphagia), itraconazole 200 mg bid for 12 weeks ± corticosteroids 60 mg with a rapid taper may be used to diminish lymph node size
Rheumatologic arthralgias	Nonsteroidal anti-inflammatory drugs (NSAIDs)
Pericarditis	NSAIDS or corticosteroids

BLASTOMYCOSIS

Blastomycosis is a systemic granulomatous disease caused by a dimorphic fungi *Blastomyces dermatitidis*. Blastomycosis mostly present as pulmonary blastomycosis, but almost every organ can be involved. It is a thermally dimorphic fungus. The yeast cells typically show broad-based budding (figure of 8 appearance) and the size of yeast cells around 8–15 μm.

EPIDEMIOLOGY

Blastomycosis is found in warm and moist soil of wooded areas, mostly reported from North America. Blastomycosis is not very uncommon in India; sporadic cases have been reported from Uttar Pradesh, Madhya Pradesh, and Maharashtra. This rise in the cases of blastomycosis in nonendemic areas may be due to the increase in international travels. Zoonotic transmission is also reported from dog bites, cat scratches etc., but it is rare.

PATHOGENESIS

After inhalation of conidia conversion to thick-walled yeast phase occurs inside the alveolar macrophages which lead to clinically apparent disease. Innate immunity and local host factors, such as lung surfactant has a very crucial role in the inhibition of this yeast phase conversion. This inhibition prevents the development of symptomatic illness. After development of the infection cellular immunity (Th1 response) is the primary host defense against *B. dermatitidis*.

CLINICAL FEATURE

Blastomycosis is most often misdiagnosed as the clinical presentation resembles with other much more common conditions such as acute bacterial community-acquired pneumonia, tuberculosis, and the extrapulmonary manifestations resembles with pyoderma gangrenosum, keratoacanthoma, or cancer. Patients often present with nonspecific complaints such as weight loss, fever, malaise, and fatigue. Pneumonia is the most common presentation of blastomycosis. Lobar infiltrate, mostly upper lobe involvement, is found in the majority of patients, miliary or reticulonodular patterns are the next most frequent pattern on radiography. Verrucous and ulcerative type of skin lesions are the next most common presentation of blastomycosis. In case of dissemination of pulmonary blastomycosis, skin is the most frequent site (40–80%) followed by bone (10–50%), genitourinary tract (10–30%), and central nervous system (CNS) (1–5%).

DIAGNOSIS

Sample for the blastomycosis depends on the site of involvement; it can be sputum, bronchial washings, pus, or biopsy material.

- *Direct microscopy*: *B. dermatitidis* is not a commensal or colonizer, its presence either in direct microscopy or culture confirms the diagnosis of blastomycosis. The fungus is most commonly identified on microscopy by its characteristic broad-based budding yeast form on KOH mount of exudate, sputum, or tissue. The organism may be visible on routine hematoxylin and eosin staining but fungal stains such as GMS and PAS allow more rapid diagnosis of the organism.
- *Culture*: For culture of blastomycosis no special media is required; it can grow on routine Sabouraud dextrose agar (SDA) media. Even if fungal stains are negative, the organism can be isolated on culture of the skin or other specimens.
- *Serology*: For the detection of antibodies against *B. dermatitidis,* initially CFT was used but due to the low sensitivity and specificity 57% and 30%, respectively this test is no longer used. ID band test utilizing the A antigen has a better sensitivity (65%) and specificity (80–100%).
- *Antigen detection assay*: This assay is most commonly done on urine specimen and the sensitivity and specificity of this assay in the urine is 92.9% and 79.3%, respectively. Cross-reactivity of the urinary antigen assay can also be seen with *H. capsulatum* because the clinical pictures for these two fungal infections can sometimes be similar.
- *Molecular methods*: Molecular techniques are not that much advanced in case of *B. dermatitidis* infection. For identification of *B. dermatitidis* in culture,

TABLE 3 Recommended treatment for blastomycosis.

Disease	Primary treatment	Alternative treatment
Pulmonary	Lipid amphotericin B, 3–5 mg/kg qd, Or Amphotericin B deoxycholate, 0.7–1.0 mg/kg qd (total dose: 1.5–2.5 g)	Itraconazole, 200–400 mg/day
Disseminated central nervous system (CNS)	Lipid amphotericin B, 3–5 mg/kg qd, Or Amphotericin B deoxycholate, 0.7–1.0 mg/kg qd (total dose: at least 2 g)	Fluconazole, 800 mg/day (if patient is intolerant to full course of amphotericin B)
Non-CNS	Lipid amphotericin B, 3–5 mg/kg qd, Or Amphotericin B deoxycholate, 0.7–1.0 mg/kg qd (total dose: 1.5–2.5 g)	Itraconazole, 200–400 mg/day (once patient's condition has stabilized)

chemiluminescent DNA probe hybridization and real-time PCR assays has been used.

TREATMENT

Therapy for blastomycosis is generally given for 6-12 months. For bone and joint disease, a 12-month course is necessary (**Table 3**).

EMERGOMYCOSIS: A CLOSE MIMIC OF HISTOPLASMOSIS

Recently a new dimorphic fungus, *Emergomyces* species, has been described that has clinical features and histopathological characters (yeast cells with narrow-based budding) similar to histoplasmosis. The genus *Emergomyces* contains *E. africanus, E. canadensis, E. europaeus, E. orientalis,* and the type species *E. pasteurianus.* Emergomycosis may present with localized clinical symptoms—cutaneous (papules, nodules, and ulcers) or pulmonary (chest X-ray abnormalities such as diffuse reticulonodular disease, consolidation, effusions, and/or lymphadenopathy) manifestations are most common, while gastrointestinal tract, liver, lymph nodes, and bone marrow are less commonly involved. All reported cases of other species have involved disseminated disease. Whether localized or disseminated, emergomycosis is almost always seen in immunocompromised patients [human immunodeficiency virus (HIV) infection, hematological malignancies, solid organ transplantation, and immunosuppressive therapy]. It is also interesting to note that since it was first described, HIV-associated emergomycosis has become the most common endemic mycosis in South Africa. Therefore, for a complete understanding of the epidemiology of endemic mycosis, it is advisable to identify all intracellular yeasts by DNA sequencing.

PNEUMOCYSTIS PNEUMONIA

INTRODUCTION

Among people with AIDS, *Pneumocystis* pneumonia (PCP) remains a common and life-threatening opportunistic infection. The incidence of PCP among patients without HIV infection has progressively increased. Non-HIV mortality rates—35-55% compared to HIV-infected—10-20%. An annual incidence of PCP with AIDS is approximately 14.7% of 1.76 million with CD4 cell count <100.

PATHOGEN AND PATHOGENESIS

Pneumocystis is an ubiquitous, obligate, and extracellular eukaryotic organism. It is host-species specific. *Pneumocystis* species does not appear to grow in standard fungal culture. A recent study from Germany: Culture *P. jirovecii* using differentiated pseudostratified respiratory epithelium (CuFi-8 cells)—trophic forms and cysts. The trophic form—tightly attached to type I pneumocytes in lung alveoli. The cyst can contain up to eight "sporozoites" and is protected by a distinctive thick cyst wall. When the wall ruptures (excystment), these "sporozoites" are released and then develop into new trophic forms.

Antibodies against *P. jirovecii* were found in majority of children under the age of 4 years. Colonization prevalence varies from 20 to 69%. Receiving anti-*Pneumocystis* prophylaxis for a long time may lead to selection of drug-resistant strains.

RISK FACTORS

Risk factors of *Pneumocystis jirovecii* infections in **Box 1**.

CLINICAL FEATURES

- HIV-infected population:
  - Subacute onset of gradual dyspnea
  - Nonproductive or minimally productive cough
  - Low grade fever and malaise
  - May be asymptomatic
- Non-HIV immunosuppressed:
  - Acute onset
  - Significant dyspnea
  - High fever and chills

Human immunodeficiency virus-infected patients have more *Pneumocystis* organisms with fewer neutrophils and correlates with a significantly higher diagnostic yield. HIV-infected patients have higher arterial oxygen tension and a lower alveolar-arterial oxygen gradient. Non-HIV patients have more likely to develop respiratory failure (40% mortality).

BOX 1	Risk factors of *Pneumocystis jirovecii* infections.
• Glucocorticoid use in patients with another cause of immunocompromised	
• Other immunosuppressive drugs such as:	
◦ Antirejection medications	
◦ Purine analogs (e.g., fludarabine)	
◦ Tumor necrosis factor-alpha inhibitors (e.g., infliximab)	
◦ Temozolomide (especially when used in combination with radiation)	
◦ Alemtuzumab	
◦ Ibrutinib	
◦ Idelalisib	
• Defects in cell-mediated immunity	
• Cancer (particularly hematologic malignancy)	
• Hematopoietic cell transplantation (HCT; especially allogeneic HCT)	
• Solid organ transplantation	
• Treatment for rejection	
• Treatment for inflammatory conditions [e.g., granulomatosis with polyangiitis (Wegener's)]	
• Severe malnutrition (especially protein malnutrition)	
• Primary immunodeficiencies (particularly severe combined immunodeficiency)	
• Prematurity	

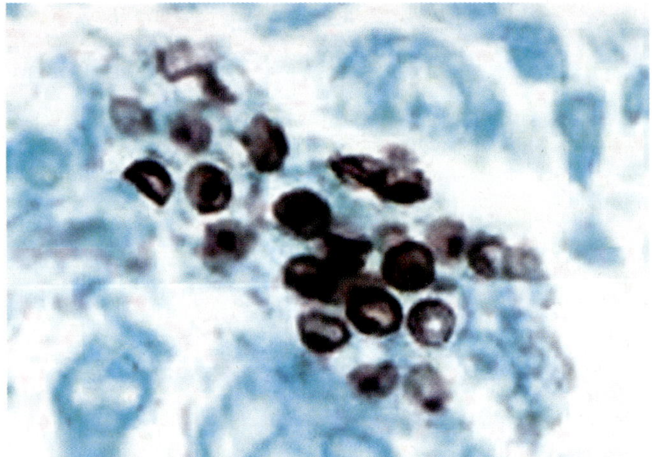

FIGURE 5: Grocott-Gomori's methenamine silver stain showing typical round and cup-shaped cysts of *P. jirovecii* (100X).

RADIOLOGICAL FEATURES

Chest radiographic findings in PCP are nonspecific. One-third of infected patients may have normal radiographic findings. High-resolution computed tomography (HRCT) "ground-glass" appearance or cystic lesions reflecting accumulation of intra-alveolar fibrin, debris, and organisms in PCP. HRCT is expensive and not cost-effective in low- and middle-income countries (LMICs).

LABORATORY DIAGNOSIS

A variety of specimens have been used for diagnosis such as lung biopsy, BAL, induced and expectorated sputum, nasopharyngeal aspirates, and oral washings. There is high morbidity associated with biopsy and BAL is the sample of choice. *Pneumocystis jirovecii* is noncultivable in vitro.

- *Microscopy*: Direct microscopy is the standard diagnostic method for PCP. The characteristic pathologic findings of lung tissue are acellular, foamy, eosinophilic, and intra-alveolar exudates seen on H&E. Fungal stains (like PAS or GMS) demonstrate cysts, allowing differentiation from alveolar proteinosis (**Fig. 5**). Immunofluorescent antibodies can be used to highlight the organism and significantly improve the sensitivity of pathologic examination.
- *Molecular diagnosis*: Superiority of PCR over microscopy both in sensitivity and in being able to analyze all sample types. Not technically and financially viable for resource-poor settings. Targets used for diagnosis: Mitochondrial large subunit (mtLSU), ribosomal ribonucleic acid (rRNA), major surface glycoprotein (MSG), ITS, dihydropteroate synthase (DHPS), dihydrofolate reductase (DHFR), and β-tubulin. Real time PCR can be performed by using commercially available kits.
- Nonspecific markers of PCP:
  - *Lactate dehydrogenase (LDH)*: Increased serum LDH levels. Underlying lung inflammatory responses and damage rather than a precise biomarker for PCP. LDH has a high sensitivity for PCP, but it is not specific.
  - *Beta-1-3-D-glucan (BDG)*: BDG is a polysaccharide—*Pneumocystis* cyst wall. Though BDG specificity for *Pneumocystis* is relatively poor, it is however highly sensitive for PCP. Due to the fact that BDG levels are also increased in other mycotic infections such as candidemia and aspergillosis. It is better used as an adjuvant test in patients with a high clinical index.

TREATMENT

Trimethoprim-sulfamethoxazole (TMP-SMX) is the preferred regimen for the treatment of PCP in patients with HIV. Therapy should be administered for 21 days. The standard dose of TMP-SMX is 15–20 mg/kg/day orally or intravenously in three or four divided doses. Dosing of TMP-SMX is based upon the TMP component and expressed as mg/kg/day of TMP. The severity of disease dictates whether oral or IV therapy should be used. Dose modifications for renal impairment may be needed. TMP-dapsone can be given as alternative therapy with patients who show allergic reactions to sulfa-containing drugs. Oral TMP is administered at a dose of 5 mg/kg (typically rounded to the nearest 100 mg) three times per day with dapsone 100 mg/day. Clindamycin-primaquine may also be used.

Use of corticosteroids: Corticosteroids given in conjunction with anti-*Pneumocystis* therapy can decrease the incidence of mortality and respiratory failure associated with PCP. It is recommended to use adjunctive corticosteroids for patients with moderate-to-severe disease. If blood gas data are available, initiate steroids in patients with:

- A partial pressure of oxygen of <70 mm Hg on room air *and/or*
- An alveolar-arterial (A-a) oxygen gradient of ≥35 mm Hg

Prophylaxis: Secondary prophylaxis is indicated in patients with prior PCP. Additionally, primary prophylaxis is recommended for people with HIV with CD4 ≤200 cells/µL or comprising <14% of total lymphocyte count, or in situations where CD4 count ≤250 cells/µL, but antiretroviral therapy (ART) cannot be initiated and q3 monthly CD4 monitoring is not possible. The preferred regimen is TMP-SMX 1 double strength (DS) PO daily. An advantage of this regiment is that it also protects against toxoplasmosis.

OTHER FUNGAL INFECTIONS

FUSARIUM SPECIES

Fusarium species cause a wide spectrum of infections in humans, including superficial infections such as onychomycosis and keratitis. Invasive and disseminated infections occur mostly in immunocompromised patients, particularly those with prolonged neutropenia etc. Among patients with hematologic malignancy, the infection predominates during periods of neutropenia, typically among patients with leukemia receiving induction chemotherapy. In contrast with aspergillosis and most other invasive mold infections, a distinct characteristic of infections due to *Fusarium* species in immunocompromised hosts is the high rates of positive blood cultures as this fungus can sporulate in vivo. *Fusarium* species may also cause allergic diseases such as rhinosinusitis and rarely mycotoxicosis following ingestion of food contaminated by toxin-producing *Fusarium* species.

In severely immunocompromised patients, two characteristics indicate towards the diagnosis of disseminated fusariosis: (1) The presence of skin lesions (either cellulitis at sites of skin breakdown caused by trauma, intertrigo, or metastatic lesions) and (2) growth of mold from blood cultures. Skin biopsy is the ideal sample in such scenario. Blood cultures should also be obtained. In individuals with lung involvement, a respiratory sample should be sent for direct microscopic examination and culture. Treatment is usually achieved with combination of antifungal agents, e.g., voriconazole plus terbinafine.

SCEDOSPORIUM AND *LOMENTOSPORA*

Scedosporium and *Lomentospora* species are commonly found in soil and polluted water and have a global distribution. These species are mainly associated with infections in immunocompromised hosts, although some localized infections have been described in immunocompetent hosts. Reported infections caused by these pathogens include pneumonia (especially near drowning), keratitis, endophthalmitis, CNS infections, soft-tissue infections, and disseminated disease.

The approach to diagnosis is individualized based upon various patient-specific factors, including site and severity of infection, as well as the immune status of the host. Whenever possible, and especially for immunocompromised hosts and/or for patients with severe disease, clinicians should aggressively pursue a diagnosis when *Scedosporium* or *Lomentospora* infection is suspected.

Histologically, *Scedosporium* and *Lomentospora*, with septated and nonpigmented hyphae branching at 45° angles, resemble the other hyaline molds such as *Aspergillus* and *Fusarium*. Definite diagnosis is made through culture. Culture is also important for testing in vitro susceptibility since these pathogens, particularly *L. prolificans*, can be resistant to multiple antifungal agents.

RECOMMENDED READINGS

1. Hage CA, Wheat LJ. Histoplasmosis. In: Jameson JL, Kasper DL, Longo DL, Fauci AS, Hauser SL, Loscalzo J (Eds). Harrison's Principle of Internal Medicine. New York: McGraw Hill; 2018. pp. 1518-20.
2. Gupta A, Ghosh A, Singh G, Xess I. A twenty-first-century perspective of disseminated histoplasmosis in India: literature review and retrospective analysis of published and unpublished cases at a tertiary care hospital in North India. Mycopathologia. 2017;182 (11-12):1077-93.
3. Deepe GS Jr. *Histoplasma capsulatum*. In: Mandell GL, Bennett JE, Dolin R (Eds). Mandell, Douglas, and Bennett's Principles and Practice of Infectious diseases. Philadelphia: Elsevier; 2015. pp. 2948-62.
4. Donnelly JP, Chen SC, Kauffman CA, Steinbach WJ, Baddley JW, Verweij PE, et al. Revision and update of the consensus definitions of invasive fungal disease from the European Organization for Research and Treatment of Cancer and the Mycoses Study Group Education and Research Consortium. Clin Infect Dis. 2020;71(6):1367-76.
5. Walzer PD, Smulian AG. *Pneumocystis* species. In: Mandell GL, Bennett JE, Dolin R (Eds). Mandell, Douglas, and Bennett's Principles and Practice of Infectious Disease. 7th edition. Philadelphia: Elsevier; 2010. pp. 3377-90.
6. Thomas CF Jr, Limper AH. Pneumocystis pneumonia. N Engl J Med. 2004;350:2487.
7. Wieruszewski PM, Barreto JN, Frazee E, et al. Early Corticosteroids for Pneumocystis Pneumonia in Adults Without HIV Are Not Associated With Better Outcome. Chest. 2018;154:636.

CHAPTER

66

Helminthic Infections

Subhash Chandra Parija, Tuhina Banerjee

ABSTRACT

Helminths are parasites with elongated flat or roundworm like bodies. They are the most common cause of infections in humans from developing countries. The global burden of these infections often outweighs other communicable diseases such as malaria and tuberculosis. Most of the helminthic infections including lymphatic filariasis, soil-transmitted helminths (STHs) including roundworms, whipworms, and hookworms, taeniasis and cysticercosis, schistosomiasis, foodborne trematode infections, echinococcosis, and dracunculiasis are enlisted as neglected tropical diseases (NTDs) by the World Health Organization (WHO). These infections affect the poorest communities of developing nations in African and Asian countries.

Helminths can be considered in three major groups. The nematodes, commonly known as roundworm include the STHs and the filarial worms that cause lymphatic filariasis and onchocerciasis. The tapeworms (also known as the cestodes) that cause cysticercosis, taeniasis, and hydatid disease and the flatworms which include the flukes (also known as trematodes) causing schistosomiasis, fascioliasis, fasciolopsiasis. The majority of these infections do not produce overt symptoms unless the worm burden becomes "heavy". This results in a huge reservoir of asymptomatic carriers in the community facilitating spread and persistence of these infections. Helminthic infections are treatable with common anthelmintic agents such as albendazole, ivermectin, and diethylcarbamazine (DEC) as detailed with the individual parasites. As these infections are highly prevalent in the tropics with unhygienic conditions, lack of access to safe water, overcrowding, and other factors, measures for prevention are of utmost importance. However, with urbanization and excessive travel due to modernization, the epidemiology of infections due to these helminths also keeps changing and thus clinical suspicion and awareness are essential for their prompt diagnosis and management.

"No matter how dark things seem to be or actually are, raise your sights and see the possibilities – always see them, for they're always there"

—Norman Vincent Peale

NEMATODES

FILARIASIS

Lymphatic filariasis is caused by filarial nematodes. These nematodes inhabit the lymphatic system in man along with skin and subcutaneous tissue. The parasite exists in two forms namely the adult worm and the larva called the microfilaria, which often exhibit periodicity in appearance. These are the diagnostic forms found in blood vessels. The disease is transmitted by the deposition of the third stage filariform larva (L3) into the skin through mosquito bite. The filarial and somatic nematodes have been summarized in **Table 1**.

Filariasis is widely prevalent throughout the globe with the bulk of the burden being borne by the Southeast Asian countries (50%) and Sub-Saharan Africa. India also accounts for nearly 40% of the global burden with most of the states being endemic for it. Both cell-mediated and humoral immune responses are seen in filariasis. **Table 2** summarizes the immune responses to filarial infection.

Clinical features:

- Recurrent high-grade fever with lymphangitis and lymphadenitis can be seen as acute presentations.
- Individuals may remain asymptomatic, especially in endemic areas.
- Chronic filariasis develops years after infection.
- Lymphedema is the most common presentation often manifesting as hydrocele, elephantiasis, and chyluria.
- Hypersensitivity reactions to microfilarial antigen might present as nocturnal paroxysmal cough and wheeze, a condition known as tropical pulmonary eosinophilia or occult filariasis.

Laboratory diagnosis: The major modes of diagnosis have been enlisted in **Table 3**.

Diethylcarbamazine provocation test: This test is done to increase the movement of the nocturnal microfilaria in the blood during the day time in order to be detected by microscopy of peripheral blood smear. Patients are administered DEC at dose 2 mg/kg and several peripheral blood smears are examined in between 15 minutes and 1 hour of ingestion of DEC.

TABLE 1 List of nematodes and site of involvement.

Filarial nematodes				Somatic nematodes
Site	**Name**	**Microfilarial periodicity and location**	**Vectors**	
Lymphatic tissue	*Wuchereria bancrofti*	Nocturnal/Blood	*Culex*	*Dracunculus medinensis*
	Brugia malayi		*Mansonia*	
	Brugia timori		*Anopheles*	
Skin and subcutaneous tissue including eye	*Loa loa*	Diurnal/Blood, adult worm in eye	*Chrysops* (deer flies)	*Trichinella spiralis*
	Onchocerca volvulus	None/Skin	*Simulium* (blackflies)	
	Mansonella streptocerca (eye not infected)		*Culicoides* (midges)	
Body cavities	*Mansonella perstans*	None/Blood	*Culicoides*	
	Mansonella ozzardi		*Culicoides* and *Simulium*	

TABLE 2 Immune response in lymphatic filariasis.

Immune response		
Early infection	**Acute infection**	**Chronic infection**
• Both TH1 and TH2 response • IL-2, IFN-γ, IL-4, and IL-5 • Eosinophilia • Raised IgE	• Mainly TH1 response • IL-4, IL-5, IL-10, and IL-13 • Eosinophilia • Parasite specific IgG4	• TH2 response • IgG1-3

(IFN-γ: interferon-γ; IgE: immunoglobulin E;IgG: immunoglobulin G; IL: interleukin;TH1: type 1 T helper; TH2: type 2 T helper)

TABLE 3 Laboratory diagnosis of filariasis.

Methods	Findings
Microscopy of PBS	Microfilaria
Serology	Antigen detection using monoclonal antibodies by ELISA or ICT
	Antibody detection by flow through assays
Molecular methods	Real-time PCR targeting several microfilarial proteins
Others	Imaging techniques like ultrasonography detecting "filarial dance sign"
	Nonspecific indicators such as eosinophilia and raised IgE

(ELISA: enzyme-linked immunosorbent assay; ICT: immunochromatographic test; IgE: immunoglobulin E; PBS: peripheral blood smear)

Treatment: The treatment strategy for management of cases as well as prevention of infection in form of "mass drug administration (MDA)" has been mentioned in **Table 4**.

INTESTINAL NEMATODES

These are among the most common infections affecting man. Majority of these infections do not manifest as prominent symptoms, thus favoring the persistence and spread of infections from asymptomatic reservoirs. The various intestinal nematodes can be enumerated as given in **Table 5**.

Man acquires infection either by ingestion of eggs contaminating food and water in infections by roundworm, pinworm, and whipworm or by skin penetration as in infections by hookworms and *Strongyloides*. Infected individuals are asymptomatic unless heavy worm burden causes significant signs and symptoms. Common presentations are:

- Abdominal pain, anorexia, and weight loss
- Iron deficiency anemia due to blood loss in hookworm and whipworm infections
- Perianal pruritus in pinworm infection
- Intestinal obstruction in cases of heavy worm burden
- Eosinophilic pneumonia (Löffler's syndrome) in roundworm infection
- Hyperinfection syndrome and disseminated strongyloidiasis: In patients with immunosuppressive conditions such as malignancy, organ transplantation, corticosteroid therapy, and *Strongyloides* infection, repeated autoinfection causes excessive burden of larvae that enter the gastrointestinal tract as well as migrate to other organs. This hyperinfection syndrome can lead to severe colitis, malabsorption, and dissemination of infection. In disseminated infection, brain abscesses, meningitis and severe central nervous system manifestations can occur, which if untreated leads to high mortality. *Strongyloides* infection is often associated with human immunodeficiency virus (HIV) infection, though disseminated infection is not a usual association.

Laboratory diagnosis: Infections by nematode can be diagnosed by the following methods as mentioned in **Table 6**. The microscopic findings in stool examination of

TABLE 4 Treatment strategy in filariasis.

Purpose	Strategy	Comment
Treatment of infection	A combination of albendazole (400 mg) with ivermectin (150–200 μg/kg) as a single dose	• Used where onchocerciasis is coendemic • Albendazole kills both microfilaria and adult worms • Ivermectin has no effect on adult worms
	A combination of albendazole (400 mg) plus diethylcarbamazine (6 mg/kg) as a single dose Or Diethylcarbamazine (DEC) at 6 mg/kg for 12 days	• Used where onchocerciasis is not coendemic • DEC kills both microfilaria and adult worms
Prevention	A combined dose of albendazole (400 mg) plus ivermectin (150–200 μg/kg) or DEC (6 mg/kg) annually	"Twin pillar strategy" for elimination of lymphatic filariasis in India encompasses administration of both albendazole and DEC in mass drug administration (MDA)

TABLE 5 Common intestinal nematodes.

Habitat	Common names	Scientific names
Small intestine	Roundworms	*Ascaris lumbricoides*
	Hookworms	*Ancylostoma duodenale*
		Necator americanus
	Military worm	*Strongyloides stercoralis*
Large intestine	Threadworm or pinworm	*Enterobius vermicularis*
	Whipworm	*Trichuris trichiura*

TABLE 6 Laboratory diagnosis of nematode infections.

Methods	Findings
Microscopy of stool	• Eggs of roundworm, hookworm, and whipworm • Special slide preparation such as cellophane tape and National Institute of Health (NIH) swab method for visualization of pinworm eggs in perianal skin • Larva in case of Strongyloides
Stool culture	• Help in differentiation of hookworm species (**Fig. 1**)
Serology	Coproantigen detection especially in *Strongyloides* infection
Molecular methods	Polymerase chain reaction (PCR) targeting intertranscriber spacer (ITS) regions

TABLE 7 Treatment of choice for common nematode infections.

Nematode infection	Treatment of choice
***Ascaris*, hookworm, *Trichuris*, and pinworm infection**	• Albendazole 400 mg once, or • Mebendazole 500 mg once, 100 mg once for children to be repeated after 2 weeks in pinworm infection
Strongyloidiasis	• Ivermectin 200 mg/kg daily for 2 days, to be extended to 7 days for disseminated infections • Albendazole, 400 mg once daily for 3 days is less preferable

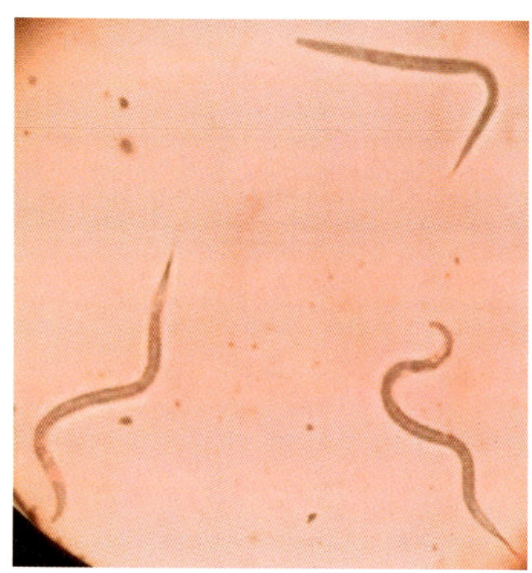

FIGURE 1: Larva of hookworm in stool culture.

few of these nematodes have been shown in **Figures 2 A to D**. As most of the infections are asymptomatic, strong clinical suspicion is required for prompt diagnosis of these infections.

Treatment: Infections by nematodes can be managed by anthelmintic agents like albendazole/mebendazole or ivermectin. The suggested treatment guidelines for the common nematode infections have been tabulated in **Table 7**.

CESTODES

INTESTINAL TAENIASIS

Cestodes are tape like segmented worms often called the tapeworm. They can be intestinal or tissue cestodes where the larval forms are found in muscles or other organs. The common tapeworms are shown in **Table 8**.

Intestinal taeniasis is caused by *Taenia solium* and *Taenia saginata* that exist in three forms. The adult worms that reside in the small intestine, the eggs that remain inside the gravid segments (proglottides) of the worm and are released outside through feces and finally the larval forms in muscles of intermediate hosts like pigs or cattle. The larval stage for *T. solium* is known as cysticercus cellulosae and for *T. saginata* is cysticercus bovis. These larval stages are

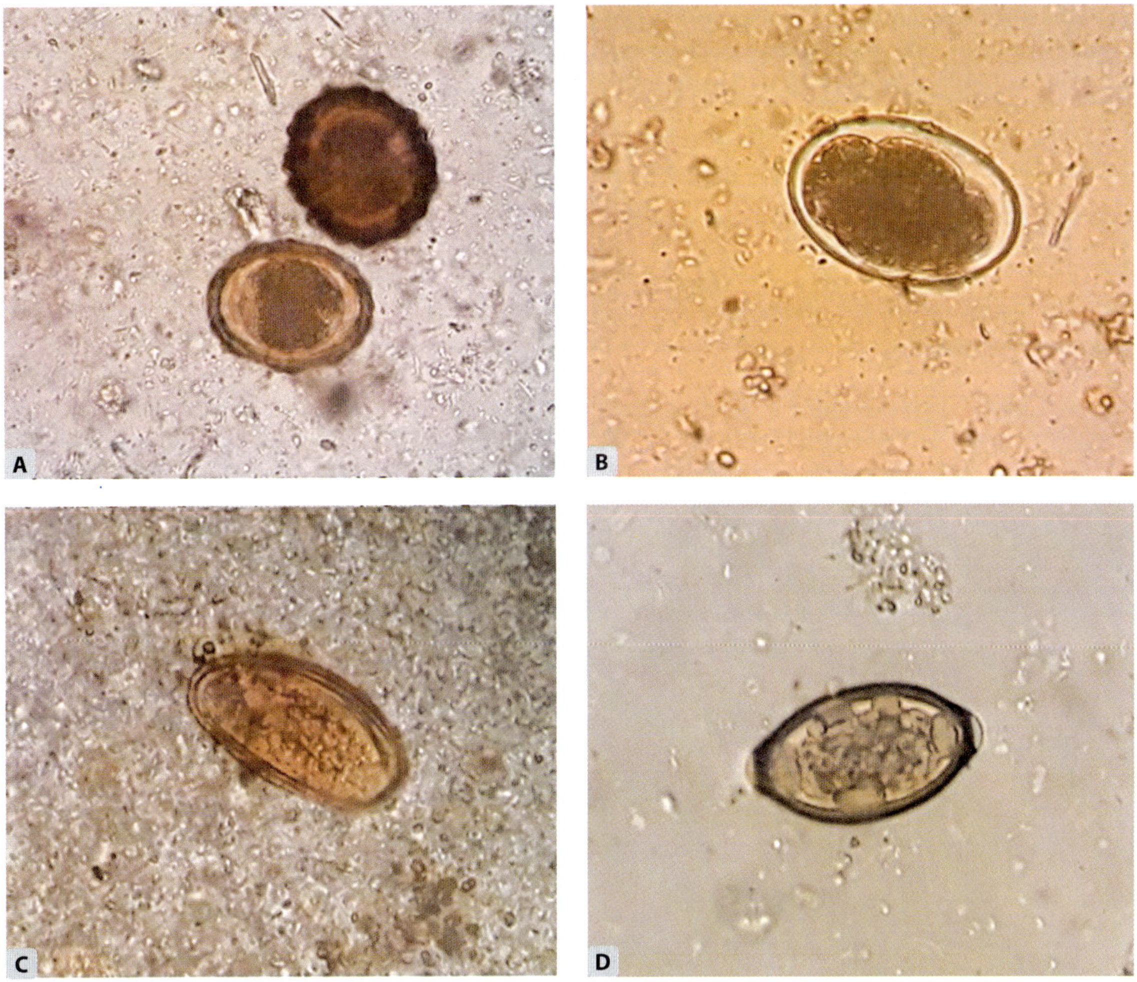

FIGURES 2 A to D: Eggs of common nematodes in stool. **(A)** Eggs of *Ascaris*; **(B)** Eggs of hookworm; **(C)** Eggs of *Enterobius*; **(D)** Eggs of *Trichuris*.

TABLE 8 List of common tapeworms causing infections.

Intestinal cestodes	Tissue cestodes
Taenia solium	*Taenia solium (cysticercosis)*
Taenia saginata	
Hymenolepis nana	*Echinococcus granulosus*
Diphyllobothrium latum	

infective in man, who acquires the infection by ingestion of improperly cooked meat (pork or beef) containing these larval stages.

Clinical features:

- Taeniasis often presents as asymptomatic passage of segments of the worm in stool, which can be motile.
- Nonspecific gastrointestinal symptoms including abdominal pain, nausea, loss of appetite, and change in bowel habits.

Laboratory diagnosis: Intestinal taeniasis can be diagnosed by stool microscopy in majority of the cases. Eggs as shown in **Figure 3** are identical between the *Taenia* species and also other cestodes. *Taenia*-specific antigen testing in stool can also be performed to detect infection.

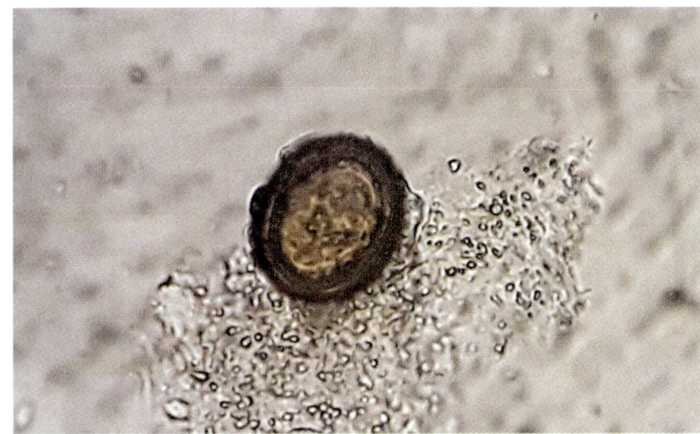

FIGURE 3: Eggs of *Taenia* species in wet mount examination of stool.

CYSTICERCOSIS

This can present with varied manifestations such as muscular, subcutaneous, and ocular forms depending upon the sites of localization of the cysts. Among them, neurocysticercosis is the most common manifestation affecting the central nervous system. It is also the most common cause of adult-onset epilepsy, seizure being the most common feature. Unlike in taeniasis, neurocysticercosis which is caused only by *T. solium* is acquired by consumption of food or water contaminated with the eggs of *T. solium* or by autoinfection whereby strong peristaltic movements of the gut introduces the mature proglottides back into one's own stomach.

Neurocysticercosis is diagnosed by a combination of indirect clinical evidences and imaging features based on Del Brutto's criteria as shown in **Table 9**.

Treatment of taeniasis and cysticercosis: The treatment for these infections has been mentioned in **Table 10**.

HYDATID DISEASE

This is caused by *Echinococcus* species, the larval form of which is called the "hydatid cyst". Infection in man can be caused by different *Echinococcus* species as listed in **Table 11**.

TABLE 9 Del Brutto's criteria for diagnosis of neurocysticercosis.

Diagnostic criteria	Features
Absolute criteria	• Histological evidence of the parasite from biopsy of a brain or spinal cord lesion • Visualization of subretinal cysticercus by fundoscopy • Neuroimaging studies demonstrating scolex within a cystic lesion
Neuroimaging criteria	• Major: ◦ Cystic lesions without a discernible scolex ◦ Enhancing lesions ◦ Multilobulated cystic lesions in the subarachnoid space ◦ Typical parenchymal brain calcifications • Confirmative: ◦ Resolution of cystic lesions after cysticidal drug therapy ◦ Spontaneous resolution of single small enhancing lesions ◦ Migration of ventricular cysts documented on sequential neuroimaging studies • Minor neuroimaging criteria: ◦ Obstructive hydrocephalus (symmetric or asymmetric) or abnormal enhancement of basal leptomeninges
Clinical/Exposure criteria	• Major: ◦ Detection of specific anticysticercal antibodies or cysticercal antigens by well-standardized immunodiagnostic tests ◦ Cysticercosis outside the central nervous system ◦ Evidence of a household contact with *T. solium* infection • Minor clinical/exposure: ◦ Clinical manifestations suggestive of neurocysticercosis ◦ Individuals coming from or living in an area where cysticercosis is endemic
Definitive diagnosis	• One absolute criterion • Two major neuroimaging criteria plus any clinical/exposure criteria • One major and one confirmative neuroimaging criteria plus any clinical/exposure criteria • One major neuroimaging criteria plus two clinical/exposure criteria (including at least one major clinical/exposure criterion), together with the exclusion of other pathologies producing similar neuroimaging findings
Probable diagnosis	• One major neuroimaging criteria plus any two clinical/exposure criteria • One minor neuroimaging criteria plus at least one major clinical/exposure criteria

TABLE 10 Management of infections caused by *Taenia* species.

Infection	Treatment modalities
Intestinal taeniasis	Single dose of praziquantel at 10 mg/kg
Cysticercosis	Albendazole at 15 mg/kg/day in two divided doses for 15 days is the better alternative Or Praziquantel (50 mg/kg/day for 15 days) Prolonged treatment required for extraparenchymal or widespread lesions
	For generalized seizures, addition of corticosteroids (albendazole 400 mg twice daily plus 6 mg dexamethasone QD for 10 days) have shown better results in trials
	Surgery is indicated for ocular or spinal lesions

This disease is widely reported in Central Asia including India. Man acquires infection by ingestion of contaminated food containing *Echinococcus* eggs in dog's feces. The eggs eventually transform into larva inside the small intestine of man and are carried through circulation to various sites such as liver (60–70%), lungs (20–30%), and others. Pressure effects due to enlarging cysts are the most common presentation while rupture of cysts can amount to severe allergic reactions.

Laboratory diagnosis: The disease is diagnosed by common modalities as mentioned in **Table 12**.

Management:
- Surgery is the definitive method depending on the number, site, and location of the cysts.
- Percutaneous aspiration followed by injection of scolicidal agents can be performed for easily accessible single cyst.
- Albendazole is the treatment of choice for reduction of cyst size prior to surgery and to prevent recurrence of infection. The usual dose of the drug for an average weight person (60 kg) is 400 mg oral tablet twice daily with meals for a period of 28 days. For those with less body weight, 15 mg/kg albendazole in two divided doses is administered. For cystic echinococcosis, this 28 days course could be repeated after 2 weeks of completion of the first cycle. A similar third cycle might be required depending upon the multiplicity of the cysts and severity of the symptoms.

TABLE 11 Infections caused by *Echinococcus* species.

Name of the species	Disease
Echinococcus granulosus	Cystic echinococcosis
Echinococcus multilocularis	Alveolar echinococcosis
Echinococcus vogeli	Polycystic hydatid disease
Echinococcus oligarthus	Unicystic hydatid disease

TABLE 12 Laboratory diagnosis of hydatid disease.

Methods	Findings
Microscopy of hydatid fluid	Brood capsules and protoscolices can be detected. Better viewed in hematoxylin eosin stain
Serology	Antibody detection by ELISA and Western blot
Molecular methods	PCR detection and genotype detection
Others	Imaging techniques like ultrasonography detecting "water-lily sign" Casoni test showing type I hypersensitivity reaction

(ELISA: enzyme-linked immunosorbent assay; PCR: polymerase chain reaction)

TREMATODES

These are infections caused by unsegmented, leaf-like flat worms called flukes. Based on habitat, these are classified as shown in **Table 13**.

SCHISTOSOMIASIS

These infections are among the NTDs that affect the rural population considerably and are the second most common cause of morbidity due to any parasitic infection following malaria. The condition is prevalent in African and Asian countries. It is rare in India limited to an endemic focus at Ratnagiri district in Maharashtra.

Schistosomiasis is acquired by penetration of the human skin by the cercaria infective form present in water. Further growth and development take place during its movement to lungs and then general circulation until its final location site at the plexus. Urinary schistosomiasis is also called bilharziasis.

Clinical features:
- In acute schistosomiasis, dermatitis occurs at the site of entry of the parasite
- Migration to lungs can manifest as cough
- Urogenital disease occurs due to deposition of eggs
- Fibrotic and ureteric obstruction
- Bladder carcinoma (squamous cell) due to chronic irritation

Laboratory diagnosis: Identification of eggs in stool or urine aids in diagnosis. Antibody and antigen detection also helps in screening. For seroepidemiology, two

TABLE 13 List of trematodes causing human infections.

Habitat	Site	Name	Disease caused/complications
Blood	Vesical venous plexus	*Schistosoma haematobium*	**Schistosomiasis**
	Rectal venous plexus	*Schistosoma mansoni*	
	Portal venous plexus	*Schistosoma japonicum*	
Liver	Liver	*Fasciola hepatica*	**Fascioliasis**
	Bile duct	*Clonorchis sinensis*	**Cholangiocarcinoma**
Lungs	Lungs	*Paragonimus westermani*	**Paragonimiasis**
Intestine	Small intestine	*Fasciolopsis buski*	**Fasciolopsiasis**

screening tests using the *Schistosoma haematobium* adult worm microsomal antigen (HAMA) in enzyme-linked immunosorbent assay (ELISA) and enzyme-linked immunoelectrotransfer blot (EITB) assays have shown appreciable results.

FASCIOLIASIS AND FASCIOLOPSIASIS

Though rare in India, fascioliasis is acquired by ingestion of water plants contaminated with metacercaria forms of *Fasciola hepatica* whereas, fasciolopsiasis by *Fasciolopsis buski*. Fascioliasis manifests as abdominal pain, hepatomegaly, and bile duct obstruction, while fasciolopsiasis present as intestinal obstruction in high worm burden. Stool microscopy is diagnostic, triclabendazole is used in treatment.

PARAGONIMIASIS

This condition is endemic in Northeastern states of India. Infection is acquired by consumption of improperly cooked crab or crayfish containing metacercaria forms of *Paragonimus westermani*. The disease manifests both as pulmonary and extrapulmonary forms. The pulmonary form is often misdiagnosed as tuberculosis infection owing to similar presentations. Pulmonary forms show eosinophilic granuloma causing cough, rusty sputum, and frank hemoptysis. Extrapulmonary forms can be cerebral or cutaneous manifestations. Sputum microscopy for parasite eggs and antibody detection in serum help in diagnosis.

PREVENTION OF INFECTIONS BY HELMINTH

The burden of infections due to helminths and the morbidity thus caused can be reduced and controlled by adopting better living conditions, health education, and awareness. Vaccines against helminth infections still have a long way to go with the most successful recombinant vaccines currently undergoing phase 1 trials are those against hookworms. Presently no vaccine is available for human use and therefore prevention is the priority. Some of the specific preventive measures can be:

- Improvement in hygienic status, both personal hygiene and sanitation
- Safe drinking and bathing water
- Food hygiene and awareness on properly cooked food
- Avoiding barefooted walking while working in fields
- Regular anthelmintic treatment
- Adhering to mass deworming programs in schools and rural centers
- Regular deworming of pets and proper disposal of feces of pets

RECOMMENDED READINGS

1. Hotez PJ, Brindley PJ, Bethony JM, King CH, Pearce EJ, Jacobson J. Helminth infections: the great neglected tropical diseases. J Clin Invest. 2008;118(4):1311-21.
2. World Health Organization. (2020). Soil transmitted helminths. [online] Available from https://www.who.int/news-room/fact-sheets/detail/soil-transmitted-helminth-infections.
3. Agrawal VK, Sashindran VK. Lymphatic Filariasis in India: Problems, Challenges and New Initiatives. Med J Armed Forces India. 2006;62(4):359-62.
4. Del Brutto OH, Nash TE, White AC Jr, Rajshekhar V, Wilkins PP, Singh G, et al. Revised diagnostic criteria for neurocysticercosis. J Neurol Sci. 2017;372: 202-10.
5. Chaya, Parija SC. Performance of polymerase chain reaction for the diagnosis of cystic echinococcosis using serum, urine, and cyst fluid samples. Trop Parasitol. 2014;4(1):43-6.
6. Sahu PS, Parija SC, Kumar D, Jayachandran S, Narayan S. Comparative profile of circulating antigenic peptides in CSF, serum & urine from patients with neurocysticercosis diagnosed by immunoblotting. Parasite Immunol. 2014;36:509-21.
7. Parija SC, Sheela Devi C. Current concepts in the diagnosis of cystic echinococcosis in humans and livestocks and intestinal echinococcosis in canine hosts. J Vet Parasitol. 1999;13:93-102.
8. Parija SC. Simple immunoassays in the serodiagnosis of hydatid disease in the field or poorly equipped laboratories. Indian J Med Microbiol. 1993;11:1-4.
9. Keiser J, Utzinger J. Food-borne trematodiases. Clin Microbiol Rev. 2009;22(3):466-83.
10. Biswal DK, Debnath M, Kharumnuid G, Thongnibah W, Tandon V. Northeast India Helminth Parasite Information Database (NEIHPID): Knowledge Base for Helminth Parasites. PLoS One. 2016;11(6):e0157459.
11. World Health Organization. (2020). Taeniasis and cysticercosis. [online] Available from https://www.who.int/news-room/fact-sheets/detail/taeniasis-cysticercosis.

MULTIPLE CHOICE QUESTIONS

To access the multiple choice questions of this Section online, kindly scan the QR code.

CHAPTER

67

Recognition and Approach to Critically ill Patient

JV Peter

ABSTRACT

Critical illness is associated with organ dysfunction that can result in significant morbidity and mortality. Except in a few situations, severe illness is often preceded by warning signs and abnormal physiology. Failure to pick up these symptoms, signs and physiological derangements could result in clinical deterioration and life-threatening events. Several systems have been proposed to evaluate such patients in order to enable early recognition of critical illness and initiate prompt treatment. The assessment of a critically ill patient may occur in the emergency department, ward, operating theatre, or in the intensive care unit (ICU). In all these situations, unlike in the assessment of a noncritically ill patient, history, examination, and treatment may need to happen in parallel with emphasis on identifying components of ABCDE (Airway, Breathing, Circulation, Disability, and Exposure) that may be life-threatening and need to be attended to immediately, even before a full history or examination is completed. Investigations would also need to be prioritized initially to those which are likely to be responsible for the physiological derangements than on investigations that would assist in arriving at a diagnosis. A rapid and systematic approach to the critically ill patient would allow appropriate initial management and better outcomes.

"Hope is being able to see that there is light despite all of the darkness"

—Desmond Tutu

INTRODUCTION

"The eye cannot see what the mind does not know".

—(Unknown).

The key elements in the successful practice of medicine involve appropriate diagnosis and prompt initiation of treatment. The diagnostic process entails detailed history taking, thorough clinical examination, and the use of relevant investigations. Although these aspects occur sequentially in most branches of medicine, in the approach to a critically ill patient, the luxury of time is lacking or limited. This is because treatment often needs to be initiated promptly when gross physiological derangements are detected in order to prevent progression to multiorgan failure that can lead to death or disability. In life-threatening situations where resuscitation becomes paramount, there may not be sufficient time to take a detailed history or do a thorough physical examination before initiating life-saving treatment and hence these may need to happen in parallel rather than sequentially. This does not obviate the need to either take a detailed history or do a thorough physical examination, which in such cases happen as treatment goes on.

INITIAL ASSESSMENT

"Patients do not die of their disease. They die of the physiological abnormalities of their disease."

—Sir William Osler

The assessment of a critically ill patient may occur in different settings—at presentation to the hospital in the emergency department, deterioration of a patient in the ward or acute deterioration during surgery or during the course of treatment in the ICU.

In the emergency department setting, particularly in well-developed health systems, hospitals have established systems to triage patients presenting to the department into various categories depending on several clinical features. The term *triage* originated from the French verb *trier* which means to sort. Its purpose is to identify patients who are in need of immediate resuscitation and to assign patients to different levels of care as appropriate. Several systems are used across the globe (**Table 1**). The most common triage system in the United States is the START (Simple Triage and Rapid Treatment) triage system. Other systems include the ATS (Australasian Triage Scale), the CTAS (Canadian

TABLE 1 Triaging systems.

START	ATS	CTAS	ESI
Pulse	Category 1: Red	I—Resuscitation	Level 1: Lifesaving intervention
Respiratory rate	Category 2: Orange	II—Emergency	Level 2: High-risk situation
Capillary refill time	Category 3: Green	III—Urgency	Level 3: Danger zone vitals
Bleeding	Category 4: Blue	IV—Less urgency	Level 4: One resource needed
Follows commands	Category 5: White	V—Nonurgency	Level 5: None needed

START—Simple Triage and Rapid Treatment triage system, intention is to triage the patients in <60 s and used primarily in mass casualty incident (MCI); it is an algorithmic approach that quickly assesses if the patient is able to walk. If they are able to, they are categorized as minor (walking wounded); subsequent assessment involves a quick assessment of respiration that includes respiratory rate and airway followed by assessment of perfusion (radial pulse and capillary refill) and mental status. This assessment categorizes patients as needing immediate care, delayed care, minor, and deceased.

ATS—Australasian Triaging Scale.

CTAS—Canadian Triage and Acuity Scale are a five-level triage system based on severity, time needed for intervention and a standardized list comprising of usual presentation and sentinel diagnosis; ^ATS and CTAS are five-level categorical scales based on patients' problems, appearance, and overview of pertinent physiological findings, described as clinical descriptors; Category 1 should be seen immediately, Category 2 within 10 min for ATS and within 15 min for CTAS, Category 3 within 30 min, Category 4 within 60 min, and Category 5 within 120 min.

ESI—Emergency Severity Index; Level 1 indicates that the patient requires immediate life-saving interventions which is determined by an assessment of the patients' airway, breath, circulation, and responsiveness. The other levels of response are determined based on clinical parameters.

Triage and Acuity Scale), the ESI (Emergency Severity Index), the MTS (Manchester Triage System), and the SATS (South African Triage Scale). In all these triaging systems, the primary objective is to recognize the sickest patient promptly and initiate treatment in a timely manner. Barring the US system, other systems have a five-level triaging which is based on severity, time needed for intervention, a list of discriminators based on clinical findings as well as the likely diagnosis. In these systems, Category 1 or Level 1 or Red (**Table 1**) are the sickest patients who need immediate attention. At the next level (Category 2, Orange), patients need to be attended to within 10–15 minutes; in Category 3 (color varying based on the system), patients would need to be seen between 30 and 60 minutes and in Category 4, it ranges from 60 to 120 minutes.

In the wards, rapid response systems (RRSs) such as the medical emergency team (MET) were introduced in hospitals to identify and treat at-risk ward patients in order to reduce the incidence of cardiac arrests, unplanned admissions to ICUs, and deaths. These were introduced on the premise that there is often a preceding period of increasing abnormalities in vital signs prior to in-hospital deterioration and cardiac arrest. These teams are multidisciplinary and have clinicians who are trained in airway management and critical illness and possess diagnostic skills. Such teams commonly employ early warning scores (EWSs) to categorize patients as critically ill. One of the most commonly used scores is the National Early Warning Score (NEWS) that was recommended by the Royal College of Physicians of London in 2012 for the initial assessment of acute illness and for continuous monitoring of all adult inpatients and modified in 2017 as NEWS2 (**Tables 2** and **3**). A score of 7 or more would categorize the patient as critically ill.

Acute deterioration can also occur in the ICU or during surgery. In the intraoperative and postoperative setting, deterioration is often due to blood loss resulting in hemodynamic instability or a cardiac event or respiratory deterioration due to unexpected pulmonary complications. In the ICU, physiological abnormalities often preclude acute deterioration, except in the situation of acute cardiac (e.g., coronary events and arrhythmia) or respiratory (pulmonary embolism, pulmonary edema, and pneumothorax) events or acute blood or fluid loss. Continuous multiparameter monitoring of patients in the ICU enable early recognition of these events.

PRIORITIZATION OF EXAMINATION

The *initial examination* should be prioritized to identify life-threatening physiological or clinical abnormalities. This would include the components of ABCDE (**Fig. 1**). In the rapid assessment of a patient, if there is airway compromise, inadequate breathing or lack of evidence of circulation, then resuscitation should be initiated promptly using the algorithms of basic life support (BLS) and advanced cardiac life support (ACLS). In the absence of cardiac or respiratory arrest, attention should be focused on identifying the extent of clinical and physiological abnormalities and the presence of any warning signs (**Table 4**). The presence of a critical trigger should alert the treating physician to assess the nature and severity of illness.

TABLE 2 The NEWS scoring system.

Physiological parameter	Score						
	3	2	1	0	1	2	3
Respiration rate (per minute)	≤8		9–11	12–20		21–24	≥25
SpO_2 scale 1 (%)	≤91	92–93	94–95	≥96			
SpO_2 scale 2 (%)	≤83	84–85	86–87	88–92 ≥93 on air	93–94 on oxygen	95–96 on oxygen	≥97 on oxygen
Air or oxygen?		Oxygen		Air			
Systolic blood pressure (mm Hg)	≤90	91–100	101–110	111–219			≥220
Pulse (per minute)	≤40		41–50	51–90	91–110	111–130	≥131
Consciousness				Alert			CVPU
Temperature (°C)	≤35.0		35.1–36.0	36.1–38.0	38.1–39.0	≥39.1	

(NEWS: The National Early Warning Score)

TABLE 3 *Aggregate score*: The risk of death from sepsis and indicates the urgency of the response.

Example of the NEWS thresholds and triggers as recommended by the Royal College of Physicians		
New score	**Clinical risk**	**Response**
Aggregate score 0–4	Low	Ward-based response
Red score Score of 3 in any individual parameter	Low-medium	Urgent ward-based response*
Aggregate score 5–6	Medium	Key thresholds for urgent response*
Aggregate score 7 or more	High	Urgent or emergency response**

*Response by a clinician or team with competence in the assessment and treatment of acutely ill patients and in recognizing when the escalation of care to a critical care team is appropriate.

**The response team must also include staff with critical care skills, including airway management.

Subsequent examination should be more detailed and would focus on determining the underlying cause for the abnormalities since a detailed examination may not have been possible in the initial stages. In the critically ill patient, repeated examinations would be required to not only determine response to treatment, but also to monitor for new events and derangements.

AIRWAY

Assessment of airway patency is vital. A quick assessment is done by asking a direct question to the patient, for example, "How are you?" The ability to respond verbally in an appropriate manner indicates a patent airway and adequate cerebral perfusion. The classical, "look, listen, and feel" approach can be adopted for a more detailed assessment. Airway compromise is suspected if there is stridor, hoarseness of voice, gurgling sounds, reduced consciousness, or evidence of neck swelling or trauma. Stridor may not be always present, particularly in severe obstruction. The presence of normal oxygen saturation does not exclude airway obstruction. The respiratory status should be assessed by respiratory rate, use of accessory muscles, oxygen saturation, hemodynamics, and arterial blood gas (ABG) estimation. Bradycardia and/or hypercarbia are late signs of respiratory failure. If airway is compromised, it should be immediately attended while simultaneously looking for a cause for airway obstruction (**Table 5**). Precious time should not be lost in trying to ascertain the cause of obstruction through detailed history and examination at the cost of securing the airway.

Airway obstruction could be a result of inability to protect the airway due to reduced consciousness, or extrinsic or intrinsic obstruction due to luminal or extraluminal causes (**Table 5**). If the airway is obstructed due to reduced consciousness, an attempt should be made to keep the airway open using the triple maneuver (**Fig. 1**) of head tilt-chin lift, jaw thrust, and open mouth. In the setting of suspected cervical spine injury, manual in-line stabilization and application of a c-spine collar would be essential before manipulating the neck. An oral or nasopharyngeal airway may help keep the airway open in patients with reduced GCS (Glasgow Coma Scale). Oral suctioning may help clear secretions and improve the patency of airway and oxygenation. If the airway is still compromised despite these initial measures, it would be prudent to take control of the airway. If a difficult airway is anticipated, it would be important to get help early and be prepared for video-assisted or bronchoscopic intubation. In some extreme situations, in the event of not being able to intubate a patient and secure the airway due to very poor view of the cords due to bleeding or edema an emergency cricothyroidotomy or tracheostomy may be required.

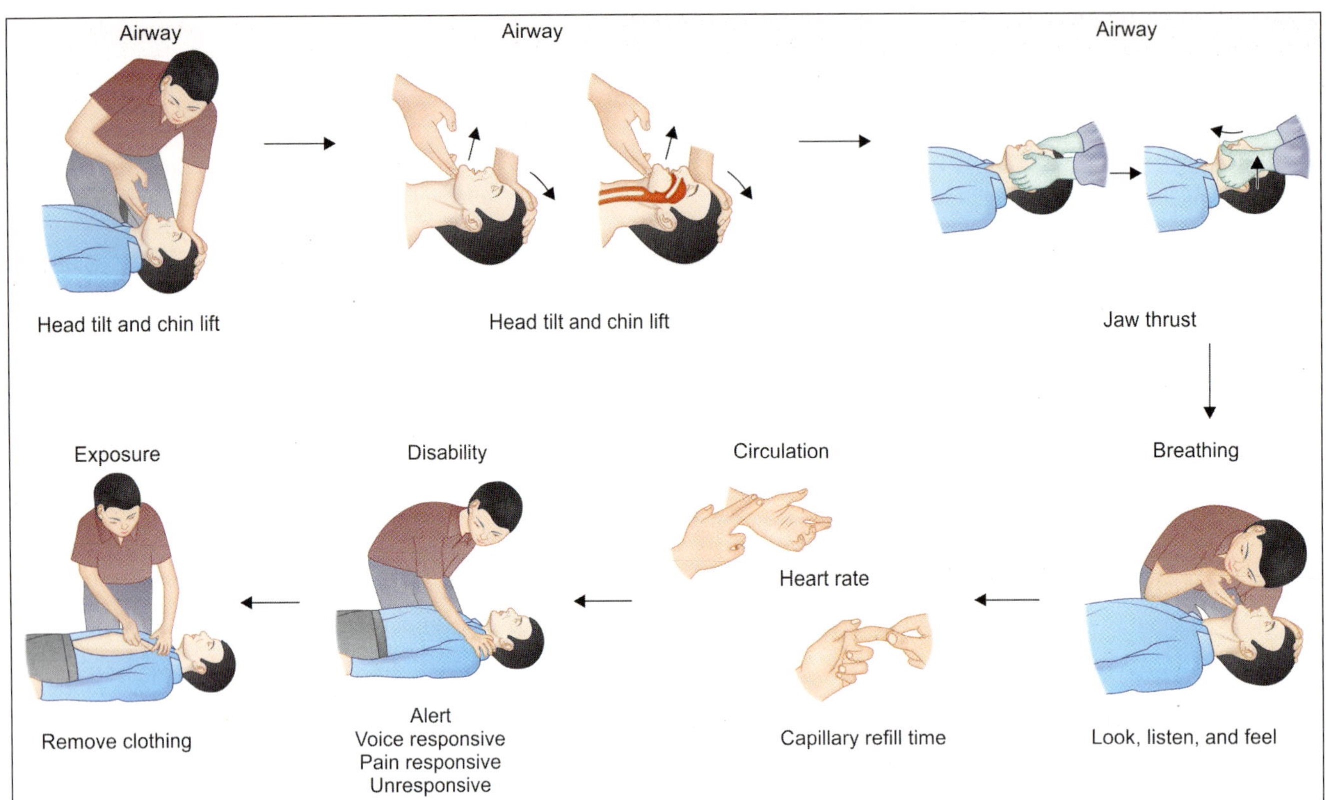

FIGURE 1: Airway, breathing, circulation, disability, and exposure (ABCDE) of assessing a critically ill patient. The initial step in a critically ill patient is to assess the patency of the airway. If the airway is compromised, then head tilt and chin lift may be attempted. If this does not open the airway, jaw thrust may also be applied. An oral or nasopharyngeal airway device may help keep the airway open. In the assessment of breathing, the look, listen, and feel approach should be adopted. Circulation may be assessed through capillary refill and assessment of heart rate, blood pressure, and the presence of peripheral pulses. Disability is assessed using the alert, voice responsive, pain responsive, unresponsive (AVPU) scale. The patient's clothing should be exposed to examine for any possible cause of critical illness.

BREATHING

The adequacy of breathing is dependent on three important components—the *pacemaker*, the *pump with the tubes,* and the *gas exchanger*. The rate and depth of respiration (tidal volume) are controlled *involuntarily* by the respiratory center in the medulla and pons and modulated through central and peripheral chemoreceptors. The motor cortex allows *voluntary* overriding of respiration.

Respiratory failure represents the failure of the lung to maintain adequate gas exchange and is characterized by abnormalities of ABG tensions. Respiratory failure may occur due to abnormalities of the pacemaker, the pump or the tubes or the gas exchanger. Pacemaker dysfunction can manifest as *reduced respiratory drive* [often due to central nervous system (CNS) depression] which results in hypoventilation or as *increased respiratory drive* (due to increased central drive or through peripheral respiratory mechanisms) that result in hyperventilation. The airway and the lungs which constitute the *pump and the tubes* affect and determine airway resistance and lung compliance. Diseases that increase airway resistance or reduce lung compliance increase the work of breathing and cause ventilatory fatigue and respiratory failure. The *gas exchanger,* which is the alveolar-capillary interface, may be involved in processes that increase the thickness of the interface (e.g., fluid and inflammation) that would impair gas transfer and result in ventilation/perfusion (V/Q) mismatch and respiratory failure.

The look, listen, and feel approach can be used to assess adequacy of breathing. Dyspnea and tachypnea are early indicators; albeit they are not specific. At the bedside, the inability to speak full sentences, use of accessory muscles, or paradoxical respiration indicate respiratory compromise. Bedside spirometry may be used to assess the nature and severity of respiratory abnormality [e.g., peak expiratory flow rate (PEFR) in acute severe asthma]. Altered mental status, cyanosis, bradycardia, and hypotension are often late signs of respiratory failure. The nature and extent of respiratory failure should be assessed using pulse oximetry and ABG.

The management of respiratory failure is dependent on the underlying etiology and whether it a hypoxic respiratory failure (type I respiratory failure) or hypercapnic respiratory failure (type II respiratory failure). The mechanisms of type I and type II respiratory failure and the common etiologies are summarized in **Table 6**. The broad management principles include treatment of the underlying condition, improving oxygenation, improving ventilation, and limiting the deleterious effects of such treatment. Hypoxic respiratory failure is treated with supplemental oxygen through fixed

TABLE 4 Warning symptoms and signs and laboratory features suggestive of a critical illness.

Parameter	Normal range (adults)	Critical illness trigger/danger signs
General		
Temperature	36–37.5°C	<32°C or >39°C
Other features	Warm extremity[‡]	Cold extremity, pallor, sweating, and skin mottling
Cardiovascular		
Perfusion[†]	Capillary refill time <2 seconds[*]; radial pulse felt	Capillary refill >2 seconds[*]; absent radial pulse
Heart rate	60–100 beats/min	<50[~] or >150 beats/min
Systolic blood pressure	100–140 mm Hg	<90 mm Hg
Mean blood pressure	>70 mm Hg	<70 mm Hg or >110 mm Hg
Respiratory		
Respiratory rate, movements	12–24 breaths/min	<8[~] or >30 breaths/min, accessory muscle use, paradoxical respiration
Oxygen saturation	≥95%	<90%
Neurological		
AVPU[†]	Conscious, alert, and awake	V, P or U in AVPU; GCS < 12, confusion, and agitation
Hematologic		
Coagulation	Normal coagulation	Thrombocytopenia, coagulopathy, clinical and bleeding
Gastrointestinal		
Bleeding	None	Hematemesis, melena, and jaundice
Renal and metabolic		
Urine output[†]	1–2 mL/kg/h	<0.5 mL/kg/h
Sodium	130–145 mEq/L	<120 mEq/L or >150 mEq/L
Potassium	3.5–5.5 mEq/L	<2.5 mEq/L or >6 mEq/L
pH	7.35–7.45	<7.2
Bicarbonate	24–27 mmol/L	<18 mmol/L

[†] Adequacy of perfusion can be assessed through the three windows: Cutaneous window (skin perfusion), neurological window (conscious level), and the renal window (urine output).

[*] Absent radial pulse and capillary refill time used in the Simple Triage and Rapid Treatment triage system.

[‡] Note that a warm extremity may not necessarily indicate adequate perfusion, particularly in distributive shock.

[~] Bradycardia or bradypnea may indicate impending cardiorespiratory arrest.

AVPU [alert (A), responds to voice (V), responds to pain (P), unresponsive (U)].

(GCS: Glasgow Coma Scale)

TABLE 5 Causes of airway obstruction.

Inability to protect airway (reduced consciousness due to)	Airway obstruction	
	Intrinsic airway obstruction	**Extrinsic airway obstruction**
• Central nervous system (CNS) suppressants (including overdose) • Alcohol • Increased intracranial pressure • Head injury (e.g., subdural hematoma) • Seizures • CNS infections • Intracranial tumors	• Intraluminal (secretions, blood, vomitus, and foreign body) • Swelling of oral structures[*] (tongue and epiglottis) • Laryngeal edema • Laryngeal muscle dysfunction • Direct trauma	• Direct (e.g., trauma and hanging) • Indirect (subcutaneous emphysema)

* Swelling due to inflammation (infection—epiglottis) and anaphylaxis.

TABLE 6 Mechanisms of respiratory failure.

Type of respiratory failure	Mechanism	Some causes
Type I respiratory failure (hypoxic respiratory failure)	Hypoxic hypoxia [inadequate arterial oxygenation due to ventilation/perfusion (V/Q) mismatch or shunt]	• Pneumonia • Pneumothorax • Pulmonary embolism • Pulmonary edema • Acute respiratory distress syndrome (ARDS)
	Anemia hypoxia (decreased oxygen carrying capacity of the blood)	• Massive hemorrhage • Carbon monoxide poisoning • Meth- or sulfhemoglobinemia
	Stagnant hypoxia (decreased oxygen transport due to inadequate circulation)	• Left ventricular failure • Pulmonary embolism • Hypovolemia • Hypothermia
	Histotoxic hypoxia (impairment of cellular metabolism)	• Alcohol intoxication • Cyanide poisoning • Arsenic poisoning
Type II respiratory failure (hypercapnic respiratory failure)	Central nervous system (CNS) depression	• Drugs and sedatives • Intracranial infections, tumor, and trauma • Cerebrovascular accident
	Peripheral nervous system abnormalities	• Spinal cord injury • Guillain–Barré syndrome
	Neuromuscular	• Myasthenia gravis • Metabolic (hypokalemia and hypophosphatemia)
	Alveolar hypoventilation	• Severe bronchospasm and airway obstruction
	Severe V/Q mismatch	• ARDS and aspiration

(e.g., Venturi mask) or variable oxygen delivery devices (e.g., nasal cannula and simple face mask). In severe cases, patients may require intubation and mechanical ventilation with titration of fixed inspired oxygen concentration [fraction of inspired oxygen (FiO_2)] and positive end-expiratory pressure (PEEP) to maintain adequate oxygenation. Hypercapnic respiratory failure is treated with invasive or noninvasive ventilation.

CIRCULATION

Rapid assessment of circulation should focus not only on blood pressure but also on tissue perfusion. It is thus more appropriate that the European Society of Intensive Care Medicine (ESICM) has redefined shock as a life-threatening and generalized form of acute circulatory failure that is associated with inadequate oxygen utilization (dysoxia) by the cells. This definition is appropriate since cellular dysoxia may be due to low cardiac output and reduced oxygen transport (cardiogenic, obstructive, and hypovolemic shock) or altered oxygen extraction (mitochondrial dysfunction) with normal or increased cardiac output (septic shock).

Clinical examination should focus on examination of extremities (cold or warm; skin mottling and capillary refill time), pulse (rate, volume, and absent pulses), blood pressure, jugular venous pressure (JVP), and cardiac examination (heart sounds and murmurs). If patient is in shock, resuscitation should commence immediately as clinical assessment is performed in parallel. A quick echocardiographic screening (if available at the bedside) may give a clue to the etiology of shock [e.g., left ventricular dysfunction with heart failure, acute right ventricular dysfunction in the setting of pulmonary embolism, collapsed inferior vena cava (IVC) suggesting hypovolemia, or absent lung sliding indicating tension pneumothorax].

The diagnosis of shock is based on a triad of features that include arterial hypotension, evidence of tissue hypoperfusion (**Table 4**), and hyperlactatemia. The adequacy of perfusion can be assessed through the three windows: Cutaneous window (skin perfusion), neurological window (conscious level), and renal window (urine output). It should be noted that although cold peripheries are generally the hallmark of circulatory shock, warm peripheries with inadequate oxygen utilization may occur in septic shock. Evidence of reduced tissue perfusion, such as cold extremities, absent radial pulses, poor capillary refill (>2 s), mottling of skin, reduced consciousness or oliguria, and metabolic acidosis (predominantly lactic acidosis), suggest the need for immediate and aggressive resuscitation.

The management principles include identification of the type of shock (**Table 7**), resuscitation, specific therapy, and monitoring clinical response. Resuscitation is focused on the "VIP" rule; V for ventilate (measures to improve oxygen delivery), I for infuse (fluid therapy to improve macro- and microvascular flow), and P for pump (use of vasoactive agents). Once the patient has stabilized, a search for the cause of shock should be undertaken.

DISABILITY AND EXPOSURE

The patient's neurological state should be assessed either using the GCS or the AVPU (Alert, Voice responsive, Pain responsive, Unresponsive) scale (**Fig. 1**). A marked reduction in consciousness would indicate either severe neurological disease or severe organ dysfunction (respiratory, hemodynamic, or metabolic). The patient should be fully exposed, maintaining dignity and examined for possible causes of critical illness. Pupillary assessment may give a clue to the etiology of altered conscious state, particularly if it is asymmetric, miosed or fully dilated. Blood sugar and temperature assessment should be done as part of the assessment. A quick and focused assessment should be done to explore for possible cause of altered conscious state (**Table 8**).

PRELIMINARY INVESTIGATIONS

"No man can hope to find out the truth without investigation."

—George F Richards

Preliminary investigations would be focused on trying to identifying the cause for the deterioration. Useful screening investigations would include ABG estimation, electrolytes, blood sugar level, electrocardiogram (ECG), renal function test, liver function tests (if clinically indicated), complete blood counts, coagulation tests, chest X-ray (if feasible), and bedside ultrasound examination, if readily available [e.g., focused assessment

TABLE 7 Types of shock and principles of management.

Type of shock	Pathophysiology	Hemodynamic changes			Treatment principles
		Central venous pressure	Cardiac output	Systemic vascular resistance	
Cardiogenic	Pump failure	High	Low	High	Improve CO (e.g., dobutamine), reduce afterload (e.g., dobutamine, PDE inhibitor, and levosimendan)[†]
Distributive	Vasodilatation	Low	High	Low	Fluids (if underfilled), vasoconstrictors (e.g., noradrenaline and vasopressin)
Hypovolemic	Loss of volume	Low	Low	High	Fluids (colloids, crystalloids, and blood), inotropes in the interim to improve BP
Obstructive	Obstruction	Variable	Low	High	Augment cardiac output (inotropes), treat underlying cause[‡]

The highlighted shaded box represents the primary changes; compensatory mechanisms are the unshaded boxes; the treatment principle indicated would include the identification and treatment of the underlying cause along with the modalities listed.

[†] Use with caution after improving blood pressure as it may further cause reductions in mean arterial pressure (MAP) due to vasodilation.

[‡] Underlying causes such as tension pneumothorax, pulmonary embolism, pericardial tamponade, and abdominal compartment syndrome.

(BP: blood pressure; CO: cardiac output; PDE: phosphodiesterase)

TABLE 8 Causes of altered conscious state.

Cerebral	Metabolic	Drugs and toxins
• Cerebrovascular accident • Intracranial infection • Trauma • Tumor • Epilepsy	*Organ failure or dysfunction* • Respiratory (hypercarbia and severe hypoxia) • Renal failure (uremia) • Hepatic encephalopathy • Sepsis (septic encephalopathy) *Electrolyte and glucose abnormalities* • Hyponatremia and hypernatremia • Hypoglycemia and severe hyperglycemia • Hypercalcemia *Endocrine abnormalities* • Severe hypothyroidism • Hypoadrenalism	• Alcohol • Sedatives and hypnotics • Narcotics • Other drug overdose • Deliberate self-harm (e.g., organophosphorus compounds)

with sonography in trauma (FAST)]. Ultrasound may also help identify a cause for cardiorespiratory arrest (e.g., pneumothorax, pericardial tamponade, and pulmonary embolism).

SUBSEQUENT ASSESSMENT AND MANAGEMENT

SUBSEQUENT HISTORY AND EXAMINATION

The subsequent assessment of a critically ill patient entails history, clinical examination, investigations, and transfer to an appropriate level of care. Preliminary history taking of the critically ill patient would have been quick and hence once the patient has been stabilized with respect to airway, breathing, and circulation, a detailed history and examination should be undertaken. This is crucial since the physiological derangements that are addressed initially reflect an underlying problem, which if not addressed, would lead to poor outcomes. Sometimes it may not be possible to elicit a full history from the patient, particularly if they are in altered conscious state or too breathless to speak, and hence one would need to obtain additional history from relatives as well as prior case notes. It is also important to assess functional status of the patient prior to this illness as well as the presence and duration of comorbidities and its control. In the postoperative setting, the anesthetist and operation notes may give insights on possible causes for clinical deterioration in the postoperative period. If the diagnosis was unclear in initial history and quick examination, a repeat examination may help identify the cause of critical illness.

ADDITIONAL INVESTIGATIONS

After the initial urgent investigations that may have been at admission, additional investigations would include liver function tests (if not already done), cardiac enzymes, calcium, phosphate, magnesium, appropriate cultures (if sepsis is suspected), and additional imaging if the patient is stable for transfer to the radiology department (e.g., CT scan or MRI of the brain).

TREATMENT

"The good physician treats the disease; the great physician treats the patient who has the disease."

—William Osler

Treatment would include supportive therapy (e.g., ventilation, vasoactive agents, or dialysis) and specific therapy. Specific therapy involves treatment of the underlying problem and this would depend on whether a diagnosis has already been reached or if subsequent evaluation is required. Depending on the severity of illness, the patient may be shifted to the ICU (if requiring organ support or needing continuous monitoring) or to the operation theatre (if requiring urgent surgery) or to a step down unit or the ward for treatment.

CONCLUSION

Patients with critical illness often present with gross alterations in physiological parameters. Such changes occur much before there is clinical deterioration. Favorable outcomes in critical illness depend on the early and rapid identification of critical illness, appropriate resuscitation and stabilization, quick and accurate diagnosis, and definitive management. A systematic approach can prevent deterioration and result in reduced mortality.

RECOMMENDED READINGS

1. Brown A, Ballal A, A-Haddad M. Recognition of the critically ill patient and escalation of therapy. Anaesth Intensive Care Med. 2019;20:1-5.
2. Yancey CC, O'Rourke MC. Emergency Department Triage. Treasure Island (FL): StatPearls Publishing; 2020.
3. Hillman K, Chen J, Cretikos M, Bellomo R, Brown D, Doig G, et al. Introduction to the medical emergency team (MET) system: a cluster-randomised controlled trial. Lancet. 2005;365:2091-7.
4. Kyriacos U, Jelsma J, Jordan S. Monitoring vital signs using early warning scoring systems: a review of the literature. J Nurs Manag. 2011;19:311-30.
5. Royal College of Physicians. National Early Warning Score (NEWS) 2: Standardizing the Assessment of Acute-illness Severity in the NHS. Updated report of a working party. London: RCP; 2017.
6. Baker T, Rylance J, Konrad D. Identifying critically ill patients: Triage, Early Warning Scores and Rapid Response Teams. Update Anaesth. 2012;28:22-6.
7. Aoyama K, Takenaka I, Sata T, Shigematsu A. The triple airway manoeuvre for insertion of the laryngeal mask airway in paralyzed patients. Can J Anaesth. 1995;42:1010-6.
8. Dupanovic M, Fox H, Kovac A. Management of the airway in multi-trauma. Curr Opin Anaesthesiol. 2010;23:276-82.
9. Peter JV. Acute respiratory failure. In: David S (Ed). Clinical Pathways in Emergency Medicine, 1st edition. New Delhi: Springer India; 2016. pp. 167-78.
10. Cecconi M, Backer DD, Antonelli M, Beale R, Bakker J, Hofer C, et al. Consensus on circulatory shock and hemodynamic monitoring. Task force of the European Society of Intensive Care medicine. Intensive Care Med. 2014;40:1795-815.
11. Peter JV, Pulicken M. Hypotension and shock. In: David S (Ed). Clinical Pathways in Emergency Medicine, 1st edition. New Delhi: Springer India; 2016. pp. 179-90.
12. Smith G, Nielsen M. Criteria for admission. BMJ. 1999;318:1544-7.

CHAPTER

68

Monitoring in Intensive Care Unit

Binila Chacko

ABSTRACT

The goal of therapy in the critically ill patient is to ensure prompt identification, prevention, and treatment of organ dysfunction and to ensure that all organs are optimally perfused and that there is adequate tissue oxygen delivery. Monitoring is an adjunct to clinical decision making and helps in determining if a patient clinical course is deviating from the expected path and therapeutic goal. In this chapter, a system-wise approach to monitor a critically ill patient will be covered.

"Prudence is precaution, prudence is protection"

—A Kalantri

INTRODUCTION

Patient management in intensive care is a resource-intensive endeavor that requires diligent process control in order to improve patient outcomes. One of the main objectives in critical care is to ensure that the vital organs have adequate tissue oxygen delivery with optimal perfusion. There is suggestion that delay in recognition of signs of organ dysfunction can result in adverse clinical outcomes. Monitoring helps in determining if a patient's clinical course is deviating from the expected path and therapeutic goal.

Every year, new devices are created to support clinicians and an array of monitoring tools is available in the market. It is important not to get sidetracked by these gadgets but to employ a scientific approach to its incorporation in routine intensive care unit (ICU) monitoring. There should additionally be no harm or lethal complications due to the device or due to errors in interpretation and resultant clinical decision making.

Monitoring is only complementary to clinical examination of the critically ill patient and cannot replace an astute clinician at the bedside.

ROLE OF MONITORING

Despite reliance on electronic monitoring systems in critical care, there is little evidence to support improved outcomes related to their use. This is because most monitoring devices, unlike pharmaceutical agents, have not had formal validation through phased clinical trials. Most devices have come up based on a physiological rationale and are used in the ICU after demonstration of its accuracy and reliability.

Given the lack of evidence, should monitoring be stopped in ICUs? One should determine whether the lack of response is due to errors in the monitoring systems, the underlying disease severity or a failure of the clinicians to interpret alarms and initiate appropriate management. Research is ongoing to assess if integrated artificial intelligent devices can improve patient outcomes. Tele-ICUs, which depend on high-intensity off-site intensivist coverage and continuous monitoring, have been associated with decreased ICU mortality and decreased ICU length of stay. One hence needs to pause and think whether the lack of benefit of monitoring devices is primarily due to failure to recognize, interpret, and take corrective action in a physiologically relevant fashion.

In this chapter, a system-wise monitoring approach of the critically ill patient will be covered with the focus on the principles, accuracy, indications, interpretation, and limitations of the monitoring device.

NEUROLOGICAL MONITORING

CLINICAL PARAMETERS

Clinical examination [Glasgow coma scale (GCS), pupillary examination, brainstem reflexes, and limb movement] is done to detect acute neurological deterioration. The reliability of information, however, depends on the availability of trained clinicians and on the ease of clinical examination (**Table 1**).

Frequency of monitoring depends on the underlying neurological disorder. For example, a patient with raised intracranial pressure (ICP) may warrant 1–2 hourly monitoring of pupils.

MONITORING OF SEDATION AND DELIRIUM

International societies have recommended monitoring of sedation in invasively ventilated critically ill patients with either the Richmond Agitation-Sedation scale (RASS) or Sedation-Agitation scale (SAS). Depth of sedation must be adapted to the patient's underlying clinical condition.

TABLE 1 Neurological monitoring.

Category	Routine or specific situational monitoring	Frequency	Clinical benefit and interpretation	Limitations
GCS, neurological examination	Routine	Depends on underlying problem	Can pick up acute neurological disorders, e.g., raised ICP and CVA	Reliability depends on trained clinicians and the ease of clinical examination
RASS	Routine	Every 2 h	Target sedation depth depends on clinical disorder. Deeper sedation warranted in raised ICP. RASS 0 to –1 recommended for most ventilated patients	Target RASS needs to be appropriately set and depends on the clinical situation
Delirium assessment CAM-ICU	Routine	Every 8 h	Positive CAM-ICU can alert the clinician to start prompt treatment for delirium and also to seek and treat the cause. (RASS should be >–3 to proceed with CAM-ICU assessment)	It has been found that medical and nursing professionals view this as a "task to be completed." Specialized education concerning significance of picking up delirium is needed
Invasive ICP monitoring	Special situations Moderate and severe TBI where neurological examination is difficult; severe TBI with abnormal CT/normal CT scan with 2 of the following (age >40, abnormal posturing, BP < 90 mm Hg	Continuous	• ICP > 20 mm Hg is elevated. P2 > P1 in the waveform suggests raised ICP. • Lundberg A waves or "plateau waves" (amplitude 50–100 mm Hg, lasting 5–20 min) seen with intracranial pathology with impending herniation. • Lundberg B waves are oscillating and up to 50 mm Hg in amplitude with a frequency 0.5–2/min indicate poor intracranial compliance. • Lundberg C waves are documented in healthy individuals (low amplitude oscillations up to 20 mm Hg in amplitude and a frequency of 4–8/min)	• Risk of hemorrhage and infection more with intraventricular drains as compared to intraparenchymal, epidural etc. • CSF cannot be drained and zero drift is a problem with the latter methods • Not reflective of global cerebral situation
Noninvasive ICP monitoring				
Optic nerve sheath diameter (ONSD)	Special situations where raised ICP can occur (TBI/medical conditions prone to increased ICP) Subarachnoid hemorrhage (SAH)	Intermittent based on clinical situation	Available evidence suggests an ONSD of 4.5–5.5 mm to be indicative of intracranial hypertension. *Trend in changes may be more helpful that absolute values*	*Limitations*: Contraindicated in orbital tumors, inflammation of eye, or diseases of the optic nerve
Transcranial Doppler			Pulsatility index (sFV-dFV/mFV) > 1.4 and dFV < 20 cm/s is suggestive of raised ICP. mFV > 120 cm/s and Lindegaard ratio > 3 indicates vasospasm in SAH	Accuracy depends on the experience of the operator and adequacy of bone window
Continuous EEG monitoring	Done in special situations (refractory status epilepticus)	Continuous		Cumbersome and needs expertise and expensive equipment

(CAM-ICU: Confusion Assessment Method ICU; CSF: cerebrospinal fluid; CVA: cerebrovascular accident; dFV: diastolic flow velocity; ICP: intracranial pressure; sFV: systolic flow velocity; mFV: mean flow velocity; RASS: Richmond Agitation Sedation Score; TBI: traumatic brain injury)

Generally, low-level sedation (RASS 0 to –1) is recommended for most mechanically ventilated patients. At present there is insufficient evidence to support use of bispectral index (BIS) monitoring for sedation in the ICU.

Delirium in ICU patients is common and has been reported in as high as 80% of mechanically ventilated patients. It has been shown to be associated with increased length of mechanical ventilation, self-extubation rates, length of hospital stay, and mortality. Confusion Assessment Method-ICU (CAM-ICU) and Intensive Care Delirium Screening Checklist are the two widely accepted delirium assessment scales in critical care. Up to 2-hourly RASS monitoring and 8-hourly CAM-ICU monitoring are recommended in ICUs.

INTRACRANIAL PRESSURE ASSESSMENT

Maintenance of cerebral perfusion pressure (CPP = MAP – ICP) >60 mm Hg helps to ensure adequate cerebral oxygen delivery. Since ICH has been shown to be associated with poor outcome and increased mortality, it is reasonable to monitor ICP in certain clinical scenarios. There are, however, no RCTs that have demonstrated that ICP-guided therapy in trauma-improved outcomes.

Intracranial pressure monitoring is recommended in traumatic brain injury (TBI) in the following situations as per the BTF (Brain Trauma Foundation) guidelines:

- Moderate to severe head injury who cannot be serially neurologically assessed
- Severe head injury (GCS < 8) with an abnormal CT scan
- Severe head injury (GCS < 8) with a normal CT if two of the following are present:
    i. Age > 40 years
    ii. BP < 90 mm Hg
    iii. Abnormal motor posturing

There may be a role for ICP monitoring in acute neurological conditions such as refractory status epilepticus, cortical venous thrombosis, hepatic encephalopathy etc.

Whilst the intraventricular drainage transducers continue to be the gold standard for monitoring ICP, complications of infection (risk of 5% after 5 days of monitoring), and hemorrhage have led to the search for *noninvasive ICP monitoring methods* such as optic nerve sheath diameters (ONSD) (**Fig. 1 A**), transcranial Doppler (TCD) (**Fig. 1 B**), jugular bulb monitoring, and imaging modalities (**Table 1**).

Interpretation: Normal ICP in adults is 5–15 mm Hg. The waveforms are pulsatile in nature and correlate with respiratory and cardiac cycle. Each wave has three components—(1) P1 (percussion wave) reflects the arterial pulses of the carotid plexus into the cerebrospinal fluid (CSF). (2) P2 (tidal wave) is considered reflective of ICP and (3) P3 wave (dicrotic notch) reflects aortic valve closure. Normally, P1 is higher than P2 (**Fig. 1 C**). In raised ICP, the waveform has an increased amplitude with a rounded form—P2 > P1. The amplitude and duration of the waves can also help to understand extent of raised ICP (Lundberg waves).

In terms of noninvasive ICP monitoring, available evidence suggests an ONSD of 4.5–5.5 mm to be indicative of ICH. *Trend in ONSD changes may be more helpful than absolute values.* Pulsatility index in TCD of the middle cerebral artery (MCA) (sFV – dFV/mFV) >1.4 and dFV <20 cm/s is suggestive of raised ICP.

In subarachnoid hemorrhage, TCD can also pick up cerebral vasospasm through estimation of mFV (mean flow velocity; normal mFV 60–80 cm/s) and Lindegaard ratio (mFV MCA/mFV extracranial ICA; normal <3). Severe vasospasm is suspected when mFV is >200 cm/s and Lindegaard ratio is >6.

These noninvasive modes, however, depend on the experience of the operator and adequacy of bone window.

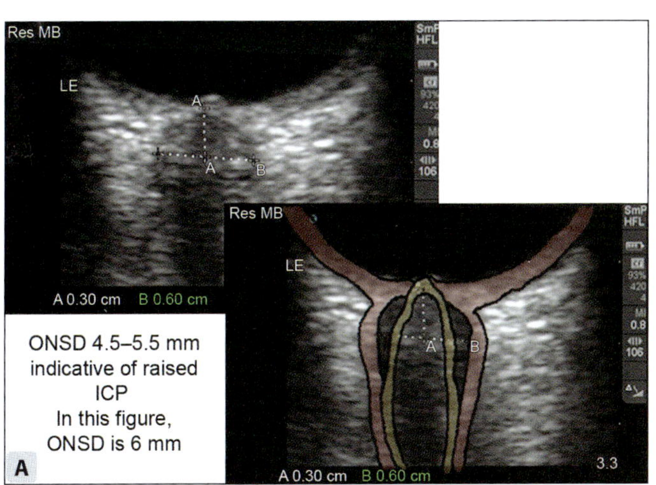

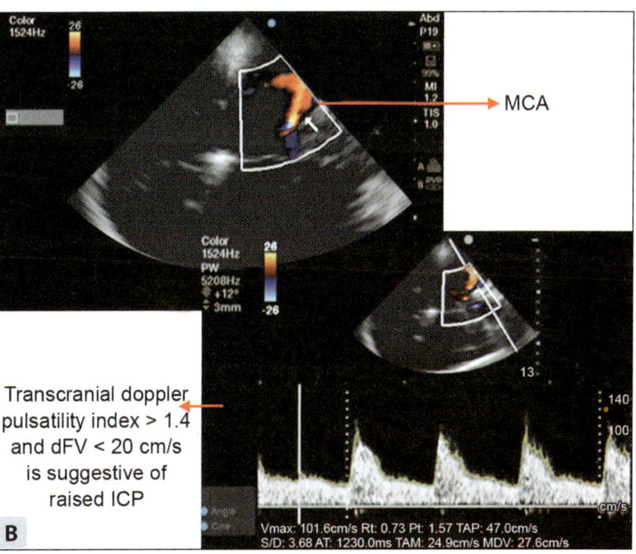

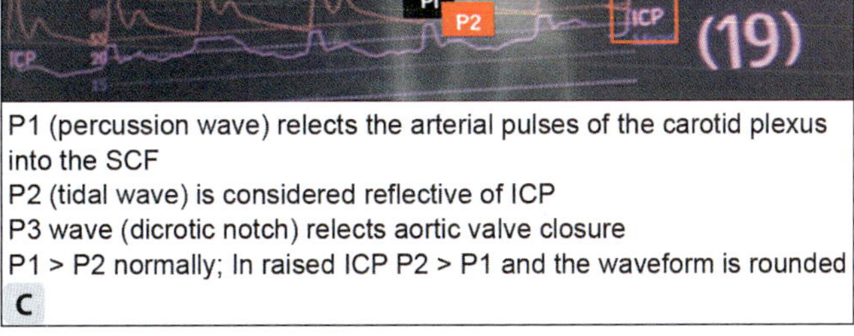

(CSF: cerebrospinal fluid; dFV: diastolic flow velocity; MCA: middle cerebral artery)

FIGURES 1 A to C: (A) Optic nerve sheath diameter (ONSD); and **(B)** transcranial Doppler; and **(C)** intracranial pressure (ICP) waveform.

Continuous electroencephalogram (EEG) monitoring is *not routinely done* in the ICU since this is cumbersome, expensive, and needs expertise. This is recommended in refractory status epilepticus since persistent seizures may worsen cerebral ischemia. Other situations where this may be beneficial include the postoperative high-risk neurosurgical patients and postcardiac arrest setting where subclinical seizures may not be evident.

CARDIOVASCULAR MONITORING

Circulatory dysfunction is a frequent presentation in ICU resulting in diminished oxygen supply to vital organs and is associated with increased mortality. Hemodynamic monitoring is therefore, addressed in several guidelines (**Table 2**).

CONTINUOUS ELECTROCARDIOGRAM AND BLOOD PRESSURE MONITORING

Blood pressure measurement is routinely done either intermittently (noninvasively) or continuously using intra-arterial lines. Invasive blood pressure monitoring is indicated in hemodynamically unstable patients for accurate recording. This is done by inserting an arterial cannula and connecting it to a calibrated transducer that converts pressure into an electrical signal.

Points to ensure accuracy (***Fig. 2***):

- Static accuracy is ensured by zeroing (opening the transducer to atmospheric pressure) and leveling to the phlebostatic axis.
- Dynamic accuracy needs to be intermittently ascertained with the fast flush test. This monitors the natural resonant frequency of the system and the extent of damping. Natural frequency of the system should be >10 harmonics over the patient's natural frequency (heart rate 60/min corresponds to 1 Hz). Most systems have a natural frequency of 30 Hz—this allows accurate blood pressure recording even at heart rates of 180/min (**Fig. 2**).

Arterial pressure wave assessment can also help in determining fluid responsiveness (FR) through pulse pressure variability (PPV) and stroke volume variability (SVV) and in estimating cardiac output (CO).

TABLE 2 Cardiovascular monitoring.

Category	Routine or specific	Frequency	Clinical benefit and interpretation	Limitations
Blood pressure	Routine	Continuous or intermittent	Can get an idea about fluid responsiveness through assessment of PPV and SVV in patients on controlled mechanical ventilation (VT 8 mL/kg) with no spontaneous respiratory effort and lung compliance >30 cm water	• Arterial blood pressure is an unreliable marker of cardiac output because systemic vascular resistance influences the latter • Need to ensure static and dynamic accuracy
Assessment of macrocirculation: Cardiac output and fluid responsiveness assessment				
PiCCO®	Not routinely used		Uses pulse contour analysis for cardiac output measurement. Requires thermodilution via a central venous catheter for calibration	• Prone to drift and inaccuracy due to indicator recirculation and dilution technique • Less VFD in the group managed with PiCCO®
FloTrac	Not routinely used		Requires only an arterial line for cardiac output determination. Pulse contour analysis is used for cardiac output measurement	Unreliable accuracy and reliability in cardiac output measurement
ECHO	Specific		• Uses Doppler principle for cardiac output determination • Non-invasive tool	Depends on operator expertise. Cannot be done often or continuously
Bioimpedance	Not routinely used in ICUs		This bioimpedance is indirectly proportional to the cardiac output	Due to limitations (interference by electro cautery, arrhythmias, patient movement, and inconsistent results of accuracy), this is not in widespread clinical use
PPV **SVV** **IVC variability**	Shock in order to assess FR	Intermittent	PPV or SVV >12% in patients on controlled mechanical ventilation (VT 8 mL/kg) with no spontaneous respiratory effort and lung compliance >30 cm water can indicate fluid responsiveness	Preconditions need to be fulfilled to accurately interpret the test
Passive leg raise			PPV or carotid blood flow velocity >12% indicates FR --this endogenous fluid challenge can be done even in the setting of spontaneous breaths	Unreliable in severely hypovolemic patients and not useful in patients with raised IAP

Continued...

Continued...

Category	Routine or specific	Frequency	Clinical benefit and interpretation	Limitations
Assessment of the microcirculation				
Direct Visualization	Not routinely done		Sublingual microcirculation is the most common site of assessment. Alterations in sublingual microcirculatory blood flow in septic shock are associated with poor outcome	Early phase of evidence
Indirect markers				
Lactate	Routine	Daily	*Lactate clearance has been shown to be a better prognostic marker* than isolated lactate values	Lactate can be influenced not only by perfusion abnormalities but also by hepatic dysfunction, drugs, and mitochondrial function
Mixed venous oxygen saturation (SvO_2)	Not routinely done		• SvO_2 between 65 and 80% indicates optimal oxygen delivery and absence of tissue hypoxia • SvO_2 < 65% indicates increased tissue extraction due to decrease in oxygen delivery • SvO_2 > 80% suggests low oxygen extraction or metabolism due to microcirculatory failure • *Central venous oxygen saturation ($ScvO_2$) can be used as a surrogate for SvO_2 given the risks associated with PAC insertion*	• PA catheter insertion is associated with harm and hence is not recommended now • Limited evidence as to whether optimizing these parameters will improve patient outcomes • There is evidence to suggest that normalization of SvO_2 has no mortality benefit in sepsis

(IAP: intra-abdominal pressure; PPV: pulse pressure variability; SVV: stroke volume variation; VT: tidal volume; SvO_2: mixed venous oxygen saturation; $ScvO_2$: central venous oxygen saturation)

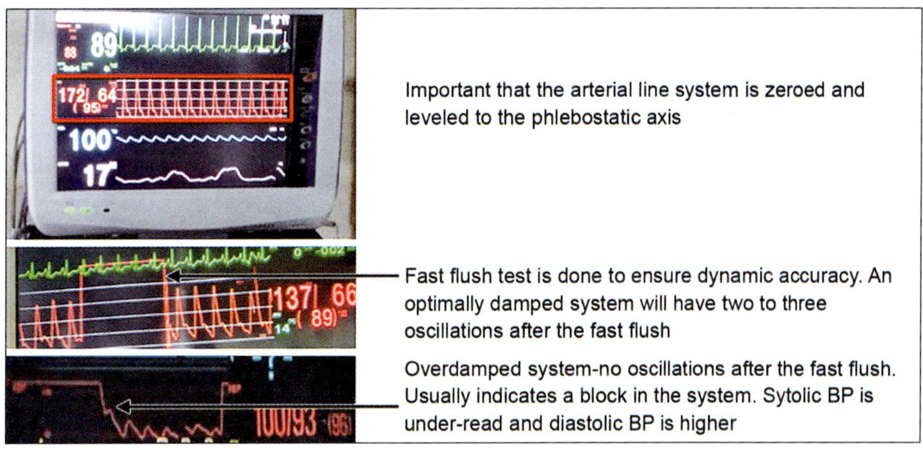

FIGURE 2: Arterial blood pressure (BP) monitoring.

Limitations:

- Arterial blood pressure is an unreliable marker of CO because systemic vascular resistance influences the latter.
- Various complications (<1%) have been reported such as digital ischemia, thrombosis, hematoma, pseudoaneurysm, arteriovenous fistula etc.

ADVANCED MONITORING

This is recommended in patients with shock to ascertain cardiac function, FR, and determine if there is supply-demand mismatch in the microcirculatory level. Therapies should be directed at optimizing the macrocirculation (upstream parameters) to meet the microcirculatory need (downstream requirements).

In order to optimize the macrocirculation, the clinician needs to rationalize use of vasoactive therapy and fluids.

ASSESSING THE MACROCIRCULATION

Monitoring tools to predict fluid responsiveness: *One needs to decide whether the patient will benefit from fluid therapy*. Static parameters such as central venous pressure (CVP), inferior vena cava (IVC) diameter, and data obtained from pulmonary artery catheters (PAC) are no longer used for hemodynamic monitoring and assessing FR in view of adverse events and inaccuracies.

There are several innovative, less invasive methods of assessing CO, and FR.

- *Arterial pressure contour analysis derived parameters such as PPV, SVV, systolic pressure variation, and sonological tests such as IVC variability.* For most of these tests, variability >12% was found to predict FR (defined as an increase in CO by >10–15%). PPV had the best performance and IVC variability was the least reliable.
  - *Limitations*: These tests are, however, limited by the number of preconditions that have to be fulfilled before the tests are done.
    - Controlled breaths with tidal volumes (VTs) of 8 mL/kg
    - No spontaneous breaths as this results in the variation in intrathoracic pressure and hence variability may not indicate FR.
    - No cardiac arrhythmias
    - Normal right heart function
    - Lung compliance > 30 mL/cm water
- *Passive leg raise (PLR) test*: To overcome the above limitations, PLR with PPV assessment is recommended.
  - This is a reversible fluid challenge of 300 mL that can be done in spontaneously breathing patients irrespective of VT and lung compliance.
  - Compared to PPV with PLR, changes in carotid blood flow velocity and in $ETCO_2$ > 5% with PLR were found to have a better area under the curve (0.85).

Monitoring cardiac output:

- *Point-of-care ultrasound* is increasingly used as a noninvasive method of assessment of CO using the Doppler principle. This is limited by operator expertise and the lack of continuous recording.
- *PiCCO®, LiDCO™, and FloTrac* use *pulse contour analysis* for determining CO. Whilst the FloTrac requires only an arterial line, PiCCO® and LiDCOTM require a central venous catheter for calibration by dilution (either thermo or lithium-based). Of the three, LiDCOTM has the best correlation with CO but needs frequent recalibration. Despite better accuracy over FloTrac, PiCCO® is being used less often in view of sources of error (due to drift and indicator recirculation) with PiCCO® and evidence of fewer ventilator free days.
- Transthoracic electrical bioimpedance measures the bioimpedance of the thorax to a high frequency, low magnitude current. This is indirectly proportional to the CO. Due to several limitations (interference by electrocautery, arrhythmias, patient movement, and inconsistent results of accuracy), this is not in widespread clinical use despite its noninvasiveness.

MONITORING THE MICROCIRCULATION

Principle: Improvement in the macrocirculation does not imply improvement in microcirculatory flow and it has been shown that patients whose microcirculation fails to improve following resuscitation are at increased mortality risk.

Tools:

- Microcirculation can be monitored either directly (through direct visualization, e.g., sublingual video-microscopy) or indirectly (more commonly used) through surrogate biochemical markers.
- *Indirect markers*:
  - Whilst lactate is the most widely studied indirect marker, there are several limitations. Lactate can be influenced not only by perfusion abnormalities but also by hepatic dysfunction, drugs, and mitochondrial function. *Lactate clearance has been shown to be a better prognostic marker*.
  - Mixed venous oxygen saturation (SvO_2) obtained from blood drawn from the PAC:
    - Venous oxygen saturation between 65 and 80% indicates optimal oxygen delivery and absence of tissue hypoxia.
    - Venous oxygen saturation <65% indicates increased tissue extraction due to decrease in oxygen delivery.
    - Venous oxygen saturation >80% suggests low oxygen extraction or low oxygen cell metabolism due to microcirculatory failure.
  - Central $ScvO_2$ can be used as a surrogate for SvO_2 given the risks associated with PAC insertion.
  - $P_{(v-a)}\,CO_2$ gap/$C_{(a-v)}\,O_2$ > 1.4 indicates tissue hypoxia

Evidence and limitations: Even though microcirculatory failure has been associated with increased mortality, more evidence is needed to ascertain whether optimizing the above parameters will be of benefit. As of now, there is evidence to suggest that normalization of SvO_2 has no mortality benefit in sepsis (**Table 2**).

RESPIRATORY MONITORING

PULSE OXIMETRY

Most guidelines recommend that pulse oximetry should be monitored in all situations when oxygen is used. This allows for simple, continuous, and noninvasive monitoring of arterial oxygen-hemoglobin saturation (SaO_2) using a finger or ear probe (**Table 3**).

Principle: Using spectrophotometric methodology, pulse oximetry measures oxygen saturation by illuminating the skin and measuring the differential absorption of red (660 nm—relatively more absorption by deoxyhemoglobin) and infrared (940 nm—more absorption by oxyhemoglobin) light in pulsatile blood flow (**Fig. 3**). A ratio R is generated based on the relative absorbance that corresponds to SaO_2 (e.g., R 0.4 corresponds to SaO_2 100% and R 1 corresponds to SaO_2 85%).

$$R = \frac{\text{Absorption of red light}}{\text{Absorption of infrared light}}$$

Accuracy: Whilst bias (difference between SpO_2 and SaO_2) and precision (standard deviation) is best when SaO_2 > 90%, reasonable accuracy and precision are still maintained as long as the SaO_2 > 75%. Pulse oximetry is reliable down to hemoglobin concentrations of 5 g/dL.

Evidence: Even though pulse oximeters may lead to a quicker treatment of serious hypoxemia, there is no evidence that pulse oximetry improves outcomes. Ear and forehead probes have, however, been shown to respond quicker that finger probes in some studies.

Limitations:
- No information is provided on adequacy of ventilation (low levels do not always indicate compromised lung function), tissue oxygen delivery, or arterial oxygenation, particularly when SaO_2 is very high or very low.

TABLE 3 **Respiratory system monitoring.**

Category	Routine or specific situational monitoring	Frequency	Clinical benefit and interpretation	Limitations
Pulse oximetry	Routine	Continuous	• It has reasonable accuracy and precision if SpO_2 > 75% • Falsely low values with methemoglobinemia and sulfhemoglobinemia • Falsely high values with carboxyhemoglobin and increased HbA1C	• Reliability decreases at SaO_2 < 75% • Requires detectable pulsatile flow • False high and low SpO_2 can be seen in specific situations

Capnography	Routine in invasively ventilated patients	Continuous	• Confirmation of intubation
			• During CPR, $P_{ET}CO_2 \geq$ 10–20 mm Hg is associated with ROSC. $P_{ET}CO_2$ < 10 mm Hg after 20 min of CPR—a low chance of ROSC
			• Dead space calculation and role in pulmonary embolism (PE):
			  ◦ ADSF = $PaCO_2 - P_{ET}CO_2/PaCO_2$
			  ◦ Normal ADSF (<0.15) with normal D-dimer can increase NPV of D-dimer in excluding PE
			• Clinical problems that can be detected include:
			  ◦ Rebreathing—phase I elevation and β > 90°
			  ◦ Bronchospasm—shark fin appearance
			  ◦ Detection of hypoventilation, malignant hyperpyrexia (increased $ETCO_2$)
			  ◦ Absent CO_2 trace with esophageal intubation, disconnection, and apnea
				• Needs calibration and zeroing as per manufacturer's recommendations
				• High volume side stream analyzers need more frequent calibration

ABG analysis	Routine	Daily	• Provides information on oxygenation and ventilation • Severity of ARDS can be assessed from PF ratio (mild ARDS: 200–300; moderate ARDS 100–200; severe ARDS < 100) • A-a gradient >15 mm Hg indicates lung involvement	• Invasive • Pain, thrombosis, digital ischemia, and hematoma

Respiratory mechanics and ventilator graphics	Routine	Hourly	• Monitors for safe ventilatory strategies (Pplat 25–30 cm water and safe VT 6–8 mL/kg PBW)
			• Volume time graph can pick up leak. VT and Ppeak drop in VCV
			• Endotracheal tube block (drop in the volume with increased peak pressure in VCV-pressures will not change in PCV)
			• Air trapping (flow-time graphic)
			• Measurement of lung compliance and resistance
			  ◦ Increase in both Ppeak and Pplat suggests poor compliance
			  ◦ High Ppeak with normal Pplat with increased airway resistance
				• Needs clinical expertise and constant attending to alarms
				• Alarms need to be appropriately set to minimize alarm fatigue

Cuff pressure monitoring	Routine	Q 6–8 h	• To be maintained between 20 to 30 cm water to decrease VAP • Check cuff pressure if evidence of leak on the ventilator	
Chest US	Special situations		To pick up pneumothorax, lung collapse, fluid overload states etc.	Depends on operator expertise

(A-a: alveolar arterial gradient; ADSF: alveolar dead space fraction; $PaCO_2$: partial pressure of arterial CO_2; $PETCO_2$: endotracheal CO_2; PF: PaO_2/FiO_2; PBW: predicted body weight; VT: tidal volume; Ppeak: peak pressure; Pplat: plateau pressure)

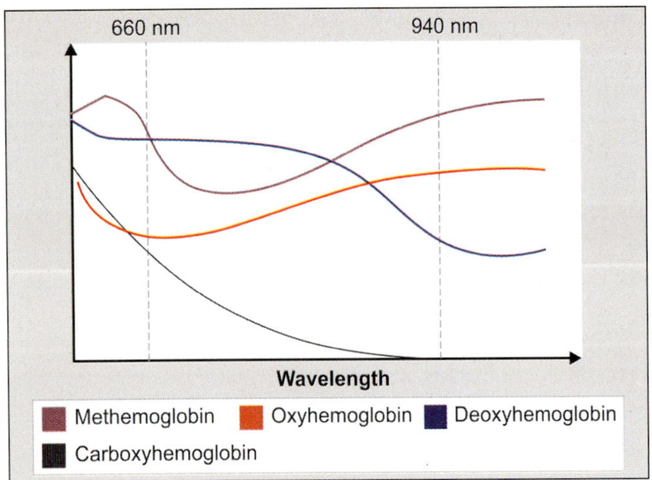

FIGURE 3: Pulse oximetry principles.

- Body movements confound readings (shivering and seizing).
- Reliability decreases at $SaO_2 < 75\%$.
- Limited by poor peripheral perfusion (shock) and nonpulsatile flow (ECMO and cardiopulmonary bypass)
- Venous pulsation can be erroneously interpreted as arterial flow.
- *Falsely low values*:
  - Methemoglobinemia absorbs both red and infrared light, thereby causing the SpO_2 to trend toward 85%.
  - Dyes such as methylene blue and indocyanine green
  - Dark fingernail polish or dark skin will cause underreading by up to 5%.
  - Sulfhemoglobin has a greater absorbance at 660 nm than oxyhemoglobin, deoxyhemoglobin, and methemoglobin. Data on 940 nm absorbance is not available. It is hence difficult to predict how this might interfere with pulse oximetry
- *Falsely high values*:
  - Carboxyhemoglobin absorbs 660 nm light to the same extent as oxyhemoglobin and hence SpO_2 is artificially high.
  - Increased glycosylated hemoglobin >7—this may be due to increased hemoglobin-oxygen affinity.

CAPNOGRAPHY

This refers to the continuous noninvasive measurement of partial pressure of carbon dioxide ($P_{ET}CO_2$) in exhaled breath over time. This can be represented graphically as a capnogram or a numeric display $ETCO_2$ (end tidal CO_2) (capnometry). This value provides information about CO_2 elimination (through alveolar ventilation and perfusion) and CO_2 production by cellular metabolism.

Principle: This works on the principle that CO_2 absorbs infrared radiation. Infrared spectroscopy is incorporated into a side stream (small fraction of exhaled gas is sampled and analyzed by a detector in the monitor) or mainstream (detector is directly in the path of the exhaled gas) analyzers. CO_2 in the expired gas leads to reduction in the infrared light falling on the sensor. This is then analyzed and the $ETCO_2$ is calculated. Mainstream analyzers are reported to give more accurate values and are less likely to be affected by water condensation like side-stream analyzers.

In heterogeneous lungs, $P_{ET}CO_2$ and $PaCO_2$ have a poor correlation due to variable alveolar emptying. In normal lungs, $P_{ET}CO_2$ is on an average 2–5 mm Hg less than $PaCO_2$

Interpretation of a capnogram: There are four phases (**Fig. 4 A**).

1. Phase I represents the inspiratory baseline that has no detectable CO_2. *Progressive elevation of this baseline suggests rebreathing.*
2. Phase II (expiratory upstroke) represents expiration of dead space gas and alveolar gas.
3. Phase III (alveolar plateau) represents expiration of alveolar gases. The slope of this phase depends on V/Q mismatch and ease of expiration. *As heterogeneity or bronchospasm increases, the slope increases in view of slower emptying of alveoli with more CO_2 slope.*
   - The alpha angle lies between phases II and III. *$\alpha > 90°$ is seen with V/Q mismatch.*
4. Phase IV (expiratory down stroke) represents the beginning of the next breath, with the CO_2 content returning rapidly to zero.
   - The beta angle lies between phases III and IV—*$\beta > 90°$ suggests rebreathing.*

Clinical utilization of capnography:

- Confirmation of intubation and monitoring endotracheal (ET) tube placement/block
- Cardiac arrest—to determine return of spontaneous circulation (ROSC) and cardiopulmonary resuscitation (CPR) adequacy. $P_{ET}CO_2 \geq 10–20$ mm Hg during CPR was strongly associated with ROSC while persistent $P_{ET}CO_2 < 10$ mm Hg after 20 minutes of CPR had low chance (0.5%) of ROSC.
- Dead space calculation and role in pulmonary embolism (PE):
  - Whilst the Bohr-Enghoff equation is the traditional equation to determine physiological dead space [uses mean exhaled carbon dioxide (P_ECO_2)], a modification of this equation has been shown to help calculate the alveolar dead space fraction (ADSF). ADSF > 0.15 could indicate hypoperfusion

$$ADSF = PaCO_2\text{-}P_{ET}CO_2/PaCO_2$$

  - Normal ADSF (<0.15) with a normal D-dimer can increase the negative predictive value of D-dimer in excluding PE regardless of clinical probability.
- Clinical conditions/problems can be detected by studying the capnogram.
  - Bronchospasm—shark fin appearance (**Fig. 4 B**)
  - Rebreathing can be detected with elevation of phase I and $\beta > 90°$ (**Fig. 4 C**).
  - Detection of hypoventilation, malignant hyperpyrexia with increased/increasing $ETCO_2$
  - Absent CO_2 trace is seen in esophageal intubation, disconnection, apnea, or airway obstruction.
- It can help to monitor alveolar recruitment with positive end-expiratory pressure (PEEP). Decrease in phase III slope can suggest improved V/Q matching.

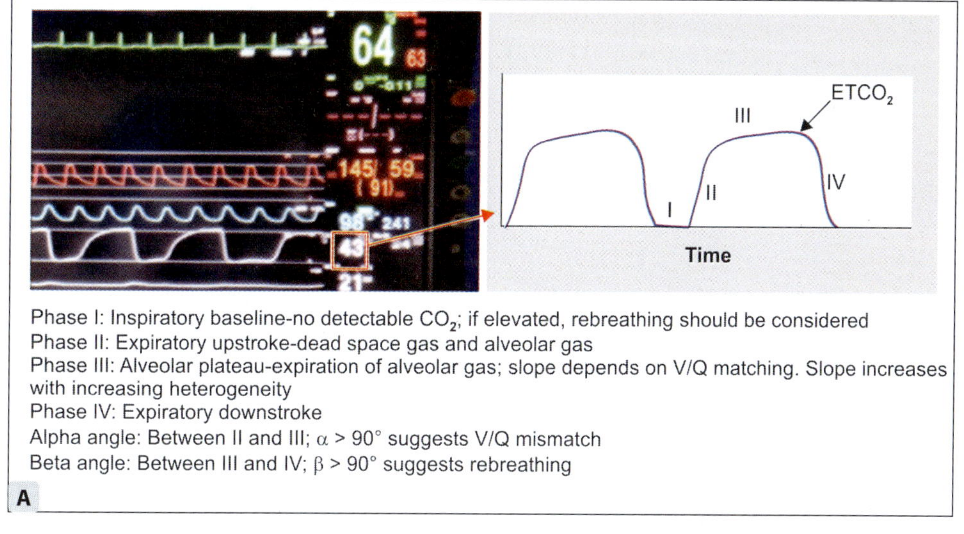

Phase I: Inspiratory baseline-no detectable CO_2; if elevated, rebreathing should be considered
Phase II: Expiratory upstroke-dead space gas and alveolar gas
Phase III: Alveolar plateau-expiration of alveolar gas; slope depends on V/Q matching. Slope increases with increasing heterogeneity
Phase IV: Expiratory downstroke
Alpha angle: Between II and III; $\alpha > 90°$ suggests V/Q mismatch
Beta angle: Between III and IV; $\beta > 90°$ suggests rebreathing

A

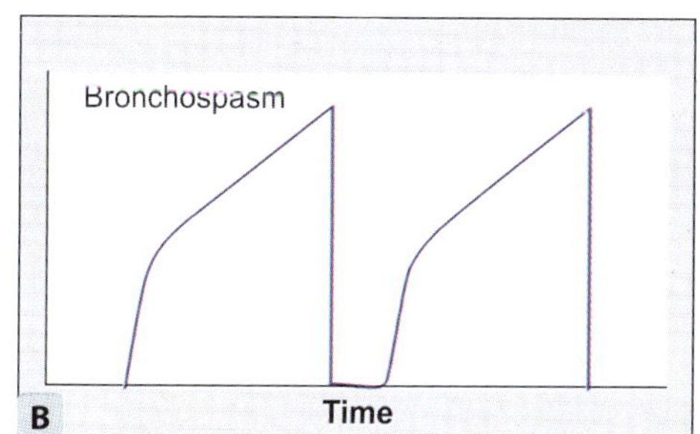

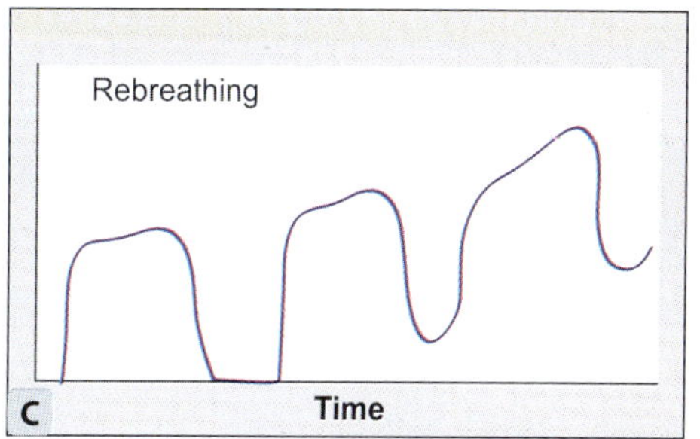

FIGURES 4 A to C: Capnography—normal capnogram; (B) bronchospasm; and (C) rebreathing.

Limitations: It needs calibration and zeroing as per manufacturer's recommendations. High volume side stream analyzers need more frequent calibration.

ARTERIAL BLOOD GAS ANALYSIS

This is done daily and during clinical deterioration in the critically ill and provides information about oxygenation and ventilation. Information about oxygenation can be obtained from the ratio of PaO_2 to the fraction of inspired oxygen (PF ratio) and the alveolar arterial (A-a) gradient. PF ratio is used to grade ARDS severity (mild: 200–300; moderate 100–200; and severe <100). A-a gradient (normal 5–15 mm Hg) monitoring gives an idea of the involvement of the lungs in respiratory failure. Higher the gradient suggests the presence of abnormal alveolar-capillary oxygen transfer. Respiratory failure with normal A-a gradient can occur with hypoventilation. Arterial blood gas (ABG) analysis can also help in picking up problems in ventilation in patients with respiratory acidosis. It is possible to distinguish pure respiratory from metabolic and mixed metabolic and respiratory causes through analysis of changes in bicarbonate and base excess (metabolic component) and the CO_2 levels.

RESPIRATORY MECHANICS

Routine monitoring of VT, peak pressures (Ppeak) and ventilator graphics is recommended. This helps to understand pathophysiology of respiratory failure and also helps to ensure that patients are safely ventilated [safe pressures—plateau pressures (Pplat) of 25–30 cm water and safe VT 6–8 mL/kg predicted body weight].

Some of the conditions that can be picked up through analysis of the graphics include:

- *Drop in VTs*:
  - Leak from the volume-time graph. The expiratory limb does not reach the baseline with loss of lung volume and pressure (**Fig. 5 A**).
  - Endotracheal tube block to be considered if Ppeak increases in volume-controlled ventilation. *Pressures will not change in pressure-controlled ventilation.*
- Air trapping (flow-time graphic-expiratory limb does not reach the baseline) can cause barotrauma. Expiratory time must be increased in this situation (**Fig. 5 B**).
- One can measure lung compliance and resistance through analysis of the Ppeak (sum of airway and alveolar pressures) and Pplat (alveolar pressures).
  - Normal compliance is 80–100 mL/cm water (compliance = VT/Pplat-PEEP)
    - In a poorly compliant lung, both Ppeak and Pplat increase (**Table 3**).
  - Resistance (R_{rs}) is calculated from the flow rate and the pressure drop across the airway. Normal R_{rs} is 10–15 cm H_2O/L/s.
    - In patients with increased airway resistance, Ppeak is high and Pplat is normal unless air trapping occurs.

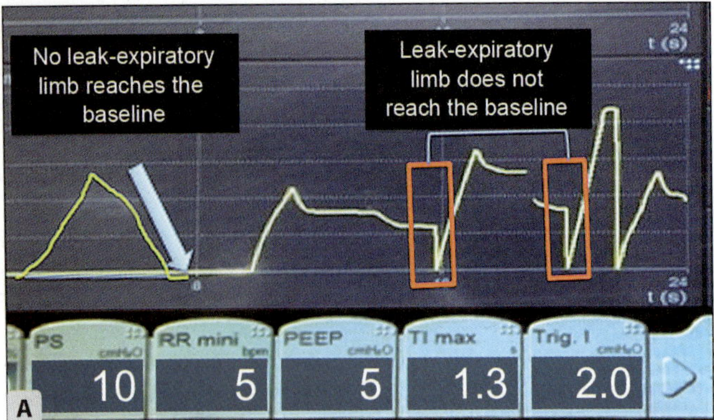

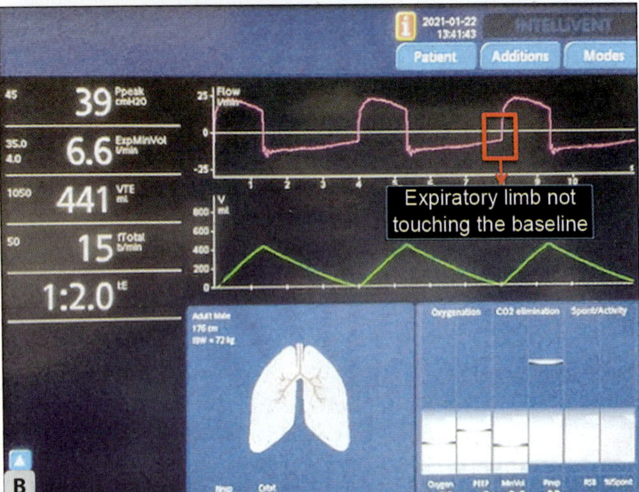

FIGURES 5 A & B: Volume-time graphic showing leak; (B) flow-time graphic showing air trapping.

ENDOTRACHEAL CUFF PRESSURE MONITORING

Maintaining cuff pressures between 20 and 30 cm water is recommended to decrease ventilator-associated pneumonia.

CHEST ULTRASONOGRAPHY

This is useful in diagnosing acute conditions such as pneumothorax, lung collapse, and pleural effusions. Lung ultrasonography can be used to estimate alveolar reaeration following recruitment with PEEP.

TRANSCUTANEOUS CO_2 MONITORING WITH EARLOBE PROBES

This is *not standard of care* given its lack of accuracy. It has been shown that the value deviates from $PaCO_2$ by as much as 15 mm Hg.

GASTROINTESTINAL AND RENAL MONITORING

INTRA-ABDOMINAL PRESSURE ANALYSIS

Even though intra-abdominal hypertension (IAH—defined as sustained intra-abdominal pressure IAP > 12 mm Hg) has been documented to occur in 35–55% of intensive care patients and abdominal compartment syndrome (ACS) in 5–10%, IAP is seldom measured by default in intensive care patients. Guidelines suggest monitoring IAP in specific patient groups (severe burns, severe trauma, severe acute pancreatitis, liver failure, abdominal surgery, excess fluid balance, or ruptured aortic aneurysms). In patients without these risk factors with PEEP < 10 cm, IAP measurements can be omitted.

The reference standard for intermittent IAP measurement is the bladder with a maximal instillation volume of 25 mL of sterile saline. IAP should be measured at *end-expiration* in *supine position* after ensuring that *abdominal muscle contractions are absent* and with the transducer zeroed at the level where the midaxillary line crosses the iliac crest.

Intra-abdominal hypertension is graded as follows:
- Grade I 12–15 mm Hg
- Grade II 16–20 mm Hg
- Grade III 21–25 mm Hg
- Grade IV >25 mm Hg

Abdominal compartment syndrome is defined as a sustained IAP > 20 mm Hg (with or without an APP < 60 mm Hg) that is associated with new organ dysfunction/failure.

Treatment should not be based on the IAH grade but on the severity and dynamics of organ dysfunction. The most extreme form of organ dysfunction in ACS is the inability to ventilate. Another frequent form of IAH-induced organ dysfunction is acute kidney injury (AKI).

RENAL MONITORING

Hourly urine output monitoring is recommended in the critically ill in order to pick up AKI. Urine output < 0.5 mL/kg/h for 6 hours indicates that the patient is at risk for AKI. As the period and severity of oliguria increase, the clinician is alerted to worsening stages of AKI. These warning signs can facilitate early detection and management even before changes in standard biochemical markers (urea and creatinine), which are well known to lag behind changes in renal blood flow and perfusion (**Table 4**).

TEMPERATURE MONITORING

The high frequency of temperature abnormalities in the critically ill and the reported negative outcome association with extremes of temperature suggest that accurate monitoring and maintenance of optimal body temperature in the ICU setting are necessary to minimize the physiological and biochemical ill effects of extremes of temperature. Either core or peripheral temperature can be monitored. Peripheral temperatures recordings have the disadvantage of being affected by the environment.

Continuous core temperature monitoring is warranted in targeted temperature management in the postcardiac arrest scenario and during cooling or rewarming for extremes of temperature. Evidence suggests that core temperature monitoring using either urinary, nasopharyngeal, or esophageal probes may be appropriate in the critically ill.

TABLE 4	Renal monitoring and KDIGO staging of AKI.	
• Increase in serum creatinine by ≥0.3 mg/dL within 48 h or • Increase in serum creatinine to 1.5 times baseline or more within the last 7 days or • Urine output < 0.5 mL/kg/h for 6 h		
	Urine output criteria	**Serum Creatinine**
Stage 1	<0.5 mL/kg/h for 6 h	1.5–1.9 times baseline or ≥0.3 mg/dL increase
Stage 2	<0.5 mL/kg/h for 12 h	2–2.9 times baseline
Stage 3	<0.3 mL/kg/h for 24 h or anuria for ≥12 h	Three times baseline or increase in serum creatinine to ≥4 mg/dL or initiation of RRT

(AKI: acute kidney injury; KDIGO: Kidney Disease Improving Global Outcomes; RRT: renal replacement therapy)

OTHER DOMAINS OF MONITORING

In hyperglycemic patients, glucose monitoring is generally recommended every 1–2 hours till stable and then 4th–6th hourly. There are several confounding factors in the critically ill that can impact point of care glucometer readings such as oxygen levels, acid-base status, hematocrit, shock, and temperature. In shock, capillary glucose levels can be falsely low due to low blood flow. It has also been shown that glucometer values can be inaccurately higher in patients with low hematocrit. The type of glucose monitoring strips is also important as glucose oxidase-based strips can be affected by oxygen levels (high oxygen can decrease glucose values and vice versa). Current recommendations are to keep blood glucose levels between 140 and 180 mg/dL in the critically ill.

Hepatic function is periodically assessed with liver function tests. Metabolic monitoring, including ABG, electrolytes, lactates, magnesium, calcium, and phosphorus, is periodically done. Therapeutic drug monitoring is another domain that is gathering momentum in the management of critically ill.

Whilst there is no evidence that nutritional assessment, monitoring, and interventions impact clinical outcomes, ICU societies across the world have come up with nutritional assessment and monitoring guidelines. The Nutrition Risk in Critically ill (NUTRIC) score is the first validated nutritional screening tool in critically ill patients that can be calculated with routine parameters [age, Acute Physiology and Chronic Health Evaluation II (APACHE II), sequential organ failure assessment (SOFA), comorbidities, time to ICU admission after coming to hospital, and interleukin-6 (IL-6)]—a score of 0–4 (if IL-6 is not available) has a low malnutrition risk. Indian Society of Critical Care Medicine practice guidelines recommend nutritional assessment by Subjective Global Assessment (SGA) when NUTRIC score > 5. Serum albumin, transferrin, and prealbumin have not been shown to be reliable in critically ill patients.

CONCLUSION

In critical care, monitoring helps in alerting the clinician to patient deterioration and in diagnosing certain clinical conditions. It is important to remember to treat the patient and not the number on the screen. Each patient needs to be managed based on the underlying clinical disorder and it is important to determine and treat the cause for deterioration.

Patient safety is paramount and hence it is important that the monitoring tools are safe, accurate, and reliable. Despite the paucity of phased clinical trials, monitoring tools are here to stay. It remains to be determined whether machine-learned algorithms and tele-ICUs would improve patient outcomes. Until then, clinicians need to understand the rationale and clinical relevance of each monitoring tool that are commonly used in critical care.

RECOMMENDED READINGS

1. Udeh C, Udeh B, Rahman N, Canfield C, Campbell J, Hata JS. Telemedicine/virtual ICU: Where are we and where are we going? Methodist Debakey Cardiovasc J. 2018;14(2):126-33.
2. Barr J, Fraser GL, Puntillo K, Ely EW, Gélinas C, Dasta JF, et al. Clinical practice guidelines for the management of pain, agitation, and delirium in adult patients in the intensive care unit. Crit Care Med. 2013;41(1):263-306.
3. Balas MC, Vasilevskis EE, Olsen KM, Schmid KK, Shostrom V, Cohen MZ, et al. Effectiveness and Safety of the Awakening and Breathing Coordination, Delirium Monitoring/Management, and Early Exercise/Mobility Bundle. Crit Care Med. 2014;42(5):1024-36.
4. Güiza F, Depreitere B, Piper I, Citerio G, Chambers I, Jones PA, et al. Visualizing the pressure and time burden of intracranial hypertension in adult and paediatric traumatic brain injury. Intensive Care Med. 2015;41(6):1067-76.
5. Chesnut RM, Temkin N, Carney N, Dikmen S, Rondina C, Videtta W, et al. A trial of intracranial-pressure monitoring in traumatic brain injury. N Engl J Med. 2012;367(26):2471-81.
6. Harary M, Dolmans RG, Gormley WB. Intracranial pressure monitoring-review and avenues for development. Sensors (Basel). 2018;18(2):465.
7. Nag DS, Sahu S, Swain A, Kant S. Intracranial pressure monitoring: Gold standard and recent innovations. World J Clin Cases. 2019;7(13):1535-53.
8. Koziarz A, Sne N, Kegel F, Nath S, Badhiwala JH, Nassiri F, et al. Bedside optic nerve ultrasonography for diagnosing increased intracranial pressure: A systematic review and meta-analysis. Ann Intern Med. 2019;171(12):896-905.
9. Robba C, Taccone FS. How I use Transcranial Doppler. Critical Care. 2019;23:420.
10. Funcke S, Sander M, Goepfert MS, Groesdonk H, Heringlake M, Hirsch J, et al. Practice of hemodynamic monitoring and management in German, Austrian, and Swiss intensive care units: the multicenter cross-sectional ICU-CardioMan Study. Ann Intensive Care. 2016;6(1):49.

11. Marik PE. Obituary: pulmonary artery catheter 1970 to 2013. Ann Intensive Care. 2013;3(1):38.
12. Monnet X, Teboul JL. Assessment of volume responsiveness during mechanical ventilation: Recent advances. Crit Care. 2013;17(2):217.
13. Vellinga NA, Boerma EC, Koopmans M, Donati A, Dubin A, Shapiro NI, et al. International study on microcirculatory shock occurrence in acutely ill patients. Crit Care Med. 2015;43(1):48-56.
14. Wouters PF, Gehring H, Meyfroidt G, Ponz L, Gil-Rodriguez J, Hornberger C, et al. Accuracy of pulse oximeters: the European multi-center trial. Anesth Analg. 2002;94(1 Suppl):S13-6.
15. Van de Louw A, Cracco C, Cerf C, Harf A, Duvaldestin P, Lemaire F, et al. Accuracy of pulse oximetry in the intensive care unit. Intensive Care Med. 2001;27(10):1606-13.
16. Paiva EF, Paxton JH, O'Neil BJ. The use of end-tidal carbon dioxide ($ETCO_2$) measurement to guide management of cardiac arrest: A systematic review. Resuscitation. 2018;123:1-7.
17. Bouhemad B, Brisson H, Le-Guen M, Arbelot C, Lu Q, Rouby JJ. Bedside ultrasound assessment of positive end-expiratory pressure-induced lung recruitment. Am J Respir Crit Care Med. 2011;183(3):341-7.
18. Conway A, Tipton E, Liu WH, Conway Z, Soalheira K, Sutherland J, et al. Accuracy and precision of transcutaneous carbon dioxide monitoring: a systematic review and meta-analysis. Thorax. 2019;74(2):157-63.
19. Bouveresse S, Piton G, Badet N, Besch G, Pili-Floury S, Delabrousse E. Abdominal compartment syndrome and intra-abdominal hypertension in critically ill patients: diagnostic value of computed tomography. Eur Radiol. 2019;29(7):3839-46.
20. De Laet IE, Malbrain MLNG, De Waele JJ. A clinician's guide to management of intra- abdominal hypertension and abdominal compartment syndrome in critically ill patients. Critical Care. 2020;24(1):97.

CHAPTER 69

Organization and Quality Indicators in Intensive Care

Subhash Todi, Saswati Sinha

ABSTRACT

Intensive care by nature is a multidisciplinary specialty and requires an organized approach for an optimum cost-effective patient care delivery. The heterogenous nature of critical care delivery makes the organizational structure complex and results in open, closed, semi-open/closed system of intensive care. Human resources needed for an optimum intensive care constitutes of multiple personnel belonging to various mainstream and support disciplines such as physicians, nurses, paramedics etc. Accreditation of this support staff is also variable and need to be customized depending on the level and complexity of care delivered.

A pivotal aspect of cost-effective critical care delivery is to maintain quality and safety in patient care. This can be provided by optimizing the structure and processes of care delivery to achieve an optimum outcome. The structural aspect consists of the quantity and quality of healthcare personnel available, appropriate availability of technology, proper space allocation etc. The processes are compliance with various policies and protocols of care. The outcome of quality care may be assessed by various quality indicators like standardized mortality ratio to compare the observed death rate to an expected death rate based on severity of patients clinical status.

"Quality means doing it right when no one is looking"

—Henry Ford

INTRODUCTION

Care provided in intensive care units (ICUs) are of high acuity, resource intensive, and involve a high cost as compared to other areas of the healthcare system. Moreover, ICUs are widely variable in terms of settings, manpower, policies, and adherence to best established evidence based practices and may have a higher rate of adverse events. The last two decades have seen a paradigm shift in focus in healthcare from a fee for service to a value for performance which makes the critical care unit one of the prime targets for initiatives directed to improve quality and safety. This can only be achieved by optimizing the organization structure and process on critical care delivery.

ORGANIZATION OF THE ICU

Critical care/intensive care/intensive therapy units are terms used interchangeably to define special areas or departments in the hospital which are equipped with highly specialized staff—(doctors, nurses, and support staff) and equipment to closely monitor and offer highly specialized treatment to patients who have potentially life-threatening single or multiple organ dysfunction. In addition, most superspeciality offer training in critical care pertaining to individual areas such as neurocritical care, organ transplant, pulmonary critical care, cardiac critical care, gastrointestinal and hepatology.

Critical care is now an independent super specialty and most countries across the world have critical care societies and professional bodies which provide training courses, certifications, and degrees. Most hospitals now have an independent department of intensive/critical care with its own administrative structure (**Box 1**).

LEVEL OF INTENSIVE CARE UNIT CARE

Depending on the setting (primary/secondary/tertiary care) and complexity of care delivery the levels of ICU care can be described as basic, intermediate, and advanced or levels I, II, and III. These levels vary depending on the human resources and technology available for care. Each intensive care should be assessed by regulatory authorities based on the availability of these resources and accredited for the level of care they can provide. Basic levels of ICU should be able to provide early resuscitative measures and stabilize the patient and have facility for triaging to higher levels in a timely manner depending on the severity of patients condition.

TYPE OF INTENSIVE CARE UNITS

Open ICU: Any physician can admit patients to the ICU. Elective consultation with intensivists could be available at the discretion of the responsible physician. Intensivists suggestions are not binding in patient care.

Closed ICU: All patients are cared for by a team of intensivists who works in collaboration with other specialty services. Only intensivists have admitting privileges to the ICU. Also called mandatory transfer where patients are transferred under the intensivist for the duration of ICU stay. All decisions made by the critical care team including transfer is binding in patient care.

Semi-closed or transitional ICU: This is a system in which may be admitted under any physician including intensivist, but there is a mandatory consultation by the intensivist in all patients. A shared decision-making between intensivist and primary care physician is made in these cases.

In India, ICUs in public sector hospitals are mostly a closed model while those in the private sector are mostly developed as transitional or open model. A gradual shift to closed model is being appreciated in this sector as well.

There has been a lot of debate regarding whether a closed ICU improves patient outcomes in comparison with an open ICU with conflicting reports on hard outcomes like mortality in various studies. A clear benefit in terms of other outcomes including better communication, family satisfaction, and resource utilization in favor of closed ICUs has been observed in many studies. As per the Indian Society of Critical Care Medicine (ISCCM) Intensivist led units (Closed units) better outcomes and resource utilization than in units without intensivist cover (open units) and a clear preference for closed model is advised to be adopted in general medical-surgical or specialty ICUs. Till the time that is feasible, semi-closed/transitional model is acceptable.

BOX 1	Organizational aspects of ICU.
• Design of ICU	
• Infection control and surveillance for infection	
• Quality of care	
• Patient safety	
• Cost-effective care	
• Outreach services	
• Legal issues in critical care	
• Physiotherapy in intensive care	
• Critical care nursing	
• Clinical information system	
• Transportation of the critically ill patients	
• Preparedness for catastrophe	

HUMAN RESOURCES

A multidisciplinary approach is key to optimum ICU care. Human resource management is one of the most important aspects of the entire process. The staff recruited for the ICU should be adequately trained, dedicated, ready to invest long hours in stressful situations, and motivated. ICU manpower includes:

- Intensivist or critical care specialist
- Resident/Junior doctors
- Nursing officers and managers
- Respiratory therapist
- Physiotherapist
- Nutritionist
- Clinical pharmacist
- Technicians
- Computer programmer and data entry operator
- Biomedical engineer
- Social worker
- Counselor (medical psychology background)
- Other support staff including security personnel

Intensivist/Critical care specialist: He/she is a medical professional trained in intensive care/critical care medicine as per the standards set by regulatory bodies. He/she should ideally be a full time consultant or spend at least 50% of his/her practicing time in the ICU. Consultants trained in other superspecialities such as pulmonary and critical care, anesthesia and organ transplant critical care, neuroanesthesia and neurocritical care, cardiology or cardiac anesthesia working in their respective specialty units can be considered intensivists in their subspecialty. There is an ongoing debate as to whether intensive care should be regarded as a primary specialty with its own training program at a postgraduate level or a subspecialty where medical professionals with postgraduate degrees in internal medicine, anesthesiology, emergency medicine, surgery, respiratory medicine, and pediatrics undergo further stipulated period of training to qualify as an intensivist. ICU director, preferably a senior intensivist plays a pivotal role in setting up policies and protocols commensurate to the resources available. Duties of consultant intensivist should include conducting one or twice daily multidisciplinary rounds with residents and other support staff and create an action plan for patient care for the day. Liaison with other specialists, family communication, end-of-life decisions, maintaining quality control through audit, teaching, and research are other duties of a consultant intensivist.

Resident doctors: Postgraduates from medicine, respiratory medicine, anesthesia as well as graduates who are exposure to critical care patients can be posted as resident doctors. The ideal recommended doctor to patient ratio in a critical unit is not clearly defined, but ISCCM guidelines recommend 1 doctor for 5 critically ill patients. So, one unit may be managed by one postgraduate and one graduate resident doctor. The duty shift of these residents are variable but efforts need to be made not to exceed 8–12 hours shift. The duties of these residents include present cases in rounds, write clinical notes, and perform procedures and proper handover.

Nursing staff: The success of any ICU is strongly dependent on the nursing team. Hence, the key lies in ensuring adequate numbers, qualification, training, and efforts to keep the team motivated.

Adequate nurse to patient ratio is essential to maintain the quality of care. Nurse to patient ratio of 1:1 for ventilated and severely ill patients with multiorgan dysfunction is desirable but at the most it can be 2:3 (2 nurses for 3 critically ill patients on organ support). Lower ratios of 1:2 or 1:3 may be acceptable for less severely ill patients not on these support.

The nursing manpower should account for leaves, offs, and attrition. A conducive working environment and financial incentives are extremely important to keep them motivated.

Support staff: *Respiratory therapist*—can form a valuable member of the team by taking care of technical aspects of ventilators, troubleshoot, and other respiratory support including adjustment of ventilatory settings under supervision, suctioning, weaning trials, bronchodilator therapy, and extubation.

Physiotherapist—regular physiotherapy and early mobilization holds the key to better outcomes in critically ill patients and hence a dedicated physiotherapist can assist the doctors and nurses.

Health assistant—assist nurses in patient care activities such as feeding, giving bath, bed-making etc.

Intensive care unit technician—there are many equipment in the ICU and an ICU technician's role is to ensure that the equipment is all functional and ready when required. They can perform simple procedures and assist in procedures in the ICU as well as patient transport. They also play a role in maintaining, calibrating, and troubleshoot different biomedical devices such as monitors and defibrillators. They ensure safe transport of these equipment and ensure proper disinfection of the equipment.

Nutritionist/dietician—nutrition is an important part of therapeutics in the ICU and has been shown to improve outcomes, reduce infectious morbidity, and promote wound healing. Dedicated ICU nutritionists add value by assessing the nutritional status, promoting early enteral nutrition, and assisting the ICU team in making a nutritional plan and is a key player in the multidisciplinary team.

Clinical pharmacist—medication errors are a common form of preventable harm in ICU and clinical pharmacist are a part of daily ward round and identify adverse drug reaction, drug dosing, and drug-drug interaction. They also ensures compliance with the hospital antibiotic policy.

Secretarial staff—they help to keep proper medical records, billing, computer entry of drugs etc. They also answer phone calls and check the laboratory and radiology report.

Data entry operator—they perform the important task of data collection, integration, preparation of reports and are a vital member of the team especially if the ICU actively collects patient data for quality assessment and research.

Housekeeping—extremely important as they help the nursing staff, perform disinfection and terminal cleaning, and keeping the ICU clean, and thereby play an important role in infection control.

Social worker—they liaise with family members and coordinate between them and ICU staff.

Other members—important members who with whom the ICU team needs to work closely which include imaging staff, laboratory personnel, microbiology and biomedical engineering department, food and beverages, and security personnel. Close collaboration and cooperation ensures smooth functioning of the department. Physician assistant and nurse practitioner are an integral part of ICU team in western countries in order to compensate for physician and nursing shortages, but these disciplines have not yet well developed in India.

Proper design and well equipped ICU is a cornerstone of executing optimal ICU care. Meticulous attention needs to be given for allocation of ICU space, bed area, and other support areas. Adequate lighting and infection control facilities should be in place. Guidelines regarding these have been developed by various professional societies, which need to be customized based on the resources available.

A well-organized ICU should have written policies and protocols in place which include antibiotic policy, infection control policy, restraint and sedation protocols, brain death declaration policy, interhospital and intrahospital transport, organ donation policy etc., to name a few.

Teaching should be an integral part of daily ICU activities. Bedside teaching, didactic lectures, procedural skill supervision, simulation activities, and journal club should be included within this program. Accredited training courses for doctors, nurses, technician etc., need to be implemented. A structured organogram depicting various activities carried out by the critical care department, personnel involved, and hierarchal structure should be developed in a properly organized ICU.

QUALITY INDICATORS

"*To Err Is Human*: Building a Safer Health System" was a landmark paper published by Institute of Medicine USA, highlighted the role of medical error as a cause of attributable mortality and morbidity in hospitalized patient. Safety of hospitalized patients has become a key factor in accreditation of hospitals worldwide. Quality and safety are two sides of the same coin and closely interlinked, quality reflects measures those should have been taken but were not taken or errors of omission, and safety reflects actions that were taken inappropriately or errors of commission. Nearly two decades ago Pronovost and coworkers in 2001 approached the area of quality management in healthcare systematically and came up with a list of core quality indicators (QI) for intensive care.

Avedis Donabedian in the "bible" of quality assurance has broadly classified three pillars of quality measurement which have been now accepted internationally as benchmark for QI (**Box 2**):

1. Structure (What we have)
2. Process (What we get)
3. Outcome (What we do)

Structure: These consist of organizational aspects, human resources, and availability of technology and is predominantly under administrative control.

Process: These consist of care given to patients by healthcare providers and is remediable and controllable. Daily check list is a suggested method to ensure compliance with the processes.

Outcome: This reflects patients mortality and morbidity parameters and is used as a benchmark for comparison among various ICUs of effectiveness of process compliance.

Based on the various processes and outcomes QIs have been proposed by international bodies. These are core quality measures (**Box 2**) and additional measures. Institutions need to adopt certain QI customized to their setting.

A uniform description of any QI should consist of a numerator which is the indicator that is to be tested and a denominator which is the patient population at risk for that indicator. The percentage of that indicator is then compared with a benchmark standard indicator to assess the quality of performance.

Examples:

Early enteral nutrition (EN): Early (within 24–48 h within ICU admission) initiation of enteral nutrition (EN) has shown reduction in infections and mortality in critically ill patients and the target population includes all patients in whom a complete oral diet is not possible and do not have a contraindication to EN.

Formula:

$$\frac{\text{Number of patients with early initiation of EN}}{\text{Number of patients with EN}} \times 100$$

Standard: 100%

Deep vein thrombosis prevention: Use of prophylaxis for venous thromboembolism during ICU stay has shown a decrease in morbidity and mortality. The target population for prophylaxis should include all patients staying in the ICU for >24 hours and prophylaxis could include unfractionated, heparin, low-molecular weight heparin, fondaparinux, or mechanical devices such as intermittent pneumatic compression.

BOX 2 Quality indicators.

Structure
- Closed model of ICU care
- ICU design
- Doctor patient ratio
- Nurse patient ratio
- 24 × 7 intensivist coverage
- Written policies and protocols
- Adequate equipment

Process
- Compliance with hand hygiene
- Compliance with ventilator bundle
- Compliance with central line insertion bundle
- End-of-life support policies
- Family conference
- Antibiotic consumption

Outcome
- Crude ICU mortality
- Risk adjusted ICU mortality
- Standardized mortality ratio
- Hospital mortality
- ICU length of stay
- Hospital length of stay
- Family satisfaction
- Ventilator associated pneumonia rate
- Central line associated blood stream infection rate
- Catheter associated urinary tract infection rate
- Surgical site infection rate
- *Clostridium (C.) difficile* infection rate
- Prevalence of multidrug resistant organism
- Device utilization days
- Cost of care

Formula:

$$\frac{\text{Number of patients receiving prophylaxis against Deep Venous Thrombosis (DVT)}}{\text{Number of patients with EN}} \times 100$$

Standard: 90%

Standardized mortality ratio: Mortality rate related to prior prediction based on severity of illness as predicted by severity of illness scores is a sensitive measure of comparison. Hence, standardized mortality ratio (SMR) or risk adjusted mortality rate allows comparison of the units performance with predicted performance based on national and international data. SMR is one of the most common indicators monitored by most countries as a core QI.

Rationale of measurement: Risk of mortality depends on severity of illness, age, and comorbidities. Hence, crude mortality rate is not useful and SMR obviates the limitations of crude mortality as it takes into account the expected mortality for other patients with similar diagnosis and risk factors using models such as acute physiology and chronic health evaluation (APACHE), simplified acute physiology score (SAPS), mortality prediction models (MPM) etc. It allows to track a unit's performance and also to compare between different units.

Formula:

$$\frac{\text{Observed hospital mortality}}{\text{Expected hospital mortality (mean value} \pm \text{confidence interval)}} \times 100$$

Observed hospital mortality: Number of patients admitted to critical care who die in the hospital/number of patients admitted to critical care by unit of time.

Expected hospital mortality: Arithmetic sum of the individual probabilities of death for each patient admitted to critical care according to the severity score/number of patients admitted to critical care.

Higher SMR in isolation does not indicate a poor quality by itself. It needs to be interpreted in context of other QI.

Benchmark: If the 95% confidence interval (CI) of the SMR includes 1, the performance is considered average. If the 95% CI does not include 1, SMRs <1 and >1 are considered to show good and poor performances, respectively.

Quality cycle: Collecting continuous patient data either electronically or manually is the cornerstone of quality performance measures. Activities which can be measured can only be improved. The quality of data itself that need to be collected should be robust and should follow the SMART rule (simple, measurable, achievable, reproducible, and time bound). The data should be properly analyzed, presented and discussed among all the stakeholders. An assessment of gaps or deficiency in performance need to be made and correctable measures planned. Review of the data after a certain stipulated time to assess improvement of performance will complete the Plan-Do-Study-Act (PDSA) cycle of quality control.

BOX 3	Adverse events.
Patient safety: Absence of the potential for, or occurrence of, healthcare-associated injury to patients	
Error: It is defined as mistakes made in the process of care that result in, or have the potential to result in, harm to patients. Mistakes include the failure of a planned action to be completed as intended or the use of a wrong plan to achieve an aim. These can be the result of an action that is taken (error of commission) or an action that is not taken (error of omission) potential to result in harm to patients	
Incident: Unexpected or unanticipated events or circumstances not consistent with the routine care of a particular patient, which could have, or did lead to an unintended or unnecessary harm to a person, or a complaint, loss, or damage	
Near miss: An occurrence of an error that did not result in harm	
Adverse event: An injury resulting from a medical intervention	
Preventable adverse event: Harm that could be avoided through reasonable planning or proper execution of an action	

Adverse events (AE) (Box 3): As mentioned earlier quality and safety are closely interlinked and continuous surveillance for adverse events (AE) need to be maintained and reported. Standardized nomenclature to describe these events have been described. Once identified certain managerial principles like root cause analysis needs to be implemented to find remediable measures. The key issue in managing such AE is to avoid fault finding in an individual but trying to identify system problem that has resulted in such an event. Rectifying this will result in a long-lasting safety performance improvement in decreasing AEs.

CONCLUSION

In the face of the rapidly changing landscape of healthcare, the role of quality and cost has become even more important in managing ICUs. In the quest for providing value for our patients, the key elements are quality and safety. It is important to choose a reasonable number of metrics covering the domains of structure, process, and outcome for each specific ICU or hospital. All the disciplines in the ICU should be aligned and take ownership of the quality program which is the fundamental factor for success.

RECOMMENDED READINGS

1. Brilli RJ, Spevetz A, Branson RD, Campbell GM, Cohen H, Dasta JF, et al. Critical care delivery in the intensive care unit: defining clinical roles and the best practice model. Crit Care Med. 2001;29(10):2007-19.
2. Haupt MT, Bekes CE, Brilli RJ, Carl LC, Gray AW, Jastremski MS, et al. Guidelines on critical care services and personnel: recommendations based on

a system of categorization of three levels of care. Crit Care Med. 2003;31(11):2677-83.

3. Society of Critical Care Medicine. Guidelines for intensive care unit design. Guidelines/Practice Parameters Committee of the American College of Critical Care Medicine. Crit Care Med. 1995;23(3):582-8.
4. Guidelines for intensive care unit admission, discharge, and triage. Task Force of the American College of Critical Care Medicine, Society of Critical Care Medicine. Crit Care Med. 1999;27(3):633-8.
5. Thompson DR, Hamilton DK, Cadenhead CD, Swoboda SM, Schwindel SM, Anderson DC, et al. Guidelines for intensive care unit design. Crit Care Med. 2012;40(5):1586-600.
6. Bauman KA, Hyzy RC. ICU 2020: five interventions to revolutionize quality of care in the ICU. J Intensive Care Med. 2014;29(1):13-21.
7. Chrusch CA, Martin CM, Project TQ. Quality improvement in critical care: selection and development of quality indicators. Can Respir J. 2016;2016:2516765.
8. Garland A. Improving the ICU: part 1. Chest. 2005;127 (6):2151-64.
9. Garland A. Improving the ICU: part 2. Chest. 2005;127 (6):2165-79.
10. Kahn JM. Bringing implementation science to the intensive care unit. Curr Opin Crit Care. 2017;23(5): 398-9.

CHAPTER 70

Chronic Critical Care

Manjunath BG, Sushmita Jakka, Sheenam Walia

ABSTRACT

Improved management in terms of organ support in modern healthcare facilities has led to increase in the number of survivors who would have otherwise succumbed to serious diseases. But most of these have prolonged dependence on life support systems and fall under the category of "chronic critical illness (CCI)," which has no universally standard definition. The identification of those who are at risk of developing CCI is very challenging. Patients having diseases with long intrinsic recovery times, conditions like sepsis and acute respiratory distress syndrome (ARDS) which have underlying severe inflammation, old age, presence of comorbidities, poor functional status before acute illness etc., have been shown to be more at risk. CCI is a complex syndrome of physiologic abnormalities, organ and immunologic dysfunctions with muscle weakness, malnutrition, brain dysfunction, pressure sore, neuroendocrine changes, neuropsychosocial changes, immunomodulation etc., as predominant clinical features.

Managing a CCI patient is essentially a multidisciplinary approach and needs a thorough discussion with the patient and family regarding the site of treatment as well as level of interventions. In most cases assisted ventilation remains the cornerstone of treatment although nutrition, managing pressure sores, physiotherapy, and rehabilitation are equally important for better outcomes.

The outcomes of CCI are not very encouraging from the point of view of long-term survival, functional capacity, and quality of life, hence the need for having a holistic approach involving all the stakeholders including family members.

"Everybody knows if you are too careful you are so occupied in being careful that you are sure to stumble over something"

—Gertrude Stein

INTRODUCTION

Once a person develops an acute critical illness and gets admitted in intensive care unit (ICU), he/she may either recover fully or succumb to illness or progress to CCI. Continuously improving management of acutely ill critical patients in modern healthcare facilities has led to increase in the number of the latter subset. These patients typically have prolonged dependence on some form of life support. The prevalence of this CCI ranges from 5 to 20% of patients admitted to the ICU.

DEFINITION OF CCI

The definition of CCI has varied across the literature (**Table 1**) and there is no *"the official definition,"* but the most standardized one till now is Research Triangle Initiative (RTI) definition which was later modified by

TABLE 1 Varied definitions of CCI used by different researchers in the literature.

Authors	Definition
Kahn et al. [Grit Care Med. 2015; 43(2):282-7]	8 or more days in an ICU with one or more of the following six conditions: MV, tracheotomy, stroke, head trauma, sepsis and serious injury
Loss et al. [Rev Assoc Med Bras (1992). 2013;59 (3):241-7]	21 days on MV or tracheotomy
Carson et al. [Crit Care Med. 2012;40(4):1171-6]	21 days on MV for at least 6 h/day
Girard and Raffin [Respir Care. 1985;30(5):339-47]	ICU patients who do not survive despite extraordinary life support for weeks to months
Douglas et al. [Am J Crit Care. 1997;6:99-105]	Patients who require long-term ventilation and intensive nursing care after receiving medical therapy for primary disease; generally, ICU stay of >2 weeks
Nasraway et al. [Crit Care Med. 2000;28:19-25]	A small subset of the ICU patients who because of underlying illness or complications suffer a prolonged and complicated ICU course; severely weakened survivors of acute illness often ventilator dependent or renal dialysis dependent
Nierman [Crit Care Clin. 2002;18:477-91]	Patients who survive a critical illness but are left with significant functional impairments and dependency on intense nursing care and advanced technology
Carson and Bach [Crit Care Clin. 2002;18:461-76]	Patients who require continued care and prolonged MV in an ICU for weeks to months; >21 days ICU stay indicates that most easily reversible conditions have been addressed
Daly et al. [Chest 2005;128:507-17]	Patients requiring MV for >72 h who survive to discharge from the index hospitalization
Nelson et al. [Grit Care Med. 2004;32:1527-34]	A syndrome of significant derangements of metabolism and of neuroendocrine, neuropsychiatric, and immunologic functions defined by performance of tracheotomy for failure to wean from MV
MacIntyre et al. [Chest 2005;128(6): 3937-54]	Prolonged MV is the need for MV for 21 consecutive days and >6 h/day
Scheinhom et al. [Chest 2007; 131 (1):76-84]	Prolonged ventilator-dependent respiratory failure
Zilberberg et al. [Crit Care Med. 2008;36:724-30]	Prolonged acute MV of >96 h

(MV: mechanical ventilation)

ProVent Study Group (**Table 2**). Basically, this definition is conceptualized to coordinate the sites of care as well as payment methods and is not meant to be a clinical definition.

TABLE 2 RTI and ProVent study group definitions of chronic critical illness.

An ICU length of stay of at least 8 days combined with at least one of the following during the hospitalization	
RTI	**ProVent study group**
Prolonged acute mechanical ventilation (i.e., mechanical ventilation for at least 96 h in a single episode)	Prolonged acute mechanical ventilation
Tracheotomy	Tracheotomy
Sepsis and other severe infections	Sepsis
Severe wounds	Severe wounds
Multiple organ failure, ischemic stroke, intercerebral hemorrhage, or traumatic brain injury	Stroke (including both ischemic stroke and intercerebral hemorrhage)
	Traumatic brain injury

(RTI: Research Triangle Initiative)

For a clinician, CCI is never a one-dimensional specific condition but a multidimensional *"not very specific"* syndrome, the concept of which is best explained by considering it as a conglomeration of the following.

- *Persistent critical illness*: Patients require intensive care because of a cascade of critical illnesses rather than for their original diagnosis at admission. In these the primary disease (such as cellulitis, poisoning, or dissecting ascending aortic aneurysm) is no longer active.
- *Medically complex patients*: Like in RTI definition
- *Diseases with long intrinsic recovery times*: For example, Guillain-Barré syndrome (GBS), where the recovery takes its own time and current medical interventions fail to speed it up. This category also includes diseases like end-stage liver or lung disorders wherein the underlying physiological derangement is too severe to sustain homeostasis, even in the absence of new complications.
- *Prolonged weaning*: Patients who require mechanical ventilation even after resolution of their other critical illnesses. This situation arises due to persistent deficits in respiratory muscle strength due to various etiologies, respiratory mechanics, gas exchange, nutrition etc. The alternative term used in literature is prolonged mechanical ventilation (PMV). Most of authors have settled on a definition for PMV as ≥21 consecutive days of mechanical ventilation for ≥6 hours per day. Inclusion of neuromuscular diseases and chronic pulmonary diseases in this group is a matter of debate and the opinions may vary (**Fig. 1**).
- *Prolonged ICU length of stay*: Purely a quantitative concept of subjective duration, wherein the reason can be anything.

RECOGNITION OF CCI

In broad terms, CCI refers to a population of patients who have survived acute critical illness but have persistent organ dysfunction after the initial insult, requiring weeks,

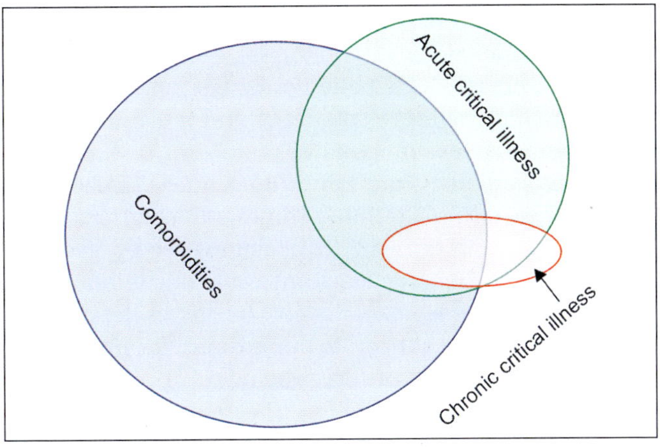

(CKD: chronic kidney disease; COAD: chronic obstructive airway disease; CTDs: connective tissue diseases; NMD: neuromuscular disease)

FIGURE 1: Representation of relationships between acute critical illness (ACI), comorbidities such as old age, diabetes, heart failure, CKD, COAD, end-stage liver disease, CTDs, and vasculitis with chronic critical illness (CCI). It shows that ACI patients with comorbidities are more prone for CCI. Also, some without comorbidities may also progress to CCI because of many other factors mainly the high inflammatory load. Some patients (like in NMDs and chronic pulmonary diseases) may land up into CCI without an obvious acute course.

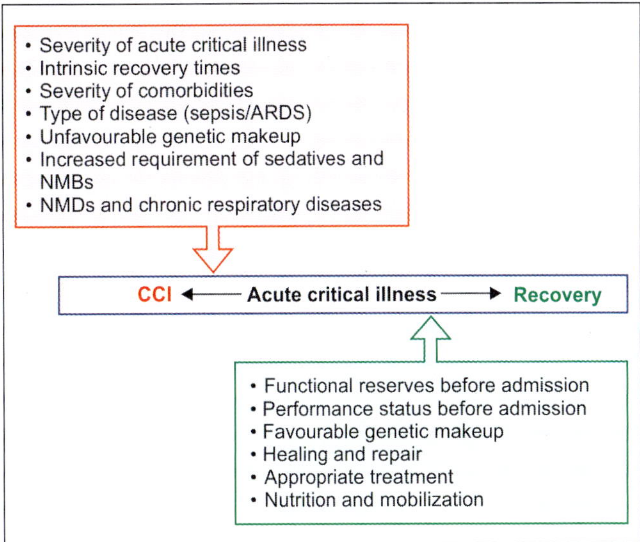

(ARDS: acute respiratory distress syndrome; CCI: chronic critical illness; NMD: neuromuscular disease; NMB: neuromuscular blockers)

FIGURE 2: Multiple simultaneously acting factors in a patient of acute critical illness which dictate the further course to either recovery or CCI.

months, or even years of specialized care. The tendency to land up into CCI is obvious in diseases with long intrinsic recovery times, but not so in other groups. There is no explanation available why few patients with similar severity and disease become chronically ill while others recover early and have normal functional status as it was pre-ICU admission. Moreover, there are no biomarkers that can assist in predicting the development of this condition.

Risk factors: The risk factors that can predict CCI are shown in **figure 2**.

Old age due to depleted functional reserves. Prevalence of CCI generally rises with age, but it declines after 80 years due to high early mortality.

Comorbidities such as diabetes, heart failure, chronic kidney disease (CKD), chronic obstructive airway disease (COAD), end-stage liver disease, and chronic diseases requiring long-term immunosuppression like connective tissue diseases (CTDs) and vasculitis. More the number of comorbidities higher are the chances of developing CCI.

Poor functional status before admission

Type of disease: Conditions like sepsis and ARDS lead to triggering of severe inflammatory response. The persistence of inflammation for long durations induces changes in the hypothalamic-pituitary-adrenal axis. This leads to variations in levels of cortisol, renin, angiotensin, and aldosterone causing derangements in metabolism processes (especially protein and bone), body composition, and vascular tone. All these lead to fluid retention, edema, loss of muscle mass, ulceration, and requirement of long-term life support systems (most important of them being ventilatory assistance).

CLINICAL FEATURES

Chronic critical illness, as distinguished from critical illness, is a complex syndrome of physiologic abnormalities, organ dysfunction, and immunologic dysfunction. It can cause protein catabolism leading to decreased respiratory muscle mass, strength, and endurance. In addition, malnutrition, in advent use of drugs, abnormal lung mechanics, all of which can contribute to impaired respiratory drive and poor respiratory muscle function, lead to chronic respiratory failure. Thus, the hallmark feature is respiratory failure requiring prolonged dependence on assisted ventilation, though it is not *sine quo non* as CCI is a syndrome comprising additional systemic features which include:

Muscle weakness: Survivors of acute illness in ICU often develop critical illness polyneuropathy (CIP) or critical illness myopathy (CIM) or most commonly a combination of these, i.e., critical illness polyneuromyopathy (CIPNM). These conditions are common in CCI and lead to functional impairment and difficulty in weaning from mechanical ventilation and mobilization. Few studies have used one common term to define these acquired disorders which is critical illness neuromuscular abnormalities (CINMAs) or ICU-acquired weakness (ICUAW). The incidence of CINMA varies significantly between various studies because of the selection of patients and defining criteria for new onset weakness. In a study, CINMAs were found in almost all patients who required mechanical ventilation for >7 days. The onset of weakness can be from few days to weeks.

Malnutrition: Malnutrition is one of the characteristic findings in CCI associated with chronic inflammation and hormonal changes. As a result of these changes, CCI patients develop (1) marasmus-type malnutrition, (2) adult kwashiorkor-like malnutrition with associated protein catabolism, hypoalbuminemia, and anasarca, (3) metabolic bone disease due to hyper-resorption and vitamin D insufficiency/deficiency, (4) hypothalamic-pituitary dysfunction, (5) various micronutrient deficiencies, and (6) stress-induced hyperglycemia. In a study, malnutrition was present in 43% of ICU population. Malnutrition reduces diaphragmatic muscle mass and strength which results in poor respiratory reserve and function. This leads to prolonged ventilator stay and vice versa. Normal albumin levels persist until very late stages when hypoalbuminemia and "third spacing" result from compromised hepatic function.

Brain dysfunction: Brain dysfunction is another common condition complicating the course of critical illness in ICU and pertaining to CCI syndrome. Nelson et al. found that more days of delirium during CCI were significantly associated with discharge to a postacute care facility as well as prolonged hospital stays and poor long-term functional status. Incidence of brain dysfunction in CCI patients is 29–69% but patients who survive may have persistent cognitive impairment. The pathophysiology of cerebral dysfunction appears to be multifactorial. Delirium seems to be related to the imbalance between dopamine production and acetylcholine depletion in controlling cognitive functions. During critical illness, inflammatory mediators cross blood brain barrier and interrupt with neurotransmitter synthesis and neurotransmission. They lead to endothelial damage and brain edema which enhance brain dysfunction. The other factors like exposure to analgesics, sedatives, and sleep deprivation also play important role in precipitating delirium.

Pressure sore: Chronically, critically ill patients are almost universally at high risk for developing pressure ulcers. CCI patients may need prolonged ventilator stay and remain immobile for long period of time that predisposes them to develop pressure sore. The pathophysiology includes poor angiogenesis and wound healing. They have poor nutritional support, increase fluid retention, and anasarca-like state which further promote pressure sore. With such strong predispositions and additional diminished sensory perception and organ failure, these patients develop pressure ulcers despite preventive care and continuous monitoring. In a study conducted by Cremasco et al. the length of ICU stay is directly related to the development of pressure ulcers.

The prevalence of pressure ulcers is estimated to be at least 10% in hospitalized patients, 20% among patients in nursing homes, and 20–30% among patients with spinal cord injury and those in rehabilitation units.

Neuroendocrine changes: Loss of pulsatile secretion of anterior pituitary hormones contribute to low target organ hormone levels and impaired anabolism.

Neuropsychosocial changes: Reports document significant distress from symptoms including pain, thirst, dyspnea, depression, and anxiety, and from inability to communicate during endotracheal intubation.

Immunomodulation: All CCI patients are susceptible for infections because of:

- Barrier breach: CCI patients always have numerous potential breaches in cutaneous and mucosal barriers owing to tracheostomy, dialysis catheter, pressure sores, urinary catheters, and intravenous lines that facilitate pathogen entry. The most commonly cited causes of barrier breach to result in infections are intravenous catheterization, tracheostomy, and decubitus ulcer. Such barrier breaches do not, by themselves, cause infection but enhance the opportunity for infection if other host defenses are overwhelmed.
- Increased organism load in CCI care environment: The CCI patients may become colonized with nosocomial pathogens, many with multidrug antibiotic resistance and increased virulence. The colonized pathogens make biofilm in trachea, feeding tube, central venous catheters, and coat body surfaces and sites of breakdown. Most of pathogens in this setting include resistant gram-negative enteric flora, methicillin-resistant *Staphylococcus aureus*, and fungal species which further slow the recovery.
- Immune exhaustion: The other major factor for susceptibility of infections is the exhaustion of immune resources in the host. Immune exhaustion is the term used to describe the potentially disabling effects of depleted, dysfunctional, or inhibited immune resources that may impair defense against pathogens. Inflammatory mediators, premorbid condition, and age are important factors which alter immune responses and make CCI patients susceptible to infections. Diabetes, chronic renal insufficiency, and pre-existing cardiopulmonary disease such as COPD alter the local and systemic defense mechanisms. Abnormal leukocyte function described in diabetes mellitus may partly explain the higher incidence of infection and increased morbidity seen in this disease. Additionally, over a prolonged ICU stay, nutritional deficiency, micronutrient deficiency, protein depletion, and use of corticosteroids further facilitate infections. Further, acute inflammatory conditions like sepsis, major surgery, and ARDS may impose defective immune responses by the transient depletion of immune resources or dysregulation of immune response. Although each CCI patient experiences a heterogeneous set of inflammatory insult, the genetic factors also play an important role in immune regulation.

MANAGEMENT

WORKUP

As almost all patients of CCI are being treated for their acute illness in some kind of ICUs most of the routine investigations such as complete hemogram, liver function tests, renal function tests, serum electrolytes levels, serum protein, and albumin levels are expected to be available, if not they are needed to be done. Apart from these following special investigations (not a complete list), as and when indicated, may be required: Thyroid profile, evaluation of other hormone levels, vitamin levels, body fluid cultures, radiology of various parts and organs, nerve conduction studies, electromyography, echocardiography, electroencephalography, muscle biopsy, pulmonary function tests etc.

PREREQUISITES

Chronic critical illness should be treated only after a thorough discussion with the patient and family regarding:

- Benefits as well as burden of treatment
- Exploration of the needs, values, preferences, and goals of the patient and family
- Education of the patient and family regarding CCI

Any choice to continue treatment should involve these additional considerations:

- Consideration of a time-limited therapeutic trial
- Periodic re-evaluation of progress
- Concomitant addressal of the palliative needs of the patient and family

FACILITY

In the western countries, especially in USA, the concept of long-term acute care (LTAC) hospitals has evolved to take care of these patients. In India the concept is still in nascent stage and no designated facilities for CCI patients are available due to various reasons especially the constraints in healthcare resources. This has led to them being treated in either hospital ICUs or high dependency units (HDUs) for prolonged periods and in few occasions at either hospital wards, hospice/palliative care facilities or homes.

TEAM

Due to vast heterogeneity in the types of CCI patients there is no *"the protocol"* or preferred approach in their treatment. Perhaps having a multidisciplinary approach is the best available option at our disposal. Team may comprise of:

- Nurse
- Physiotherapists
- Dieticians
- Occupational therapists
- Speech and language therapists
- Pharmacists
- Social workers
- Psychologists
- Intensivists
- Specialists on need base

ASSISTED VENTILATION

Subjective findings as well as objective tests determine, if ventilation needs assistance. Those with cardiopulmonary arrest, marked blood gas derangements, aspiration due to bulbar dysfunction, and poor GCS (Glasgow Coma Scale) need immediate mechanical ventilation, while for the rest of the patients, overall clinical status dictates the need for it. In neuromuscular disease (NMD) patients a rule of "20–30–40" has been proposed although serial measurements give better idea of the requirement of mechanical ventilation (**Box 1**). Once it is decided to assist the ventilation the options are noninvasive ventilation (NIV) or invasive mechanical ventilation (IMV).

The role of NIV in patients with CCI in general is not clear. Its use can be mostly extrapolated from patients such as chronic obstructive pulmonary disease (COPD) and NMD. NIV may avoid intubation in patients with acute exacerbations of COPD and patients with chronic progressive NMDs. Appropriate ventilator, ventilatory settings, and interface selection are keys to the success of NIV. NIV may benefit in the following situations:

- Continuous mechanical ventilation for short duration like in GBS
- Intermittent mechanical ventilation for longer duration like in nocturnal hypoventilation and early chronic respiratory failure

Any other patient requiring assisted ventilation needs to be put on IMV. Using lung protective ventilation strategies [tidal volumes in the 4–8 mL/kg (ideal body weight) range and plateau pressures <30 cm H_2O] during acute illness is associated with improved survival and also fewer ventilator days and ICU stay. Daily awakening trials and daily spontaneous breathing trials (SBTs) also improve survival and reduce ICU stay. Early tracheostomy should be considered once the risk for CCI is noted (**Box 2**). People are trying to use NIV through tracheotomy tubes with some amount of success thus reducing cost of assisted ventilation.

WEANING

Identifying the underlying cause leading to difficulty in liberation from ventilator is the important step in these patients. All the potential treatable causes such as drugs, electrolyte imbalance, and nutritional status should be managed. Initiation of weaning should be done only after the underlying cause of respiratory failure has improved, hemodynamic stability has been achieved, and the patient is able to initiate adequate respiratory effort. Weaning should be gradual in patients requiring PMV.

NUTRITION

Nutritional management plays a key role in the management of patients with CCI as major contribution of the

BOX 1	Assessment of need for mechanical ventilation in NMD patients.
Mechanical ventilation indicated if one or more of the following are present*	
FVC < 50% of the predicted	
MIP > -30 cmH_2O	
MEP < 40 cmH_2O	
Vital capacity either < 20 mL/kg /60% predicted /1 L	

* None is superior to other.

20-30-40 rule: MV indicated when VC < 20 mL/kg or MIP > -30 cmH_2O or MEP < 40 cmH_2O.

(FVC: forced vital capacity; MEP: maximal expiratory pressure; MIP: maximal inspiratory pressure; MV: mechanical ventilation; NMD: neuromuscular disease)

disease process revolves around persistent catabolism, malnutrition, and neuroendocrine imbalances. The goal of nutritional management in these patients is to strike the balance between benefit of providing metabolic substrates to minimize further loss of lean body mass against adverse consequences of overfeeding and other risks. Those patients without any gastrointestinal intolerance, enteral feeding should be started as soon as possible. Recommendations range from 20 to 25 kcal/kg/day, high protein levels (1.2–2 g/kg/day), and high vitamins and trace elements. The need for vitamins and trace elements is greater in these patients due to loss through the capillary membrane. There is no recommended amount for these substrates. Hyperglycemia related to stress or other related causes may require insulin therapy preferably subcutaneous NPH (neutral protamine Hagedorn). Diarrhea is common in these patients and may be present in one-third, which should be managed with the addition of soluble fiber (15–20 g/day) and probiotics.

MANAGEMENT OF PRESSURE INJURIES

Prevention is the most cost-effective approach in the management of pressure sores. Proper positioning, together with regular repositioning, paying particular attention to vulnerable tissue overlying bony prominences, is an integral component of pressure sore prevention. Early mobilization, prompt treatment of hypotension, limiting the use of vasopressors, and improving cardiac contractility are effective ways in improving skin perfusion. Keeping the pressure areas dry and timely application of topical medications can prevent secondary infections. Osteomyelitis should not be missed in deep wounds and signs of systemic inflammation without an obvious site.

PHYSIOTHERAPY

Patients with CCI have gross functional deficits that interfere with self-care and mobility. These deficits need to be addressed early and managed aggressively. Minimal sedation along with early mobilization should be done as soon as possible, ideally on the first ICU day, if the patient is stable from a cardiovascular, respiratory, and neurologic standpoint. The goal of physical rehabilitation is to achieve the near complete restoration of physical, psychologic, social, vocational, recreational, and economic functions within the limits imposed by the illness and the physical/mental impairment. Patients, bedridden for longer duration, are at increased risk for developing joint contractures. The most frequently involved areas are neck in flexion, shoulders in adduction and internal rotation, elbows in flexion, wrists in flexion, fingers in flexion, hips in flexion and external rotation, knees in flexion, and ankles in plantar flexion. These contractures may be painful and they interfere in positioning and mobilization leading to pressure sores and vice versa. Regular physiotherapy helps in alleviating contractures and therefore, improves patient's mobility at hospital discharge and shortening the length of hospital stay.

Patients with CCI have a tendency for pooling of mucus in the airways, which predisposes the patient to mucous plugging, atelectasis, and pneumonia. This is aggravated by a decrease in respiratory activity and an impaired cough mechanism. Impaired mucociliary function and respiratory muscle weakness contribute to ineffective cough in these patients. Regular change in position, aggressive mobilization, incentive spirometry, deep breathing, coughing, and pulmonary toilet help in optimizing the pulmonary function and preventing aspiration and atelectasis. For all patients with ineffective cough, following methods either singly or in combination will be required.

- Mechanical insufflation-exsufflation
- Manually assisted cough
- Hyperinflation maneuvers
- High frequency chest wall oscillation
- Intrapulmonary percussive ventilation

BOX 2	Indications for tracheostomy in CCI patients.
• Difficulty in clearing secretions due to either poor GCS or NMD	
• Requiring long-term mechanical ventilation/ prolonged mechanical ventilation	
• Requiring intermittent long-term mechanical ventilation with contraindications to NIV	
• Hypertension	
• NIV failure due to worsening chronic respiratory failure	
• Failure to wean from IMV	

(CCI: chronic critical illness; GCS: Glasgow Coma Scale; IMV: invasive mechanical ventilation; NIV: noninvasive ventilation; NMD: neuromuscular disease)

OTHER SUPPORTIVE INTERVENTIONS

Many other measures may be required to tackle the complications of prolonged illness. Long-term oxygen therapy may be indicated in chronic respiratory patients. The goals of oxygen saturation in such cases must be individualized. Administration of nonsteroidal anabolic agents may be considered in patients with clear hypogonadism and/or severe cachexia. Periodical screening for osteopenia and osteoporosis using radiological techniques and clinical analysis (calcium, vitamin D, and parathyroid hormone) is required and may need treatment with calcium and vitamin D. Occasionally patients may also require either iron or blood product infusions. Management of secondary infections by early identification and appropriate antimicrobials needs no mention. Antidepressants/antipsychotics and psychological support will mostly be required to manage depression and other mental changes.

Encouragement to get out of bed, even if receiving ventilatory support, active or passive muscle rehabilitation strategies are important. Physical activity programs including walking tests in the ICU, electrostimulation, and exercise should be administered and monitored by specialized professionals.

The physical educators, occupational therapists, and social workers should be involved in all patients who are undergoing rehabilitation. Family training is the most important component and key to success in rehabilitating the patient.

OUTCOMES

Eventual functional recovery of any CCI patient is always an uncertainty. The long-term prognosis of CCI patients looks grim which was confirmed in the meta-analysis by Damuth et al. (39 studies from 16 countries) showing a pooled mortality rate at hospital discharge of 29% and 59% at 1 year rising to 74% in those requiring any assisted ventilation at home. The 1-year mortality is as high as 95% in those over 75 years old and over 65 years old with impaired functional capacity. The 5-year mortality in all CCI patients is around 80%.

The quality of life of CCI patients remains dismal even if discharged to home. The functional capacity remains poor compared to general population. Cognitive impairment and psychiatric illness are much more common in these patients. The long-term intensive care required in these patients is very taxing to the family in terms of workload and finances.

CONCLUSION

Critically ill patients are at risk for CCI which is characterized by long hospitalization, high costs, and reduced survival and intense suffering. A set of features to identify those at risk, steps to prevent, and therapies focused on restoring organ function, nutritional status, mobility, mental health, quality of life, and socioeconomic status have been proposed. Still the prevalence of CCI remains high, treatment costly, and prognosis poor. High quality research is the need of the hour to decrease its incidence, identify those who may benefit from care, and improve outcomes.

RECOMMENDED READINGS

1. Kandilov AM, Ingber MJ, Morley M, Coomer N, Dalton K, Gage B, et al. Chronically Critically Ill Population Payment Recommendations. Research Triangle Park, NC: RTI International; 2014.
2. Kahn JM, Le T, Angus DC, Cox CE, Hough CL, White DB, et al.; ProVent Study Group Investigators. The epidemiology of chronic critical illness in the United States. Crit Care Med. 2015;43(2):282-7.
3. Iwashyna TJ, Hodgson CL, Pilcher D, Orford N, Santamaria JD, Bailey M, et al. Towards Defining Persistent Critical Illness and Other Varieties of Chronic Critical Illness. Crit Care Resusc. 2015;17(3):215-8.
4. MacIntyre NR, Epstein SK, Carson S, Scheinhorn D, Christopher K, Muldoon S; National Association for Medical Direction of Respiratory Care. Management of patients requiring prolonged mechanical ventilation: report of a NAMDRC consensus conference. Chest. 2005;128(6):3937-54.
5. Macintyre NR. Chronic Critical Illness: The Growing Challenge to Health Care. Respiratory Care. 2012;57(6):1021-7.
6. Theaker C, Mannan M, Ives N, Soni N. Risk factors for pressure sores in the critically ill. Anaesthesia. 2000;55:221-4.
7. Mehta S. Neuromuscular disease causing acute respiratory failure. Respir Care. 2006;51:1016.
8. Brower RG, Matthay MA, Morris A, Schoenfeld D, Thompson BT, Wheeler A. Ventilation with lower tidal volumes as compared with traditional tidal volumes for acute lung injury and the acute respiratory distress syndrome. N Engl J Med. 2000;342(18):1301-8.
9. Girard TD, Kress JP, Fuchs BD, Thomason JW, Schweickert WD, Pun BT, et al. Efficacy and safety of a paired sedation and ventilator weaning protocol for mechanically ventilated patients in intensive care (Awakening and Breathing Controlled trial): a randomised controlled trial. Lancet. 2008;371(9607):126-34.
10. Durbin CG, Jr. Indications for and timing of tracheostomy. Respir Care. 2005;50(4):483-7.
11. Damuth E, Mitchel JA, Bartock JL, Roberts BW, Trzeciak S. Long-term survival of critically ill patients treated with prolonged mechanical ventilation: a systematic review and meta-analysis. Lancet Respir Med. 2015;3(7):544-53.
12. Bigatello LM, Stelfox HT, Berra L, Schmidt U, Gettings EM. Outcome of patients undergoing prolonged mechanical ventilation after critical illness. Crit Care Med. 2007;35(11):2491-7.
13. Hartl WH, Wolf H, Schneider CP, Küchenhoff H, Jauch KW. Acute and long-term survival in chronically critically ill surgical patients: a retrospective observational study. Crit Care. 2007;11(3):R55.
14. Mikkelsen ME, Still M, Anderson BJ, Bienvenu OJ, Brodsky MB, Brummel N, et al. Society of Critical Care Medicine's International Consensus Conference on Prediction and Identification of Long-Term Impairments After Critical Illness. Crit Care Med. 2020;48(11):1670-9.
15. Fan E, Cheek F, Chlan L, Gosselink R, Hart N, Herridge MS, et al. An official American Thoracic Society Clinical Practice guideline: the diagnosis of intensive care unit-acquired weakness in adults. Am J Respir Crit Care Med. 2014;190(12):1437-46.
16. Schmidt GA, Girard TD, Kress JP, Morris PE, Ouellette DR, Alhazzani W, et al. Official Executive Summary of an American Thoracic Society/American College of Chest Physicians Clinical Practice Guideline: Liberation from Mechanical Ventilation in Critically Ill Adults. Am J Respir Crit Care Med. 2017;195(1):115-9.
17. Mehlhorn J, Freytag A, Schmidt K, Brunkhorst FM, Graf J, Troitzsch U, et al. Rehabilitation interventions for postintensive care syndrome: a systematic review. Crit Care Med. 2014;42(5):1263-71.
18. Calvo-Ayala E, Khan BA, Farber MO, Ely EW, Boustani MA. Interventions to improve the physical function of ICU survivors: a systematic review. Chest. 2013;144(5):1469-80.
19. Lone NI, Gillies MA, Haddow C, Dobbie R, Rowan KM, Wild SH, et al. Five-Year Mortality and Hospital Costs Associated with Surviving Intensive Care. Am J Respir Crit Care Med. 2016;194(2):198-208.

CHAPTER 71 Fluid Assessment and Management in Critically ill Patients

Sheila Nainan Myatra, Nishanth Baliga

ABSTRACT

Fluid therapy in intensive care unit (ICU) is indicated for resuscitation, maintenance, and replacement. Fluids are cornerstone for therapy in patients with circulatory shock when etiology is hypovolemia or sepsis. During resuscitation the goal of fluid therapy is to increase the preload by increasing venous return leading to increase in cardiac output and hence tissue oxygenation. After initial fluid resuscitation further fluid therapy should be guided by determination of fluid responsiveness. The gold standard for assessment of fluid responsiveness is a conventional fluid challenge with 500 mL of crystalloid given over 30 minutes and looking for increase in stroke volume or cardiac output. However, as a fluid bolus is irreversible it can potentially be harmful in fluid nonresponsive patients.

Predictors of fluid responsiveness include both static and dynamic parameters. Static parameters are based on ventricular volume or pressures. Dynamic measures of fluid responsiveness include those based on heart–lung interactions during mechanical ventilation and the passive leg raising test (PLRT), an autofluid challenge not based on heart–lung interactions. Dynamic parameters are more reliable for prediction of fluid responsiveness compared to the static parameters. Fluid responsiveness does not equate to fluid administration in all patients and there should be indication for fluid loading. Effectiveness of fluid loading should be judged by improvement in tissue oxygenation and not by hemodynamic parameters alone. Excessive fluid therapy leading to hypervolemia can lead to complications such as edema, pulmonary edema, gut edema, and abdominal compartment syndrome. Excessive fluid loading is associated with increased complications, mortality, and length of ICU stay.

"Intellectuals solve problems, geniuses prevent them"

—Albert Einstein

INTRODUCTION

Intravenous fluid therapy is a common intervention in critically ill patient. Indications for fluid therapy in ICU are resuscitation in shock, maintenance, and replacement therapy. The goal of fluid therapy is to improve tissue oxygenation in patients with acute circulatory failure. Resuscitation fluids are used to correct acute hypovolemia or an intravascular volume deficit. Maintenance fluids are given to patients who are not able to take orally but do not have hypotension or ongoing losses. The basic daily needs are water about 25–30 mL/kg of body weight, 1 mmol/kg potassium, 1–1.5 mmol/kg sodium, and glucose 1.4–1.6 g/kg. Replacement fluids are fluids given to replace losses such as gastrointestinal loss, drains, polyuria, and excessive sweating.

Common types of fluids used in critical care unit are crystalloids and colloids. Crystalloids are solutions of salts or dextrose. Examples of crystalloids are 0.9% saline, Ringer's lactate, 5% dextrose, dextrose normal saline etc. Colloids are solutions containing large insoluble molecules. Examples of colloids are albumin, dextran, gelatin, and starches.

The goal of fluid therapy during resuscitation is to increase the preload by increasing venous return leading to increase in cardiac output and hence tissue oxygenation. Inadequate fluid therapy can lead to nonresolution of shock, inappropriate excessive vasopressors, and poor tissue oxygenation which can worsen outcome. However, fluid therapy is not without complications. Recent evidence suggests hypervolemia leads to edema of various organs and is associated with increased mortality, complications, length of hospital, and ICU stay. Hence fluid therapy should be treated like any other drug and its administration should be tailored to patient's needs. Fluid should only be administered to a fluid responder. Thus predicting fluid responsiveness is essential, as fluid administration in a fluid nonresponder is not beneficial and may even cause harm.

FLUID RESPONSIVENESS

Fluid responsiveness or *volume responsiveness* is a state where administration of fluid will lead to improvement in the stroke volume and hence the cardiac output. According to the Frank–Starling law of the heart, stroke volume is dependent on end-diastolic volume and forms a curvilinear shape. Increase in stroke volume is seen when preload increases when the ventricle is functioning on steep part of the curve (fluid responder), whereas increase in preload

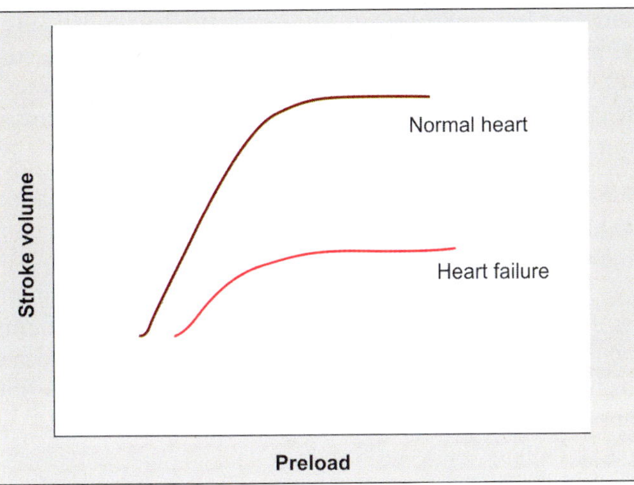

FIGURE 1: Frank–Starling curve showing the relationship between end-diastolic left ventricular volume, i.e., preload with stroke volume in the normal heart and in patients with heart failure.

leads to minimal change in stroke volume when the ventricle lies in flat portion of curve (fluid nonresponder). In patients with normal left ventricular function, usually both ventricles operate on steep portion of Frank–Starling curve. Patients with depressed left ventricle function as in failure, this curve is flatter and hence giving fluids in such patients will not lead to increase in stroke volume (**Fig. 1**). Echocardiography can be done at the bedside to determine the left ventricular function prior to administration of fluids.

During initial phase of hypovolemic or septic shock, most patients have some degree of intravascular fluid deficit and usually respond to fluid bolus. The Surviving Sepsis Campaign recommends an initial volume of 30 mL/kg body weight of fluids for a patient with septic shock. When patient continues to remain in shock despite resuscitation, further fluid therapy should be guided by assessment of fluid responsiveness.

The gold standard to assess fluid responsiveness is to give fluid bolus and see the changes in stroke volume or cardiac output. A fluid responder is one whom there is an increase in the stroke volume or cardiac output by >10–15% on administration of fluid bolus. Conventional fluid bolus consists of giving 500 mL of fluid over 30 minutes. The increase in stroke volume or cardiac output is assessed by real-time measurement as blood pressure may not reliably track changes in cardiac output. However, repeated fluid boluses in a nonresponder can lead to fluid overload and lead to complications like increase in extravascular lung water (EVLW), cor pulmonale etc.

Mini-fluid challenge was proposed to avoid administration of large volume and consists of administration of 100 mL of colloid over 1 minute and observing changes in left ventricular outflow tract (LVOT) velocity time integral (VTI). LVOT VTI change >10% predicts fluid responsiveness with 95% sensitivity and 78% specificity. As the volume given is less, only small changes in cardiac output are observed. Thus this needs an expert echocardiographer to assess the response. In addition, repeated assessments with mini-fluid challenge can also lead to fluid overload. Hence it is better to be able to predict fluid responsiveness, rather than give fluid boluses to assess fluid responsiveness.

PREDICTING FLUID RESPONSIVENESS

Fluid responsiveness can also be predicted by using various static and dynamic parameters which suggest that patient ventricle may lie in steep portion of Frank–Starling curve and will respond to fluid bolus with increase in stroke volume.

STATIC INDICES OF FLUID RESPONSIVENESS

Static parameters are based on the evaluation of cardiovascular pressures and volumes. Central venous pressure (CVP) and pulmonary artery occlusion pressure (PAOP) are the commonly used static parameters which are markers of right ventricular and left ventricular preload, respectively. Absolute values of CVP and PAOP do not determine fluid responsiveness accurately. Studies which looked at CVP and PAOP as predictors of fluid responsiveness found that baseline CVP was similar in responders and nonresponders. Hence it was concluded that CVP correlated poorly with intravascular volume and it should not be used for fluid administration. Studies which looked at PAOP found that no specific value of PAOP was able to predict if patient would be fluid responder. Ventricular volumes such as left ventricular end-diastolic volume and area have also been used as static measures of fluid responsiveness. However, these measures are dependent on ventricular compliance and hence are not accurate.

DYNAMIC INDICES OF FLUID RESPONSIVENESS BASED ON HEART–LUNG INTERACTIONS

These are dynamic tests used to predict fluid responsiveness which is based on the changes in preload during mechanical ventilation. In mechanically ventilated patient, changes in preload occur due to heart–lung interactions. The intrathoracic and transpulmonary pressures increase during inspiration in a mechanically ventilated patient which leads to decrease in venous return and increase in right ventricular afterload, with a consequent fall in right ventricular output. The pulmonary vessels are squeezed which leads to increased left ventricular preload and decrease in transmural pressure (pressure inside ventricle-pressure outside ventricle) and hence afterload which leads to increased stroke volume. After two or three beats, the previous fall in right ventricular output will produce a decrease in left ventricular preload and hence output in the expiratory phase. Cyclical changes in left ventricle stroke volume with maximum during inspiration and minimum during expiration are seen. When the patient is preload dependent these changes are greatly increased.

Pulse pressure variation and stroke volume variation: Pulse pressure variation (PPV) is the difference between the maximum and minimum pulse pressure value over one ventilatory cycle, divided by the average of the two values. Stroke volume variation (SVV) can be determined by analysis of arterial pressure waveform. Cardiac output monitors both calibrated and uncalibrated can determine SVV. PPV and SVV are usually high in fluid responsive patients whereas low values are seen in fluid unresponsive patient. Studies have shown that SVV > 10% predicts fluid responsiveness with high sensitivity and specificity whereas the cut-off value for PPV is 12–13% in mechanically ventilated patient with tidal volume (Vt) > 8 mL/kg. PPV and SVV are not reliable in patients with spontaneously breathing, low Vt ventilation, arrhythmias, open thorax, and increased intra-abdominal pressures.

Tidal volume challenge test: During low Vt ventilation [Vt ≤ 6 mL/kg PBW (predicted body weight)], the dynamic indices like PPV and SVV are not reliable in predicting fluid responsiveness. A low Vt may not be sufficient to produce significant change in the intrathoracic pressure, thus making these indices indicate a fluid nonresponsive state even in a fluid responder. This may limit the use of PPV and SVV during low tidal ventilation. To overcome this limitation, a new test called the "tidal volume challenge (TVC)" was proposed. This test can improve the reliability of PPV and SVV during low Vt ventilation. The test is performed by transiently increasing Vt from 6 mL/kg PBW to 8 mL/kg PBW for 1 minute and observing the change in PPV (ΔPPV6–8) and SVV (ΔSVV6–8) from baseline to that at 8 mL/kg PBW. A change in PPV of 3.5% or SVV of 2.5%, after performing the Vt challenge, reliably predicted fluid responsiveness. This test is very simple to perform at the bedside without changing the position of the patient. When used with PPV, cardiac output monitoring is not required, making this test applicable for use even in resource-limited settings.

Echocardiographic assessment of inferior vena cava: Echocardiography can be utilized to visualize great vessels and assess their variability with respiration. In patients who are mechanically ventilated, inspiration leads to distension of inferior vena cava (IVC) and the distensibility index = maximum diameter – minimum diameter/minimum diameter is calculated. A *distensibility index* >18% indicates fluid responsiveness. Superior vena cava (SVC) collapsibility in the thorax during mechanical ventilation can be assessed using a transesophageal echocardiography; a value >36% suggests fluid responsiveness. This is unreliable in spontaneously breathing patients and low Vt ventilation, however, it is reliable in patients with arrhythmias.

End-expiratory occlusion test: End-expiratory occlusion test (EEOT) is performed in a mechanically ventilated patient by giving a 15-second hold at the end of expiration. There is prevention of increase in intrathoracic pressure with application of expiratory hold which will lead to increase in venous return and hence preload which leads to increase in stroke volume and cardiac output. The cut-off value for prediction of fluid responsiveness is increase in cardiac output >5%. This test requires continuous cardiac output monitoring.

Plethysmographic variability index: Respiratory variation in plethysmographic reading is plethysmographic variation index. The cut-off for prediction of fluid responsiveness in mechanically ventilated patients is 14–17%. Main limitation of this technique is inadequate signal capture in patients whose peripheries are cold as in shock. It has been found to be unreliable in patients on vasopressors. Hence the applicability of plethysmographic variability index (PVI) in ICU patients in shock is limited.

DYNAMIC TEST OF FLUID RESPONSIVENESS INDEPENDENT OF HEART–LUNG INTERACTIONS

Passive leg raising test (PLRT): This test is a dynamic measure of fluid responsiveness which is not dependent on heart–lung interactions. This test involves transiently raising the legs to 45° from the horizontal. This leads to autotransfusion of blood from the limbs and splanchnic circulation into the heart leading to increase in preload and hence cardiac output. Cut-off value for prediction of fluid responsiveness with PLRT is an increase in cardiac output by 10%. Since this test does not depend on heart–lung interactions, it is not limited by the presence of low Vt ventilation, arrhythmias, or an open thorax. This test can be performed in ventilated or spontaneously breathing patients. The main advantage of this test is its completely reversible on changing patient position. PLRT is contraindicated in patients with raised intra-cranial pressure, raised intra-abdominal pressure and in those who require immobilization.

Several studies suggest superiority of dynamic parameters over static parameters. Surviving sepsis campaign guidelines suggest use of dynamic parameters over static parameters for assessment of fluid responsiveness. Even though these tests predict fluid responsiveness with reasonable accuracy, it is important to note that fluid responsiveness does not equate to hypovolemia and is not an indication for fluid therapy.

CRITERIA FOR FLUID ADMINISTRATION

- *The patient should have acute circulatory failure*: Fluid therapy should be initiated only when a patient is in acute circulatory failure. A normal patient may also be fluid responsive, but this is not an indication to administer fluids.
- *The patient should be fluid responsive*: Fluid responsiveness is defined as increase in cardiac output following fluid administration.
- *There should be no risk of giving fluids*: Patient with conditions such as cardiac dysfunction, acute respiratory distress syndrome (ARDS), and renal

failure may be at high risk of complications with fluid administration. In such patient fluid administration is avoided even if the patient is a fluid responder, if the risk of administering fluids is high.

EFFECTIVENESS

Effectiveness of fluid administration should not be judged by an increase in cardiac output alone, rather from an improvement in tissue oxygenation. The resolution of organ failure caused by shock, like acute kidney injury, indicates that tissue perfusion has improved. Improvement in oxygenation should be assessed using indices like lactate, central/mixed venous oxygen saturation ($ScvO_2/SvO_2$) and the ratio of partial pressure of carbon dioxide (pCO_2) gap (venoarterial difference in carbon dioxide pressure), and the arteriovenous difference in oxygen content, as this reflects anaerobic metabolism more directly (pCO_2 gap/O_2 content difference). It is as reliable as lactate to indicate that tissue oxygenation improves with fluid therapy, with the potential advantage of decreasing more rapidly than lactates.

COMPLICATIONS

Excessive fluid administration can lead to edema which in turn results in altered organ function. Altered capillary permeability and hypo-oncocity can lead to edema formation even when circulating blood volume is not increased. Hypervolemia can lead to pulmonary edema which results in altered gas exchange. Edema in other organs can lead to raised intracranial pressure, abdominal wall edema, hepatic congestion, gut edema, abdominal compartment syndrome, renal interstitial edema, and impaired wound healing. Excessive fluid loading leading to positive balance is associated with increased complications, mortality, and length of ICU stay. Fluids should be given with caution in patients with ARDS, underlying pulmonary parenchymal disease, cardiac failure, and renal dysfunction. Alternative therapies like use of vasopressors should be considered for the treatment of shock, even in fluid responders, when the risk of giving fluids is high.

Fluid overload can be assessed clinically and on examination using chest radiography (features suggestive of pulmonary edema), lung ultrasound (appearance of B-lines), and using advanced hemodynamic monitoring indices like EVLW and pulmonary vascular permeability index (PVPI) which are obtained using transpulmonary thermodilution devices like VolumeView™ and PiCCO™. EVLW is the fluid that accumulates in the interstitial and alveolar spaces. The value increases in case of hydrostatic pulmonary edema like in ARDS. PVPI is the ratio of EVLW over pulmonary blood volume, i.e., the ratio of the fluid volume that is out of the vessels over the fluid volume that remains in the vessels. High value of EVLW along with PVPI indicates that fluid therapy should be withheld, even if the patient is fluid responsive.

RECOMMENDED READINGS

1. Pinsky MR, Brophy P, Padilla J, Paganini E, Pannu N. Fluid and volume monitoring. Int J Artif Organs. 2008;31:111-26.
2. Jozwiak M, Hamzaoui O, Monnet X, Teboul JL. Fluid resuscitation during early sepsis: a need for individualization. Minerva Anestesiol. 2018;84:987-92.
3. Cecconi M, Parsons AK, Rhodes A. What is a fluid challenge? Curr Opin Crit Care. 2011;17:290-5.
4. Vincent JL, Weil MH. Fluid challenge revisited. Crit Care Med. 2006;34:1333-7.
5. Monnet X, Marik P, Teboul JL. Prediction of fluid responsiveness: an update. Ann Intensive Care. 2016;6:111.
6. Michard F, Teboul JL. Using heart lung interactions to assess fluid responsiveness during mechanical ventilation. Crit Care. 2000;4:282-9.
7. Myatra SN, Monnet X, Teboul JL. Use of 'tidal volume challenge' to improve the reliability of pulse pressure variation. Crit Care. 2017;21:60.
8. Myatra SN, Prabu NR, Divatia JV, Monnet X, Kulkarni AP, Teboul JL. The Changes in Pulse Pressure Variation or Stroke Volume Variation After a "Tidal Volume Challenge" Reliably Predict Fluid Responsiveness During Low Tidal Volume Ventilation. Crit Care Med. 2017;45:415-21.
9. Vignon P, Repessé X, Begot E, Léger J, Jacob C, Bouferrache K, et al. Comparison of echocardiographic indices used to predict fluid responsiveness in ventilated patients. Am J Respir Crit Care Med. 2017;195(8):1022-32.
10. Monnet X, Teboul JL. Passive leg raising. Intensive Care Med. 2008;34:659-63.
11. Monnet X, Teboul JL. Passive leg raising: five rules, not a drop of fluid! Crit Care. 2015;19:18.

CHAPTER 72

Oxygen Therapy

Pawan Kumar Singh, Dhruva Chaudhry

ABSTRACT

Oxygen is one of the most commonly prescribed drugs. And just like any other drug, it has its own indications, doses, and adverse effects. Oxygen therapy prescription is a commonly ignored learning exercise. This lack of knowledge of prescription practice adds to the overuse of oxygen therapy. In this chapter, the details of oxygen therapy and the methods of its prescription are discussed. In addition, the target of this chapter is to make its reader (postgraduate students) more familiar with oxygen generating as well as delivery devices. The different setting and types of oxygen therapy have been elaborated. And in the end, the adverse effects of oxygen therapy have been touched upon. It is intended that by the end of this chapter, the students must be able to justify, write, and prescribe oxygen therapy in a more efficient and evidence-based manner.

"The trick to life is to just keep breathing"

—Johnny Lung

INTRODUCTION

Labeling *oxygen* as a drug is not just a matter of semantics but also highlights its properties. Like any other drug, oxygen, is supplemented to the needed, is prescribed in dose-dependent manner, it saves lives and what is most important is, *oxygen* causes adverse events when used inappropriately. Common misconception of oxygen being harmless had been embedded into practice for decades. *Oxygen can be never be given enough* has been the traditional thinking. This has been despite various authors having documented the adverse effects of oxygen in chronic obstructive pulmonary disease (COPD) as well as other disease.

Oxygen constitutes nearly 20% of the ambient atmosphere at sea level. There have been several documented uses of oxygen supplementation but very few of them are therapeutic. In most of the cases, oxygen is supplemented in subjects where it is deficient, like in vitamin deficiencies. The duration of supplementation as well as the route of supplementation is guided by the clinical condition. Therapeutic uses of oxygen are limited like diabetic ulcer management, carbon monoxide poisoning, arterial gas embolism, and decompression sickness. Similarly, injudicious oxygen supplementation has been associated with some of the severe and glaring adverse events especially in neonatal age group like bronchopulmonary dysplasia and retinopathy of prematurity. In this chapter, we will be focusing mainly on the art of prescribing oxygen supplementation (**Box 1**). Subjects having medium (noninvasive ventilation) or high dependency (invasive positive-pressure ventilation) on oxygenation or ventilation will not be discussed here.

BOX 1	Aims of this chapter.
After reading this chapter, one must know:	
• How to write a prescription of oxygen supplementation?	
• How to choose oxygen delivery device interface?	
• How to choose a device for domiciliary oxygen therapy?	
• Patient-friendly and pocket-friendly judicious use of oxygen therapy	

INDICATIONS

The most common indication of oxygen therapy is its deficiency, i.e., hypoxia. Discussion on hypoxia is beyond the scope of this chapter. There are five types of hypoxias [(1) atmospheric hypoxia, (2) hypoventilation hypoxia, (3) hypoxia caused by impaired alveolar membrane diffusion, (4) hypoxia due to abnormal transport, and (5) finally hypoxia due to impaired tissue utilization]. The benefits as well as harms of use of oxygen therapy in each type of hypoxia are not uniform.

Atmospheric hypoxia: This is one of the most empiric uses of oxygen therapy. The mechanism is simple and lies in the mechanism of hypoxia. Partial pressure and concentration of oxygen in the ambient air are lower than physiological requirement and hence it is met by external supplementation.

Hypoventilation hypoxia: This type of hypoxia is usually due to lack of respiratory drive or due to lack of adequate ventilation of the terminal alveoli. There is usually no fallacy in the ambient atmospheric oxygen supplementation or the alveolar membrane oxygen diffusion. This type of hypoxia is usually accompanied with rise in partial pressure of carbon dioxide in the arterial blood. Most common causes of such hypoxias are sleep-related breathing disorders. Oxygen supplementation is usually not recommended in such cases and improvement in ventilation is the primary modality of management, either with pharmacological approach or positive ventilation therapies.

Hypoxia due to impaired alveolar diffusion: It is the most common indication of oxygen supplementation. Common diagnosis in such types of hypoxia is pulmonary edema, acute respiratory distress syndrome (ARDS), and emphysema. Most of the indications in this category are acute and temporary but some of them are chronic, requiring domiciliary oxygen therapy. In acute settings, oxygen therapy can be lifesaving as well as time buying especially in ARDS and pulmonary edema. In COPD and other end-stage pulmonary disease, oxygen therapy improves quality of life as well as survival.

Abnormalities in oxygen transport: Oxygen therapy has also been used for hypoxia, etiology of which has been related to abnormalities in oxygen transport. Transport-related abnormalities can be due to poor pulmonary circulation, hemoglobin deficiencies or structural abnormalities, and poisonings like carbon monoxide and methemoglobinemia. Given the heterogeneity of etiologies in this category, the individual treatments also are varied and so is the role of oxygen therapy. Hyperbaric oxygen therapy has been used as therapeutic modalities in carbon monoxide and methemoglobinemia.

Tissue level hypoxias: They have a limited role of oxygen therapy. This is due to inability of tissues to utilize oxygen even when the blood levels of oxygen are by far near normal. Various etiologies falling into this category are cyanide poisoning, sepsis etc. Extraction of oxygen from the blood is abnormal in these conditions and it is reflected in the rising level of venous oxygenation.

TYPES OF OXYGEN THERAPY

Broadly, oxygen therapy can be categorized based on two parameters (1) Place of administration and (2) Flow of administration. Currently, oxygen therapy is not restricted to hospitals or even acute conditions. With the advent of technologies and availability of oxygen, the benefits derived from this therapy can be numerous and hence its application.

BASED ON PLACE OF ADMINISTRATION

Hospital setting: Predominantly used in acute conditions, oxygen therapy finds its use in various indications. Oxygen therapy is mostly used in emergency departments, intensive care units, and high dependency unit. Also, hospital setting is a place where oxygen is most over-used and ill-prescribed. In a review on prescription and administration practices of oxygen therapy, it was found that only 55% of the patients had a valid prescription for oxygen. Administration practices were even poorer. Since the release of 2008 British Thoracic Society (BTS) guidelines on acute oxygen administration, there has been a consistent improvement in the administration practices, but prescription trends are still below par.

Domiciliary oxygen therapy: In advanced stage of COPD, long-term oxygen therapy has been proven to improve survival. This has been translated into various other trials to expand the scope of home oxygen therapy prescription. Different indications like interstitial lung diseases, bronchiectasis, and penultimate stages of COPD have been studied to be an indication of home oxygen therapy. Oxygen therapy has been found to improve survival, quality of life, exercise tolerance as well as dependence on caregivers. The spectrum of indications of domiciliary oxygen therapy has seen a recent expansion due to the pandemic of coronavirus disease 2019 (COVID-19). Apart from steroids, only lifesaving proven medication was found to be oxygen. And with sudden spurt in number of hypoxic cases and unwarranted strain on the healthcare system, it was observed that a large section of hemodynamically stable but hypoxic patients were discharged with domiciliary oxygen therapy. This practice has not only allowed decongestion of emergency departments but also has contributed to fall in overall mortality rate.

BASED ON FLOW OF ADMINISTRATION

A more scientific and practical way of classifying oxygen therapy is based on flow with which oxygen is provided. In all spontaneously breathing hypoxic patients in whom oxygen therapy is being prescribed, the flow is based on degree of hypoxia, diagnosis, and ancillary factors like cost and comfort. Among low dependency systems, the flow of oxygen supplied can be either fixed performance or variable performance.

Low-flow devices: Oxygen supplied through these devices provides a variable performance. Performance here means the fraction of oxygen in inspired air. For example, a subject inhaling oxygen through nasal prongs at 2 liters per minute (LPM) with a minute ventilation of 10 LPM (respiratory rate of 20 breaths/min with tidal volume of 500 mL) is inhaling 8 liters of room air and 2 liters of 100% oxygen at any given time. Similarly, if the minute ventilation of same subject changes, the fraction of inspired oxygen (FiO_2) will also change. This way nasal prongs can provide a variable performance despite a consistent flow. Examples of such devices are nasal cannula, face masks, rebreathing masks etc.

These devices are commonly used in patients where oxygen demand is low (acute exacerbation of COPD and end-stage lung diseases) and in domiciliary oxygen therapy where the wastage of oxygen must be prevented.

High-flow devices: As the name suggests, these devices provide a consistent oxygen flow and can maintain a consistent FiO_2. There can be two main mechanisms through which consistent FiO_2 can be maintained—first, inhalation is done from a reservoir where there is no mixing with exhaled air (for example Hudson mask and oxygen mask with nonreservoir bags) and second, oxygen flow is high enough to meet the minute ventilation demand of the patient and hence whatever patient is inhaling has minimum mixing with room air. Examples of such devices are high-flow nasal cannula (HFNC), Hudson mask, and venturi mask with jet mixing.

High-flow devices are used only in acute care, hospital settings as they require consistent and high level of oxygen back-up supply. Such high demands are seen in patients of ARDS, pulmonary edema, and sepsis.

The differences in two types of devices are outlined in **Table 1**.

PRESCRIPTION

In the field of oxygen therapy, one of the most ignored fields is prescription of oxygen therapy. This practice is consistently flawed even in the best of centers. There are two main aims of any prescription are:

1. To document the administration of any drug
2. To set up an auto mode of treatment, which can be carried on by the nurses.

And like any treatment chart, it requires continuous checks, modifications, and a course of treatment. Empirically giving oxygen can only be short outcome measure in emergency department but not a uniform policy.

There are three components of any therapy prescription—(1) dose or rate, (2) route, and (3) target variable assessment. The easiest way of understanding is considering an example of noradrenaline infusion, started in order to maintain mean arterial pressure above a certain prespecified limit (target variable). To achieve the target variable, it is given at a certain rate and dilution (dose) and in a manner of intravenous infusion (route). Similarly, the prescription of oxygen therapy must contain these elements:

Target variable: Oxygen saturation is easily measurable variable. Due to significant linear correlation between partial pressure of oxygen and arterial saturation, there is hardly any indication of continuous arterial pricks (except for methemoglobinemia). The aim of saturation varies with diagnosis and other clinical parameters. In a resting state of acute illness, the commonly used saturation target is 92–94%, especially in ARDS. Similarly, in COPD the target is even lower due to several adverse effects of oxygen in patients of acute exacerbation of COPD. Target of 88% in resting state and 94% in ambulatory state is considered adequate in patients of COPD. Reaching of target for a finite period like 2 hours must be followed by decrease in flow and vice versa. This is just like a timely monitoring of vital to adjust the dose of inotropes.

Route (device) of administration: Route of oxygen administration is inhalation (except for in cases of extracorporeal oxygenation, where it is given intravenous) but this subheading must also consider the device of administration. As will be covered in the upcoming subsection, there are several devices for oxygen supplementation mainly based on the requirement and comfort for the patient.

Dose/rate of administration: Like any drug, the prescription of oxygen therapy must contain the rate of administration. Preferable there should be narrow range provided for the flow. It gives a working independence to the caregivers to modify the flow according to the target. This flow must also take into consideration the device which is being used for oxygenation.

Table 2 gives examples of both flawed and accurate oxygen therapy prescriptions. It must be remembered that writing a prescription does not end with the advice but requires continuous modifications according to the clinical status of the patient. It is also mandatory to train the ground level workers (nurses, attendants, and caregivers) on how to measure and change the oxygen flow.

TABLE 1 The types of devices for oxygen therapy.

Low-flow oxygen devices	High-flow oxygen devices
Unable to deliver a consistent FiO_2	Maintains a consistent flow
Flow 2–8 L/min	Flow more than the minute ventilation
Mixing of oxygen with room air	Minimal mixing
FiO_2 varies with the tidal volume	FiO_2 remains consistent
Used in cases where FiO_2 requirement is low, e.g., COPD, ILD etc.	Used in cases where minute ventilation and hypoxia are severe, e.g., ARDS, and pulmonary edema
Example: Nasal cannula and face masks	*Example*: HFNC, Hudson mask, and venturi-mask

(FiO_2: fraction of inspired oxygen; ILD: interstitial lung disease; HFNC: high-flow nasal cannula)

TABLE 2 Examples of correct and incorrect methods of oxygen prescription.

Domiciliary setting		
	Oxygen supplementation at 2 LPM through nasal prongs from oxygen concentrator for at least 16 hours a day	Target saturation 88–92% (resting) (Increase flow during exercise/exertion or fall in saturation)
Acute care setting		
Wrong prescription	Oxygen at 8 LPM	
Correct prescription	Oxygen supplementation at 8 LPM from wall mount though venturi mask throughout the day	Avoid exertion, bedside toiletry to be arranged

(LPM: liters per minute)

DEVICES

There are three types of oxygen-generating devices commonly available and used. The use of such devices is dependent upon setting, availability, and cost of usage. In acute care settings, there was dominance of liquid oxygen cylinders for meeting up the hospital needs and requirements but recently there has been surge of use of on-site gas generation systems.

HOSPITAL SETTING

Liquid oxygen cylinder: Oxygen plants in hospital commonly have 10,000 liter cylinders (**Fig. 1**). These types of cylinders are used for continuous supply all over the hospital. Cylinders are refilled on-demand basis.

On-site gas systems: On-site oxygen and nitrogen generation plants use electricity and ambient air to provide purified oxygen/nitrogen. It is being realized that not only it is more reliable but also is more economical (**Fig. 2**).

Compressed gas cylinder: Rarely in remote location and small hospitals, compressed oxygen is supplied using type H cylinders. They are usually seen in low-capacity centers and daycare units.

DOMICILIARY OXYGEN THERAPY

Oxygen cylinder: One of the most used devices for home oxygen supply is the crude cylinder containing compressed gas. They come in various sizes and require to be refilled frequently. They have benefits of not being dependent on electricity and a low installation cost with portability. But the overall cost which includes refilling and transportations comes out to be high. The commonly used cylinder is type E and C cylinders with capacity of 680 liter and 170 liters, respectively.

Liquid oxygen: Compressed and cooled oxygen acts like a cryogenic fluid with a boiling point of –183°C. As per the expansion ratio, one liter of liquid oxygen expands to occupy 860 liters of oxygen at room air. Maintaining a purity of >99%, it is one of the most cost-effective and portable types of oxygen supply at home. It does not require electricity to be operational. In cases where there is high-flow requirement, there can be icing at the outlet nozzles and intermittent de-icing or warming may be needed. Otherwise, low-flow oxygen supplementations do not require humidification or warming. Compressed liquid oxygen chamber can even provide prolonged ambulation and mobility. Refill is easy and less frequently needed than compressed oxygen cylinders.

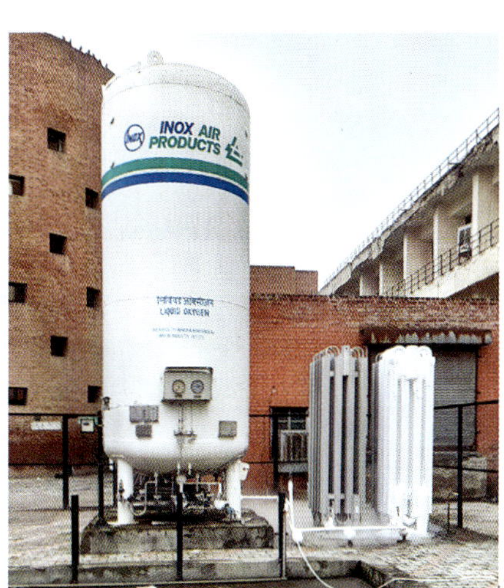

FIGURE 1: Liquid oxygen 10,000 liter cylinder in gas plant of a tertiary care hospital.

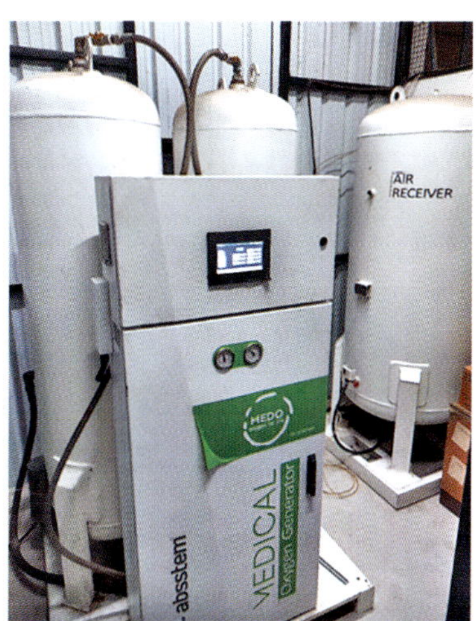

FIGURE 2: On-site oxygen generation using the oxygen concentrator technology, catering to entire hospital.

TABLE 3 Devices commonly available for domiciliary oxygen therapy with their characteristics.

	Oxygen concentrators	Compressed oxygen cylinders	Liquid nitrogen
Power source	Yes	No	No
Refilling required	No	Frequently	Yes but less frequently
Availability	Easily	Easily	Difficult outside major cities
Mobility	Limited	Yes	Yes
Exhaustible supply	No	Yes	Yes
Installation cost	Significant	Minimal	Minimal
Maintenance	Minimal	None	Minimal
Operational cost	Minimal	Significant transportation and refill charges	Infrequent but refill charges are present

Oxygen concentrators: Commonly available and frequently recommended nowadays, oxygen concentrators (**Fig. 3**) provide a rich, safe, and continuous source of oxygen at home. They work on principle of adsorption of nitrogen and other gases following filtration. Only limitation is continuous dependence on electricity, even though battery operated, and mobile units are also emerging, but cost is prohibitive for some patients.

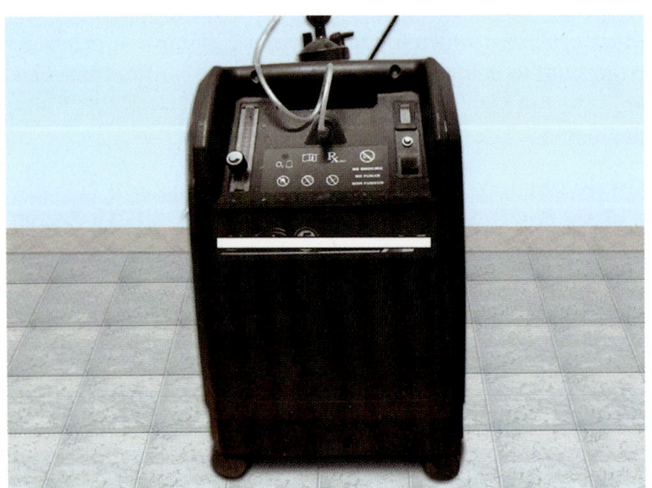

FIGURE 3: Oxygen concentrator with flowmeter for domiciliary use.

Comparison between the three modes of oxygenation is provided in **Table 3**.

INTERFACE DEVICES

The most common devices used in domiciliary settings are nasal prongs, which can provide, mobility and less obstructive toward communication, eating, and drinking. There are several other types of interface devices which are compatible with various ranges of oxygen flows (**Figs. 4 A** to **D**).

Nasal cannula: They are the most common devices and are suitable to provide 1–6 LPM of oxygen flow. Oxygen accumulates in the nasopharynx and the concentrated oxygen is inhaled subsequently. Nasal prongs can provide FiO_2 of up to 40–45%. They have an added advantage of being convenient to the patients. Patients with nasal polyps and deviated nasal spectrum might find it difficult for use.

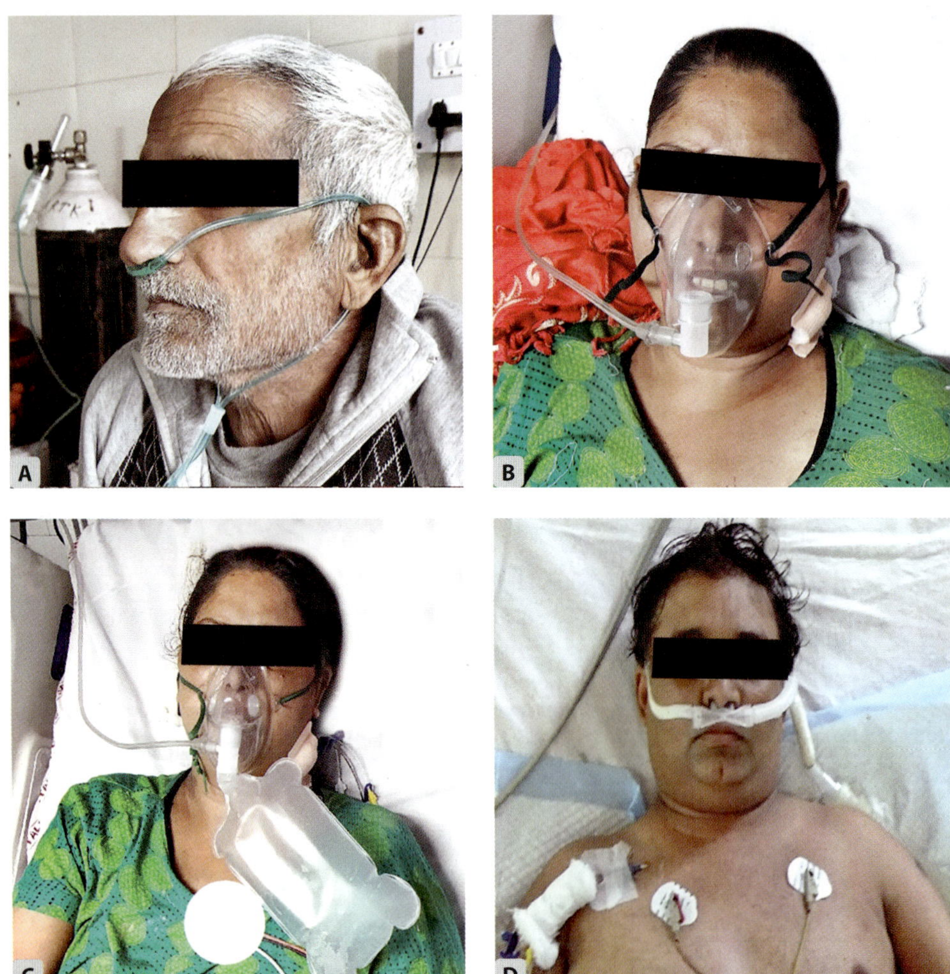

(ARDS: acute respiratory distress syndrome; ICU: intensive care unit)

FIGURES 4 A to D: Images of different devices used as interface in oxygen therapy. **(A)** Nasal prongs with correct technique of usage so that the joint is in front of neck and not behind the head. **(B)** Face mask on patient in ward. **(C)** Nonrebreathing mask with reservoir bag. **(D)** High-flow nasal cannula in a patient of ARDS in ICU.

Simple face mask: Higher flow of 5–10 LPM may require additional chamber for oxygen accumulation which is provided by simple face mask. Simple face mask has side ports for exhalation as well as mixing of room air with oxygen. FiO_2 varies with the flow, minute ventilation and the tight fitting of the face mask.

Venturi masks: These masks provide oxygen through a jet and using the side ports (the size of which can be calibrated) and allow mixing of room air with oxygen using Bernoulli's principle. FiO_2 as high as 50% can be delivered depending upon patients' minute ventilation. There are two side ports with valves in the mask for exhalation. Usually, there are marking or color coding to provide accurate FiO_2 to the patients as per the requirement (**Figs. 5 A** and **B**).

Masks with reservoir bags: Oxygen flow in continuous when connected with masks, even in expiration. To counter this wastage of oxygen, reservoir bags are connected in between the mask and oxygen inlet. This bag fills with oxygen during expiration and inhalation takes place from the oxygen in the bag, this way a higher FiO_2 can be provided, while at the same time avoiding the wastage of oxygen. There are two types of mask with reservoir bags:

1. *Rebreathing:* As the name suggests, there is no valve between mask and reservoir bag. This allows mixing of exhaled air and oxygen, therefore diluting the final mixture of inhaled oxygen.
2. *Nonrebreathing:* In this type of device, there is a valve which prevents the entry of exhaled air into the reservoir bag and hence nearly 100% oxygen is inhaled by the patient.

High-flow nasal cannula: Though a part of oxygen therapy, HFNC has become a hot topic of discussion. The umbrella of indication of use of HFNC is expanding day by day. The recent COVID-19 pandemic has seen a major surge in the use of HFNC. Basically, it is a device which can provide heated, humidified, oxygen at unconventionally high-flow rates. It consists of flow generator, air and oxygen blender, a humidifier, and specialized nasal cannulas. Modern HFNC machines can provide a flow of as high as 60–80 LPM with nearly 100% FiO_2. The evidence and use of HFNC are beyond the scope of this chapter but in summary, currently HFNC can be used in hypoxemic nonhypercapnic respiratory failures of mild-to-moderate severity.

ADVERSE EFFECTS

As has been reiterated previously, oxygen like any other drug is not free of adverse effects. This concept is being recognized more commonly nowadays and is being labeled as *oxygen toxicity*. The common mechanism of this toxicity is:

Generation of free radicals: Hyperoxemia caused due to high FiO_2 leads to formation of free radicals from mitochondria (hydroxyl and superoxide). Intense production of these reactive oxygen species leads to oxidative stress which is manifested at molecular level in form of damage to nucleic acids and protein denaturation. At clinical level, this is translated into worsening of ARDS and subsequent fibrosis.

Cardiovascular effects: Oxygen acts on peripheral chemoreceptors and starts a cascade which causes diverse physiological changes like vasoconstriction, decrease in cardiac output, and fall in heart rate.

Central nervous system (CNS): It is also known as Bert effect; CNS manifestations of oxygen toxicity are mainly seen in cases of hyperbaric oxygen therapy. It manifests in form of headaches, seizures, nausea, dizziness, visual, or auditory symptoms.

Hypercapnia: Rise in pCO_2 in arterial blood is one of the most common and well-described side effects of oxygen therapy. It is commonly observed in cases of COPD and its acute exacerbation. The mechanisms are Haldane effect (liberation of CO_2 from hemoglobin in presence of oxygen), ventilation perfusion mismatch worsening secondary to pulmonary vasodilation on exposure to oxygen, absorption atelectasis, and minor contribution of withdrawal of hypoxic stimulus of respiratory center.

Delay in recognition of clinical deterioration: Due to the sigmoid shape of oxygen-hemoglobin curve, even when

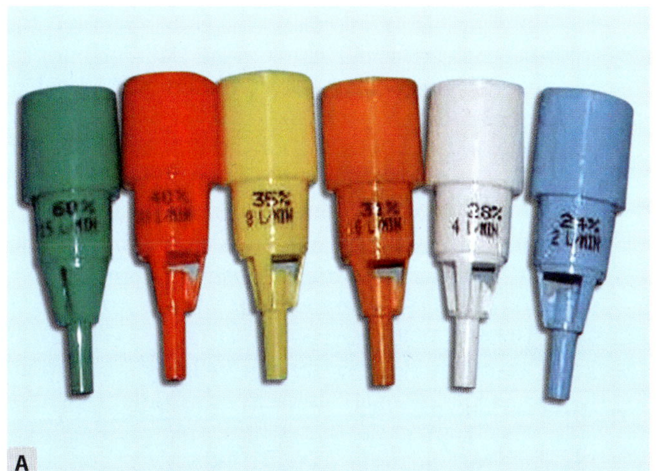

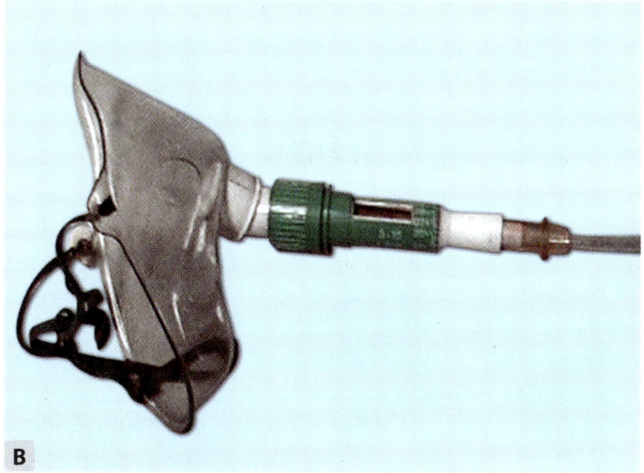

FIGURES 5 A & B: Two types of venturi mask: (A) Color coded; and (B) Port rotatory mask.

there is fall in PaO_2, the saturation may stay to be persistently high. This happens when there is clinical worsening of ARDS. Fall of saturation from 100 to 96% is rarely recognized but the same fall from 92 to 88% is easily picked up and is more representative of clinical worsening. Hyperoxia prevents timely acknowledgment of clinical deterioration.

High mortality rates: High oxygen supplementation has been associated with higher mortality among CPR survivors and poisoning cases. This has been attributed to coronary vasoconstriction as a result of supranormal oxygen supplementation and reactive oxygen species formation.

SPECIAL MENTIONS

HYPERBARIC OXYGEN THERAPY

Hyperbaric oxygen therapy has been found to be beneficial in treatment of diabetic ulcers, radiation injuries, gangrenes, air or gas embolism, decompression sickness, and other types of anaerobic infections and arterial insufficiencies. Correction of partial pressure of oxygen is not the primary mechanism of action but depends on the etiology as well. Decompression sickness utilizes the physical properties of gas to reduce the formation of air bubbles in vessels and wound healing utilizes the effects of hyperoxia on tissues which reduces inflammation, causes angiogenesis and other ancillary mechanisms. The details of use, mechanism, indication, and adverse effects can be found in other chapters.

HIGH-FLOW NASAL CANNULA

High-flow nasal cannula is specialized form of oxygen therapy which utilizes very high flows of heated and humidified oxygen for management. Currently, it is being mainly recommended for nonhypercapnic respiratory failures, but the use is being evaluated in hypercapnic respiratory failures are well. Such high-flow rates can generate minimal positive end-expiratory pressures, increased mucociliary clearance, and decrease in dead space with decreased work of breathing. These effects are, theoretically, responsible for added benefits of HFNC therapy. The details of setting up, indication, and evidence are provided elsewhere. Some specific adverse effects are the nasal mucosal damage (if humidification is lost), delay in intubation or noninvasive mechanical ventilation (NIV) application, and adverse effects of hyperoxia.

WEANING FROM OXYGEN

Taking a patient off oxygen therapy is as important as is putting him on. It is vital to monitor the oxygen requirement and identify the point when the oxygen requirement can be tapered. Following is an outline to taper the oxygen supplementation:

- Recovered or recovering basic condition for which oxygen was started.
- Maintenance of oxygen saturation for a prerequisite time period (like 2 hours or more) (targets in nonhypercapnic respiratory failure 92–94% and hypercapnic respiratory failure is 88–92%)
- Hemodynamic and respiratory stability
- Oxygen interface device suitable for low flows as well (for example nonrebreathing mask cannot be used for low flow of oxygen therapies and nasal cannula is incompatible with higher flows).
- Stepwise reduction in oxygen supplementation with decrease in flow (usually done in a multiple of 2).
- Take off oxygen therapy when flow is <2 LPM and rest of the criteria are fulfilled.
- Weaning is best done when it is possible to monitor the subject and deterioration can be picked up. It should be avoided in evening or night-time when the staff strength is low.

CONCLUSION

Oxygen therapy is one of the most commonly utilized modalities of supportive care. It has stood the test of time and its use and availability is only rising. Despite such high availability, the awareness about its prescription, use, and adverse effects is distressingly poor. Oxygen therapy not only adds to the cost of therapy but also is responsible for some side effects. Not only this with advancement of technology, but there are several types of devices for source and interface of oxygen therapy also. It is vital for any healthcare worker to know the types, their indication along with advantages and disadvantages so that prescription can be informed and adjusted as per the requirement of the patient.

RECOMMENDED READINGS

1. Tejada S, Batle JM, Ferrer MD, Busquets-Cortés C, Monserrat-Mesquida M, Nabavi SM, et al. Therapeutic effects of hyperbaric oxygen in the process of wound healing. Curr Pharm Des. 2019;25(15):1682-93.
2. Kirby JP. Hyperbaric oxygen therapy as an elective treatment. Mo Med. 2019;116(3):184-7.
3. Jobe AH. Mechanisms of lung injury and bronchopulmonary dysplasia. Am J Perinatol. 2016; 33(11): 1076-8.
4. Higgins RD. Oxygen saturation and retinopathy of prematurity. Clin Perinatol. 2019;46(3):593-9.
5. John E. Hall MEH. Respiratory Insufficiency—Pathophysiology, Diagnosis, Oxygen Therapy. In: John E. Hall MEH (Eds). Guyton and Hall Textbook of Medical Physiology, 14 edition. Netherlands: Elsevier; 2021. pp. 541-9.
6. Cousins JL, Wark PAB, McDonald VM. Acute oxygen therapy: a review of prescribing and delivery practices. Int J Chron Obstruct Pulmon Dis. 2016;11:1067-75.
7. Continuous or nocturnal oxygen therapy in hypoxemic chronic obstructive lung disease: a clinical trial. Nocturnal Oxygen Therapy Trial Group. Ann Intern Med. 1980;93(3):391-8.
8. Long term domiciliary oxygen therapy in chronic hypoxic cor pulmonale complicating chronic bronchitis and emphysema. Report of the Medical Research Council Working Party. Lancet. 1981;1(8222):681-6.

9. Chailleux E, Fauroux B, Binet F, Dautzenberg B, Polu JM. Predictors of survival in patients receiving domiciliary oxygen therapy or mechanical ventilation. A 10-year analysis of ANTADIR Observatory. Chest. 1996;109(3):741-9.
10. Bell EC, Cox NS, Goh N, Glaspole I, Westall GP, Watson A, et al. Oxygen therapy for interstitial lung disease: a systematic review. Eur Respir Rev. 2017;26(143):160080.
11. Khor YH, Goh NS, Glaspole I, Holland AE, McDonald CF. Exertional desaturation and prescription of ambulatory oxygen therapy in interstitial lung disease. Respir Care. 2019;64(3):299-306.
12. Sardesai I, Grover J, Garg M, Nanayakkara PWB, Di Somma S, Paladino L, et al. Short Term Home Oxygen Therapy for COVID-19 patients: The COVID-HOT algorithm. J Family Med Prim Care. 2020;9(7):3209-19.
13. Girardis M, Busani S, Damiani E, Donati A, Rinaldi L, Marudi A, et al. Effect of conservative vs conventional oxygen therapy on mortality among patients in an intensive care unit: The oxygen-ICU randomized clinical trial. JAMA. 2016;316(15):1583-9.
14. Branson RD. Oxygen therapy in COPD. Respir Care. 2018;63(6):734-48.
15. Hardavella G, Karampinis I, Frille A, Sreter K, Rousalova I. Oxygen devices and delivery systems. Breathe (Sheff). 2019;15(3):e108-e16.
16. Gürün Kaya A, Öz M, Erol S, Çiftçi F, Çiledağ A, Kaya A. High flow nasal cannula in COVID-19: a literature review. Tuberk Toraks. 2020;68(2):168-74.
17. Manning EP. Central nervous system oxygen toxicity and hyperbaric oxygen seizures. Aerosp Med Hum Perform. 2016;87(5):477-86.
18. O'Driscoll BR, Howard LS, Earis J, Mak V. British Thoracic Society Guideline for oxygen use in adults in healthcare and emergency settings. BMJ Open Respir Res. 2017;4(1):e000170.
19. Choudhury R. Hypoxia and hyperbaric oxygen therapy: A review. Int J Gen Med. 2018;11:431-42.
20. Helviz Y, Einav S. A systematic review of the high-flow nasal cannula for adult patients. Crit Care. 2018;22(1):71.

CHAPTER 73 Mechanical Ventilation: Principles and Strategies

Satya Ranjan Sahu, Kunal Ahuja, GC Khilnani

ABSTRACT

Mechanical ventilation is required in acute respiratory failure when patient is unable to maintain adequate oxygenation and/or removal of carbon dioxide with other noninvasive measures. They work by applying a positive pressure breath which is different from the natural negative pressure ventilation. This can alter the patient's hemodynamic status.

Modern day ventilators are highly advanced, and one can provide various modes of ventilation depending on the underlying disease. The assisted controlled mandatory ventilation (ACMV) is the most commonly used mode of mechanical ventilation. It can be delivered with a preset volume or pressure. Operator can adjust various parameters like the tidal volume (TV), rate, inspiratory flow rate (IFR), and the positive end-expiratory pressure (PEEP).

The mechanically ventilated patient needs continuous monitoring of hemodynamics and oxygenation. It needs a team approach for overall care of the patient and the underlying disease. The weaning protocol should be followed, and effort should be to use it for only as long as it is required. Once the reversible factors are controlled patients should be weaned off the mechanical ventilation.

"Formula for success: Under promise and over deliver"

—Thomas J Peters

INTRODUCTION

Mechanical ventilation is "a necessary evil": A lifesaving technique but with many potential complications which at times are life-threatening. The first description of endotracheal intubation and artificial ventilation was made in the 16th century, by Andreas Vesalius by insertion of a tube of reed into the trachea of animals and blowing air into its lungs to keep it alive. The first negative pressure ventilator was successfully used in clinical practice in the 20th century known as the "iron lungs." During the poliomyelitis epidemics of early 1950s, positive pressure ventilator techniques were developed on principle similar to techniques of Vesalius. The first efficient mechanical ventilators were developed by Claus Bang, a Danish physician and Carl Gunner Engstrom, a Swedish anesthesiologist. In 1972, the Servo 900A was released which was the first mechanical ventilator with PEEP, and Servo valves. The control of flow allowed the introduction of new modes of ventilation, such as pressure-controlled ventilation and pressure support ventilation (PSV). Subsequently the ventilators became progressively more compact, user friendly, and electronically based with advanced monitoring capabilities.

INDICATIONS

Mechanical ventilation is indicated in patients with acute respiratory failure when they are unable to maintain adequate oxygenation and/or remove carbon dioxide.

In critical care setting, the indications for using mechanical ventilation are primarily as follows:

- Protection of airways in a patient who is obtunded or has a dynamic airway, e.g., from trauma or oropharyngeal infection.
- Hypercapnic respiratory failure due to a decrease in minute ventilation.
- Hypoxemic respiratory failure due to a failure of oxygenation.
- Cardiovascular distress whereby mechanical ventilation can decrease the load of energy requirements of breathing.

PRINCIPLES

Mechanism: Mechanical ventilation works by applying a positive pressure breath and is dependent on the compliance and resistance of the airway system. This is affected by how much pressure must be generated by the ventilator to provide a given TV or predefined pressure. Compliance and resistance are dynamic and can be affected by the disease state(s) that led to the intubation. Understanding the changes in compliance and resistance will allow to pick the proper ventilator strategies.

Stages: There are four stages of mechanical ventilation namely the trigger phase, the inspiratory phase, the cycling phase, and the expiratory phase. The trigger phase is the initiation of an inhalation which is triggered by an effort from the patient or by set parameters by the mechanical ventilator. The inhalation of air into the patient defines the inspiratory phase. The cycling phase is the brief moment when inhalation has ceased but before exhalation has begun. The expiratory phase is passive and leads to exhalation of air from the lungs (**Fig. 1**).

Issues of concern: There is a change in the natural negative pressure ventilation to one of positive pressure ventilation when placing a patient on mechanical ventilation which will affect the heart-lung physiology and can alter the patients hemodynamic status. There is increase in the intrathoracic pressure after the addition of positive pressure ventilation. The increase in intrathoracic pressure will lead to a decrease in right ventricular preload and left ventricular preload and afterload. It will also increase the right ventricular afterload. These effects could have a minimal change on a healthy person's hemodynamics, but in critically ill patients it can cause profound alterations in the hemodynamics. For example, a patient in acute pulmonary edema will benefit from the reduced preload while someone in septic shock would not.

MODES OF VENTILATION

- Once the decision is made to place a patient on mechanical ventilation, the clinician may be presented with multiple options on how to set up the ventilator. There are many modes of ventilation, such as assist-control (AC), synchronized intermittent mechanical ventilation (SIMV), PSV, and others.
- Depending on the clinical state of patient and use of patient's effort for triggering the ventilator, the ventilatory support can be controlled mandatory ventilation (CMV) or ACMV.
- In CMV mode, the patient's ventilation is totally controlled by the ventilator and the patient cannot trigger the ventilator, while ACMV delivers controlled

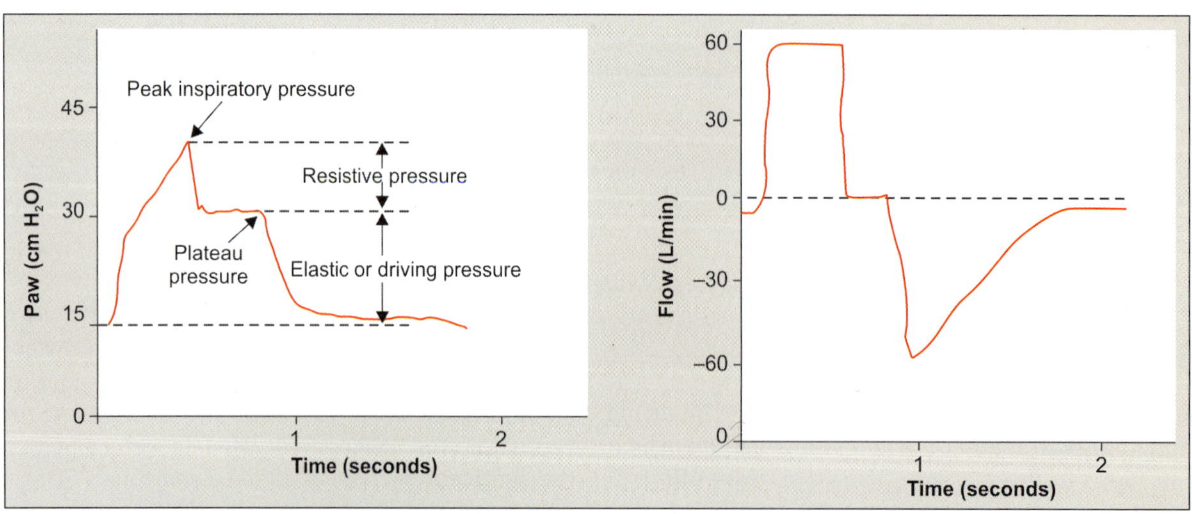

FIGURE 1: Ventilatory wave forms (pressure time and flow time wave forms). (Paw: airway pressure)

TABLE 1 Commonly used modes of ventilation with their special features.

Mode	Type of breath	Triggering mechanism	Cycling mechanism	Comments
CMV	Each breath delivers a preset mechanical tidal volume or pressure	Time	Inspiration is terminated by delivery of preset tidal volume or by time in pressure-controlled	Used in patients who have no respiratory effort
ACMV	Each breath, assist or control, delivers a preset mechanical tidal volume or pressure	Either patient-triggered (assist) or time-triggered (controlled)	Inspiration is terminated either by delivery of preset tidal volume (volume-controlled) or by high pressure limit or by time in pressure-controlled	Alveolar hyperventilation may be a potential hazard
SIMV	Mechanical tidal breath at preset rate and the patient may breathe spontaneously between mandatory breaths	Mandatory breath may be time-triggered or patient-triggered	Mandatory breaths are volume- or time-cycled; patient controls spontaneous rate and volume	It provides an interval (synchronization window) just prior to triggering during which the ventilator is responsive to patient's effort and supports spontaneous breath
PSV	Pressure-support breaths are considered as spontaneous	Patient-triggered	The breaths are flow cycled by a set flow threshold, which is generated by the patient	This a commonly used mode for weaning

(ACMV: assisted controlled mandatory ventilation; CMV: controlled mandatory ventilation; IMV: intermittent mandatory ventilation; SIMV: synchronized intermittent mechanical ventilation; PSV: pressure support ventilation)

breaths as well as assists patient-triggered breath. There is always a backup ventilation in case the patient does not trigger the breath.

- Assisted controlled mandatory ventilation is the most commonly used mode of mechanical ventilation and can be used to deliver either volume-preset or pressure-preset ventilation.
- In volume-preset ACMV, a preset TV is delivered, irrespective of inspiratory pressure (Pinsp).
- In pressure-preset ACMV, a fixed Pinsp is applied to the respiratory system. The TV is determined by lung (and chest wall) compliance and airway resistance.
- Although both volume-set and pressure-set ACMVs can achieve the same levels of ventilation, volume-preset ACMV is more frequently used. The various modes of ventilation are described in **Table 1**.

VENTILATORY SETTINGS

After choosing the mode of ventilation, the rest of the parameters have to be set on the ventilator. These parameters are the respiratory rate (RR), IFR, the fraction of inspired oxygen (FiO_2), and PEEP. In ACMV mode, RR is a "back up" rate in case the patient does not trigger the ventilator (insufficient effort or paralysis). The IFR is a measure of how fast the inspiration is provided. Generally, it is expressed in liters/minute. FiO_2 is the fraction of inspired air and should be set to the lowest level to achieve an SpO_2 of 92–96%, as hyperoxemia has been shown to increase mortality in critically ill patients. PEEP is used to increase the functional residual capacity, and to stent open collapsible alveoli thus reducing atelectatic trauma. Finally, all patients on mechanical ventilation should have the head of the bed elevated to at least 30° (unless contraindicated) and have continuous waveform monitoring. **Table 2** depicts initial settings to be made when a patient is put on a ventilator and changes to be done when the patient is stabilized after sometime. **Table 3** shows the differences in the ventilatory settings which are to be made depending on the underlying disease.

TABLE 2 Ventilatory setting: Initially and once the patient stabilizes.

Initial setting (assist/control; volume/pressure)	
Plateau pressure	<30 cm H_2O
Tidal volume	8 mL/kg ideal body weight (also see **Table 3**)
Inspiratory time	0.7–1.2 second
Rate	10–12 breaths/min
PEEP	4 cm H_2O
FiO_2	1.0
Once the patient is stabilized	
FiO_2	To maintain PaO_2 > 60 mm Hg
PEEP	Set according to FiO_2 requirements (predetermined according to the degree of hypoxemia)
Plateau pressure	Recheck in an attempt to keep plateau pressure below 30 cm H_2O
Tidal volume	Maintain 6 mL/kg of ideal body weight

(FiO_2: fraction of inspired oxygen; PEEP: positive end-expiratory pressure)

CLINICAL STRATEGIES

Three clinical strategies may be chosen to assist in ventilator management. An intermediate strategy is also used and mentioned here.

LUNG PROTECTIVE STRATEGY

Lung protective strategy should be used for any patient with the potential to develop acute lung injury (ALI) or whose disease state risks progression to acute respiratory distress syndrome (ARDS). The principle of this strategy was based on providing low tidal volume (LTV) which was developed after the landmark ARDS net trials which showed that LTV ventilation in patients with ARDS improved mortality. This method is used to avoid barotrauma, volume trauma, and atelectatic trauma. All patients with acute lung or ARDS should be managed with the LTV strategy.

The ideal body weight is first calculated and the TV should be initially set at 6 mL/kg based upon ideal body weight. As patients develop ALI and progress into ARDS, their lungs become progressively recruited and develop shunts, which leads to decreased functional lung volume. A LTV strategy offsets the decreased functional lung volume. TV should not be adjusted based on minute ventilation goals. RR is adjusted based upon minute ventilation goals and the acid-base status of the patient. To achieve normocapnia an initial rate of 16 breaths/min is appropriate for most patients. A blood gas should be done approximately 30 minutes after initiation of mechanical ventilation and RR adjusted based upon the acid-base status and $PaCO_2$ of the patient. Normocapnia is a $PaCO_2$ of 35–45 mm Hg. It is the pH rather than pCO_2 which is important for adjusting the minute ventilation. The IFR should be set at 60 L/min. If the patient appears to be trying to inhale more during the initiation of inspiration, then it can be increased.

After intubating patient and initiation of mechanical ventilation immediately an attempt should be made to reduce the FIO_2 to 40% to maintain a SpO_2 of around 90%. From there, adjustments of the FIO_2 and PEEP are simultaneously controlled in the lung-protective strategy. In ALI and ARDS, difficulty in oxygenation is due to derecruited alveoli and physiological shunt. To counteract this, one should increase the FiO_2 and PEEP together. The oxygenation goal of 88–95% should be followed. The ARDSnet protocol for simultaneous increase in PEEP and FiO_2 to achieve this goal is shown in **Table 4**.

After connecting a patient to mechanical ventilation, it is essential to frequently reassess its effects on various parameter, including the heart rate and blood pressure. This assessment is done by examining the plateau pressure and driving pressure. The plateau pressure is the pressure applied to small airways and alveoli and the target pressure should be under 30 cm of H_2O, to prevent volume trauma. The protocol to be followed to achieve the plateau pressure goal of 30 cm of H_2O is shown in **Box 1**.

To obtain the plateau pressure, one must perform an inspiratory pause. The driving pressure is the ratio of the TV to the compliance of the lung, providing an approximation of the "functional" amount of lung that has not been

TABLE 3 Difference in desired ventilatory settings for patients with different diseases.

	Tidal volume	RR	I:E ratio	PEEP	FiO_2
Normal lung	8 mL/kg	10–12	1:2	4	1.0
Asthma/COPD	6 mL/kg	5–8	1:4	4	1.0
ARDS	6 mL/kg	10–12	1:2	4–15	1.0
Hypovolemia	6 mL/kg	10–12	1:2	0–4	1.0

(FiO_2: fraction of inspired oxygen; I:E: inspiratory:expiratory; PEEP: positive end-expiratory pressure; RR: respiratory rate)

BOX 1 Protocol for plateau pressure (Pplat) goal of ≤30 cm H_2O.

Check Pplat (0.5 second inspiratory pause) at least q4h and after each change in PEEP or TV

- **If Pplat > 30 cm H_2O:** Decrease TV by 1 mL/kg steps (minimum 4 mL/kg)
- **If Pplat < 25 cm H_2O and TV < 6 mL/kg:** Increase TV by 1 mL/kg until Pplat > 25 cm H_2O or TV > 6 mL/kg
- **If Pplat < 30 cm H_2O and breath stacking or desynchrony occurs:** May increase TV in 1 mL/kg increments up to 7–8 mL/kg if Pplat remains ≤30 cm H_2O

(TV: tidal volume)

TABLE 4 ARDSnet protocol for increase of PEEP/FiO_2 to achieve the oxygenation goal of PaO_2 of 55–80 or SpO_2 of 88–95%.

Lower PEEP/higher FiO_2								
FiO_2	0.3	0.4	0.4	0.5	0.5	0.6	0.7	0.7
PEEP	5	5	8	8	10	10	10	12
FiO_2	0.7	0.8	0.9	0.9	0.9	1.0		
PEEP	14	14	14	16	18	18–24		
Higher PEEP/lower FiO_2								
FiO_2	0.3	0.3	0.3	0.3	0.3	0.4	0.4	0.5
PEEP	5	8	10	12	14	14	16	16
FiO_2	0.5	0.5–0.8	0.8	0.9	1.0	1.0		
PEEP	18	20	22	22	22	24		

Note: Use a minimum PEEP of 5 cm H_2O. Consider use of incremental FiO_2/PEEP combinations such as shown below to achieve goal.

derecruited or shunted and can be calculated simply by subtracting the amount of PEEP from the plateau pressure. The driving pressure should remain below 14. If plateau and driving pressures start to exceed these limits, then decrease the TV to 4 mL/kg. RR can be increased to compensate for the decrease in minute ventilation, though permissive hypercapnia might be necessary. Permissive hypercapnia is a ventilation strategy to allow for an unphysiologically high partial pressure of carbon dioxide (pCO_2) to permit lung-protective ventilation with LTVs.

STRATEGY FOR OBSTRUCTIVE AIRWAY DISEASES

Patients with obstructive lung disease (OLD), such as asthma and chronic obstructive pulmonary disease (COPD), are often treated with noninvasive ventilation. However, they sometimes require intubation and placement on mechanical ventilation. OLD is characterized by narrowed airways and the collapse of the small airways on expiration. This leads to increased airflow resistance and decreases the expiratory flow, resulting in more time required to exhale the TV fully. If inhalation begins before the full TV has been exhaled, then there is some residual air left inside the chest. The intrathoracic pressure increases as more and more air get trapped inside the alveoli which is termed auto-PEEP, and this pressure must be overcome during inhalation. As the amount of air trapped inside the chest increases, there is flattening of the diaphragm and expansion of the lungs which decreases its compliance. This is called as dynamic hyperinflation. Due to this there is an increased work of breathing, decreased efficiency of inhalation, and potential for hemodynamic instability due to the high intrathoracic pressures (auto-PEEP). Given these unique circumstances in OLD, the ventilator strategy employed must offset these pathologically increased intrathoracic pressures by applying external PEEP. Furthermore, ventilatory management must be combined with maximal medical therapy such as in-line nebulizers to reverse the obstructive process.

The most important thing to achieve when managing the ventilator for an obstructive patient is to increase the expiratory phase, which will allow for more time to exhale, which in turn will reduce auto-PEEP and dynamic hyperinflation. Most patients will require deep sedation in order not to over-breathe the ventilator and inspire too often. The initial TV should be set at 8 mL/kg, while the RR should start at 10 breaths/min. These settings will allow for ample time for a full expiration and hence decreased auto-PEEP which tends to employ the above-described permissive hypercapnia strategy by focusing on lowered TVs and oxygenation over elevated $PaCO_2$. IFR should be set at 60 L/min. FiO_2 should be set at 40% after the initiation of ventilation. In OLD, there is typically a problem with ventilation and not one of oxygenation, so the FiO_2 should not be increased. Minimal PEEP should be employed. Some studies advocate for a PEEP of zero (in acute severe asthma), while some advocate for a small amount of PEEP to help overcome the auto-PEEP (COPD). The plateau pressure should be <30.

The ventilator waveform requires careful assessment. If the waveform does not reach zero by the beginning of the new breath, then the RR must be decreased, or else hyperinflation and auto-PEEP will rise. A close monitoring of all parameters is always required. Pneumothorax is a complication of positive pressure ventilation which would lead to drop in oxygen and increase in peak airway pressures. This should always be looked for by clinical examination and confirmed by X-ray and ultrasound examination.

INTERMEDIATE STRATEGY

In a patient who is being placed on mechanical ventilation and has no obstructive physiology or risk to develop ALI, then an intermediate TV strategy using 8–10 mL/kg could be employed. The PReVENT (Prevention of Recurrent Venous Thromboembolism) trial showed no difference in an intermediate TV strategy (10 mL/kg) versus a LTV strategy (6 mL/kg) in patients without ARDS. Generally, as this patient would not have oxygenation or ventilation difficulties, minimal ventilator settings could be employed. Starting with a TV of 8 mL/kg, RR of 16, IFR of 60 L/min, FiO_2 of 40%, and PEEP of 5, with titration as needed, is a reasonable starting point.

AIRWAY PRESSURE RELEASE VENTILATION

Airway pressure release ventilation (APRV) was previously considered a rescue strategy, but has recently gained acceptance as a primary ventilatory mode by some experts. APRV is a form of continuous positive airway pressure (CPAP) that is characterized by a timed pressure release while allowing for spontaneous breathing. Its indications for ALI, ARDS, multifocal pneumonia, and severe atelectasis make it a very attractive ventilatory option.

Airway pressure release ventilation functions by providing a continuous pressure to keep the lungs open with a timed-release to a lower set pressure. The continuous pressure phase of APRV transmits pressure to the chest wall which allows for the recruitment of both proximal and distal alveoli. The prolonged continuous pressure phase with the short release phase avoids the continuous cycles of recruitment-derecruitment that occur in pressure/volume control settings. This strategy helps to avoid atelectrauma and barotrauma, resulting in reduced ventilator-induced lung injury. The timed release allows for a passive exhalation and improved clearance of CO_2. APRV requires less sedation compared to conventional modalities as it relies upon spontaneous ventilation and thus mitigating adverse events due to sedation. Spontaneous breathing has the benefit of increasing end-expiratory lung volume, decreasing atelectasis, and improves ventilation to the dependent lung regions. Spontaneous breathing, further improves the hemodynamic profile by decreasing intrathoracic pressure, thus improving preload and cardiac output.

GENERAL CARE OF VENTILATOR PATIENT

In critical care settings before initiating mechanical ventilation one should also consider what medications to provide for postintubation pain control and sedation. An "analgesia first" sedation strategy is recommended with the most commonly used agent being fentanyl as it has minimal hypotension-inducing hemodynamic properties. If the patient is still agitated while getting an analgesia sedation regimen then additional agents, such as propofol, can be added dependent on the patient's hemodynamics and clinical needs. A chest X-ray and a blood gas should be obtained to determine proper endotracheal placement and to assess minute ventilation. Many centers are now utilizing ultrasound to confirm endotracheal tube (ETT) placement; however, its use has not become standard of care. Plateau pressures should be checked frequently to assess alveolar integrity.

If the patient suddenly desaturates: The DOPES mnemonic should be followed to determine the causes of the problem. DOPES stands for displacement, obstruction of the ETT or airways, pneumothorax/pulmonary embolism/pulmonary edema, equipment failure, and stacked breaths. The patient should immediately be disconnected from the ventilator and switched to a bag valve mask. The person bagging should ventilate calmly and allow for a full exhalation. Following this, a systematic approach should be followed. Does the patient still have a good waveform on their $EtCO_2$. If not, then the ETT may have become dislodged. Does the patient bag easily or with difficulty. If bagging is difficult, this will indicate some acute problem such as an obstructed ETT, pneumothorax, or severe bronchospasm. If the patient bags easily and SpO_2 rises rapidly then it points to equipment failure. While this is under evaluation, another provider should be assessing the patient with an ultrasound of the lungs and heart, and a chest X-ray should be obtained. Pulmonary embolism should be a consideration if no other cause of the desaturation is found.

Healthcare team approach: The management for a patient on mechanical ventilation requires an interprofessional team involving physicians, nurses, and respiratory therapists. Good communication among the team is essential for optimum outcome. Respiratory therapists (whenever available) provide a crucial role in managing the ventilated patient, and their expertise should be utilized extensively. Finally, only one dedicated professional should be incharge of the ventilator and nonemergent changes in setting should not be made without communication with the incharge of the patient.

Mechanical ventilation is a dynamic process. Understanding of pulmonary physiology is essential for providing safe and effective ventilation. A team approach with perfect coordination goes a long way in attaining a good outcome.

RECOMMENDED READINGS

1. Engstrom CG. Treatment of severe cases of respiratory paralysis by the Engström universal respirator. Br Med J. 1954;2(4889):666-9.
2. Ingelstedt S, Jonson B, Nordström L, Olsson SG. A servo-controlled ventilator measuring expired minute volume, airway flow and pressure. Acta Anaesthesiol Scand Suppl. 1972;47:7-27.
3. Pham T, Brochard LJ, Slutsky AS. Mechanical Ventilation: State of the Art. Mayo Clin Proc. 2017;92(9):1382-400.
4. Girardis M, Busani S, Damiani E, Donati A, Rinaldi L, Marudi A, et al. Effect of Conservative vs Conventional Oxygen Therapy on Mortality Among Patients in an Intensive Care Unit: The Oxygen-ICU Randomized Clinical Trial. JAMA. 2016;316(15):1583-9.
5. Grübler MR, Wigger O, Berger D, Blöchlinger S. Basic concepts of heart-lung interactions during mechanical ventilation. Swiss Med Wkly. 2017;147:w14491.
6. Brower RG, Matthay MA, Morris A, Schoenfeld D, Thompson BT, Wheeler A. Ventilation with lower tidal volumes as compared with traditional tidal volumes for acute lung injury and the acute respiratory distress syndrome. N Engl J Med. 2000;342(18):1301-8.
7. Sutherasan Y, Vargas M, Pelosi P. Protective mechanical ventilation in the non-injured lung: review and meta-analysis. Crit Care. 2014;18(2):211.
8. Brower RG, Lanken PN, MacIntyre N, Matthay MA, Morris A, Ancukiewicz M, et al. National Heart, Lung, and Blood Institute ARDS Clinical Trials Network. Higher versus lower positive end-expiratory pressures in patients with the acute respiratory distress syndrome. N Engl J Med. 2004;351(4):327-36.
9. Needham DM, Colantuoni E, Mendez-Tellez PA, Dinglas VD, Sevransky JE, Dennison Himmelfarb CR, et al. Lung protective mechanical ventilation and two year survival in patients with acute lung injury: prospective cohort study. BMJ. 2012;344:e2124.
10. Amato MB, Meade MO, Slutsky AS, Brochard L, Costa EL, Schoenfeld DA, et al. Driving pressure and survival in the acute respiratory distress syndrome. N Engl J Med. 2015;372(8):747-55.
11. Fuchs H, Rossmann N, Schmid MB, Hoenig M, Thome U, Mayer B, et al. Permissive hypercapnia for severe acute respiratory distress syndrome in immunocompromised children: A single center experience. PLoS One. 2017;12(6):e0179974.
12. Simonis FD, Serpa Neto A, Binnekade JM, Braber A, Bruin KCM, Determann RM, et al. Effect of a Low vs Intermediate Tidal Volume Strategy on Ventilator-Free Days in Intensive Care Unit Patients Without ARDS: A Randomized Clinical Trial. JAMA. 2018;320(18):1872-80.
13. Zhou Y, Jin X, Lv Y, Wang P, Yang Y, Liang G, et al. Early application of airway pressure release ventilation may reduce the duration of mechanical ventilation in acute respiratory distress syndrome. Intensive Care Med. 2017;43(11):1648-59.
14. Barr J, Fraser GL, Puntillo K, Ely EW, Gélinas C, Dasta JF, et al. American College of Critical Care Medicine. Clinical practice guidelines for the management of pain, agitation, and delirium in adult patients in the intensive care unit. Crit Care Med. 2013;41(1):263-306.
15. Kollef MH. Evaluating the Value of the Respiratory Therapist: Where Is the Evidence? Focus on the Barnes-Jewish Hospital Experience. Respir Care. 2017;62(12):1602-10.

CHAPTER

74 Acute Respiratory Distress Syndrome

Rupali Patnaik, Shreyas H Gutte, Mohan Gurjar

ABSTRACT

Acute respiratory distress syndrome (ARDS) is a life threatening condition characterized by acute and diffuse inflammatory lung injury which manifests clinically as hypoxemia and presence of bilateral lung infiltrates due to noncardiogenic pulmonary edema. Since its first description, multiple attempts have been made to understand this heterogeneous syndrome. There is huge variability in the reported incidence of ARDS worldwide. Though, recent Berlin definition of ARDS addressed important shortcomings of older definitions, there are still multiple areas of uncertainty.

Managing ARDS is a multifaceted approach with a primary goal to correct hypoxemia. Simultaneously minimizing ongoing insult to already damaged lungs, due to mechanical ventilation (MV), is required for better outcome. Noninvasive approaches available for mild to moderate ARDS are noninvasive positive pressure ventilation and high flow nasal cannula (HFNC). As respiratory parameters worsen, they need invasive MV, where lung protective ventilation with optimal positive end-expiratory pressure (PEEP) is highly recommended. Various rescue strategies available are recruitment maneuver, prone ventilation, and extracorporeal membrane oxygenation. Conservative fluid strategy and appropriate nutritional therapy are associated with better outcome. Readiness for weaning should be evaluated early in course of MV. Various pharmacological therapies have been proposed, with limited success till date. While treating patients with ARDS with sepsis and organ dysfunction, physician should focus on appropriate monitoring and timely interventions, to tackle multi-organ dysfunction syndrome. Current reported incidence of mortality in ARDS is 30–60%. Survivors of ARDS have been found to have significant reduction in physical function, decreased quality of life, cognitive impairment, and post-traumatic stress disorder.

"Instead of giving up, try a different approach"

—Anonymous

INTRODUCTION

Acute respiratory distress syndrome (ARDS) is a life threatening condition characterized by acute and diffuse inflammatory lung injury, which manifests as hypoxemia and presence of bilateral lung infiltrates due to non-cardiogenic pulmonary edema.

The first description of ARDS, which was not coined as a term at that time, goes back to 1821, when Laennec described it as fatal idiopathic pulmonary edema. Later on, similar description found in traumatic injuries during first and second world war, defined "shock lung" or "wet lung" to the unexplained pulmonary edema. It was first time in 1967, when Ashbaugh and colleagues, coined the term "adult respiratory distress syndrome" as acute onset dyspnea, tachypnea, hypoxemia, and cyanosis not responsive to oxygen therapy with loss of lung compliance and diffuse bilateral infiltrates on chest radiograph, in a series of 12 adult patients. Subsequently, in the literature, the word "adult" had been replaced by "acute"; and currently terminology "acute respiratory distress syndrome" is being used.

EPIDEMIOLOGY

There is huge variability in the reported incidence of ARDS worldwide ranging from 3.65 to 81 per 100,000 populations per year/percentage over the data from last 50 years. Different definitions of ARDS over time points with lack of public reporting could be the contributing factors which affected the epidemiology. ARDS remains under-recognized not only in resource limited countries, but also in high income countries. Recent observational trial of largest data involving 459 intensive care units (ICUs) in 50 countries has suggested an incidence of ARDS as 10.4%. ARDS contributed to 10% of ICU admissions and 24% of patients needing mechanical ventilator support. Clinical recognition rate of ARDS ranged from 51.3% in mild to 78.5% in severe ARDS and mortality rate ranged from 27% for mild ARDS to 32% and 46% for those with moderate and severe ARDS respectively.

DIAGNOSIS

Acute respiratory distress syndrome is a syndrome and not a disease per se, which is the common endpoint of various predisposing factors along with potential direct and/or indirect insult to the lung.

DEFINITIONS

Older definitions: After initial description by Ashbaugh (1967), Murray and colleagues (1988) proposed a definition called expanded definition of ARDS comprising four different variables, i.e., the chest roentgenogram score describing the amount of pulmonary consolidation of the four quadrants, hypoxemia stratified according to PaO_2/FiO_2, PEEP level and compliance of the respiratory system. Each variable was assigned a score varying from 0 to 4 as per severity. The authors coined the final score as the "Murray Lung Injury Score" calculated as the sum of the single component score divided by the number of the accounted variables. Severity was defined as absence of lung injury (0), mild-to-moderate lung injury (score 1–2.5), and severe lung injury (score >2.5).

In 1994, the American European consensus conference (AECC) definition was established. AECC defined acute lung injury (ALI) and ARDS as respiratory failure with: Acute onset hypoxemia, presence of bilateral infiltrates at chest radiograph, and no clinical evidence of left atrial hypertension (pulmonary artery wedge pressure ≤18 mm Hg when measured to rule out cardiogenic cause of lung edema). Severity of hypoxemia was defined as ALI with PaO_2/FiO_2 ratio ≤300 or ARDS with PaO_2/FiO_2 ratio ≤200. AECC definition differed from Murray score by exclusion of cardiogenic cause of edema, but did not include respiratory system compliance and PEEP level.

Newer definition: After 18 years of AECC definition, European Society of Intensive Care Medicine (ESICM), endorsed a task force to revise the ARDS definition. "Berlin definition (2012)" was proposed and was also endorsed by the American Thoracic Society (ATS) and Society of Critical Care Medicine (SCCM). Berlin definition eliminates the use of term "acute lung injury". All limitations of AECC definition were updated and clarified in Berlin definition which include lack of exact criteria for timing, poor inter-observer reliability of chest radiograph, difficulties with excluding volume overload or congestive heart failure as the primary cause of respiratory failure and use of PaO_2/FiO_2 ratio only to define ARDS but no specification of it with respect to PEEP.

Berlin definition includes:

- *Timing*: The acute onset, established within 1 week of known clinical insult or new or worsening respiratory symptoms.
- *Chest radiograph*: Bilateral opacities not fully explained by effusions, lobar/lung collapse, or nodules.
- Respiratory failure not fully explained by cardiac failure or fluid overload. Need objective assessment (e.g., echocardiography) to exclude hydrostatic edema, if no risk factors present.
- Standardization of the hypoxemia with PEEP or continuous positive airway pressure (CPAP) ≥5 cmH_2O and classification of severity as described in **Table 1**.

In the resource limited settings, "Kigali modification" of Berlin definition with measurement of SpO_2/FiO_2 ratio in place of PaO_2/FiO_2 along with lung ultrasound can be a promising alternative.

RADIOLOGICAL FEATURES

Chest radiograph: Typically, in ARDS, there are bilateral airspace opacities more or less involving all the zones and usually persistent over days to weeks (**Fig. 1 A**). As the bilateral infiltrates can be obscured by atelectasis, effusion, and isolated lower lobe involvement, recent Berlin criteria define that these bilateral airspace opacities are not being explained by effusion, lobar collapse, or nodules.

Computed tomography scan of lung: Heterogeneous and patchy distributions with areas of normal aerated lung interspersed with areas of ground glass opacities and consolidation are predominant findings in ARDS (**Fig. 1 B**).

TABLE 1 Severity of ARDS as per Berlin definition.

Severity	PaO_2/FiO_2 (mm Hg)	PEEP or CPAP (cmH_2O)
Mild ARDS	≤300 to >200	≥5
Moderate ARDS	≤200 to >100	≥5
Severe ARDS	≤100	≥5

(PEEP: positive end expiratory pressure; CPAP: continuous positive airway pressure)

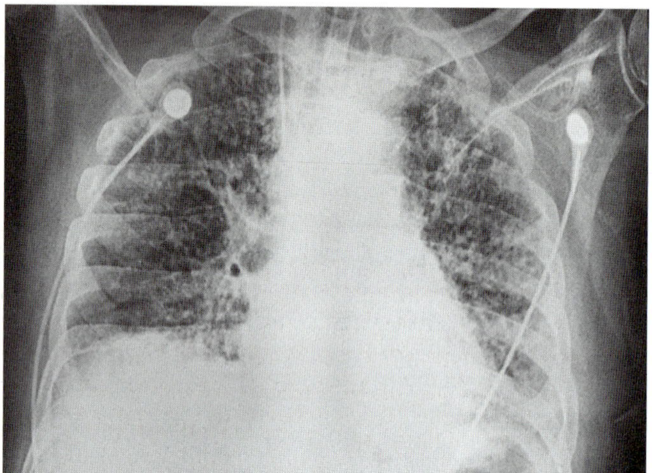

FIGURE 1 A: Chest X-ray in acute respiratory distress syndrome.

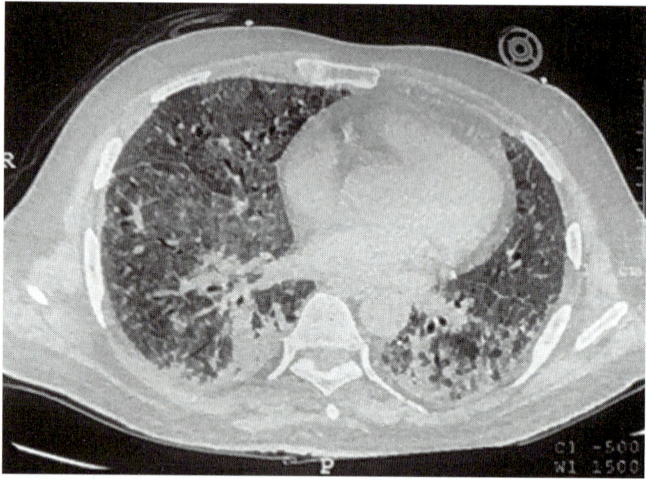

FIGURE 1 B: CT scan of the lung in acute respiratory distress syndrome.

BOX 1	Conditions mimicking ARDS.
ARDS mimics	
• Congestive cardiac failure with cardiogenic pulmonary edema	
• Negative pressure pulmonary edema	
• Interstitial lung disease (acute interstitial pneumonia, nonspecific interstitial pneumonitis, cryptogenic organizing pneumonia, acute eosinophilic pneumonia, hypersensitivity pneumonia, and pulmonary alveolar proteinosis)	
• Connective tissue diseases	
• Diffuse alveolar hemorrhage	
• Drug induced (bleomycin or amiodarone)	
• Cancer (lymphoma or metastatic carcinoma)	
• Endobronchial tuberculosis	

(ARDS: acute respiratory distress syndrome)

TABLE 2 Direct and indirect risk factors for ARDS.

Direct risk factors	Indirect risk factors
• Pneumonia • Aspiration • Pulmonary contusion • Chest trauma • Inhalational injury • Near drowning • Fat emboli • Reperfusion injury after lung transplant or embolectomy	• Sepsis and systemic inflammatory response syndrome • Prolonged hypotension/shock • Multisystem trauma • Acute pancreatitis • Transfusion of plasma and other blood products • Disseminated intravascular coagulation • Drug overdose • Cardiopulmonary bypass • Elevated intracranial pressure (traumatic brain injury, and intracerebral hemorrhage)

Lung ultrasound: Focused cardiac and thoracic ultrasound is of utmost importance in assessing ventricular function, hemodynamic assessment, and to rule out other differential diagnosis. Ultrasound lung suggest irregular thickened and coarse pleural line with spared areas of B lines. Shred sign and tissue like signs are evident on areas of consolidation.

ARDS MIMICKING CONDITIONS

Appropriate history and clinical examination along with laboratory parameters are of immense help in diagnosis of ARDS and differentiating it from other clinical conditions. Arterial blood gas findings of hypoxemia and/or associated hypercapnia along with parameters of noninvasive and invasive MV typical of ARDS are of immense help. Conditions mimicking ARDS are mentioned in the **Box 1**.

RISK FACTORS

Acute respiratory distress syndrome is a condition, triggered by injury to alveolar epithelium and/or capillary endothelium. Risk factors bring injury either directly or indirectly. Direct and indirect risk factors are described in **Table 2**.

These risk factors act synergistically rather than being additive. Sepsis is most commonly identified cause of ARDS (5–40%) and is associated with worst outcome, while trauma ARDS has significantly lower mortality. Other factors such as genetic susceptibility, virulence factor of the pathogen, coexisting conditions (immunosuppressed status, pneumococcal pneumonia after splenectomy), environmental exposures (use of alcohol and smoking) add up to the risk factors.

PATHOPHYSIOLOGY

Damages to pulmonary alveolar epithelial and/or capillary endothelial cells are the initiating changes in the development of ARDS. Direct lung injury leads to initial insult to alveolar epithelial cells; whereas indirect leads to initial insult of capillary endothelial cells. Ultimately, both injuries coincide and at the time of presentation, there is involvement of both epithelium and endothelium. *Widespread pulmonary epithelial and endothelial injury* is the hallmark of ARDS pathology. There is sloughing and apoptosis of type I alveolar epithelial cells. Receptor for advanced glycosylation end product (RAGE) is highly expressed on type I alveolar cells which is an important marker of ARDS and its prognosis. Type II alveolar cells, when involved lead to surfactant dysfunction. Widespread endothelial injury leads to release of inflammatory molecules, expression of cell surface adhesion molecules, and neutrophilic infiltration. Neutrophils release variety of proteases such as elastase, collagenase and gelatinase, reactive oxygen species along with proinflammatory cytokines, and chemokines, thereby further recruitment of neutrophils.

Activated leukocytes and endothelial cells, activates *proinflammatory and procoagulant pathway* resulting in dysregulated intravascular and extravascular coagulation. Increased expression of tissue factor and other procoagulant factors lead to thrombus formation within microvasculature and airspace with suppression of fibrinolysis, thereby perpetuation of microthrombi and fibrinous exudates typical of ARDS.

Alveolar edema fluid and protein accumulate with in the alveoli and there is development of physiologic shunt as perfusion occurs to the alveoli which are either filled with edema fluid or collapsed from increased surface tension. Consequences manifest as refractory hypoxemia and decreased pulmonary compliance thereby prone for alveolar closure. Hypoxic pulmonary vasoconstriction (HPV) is a protective reflex by which vasoconstriction diverts capillary blood away from poorly ventilated lungs to match perfusion with ventilation. Pulmonary hypertension develops due to HPV along with local production of endothelin and thromboxane A2. Increased vasoconstriction along with scattered micro and macrothrombi contribute to worsening of physiologic dead space.

Recently, coronavirus disease 2019 (COVID-19) caused by novel severe acute respiratory distress syndrome coronavirus (SARS-CoV-2) emerged as a pandemic affecting all over the globe. Apart from ventilation perfusion mismatch and shunt in ARDS occurs, various other pathophysiologic mechanisms proposed are: Angiotensin-converting enzyme 2 (ACE-2) receptor mediated endothelial injury, intravascular micro and macro thrombi, concept of silent hypoxemia in earlier stage, and patient self-inflicted lung injury.

PHASES OF ARDS

The typical histopathological finding of ARDS is diffuse alveolar damage. It is a continuum of changes which divided into exudative, proliferative, and fibrotic phases between which considerable overlap exists.

- *Exudative phase*: It is the earliest phase occurring in first week of illness. During this phase, epithelial, endothelial injury, neutrophilic infiltration, platelet fibrin thrombi, and interstitial edema followed by accumulation of exudates within airspaces consisting of protein, edema fluid, and cellular debris which organize to form hyaline membrane.
- *Proliferative phase*: This phase usually occurs in 7–14 days of insult, during which there is organization of exudates and proliferation of fibroblasts.
- *Fibrotic phase*: When disease process continues beyond 2–3 weeks, chronic inflammation sets in leading to fibrosis of alveoli. Fibrotic response to ARDS has been documented as early as 24 hours from presentation. Fibrotic and proliferative phases often overlap and described as fibroproliferative phase.

BIOMARKERS OF ARDS

Various biomarkers pertaining to pathophysiology of ARDS have been detected in plasma and/or bronchoalveolar lavage fluid (BALF).

- *Inflammatory markers*: Interleukins (IL); IL-1β, IL-6, and tumor necrosis factor-α (TNF-α)
- *Endothelial injury markers*: Angiopoietin-2 (Ang-2), intercellular adhesion molecule (I-CAM), and von Willebrand factor (VWF)
- *Epithelial injury markers*: Clara cell protein (CC-16), vascular endothelial growth factor (VEGF), soluble receptor for advanced glycosylation end product (sRAGE), and surfactant proteins (SP)
- *Markers of impaired coagulation*: Plasminogen activator inhibitor-1 (PAI-1), and protein C

PHENOTYPES OF ARDS

There has been continuous attempt to understand this heterogeneous syndrome by classifying ARDS as per, clinical, biologic, and physiologic criteria with proposed phenotypes. Clinically, ARDS has been classified as direct and indirect, depending on the initiating factor leading to lung injury. Biologically, as per level of inflammatory biomarkers, it has been classified as hyper- and hypoinflammatory phenotypes with proposed pharmacological therapies. As per physiologic criteria, *severity has been classified according to PaO_2/FiO_2 ratio of Berlin definition.* A time-related disease spectrum with two primary "phenotypes": with Type L presenting early in disease course characterized by low elastance (i.e., high compliance), low ventilation to perfusion ratio, low lung weight, and low recruitability and Type H presenting later in disease course as severe ARDS characterized by high elastance, high right-to-left shunt, high lung weight, and high recruitability have been proposed in COVID-19 ARDS.

MANAGEMENT

Managing ARDS is a multifaceted approach with a primary goal to correct hypoxemia; while during same time minimizing ongoing insult to already damaged lungs by both initiating risk factor as well as possible damage due to MV is required for better outcome (**Table 3**).

Over last two decades, various interventions/therapies (**Table 4**) had been tried in the ARDS patients. **Table 5** summarizes recent important trials in the COVID-19 related ARDS.

Here, ARDS management is being described under these three aspects:

1. Mechanical ventilation
2. Rescue strategies for severe hypoxemia
3. Pharmacological therapies.

MECHANICAL VENTILATION

Invasive mechanical ventilation: Almost all patients with ARDS need oxygen therapy, with significant proportion needing invasive MV. MV does not cure ARDS but simply buys time by maintaining a gas exchange sufficient for survival. This benefit is provided by taking over the function of the respiratory muscles. Goal is to maintain adequate gas exchange, give rest to respiratory muscles and protect lungs from deleterious effects of ventilation induced lung injury (VILI) which perpetuates morbidity and mortality of ARDS patients. Excessive stress, tidal volume, driving pressure, respiratory rate, and gas flow are risk factors for VILI. Aim should be limitation of tidal stress, i.e., limitation of excessive volume or pressure with which lungs are ventilated (volutrauma), and limitation of cyclic tidal recruitment at the interface between collapsed and aerated lung regions (atelectrauma) by providing optimal PEEP.

Concept of baby lung: The concept of "baby lung" was put-forward by Gattinoni et al. where lung of an ARDS patient is modeled as a small aerated lung. Appearance of lung tissue is heterogenous on CT scan. Lungs comprised of normally aerated, poorly aerated, and nonaerated region. On quantitative estimation from CT images, volume of normally aerated lungs in adult patients with severe ARDS is equivalent to the normally aerated lung of a healthy boy of 5–6 years of age. Respiratory system compliance in these patients is linearly related to baby lung dimension. Size of the baby lung determines the susceptibility for VILI.

TABLE 3 Management overview for ARDS patient.

Primary aim	Core aspects	Other aspects
Maintain adequate oxygenation and Minimize ongoing lung injury	**Before intubation** • Intensive monitoring to avoid catastrophic event • Take timely decision for endotracheal intubation **During mechanical ventilation** • Avoid ventilator-induced lung injury (VILI) • Individualized and periodic optimization of various ventilator parameters • Targets: Low tidal volume (4–8 mL/kg); Pplat < 30 cmH_2O, Driving pressure < 15 cmH_2O • Achieve synchronize ventilation • Consider prone positioning, if no contraindication present **Rescue strategies** • ECMO • $ECCO_2R$ • NMB **Weaning from mechanical ventilation** • Consider daily assessment of readiness for spontaneous breathing trial (SBT), if no contraindication present • Weaning from ventilator as early as possible, once primary indication for intubation resolved	• Try to achieve conservative fluid strategy over liberal • Avoid over sedation • Maintain target glucose between 140 and 180 mg/dL • Adequate calorie and protein supplementation; prefer enteral route • **FAST HUGS BID** (***F***eeding, ***A***nalgesia, ***S***edation, ***T***hromboembolic prophylaxis, ***H***ead of bed elevation, stress, ***U***lcer prevention, ***G***lucose control, ***S***pontaneous breathing trial, ***B***owel function, ***I***ndwelling catheter removal, ***D***e-escalation of antibiotics)

($ECCO_2R$: extracorporeal carbon dioxide removal; NMB: neuromuscular blockade; ECMO: extracorporeal membrane oxygenation)

TABLE 4 Landmark trials related to mechanical ventilation for ARDS.

Intervention	Primary finding (in simple language)	Author/Journal/Year
Tidal volume		
Low tidal volume ventilation	6 mL/kg PBW and Pplat < 30 cm H_2O associated with mortality benefit	ARMA trial Brower/NEJM/2000
Positive end-expiratory pressure (PEEP)		
Higher versus lower PEEP	Higher versus lower PEEP no significant difference in mortality	ALVEOLI trial Brower/NEJM/2004
PEEP with recruitment	PEEP aimed to increase recruitment and limiting hyperinflation associated with no mortality benefit	Express trial Mercat/JAMA/2008
Driving pressure		
Driving pressure < 15 cmH_2O	Driving pressure independent predictor of survival	Amato/NEJM/2015
Prone ventilation		
Prone ventilation	Prone ventilation associated with mortality benefit	PROSEVA trial Guerin/NEJM/2013
Fluid management		
Conservative fluid strategy	Conservative fluid therapy improved lung function and shortened MV days	FACTT trial Wiedemann/NEJM/2006
Neuromuscular blockers		
NMB started within 48 h	Mortality reduction and increased ventilator free days	ACURASYS trial Papazian/NEJM/2010
NMB and sedation compared to usual care	No mortality difference when NMB with heavy sedation versus usual care without NMB and lighter sedation	ROSE trial PETAL network/NEJM/2019
ECMO		
Outcome of referral to ECMO center	ECMO patients have significantly better chance of survival	CESAR trial Peek/Lancet/2009
Conventional ventilation with ECMO as rescue	No survival benefit of ECMO from conventional ventilation with ECMO as rescue strategy	EOLIA trial Combes/NEJM/2018

(ALVEOLI: Assessment of Low Tidal Volume and Elevated End-Expiratory Pressure to Obviate Lung Injury; PROSEVA: Proning Severe ARDS Patients; FACTT: Fluid and Catheter Treatment Trial; ACURASYS: ARDS et Curarisation Systematique; PETAL: Prevention and Early Treatment of Acute Lung Injury; ROSE: Re-evaluation of Systemic Early Neuromuscular Blockade; ECMO: extracorporeal membrane oxygenation; CESAR: Conventional ventilatory support versus Extracorporeal Membrane Oxygenation for Severe Adult Respiratory Failure; MV: mechanical ventilation)

TABLE 5 Recent important trials related to COVID-19 ARDS (updated till January, 2021).

Intervention	Primary finding (in simple language)	Author/Journal/Year
Steroids		
Dexamethasone 6 mg once daily for 10 days	• **Significant reduction of 28-day mortality** • Effect best demonstrated in mechanically ventilated patients	RECOVERY trial, UK Horby/NEJM/2020
Remdesivir		
Remdesivir 200 mg IV LD on day 1 F/B 100 mg maintenance OD on days 2–10	**Significant shorter time** to recovery in remdesivir arm (11 days vs. 15 days, $p < 0.001$) than usual care	ACTT-1 trial Beigel/NEJM/2020
Hydroxychloroquine		
Hydroxychloroquine 800 mg orally at baseline and at 6 h F/B 400 mg start 12 h after initial dose then twice daily for next 9 days	**No difference** in 28-day mortality compared to usual care	RECOVERY: Hydroxychloroquine Horby/NEJM/2020
Lopinavir-Ritonavir		
Lopinavir 400 mg-Ritonavir 100 mg orally 12 hourly for 10 days	**No difference** in 28-day mortality compared to usual care	RECOVERY: Kaletra Horby/Lancet/2020

(COVID-19: coronavirus disease-2019; RECOVERY: Randomized Evaluation of Covid-19 Therapy; ACTT: Adaptive COVID-19 Treatment Trial)

Ventilation of the "baby lung" implies the use of stress (tidal volume) and strain (driving pressure) that is excessive for the dimensions of the residual ventilated lung. Therefore, ARDS lung is not stiff but small. As per severity of ARDS, the mechanical stress imposed on the "baby lung" may be such as to alter the extracellular matrix and thereby trigger further inflammation. "Baby lung" is more a functional concept than an anatomical one.

Lung protective ventilation strategies:

Low tidal volume and plateau pressure: Low tidal volume ventilation (6 mL/kg predicted body weight and plateau pressure <30 cmH_2O g) lead to mortality benefit and increased ventilator free days compared to traditional tidal volume group of 12–15 mL/kg. Despite available evidences use of low tidal volume still not ubiquitous.

Permissive hypercapnia: Protective lung ventilation with low tidal volume lead to hypercapnia and respiratory acidosis. This rise in CO_2 is accepted coined as the term permissive hypercapnia as long as there is no harm with this respiratory acidosis. Though limits for PCO_2 and pH are not clear, clinical data suggest safety up to PCO_2 of 60–70 mm Hg and pH of 7.20–7.25.

Optimal positive end-expiratory pressure: Ideal PEEP is an issue which is difficult to resolve. While low PEEP leads to alveolar collapse, excessive PEEP generate dead space and tissue stretch. When in earlier days PEEP was considered a tool for increase oxygenation, now a days it is considered a tool to avoid repetitive alveolar opening and closing during respiratory cycle thereby maintaining lung protective ventilation. Individual response to PEEP is variable and titration is based on lung recruitability. Various approaches are there for selection of optimal PEEP. Titration based on PEEP/FiO_2 table to achieve target level of oxygenation (LOV study) and/or maintaining inspiratory plateau pressure between 28 and 30 cmH_2O, through stepwise increase in PEEP and maintaining constant tidal volume. PEEP can be titrated to obtain stress index coefficient of 1. Another approach is to set PEEP to target driving pressure <15 cmH_2O.

Driving pressure: Airway driving pressure is the ratio between tidal volume and static respiratory system compliance better defines lung strain (deformability). It is also equal to plateau airway pressure minus PEEP. Normalizing tidal volume to respiratory system compliance takes into account the reduced proportion of lung available for ventilation (size of "baby lung"), rather than traditional scaling to lung size using predicted body weight. Driving pressure = Vt/Crs = Pplat – PEEP. When there is recruitment due to increase in tidal volume or PEEP, it is reflected as decrease in driving pressure, whereas over-distention leads to increase in driving pressure. In the recent study by Amato et al. driving pressure was found to be an independent predictor of survival with target <15 cmH_2O.

Pressure/volume (p/v) loops and stress index: Pressure/volume (P/V) loops with volume on Y-axis and pressure on X-axis represent relation between pressure and volume with inflation and deflation of lungs. The lower inflection point is the point where alveolar recruitment starts and upper inflection point is the pressure beyond which there is over-distention. Amato et al. proposed the concept of setting optimal PEEP based on P/V loop with recommendations of setting PEEP 2 cmH_2O more than the lower inflection point. However, both inflection points are difficult to identify and to get a correct P/V loop there is always need of deep sedation and/or paralysis.

Transpulmonary pressure: It is a surrogate marker of lung stress in ARDS patients. It is difference between airway pressure (Paw in dynamic conditions) or pressure inside the alveoli (Palv = Pplat + total PEEP, in static condition) and pleural pressure. Pleural pressure corresponds to esophageal pressure measured with esophageal catheter. Optimal PEEP titration to get transpulmonary pressure of

0–10 cmH_2O is desirable. If less than zero, there is chance of atelectasis and when value exceeds >25 cmH_2O, there is over-distention and increased stress.

Mechanical energy and power: Mechanical energy is the mechanics which is transferred from ventilator to lungs. It is the area under transpulmonary pressure and volume curve (Y axis). VILI results due to excessive mechanical power (energy per unit time) applied to the lung tissue where "excessive" is relative to the "baby lung" dimensions. The mechanical power depends on tidal volume, driving pressure, and respiratory rate. Animal study has shown that higher chances of VILI when mechanical power exceeds 12 J/min. Disappointing results of high frequency oscillatory ventilation (HFOV) could be attributed to high mechanical power.

Mode of mechanical ventilation: Volume controlled modes allow better measurement of respiratory mechanics and pressure controlled modes have advantage of decelerating flow curve. But studies have found no advantage of one over other and a recent systematic review did not suggest difference in clinical outcome between two modes of MV. Airway pressure release ventilation (APRV), a partial ventilator mode, allows spontaneous ventilation by providing high airway pressure and intermittent pressure release. High pressure helps in recruitment of alveoli and spontaneous breathing recruits caudal and dorsal lung regions. Though this mode is helpful in improving oxygenation, there is no mortality benefit. During spontaneous breathing, high transalveolar distending pressure can lead to VILI.

Weaning from mechanical ventilation: Readiness to wean should be suspected early in course of MV and assessed by objective weaning criteria. Once the readiness to wean has been confirmed as per objective criteria, spontaneous breathing trials (SBT) should be conducted followed by liberation from MV.

Noninvasive approach to ventilation:

Noninvasive positive pressure ventilation (NIPPV or NIV): It reduces work of breathing and extent of intrapulmonary shunt, thereby improving gas exchange and can be considered in patients with less severe hypoxemia. When increased levels of PEEP required as per degree of hypoxemia, helmet interface can be an alternative to face mask interface to facilitate reduced air leak and permit delivery of higher PEEP with greater patient tolerance. In a single-center randomized controlled trial (RCT), patients with ARDS in the helmet noninvasive ventilation group had a significantly lower rate of intubation than facemask NIPPV. Rapidly deteriorating hypoxemia, P/F ratio <150 and multi-organ involvement itself are contraindications for NIPPV.

High flow nasal cannula oxygen therapy: High flow nasal cannula delivers heated humidified gas up to 37°C at high flows through nasal cannulae using an air/oxygen blender. Most commercial devices deliver air/oxygen mixtures up to a flow of 60 L/min at an adjustable fraction of inspired oxygen (FIO_2) of 0.21 (room air) to 1.0 (100% oxygen). HFNC, washes out anatomical dead space and reduces rebreathing of expired carbon dioxide, thereby, reducing work of breathing. It prevents supraglottic collapse, decreases nasopharyngeal resistance which creates CPAP effect (with closed mouth generation of PEEP 0.7 mm Hg for every 10 L/min flow). It improves mucociliary clearance and maintains immune function of mucosal surfaces. Moreover, it is more comfortable, easy to apply, and better tolerant than NIPPV. As per "High Flow Oxygen through Nasal Cannula in Acute Hypoxemic Respiratory Failure" (FLORALI) trial, there was no difference in need for endotracheal intubation when HFNC was compared with standard facemask or NIPPV. However, there was significant reduction of 90-day mortality in HFNC group.

RESCUE STRATEGIES FOR SEVERE HYPOXEMIA

Recruitment maneuvers: This maneuver recruits collapsed but potentially recruitable alveoli. Recruitment can be done either with sustained inflation or stepwise increase in PEEP or using sigh of mechanical ventilator. Lung recruitment maneuver followed by appropriate PEEP prevents risk of VILI by reducing regional heterogeneity. Prone positioning also facilitates recruitment.

Prone positioning: It has numerous benefits in ARDS patients. It decreases ventilation heterogeneity, ventilates dorsal lung regions, improves ventilation-perfusion matching, decreases compression effect of heart on lung parenchyma, avoids influence of intra-abdominal pressure, and enhances secretion clearing. Mortality benefit has been observed in landmark trial "Prone Positioning in Severe Acute Respiratory Distress Syndrome" (PROSEVA). Patients in the early stages of ARDS are good candidates for prone positioning and should be instituted as early as possible, when progress to moderate-to-severe ARDS and have refractory hypoxemia with partial pressure of arterial oxygen (PaO_2)/FiO_2 ratio <150 mm Hg.

High frequency oscillatory ventilation: It provides small tidal volume (1–3 mL/kg) at very high frequency (100–600/min or 2–10 Hz) and high airway pressure for recruitment. Landmark trials have suggested that, patients ventilated with HFOV, need more neuromuscular blocker, vasopressor support, and higher doses of sedatives without survival benefit. Therefore, HFOV should be reserved as a rescue strategy rather than using routinely as a primary mode of ventilation.

Extracorporeal carbon dioxide removal: Low tidal volume causes less VILI, but it is limited by resultant hypercapnia and acidosis. Extracorporeal carbon dioxide removal ($ECCO_2R$) takes CO_2 out of blood through an extracorporeal gas exchanger, thereby facilitating the application of ultraprotective ventilation.

Extracorporeal membrane oxygenation (ECMO): It removes blood from the body using mechanical pump, oxygenates and removes CO_2 using oxygenator then returns it back to body. Severe ARDS with anyone of P/F ratio <80 or P/F ratio in the range of 50 for 3 hours, despite high PEEP of 15–20 cmH_2O, uncompensated hypercapnia and academia despite appropriate ventilation, excessive end inspiratory plateau pressures (>35–45 cmH_2O) are indications for ECMO in ARDS. Contraindications are conditions precluding use of anticoagulants, high pressure ventilation and high FiO_2 requirement for >7 days, limited vascular access and conditions, limiting benefit from ECMO like irreversible brain injury. Use of veno-venous ECMO in patients with ARDS has increased dramatically since the influenza A (H1N1) pandemic in 2009. Though, previous landmark trials showed survival benefit which results could not be reflected in the recent multicenter trial. Therefore, currently, it is not possible to conclude for a superiority of ECMO with respect to conventional MV.

PHARMACOLOGICAL THERAPIES

Steroids: Role of inflammatory response in pathogenesis of ARDS is rationale for corticosteroids as a therapy in ARDS. Several trials investigated corticosteroids use but with heterogeneous results.

Low dose steroid methylprednisolone (1 mg/kg bolus followed by 1 mg/kg/day) infusion for 14 days or extubation then tapered over next 14 days has been associated with significant improvement in pulmonary outcome with dramatic increase in ventilator free days with variable result on survival benefit. Steroids are found to be harmful in late stage of ARDS. Therefore, there are no recommendations for routine use of steroids. Steroids may only be effective if supplemented in early lung injury and should not be started after 14 days of diagnosis of ARDS. Critically ill ARDS patients should be monitored for hyperglycemia, worsening neuromuscular weakness, and infectious morbidity while on steroid therapy.

Neuromuscular blockade agents: These agents avoid patient ventilator dys-synchrony, reduces excessive transpulmonary pressures, reduces work of breathing, prevent breath stacking due to inspiratory effect and derecruitment by expiratory effort, thereby preventing VILI. Though survival benefit was proposed as per ACURASYS trial, recently a multicenter trial [Re-evaluation of Systemic Early Neuromuscular Blockade (ROSE)] found no survival benefit and promoted usual care approach without neuromuscular blockade and lighter sedation targets. Due to numerous side effects, these drugs should be restricted for severe form of ARDS (P/F ratio <150) and during first 48 hours.

Fluid management: Conservative fluid strategy should be targeted rather than liberal and has been associated with improved lung function and shortened duration of MV without increase in nonpulmonary organ failure.

Inhaled pulmonary vasodilators: Endothelial injury, physiologic shunt, and pulmonary hypertension as pathophysiologic abnormality of ARDS, led to search for pulmonary vasodilators as a therapeutic option. Therapy with inhaled nitric oxide (iNO) is associated with transient and modest improvement in oxygenation rather than consistency, without being associated mortality benefit or improvement in ventilator free days. Adverse consequences such as methemoglobinemia, pulmonary hypertension, and renal impairment have been documented with the therapy. Inhaled NO is not currently recommended for treatment, expect for rescue therapy at some centers. Similar to inhaled NO, inhaled prostacyclin (Iloprost) is associated with transient improvement in oxygenation without mortality and morbidity benefit. Contrary to inhaled NO, it does not need sophisticated devices for delivery and without adverse effects on systemic hemodynamics.

Nutritional supplementation: Though various immune-nutrition including omega-3 fatty acid and benefit of high fat with low carbohydrate diet have been investigated in ARDS patients, none of them are associated with improved outcome. Nothing other than standard enteral nutrition support without overfeeding is recommended at present in patients with ARDS.

Other pharmacological therapies with no proven benefits: Various other drugs had been studied with no proven benefit in ARDS, such as beta-2 agonist, keratinocyte growth factor, statins, and aspirin.

PROGNOSIS

Reported incidence of mortality rate in patients with ARDS has decreased from 60–90% in the past to 30–60% as per the current trials. Most common cause of death remains multi-organ dysfunction and sepsis. Survivors of ARDS subject to persistent abnormalities in pulmonary function, disruption in quality of life, and neurocognitive dysfunction. Though majority of patients show initial improvement in pulmonary function within 3–6 months, when observed over next 5 years, their pulmonary function showed residual abnormalities as restrictive pulmonary defect and reduction in carbon monoxide diffusion capacity. These manifest as exercise desaturation and decrease in timed walked distance. Survivors of ARDS have been found to have clinical significant reduction in physical function, decreased quality of life, insomnia, depression, anxiety, cognitive impairment, and post-traumatic stress disorder.

In future, with the advancement in molecular biology and genetics, individuals with increased risk of ARDS can be identified. With growing knowledge, the genetic makeup of an individual can be modified and transcription can be regulated with effect on various proteins. Studies on mesenchymal stem cells in rodents can be potential promise for future therapy.

CONCLUSION

Acute respiratory distress syndrome is a syndrome with substantial heterogeneity, which is characterized by inflammatory lung injury leading to increased pulmonary capillary permeability, damage to alveolar epithelium, and capillary endothelium with accumulation of protein-rich fluid inside the alveoli. Clinical consequences manifest as profound hypoxemia, decreased lung compliance, increased intrapulmonary shunt, and dead space.

Despite enormous research on understanding of pathophysiology, clinical management emphasizes primarily on correcting hypoxemia and underline initiating conditions; while avoiding further lung injury through protective MV strategies, as ARDS contribute to significant morbidity and mortality in critically ill patients.

RECOMMENDED READINGS

1. Bellani G, Laffey JG, Pham T, Fan E, Brochard L, Esteban A, et al. Epidemiology, patterns of care, and mortality for patients with acute respiratory distress syndrome in intensive care units in 50 countries. JAMA. 2016;315(8):788-800.
2. Ranieri VM, Rubenfeld GD, Thompson BT, Ferguson ND, Caldwell E, Fan E, et al. Acute respiratory distress syndrome: the Berlin definition. JAMA. 2012;307(23): 2526-33.
3. Acute respiratory distress syndrome Network, Brower RG, Matthay MA, Morris A, Schoenfeld D, Thompson BT, Wheeler A. Ventilation with lower tidal volumes as compared with traditional tidal volumes for acute lung injury and the acute respiratory distress syndrome. N Engl J Med. 2000;342(18):1301-8.
4. Amato MB, Meade MO, Slutsky AS, Brochard L, Costa EL, Schoenfeld DA, et al. Driving pressure and survival in the acute respiratory distress syndrome. N Engl J Med. 2015;372(8):747-55.
5. Guerin C, Reignier J, Richard JC, Beuret P, Gacouin A, Boulain T, et al. Prone positioning in severe acute respiratory distress syndrome. N Engl J Med. 2013; 368(23):2159-68.
6. Gattinoni L, Vasques F, Quintel M. Use of ECMO in ARDS: does the EOLIA trial really help? Crit Care. 2018;22(1):171.
7. Wiedemann HP, Wheller AP, Bernard GR, Thompson BT, Hayden D, deBoisblanc B, et al. Comparison of two fluid-management strategies in acute lung injury. N Engl J Med. 2006;354(24):2564-75.
8. Gattinoni L, Pesenti A. The concept of "baby lung". Intensive Care Med. 2005;31(6):776-84.
9. Kulkarni AP, Divatia JV. Ventilator-induced lung injury. In: Vineet Nayar, Peter JV, Roop Kishen, Srinivas S, (Eds). Critical Care Update. Mumbai: Jaypee Brothers Medical Publishers; 2009. pp. 48-58.
10. Moss M, Huang DT, Brower RG, Ferguson ND, Ginde AA, Gong MN, et al. Early neuromuscular blockade in the acute respiratory distress syndrome. N Engl J Med. 2019;380(21):1997-2008.
11. Papazian L, Aubron C, Brochard L, Chiche JD, Combes A, Dreyfuss D, et al. Formal guidelines: management of acute respiratory distress syndrome. Ann Intensive Care. 2019;9(1):69.
12. Fan E, Del Sorbo L, Goligher EC, Hodgson CL, Munshi L, Walkey AJ, et al. An Official American Thoracic Society/European Society of Intensive Care Medicine/Society of Critical Care Medicine Clinical Practice Guideline: Mechanical Ventilation in Adult Patients with Acute Respiratory Distress Syndrome. Am J Respir Crit Care Med. 2017;195(9): 1253-63.
13. Wahab A, Donthi S, Surani S, Kashyap. Lung recruitment maneuvers. In: Gurjar M (Ed). Textbook of Ventilation, Fluids, Electrolytes and Blood Gases, Ist edition. New Delhi: Jaypee Brothers Medical Publishers (P) Ltd; 2020. pp. 121-7.
14. Mendes RS, Silva PL, Pelosi P, Rocco PRM. Ventilator-induced lung injury. In: Gurjar M (Ed). Textbook of Ventilation, Fluids, Electrolytes and Blood Gases, Ist edition. New Delhi: Jaypee Brothers Medical Publishers (P) Ltd; 2020. PP. 151-60.

CHAPTER 75 Approach to Hemodynamic Instability and Shock

Atul Prabhakar Kulkarni, Ruchira Wasudeo Khasne

ABSTRACT

Shock is a life-threatening generalized form of acute circulatory failure associated with inadequate oxygen utilization by the cells. A diagnosis of shock is based on clinical signs of tissue hypoperfusion (through the three "window" approach: Skin, kidney, and brain), hemodynamic instability (hypotension), and laboratory abnormalities (raised lactates). Based on pathophysiology, shock is divided into four types: Three with a low flow state (hypovolemic, cardiogenic, obstructive) and one with hyperkinetic state (distributive shock). Treatment strategy comprises a multidisciplinary team approach with rapid clinical evaluation combined with the point-of-care ultrasound (rapid ultrasound for shock and hypotension: RUSH) protocol. Based on hemodynamic profile and results of the diagnostic test, resuscitation of the patient is initiated with crystalloids (and early vasopressors if needed) with goals to restore mean arterial pressure (MAP > 65–70 mm Hg) and central venous O_2 saturation ($ScvO_2$) > 70%. A downward trend in arterial lactate confirms the success of the resuscitation strategy. Simultaneously, specific management strategies should be implemented as needed for the etiology of shock. Achieving normalization of macrocirculation and microcirculation, however, does not guarantee that cellular hypoxia has been alleviated. This disparity between the three levels of circulation is termed as hemodynamic coherence. The future research is likely to be directed toward strategies aimed at achieving hemodynamic coherence.

"The cell never acts, it reacts"

—Ernst Haeckel

INTRODUCTION

Hemodynamic instability is defined as perfusion failure, evidenced by presence of circulatory shock and/or advanced cardiac failure. Shock is life-threatening, generalized form of acute circulatory failure associated with inadequate oxygen utilization by the cells. This may be caused by decreased oxygen delivery or increased oxygen consumption and/or failure of oxygen utilization by cells. The presence of shock thus three components: (1) Clinical signs of tissue hypoperfusion (mental obtundation, oliguria); (2) hemodynamic instability (hypotension); and (3) laboratory abnormalities (raised lactate) (**Fig. 1**). Left untreated, circulatory shock will result in multiorgan failure and death. In the Sepsis Occurrence in Acutely III Patients (SOAP) study, nearly 30% patients had shock during their intensive care unit (ICU) stay. In a subsequent study, comparing dopamine versus noradrenaline in shock patients, septic shock was the most common reason for shock (62%), followed by cardiogenic shock (17%) and hypovolemic (hemorrhagic) shock (16%), others such as anaphylactic, neurogenic etc. made up the rest (5%). Shock is an emergency and must be approached and managed as such. In this chapter, we discuss the approach to assessment, diagnosis, and management of the hemodynamically unstable patients.

TYPES OF SHOCK

Shock can be divided into four types depending on the etiology and associated hemodynamic patterns. The European Society of Intensive Care Medicine task force divided shock in to four types as follows, based on the primary pathophysiology: Three types associated with a low flow state (hypovolemic, cardiogenic, obstructive) and one associated with a hyperkinetic state (distributive) (**Table 1**).

In a patient with shock while one etiology may predominate, there can be more than two processes involved giving a picture of "mixed shock". For example, a patient with septic shock may have pre-existing myocardial dysfunction or the patient may develop sepsis induced myocardial depression and may respond differently to fluid resuscitation as compared to a patient with pure septic shock.

PATHOPHYSIOLOGY OF OXYGEN DELIVERY AND CONSUMPTION

In a healthy individual, the left ventricle supplies 1,000 mL of O_2 to the tissues/min (Oxygen Flux). The delivery of O_2 (DO_2) depends on the cardiac output (CO) and the oxygen content of the arterial blood (CaO_2), which is the sum of O_2 carried by the saturated hemoglobin (Hb × 1.39 × SaO_2) and O_2 dissolved in plasma (PaO_2 × 0.03).

$$DO_2 = CO \times [(Hb \times 1.39 \times SaO_2) + (PaO_2 \times 0.03)]$$

Normally, tissues will extract 25–30% O_2 (O_2 extraction ratio 0.25–0.3) and therefore the venous blood returning to the heart will have SvO_2 of 70–75%.

Reduction in either CO or arterial oxygen content will lead to reduced O_2 delivery to the tissues, and the tissues

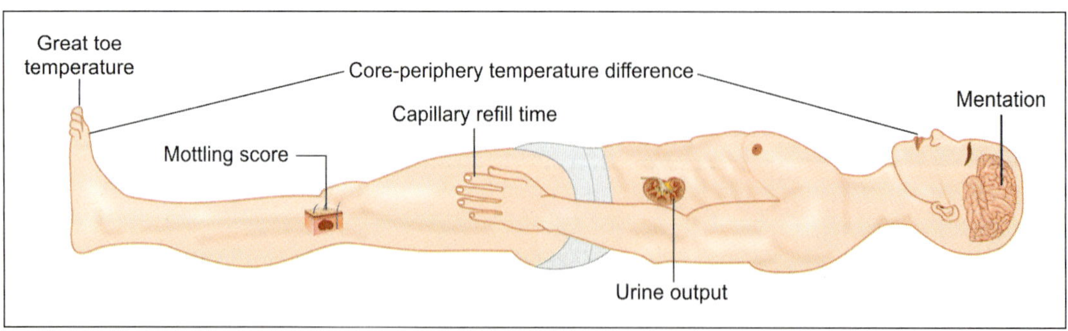

(CRT: capillary refill time)

FIGURE 1: Windows for assessing circulation. Mentation, urine output and skin as windows to circulation, mental obtundation, decreased urine output and assessment of skin temperature, CRT and temperature gradients allow determination of presence of shock (See **Table 2** for details).

TABLE 1 Types of shock and common etiologies.

Type of shock	Common etiologies
Hypovolemic	Hemorrhage, gastrointestinal losses, burns, diabetic ketoacidosis, diabetes insipidus
Cardiogenic	Myocardial infarction, cardiomyopathy, myocarditis, arrhythmia, severe valvular insufficiency (aortic, mitral)
Distributive	Septic shock, pancreatitis, severe burns, anaphylactic shock, neurogenic shock, endocrine shock, adrenal shock
Obstructive shock	Tension pneumothorax, cardiac tamponade, restrictive pericarditis, pulmonary embolism, aortic dissection

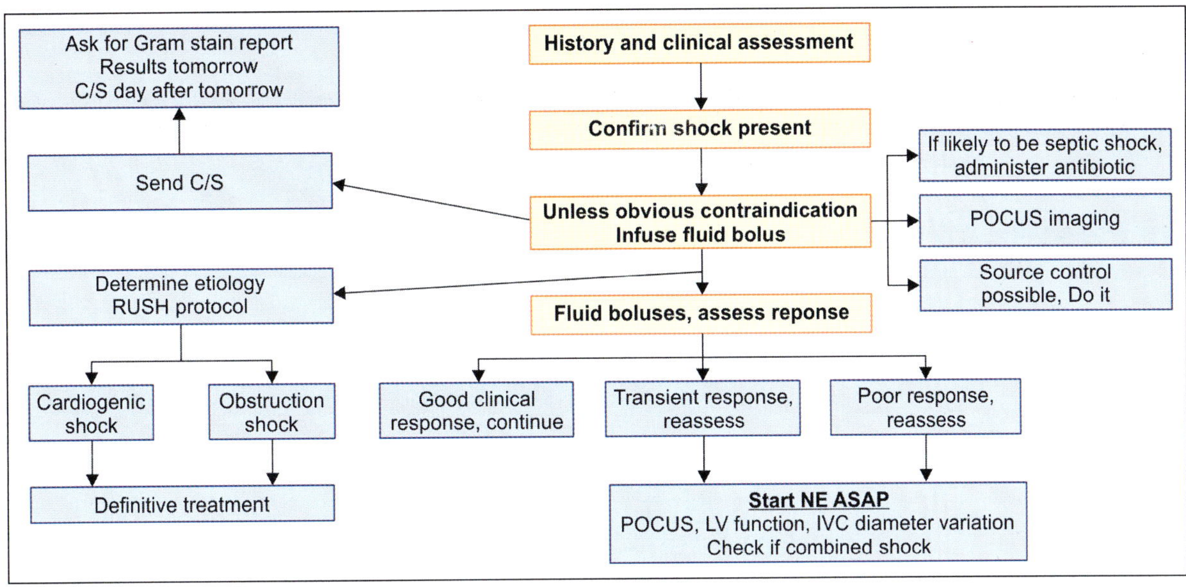

(POCUS: point-of-care ultrasound; IVC: inferior vena cava; LV: left ventricular; RUSH: rapid ultrasound in shock and hypotension)

FLOWCHART 1: Algorithmic approach to patient with hemodynamic stability and shock.

will be forced to extract more O_2 from the blood reaching them and the O_2 extraction ratio will increase, leading to a drop in saturation of venous blood reaching back to the heart (mixed venous oxygen saturation < 65% or central venous oxygen saturation < 70%). At the same time since the O_2 delivery is low, the tissues will switch to anaerobic metabolism to generate at least a few adenosine triphosphates (ATPs), leading increased lactate levels, and ultimately to lactic acidosis.

CLINICAL ASSESSMENT AND LABORATORY ABNORMALITIES

It is worth re-emphasizing that circulatory shock is an emergency and we should aim to normalize the tissue perfusion as soon as possible (ASAP). Therefore history, clinical assessment point-of-care laboratory testing, and therapy should occur simultaneously. A multidisciplinary "Shock Team" based care has been shown to improve outcomes in patients with refractory cardiogenic shock and it is easy to understand the benefits of using similar approach in other types of shock. Involvement of multiple team members with varied skillsets will also allow assessment and therapy to progress simultaneously (**Flowchart 1**).

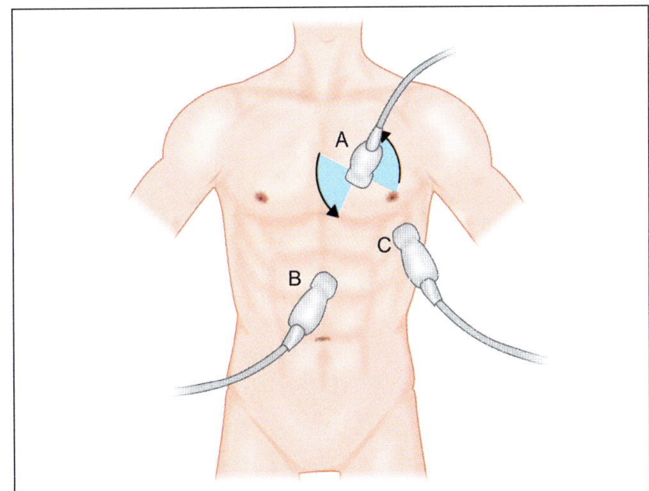

(RUSH: rapid ultrasound for shock and hypotension)

FIGURE 2: RUSH examination: Step 1. Probe positions for evaluation of the "pump". Probe positions for (**A**) Parasternal long and short-axis views; (**B**) Subxiphoid view; (**C**) Apical view.

A quick but careful history taking will generally lead to a prompt diagnosis of the type of shock the team is dealing with and will suggest the way forward. The clinical examinations should be combined with bedside ultrasonography to assess the patient the RUSH protocol (**Fig. 2**). Apart from assessing the routine vital signs, i.e., pulse, blood pressure, respiratory rate and temperature, and clinical examination involves examination of the peripheries for pulse rate volume, turgor, moistness or dryness of skin and mucosa, pallor, icterus, peripheral edema, obvious bleeding, presence of petechiae, ecchymosis, level of consciousness etc., and other clinical parameters and point of testing can provide further information about the patient's clinical condition (**Table 2**). Clinical examination and the point of care tests can be repeated to assess the response to therapy. Use of bedside portable ultrasound machine, in addition to the clinical assessment, allows rapid confirmation of diagnosis (e.g., pneumothorax or hemothorax in trauma, myocardial infarction by visualizing akinetic segments of myocardium etc.), and also allows therapies such as insertion of intercostal drains, fluid or blood transfusion in case of hemoperitoneum or collapsed inferior vena cava (IVC) etc., (**Fig. 3**). Rapid ultrasound in shock (RUSH) protocol is a three-step ultrasonography protocol for quick

TABLE 2 Clinical assessment and point-of-care (POC) laboratory tests in patients with shock.

Variable	Assessment	Interpretation
Clinical assessment		
Peripheral temperature		
	Cold, clammy extremities	Suggest reduced cardiac output, decreased tissue perfusion
	Peripheral temperature <27°C	Indicates low cardiac index (<2 L/m^2/min)
Core-periphery temperature difference		
	Forearm-to-fingertip >4°C	Suggests decreased tissue perfusion due to reduced cardiac output
	Core-great-ambient temperature >3°C	• Suggests poor perfusion due to reduced cardiac output • Associated with increased mortality
	Knee-ambient temperature	Suggests poor perfusion, associated with increased mortality
Capillary refill time (2–7 Newton pressure applied to fingertip or sternum)		
	Normal <2 s varies with age	Delayed CRT correlates with tissue hypoperfusion, lactate levels, may be associated with increased mortality. Decreasing CRT suggests improving perfusion
Mottling score#	Score 0–5	Strongly correlates with lactate levels and 14-day mortality. Mottling score will reduce when perfusion improves and vice versa
Laser Doppler imaging	Can visualize the circulation around the knee area	Correlates well with skin mottling score. Reduced perfusion evidence of reduced tissue perfusion. Can be used in dark skinned people
Pedal edema, ascites is generally seen late in CHF	Pitting edema of foot and ankle	Suggest presence of cardiac failure in absence of liver or renal failure
Urine output	Oliguria	Suggests reduced cardiac output in absence of diuretics or renal failure
Mental obtundation	Altered level of consciousness	Suggests reduced cardiac output in previously healthy individual, mentation will improve once perfusion is restored, unless another pathology is present
Laboratory parameters		
Serum lactate levels (arterial)	N ≥ 2 mmol/L	Suggests hypoperfusion. If lactate levels are high in presence of normal blood pressure, then it is called occult hypoperfusion. Decreasing lactate levels suggest improving perfusion
Central venous oxygen saturation$	>70%	Reduction in $ScvO_2$ suggest increased O_2 extraction by tissues due to decreased delivery (low CO state, anemia etc.). Increase in $ScvO_2$ after intervention suggest improvement in O_2 delivery
CO_2 gap%	N ≥ 5 mm Hg	A widened pCO_2 gap suggests hypoperfusion, indicating the inability of venous circulation to washout the CO_2 produced in peripheral tissues

#Heterogeneous vasoconstriction of the microcirculation is classically described as an erythematous-violaceous hue of the skin that starts around the knees and progressively spreads both upward and downward. Seen in fair skinned individuals, difficult to assess in with dark skinned people.

$Central venous oxygen saturation, $ScvO_2$ (sample collected from central venous catheter) is a surrogate for mixed venous oxygen saturation, MvO_2 (sample collected from distal port of pulmonary artery catheter).

%CO_2 gap: Central venous-to-arterial CO_2 difference (ΔPCO_2) blood collected simultaneously from the central venous catheter and arterial catheter, is a surrogate for mixed venous-to-arterial carbon dioxide (CO_2) tension difference [P(v - a)CO_2].

(CHF: congestive heart failure)

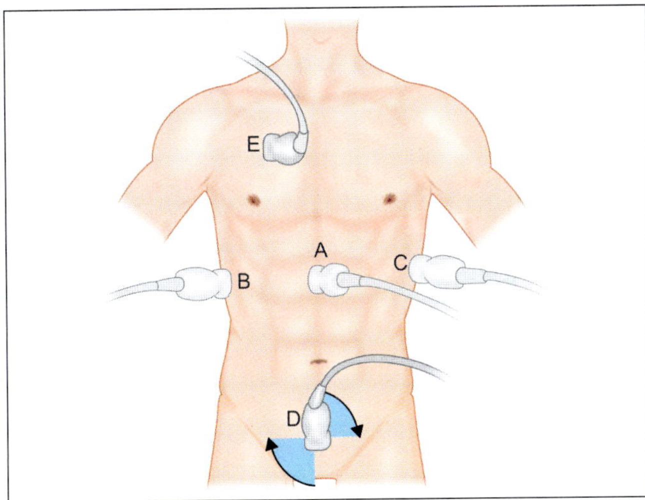

(FAST/LUQ: focused assessment with sonography for trauma/left upper quadrant view; FAST/RUQ: focused assessment with sonography for trauma/right upper quadrant; IVC: inferior vena cava; RUSH: rapid ultrasound for shock and hypotension)

FIGURE 3: RUSH examination: Step 2. Evaluation of "the tank". Probe positions for (**A**) IVC view; (**B**) FAST/RUQ, add pleural view; (**C**) FAST/LUQ, add pleural view; (**D**) Fast/Pelvis; (**E**) Lung views.

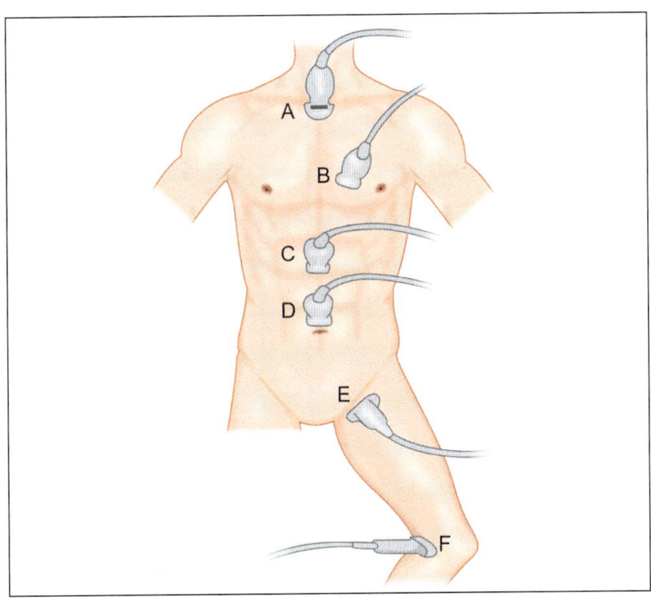

(DVT: deep vein thrombosis; RUSH: rapid ultrasound for shock and hypotension)

FIGURE 4: The RUSH examination: Step 3. Evaluation of "the pipes". Probe position for (**A**) Suprasternal aorta; (**B**) Parasternal aorta; (**C**) Epigastric aorta; (**D**) Supraumbilical aorta; (**E**) Femoral DVT; (**F**) Popliteal DVT.

assessment of a patient with hypotension. Once the type of shock is diagnosed specific therapies can be initiated (**Table 3** and **Fig. 4**).

Once MAP is restored, additional hemodynamic monitoring can be instituted, which will allow confirmation of type of shock by assessing hemodynamic profile and guide further therapy (**Table 4**).

TABLE 3 Urgent targeted therapeutic interventions for specific types of shock.

Type of shock	Specific interventions
Distributive shock (septic)	• Measure (arterial) lactate level. Remeasure if initial lactate is > 2 mmol/L[!] • Obtain blood cultures prior to administration of antibiotics • Administer broad-spectrum antibiotics[*] • Rapidly administer 30 mL/kg crystalloid for hypotension or lactate ≥ 4 mmol/L • Apply vasopressors if patient is hypotensive during or after fluid resuscitation to maintain MAP ≥ 65 mm Hg[**] • Source control by surgical or radiological intervention, removal of infected devices, if present
Cardiogenic shock	• Immediate revascularization with PCI or CABG or thrombolysis[#] • Mechanical circulatory support (IABP, LVAD)
Hypovolemic (hemorrhagic)[$] shock	• Activate massive transfusion protocol • Measure lactate or base deficit upon arrival • Transfuse packed red blood cells, plasma, and platelets in a 1:1:1 ratio • Measure coagulopathy using viscoelastic methods upon arrival • Do not use large volume crystalloid resuscitation (no >3 L over 6 hours) • *Stop bleeding*: Damage control surgery, interventional radiology, external compression, correction of coagulopathy if present
Obstructive shock	• Fluid therapy[^] and vasopressors to maintain perfusion pressure • Etiology specific interventions, e.g., pericardiocentesis for cardiac tamponade, thrombolysis (pharmacological or mechanical) for pulmonary embolism etc.

All patients will need immediate intravenous (IV) access (2 large cannulas, in particular for hemorrhagic shock)

[!]Arterial cannulation should be performed early, as it will help in collecting repeated ABG and lactate samples, apart from giving continuous accurate blood pressure measurement.

[*] Do not delay administration of antibiotics, for obtaining blood for culture.

[**] Start vasopressors early rather than late, as each hour's delay in restoring MAP may lead an increased mortality/hour.

[#]Due to newly added third arm of inflammatory cascade, even with cardiogenic some patients may need cautious fluid infusion.

[$]This only pertains to managing hemorrhagic shock, and not other aspects of trauma.

[^]The response to fluid in patients with obstructive shock is likely to be transient.

(CABG: coronary artery bypass graft; IABP: intra-aortic balloon pump; LVAD: left ventricular assist device; MAP: mean arterial pressure; PCI: percutaneous coronary intervention)

TABLE 4 Hemodynamic profile in different types of shock.

Type of shock	CO/CI	SvO_2	CVP	PAOP	SVR	Echocardiographic signs
Hypovolemic shock	Low	Low	Low	Low	Normal/High	Small volumes of the cardiac chambers and normal or high contractility
Cardiogenic shock	Low	Low, acute VSD step-up in O_2 saturation between RA and RV	High	• High • RV failure • Normal or low	High	Diagnostic value by assessing regional wall motion abnormality, structural problems such as valve dysfunction, septal defects, cardiac contractility, and dilated ventricles
Distributive	• Normal/ High • Late stage • Normal/ Low	High or low	Low	Low/normal	Low	Echocardiography in general shows normal cardiac chambers and preserved or increased contractility (unless septic cardiomyopathy occurs)
Obstructive shock	Low	Low	High	• High • Equalization of diastolic pressure in tamponade	High	Tamponade is characterized by pericardial effusion, small RV and LV, and dilated inferior vena cava (IVC); in pulmonary embolism, dilated RV and small LV are present; in tension pneumothorax, the hallmark is the compression of the RV, LV with small cardiac chambers

(CI: cardiac index; PAOP: pulmonary artery occlusion pressure; SvO_2: mixed venous O_2 saturation)

TABLE 5 Specific diagnostic tests for different types of shock.

Specific tests	Significance
• ECG • Cardiogenic shock secondary to MI, pulmonary embolism (obstructive shock)	Arrhythmias, ST elevation and reciprocal ST depression, sinus tachycardia, S1, Q3,T3 pattern, reduced voltage with electrical alternans
• Biomarkers • Creatinine kinase MB fraction (CKMB), myocardial stretch (BNP) myocardial injury (troponin C and I), oxidative stress (myeloperoxidase)	Ischemia, myocarditis, pulmonary embolism due to myocardial damage
Blood, urine, sputum cultures, imaging appropriate to the organ system involved, e.g., X-ray chest or standing X-ray abdomen, CT thorax, abdomen or lumber puncture with CSF culture, CT head	Septic shock
Elevated alkaline phosphatase	Biliary obstruction/cholangitis, septic shock
Fractional excretion of sodium/urea	Hypovolemic shock
X-ray chest (there is no time for this, rely on clinical diagnosis)	Obstructive shock due to pneumothorax

(BNP: brain natriuretic peptide)

The additional monitoring includes central venous catheterization (CVC) and central venous pressure (CVP) measurement, pulmonary artery catheter insertion for monitoring systolic and diastolic pulmonary artery pressure and pulmonary artery occlusion pressure (PAOP), and CO measurement. There are now less invasive ways to measure CO such as Flo Trac (Edwards Lifesciences), PiCCO and volume view, LiDCO etc. The newer systems also allow measurement of parameters such as Global end-diastolic volume (GEDV), a measure of preload and extravascular lung water (EVLW), and a measure of fluid in the lung. Other parameters to assess fluid responsiveness such as pulse pressure variation (PPV), systolic pressure variation (SPV), stroke volume variation (SVV) etc., are also available. Apart from this, hourly urine output (called poor man's CO monitor) should be measured.

Diagnostic tests and imaging: Additional imaging appropriate for suspected system involvement, sampling for culture sensitivity from the suspected site of infection, various biomarkers, and biochemical tests as appropriate should be carried out (**Table 5**).

MANAGEMENT

Primary goal of initial resuscitation is not just to restore blood pressure but to improve tissue oxygenation. Once the cause is identified measures should be taken to correct it. Prompt venous access with wide bore peripheral cannula, followed by arterial catheter placement for accurate measurement of blood pressure and lactate should be achieved ASAP. Proximally cited single lumen large bore venous catheters (16G/18G) are preferred over multilumen central venous catheters since they allow faster infusion of fluids. Similarly, short cannula is preferred over longer cannulas. Placement of CVC is not urgent and may be indicated if vasopressors are needed, however, this can wait, and vasopressors can be given through peripheral veins for a short period of time, till CVC can be paced. Urinary catheter for monitoring hourly urine output and nasogastric/ orogastric tube placement should be done promptly [for suspected upper gastrointestinal (GI) bleeding].

INITIAL RESUSCITATION

Fluid therapy: It is the cornerstone in the management of patients with septic and hypovolemic shock. Initial large bolus of 30–40 mL/kg of crystalloid may be followed by slower infusion rates as per patient response. In case of hemorrhagic shock, massive transfusion protocol should be activated early and noncross-matched O negative blood products followed by cross-matched blood and blood products infused. Even patients with obstructive shock and cardiogenic shock cautious fluid administration may be attempted, some patients may respond to this.

In general, the fluid therapy should be given in a "goal-directed manner" and targeted to physiologic needs of individual patients. Restoration of MAP (65–70 mm Hg) and $ScvO_2 > 70\%$ is the initial goal of resuscitation. Crystalloids are the preferred fluids in resuscitation; however, when large volumes of fluids are needed, the surviving sepsis campaign (SSC) guidelines suggest addition of albumin to crystalloid as excessive crystalloid infusion can lead to abdominal compartment syndrome (ACS). Glucose-containing fluid should not be used to correct intravascular volume deficit or acute hypovolemia. If after initial resuscitation patient continues to be hemodynamically unstable, further fluid therapy should be guided by assessing fluid responsiveness. (See the chapter Fluid Assessment and Management in Critically Ill).

Though fluid resuscitation is touted as the cornerstone of resuscitation, there may be problems caused by overzealous fluid therapy. The response to fluids is transient and may delay optimization, though fluid administration results in 25–30% increase in blood volume, but only 10–15% persists at the end of 4 hours in contrast, in patients with sepsis only <5% of crystalloids stay at end of 1 hour. The benefits increase in MAP and stroke volume (SV) with fluids are short lived. Fluid administration may lead to interstitial edema, increased filling pressures, and high EVLW, and increased organ dysfunction. Fluid infusion may not always increase MAP; fluid overload may cause adverse outcomes.

Aggressive fluid resuscitation causes vasodilatation, damage to endothelial glycocalyx, increased tissue edema thereby further aggravating tissue hypoperfusion and adverse outcomes.

Vasopressor therapy: There is some rationale in starting vasopressors early, instead of waiting for completion of fluid resuscitation to be complete. The hypoperfusion in shock in general and septic shock in particular is multifactorial, so fluid therapy alone is not the answer. The hemodynamic targets cannot be achieved always by fluid only approach thus addition of vasopressors early will help to achieve quickly the safe perfusion pressure particularly in case of life-threatening hypotension. We can administer noradrenaline through a peripheral line for a short period. Though noradrenaline is traditionally given via central venous route, the incidence of complication was found to be more in peripherally inserted intravenous cannulas (hand and feet) and if administered for long time (>6 h). Prolonged hypotension and the degree of hypotension are associated with increased mortality.

Low diastolic pressure reflects low vasomotor tone and is an independent predictor of mortality. It reflects severe vasoplegia and warrants emergency noradrenaline infusion to maintain organ perfusion. Studies show that early initiation of vasopressors is associated with improved survival and better outcome. There is some evidence that early administration of noradrenaline increases preload and CO. Noradrenaline causes both arterial and venoconstriction thus increasing mean systemic filling pressure and venous return. Noradrenaline increases the preload probably by converting unstressed volume into stressed volume. Early administration of noradrenaline improves microcirculation in severely hypotensive patients. Finally, early administration of noradrenaline reduces fluid requirements and may prevent harmful fluid overload.

MANAGEMENT BASED ON TYPE OF SHOCK

Here we discuss aspects of management specific to the type of shock (**Table 3**).

Hypovolemic shock: It is due to internal or external fluid loss. Trauma is the leading cause of hemorrhagic shock. Advanced Trauma Life Support (ATLS®) has divided shock in four classes depending in vital signs (i.e., pulse rate, blood pressure, pulse pressure, respiratory rate, mental status, hourly urine output and mentation) and estimated blood loss. (Class I < 15%, class II 15–30%, class III 30–40%, and class IV > 40%). For patients with class I and II shock, crystalloids may be enough to optimize hemodynamics, provided no further bleeding occurs.

The European guidelines on management of major bleeding and coagulopathy recommend that fluid therapy using isotonic balanced salt solutions (over salt solutions) should be used in these patients. Further, they suggest avoiding hypotonic solutions such as Ringer's lactate (RL) in patients with severe traumatic brain injury (TBI). The United States Food and Drug Administration (USFDA) advises that starches should not be used in critically ill adults, including those with sepsis, and those with pre-existing renal dysfunction. If used, they should be discontinued at first sign of renal injury or coagulopathy. Damage control surgery or interventional radiological procedures as needed should be done to control bleeding.

Cardiogenic shock: It is defined as a state of ineffective CO due to a primary cardiac dysfunction resulting in inadequate end-organ perfusion. The aim is to attain euvolemia, by cautious administration of 250 mL aliquots or using fluid challenge with reassessment at every stage, unless there is obvious fluid overload. Optimal blood pressure value is not known and should be individualized. Noradrenaline remains the first choice vasopressor, since the SOAP II trial found increased incidence of arrhythmias with the use of dopamine in these patients. Presence of right ventricle (RV) failure poses a challenge and it is important to not to volume overload RV as it can hamper left ventricular function by impairs left ventricular filling due to ventricular interdependence and reduce CO. Shock related to mechanical causes like valvular dysfunction should be immediately treated by surgical interventions.

Distributive shock: In septic shock, the most common distributive shock the concept of "Four Ds" is now advocated as part of "Fluid stewardship". The four Ds represent drug, duration, dosing, and de-escalation. It should go hand in hand with fluid strategies called "ROSE" (resuscitation, optimization, salvage, and evacuation) or "SOSD" (salvage, optimization, stabilization, and de-escalation). These concepts represent the dynamic aspects of fluid administration in different phases of septic shock. When the patient needs urgent fluids or is getting stabilized fluids are required to correct hypovolemia, then to maintain stability and lastly just as replacement. Once this has been achieved, and patients start getting better, if they do not have spontaneous diuresis, fluid need to be actively removed for achieving net negative balance. Neurogenic shock occurs secondary to a disruption of the sympathetic pathway with unopposed parasympathetic excitation, presenting as hypotension and bradycardia. Anaphylactic shock needs removal of offending agent, adrenaline bolus and infusion, fluid resuscitation and supportive measures.

Obstructive shock: It is less frequent than other types of shock. The treatment is directed at correcting the underlying etiology, which obstructs cardiopulmonary flow. Fluid administration should be attempted in all patients with a critical alteration of tissue perfusion in order to increase preload, even though clinical benefit is unlikely. Aortic dissection with cardiac tamponade may require urgent surgery.

FUTURE DIRECTIONS

We always worry about the global hemodynamics and macrocirculation (systolic blood pressure and MAP etc.); however, this may not reflect what is happening at the cellular level. Even after restoring macrocirculation to apparent "normal levels", tissue perfusion may be inadequate and hypoxia may persist at the cellular levels. This loss of coherence between global and tissue perfusion is called hemodynamic incoherence (**Table 6**). We expect that this may be the direction of future research.

CONCLUSION

Shock is a complex, heterogeneous clinical syndrome with high mortality. It requires multidisciplinary approach with ongoing resuscitation with simultaneous identification of etiology and implementation of definitive therapy. Immediate recognition of the problem with clinical assessment, point-of-care testing, and restoration of organ perfusion are the goals of therapy. After diagnosis, prompt corrective therapy directed toward specific etiology will go a long way toward improving patient outcomes. We expect future research to take the direction toward reducing hemodynamic incoherence.

TABLE 6 Resuscitation incoherence.

Item	Type 1	Type 2	Type 3	Type 4
Macro: Maintained	• MAP $\geq$ 65 mm Hg (or usual level) • $ScvO_2 \geq 70\%$ • $P(v\text{-}a)CO_2 \leq 6$ mm Hg • CI > 2.2 L/m^2			
Micro: Normal	• Severely impaired microcirculation with macro -micro decoupling • CRT >5 s, PI < 0.6 • PPV < 60%, MFI < 2 • Mottling score > 2 • Cold extremities, • UO < 0.3 mL/kg/min	• Mildly impaired • CRT 2–5 s, PI 0.6–1.4 • PPV 60–80%, MFI 2–3 • Mottling score 0–2 • Cold extremities, • UO 0.3–0.5 mL/kg/min	• Normal micro circulation • CRT $\leq$ 2 s, PI $\geq$ 1.4 • PPV $\geq$ 80%, MFI $\geq$ 3 • Mottling score 0 • Warm extremities, • UO > 0.5 mL/kg/min	• Severely impaired microcirculation and micro -macro decoupling • CRT >5 s, PI < 0.6 • PPV < 60%, MFI < 2 • Mottling score > 2 • Cold extremities, • UO < 0.3 mL/kg/min

Continued...

Continued...

Item	Type 1	Type 2	Type 3	Type 4
Cellular hypoxia	• Hypoxia dependent on microcirculatory perfusion. Abnormalities may reduce once microcirculation improves. • Lactate > 2 mmol/L • $P(v\text{-}a)CO_2/C(a\text{-}v)O_2 > 1.6$ etc.	• Compensatory mechanisms maintaining cellular oxygen demand. However, if demand rises, hypoxia ensues. • Lactate < 2 mmol/L • $P(v\text{-}a)CO_2/C(a\text{-}v)O_2 < 1.6$ etc.	• Cellular hypoxia due to cytopathy. Circulatory changes do not affect the cells. No manipulation of macro or microcirculation can help. • Lactate > 2 mmol/L • $P(v\text{-}a)CO_2/C(a\text{-}v)O_2 > 1.6$ etc.	• Microcirculatory abnormalities mask an underlying cytopathy. Even after correction of microcirculation, tissue hypoxia does not improve due to coexisting mitochondrial dysfunction. • $P(v\text{-}a)CO_2/C(a\text{-}v)\ O_2 < 1.6$ etc.

Type 1: Macro-micro incoherence + impaired cell; **Type 2:** Macro-micro incoherence + normal cell; **Type 3:** Micro-cell incoherence + normal micro; **Type 4:** "Macro-micro + Micro-cell" incoherence.

[$C(a\text{-}v)O_2$: difference in arterio-veous oxygen saturation; CI: cardiac index; CRT: capillary refill time; Macro: macrocirculation; MAP: mean arterial pressure; MFI: microvascular flow index; Micro: microcirculation; $P(v\text{-}a)CO_2$ - PCO_2 gap; $P(v\text{-}a)CO_2/C(a\text{-}v)O_2$: central venous-arterial carbon dioxide difference/arterial-central venous oxygen difference; PI: peripheral perfusion index; PPV: proportion of perfused vessels); $ScvO_2$: central venous oxygen saturation]

Source: Adapted from He HW, Long Y, Liu DW, Ince C. Resuscitation incoherence and dynamic circulation-perfusion coupling in circulatory shock. Chin Med J (Engl). 2019;132(10):1218-27.

RECOMMENDED READINGS

1. Weil MH. Defining hemodynamic instability. In: Pinsky MR, Payen D, (Eds). Functional hemodynamic monitoring. Update in intensive care and emergency medicine. Berlin, Heidelberg: Springer; 2005.
2. Cecconi M, De Backer D, Antonelli M, Beale R, Bakker J, Hofer C, et al. Consensus on circulatory shock and hemodynamic monitoring. Task force of the European Society of Intensive Care Medicine. Intensive Care Med. 2014;40(12):1795-815.
3. Standl T, Annecke T, Cascorbi I, Heller AR, Sabashnikov A, Teske W. The Nomenclature, Definition and Distinction of Types of Shock. Dtsch Arztebl Int. 2018;115(45):757-68.
4. Levy MM, Evans LE, Rhodes A. The Surviving Sepsis Campaign Bundle: 2018 update. Intensive Care Med. 2018;44(6):925-8.
5. Tehrani BN, Truesdell AG, Sherwood MW, Desai S, Tran HA, Epps KC, et al. Standardized Team-Based Care for Cardiogenic Shock. J Am Coll Cardiol. 2019;73(13):1659-69.
6. Spahn DR, Bouillon B, Cerny V, Duranteau J, Filipescu D, Hunt BJ, et al. The European guideline on management of major bleeding and coagulopathy following trauma: fifth edition. Crit Care. 2019;23(1):98.
7. Thiele H, Ohman EM, Desch S, Eitel I, de Waha S. Management of cardiogenic shock. Eur Heart J. 2015;36(20):1223-30.
8. Seif D, Perera P, Mailhot T, Riley D, Mandavia D. Bedside ultrasound in resuscitation and the rapid ultrasound in shock protocol. Crit Care Res Pract. 2012;2012:503254.
9. Shafi S, Collinsworth AW, Richter KM, Alam HB, Becker LB, Bullock MR, et al. Bundles of care for resuscitation from hemorrhagic shock and severe brain injury in trauma patients-Translating knowledge into practice. J Trauma Acute Care Surg. 2016;81(4):780-94.
10. Waechter J, Kumar A, Lapinsky SE, Marshall J, Dodek P, Arabi Y, et al; Cooperative Antimicrobial Therapy of Septic Shock Database Research Group. Interaction between fluids and vasoactive agents on mortality in septic shock: a multicenter, observational study. Crit Care Med. 2014;42(10):2158-68.
11. Monnet X, Jabot J, Maizel J, Richard C, Teboul JL. Norepinephrine increases cardiac preload and reduces preload dependency assessed by passive leg raising in septic shock patients. Crit Care Med. 2011;39(4):689-94.
12. He HW, Long Y, Liu DW, Ince C. Resuscitation incoherence and dynamic circulation-perfusion coupling in circulatory shock. Chin Med J (Engl). 2019;132(10):1218-27.

CHAPTER
76
Fever in Intensive Care Unit

Rajesh Chawla, Roseleen Kaur Bali, Aakanksha Chawla Jain

ABSTRACT

Fever is a very common occurrence in intensive care unit (ICU). Fever can occur in up to 26–88% of ICU admissions. This will vary depending on the ICU patient population and definition used. The joint task force of American College of Critical Care Medicine (ACCM) and Infection Disease Society of America (IDSA) defined fever in ICU as body temperature of 38.3°C (101°F) or higher. In the ICU, patient may be admitted with fever or it may develop during the stay in the ICU. A variety of methods have been used to measure body temperature. This can be measured from a peripheral or from core sites.

The beginning of new onset fever in ICU most often leads to performance of unfocused diagnostic investigations and initiation of multiple empirical antimicrobial therapy. This kind of approach leads to patient discomfort, unnecessary diagnostic tests, antibiotics resistance, and cost to the ailing patient. Most common causes of infectious fever in ICU include ventilator-associated pneumonia (VAP), nasal sinusitis, catheter-related sepsis, *Clostridioides difficile,* diarrhea, abdominal sepsis, and complicated wound infections. The diagnostic approach to a new onset fever in ICU should be focused. All patients with new onset fever in ICU above 38.3°C (101°F) should be investigated. These patients of fever need comprehensive and systemic diagnostic approach to reach the correct diagnosis and start appropriate treatment.

"Be sure you put your feet in the right place, then stand firm"

—Abraham Lincoln

INTRODUCTION

Fever is a very common occurrence in ICU. This may occur as a response to infection or it may occur as a nonspecific physical sign accompanying serious illness like in postoperative patients. In the ICU, patient may be admitted with fever or it may develop during the stay in the ICU. This chapter will restrict discussion to new onset fever in ICU.

The beginning of new onset fever in ICU most often leads to performance of unfocused diagnostic investigations and initiation of multiple empirical antimicrobial therapy. This kind of approach leads to patient discomfort, unnecessary diagnostic tests, antibiotics resistance, and cost to the ailing patient. These patients of fever need comprehensive and systemic diagnostic approach to reach the correct diagnosis and start appropriate treatment.

This article outlines the systemic approach to new onset fever in ICU and their evaluation and treatment.

DEFINITION

Normal body temperature is approximately 37°C (98.6°F). It can range from 36 to 37.5°C depending on which time of the day it is recorded and the method of temperature measurement used. The joint task force of ACCM and IDSA defined fever in ICU as body temperature of 38.3°C (101°F) or higher. This definition is arbitrary but most of the studies have used this threshold to define fever.

Hyperthermia is any fever which exceeds 41°C (105.8°F). These are often noninfectious and can rapidly deteriorate and their treatment differs from that of regular fever in ICU.

TEMPERATURE MEASUREMENT

All patients in the ICU should have an hourly temperature recorded and charted in nursing record. A variety of methods have been used to measure body temperature. This can be measured from a peripheral or from core sites.

Core sites such as intravascular pulmonary artery catheter (PAC) and intravesicular (urinary bladder) are considered the most appropriate site for measurement of core temperature. This requires placement of PAC which is not practiced frequently nowadays. Another method is rectal core temperature which is measured either with thermometer or rectal probe, which is tenth of a degree higher than core temperature. Some other methods which are less accurate include temporal artery and tympanic sites.

However, most popular methods are peripheral which include oral and axillary temperature measurements and have limitations such as oral is influenced by eating, drinking, and presence of respiratory devices delivering warm gases. Axillary measurements underestimate core temperature. So ideally, all ICU should have an access to core temperature (rectal and tympanic) properly calibrated and sterilized.

PATHOGENESIS

Fever can occur in up to 26–88% of ICU admissions. This will vary depending on the ICU patient population and definition used.

Almost 50% of fevers in ICU are due to infections. Most of the patients in the ICU have devices such as central venous catheter (CVC), arterial lines, urinary catheter, endotracheal tube, and nasogastric tube. These devices bypass the natural host defenses and provide easy access to microorganisms. Fever is an adaptive response that helps the host to get rid of pathogens and increase in temperature results in antibody production, T-cell activation, cytokines production, and increase in neutrophil and macrophage functions.

The cytokines released by monocyte cells are the most important cells in the genesis of fever. The cytokines primarily involved in the development of fever include interleukin-1 (IL-1), IL-6, and tumor necrosis factor-α (TNF-α).

These cytokines bind to receptors located in anterior hypothalamus. Here cytokines receptor interaction activates phospholipase A2 which liberates arachidonic acid as substrate for cyclooxygenase pathway. Some cytokine increases cyclooxygenase expression directly which leads to the release of prostaglandin E2. This small lipid mediator diffuses across the blood-brain barrier to decrease the fire up of phosphate warm sensitive neurons which leads to activation of response to decrease heat loss and increase heat production.

Many noninfectious conditions also release proinflammatory cytokines which lead to a febrile response.

Causes of infectious and noninfectious fever in the ICU are given in **Table 1**. Out of these most common causes of infectious fever in ICU include VAP, nasal sinusitis, catheter-related sepsis, *Clostridioides difficile*, diarrhea, abdominal sepsis, and complicated wound infections.

DIAGNOSTIC APPROACH

The process of fever in ICU leads to initiation of a large number of unnecessary tests that are costly and expose the patient to lot of risks with inconclusive results. So, it is important that fever in ICU should be systematically evaluated in systematic and clinically appropriate manner to reach a diagnosis and start treatment.

The diagnostic approach to a new onset fever in ICU should be focused. All patients with new onset fever

TABLE 1 Causes of infectious and noninfectious fever.

Site	Infectious	Noninfectious
Pulmonary	• Ventilator-associated tracheobronchitis • Ventilator-associated pneumonia • Empyema	• Pulmonary embolism • ARDS
Head and neck	• Meningitis • Otitis media • Sinusitis • Infection	• Cerebrovascular accident • Seizure disorder • Traumatic brain injury
Cardiac	• Infective endocarditis	• Myocardial infarction • Pericarditis
Skin	• Cellulitis • Infected pressure ulcer • Surgical site infection	• Drug eruptions
Abdomen	• Intra-abdominal infections (e.g., SBP and abscesses) • *Clostridium difficile* infection • Pyelonephritis • Catheter-related UTI • Perineal or perianal abscess	• Pancreatitis • Acalculous cholecystitis • Mesenteric ischemia • Ischemic colitis
Extremities	• CVC-related bloodstream infection • Femoral line/PICC-related bloodstream infection • Septic arthritis	• Gout • DVT
Miscellaneous		• Postoperative fever • Drugs • Transfusion reactions • Endocrine disorders (e.g., thyrotoxicosis and adrenal insufficiency) • Malignancy • Inflammatory disorders

(CVC: central venous catheter; DVT: deep vein thrombosis; PICC: peripherally inserted central catheter; SBP: spontaneous bacterial peritonitis; UTI: urinary tract infection)

in ICU above 38.3°C (101°F) should be investigated. In many patients with low grade fever <38.3°C that appear during ICU course are not investigated unless patient is immunocompromised.

TAKE DETAILED HISTORY

Take proper history from bedside nurse and resident doctor and do a thorough chart review.

- Enquire about medications, blood transfusions, rash, new procedure, dressing changed, any catheter or line manipulation, and dialysis. Inquire about duration of mechanical ventilation, indwelling urinary catheter, central line and arterial line placements, chest drains, and abdominal drains.
- Assess previous microbiologic history and antimicrobial therapy given for these conditions.
- Enquire about diarrhea to rule out the possibility of *Clostridioides* (formerly *Clostridium*) *difficile* infection.

PERFORM FOCUSED CLINICAL EXAMINATION

This should be performed from head to toe to look for various causes which can cause fever (**Table 1**).

- Look for any wound infection in the scalp, purulent nasal discharge, and sinus tenderness.
- Examine parotid swelling and oral hygiene.
- Look for neck rigidity.
- The treating physician should look for quality of sputum, endotracheal secretions (color, amount, and thickness), and perform detailed chest examination to look for pneumonia.
- Cardiac examination should be done to look for heart sounds with new onset murmur suggesting infective endocarditis or pericardial rub suggesting pericarditis.
- Clinical examination of abdomen should be done to look for evidence of liver abscess, acalculous cholecystitis, pancreatitis, mesenteric ischemia, or possibility of spontaneous bacterial peritonitis.
- Examine skin, joints, and lower limbs for evidence of wound infections, cellulites, lymphadenitis, septic arthritis, osteomyelitis, erythema, swelling, or tenderness to indicate deep venous thrombosis.
- Examine all vascular devices for duration, purulence, and erythema at insertion site.
- Examine urinary catheter site.

All infections when deteriorate have the capability to progress to septic shock which is distributive type of shock. Some noninfectious causes of fever can also result in distributive shock such as adrenal crises, thyroid storm, and acute hemolytic transfusion reaction.

INVESTIGATIONS

There are no guidelines to suggest set of investigations to find out the cause of fever. Do investigations which are clinically driven and cost effective. Commonly the following tests are suggested to target the common causes of infections.

- If the examination does not suggest noninfectious cause and fever is above 101°F or patient is hemodynamically unstable or has developed new organ dysfunction or immunosuppressed, two sets of blood culture should be sent. All blood cultures should be obtained after skin disinfection with 2% chlorhexidine or 2% iodine. All samples should be taken from two peripheral venepunctures or one from distal lumen of the central line and another from periphery. If blood cannot be taken from peripheral vein, then blood can be drawn from the different lumen of multi-lumen catheter. Minimum two sets, each set containing two bottles (one aerobic and another anaerobic), at least 10 mL in each bottle to be inoculated directly into culture bottle.
- If clinically infection is suspected, the following tests should be sent:
    - Routine blood count, liver function tests, and kidney function tests.
    - C-reactive protein, procalcitonin when presence of infection is not clear.
    - Chest imaging such as chest skiagram which can detect a new or progressive pulmonary infiltrate. This could also detect pleural effusion or empyema as a cause of fever. Patients who have got already abnormalities in chest skiagram such as acute respiratory distress syndrome (ARDS) and interstitial lung disease, then CT chest is advised in such cases.
- *Urine analysis and culture sensitivity*: This should be done in all cases, particularly those with catheter or who have renal disease such as stone, trauma, or are immunosuppressed.
- Sputum, endotracheal aspiration, nonbronchoscopic bronchoalveolar lavage (NBAL), or bronchoscopy BAL should be sent for Gram stain and quantitative aerobic culture, acid-fast bacilli (AFB) stain, if there is suspicion of nosocomial pneumonia/VAP.
- *Sampling from suspected site of infection*: Many patients have several potential areas which can get infections. Appropriate samples should be obtained from sites such as the wounds, catheters, fluid collection sites, joints, or stool (for *Clostridioides*).
- Abdominal imaging such as ultrasound and computed tomography (CT) should be done in the following conditions:
    - Abdominal distress, tenderness, and absent bowel sounds
    - Recent abdominal surgery
    - Laboratory testing suggest intra-abdominal pathology
    - No alternate source of fever identified
- Sinus evaluation should be done if there is purulent nasal discharge.
- Avoid sending culture from urinary catheter tips, superficial wound swabs, and from drains which have been there for > 48 hours.

COMMON CAUSES

CENTRAL LINE-RELATED BLOODSTREAM INFECTION

Central venous catheter infection as a cause of fever implies colonization of catheter with bacteria with accompanying clinical manifestations suggestive of infection. Catheter-related bloodstream infection (CRBSI) is laboratory confirmed BSI in a patient with intravascular access device and has at least positive culture obtained from peripheral vein, clinical manifestation of infection, and no other apparent cause of infection identified and have in addition one of the following features:

- Positive semiquantitative culture >15 colony-forming unit (CFU)/catheter segment with the same organisms.
- Positive quantitative culture (>10^5 CFU/catheter segment) with same organisms.
- Simultaneous quantitative culture with a ≥5:1 ratio CVC versus peripheral blood culture.
- *Differential to the positivity*: Central line culture is positive at least 2 hours earlier than peripheral blood culture.

Once you suspect catheter-related infection, first of all examine CVC insertion site for any discharge and erythema. After this, blood culture should be sent from the catheter and peripheral blood. After obtaining specimens, start empirical antibiotics and change or de-escalate later based in the culture and sensitivity report.

VENTILATOR-ASSOCIATED PNEUMONIA

When a patient on ventilator support develops a new or progressive infiltrate in the chest X-ray along with fever and leukocytosis, it indicates VAP. New infiltrates in chest skiagram must be differentiated from noninfectious causes of infiltrate such as atelectasis, aspiration, pulmonary embolism, cardiogenic pulmonary edema, ARDS, drug reaction, and fluid overload.

If pneumonia is suspected, blood culture should be sent in all cases. Endotracheal aspiration, nonbronchoscopic, or bronchoscopic bronchoalveolar lavage specimen should be sent for Gram stain and aerobic culture before starting antimicrobial treatment. The choice of initial antibiotic will depend on the Gram stain and the local epidemiology of the ICU. Once culture results are available, then antibiotic can be modified or de-escalated based on culture result.

URINARY TRACT INFECTION

Most of the infections in the ICU are catheter related with an estimate incidence of the 11 per 1,000 catheter days. Urinary tract infection (UTI) is associated with increase length of stay and increase mortality. Generally, common symptoms of UTI include dysuria, urgency, pelvic discomfort, or flank pain. These are not seen commonly in catheterized patient. Routine microscopic examination of urine is insensitive but specific test. Urine culture should be restricted to patients who do not have another source of infection. The sampling should be done from port of the urinary catheter rather than urinary bag. The culture threshold criteria for positive urine culture are 10^5 CFU/mL. Antibiotics should be started when urine culture is positive and patient has no other source of infection identified. Antibiotics should also be started in immunosuppressed patient.

CLOSTRIDIOIDES DIFFICILE INFECTION

Clostridium difficile infection is now called *Clostridioides* (new name) *difficile* infection (CDI). If a patient with new onset of fever in ICU has developed diarrhea, then this diagnosis should be suspected. Severe CDI may also present with abdominal pain, ileus, and systemic inflammatory symptoms. The test commonly advised toxin A and toxin B by enzyme-linked immunosorbent assay (ELISA) are widely available, but it is an insensitive test. Real-time polymerase chain reaction for toxin A and toxin B gene is rapid, accurate, and is now the preferred option. In severe cases, endoscopy and CT scan are advised. Oral vancomycin alone or with metronidazole is recommended for initial treatment.

MANAGEMENT

The most important aspect of management of fever in ICU is to treat the underlying cause of fever. Empiric antibiotic may be started in some patients and in some it may be delayed. Commonly, it is suggested to start antibiotic after obtaining cultures if fever is above 38.3°F and/or patients have sepsis or septic shock, neutropenia, immunosuppressed, and have devices.

REMOVING CENTRAL CATHETERS

The decision to remove the catheter is considered based on severity of illness, age, probability of it being causes of fever, and its consequences. Catheter removal is considered in following conditions:

- Site looks infected and catheter is in situ >48 hours.
- Catheter is known to be infected and have evidence of metastatic infection.
- Persistent bacteremia or fungemia particularly with *Staphylococcus aureus*, *Pseudomonas aeruginosa*, and *Candida*.

TREATMENT OF FEVER

This is the choice of clinician. Some clinicians do not routinely treat fever, but some treat it with antipyretic (paracetamol) on initial presentation. Protocols to treat fever symptomatically have not been found to be of benefit. When treating fever, choose acetaminophen rather than nonsteroidal anti-inflammatory drugs (NSAIDs) or aspirin.

Always prefer enteral route if patient is able to tolerate enteral administration. Aggressive or prolonged cooling with external cooling devices like blankets or ice pack is not generally indicated unless the fever is considered harmful like temperature above 41°C (>105.8°F). The effort to find out the cause of fever is ongoing while you treat with empirical antimicrobials. An approach to such a patient is summarized in **Flowchart 1**.

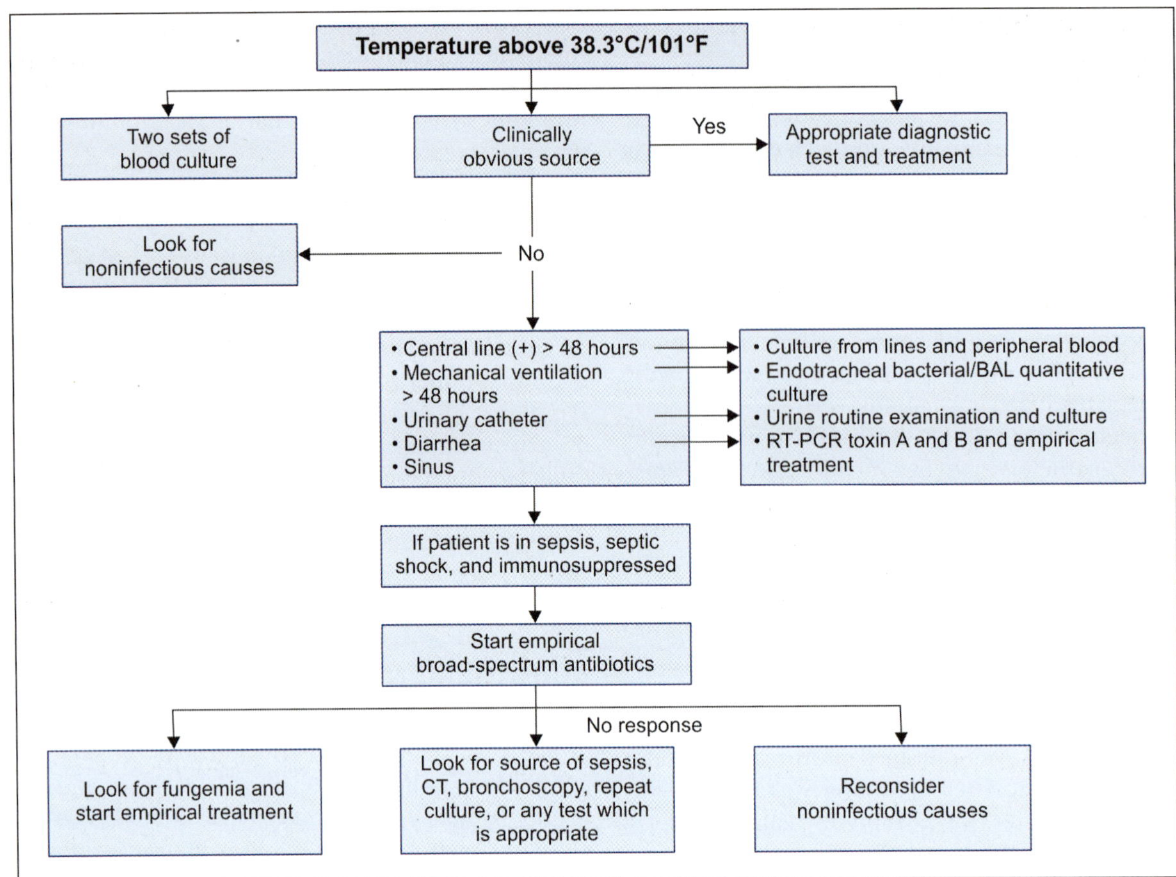

(BAL: bronchoalveolar lavage; CT: computed tomography; ICU: intensive care unit; RT-PCR: reverse transcription-polymerase chain reaction)

FLOWCHART 1: An approach to new onset fever in ICU.

RECOMMENDED READINGS

1. Meduri GU, Mauldin GL, Wunderink RG, Leeper KV Jr, Jones CB, Tolley E, et al. Causes of fever and pulmonary densities in patients with clinical manifestations of ventilator-associated pneumonia. Chest. 1994;106:221-35.
2. O'Grady NP, Alexander M, Burns LA, Dellinger EP, Garland J, Heard SO, et al. Guidelines for the prevention of intravascular catheter-related infections. Clin Infect Dis. 2011;52(9):e162-93.
3. O'Grady NP, Barie PS, Bartlett JG, Bleck T, Carroll K, Kalil AC, et al. Guidelines for evaluation of new fever in critically ill adult patients: 2008 update from the American College of Critical Care Medicine and the Infectious Diseases Society of America. Crit Care Med. 2008;36:1330-49.
4. Fallis WM. Monitoring urinary bladder temperature in the intensive care unit: state of the science. Am J Crit Care. 2002;11:38-45.
5. Giuliano KK, Scott SS, Elliot S, Giuliano AJ. Temperature measurement in critically ill orally intubated adults: a comparison of pulmonary artery core, tympanic, and oral methods. Crit Care Med. 1999;27:2188-93.
6. Egi M, Morita K. Fever in non-neurological critically ill patients: a systematic review of observational studies. J Crit Care. 2012;27:428-33.
7. Mackowiak PA. Concepts of fever. Arch Intern Med. 1998;158:1870-81.
8. Saper CB, Breder CD. The neurologic basis of fever. N Engl J Med. 1994;330:1880-6.
9. Dinarello CA, Cannon JG, Mancilla J. Interleukin-6 as an endogenous pyrogen: induction of prostaglandin E2 in brain but not in peripheral blood mononuclear cells. Brain Res. 1991;562:199-206.
10. Dinarello CA, Wolff SM. The role of interleukin-1 in disease. N Engl J Med. 1993;328:106-13.
11. Dinarello CA, Cannon JG, Mier JW, Bernheim HA, LoPreste G, Lynn DL, et al. Multiple biological activities of human recombinant interleukin 1. J Clin Invest. 1986;77:1734-9.
12. Dinarello CA. Interleukin-1 and the pathogenesis of the acute-phase response. N Engl J Med. 1984;311:1413-8.
13. Fontana A, Weber E, Dayer JM. Synthesis of interleukin 1/endogenous pyrogen in the brain of endotoxin-treated mice: a step in fever induction? J Immunol. 1984;133:1696-8.
14. Gourine AV, Rudolph K, Tesfaigzi J, Kluger MJ. Role of hypothalamic interleukin-1 beta in fever induced by cecal ligation and puncture in rats. Am J Physiol. 1998;275:R754-61.
15. Leon LR, White AA, Kluger MJ. Role of IL-6 and TNF in thermoregulation and survival during sepsis in mice. Am J Physiol. 1998;275:R269-77.
16. Klir JJ, Roth J, Szelenyi Z, McClellan JL, Kluger MJ. Role of hypothalamic interleukin-6 and tumor

necrosis factor-alpha in LPS fever in rat. Am J Physiol. 1993;265(3 Pt 2):R512-7.
17. Mackowiak PA, Bartlett JG, Borden EC, Goldblum SE, Hasday JD, Munford RS, et al. Concepts of fever: recent advances and lingering dogma. Clin Infect Dis. 1997;25:119-38.
18. Ferrara JL. The febrile platelet transfusion reaction: a cytokine shower. Transfusion. 1995;35:89-90.
19. Chen CC, Wang SS, Lee FY, Chang FY, Lee SD. Proinflammatory cytokines in early assessment of the prognosis of acute pancreatitis. Am J Gastroenterol. 1999;94:213-8.
20. Laupland KB, Bagshaw SM, Gregson DB, Kirkpatrick AW, Ross T, Church DL. Intensive care unit-acquired urinary tract infections in a regional critical care system. Crit Care. 2005;9(2):R60-5.

CHAPTER
77

Sepsis and Septic Shock

Mradul Kumar Daga, J Aarthi, Raghu RV

ABSTRACT

Sepsis is the consequence of a dysregulated inflammatory response to an infectious insult. Sepsis exists on a continuum of severity ranging from infection (invasion of sterile tissue by organisms) and bacteremia (bacteria in the blood) to sepsis and septic shock, which can lead to multiple organ dysfunction syndrome (MODS) and death.

A constellation of clinical, laboratory, radiologic, physiologic, and microbiologic data is typically required for the diagnosis of sepsis and septic shock. The diagnosis is often made empirically at the bedside upon presentation, or retrospectively when follow-up data return or a response to antibiotics is evident. Importantly, the identification of a culprit organism, although preferred, is not always feasible due to antibiotics administered prior to blood cultures being set.

Sepsis has a high mortality rate that appears to be decreasing. Sepsis and particularly septic shock should be recognized as medical emergencies in which time matters. It requires prompt recognition, appropriate broadspectrum antibiotics, fluid administration, careful hemodynamic support, and controlling the source of infection. Newer therapies are under investigation and warrants larger randomized clinical trials (RCTs) to prove its role.

"Wise and humane management of the patient is the best safeguard against infection"

—Florence Nightingale

INTRODUCTION

Sepsis remains in the top 10 leading causes of death. It is estimated to affect at least 19 million patients worldwide. The contribution of various infectious organisms to the burden of sepsis has changed over time. Gram positive bacteria are being frequently identified in patients with sepsis now, although the cases of gram negative sepsis remains substantial. The incidence of fungal sepsis has increased over the past decade, but remains lower than bacterial sepsis. The organism is not identified in half of the cases.

In a point prevalence study Indian Intensive Care Case Mix and Practice Patterns (INDICAPs) conducted in 120 intensive care units (ICUs) across India, reported a prevalence of severe sepsis of 28.3% out of which 20.5% were ICU acquired.

In a prospective study of 5 years conducted in India, severe sepsis (now termed "sepsis") was noted in 6% of the study group. The most frequent site of infection among severe sepsis patients was respiratory tract. Majority of infections were caused by gram-negative organisms (73%).

Reasons for a possible increased rate of sepsis include advancing age, immunosuppression, and multidrug-resistant infection.

DEFINITIONS AND SCORES

Sepsis exists on a continuum of severity ranging from infection and bacteremia to sepsis and septic shock, which can lead to MODS and death. The definitions of sepsis and septic shock have rapidly evolved since the early 1990s.

Early sepsis: Infection and bacteremia may be early forms of infection that can progress to sepsis. However, there is no formal definition of early sepsis.

Identification of early sepsis (qSOFA, NEWS): Societal guidelines emphasize the early identification of infected patients. The two most commonly used scores are the quick Sequential (Sepsis-related) Organ Failure Assessment score (qSOFA) and the National Early Warning Score (NEWS).

This qSOFA score is a modified version of the Sequential (Sepsis-related) Organ Failure Assessment score (SOFA). A score ≥2 is associated with poor outcomes due to sepsis.

TABLE 1 The sequential organ failure assessment score (SOFA score).

System	0	1	2	3	4
Respiration PaO_2/FIO_2 mm Hg (kPa)	≥400 (53.3)	<400 (53.3)	<300 (40)	<200 (26.7) with respiratory support	<100 (13.3) with respiratory support
Coagulation Platelets × 10^3/µL	≥150	<50	<100	<50	<20
Liver Bilirubin mg/dL (µmol/L)	<1.2 (20)	1.2–1.9 (20–32)	2.0–5.9 (33–101)	6.0–11.9 (102–204)	>12.0 (204)
Cardiovascular	MAP ≥70 mm Hg	MAP <70 mm Hg	Dopamine <5 or Dobutamine (any dose)	Dopamine 5.1–15 or Epinephrine ≤ 0.1 or Norepinephrine ≤ 0.1	Dopamine >15 or Epinephrine >0.1 or Norepinephrine >0.1
CNS GCS score	15	13–14	10–12	6–9	<6
Renal creatinine, mg/dL (µmol/L) Urine output, mL/day	<1.2 (110)	1.2–1.9 (110–170)	2.0–3.4 (171–299)	3.5–4.9 (300–440)	> 5.0 (440) <200

Catecholamine Doses = µg/kg/min for at least 1 hour

The qSOFA score is easy to calculate at bedside with each component easily identifiable.

- Respiratory rate ≥ 22 breaths per minute
- Altered mentation
- Systolic blood pressure (SBP) ≤ 100 mm Hg

NEWS is an aggregate scoring system derived from six physiologic parameters (**see Table 2 in chapter 67**).

The aggregate score represents the risk of death from sepsis and indicates the urgency of the response (**see Table 3 in chapter 67**).

A 2016 task force from the Society of Critical Care Medicine and European Society of Intensive Care Medicine (SCCM/ESICM) define sepsis and septic shock as the following:

- *Sepsis*—is defined as life-threatening organ dysfunction caused by a dysregulated host response to infection.
- *Severe sepsis*—is defined as sepsis associated with organ dysfunction, hypoperfusion abnormality, or sepsis-induced hypotension. Hypoperfusion abnormalities include lactic acidosis, oliguria, and acute alteration of mental status. Organ dysfunction is defined as an increase of two or more points in the SOFA score.
- *Sepsis-induced hypotension*—is defined by the presence of a SBP of < 90 mm Hg or its reduction by 40 mm Hg or more from baseline in the absence of other causes for hypotension (e.g., cardiogenic shock).
- *Septic shock*—can be clinically identified as patients who fulfill the criteria for sepsis who, despite adequate fluid resuscitation, require vasopressors to maintain a mean arterial pressure (MAP) ≥65 mm Hg and have a lactate >2 mmol/L (>18 mg/dL).

In 2016, *the sepsis-three committee* issued the following new definitions:

- *Sepsis*—a life-threatening condition caused by a dysregulated host response to infection, resulting in organ dysfunction.
- *Septic shock*—circulatory, cellular, and metabolic abnormalities in septic patients, presenting as fluid-refractory hypotension requiring vasopressor therapy with associated tissue hypoperfusion (lactate >2 mmol/L).
- *The classification of severe sepsis was eliminated.*

However, clinicians should be aware that SCCM/ESICM definitions are not unanimously accepted. For example, the center for medicare and medicaid services (CMS) still continues to support the previous definition of systemic inflammatory response syndrome (SIRS), sepsis, and severe sepsis.

SEQUENTIAL ORGAN FAILURE ASSESSMENT SCORE

The SOFA score was initially designed to sequentially assess the severity of organ dysfunction in patients who were critically ill from sepsis. SOFA uses simple measurements of major organ function to calculate a severity score. The scores are calculated 24 hours after admission to the ICU and every 48 hours thereafter (thus, the term "Sequential" Organ Failure Assessment). The mean and the highest scores are most predictive of mortality (**Table 1**).

Systemic inflammatory response syndrome: The use of SIRS criteria to identify those with sepsis has fallen out of favor since it is considered by many experts that SIRS criteria are present in many hospitalized patients who do not develop infection such as vasculitis, burns etc., and their ability to predict death is poor when compared with other scores such as the SOFA score. It was previously defined as two or more abnormalities in temperature, heart rate, respiration, or white blood cell count.

PATHOPHYSIOLOGY OF SEPSIS

The pathophysiology of sepsis is extremely complex. The sepsis manifestations depend on the virulence of the invading pathogen (microbial factors) as well as the ability of host to produce an appropriate immune response (host

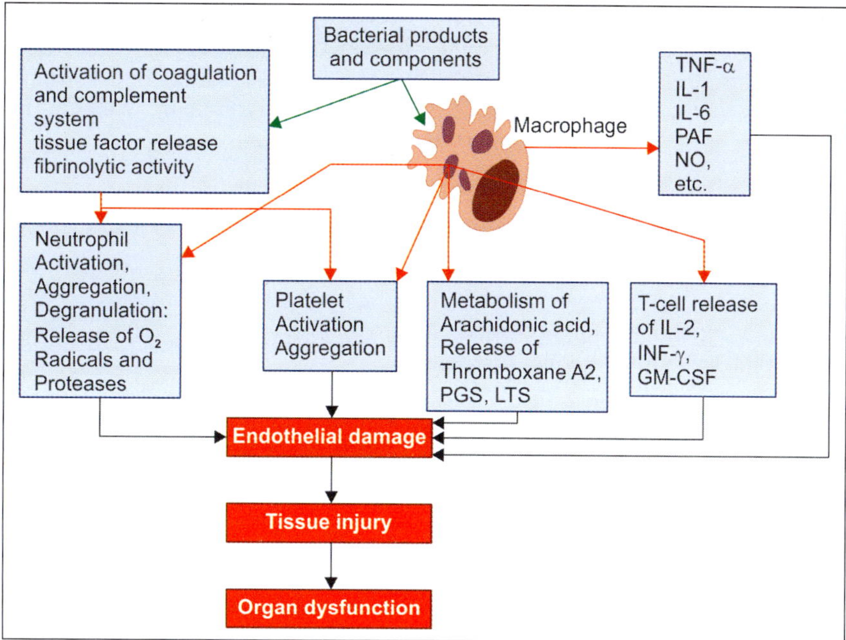

(TNF-α: tumor necrosis factor alpha; PGs: prostaglandins; LTS: leukotrienes; IL: interleukins; INF-γ: interferon-gamma; GM-CSF: granulocyte-macrophage colony-stimulating factor; PAF: platelet-activating factor)

FLOWCHART 1: The sepsis cascade.

factors). There may be an early phase of sepsis in which the immunomodulatory markers predominate as well as a late phase of prolonged immune suppression.

The host response evolves over time with the patient's clinical course. Proinflammatory reactions (directed at eliminating pathogens) are responsible for tissue damage in sepsis, whereas anti-inflammatory responses are implicated in the enhanced susceptibility to secondary infections that occurs later in the course.

Pathogens activate immune cells by an interaction with pattern recognition receptors. The recognition of structures is conserved across microbial species—pathogen-associated molecular patterns (PAMPs). These receptors result in upregulation of inflammatory gene transcription and initiation of innate immunity. A common PAMP is the lipid A moiety of lipopolysaccharide (LPS or endotoxin), which attaches to the LPS-binding protein on the surface of monocytes, macrophages, and neutrophils. LPS is transferred to and signals via toll-like receptor-4 (TLR4) to produce and release cytokines such as tumor necrosis factor (TNF) that grow the signal and alert other cells and tissues.

These receptors also sense endogenous molecules released from injured cells—damage-associated molecular patterns (DAMPs), such as high-mobility group protein B1, S100 proteins, and extracellular ribonucleic acid (RNA), deoxyribonucleic acid (DNA), and histones. Immune cells generate the proinflammatory cytokines (TNF, IL-1 and IL-6), and these produce systemic inflammation by activating circulating polymorphonuclear leukocytes (PMNs) and stimulating the liver to produce C-reactive protein (CRP). Procalcitonin and chemokines also are produced locally (**Flowchart 1**).

BOX 1 | Risk factors of sepsis.

- **Intensive care unit admission:** Approximately, 50% of intensive care unit (ICU) patients have a nosocomial infection and are, therefore, intrinsically at high risk for sepsis
- **Bacteremia:** Patients with bacteremia often develop systemic consequences of infection
- **Advanced age** (>65 years)
- **Immunosuppression**
- **Diabetes and obesity:** Diabetes and obesity may alter the immune system, resulting in an elevated risk for developing sepsis
- ***Cancer:*** Malignancy is one of the most common comorbidities among patients with sepsis
- Community acquired pneumonia
- **Previous hospitalization:** Hospitalization is thought to induce an altered human microbiome, particularly in patients who are treated with antibiotics
- **Genetic factors:** Both experimental and clinical studies have confirmed that genetic factors can increase the risk of infection

RISK FACTORS

Vulnerability of sepsis appears to be growing. Those at the highest risk of developing sepsis include people with chronic illness and those who have an impaired immune system. The other risk factors are mentioned in **Box 1**.

CLINICAL PRESENTATION

The symptoms and signs of sepsis are nonspecific but may include the following:

- Symptoms and signs specific to an infectious source (e.g., cough and dyspnea may suggest pneumonia, pain and purulent exudate in a surgical wound may suggest an underlying abscess).
- Arterial hypotension (e.g., SBP < 90 mm Hg, MAP < 70 mm Hg, and SBP decrease > 40 mm Hg, or less than two standard deviations below normal for age).
- Temperature > 38.3 or < 36°C.
- Heart rate > 90 bpm or more than two standard deviations above the normal value for age.
- Tachypnea, respiratory rate > 20 breaths per minute.
- *Signs of end-organ perfusion*: Warm, flushed skin may be present in the early phases of sepsis. As sepsis progresses to shock, the skin may become cool due to redirection of blood flow to core organs. Decreased capillary refill, cyanosis, or mottling may indicate shock.
- Additional signs of hypoperfusion include altered mental status, obtundation or restlessness, and oliguria or anuria.
- Ileus or absent bowel sounds are often an end-stage sign of hypoperfusion.

LABORATORY FINDINGS

Laboratory features are non-specific. Certain hematological, biochemical, and microbiological tests which aids in the diagnosis are mentioned in **Box 2**. Various biomarkers of sepsis are being studied. Commonly used biomarkers include procalcitonin and C-reactive protein. Other emerging useful markers are serum amyloid A (SAA), interferon gamma inducible protein-10 (IP-10), soluble triggering receptor expressed on myeloid cell-1 (sTREM-1), mannan (Mn) and antimannan (A-Mn) antibodies.

BOX 2 Laboratory findings of sepsis.
• Leukocytosis [white blood cell (WBC) count >12,000 µL-1] or leukopenia (WBC count <4,000 µL-1)
• Normal WBC count with >10% immature forms
• Hyperglycemia (plasma glucose >140 mg/dL) in the absence of diabetes
• Plasma C-reactive protein more than two standard deviations above the normal value
• Arterial hypoxemia [arterial oxygen tension (PaO_2)/fraction of inspired oxygen (FiO_2) <300]
• Acute oliguria [urine output <0.5 mL/kg/h for at least 2 h despite adequate fluid resuscitation]
• Creatinine increase >0.5 mg/dL or 44.2 mmol/L
• Coagulation abnormalities [international normalized ratio (INR) >1.5 or activated partial thromboplastin time (aPTT) >60 s]
• Thrombocytopenia (platelet count <100,000 µL-1)
• Hyperbilirubinemia (plasma total bilirubin >4 mg/dL or 70 mmol/L)
• Adrenal insufficiency (e.g., hyponatremia, hyperkalemia), and the euthyroid sick syndrome can also be found in sepsis
• Hyperlactatemia (e.g., >2 mmol/L)
• Plasma procalcitonin more than two standard deviations above the normal value
• Elevated mid-regional proadrenomedullin (MR-proADM)
• The identification of an organism in culture in a patient who fulfils the definition of sepsis is highly supportive of the diagnosis of sepsis but is not necessary

MANAGEMENT

Sepsis and septic shock should be recognized as medical emergencies in which time matters, as in stroke and acute myocardial infarction. Early recognition and rapid institution of resuscitative measures are critical.

IMMEDIATE EVALUATION AND MANAGEMENT

Stabilize respiration—supplemental oxygen should be supplied to all patients with sepsis and hypoxia. Intubation and mechanical ventilation may be required to support the increased work of breathing, or for airway protection since encephalopathy and a depressed level of consciousness frequently complicate sepsis.

Establish venous access—while peripheral venous access may be sufficient in some patients, the majority will require central venous access at some point during their course.

Initial investigations: Quickly obtaining the following is preferable (within 45 minutes of presentation) but *should not delay the administration of fluids and antibiotics*:

- Complete blood counts, liver function tests, and coagulation studies including D-dimer level.
- *Serum lactate*: An elevated serum lactate may indicate the severity of sepsis and is used to follow the therapeutic response.
- Peripheral blood cultures, urinalysis, and microbiologic cultures from suspected sources. If blood cultures are drawn from an intravenous line, a second specimen should be drawn from a peripheral venipuncture site.
- Arterial blood gas (ABG) analysis.
- Imaging targeted at the suspected site of infection is warranted (e.g., chest radiography, computed tomography of chest and/or abdomen).
- *Procalcitonin*: The diagnostic value of procalcitonin in patients with sepsis is poorly supported by evidence.

Initial resuscitation: The cornerstone of initial resuscitation is the rapid restoration of perfusion and the early administration of antibiotics.

- Tissue perfusion is predominantly achieved by the aggressive administration of intravenous fluids (IVF), usually crystalloids (balanced crystalloids or normal saline) given at 30 mL/kg (actual body weight), started by 1 hour and completed within the first *3* hours following presentation.
- Empiric antibiotic therapy is targeted at the suspected organisms and sites of infection and preferably administered within the 1st hour.

Hour-1 bundle (Fig. 1): The most important change in the revision of the surviving sepsis campaign (SSC) bundles

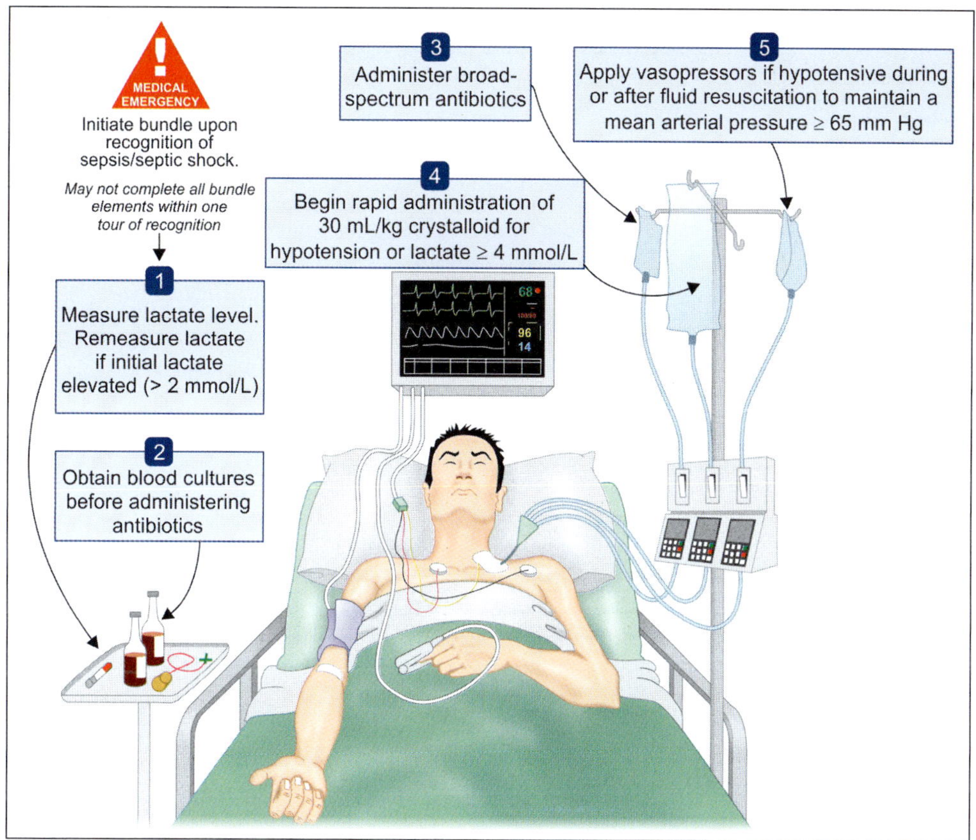

FIGURE 1: Hour-1 bundle.

TABLE 2 Bundle elements with strength of recommendations.

Bundle element	Grade of recommendation and level of evidence
Measure lactate level. Remeasure if initial lactate >2 mmol/L	**Weak recommendation**
Obtain blood cultures before administration of antibiotics	**Best practice statement**
Administer broad-spectrum antibiotics	**Strong recommendation**
Rapidly administer 30 mL/kg crystalloid for hypotension or lactate ≥4 mmol/L	**Strong recommendation**
Apply vasopressors if patient is hypotensive	**Strong recommendation**

is that the 3- and 6-hours bundles have been combined into a single "hour-1 bundle" with the explicit intention of beginning resuscitation and management immediately. More than 1 hour may be required for resuscitation to be completed (**Table 2**).

Intravenous fluids: Rapid, large volume infusions of IVF (30 mL/kg) are indicated as initial therapy for severe sepsis or septic shock, unless there is convincing evidence of significant pulmonary edema.

Overzealous fluid administration can result in pulmonary edema, hypoxemic respiratory failure, organ edema, intra-abdominal hypertension, prolonged ICU stay and time on mechanical ventilation, and even increased risk of death (**Fig. 2**).

Choice of fluid: Crystalloid solutions (isotonic saline or balanced crystalloids) are recommended for volume resuscitation in sepsis and septic shock.

No proven benefit from colloids. One can consider using albumin in sepsis if a significant amount of resuscitative fluid is required to restore intravascular volume. But have found no benefit in terms of morbidity or mortality.

Empiric antibiotic therapy (1st hour)—prompt identification and treatment of the site of infection. Appropriate antimicrobials should be initiated within the 1st hour of recognizing sepsis, after obtaining relevant samples for culture. The initial antimicrobial drugs should be broad-spectrum, covering all likely pathogens. The empiric choice of antimicrobials should consider the site of infection, previous antibiotic use, local pathogen susceptibility patterns, immunosuppression, and risk factors for resistant organisms. Double coverage for gram-negative organisms and for methicillin-resistant *Staphylococcus aureus* (MRSA) should be considered for patients with a high likelihood of infection with such pathogens. Double gram-negative coverage may be appropriate when a high degree of suspicion exists for infection with multi-drug-resistant organisms such as *Pseudomonas* or *Acinetobacter*. If a nosocomial source of infection is suspected to be the cause of sepsis, anti-MRSA agents are recommended. An initial

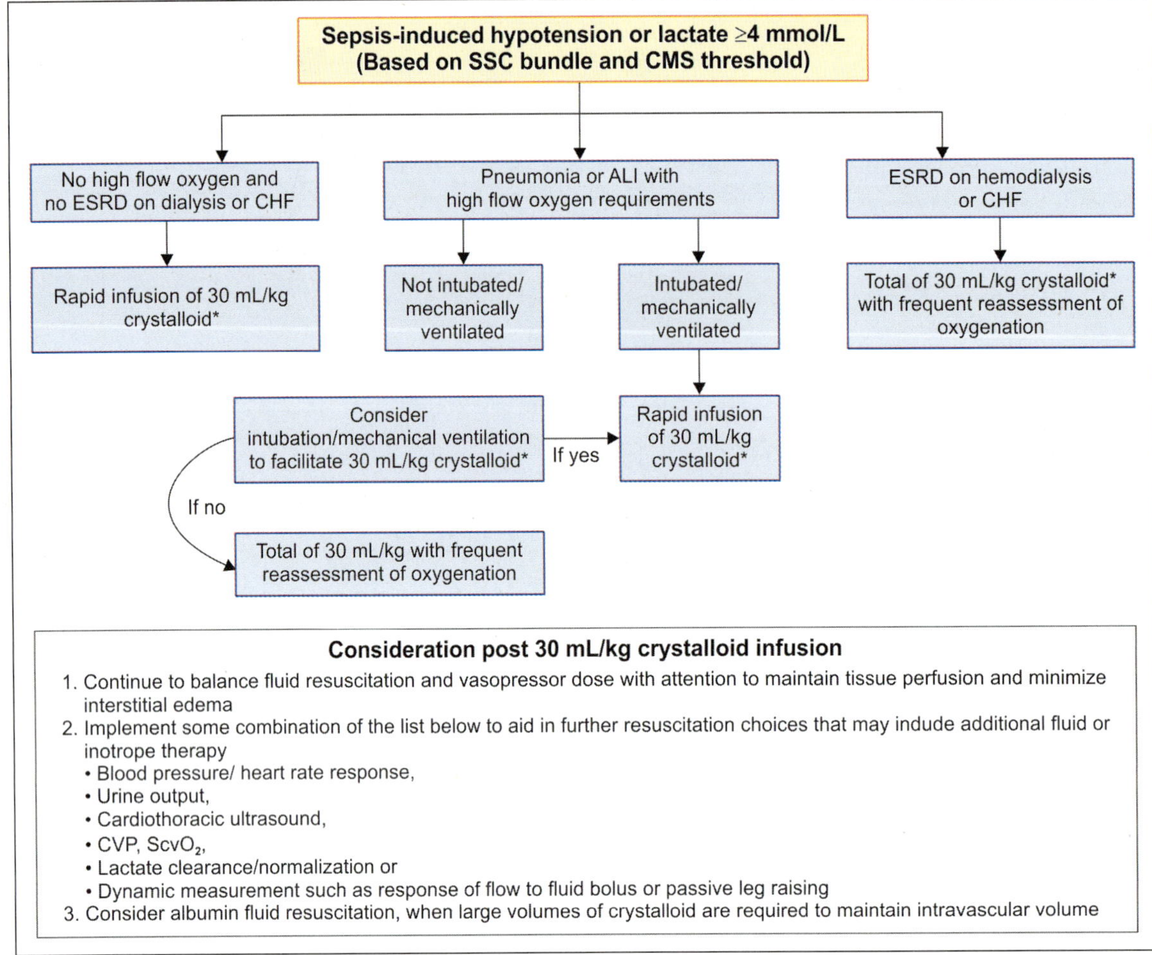

* Administer 30 mL/kg crystalloid within first 3 hours.

(SSC: surviving sepsis campaign; ESRD: end-stage renal disease; CHF: congestive heart failure; ALI: acute lung injury; CVP: central venous pressure; CMS: US Centers for Medicare and Medicaid Services; $ScvO_2$: superior vena cava oxygen saturation)

FIGURE 2: This figure explores the nuancing of initial administration of 30 mL/kg crystalloid for sepsis induced hypoperfusion based on patient characteristics. It also draws attention to reassessment tools following the initial fluid dose as an influence on further fluid administration or inotropic therapy.

higher loading dose may be the best strategy to achieve the therapeutic blood level (**Table 3**).

Consider antifungals: Antifungals should be considered for patients such as those who have had total parenteral nutrition, recent broad-spectrum antibiotic exposure, perforated abdominal viscus, or immunocompromised status, or when clinical suspicion of fungal infection is high. If invasive *Candida* or *Aspergillus* infection is suspected, serologic assays for 1,3 beta-D-glucan, galactomannan, and anti-mannan antibodies may provide early evidence of these fungal infections.

Early source control: Inadequate source control may lead to worsening organ function and hemodynamic instability despite appropriate resuscitative measures. If appropriate, source control should be achieved within 6–12 hours of diagnosis, once initial resuscitation is completed.

MONITOR RESPONSE

After fluids and empiric antibiotics have been administered, the therapeutic response should be assessed frequently.

Clinical: All patients should be followed clinically for improved MAP, urine output, heart rate, respiratory rate, skin color, temperature, pulse oximetry, and mental status. Among these, a MAP ≥ 65 mm Hg and urine output ≥0.5 mL/kg/h are common targets used in clinical practice.

Monitoring catheters: A central venous catheter (CVC) may be placed if the infusion of large volumes of fluids or vasopressors are anticipated, peripheral access is poor, or the central venous pressure (CVP) or the central venous oxyhemoglobin saturation ($ScvO_2$) is chosen as methods of monitoring the hemodynamic response.

Hemodynamic:

- *Static*: In addition to MAP, the following static CVC measurements were used to determine adequate fluid management:
  - Central venous pressure at a target of 8–12 mm Hg
  - Central venous oxyhemoglobin saturation ≥70%
- *Dynamic*: Respiratory changes in the vena caval diameter, radial artery pulse pressure, aortic blood flow peak velocity, left ventricular outflow tract velocity-time integral, and brachial artery blood flow velocity are

TABLE 3 Initial antimicrobial therapy for severe sepsis with no obvious source in adults with normal renal function.

Clinical condition	Antimicrobial regimens[a]
Septic shock (immunocompetent adult)	The many acceptable regimens include (1) piperacillin-tazobactam (3.375–4.5 g), (2) cefepime (2 g q12h), or (3) meropenem (1 g q8h) or imipenem-cilastatin (0.5 g q6h). If the patient is allergic to β-lactam antibiotics, use (1) aztreonam (2 g q8h) or (2) ciprofloxacin (400 mg q12h) or levofloxacin (750 mg q24h). Add vancomycin (loading dose of 25–30 mg/kg, then 15–20 mg/kg q8-12h) to each of the above regimens
Neutropenia (<500 neutrophils/μL)	Regimens include (1) cefepime (2 g q8h), (2) meropenem (1 g q8h) or imipenem-cilastatin (0.5 g q6h) or doripenem (500 mg q8h), or (3) piperacillin-tazobactam (3.375 g q4h). Add vancomycin (as above) if the patient has a suspected central line-associated bloodstream infection, severe mucositis, skin/soft tissue infection, or hypotension. Add tobramycin (5–7 mg/kg q24h) plus vancomycin (as above) plus caspofungin (one dose of 70 mg, then 50 mg q24h) if the patient has severe sepsis/septic shock
Splenectomy	Use ceftriaxone (2 g q24h, or in meningitis —2 g q12h). If the local prevalence of cephalosporin-resistant pneumococci is high, add vancomycin (as above). If the patient is allergic to β-lactam antibiotics, use levofloxacin (750 mg q24h) or moxifloxacin (400 mg q24h) plus vancomycin (as above)

[a] All agents are administered by the intravenous route.

Source: Adapted in part from DN Gilbert et al. The Sanford Guide to antimicrobial therapy, 47th edition, 2017; and from RS Munford: Sepsis and septic shock, in DL Kapsper (Eds). Harrison's Principles of Internal Medicine, 19th edition. New York: McGraw-Hill; 2015. pp. 1757.

considered dynamic measures of fluid responsiveness. For actively breathing patients or those with irregular cardiac rhythms, an increase in the cardiac output in response to a passive leg-raising maneuver (measured by echocardiography, arterial pulse waveform analysis, or pulmonary artery catheterization) also predicts fluid responsiveness. Passive leg raising maneuver may be the most accurate and broadly available.

Laboratory:

- *Lactate clearance*: Ideally, every 6 hours it should be measured.

  The lactate clearance is defined by the equation [(initial lactate - lactate > 2 h later)/initial lactate] × 100. The lactate clearance and interval change in lactate over the first 12 hours of resuscitation has been evaluated as a potential marker for effective resuscitation.
- *Arterial blood gases*: It is prudent to follow worsening or resolution of arterial blood gas parameters including the arterial partial pressure of oxygen:fraction of inspired oxygen ratio as well as severity and type of acidosis. Worsening gas exchange may be a clue to the presence of pulmonary edema, pneumothorax acute respiratory distress syndrome (ARDS) or thromboembolism.
- *Routine laboratories*: Follow-up laboratory studies are often performed (e.g., every 6 h) until values have reached normal or baseline. Hyperchloremia should be avoided, but if it occurs, switching to low chloride-containing (i.e., buffered) solutions may be indicated.
- *Microbiology*: Follow-up indices of infection are indicated. Results should prompt alteration of antibiotic choice if a better and safer regimen can be substituted and/or investigations directed toward source control.

PATIENTS WHO FAIL INITIAL THERAPY

Persistent hypoperfusion is caused by loss of normal sympathetic vascular tone, leading to vasodilation, neurohormonal imbalances, myocardial depression, microcirculatory dysregulation, and mitochondrial dysfunction.

A higher MAP goal of 80–85 mm Hg may help patients with chronic hypertension, while a lower target may be better tolerated in patients with reduced systolic function, older patients, and patients with end-stage liver disease.

Vasopressors:

- First agent *norepinephrine* remains the preferred vasopressor for achieving the target MAP and is strongly recommended by the SSC guidelines, albeit supported by only moderate-quality data.
- *Additional agents*:

A second vasopressor is routinely added when norepinephrine doses exceed 40 or 50 μg/minute.

Vasopressin: Septic shock involves relative vasopressin deficiency. Adding vasopressin as a replacement hormone has been shown to have a sparing effect on norepinephrine.

Epinephrine: Is recommended by the SSC guidelines as a second-line vasopressor. Use of epinephrine is limited by significant risk of tachycardia, arrhythmia, and transient lactic acidosis.

Dopamine: Use is discouraged in sepsis owing to its propensity to induce tachyarrhythmia and significantly worsen outcomes in this setting.

Phenylephrine: Is a pure alpha-adrenergic agonist that is routinely used in septic shock, albeit with limited data on its efficacy and safety. Phenylephrine use should be limited to septic shock complicated by significant tachyarrhythmia or as an adjunct for refractory vasodilatory shock.

Angiotensin II: Activates angiotensin type 1a and 1b receptors to increase intracellular calcium in smooth muscle, promoting vasoconstriction. The data are still sparse on its safety.

Inotropic agents: May be required for patients with inadequate cardiac output after fluid resuscitation due to sepsis-induced cardiomyopathy or combined shock. *Epinephrine* and *dobutamine* are most commonly used (**Fig. 3**).

Glucocorticoids: Corticosteroids downregulate the maladaptive inflammatory response seen in sepsis and help address relative adrenal insufficiency caused by adrenal suppression or glucocorticoid tissue resistance. In septic shock, they have a vasopressor-sparing role and reduce the duration of shock, ventilator use, and ICU stay.

Current guidelines recommend hydrocortisone 200 mg/d intravenously as a continuous drip or 50 mg bolus in 4 divided doses for at least 3 days, based on a systematic review showing a longer course of low-dose steroids is associated with a lower mortality rate. In most cases, steroids are stopped after cessation of vasopressors.

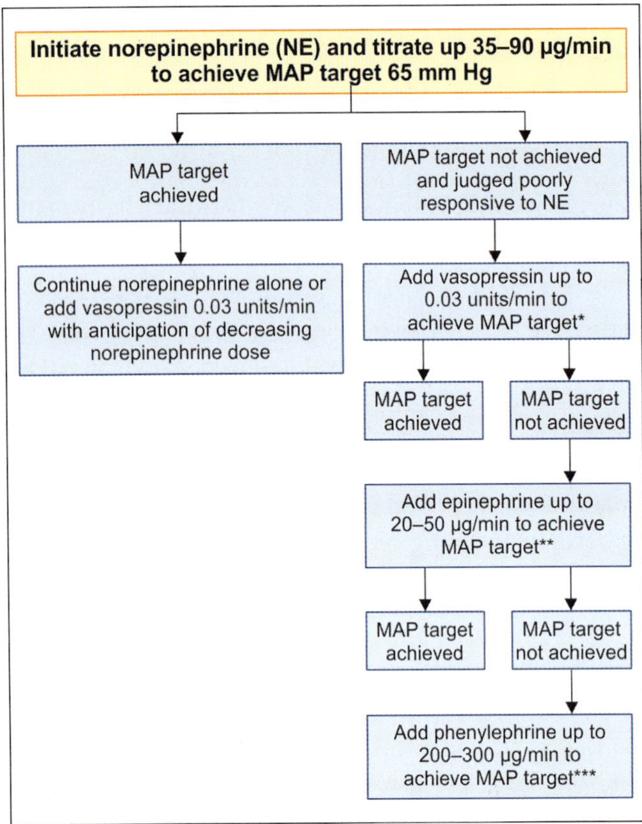

* Consider IV steroid administration

** Administer IV steroids

*** SSC guidelines are silent on phenylephrine

Notes:
- Consider dopamine as niche vasopressor in the presence of sinus bradycardia
- Consider phenylephrine when serious tachyarrhythmias occur with norepinephrine or epinephrine
- Evidence based medicine dose not allow the firm establishment of upper dose ranges of norepinephrine, epinephrine and phenylephrine and the dose ranges expressed in this figure are based on the authors interpretation of the literature that dose exist and personal preference/experience. Maximum doses in any individual patient should be considered based on physiologic response and side effects

FIGURE 3: This demonstrates how the guideline recommendations on vasopressor and steroid use can be molded into a flow diagram approach to the management of septic shock.

Source: Dellinger RP, Schorr CA, Levy MM: User's guide to the 2016 surviving sepsis guidelines.

Red blood cell transfusions: Reserve red blood cell transfusion for patients with a hemoglobin level ≤ 7 g/dL. Exceptions include suspicion of concurrent hemorrhagic shock or active myocardial ischemia.

PATIENTS WHO RESPOND TO THERAPY

Identification and control of the septic focus: Further efforts aimed at identifying and controlling the source of infection should be done if the initial evaluation and investigations fail to identify a source.

De-escalation fluids: Patients who respond to initial fluid therapy should have the rate of fluid administration reduced or stopped, vasopressor support weaned.

De-escalation and duration of antibiotics: It is appropriate that de-escalation and duration of antimicrobial agents be assessed daily.

After culture and susceptibility results return and/or after patients clinically improve, we recommend that antimicrobial therapy be narrowed.

The duration of antibiotics should be individualized. For most patients, it is typically 7–10 days. However, longer courses are appropriate in patients who have a slow clinical response, an undrainable focus of infection, bacteremia with *S. aureus*, some fungal (e.g., deep *Candida* infections) or viral infections (e.g., herpes or cytomegalovirus), endocarditis, osteomyelitis, large abscesses, highly resistant gram-negative pathogens with limited sensitivities, neutropenia, or immunologic deficiencies. Similarly, shorter courses may be acceptable in patients with negative cultures and rapid resolution of sepsis and laboratory studies.

GENERAL SUPPORTIVE CARE

After fluids and antibiotics administration, response should be assessed and certain general supportive measures are taken as mentioned in **Box 3**.

NEWER THERAPIES

Anticoagulants: Organ dysfunction in sepsis can be regarded as the consequence of uncontrolled inflammatory and procoagulant response to infection.

- *Activated protein C*: Drotrecogin alpha activated (DAA), trade name Xigris, is a recombinant human protein which showed promising results in PROWESS trial (**Fig. 4**).

  It was later withdrawn due to failure to show a survival benefit in further studies.
- *Antithrombin (AT)*: Is a natural inhibitor of thrombin as well as factors VIIa, IXa, Xa, XIa, XIIa. AT also suppresses the proinflammatory reactions. However, large-scale randomized trials have failed to demonstrate any mortality benefit in patients treated with AT concentrate.

BOX 3	General supportive care.
• Patients requiring a vasopressor should have an arterial catheter placed as soon as is practical	
• Hydrocortisone is not suggested in septic shock if adequate fluids and vasopressor therapy can restore hemodynamic stability	
• Continuous or intermittent sedation should be minimized in mechanically ventilated sepsis patients, with titration targets used whenever possible	
• A protocol-based approach to blood glucose management should be used in ICU patients with sepsis, with insulin dosing initiated when two consecutive blood glucose levels are >180 mg/dL	
• Continuous or intermittent renal replacement therapy should be used in patients with sepsis and acute kidney injury	
• Pharmacologic prophylaxis (unfractionated heparin or low-molecular-weight heparin) against venous thromboembolism should be used in the absence of contraindications	
• Stress ulcer prophylaxis should be given to patients with risk factors for gastrointestinal bleeding	
• The goals of care and prognosis should be discussed with patients and their families	

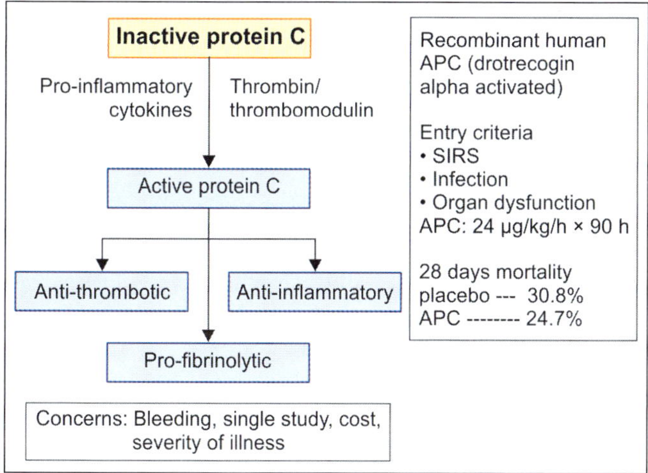

FIGURE 4: Activated protein C.

- *Thrombomodulin (TM)*: Plays a vital role in maintaining intravascular patency due to its anticoagulant, anti-inflammatory, and cytoprotective properties. The effect of externally administered rTM has long been examined through the clinical trials and practice, further clinical study is required to prove its efficacy.
- *Heparin*: Unfractionated heparin (UFH) acts by way of maximizing the effect of antithrombin, decreases platelet aggregation and prevents platelet-histone interaction. Overall impact of heparin use in septic patients remains uncertain and more research is needed.

Angiotensin II: In December 2017, GIAPREZA (angiotensin II) was approved by the United States Food and Drug Administration (US FDA) as a vasoconstrictor indicated in refractory septic shock based on the results of

TABLE 4	Features and benefits of cilengitide.
Features	**Benefits**
Inhibition of bacterial binding to endothelial cells	Prevents endothelial injury thus preventing the infection from progressing to septic shock and multi-organ failure
Nonantibiotic mechanism	Avoids selection for multi-drug resistance strains
Prophylactic use	Allows early intervention to prevent serious infection progressing to sepsis
Repositioned drug	Cilengitide previously taken into Phase III by Merck KGaA for Glioblastoma. Lower development risks as safety and toxicity profile are known
Freedom to operate	Cilengitide is off-patent for its original indication and a new patent has been filed by RCSI for its use in sepsis

(RCSI: Royal College of Surgeons in Ireland)

ATHOS-3 (Angiotensin II for the Treatment of High Output Shock) trial. Most common adverse reaction reported was thromboembolic events, so concurrent thromboembolism prophylaxis to be used.

Cilengitide: A potent inhibitor of αVβ3 integrin signaling, has been shown to inhibit bacterial binding to the vascular endothelium as per preclinical trials conducted by Royal College of Surgeons in Ireland (RCSI) (**Table 4**).

Further studies are required to validate its use in sepsis.

Immune stimulation: Sepsis initiates a complex immune response that varies over time, most patients with sepsis rapidly display signs of profound immunosuppression, which is associated with deleterious consequences.

Targets of immune stimulation:

- To help bacterial killing at primary focus of infection.
- To prevent development of nosocomial infections.
- To prevent reactivation of dormant viruses.

Intravenous immunoglobulin (IVIG): Role as adjunctive therapy due to its immunomodulatory property and enhanced bacterial clearance has been proposed. Currently, only toxin mediated bacterial diseases are considered as indication of IVIG.

Interferon gamma: Associated with improved immune functions and increased human leukocyte antigen (HLA-DR) expression.

Granulocyte-macrophage colony-stimulating factor (GM-CSF): Stimulates the production of neutrophils and monocytes and is also a potent stimulant of monocyte survival and functions.

Interleukin-7 (IL-7): Helps in growth, differentiation, and effector functions of T cells, hence useful in lymphopenia caused by sepsis.

Immune checkpoint inhibitors: One of the immune checkpoint pathways is the programmed cell death protein-1 (PD-1)/programmed cell death-ligand 1 (PD-L1) pathway. PD-1 and PD-L1 are also up-regulated on immune cells of patients with sepsis, and higher expression of these proteins is associated with increased mortality. Two case reports describe the use of a single dose of nivolumab (anti-PD1 blocking monoclonal antibody) as adjunctive therapy which showed positive outcome.

Extracorporeal therapies: Extracorporeal blood purification therapies helps removing both inflammatory and anti-inflammatory mediators and hence preventing immunosuppression.

Immunostimulation therapy is under study and warrants larger RCTs to prove its role in sepsis.

RECOMMENDED READINGS

1. Rhodes A, Evans LE, Alhazzani W, Levy MM, Antonelli M, Ferrer R, et al. Surviving Sepsis Campaign: International Guidelines for Management of Sepsis and Septic Shock: 2016. Crit Care Med. 2017;45(3):486-552.
2. Seymour CW, Liu VX, Iwashyna TJ, Brunkhorst FM, Rea TD, Scherag A, et al. Assessment of Clinical Criteria for Sepsis: For the Third International Consensus Definitions for Sepsis and Septic Shock (Sepsis-3). JAMA. 2016;315(8):762-74.
3. Seymour CW, Angus DC. Sepsis and Septic Shock. In: Kasper DL, Fauci AS, Hauser S, Hauser SL, Longo DL, Loscalzo J. (Eds). Harrison's principles of internal medicine, 20th edition. New York: The McGraw-Hill Companies; c2018. pp. 2044-52.
4. Divatia JV, Amin PR, Ramakrishnan N, Kapadia FN, Todi S, Sahu S, et al. Intensive care in India: the Indian intensive care case mix and practice patterns study. Indian J Crit Care Med. 2016;20(4):216-25.
5. Chatterjee S, Bhattacharya M, Todi SK. Epidemiology of adult-population sepsis in India: a single center 5 year experience. Indian J Crit Care Med. 2017;21(9): 573-7.
6. Neviere R, Parsons PE, Finlay G (Eds). (2021). Sepsis syndromes in adults: Epidemiology, definitions, clinical presentation, diagnosis, and prognosis. In. UptoDate [online]. Available from https://www.uptodate.com/contents/sepsis-syndromes-in-adults-epidemiology-definitions-clinical-presentation-diagnosis-and-prognosis?topicRef=1613&source=see_link
7. Schmidt GA, Mandel J, Parsons PE, Sexton DJ, Hockberger RS, (Eds). (2021). Evaluation and management of suspected sepsis and septic shock in adults. In UptoDate [online]. Available from https://www.uptodate.com/contents/evaluation-and-management-of-suspected-sepsis-and-septic-shock-in-adults
8. Dugar S, Choudhary C, Duggal A. Sepsis and septic shock: Guideline-based management. Clev Clin J Med. 2020;87(1):53-64.
9. Scarlatescu E, Tomescu D, Arama SS. Anticoagulant Therapy in Sepsis. The Importance of Timing. J Crit Care Med. 2017;3(2):63-9.
10. Senatore F, Jagadeesh G, Rose M, Pillai VC, Hariharan S, Liu Q, et al. FDA Approval of Angiotensin II for the Treatment of Hypotension in Adults with Distributive Shock. Am J Cardiovasc Drugs. 2019;19(1):11-20.
11. John D. InnovoSep: A Non-Antibiotic Approach for Treating or Preventing Severe Bloodstream Infection. Principal Investigator: Prof. Steve Kerrigan Cardiovascular Infection Research Group RCSI [online]. Available from file:///C:/Users/Vertika.kaushik/Downloads/InnovoSep%20A%20Non-Antibiotic%20Approach%20for%20Treating%20or%20Preventing%20Severe%20Bloodstream%20Infection%20(3).pdf

CHAPTER 78 Antibiogram and Molecular Diagnostic Tests in an Intensive Care Unit: Interpretation and Relevance

Shaoli Basu, Camilla Rodrigues

ABSTRACT

Ever-increasing antimicrobial resistance (AMR) remains a global crisis. The Centers for Disease Control and Prevention (CDC) estimated that >2.8 million antibiotic-resistant infections occur in the United States each year accounting for > 35,000 deaths. The intensive care units (ICUs) in the Western world are predominated by gram-positive bugs while gram-negative organisms dominate the Indian ICUs.

An antibiogram shows the susceptibility of pathogens to specific antibiotics. Hospital-based antibiogram is a periodic summary of antimicrobial susceptibilities of local bacterial isolates. Hospital antibiogram is used to formulate the antibiotic policy and guides empiric treatment. The Indian Council of Medical Research (ICMR) initiated the Antimicrobial Resistance Surveillance and Research Network (AMRSN) in 2013 to collate nationwide representative data. It has been used for formulation of national treatment guidelines.

Blood culture, the gold standard for diagnosing sepsis, is too slow with low yield and is cumbersome to influence the initial management of patients. Rapid diagnostic tests that are capable of ruling out the bacterial cause of sepsis and help profiling AMR must be added into the initial 1–3-hour diagnostic window to help decide the appropriate antibiotics and improve patient outcomes. A variety of tests are commercially available to detect carbapenemase activity or the genes encoding these proteins such as colorimetric-based assays, phenotype-based assays, immunochromatographic assays, MALDI-ToF (matrix-assisted laser desorption ionization-time of flight), carbapenem hydrolysis assays, and polymerase chain reaction (PCR)-based methods. The exact resistance mechanism will optimize the use of the newer antibiotics. Molecular diagnostics from whole blood will also add to the armamentarium to combat AMR.

"Without laboratories men of science are soldiers without arms"

—Louis Pasteur

INTRODUCTION

The World Health Organization (WHO) has declared AMR in the top 10 global public health threats. AMR also significantly impacts the economy due to death, disability, prolonged hospital stays, need for more expensive medicines, and financial challenges for those impacted. "Antimicrobials: handle with care" was the slogan for World Antimicrobials Awareness Week (WAAW) 2020 whereas the theme for human health was "United to preserve antimicrobials." The President of the UN General Assembly stated in December 2020, "AMR threatens to unwind a century of medical progress, and send us back to the pre-antibiotic era, when routine infections could mean death." The main driver in the development of drug-resistant pathogens is irrational use of antimicrobials.

The CDC estimated that >2.8 million antibiotic-resistant infections occur in the United States each year accounting for >35,000 deaths. It is estimated that by the year 2050, Asia will have 4.7 million deaths that could be directly attributed to AMR. It is important to optimize the use of antimicrobials. While antibiotic development has slowed, antibiotic resistance has not.

The Western ICUs are burdened with gram-positive bugs such as methicillin-resistant *Staphylococcus aureus* (MRSA), vancomycin-resistant enterococci (VRE), and *Clostridium difficile* colitis. However, in India and other Asian countries, it is predominantly gram-negative bacteria with extended-spectrum beta-lactamase (ESBLs), AmpCs, and carbapenemases. The Extended Prevalence of Infection in Intensive Care (EPIC) II demonstrates this difference as shown in **Table 1**.

ANTIBIOGRAM

Antimicrobial resistance augments health and economic burden on the patient as well as on the healthcare system. The global rise of AMR makes it imperative to monitor emerging trends in drug resistance at the local level to guide clinical decision-making and contain the ever-increasing antimicrobial-resistance issues.

An *antibiogram* shows the susceptibility of pathogens to specific antibiotics. It can be patient specific or hospital based.

- *Patient-specific antibiogram* determines the susceptibility pattern of a given microorganism to a range of antibiotics. It helps decide the definitive treatment for the patient.
- *Hospital-based antibiogram* is a periodic summary of antimicrobial susceptibilities of local bacterial isolates, usually made annually.

It is important to classify it appropriately as microbial flora and their resistance pattern differs in the community and hospital, wards, and ICU. It can be categorized as per the site and type of infection, location, and type of patient (history of hospitalization, comorbidities, antibiotic usage, presence of invasive devices). Hospital antibiogram is used to formulate the antibiotic policy and guides empiric treatment. The formulation of an antibiotic policy is also mandatory for accreditation.

The ICMR, New Delhi, initiated AMRSN in 2013 to collate nationwide representative data. The main goals of ICMR-AMRSN include the following:

- Development of a network of hospitals and monitor trends in the antimicrobial susceptibility profile of clinically important bacteria and fungi in alignment with the 2017 WHO priority pathogen list
- Detection of clonality of drug-resistant pathogens and their transmission dynamics with the help of molecular studies. This will aid better understanding of the AMR pattern in India and develop appropriate interventions.
- Dissemination of the collated AMR data to suitable stakeholders and promote interventions to reduce AMR
- Creating web-based data management system for data collection and analysis

This nationwide ICMR surveillance study showcased the dominance of gram-negative bacteria which is contrary to the Western data. It also documented nonsusceptibility to the broad-spectrum antibiotics, such as third-generation cephalosporins and fluoroquinolones, which was 75–80% in *Escherichia coli*, 65–77% in *Klebsiella pneumoniae*, 73–87% in *Acinetobacter baumannii*, and approximately

TABLE 1 Prevalence of microbiologic isolates from intensive care units (ICUs) of different geographical areas as depicted by EPIC II.

N (%)	All ICUs N (%)	Western European ICUs N (%)	North American ICUs N (%)	Asian ICUs N (%)
Positive isolate	4,947 (69.8)	2,678 (72.7)	457 (75.3)	478 (67.6)
Gram positive	2,315 (46.8)	1,311 (49.0)	252 (55.1)	163 (34.1)
Gram negative	3,077 (62.2)	1,573 (58.7)	228 (49.9)	355 (74.3)
Anaerobes	222 (4.5)	142 (5.3)	36 (7.9)	14 (2.9)
Fungi	963 (19.4)	548 (20)	105 (23)	84 (17.5)
Parasite	34 (0.7)	18 (0.7)	3 (0.7)	3 (0.6)
Others	192 (3.9)	122 (4.6)	22 (4.8)	14 (2.9)

Note: Percentages do not necessarily equal 100, because patients may have had more than one type of infection or microorganism.

40% in *Pseudomonas aeruginosa.* It also showed increasing resistance to high-end antibiotics such as carbapenems. Nonsusceptibility to meropenem was highest in *A. baumannii* isolates and was observed in 69.8%, 81.3%, and 80.1% of them followed by *K. pneumonia* (48.6%, 51.8%, and 50.4%), *P. aeruginosa* (32.9%, 31.3%, and 30.9%), and *E. coli* (13%, 21%, and 23%) in 2016, 2017, and 2018, respectively. Metallo-β-lactamases [MBLs; New Delhi metallo-β-lactamases (NDMs) and Verona Integron-encoded metallo-β-lactamases (VIMs)] and carbapenem hydrolyzing class D β-lactamases [oxacillinases (OXA-48)-like] contributed predominantly to carbapenem resistance. This data has been used to develop national treatment guidelines. This will enable harmonizing treatment practices nationwide in the various tertiary care hospitals.

DIAGNOSIS OF SEPSIS

Blood culture still remains the gold standard for diagnosing sepsis. Conventional blood culture is slow, offers a low yield, is cumbersome, and prone to contamination. However, automated blood culture systems have value added significantly in the diagnosis of sepsis. Various other factors such as volume of blood, number of blood culture sets (aerobic and anaerobic), and timing of collection play a significant role to markedly increase the yield. It is recommended that two to three sets (four to six bottles) of blood cultures prior to initiating antimicrobial therapy should be collected. The American Society for Microbiology/Infectious Diseases Society of America (ASM/IDSA) 2018 joint guidelines for adults recommend 20–30 mL of blood per culture set. Skin should be prepared meticulously prior to venepuncture preferably with chlorhexidine (2% w/v) in ethanol (80%) to avoid contamination with skin commensals.

There are various methods currently available for detection of microorganisms in a clinical microbiology setup. Conventional biochemical tests and traditional Kirby–Bauer disc diffusion techniques for antimicrobial drug susceptibility testing (DST) have been replaced by automated identification and DST by automated systems such as VITEK and Phoenix.

MALDI-ToF mass spectrometry (MS) helps rapid, reliable, sensitive microbial identification of bacteria, viruses, and fungi. In the ionization phase, samples are fixed in a crystalline matrix and are bombarded with laser. The sample molecules vaporize into the vacuum while being ionized simultaneously. The ions are separated as per their mass-to-charge ratio by the time they reach the detector in the time-of-flight phase. The mass spectrum is compared to well-characterized organisms available in the reference library database and isolate is identified accordingly. Aerobic actinomycetes, *Nocardia*, and mycobacteria have complex cell walls; thus they require a modified processing technique prior to subjecting them to MALDI-ToF MS. However, this test also has its own limitations as it can identify new isolates only if the specific peptide mass fingerprints (PMF) are present in the spectral database.

The advantages and disadvantages of the various methods for microbial detection are depicted in **Table 2**.

Rapid diagnostic tests that are capable of ruling out the bacterial cause of sepsis and help profiling AMR must be added into the initial 1–3-hour diagnostic window to help decide the appropriate antibiotics and improve patient outcomes.

White blood cell (WBC), *C-reactive protein* (CRP), *lactate dehydrogenase* (LDH), and *interleukins* (IL-1, IL-6) are the conventional markers used for the diagnosis of sepsis. A biomarker such as *procalcitonin* (PCT) is a useful diagnostic and prognostic tool for sepsis. PCT also helps differentiate between infective and noninfective causes of systemic inflammation. Use of antibiotics is strongly encouraged with PCT > 0.5 ng/mL while they are strongly discouraged if PCT < 0.1 ng/mL. Thus, it also helps in antimicrobial stewardship by early de-escalation of broad-spectrum antibiotics.

Rapid and accurate diagnosis of invasive fungal infections (IFI) is critical but challenging as clinical-radiological findings are nonspecific. Also, conventional culture and histopathology have low sensitivity with the

TABLE 2 Various methods for detection of microorganisms in clinical microbiology.

Detection method	Advantages	Disadvantages
Conventional; culture biochemical tests	• Sensitive • Cost-effective	• Lengthy and time-consuming process • Requires 24–48 hours
Immunological-based methods	• Faster than conventional methods • Can detect both contaminating organisms and their toxins	• Sensitivity and specificity lower than nucleic-acid based detection methods • Require large amounts of antigen • Only few microorganisms covered in this assay
Fluorescent in situ hybridization (FISH)	• Rapid detection and identification directly from slide smears • Easy but as specific as molecular methods	• Limited antigens available for detection
Molecular-based methods • **Real-time PCR** • **Multiplex-PCR**	• Can be done directly from sample • Specific, sensitive, rapid and accurate • Minimal chances of contamination due to closed-tube system • Can detect many pathogens simultaneously	• A highly precise thermal cycler is needed • Trained laboratory personnel required for performing the test
DNA sequencing	• 16S rDNA and 18S rDNA sequencing are the gold standards • Can identify fastidious and uncultivable microorganisms	• Trained laboratory personnel and powerful interpretation software are required • Expensive • Not suitable for routine clinical use
Microarrays	• Large-scale screening system for simultaneous diagnosis and detection of many pathogens	• Expensive • Trained laboratory personnel required
Loop-mediated isothermal amplification (LAMP) assay	• Can generate large copies of DNA in less than an hour • Easy to use • No sophisticated equipment is required	• Developed for only a small number of microorganisms as yet
Metagenomic assay	• Useful for random detection of pathogens	• Data acquisition and data analysis is time consuming • Trained laboratory personnel required
MALDI-ToF MS	• Fast and accurate • Less expensive than molecular and immunological-based detection methods • Trained laboratory personnel not required	• High initial cost of the MALDI-ToF equipment

(MALDI-TOF MS: matrix-assisted laser desorption ionization-time of flight mass spectrophotometry; PCR: polymerase chain reaction)

need for invasive sampling. Hence, the need for nonculture-based fungal biomarkers arises.

Galactomannan (GM) assay (Platelia *Aspergillus*, Bio-Rad) is validated only for use in serum and bronchoalveolar lavage (BAL) fluid; however, detection of GM in plasma and CSF should support a diagnosis of invasive aspergillosis (IA) as per the European Organization for Research and Treatment of Cancer/Mycoses Study Group Education (EORTC/MSG) 2020. However, exposure to mold active antifungals compromises the utility of the GM test for IA. EORTC/MSG also recommends a single threshold (>80 pg/mL) of *(1–3)-β-d-glucan* using the Fungitell test (Associates of Cape Cod, Falmouth, MA) for the diagnosis of probable invasive fungal diseases in an appropriate clinical setting.

OPTIMIZING TREATMENT BASED ON RESISTANCE MECHANISM

A delay in initiating the right antibiotic could lead to over- or underutilization. The need is to rapidly detect, prevent spread, and innovate against antibiotic resistance.

Carbapenem-resistant Enterobacterales (CRE) may or may not be carbapenemase producers. Other resistance mechanisms include efflux pump, porin channels etc. These can be differentiated by phenotypic tests such as the modified carbapenem inactivation method and the Carba NP test.

The five most common carbapenemases include New Delhi metallo-β-lactamases (NDMs), Verona Integron-encoded metallo-β-lactamases (VIMs), Imipenem-hydrolyzing metallo-β-lactamases (IMPs), and oxacillinases (e.g., OXA-48-like) carbapenemases. In the Western world, *K. pneumoniae* carbapenemases (KPCs) are the most frequent carbapenemase detected. In South East Asia, MBLs such as NDM and OXA-48-like are the most frequent. It is essential to know the specific carbapenemases that are operational as it dictates the specific treatment in carbapenem-resistant infections. For example, ceftazidime-avibactam (CAZ-AVI) can be effectively used for KPC or OXA-48 producers but is ineffective for MBLs such as NDM. For MBLs or coproducers with NDM and OXA-48-like, aztreonam has to be added to CAZ-AVI to overcome the MBL.

It is essential to optimize treatment based on the susceptibility pattern with or without access to molecular methods. Most carbapenem-resistant organisms may be resistant to other drugs such as fluoroquinolones, aminoglycosides, and trimethoprim-sulfamethoxazole. Treatment for CRE is summarized in **Table 3**. For difficult-to-treat *P. aeruginosa*, drugs such as ceftolozane-tazobactam, ceftazidime-avibactam, imipenem-cilastatin-relebactam, cefiderocol, or polymyxins can be used based on in vitro susceptibility. Minocycline, high-dose sulbactam, or polymyxins are good alternatives for the treatment of *A. baumannii.*

Similarly, many newer drugs have action against certain specific β-lactamases as shown in **Table 4**.

NEWER DIAGNOSTIC METHODS

A variety of tests are commercially available to detect carbapenemase activity or the genes encoding these proteins such as colorimetric-based assays, phenotype-based assays, immunochromatographic assays, MALDI-ToF, carbapenem hydrolysis assays, and PCR-based method, but only a few of them have been evaluated directly on biological samples.

The *Carba NP test (BioMérieux)* is a rapid manual colorimetric carbapenemase confirmatory test. It is used when carbapenems are resistant by the routine drug susceptibility test. This test has a high level of sensitivity (>90%) and specificity (>90%) in detecting KPC, NDM, VIM, IMP, São Paulo metallo-β-lactamase (SPM), and Serratia marcescens enzyme (SME)-type carbapenemases in Enterobacterales and *P. aeruginosa* isolates. However, the ability of this test to detect OXA-48-like producers is poor. Carba NP showed poor sensitivity to *Acinetobacter* species (21.3% for *A. baumannii*); hence, this test is not recommended by the Clinical and Laboratory Standards Institute (CLSI) 2020 for *Acinetobacter* species. Another drawback of this test is that it cannot classify the type of carbapenemase produced.

BD Phoenix CPO Detect is a qualitative, confirmatory, growth-based phenotypic test that detects carbapenemase production in isolates of Enterobacterales, *P. aeruginosa*, and *A. baumannii* when the Phoenix Automated Microbiology System is used. A study by Whitley et al. showed that the positive and negative percentages of agreement (PPA and NPA) values for CPO detect were similar across organism types and ranged from 95.9 to 98.5% and from 92.3 to 97.2%, respectively, when compared to reference methods. It provides advantages of automated carbapenemase detection, inclusion in susceptibility panels to eliminate delays and subjectivity in initiating carbapenemase tests, and classification of most carbapenemases.

Immunochromatographic assays are based on murine monoclonal antibodies. They detect VIM, NDM, KPC, and OXA-48 carbapenemases in 5 minutes directly from cultured bacterial colonies.

TABLE 3 Treatment options for ESBL and Carbapenemase producing Enterobacteriaceae.

Phenotypic Susceptibility	Possible resistance mechanism	Recommended treatment (when other drugs cannot be used)	Alternative drugs for site specific infections
Ceftriaxone resistant	Extended spectrum β-lactamase producer (ESBL): CTX-M, SHV, TEM etc.	Carbapenem	Fosfomycin for urosepsis
Carbapenem resistant	Carbapenemase producing CRE		Tigecycline for intra-addominal infections
	MBL (NDM, IMP, VIM)	Ceftazidime-avibactam + aztreonam or cefiderocol or polymyxins	
	OXA-48 like	Ceftazidime-avibactam or cefiderocol or polymyxins	
	NDM + OXA 48	Ceftazidime-avibactam + aztreonam or cefiderocol or polymyxins	
	KPC	Ceftazidime-avibactam or meropenem-vaborbactam or imipenem-cilastatin-relebactam or polymyxins	

TABLE 4 Expected activity of newer antimicrobials (derived from WHO/IDSA).

Drug	CRE		CRPA	CRAB
	Active against	Not active against		
Ceftazidime-avibactam	ESBLs, AmpC, KPC-2, OXA-48 like	MBL (NDM), KPC-3	YES	No
Meropenem-vaborbactam	ESBLs, AmpC, KPC	MBL (NDM), *OXA-48 like	No	No
Imipenem-cilastin-relebactam	ESBLs, AmpC, KPC	MBL (NDM), *OXA-48 like	YES	No
Cefiderocol	ESBLs, AmpC, KPC, MBL (NDM), OXA-48 Like		YES	Data awaited

*Limited to no activity.

(CRAB: carbapenem-resistant *Acinetobacter baumannii*; CRE: carbapenem resistant Enterobacterales; CRPA: carbapenem-resistant *Pseudomonas aeruginosa*; ESBL: extended-spectrum beta-lactamase; KPC: *Klebsiella pneumoniae* carbapenemase; MBL: metallo-β-lactamase; NDM: New Delhi metallo-β-lactamase; OXA-48: oxacillinase)

MALDI-ToF MS uses freshly prepared bacterial cultures with mixture of carbapenem solutions such as ertapenem or meropenem which are incubated for 2–4 hours at 35–37°C. The mixture is then centrifuged and the mass spectrometry is used to measure the supernatant. The degradation products and sodium salt of the carbapenem molecule are visible in spectra in case of carbapenemase hydrolysis.

Xpert Carba: The Xpert Carba-R Assay, performed on the GeneXpert® Instrument Systems, detects and differentiates five genes (bla_{KPC}, bla_{NDM}, bla_{VIM}, $bla_{OXA\text{-}48}$, and bla_{IMP}) responsible for carbapenem resistance in gram-negative bacteria from pure colonies and rectal/perirectal swabs. However, a study by Aurélie Cointe et al. showed that it also allowed carbapenemase-producing (CP) Enterobacteriaceae (CPE) detection directly on positive blood vials, with a rapid turnaround time of <1 hour.

BioFire® FilmArray® Blood Culture Identification (BCID) panel helps rapid identification of the causative organism. Antimicrobial usage, length of stay (LOS), mortality, and/or cost may be reduced through use of rapid blood culture diagnostic tests. A study by Fiori et al. showed that the median time to final ID (TFI) from a blood culture bottle reaching the laboratory was 19.5 hours [interquartile range (IQR), 14.3–26.5 h] for the direct method (MALDI-ToF MS and/or FilmArray BCID panel) in contrast to the TFI of 41.7 hours (IQR, 35.5–53.0 h) for the culture-based reference method ($p < 0.001$). This indicates that use of MALDI/BCID led to a significantly shortened TFI by 22.2 hours compared with the conventional culture method. Additionally, BCID also provides the mechanism of resistance.

The upgraded version, i.e., *BCID2* panel, covers 26 bacterial pathogens, 7 fungal pathogens (including *Candida auris* and *Cryptococcus neoformans*), and 10 AMR genes from positive blood culture (PBC) specimens in about an hour. The AMR genes detected now address the Indian concerns of CTX-M, NDM, IMP, VIM, and OXA-48-like along with the previous ones which catered mainly to the West such as KPC, mecA/C, and Van A, B. This will also aid the antimicrobial stewardship program (ASP) by guiding the use of appropriate antibiotics early and faster de-escalation. A study by MacVane et al. showed that addition of BCID to an established ASP shortened the time to effective therapy [5 h in the BCID arm vs. 13 h in only ASP arm ($p < 0.001$)] and also improved antimicrobial use [48 h to de-escalation in the BCID group compared to 61 h in ASP alone ($p = 0.034$)], even in a setting of low AMR rates.

EMERGING MOLECULAR DIAGNOSTICS

Nucleic acid amplification technologies (NAATs) function by rapidly creating copies of DNA or RNA originating from pathogen or host cell by amplifying the nucleic acid sequences to a detectable level. NAAT is widely used for viral pathogens for qualitative and quantitative detection, but it is yet to revolutionize the diagnosis of sepsis. This is probably attributed to the fact that the bacteria are present in low numbers with a high background of human DNA in complex samples like blood; thus, it is difficult to reliably capture and amplify the pathogen nucleic acid. Few emerging molecular diagnostic tests from whole blood have been summarized in **Table 5**.

MACHINE LEARNING-BASED ALGORITHMS

A single biomarker may not suffice to guide optimal treatment. Powerful algorithms applied to large clinical data sets enable technologies to learn site-specific contexts and novel relationships. Proposed algorithm by several groups combines optimal subsets of biomarkers with rich electronic medical record (EMR) data. Two of these promising approaches, which are under commercial development, include HeRO score and InSight, respectively.

- HeRO uses signal processing and machine learning to identify subtle irregularities in heart rate variability. It may be a value-added technology that could provide synergy in an integrated format with other diagnostic measures for septic patients.
- The InSight algorithm score demonstrated a sensitivity and a specificity of 83% and 96%, respectively, for sepsis. Thus, it shows promising results for early detection of sepsis in adult and pediatric patients.

TABLE 5 Emerging molecular diagnostics from whole blood.

Assay (manufacturer)	Technique	Volume of sample	TAT (h)	Detection limit	Sensitivity/ Specificity (%)	Breadth of detection and ability to expand	Quantification of load	Antimicrobial resistance markers
Iridica Plex ID (Abbott Molecular)	Multiplex broad-range PCR/ ESI-MS	5 mL	6	0.25–128 CFU/mL	45–83/69–94	780 bacteria and *Candida*; highly expandable	Semi-quantification	*mecA*, *vanA*, *vanB* and *bla*$_{KPC}$
SeptiFast (Roche Diagnostics)	Multiplex target-specific real-time PCR/in situ hybridization/ melt analysis	1.5 mL	4–6	3–100 CFU/mL	63–83/83–95	>16 bacteria, *Candida*, and *Aspergillus fumigatus*; low expandability	Semi-quantification	*mecA* (after positive test for *Staphylococcus aureus*
SepsiTest (Molzyme)	Universal PCR/ sequencing	1 mL	8–10	10–80 CFU/mL	11–87/83–96	>345 bacteria and 13 fungi; highly expandable	No	None
Mini Ion (Oxford Nanopore Technologies)	Nanopore sequencing	10 ng high-molecular-weight DNA (not validated for whole blood)	4–6	~100 copies/mL	NA/97–100	Initial validation on few viruses and bacteria; highly expandable	Yes	Can be added in the future
U-dHRM	Digital PCR/high resolution melt	1 mL	<4	Single cell	Single cell/99.9	37 bacteria; highly expandable to include other bacteria, viruses, and fungi	Yes	Can be added in the future
SeptiCyte (Immunexpress)	RT-qPCR to quantify the host response of 4 RNA biomarkers; machine learning	2.5 mL	1–6	NA	NA/95	All pathogens	NA	None
Loop-mediated isothermal amplification (LAMP) technology	LAMP	Varies ~30 µL to a few mL	1	Single cell	Single cell/100	No integrated platfrom for broad-based detection (1 pathogen/ sample)	Limited	Can detect 1 resistance gene at a time in a separate sample
Integrated comprehensive droplet digital detection technology (IC 3D) (Velox Biosystems	DNAzyme-based sensor droplet microencapsulation 3D particle counter system	µL to mL	1–4	Single cell	Single cell	No integrated platfrom for broad-based detection (1 pathogen/ sample)	Limited	Can be added in the future; limited by number of fluorescence channels

(PCR: polymerase chain reaction; ESI-MS: electrospray ionization mass spectrometry; RT-qPCR: quantitative reverse transcription PCR)

Machine learning techniques use heterogeneous data sets to inform clinical decisions. The future beholds incorporation of EMR data with broad-based molecular detection technologies and clinical data. This integrated approach may overcome the limitations of each technology when used in isolation and will facilitate targeted antibiotic use and optimum patient management.

CONCLUSION

The new exciting era of molecular diagnostics is going to change the face of microbiology. Rapid diagnosis of the pathogen with its mechanism of resistance will facilitate clinicians to use targeted antibiotics. Optimizing the use of antibiotics will assist the ASP and will enable us to combat AMR. As someone rightly said, "Antimicrobial stewardship is a team game with the patient at the center and it is our teamwork that makes the dream work."

RECOMMENDED READINGS

1. World Health Organization. (2020). Antimicrobial resistance. [online] Available from https://www.who.int/news-room/fact-sheets/detail/antimicrobial-resistance
2. World Health Organization. (2020). World Antimicrobial Awareness Week 2020. [online] Available from https://www.who.int/news-room/events/detail/2020/11/18/default-calendar/world-antimicrobial-awareness-week-2020
3. CDC. Antibiotic Resistance Threats in the United States, 2019. Atlanta, GA: U.S. Department of Health and Human Services, CDC; 2019. [online] Available from www.cdc.gov/DrugResistance/Biggest-Threats.html
4. Indian Council of Medical Research. Treatment Guidelines for Antimicrobial Use in Common Syndromes, 2nd edition. New Delhi: ICMR; 2019.
5. Vincent JL, Rello J, Marshall J, Silva E, Anzueto A, Martin CD, et al. for the EPIC II Group of Investigators. International study of the prevalence and outcomes of infection in intensive care units. JAMA. 2009; 302(21):2323-9.
6. Walia K, Madhumathi J, Veeraraghavan B, Chakrabarti A, Kapil A, Ray P, et al. Establishing antimicrobial resistance surveillance and research network in India: Journey so far. Indian J Med Res. 2019;149:164-79.
7. Singhal N, Kumar M, Kanaujia PK, Virdi JS. MALDI-TOF mass spectrometry: an emerging technology for microbial identification and diagnosis. Front Microbiol. 2015;6:791.
8. Donnelly JP, Chen SC, Kauffman CA, Steinbach WJ, Baddley JW, Verweij PE, et al. Revision and update of the consensus definitions of invasive fungal disease from the European Organization for Research and Treatment of Cancer and the Mycoses Study Group Education and Research Consortium. Clin Infect Dis. 2020;71(6):1367-76.
9. Tamma PD, Aitken SL, Bonomo RA, Mathers AJ, van Duin D, Clancy CJ. Infectious Diseases Society of America Guidance on the treatment of antimicrobial resistant gram-negative infections. A Focus on Extended-Spectrum β-lactamase Producing Enterobacterales (ESBL-E), Carbapenem-Resistant Enterobacterales (CRE), and Pseudomonas aeruginosa with Difficult-to-Treat Resistance (DTR-P. aeruginosa). IDSA 2020.
10. World Health Organization. Antibacterial agents in clinical development: an analysis of the antibacterial clinical development pipeline. Geneva: World Health Organization; 2019.
11. CLSI. Performance Standards for Antimicrobial Susceptibility Testing, 30th edition. CLSI supplement M100. Wayne, PA: Clinical and Laboratory Standards Institute; 2020.
12. Whitley V, Kircher S, Gill T, Hindler JA, O'Rourke S, Cooper C, et al. Multicenter evaluation of the BD Phoenix CPO detect test for detection and classification of carbapenemase-producing organisms in clinical isolates. J Clin Microbiol. 2020;58:e01752-19.
13. Thomson G, Turner D, Brasso W, Kircher S, Guillet T, Thomson K. High stringency evaluation of the automated BD Phoenix CPO Detect and Rapidec Carba NP tests for detection and classification of carbapenemases. J Clin Microbiol. 2017;55:3437-43.
14. Cointe A, Walewski V, Hobson CA, Doit C, Bidet P, Dortet L, et al. Rapid carbapenemase detection with Xpert Carba-R V2 directly on positive blood vials. Infect Drug Resist. 2019;12:3311-6.
15. Fiori B, D'Inzeo T, Giaquinto A, Menchinelli G, Liotti FM, de Maio F, et al. Optimized use of the MALDI BioTyper system and the FilmArray BCID panel for direct identification of microbial pathogens from positive blood cultures. J Clin Microbiol. 2016;54:576-84.
16. MacVane SH, Nolte FS. Benefits of adding a rapid PCR-based blood culture identification panel to an established antimicrobial stewardship program. J Clin Microbiol. 2016;54:2455-63.
17. Sinha M, Jupe J, Mack H, Coleman TP, Lawrence SM, Fraley SI. Emerging technologies for molecular diagnosis of sepsis. Clin Microbiol Rev. 2018;31:e00089-17.

CHAPTER 79 Antimicrobial Stewardship

Apurba Sankar Sastry, Deepashree R, Haritha Madigubba

ABSTRACT

Antimicrobial stewardship (AMS) is defined as use of the right antimicrobial agent, for the right patient, at the right time, with the right dose, route and frequency, causing the least harm to the patient and future patients. Antimicrobial stewardship program (AMSP) in a hospital is required for various reasons: (1) increased antimicrobial resistance (AMR), (2) misuse and overuse of antimicrobials, (3) widespread use of antimicrobials in other sectors, and (4) poor antimicrobial research.

Implementation of AMSP involves six important steps: (1) administrative support (leadership), (2) formulating AMS team, (3) infrastructure support, (4) framing antimicrobial policy, (5) implementing AMS strategies which include front-end strategy (formulary restriction) and back-end strategy (prospective audit and feedback), and (6) education and training.

Monitoring the compliance to AMSP is essential, which involves several indicators such as: (1) policy adherence indicator, (2) antimicrobial usage outcome indicators such as defined daily dosage (DDD) and days of therapy (DOT), (3) AMR outcome indicator, (4) clinical outcome indicators such as morbidity and mortality indicators, and (5) financial outcome indicators.

When prescribing antimicrobial agents, the clinicians should consider the following advices: (1) antibiotics should be prescribed only when it is indicated, (2) antibiotics should always be started only after site-specific specimens are collected for culture, (3) empirical therapy should be modified based on susceptibility test report; which may be of two types—escalation or de-escalation, (4) antimicrobials must be administrated at the correct dose, frequency, and duration, (5) minimum inhibitory concentration (MIC)-guided therapy should be preferred over disk diffusion test as MIC helps to select the most appropriate antibiotic, (6) therapeutic drug monitoring may be performed if feasible, and (7) antimicrobial must be stopped at appropriate time.

"Goodness is like antibiotics nowadays. Normal dose heals, Overdose kills"

—Yash S Yawalkar

INTRODUCTION

Antimicrobial stewardship program provides strategies for rationalizing the use of antimicrobials in the hospital.

Centers for Disease Control and Prevention (CDC) has defined AMS as use of the right antimicrobial agent, for the right patient, at the right time, with the right dose, route and frequency, causing the least harm to the patient and future patients.

WHY AMSP IS NEEDED

Antimicrobial stewardship program in a hospital is required for the following reasons.

Antimicrobial resistance: Antimicrobial resistance is a rising threat across the globe. The multidrug-resistant organisms (MDROs) are prevalent in every country though the extent and the severity of the problem varies. Extensive use of antimicrobials is the single most important factor for the bacteria to undergo mutation, which leads bacteria to become resistant to antimicrobials and then the resistant strain flourish exponentially in the presence of selective pressure of antimicrobials.

Misuse and overuse of antimicrobials: The last eight decades, since the discovery of penicillin, witnessed the saving of millions of lives due to use of antimicrobials in treating infections. However, at the same time, this has also led to their misuse through various ways—(1) use without a prescription, (2) overuse for self-limiting infections and nonbacterial infections, and (3) treatment of colonizer/contaminant.

Widespread use in other sectors: World's largest antimicrobial use occurs for animal nontherapeutic purpose (70%), followed by animal therapeutic purpose (15%). Human use accounts only 15% of total antimicrobial consumption, out of which only 9% is being used for human therapeutic purpose. This data explains that just bringing in stewardship program in healthcare facility would not bring down antimicrobial use dramatically. A robust plan should also be in place for control of antimicrobial use in animals.

Poor antimicrobial research: Research in the development of new antimicrobial is a huge investment for the pharmaceutical industry. More so, soon after the discovery of an antimicrobial, the bacteria develop resistance mechanisms to tackle the antimicrobial. As a result, investment goes waste. It is also hypothesized that there could be a return to the preantibiotic era, where many people could suffer or die from untreatable bacterial infections.

IMPLEMENTATION OF AMSP

The key steps of implementation of AMSP in a hospital are as follows.

ADMINISTRATIVE SUPPORT

The most important prerequisite for implementing AMSP is a strong administrative support. They should be publicly committed to the program and provide necessary funding and infrastructure support.

TEAM

Antimicrobial stewardship team is a multidisciplinary committee which is responsible for framing, implementing, and monitoring the compliance to antimicrobial policy of the hospital.

- AMS team is led by the antimicrobial steward who may be an infectious disease physician or infection control officer or clinical microbiologist.
- *Antimicrobial steward* is the central driving force behind this program. A larger hospital may require more than one antimicrobial steward.
- Other members of AMS team include stewardship nurses, clinical pharmacists, and officer-in-charge of pharmacy.

INFRASTRUCTURE

Infrastructure support is essential to initiate appropriate pathogen-directed antimicrobial agent at the earliest.

- *Support from the microbiology laboratory*:
  - *Automations*: Facility for automated culture (e.g., BACTEC, BacT/ALERT, or Virtuo), identification [matrix-assisted laser desorption/ionization-time-of-flight (MALDI-TOF)] and sensitivity (e.g., VITEK) should be available. This reduces the turnaround time to 24–48 hours; compared to conventional cultures which takes 2–5 days.
  - *Biomarkers*: Facility for testing biomarkers such as procalcitonin (PCT) and C-reactive protein (CRP) must be available (discussed subsequently).
  - *Molecular tests*: Facility to perform rapid molecular tests must be available; e.g., BioFire FilmArray multiplex PCR.
  - *Emergency laboratory*: Emergency laboratory functioning round the clock is a marker of a quality microbiology laboratory.
- *Hospital information system (HIS)*: Fully functional HIS including laboratory information system will augment the stewardship program by many folds.
- Supporting manpower availability.

FRAMING POLICY

Every hospital should frame their own hospital antimicrobial policy, which is usually a pocket handbook comprising of system/syndrome-wise indications for antimicrobial choice and their dosage.

- It should be prepared by AMS team after discussing with all the clinicians, microbiologists, and administrators.
- The policy must be compliant to the standard national and international antimicrobial guidelines and local antibiogram pattern.
- Common consensus between all clinicians must be arrived, before framing the policy; which facilitates better adherence to policy.

STRATEGIES

Two types of strategies are available for implementing AMSP:

1. Front-end strategies (formulary restriction)
2. Back-end strategies (prospective audit and feedback)

Front-end strategy (formulary restriction): This involves classifying antimicrobial agents into restricted, semi-restricted, and nonrestricted antimicrobials with indications for their use combined with an approval system regulated by the AMS team (**Table 1**).

- This strategy sounds more attractive, impact is immediate and appears to be the most ideal way to achieve AMS, but practically implementing formulary restrictions is challenging and a difficult task.
- It creates a lot of confusion as it directly compromises the clinician's freedom to choose antimicrobials.
- More so availability of the AMSP consultants to give approval all the time further complicates the problem, especially in emergency situations.

Back-end strategy: This is carried out by *prospective audit and feedback*. Though difficult to perform, but it is the most effective strategy to implement AMSP.

- The AMS team goes for stewardship round during which they discuss with the clinical team in detail about the compliance to the antimicrobial policy in terms of

TABLE 1 Proposed formulary restriction.

Restricted antimicrobials	Semirestricted antimicrobials	Unrestricted antimicrobials
Supply		
Pharmacy supply of >1 days requires prior approval by antimicrobial stewardship (AMS) team	Pharmacy supply of >3 days requires prior approval by AMS team	Pharmacy supply does not require AMS team approval
Agents		
• Colistin • Carbapenem • Tigecycline	• Teicoplanin, vancomycin, daptomycin • Linezolid • Third- and fourth-generation • Cephalosporins	• First- and second-generation cephalosporins • Cotrimoxazole • Azithromycin • Clarithromycin • Fluoroquinolones

appropriateness of the antimicrobials used, dosage with renal adjustment, compliance to susceptibility report etc. The clinical team gives justification about the noncompliance occurred, if any.

- The prospective audit and feedback is a mutually agreed upon constructive discussion between AMS team and the clinical team on the cases with daily follow-up.
- Although the back-end strategy is more labor-intensive, it has several advantages:
  - It is more widely practiced.
  - It is more easily accepted by clinicians.
  - It provides a higher opportunity for educating and training healthcare professionals.
  - Impact is delayed but sustainable improving the overall quality of antimicrobial prescribing practice.

EDUCATION AND TRAINING

Similar to any other healthcare program, AMSP also needs continuous education, training, motivation, and assessment of the healthcare providers. Developing AMS is a behavioral change within the person. Hence, adequate motivational education is a must to bring in such change.

MONITORING THE COMPLIANCE

It is said that "If you cannot measure it, you cannot improve it". Measurement of the compliance to AMSP is achieved by looking at both process and outcome indicators.

- *Policy adherence indicator (process indicator)*: This is achieved by conducting AMS audit as described under backward strategy. Both prescription and administrative compliance can be calculated.

  Indicators of prescription compliance

  Examples of prescription compliance indicators include:
  - Percentage of time the empirical antibiotic given is according to the infective syndrome suspected.
  - Percentage of time the empirical antibiotic is modified according to antimicrobial susceptibility report.
  - Percentage of time cultures is taken before the start of antibiotics.
  - Percentage of time the choice of surgical antimicrobial prophylaxis given is according to the policy.

  Indicators of administrative compliance

  Examples of administrative compliance indicators include:
  - Percentage of time the antibiotic is administrated in correct dose, correct frequency, and correct route [intravenous (IV), oral, or infusion].
  - Percentage of time the surgical antimicrobial prophylaxis is administrated in correct dose, correct time, and correct frequency.
- *Antimicrobial usage outcome indicators* such as DDD and DOT. These indicators are used to estimate the antibiotic consumption. They are discussed below.
- *AMR outcome indicator*: The change in AMR pattern is analyzed by conducting periodic AMR surveillance.
- *Clinical outcome indicators* such as morbidity (e.g., length of stay) and mortality (e.g., infection-related deaths) indicators.
- *Financial outcome indicators* such as antimicrobial cost per patient day or per year or per admission.

DEFINED DAILY DOSAGE

Defined daily dosage is the average maintenance dose per day for a drug used for its main indication in adults.

- Therapeutic dose should not be used for calculating antibiotic usage because it varies between the persons depending upon the weight, disease type, and associated factors such as renal adjustment etc. Therefore, DDD is a better indicator to calculate the antimicrobial consumption.
- The World Health Organization (WHO)-assigned DDDs are available in website, which should be used while calculating the number of DDDs consumed.
- DDD cannot be used for estimating antibiotic consumption in patients with renal failure and pediatric patients, because the daily dose actually prescribed is typically lower than the average dose defining the DDD.

Calculation of DDDs

No. of DDDs = Therapeutic dose (No. of tablets/vials used × g per tablet/vial)

WHO-defined DDD of the antimicrobial agent

Example

Levofloxacin is administered as 750 mg PO daily for 7 days. The WHO-assigned DDD for levofloxacin is 0.5 g.

Therefore, the number of DDD is calculated as:

(0.75 g dose × 7 days/0.5 g DDD) = 10.5 DDDs

DAYS OF THERAPY

Days of therapy of an antibiotic is the number of days that patient receives at least one dose of that antibiotic. It can be used for estimating antibiotic consumption in patients with renal failure, pediatric patients, and therefore is preferred over DDDs.

Examples include:

- A patient has received meropenem 1 g, twice daily for 3 days; the DOT is 3
- A patient has received meropenem 0.5 g, thrice daily for 3 days; the DOT is 3
- A patient has received meropenem 1 g, twice daily and vancomycin 1 g thrice daily for 3 days; the DOT is 3 + 3 = 6

RATIONAL USE OF ANTIMICROBIAL AGENTS

When prescribing antimicrobial agents, the clinicians should consider the following advice.

PRESCRIBE ONLY WHEN INDICATED

Prescribe antibiotics only when it is indicated. There are various conditions where antibiotics are not required.

- *Diarrhea*: Oral rehydration solution is the mainstay of treatment, not antibiotics. More so, the most common cause of diarrhea is of viral etiology.
- *Upper respiratory tract infections* such as common cold and sore throat, where the primary cause is viral infections (except when bacterial infections such as streptococcal sore throat or diphtheria are strongly suspected).
- When an *alternative diagnosis* is suspected/confirmed such as dengue, chikungunya, and malaria.
- *Prophylaxis*: Routine antibiotic prophylaxis should not be given to prevent infection, except for particular situations such as cotrimoxazole prophylaxis in HIV-infected individuals.

CULTURE OF CULTURES

Antibiotics should always be started only after site-specific specimens are collected for culture. If specimens are collected after antibiotic start, then cultures become false negative and thus it will not help in targeted therapy.

EMPIRICAL VERSUS TARGETED THERAPY

Empirical therapy: Empirical antibiotic should not be given randomly, but based on three important elements:

1. The infective syndrome likely to be present
2. The common etiological bacterial agents for that infective syndrome
3. The local antibiogram for those organisms, indicating the AMR pattern

Targeted or pathogen-directed therapy: The empirical therapy should be modified subsequently, based on antimicrobial susceptibility test (AST) report. The modifications may be of two types—escalation or de-escalation.

ESCALATION VERSUS DE-ESCALATION APPROACH

There are two approaches by which antimicrobial agents are prescribed—escalation and de-escalation.

- The approach needs to be chosen based on local AMR pattern and the spectrum of activity of the antibiotic.
- Antibiotics prescribed for an organism can be ranked based on their spectrum of activity and local AMR pattern.
- For example; in hospital X, the antibiotics given for gram-negative organisms such as *Escherichia coli* are ranked according to decreasing order of susceptibility: colistin (rank-1) → tigecycline → carbapenems → piperacillin-tazobactam → cefoperazone sulbactam → amikacin → cefepime → ceftazidime → cotrimoxazole → ceftazidime → ciprofloxacin → ceftriaxone (lowest rank).

Escalation approach: This approach is chosen if local AMR pattern is unlikely and/or the patient is clinically stable. The empirical therapy is started with a narrow-spectrum antibiotics (e.g., ceftriaxone for *E. coli*). If AST report shows resistance, then can be escalated to a higher rank antibiotic subsequently (e.g., meropenem for *E. coli*).

De-escalation approach: This approach is chosen if local AMR pattern is expected to be high and/or patient is critically ill. Empirical therapy is started with broad-spectrum antibiotics (e.g., meropenem for *E. coli*). If AST report shows susceptible, it can be de-escalated to a narrow-spectrum antibiotic subsequently (e.g., ceftriaxone for *E. coli)*. However, the reserved/restricted antimicrobials such as colistin and tigecycline should not be given as empirical therapy even under de-escalation strategy. They should be prescribed only when AST report is available and shows resistant results to all other antimicrobials tested.

SITE-SPECIFIC ANTIMICROBIALS

Only those antimicrobials should be prescribed which are active at the infection site. The following antimicrobials are not active at the respective sites and therefore should be excluded from treatment.

- *Lungs*: Daptomycin is not active at respiratory site as it gets inactivated by pulmonary surfactants.
- *Cerebrospinal fluid (CSF)*: Any oral antibiotic, first- and second-generation cephalosporins, tetracyclines, macrolides, quinolones, and clindamycin are not active in CSF.
- *Urine*: Antibiotics such as chloramphenicol, macrolide, and clindamycin should be avoided in urinary tract infection (UTI); as they do not achieve adequate urinary concentrations.

AVOID ADMINISTRATION ERRORS

Antimicrobials must be administrated at the correct dose (as per the age/body weight), and frequency and duration of therapy.

- *Loading dose*: Certain concentration-dependent antimicrobials such as aminoglycoside, vancomycin, and colistin should be administered with a loading dose.
- *Infusion*: The efficacy of certain antimicrobials such as vancomycin is better when mixed with saline and given as an IV infusion over 2–3 hours.
- *Renal adjustment*: The dosage of the nephrotoxic drugs (such as aminoglycoside, vancomycin, and colistin) should be adjusted according to the creatinine clearance.

MINIMUM INHIBITORY CONCENTRATION-GUIDED THERAPY

The AST can be performed by disk diffusion or by MIC-based method; the latter being more accurate and reliable. There are certain situations where the antibiotic treatment is MIC guided.

- Clinical conditions such as endocarditis and pneumococcal meningitis/pneumonia
- *Vancomycin for Staphylococcus aureus*: Vancomycin should be avoided if MIC is >1 µg/mL.

Minimum inhibitory concentration helps to select the most appropriate antibiotic. Lower is the MIC, better is the therapeutic efficacy. If >1 antimicrobial agents are found susceptible, then the antibiotic having the lowest MIC (when compared with the susceptibility breakpoint) should be chosen for therapy. This is better guided by calculating the *therapeutic index*.

Therapeutic index

It is the ratio of susceptibility breakpoint divided by MIC of the test isolate.

Therapeutic index = Susceptible breakpoint/test MIC

Higher the therapeutic index better is the efficacy of the antimicrobial agent.

For example, if a clinical isolate of *E. coli* is susceptible to both meropenem (MIC 1 µg/mL) and amikacin (MIC 8 µg/mL), then meropenem falsely appears to be more efficacious as its absolute MIC value is lower than amikacin. However, the MIC value compared with the standard susceptibility breakpoint (and not the absolute MIC value) determines therapeutic efficacy.

Susceptible breakpoints of meropenem and amikacin for *E. coli* are 1 µg/mL and 16 µg/mL, respectively, according to Clinical and Laboratory Standards Institute (CLSI) guideline 2020.

The therapeutic index is calculated as:

- Therapeutic index of meropenem = 1/1 = 1
- Therapeutic index of meropenem = 16/8 = 2

Therefore, in this case, amikacin is superior to meropenem.

THERAPEUTIC DRUG MONITORING

Therapeutic efficacy is not only relies on in vitro susceptibility result (MIC), but also dependent on in vivo activity which is in turn dependent on pharmacokinetic and pharmacodynamics (PK/PD) parameters of the antimicrobial agent.

- Therefore, therapeutic drug monitoring is necessary to find out how the drug behaves in vivo.
- It is particularly important for antibiotic such as vancomycin, amikacin, and colistin. Depending up on PK/PD parameters, antibiotics are classified as:
  - *Concentration-dependent antibiotics, e.g., aminoglycosides*: They work better if the drug concentration in serum is much higher than the MIC of the drug (determined in vitro). They are usually given as a loading dose so that the drug concentration reaches its peak immediately.
  - *Time-dependent antibiotics, e.g., beta-lactams*: Here, the efficacy of the drug is dependent upon how much time the drug concentration remains higher than the MIC. Therefore, these drugs are given in frequent intervals (e.g., thrice daily) so that the drug level in serum would remain always higher than the MIC.

TIMELY STOPPAGE OF ANTIMICROBIAL

Antimicrobial agent must be stopped at appropriate time, which may be determined by clinical improvement or after obtaining negative culture or by use of biomarkers.

BIOMARKERS-GUIDED THERAPY

Biomarkers such as PCT or CRP may be used for predicting bacterial infection. PCT is more reliable marker than CRP.

Procalcitonin: It is a peptide precursor of the hormone calcitonin secreted at very low level (<0.05 ng/mL) normally by the body, but the level goes up by manifolds in bacterial infection. The various diagnostic application of PCT includes:

- To differentiate bacterial versus viral infection
- For predicting bacterial infections such as local or systemic infection (e.g., bacterial sepsis or bacterial pneumonia), depending upon PCT level and associated clinical presentation
  - 0.05–2.0 ng/mL indicates possible local infection
  - 2–10 ng/mL indicates systemic infection
  - >10 ng/mL indicates septic shock
- Helps to decide whether to continue antibiotics in culture negative cases
- Helps to decide whether to stop antibiotics
- *Severity*: PCT levels parallel with the severity of the bacterial infections; higher the PCT level, severe is the infection. Therefore, PCT can be used as prognostic indicator. However, PCT should not be used alone, but should always be used in adjunct with cultures.

AVOID MISUSE OF ANTIMICROBIALS

The following are the common examples of misuse of antimicrobials which should be avoided.

- *Avoid overlapping spectra*: Meropenem and piperacillin-tazobactam combination therapy for double gram-negative coverage should be avoided as both these drugs belong to beta-lactam group of antimicrobials and therefore share similar antibacterial spectra.
- *Redundant antibiotic*: Meropenem and metronidazole combination therapy for suspected gram-negative/anaerobic sepsis should be avoided as meropenem is active against anaerobes in addition to gram-negative bacteria. Therefore, metronidazole can be withdrawn from therapy.
- *Ineffective antibiotic*: Cloxacillin in methicillin-resistant *S. aureus* (MRSA) infection is ineffective and therefore, should be avoided. Vancomycin is the drug of choice for MRSA.
- *Inferior antibiotic*: Vancomycin is an inferior cell wall acting agent compared to cloxacillin for methicillin-susceptible *S. aureus* (MSSA) infection.

HOSPITAL ANTIBIOGRAM

An *antibiogram* is an overall profile of AST results of a specific microorganism to a battery of antimicrobial agents (**Table 2**). It is the responsibility of the department of microbiology to construct a hospital antibiogram and share it with clinicians. It has the following uses:

- Antibiogram guides the clinicians in selecting the best empirical antimicrobial treatment in the event of pending culture and susceptibility results.

TABLE 2 Hospital antibiogram of gram-negative bacteria for the year 2020, expressed in terms of susceptibility rate.

	Ciprofloxacin	Amikacin	Ceftazidime	Piperacillin-tazobactam	Meropenem	Colistin
Escherichia coli	25	85	55	75	82	99
Klebsiella	15	75	35	65	70	85
Pseudomonas	32	80	60	80	80	99
Acinetobacter	29	70	10	18	20	99

- It is also an useful tool for detecting and monitoring trends in AMR within the hospital.
- Antibiogram can also be used to compare susceptibility rates across institutions and track resistance trends and thereby contributing to national AMR surveillance database.

FUTURE DIRECTIONS

The Indian Ministry of Health (MOH) needs to take urgent initiatives to implement and monitor the implementation of national policy to control the rising trend of AMR.

- *Implementable AMSP*: India needs an implementable AMSP policy, and not a perfect policy. The best method is to introduce step-by-step regulation of antimicrobial usage, concentrating on higher end antimicrobials first and then slowly extending the list to second- and first-line antimicrobials.
- *Drugs Controller General of India (DGCI)*: The DCGI will need to formulate and implement a policy on rationalizing antimicrobial usage in the country, both in hospitals and over the counters, after consultation with stake holders and experts in the field.
- *H1 drugs*: Implementation of H1 drugs with red line need to be strictly monitored to control the over the counter sale of antimicrobials.
- *Hospital Infection Control Committee (HICC)*: Structured and fully functioning HICC must be made mandatory in all hospitals. Regulatory authorities and accreditation agencies [National Accreditation Board for Hospitals and Healthcare Providers (NABH) and International Organization for Standardization (ISO)] must insist on a functioning HICC, during the licensing, and accreditation process. State department of health should take initiatives in organizing regional and state infection control committees to supervise the functioning of hospital HICC.
- *National task force* has to be appointed to oversee implementation. The officers appointed for monitoring the implementation need to adequately trained so as to improvise the quality of monitoring and to bring in uniformity.
- *Fund*: The most important step toward control of AMR is availability of funds. The Government of India (GOI) should provide fund for manpower, improved diagnostics, and development of information technology.
- *Answerability*: There should be chain of unidirectional monitoring of implementation of various activities so that everyone in the chain will compile to the policy and produce maximum output.

  GOI → State → Directors of institutes → AMSP team → stake holders (clinical and laboratory consultants)
- *Non-governmental organizations (NGOs)*: National and international have played a pivotal role in disseminating public information and funding research in diseases such as cancer and cardiac diseases. They should come forward with similar enthusiasm to tackle AMR issue, with the same vigor.
- *National Accreditation Board of Hospitals* is required to insist on strict implementation of hospital antimicrobial and infection control policy, during hospital accreditation, and reaccreditation processes. Hospitals without compliance with the policy should not be given accreditation.
- *Indian Council of Medical Research (ICMR)*: The ICMR should broaden the AMR surveillance, HAI and AMSP networks, incorporating hospitals from both the government and private sector. ICMR will need to provide funds for research on AMR, drug development, and vaccines.
- *WHO India*: The Indian division of the WHO should step-up interaction with the government on issues related to drug resistance, antimicrobial policy, and infection control.
- *Medical Council of India (MCI)*: The MCI will need to make necessary curriculum changes so as to include a structured training on AMS and infection control at the undergraduate and postgraduate level.
- *Improved laboratory stewardship*: There is an urgent need to standardize microbiology laboratories in India. Hospitals must have good quality microbiology laboratory or should be willing to outsource specimens, in the absence of a standardized laboratory. Technician-equipped emergency microbiology laboratory should be made compulsory.
- *Increased awareness and education*:
  - Medical journals and medical educational forums should focus more on AMR and AMSP
  - Public awareness through electronic and print mass media
  - AMSP at district level
- *Animal use*: Control of antimicrobial use in animals and poultry (nontherapeutic use) through appropriate legislation.

- *Research*: The GOI should look for promotion of research on new antimicrobials and AMSP.

ACKNOWLEDGMENT

We are thankful to Dr Ketan Priyadarshi, Fellow ID (AIIMS), Fellow HIC (First year), JIPMER, Puducherry for helping us prepare this chapter.

RECOMMENDED READINGS

1. bioMérieux. (2019). Antimicrobial stewardship—A practical guide to implementation in hospitals. [online] Available from https://www.biomerieuxindia.in/sites/clinic/files/antimicrobial_stewardship_booklet_9305408_010-gb-a_final.pdf.
2. Pollack LA, Srinivasan A. Core elements of hospital antimicrobial stewardship programs from the Centers for Disease Control and Prevention. Clin Infect Dis. 2014;59(suppl 3):S97-100.
3. Dellit TH, Owens RC, McGowan JE, Gerding DN, Weinstein RA, Burke JP, et al. Infectious Diseases Society of America and the Society for Healthcare Epidemiology of America guidelines for developing an institutional program to enhance antimicrobial stewardship. Clin Infect Dis. 2007;44(2):159-77.
4. Barlam TF, Cosgrove SE, Abbo LM, MacDougall C, Schuetz AN, Septimus EJ, et al. Implementing an antimicrobial stewardship program: guidelines by the Infectious Diseases Society of America and the Society for Healthcare Epidemiology of America. Clin Infect Dis. 2016;62(10):e51-77.
5. Sinha M, Jupe J, Mack H, Coleman TP, Lawrence SM, Fraley SI. Emerging technologies for molecular diagnosis of sepsis. Clin Microbiol Rev. 2018;31(2):e00089-17.
6. Brown EM, Nathwani D. Antimicrobial cycling or rotation: a systematic review of the evidence of efficacy. J Antimicrob Chemother. 2005;55(1):6-9.
7. Magiorakos AP, Srinivasan A, Carey RB, Carmeli Y, Falagas ME, Giske CG, et al. Multidrug-resistant, extensively drug-resistant and pandrug-resistant bacteria: an international expert proposal for interim standard definitions for acquired resistance. Clin Microbiol Infect. 2012;18(3):268-81.
8. WHO. (2017). National Action Plan on Antimicrobial Resistance (NAP-AMR) 2017-2021. [online] Available from https://ncdc.gov.in/WriteReadData/l892s/File645.pdf.
9. Kakkar M, Walia K, Vong S, Chatterjee P, Sharma A. Antimicrobial resistance and its containment in India. BMJ. 2017;358:j2687.
10. Ghafur A. The Chennai Declaration: a solution to the antimicrobial resistance problem in the Indian subcontinent. Clin Infect Dis. 2013;56(8):1190.

CHAPTER
80

Cytokine Release Syndrome

Harpreet Singh, Ritu Sangwan, Prabhudev

ABSTRACT

Cytokine release syndrome (CRS) is a superphysiological response of the immune system to a trigger (pathogens, autoimmune diseases, and immunotherapy) resulting in acute inflammatory syndrome. The dysregulated immune response leads to inflammation/dysfunction of multiple organs due to collateral damage to the host. The innate as well as adapted immune cells participate through a complex network of cytokines and signaling pathways culminating into a hyperproinflammatory response. Spectrum of clinical presentation can vary from mild ones (fever and fatigue) to severe systemic involvement [acute respiratory distress syndrome (ARDS) and multiple organ dysfunction syndrome (MODS)] to even death.

When suspected, early identification is the key to the management of CRS by evaluation of the trigger (detail history and clinical examination) along with laboratory investigations [especially rise in inflammatory markers: interleukin-6 (IL-6), C-reactive protein (CRP), and ferritin]. The management of CRS is as per severity grading. The mild CRS is symptomatically treated whereas severe CRS is managed using corticosteroids with tocilizumab (IL-6 receptor blocker). Additionally, aggressive intensive care management for hypotension, hypoxemia, cardiac arrhythmias, infections, and associated complications [heart failure/disseminated intravascular coagulopathy (DIC)] can be tried. In patients with unresolving/partial response to therapy, alemtuzumab, antithymocyte globulins (ATGs), cyclophosphamide, ruxolitinib, and ibrutinib have been tried.

"The most powerful therapeutic in the world is our own immune system"

—Francis deSouza

INTRODUCTION

Cytokine release syndrome is an acute inflammatory syndrome with a supraphysiologic response by the immune system to various triggers that activate or engage T cells or other immune effector cells like macrophages and endothelial cells. The first use of this term appeared in context of graft-versus-host disease (GVHD) in 1993. CRS represents the classical double-edged sword effect of normal physiological response of host's immune system triggered by pathogens, autoimmune disease, and therapies (**Box 1**) where in immune system overshoots its response causing collateral damage to host. Due to the dysregulated immune response in CRS there is a massive upsurge of cytokine release which results in inflammation/dysfunction of multiorgans. The ongoing pandemic of COVID-19 has resurrected this concept. CRS has prognostic and therapeutic implications so should be identified by clinician for early management.

PATHOPHYSIOLOGY

Physiologically, the activated immune system should produce sufficient cytokines to eliminate the trigger, thereafter the negative feedback mechanism to the immune system brings back the hyperinflammatory response to basal state so as to avoid/minimize collateral damage (if any). CRS is a result of imbalance between overloaded "pro" and under loaded "anti" inflammatory states.

The CRS may result due to inappropriate danger sensing response despite absence of pathogens (e.g., Castleman disease); ineffective response to overwhelming pathogen burden (e.g., sepsis); exaggerated effector response [e.g., chimeric antigen receptor (CAR) T-cell therapy]; and prolonged immune response due to failure to resolve [hemophagocytic lymphohistiocytosis (HLH)].

BOX 1	Clinical causes of cytokine release syndrome.
Iatrogenic:	
• CAR T-cell therapy	
• Blinatumomab	
Pathogen-induced:	
• Bacterial sepsis	
• EBV-associated HLH	
• HHV-8-associated MCD	
• COVID-19	
Monogenic and autoimmune:	
• Primary HLH	
• Secondary HLH/MAS	
• Autoinflammatory disorders	
• Idiopathic MCD	

(CAR: chimeric antigen receptor; EBV: Epstein–Barr virus; HHV-8: human herpesvirus 8; HLH: hemophagocytic lymphohistiocytosis; MAS: macrophage activation syndrome; MCD: multicentric Castleman disease)

The inadequate negative feedback to activated immune response, i.e., anti-inflammatory arm involving regulatory T cells, mesenchymal stem cells, decoy receptor (IL-1 receptor antagonist), and anti-inflammatory cytokine (IL-10), may be responsible for CRS as well.

A complex, interconnected network of cell types, cytokines, and signaling pathways is involved in CRS disorders (**Fig. 1**). Both the innate [neutrophils, macrophages, and natural killer (NK) cell] as well as adaptive immune cells (T cells) play a key role in the CRS. Neutrophils produce neutrophil extracellular traps (NETs), cytokines, and stored granules while the macrophages bring about phagocytosis. The NK cells being cytolytic through their perforins and granzyme production can contribute to tissue destruction.

The activated driver cells (antigen-presenting cells and T cells) release cytokines such as ILs (IL-1, 5, 6, 8, 10, 18), interferon (IFN)-gamma, tumor necrosis factor (TNF), vascular endothelial growth factor (VEGF), granulocyte-macrophage colony-stimulating factor (GM-CSF), and several others. These cytokines activate the several T cell subgroups (Th1, Th2, Th17, and cytotoxic T cells) which in

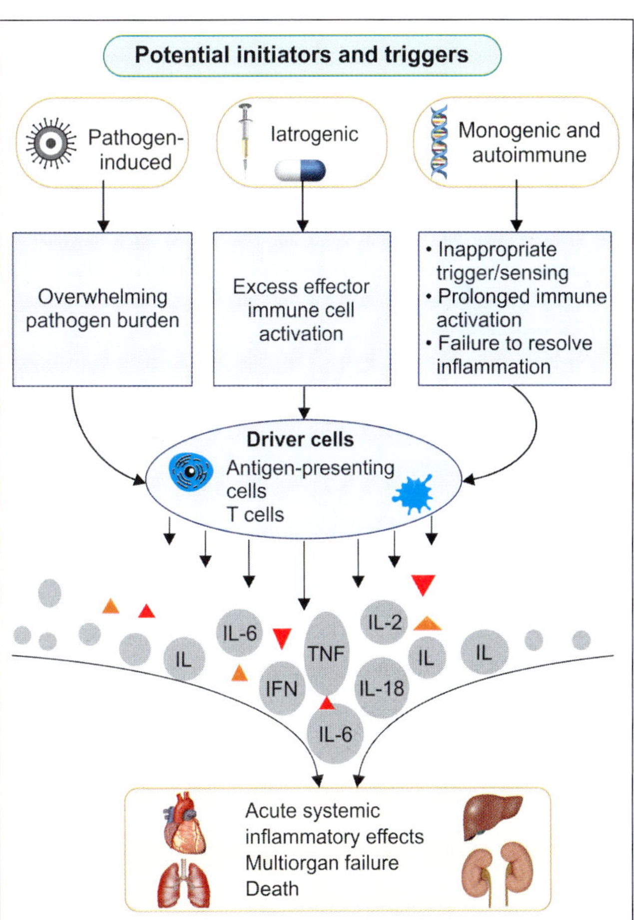

(IFN: interferon; IL: interleukin; TNF: tumor necrosis factor)

FIGURE 1: Underlying pathophysiology of cytokine release syndrome.

turn activate the neutrophils, macrophages, eosinophils, and several other cells through their released cytokines contributing to capillary leakage and coagulopathy thus amplifying the immune response and forming a continuous vicious cycle with no "anti-inflammatory brake" to stop the "hyperinflammatory wheel."

PROINFLAMMATORY ARM

Interleukin-6 is produced both by immune cells (via cis pathway) and nonimmune cells (via trans pathway) that have inflammatory effects wherein the trans pathway dominates over cis pathway in cytokine production. Consequently, the amount of cytokine production via the trans signaling (pathological response) is huge compared to the cis signaling (physiological response) so mediating cytokine production to be metaphorically called as cytokine "storm." IL-6 is associated with vascular leakage, activation of complement and coagulation cascade, DIC, and cardiomyopathy.

Interferon-gamma is associated with fever, chills, headache, dizziness, and fatigue.

Tumor necrosis factor-alpha causes flu-like symptoms with fever, malaise, watery diarrhea, vascular leakage, cardiomyopathy, lung injury, and production of acute phase proteins.

Chemokines (CXCL8, CXCL9, CXCL 10 etc.) and plasma proteins (CRP, ferritin, and complements) also contribute to the pathogenesis of CRS.

ANTI-INFLAMMATORY ARM

Interleukin-10 is the main anti-inflammatory cytokine which suppresses the activity of Th1 cells, NK cells, and macrophages by inhibiting major histocompatibility complex (MHC) class II and costimulatory molecule B7-1/B7-2 expression on monocytes and macrophages and limits the production of proinflammatory cytokines (including IL-1, IL-6, IL-12, IL-18, and TNF) and chemokines.

Apart from IL-10, the negative feedback mechanism is also mediated by the regulatory T cells, mesenchymal stem cells, and decoy cytokine receptors (IL1RA).

CLINICAL FEATURES

Cytokine release syndrome is an amalgam of constitutional symptoms (fever, fatigue, and anorexia), systemic inflammation, and multiorgan dysfunction.

Cough and dyspnea are the chief respiratory symptoms which can progress to ARDS with hypoxemia requiring mechanical ventilation. Headache, dizziness, and fatigue are commonly reported. Other manifesting features are skin rashes, edema, vasculitis, arthritis/arthralgias, gastro-intestinal manifestations—nausea, vomiting, diarrhea—and ascites.

In severe cases, renal failure, acute liver injury or cholestasis, and a stress-related or Takotsubo cardiomyopathy may develop.

Immune effector cell-associated neurotoxicity syndrome/CRS-associated encephalopathy due to T-cell immune therapy may develop over several days after onset of CRS and manifests as confusion, delirium, aphasia, and seizures.

Cases can progress rapidly to DIC (vascular occlusion or catastrophic hemorrhages), persistent hypoxemia, hypotension, hemostatic imbalance, vasodilatory shock, and death.

EVALUATION

The evaluation of patient with suspected CRS should promptly establish presence and severity of CRS along with identification of underlying cause (**Box 1**). This should include thorough vigilant physical examination, laboratory tests, and imaging.

History should cover the nature and time course of CRS and associated clinical findings including constitutional symptoms (fever myalgia headache fatigue, dyspnea, confusion, rash, arthralgia, and baseline neurological function). The underlying disease status and treatment history should be noted. The physical examination should document vitals including blood pressure, temperature, oxygen status, examination of skin; heart, lungs, and mental status to assess for organ dysfunction.

The *laboratory evaluation* should include complete blood count, coagulation profile [prothrombin time (PT), activated partial thromboplastin time (aPTT), and D-dimer], biochemical parameters [liver function test (LFT), renal function test (RFT), serum electrolytes, triglycerides, uric acid, and lactate dehydrogenase (LDH)], arterial blood gas analysis, markers of inflammation (CRP, ferritin, cytokine levels), and additional tests such as imaging modalities (chest X-ray and CT of chest), cardiac evaluation [brain natriuretic peptide (BNP), electrocardiography (ECG), echocardiography], and bronchoalveolar lavage (BAL) are often needed to identify other contributing processes like sepsis, heart failure, thromboembolism, and HLH/macrophage activation syndrome (MAS).

The laboratory findings are variable and are influenced by underlying cause. The nonspecific markers of inflammation such as CRP and serum ferritin are universally elevated and correlate with severity. Many others may have hypertriglyceridemia, increased LDH, blood count abnormalities such as leukocytosis/leukopenia, lymphopenia (COVID 19), anemia, thrombocytopenia, and deranged coagulation profile. Elevation in serum cytokine levels such as IFN-γ, IL-6, IL-10, soluble IL-2α receptor (marker of T-cell activation) is present. Deranged RFT and LFT, serum electrolytes, and blood gas analysis may suggest severity.

APPROACH TO DIAGNOSIS

Cytokine release syndrome manifests as an initial fever and a constellation of nonspecific clinical findings that may also be caused by infection/sepsis and disease progression. A high index of suspicion is necessary to diagnose CRS and to distinguish it from other conditions.

CRS should be suspected in a patient with fever, which may be accompanied by tachypnea, tachycardia, hypotension, and hypoxia. CRS is most commonly seen after treatment with antigen-specific CAR T-cell therapy, but it also occurs following treatment with a therapeutic antibody (e.g., blinatumomab), after haploidentical allogeneic hematopoietic cell transplantation and viral infections.

In a patient suspected to have a CRS, a three-modal approach to diagnosis is:

1. Identifying the underlying disease (ruling out disorders that may mimic CRS)
2. Establishing severity
3. Determining the clinical progress trajectory

Identifying the underlying disorder can be challenging as it is not a diagnosis of exclusion and can encompass many disorders. It is important to differentiate between CRS due to an iatrogenic cause such as CAR T-cell therapy and CRS due to systemic infection, since use of immune suppressives could be detrimental if used in patients with septicemia.

Based on clinical features, it is difficult to distinguish CRS due to sepsis from the CRS due to CAR T-cell therapy. Levels of serum cytokines, most prominently IFN-γ, are often more elevated in patients with CRS due to CAR T-cell therapy while higher levels of circulating IL-1β, procalcitonin, and markers of endothelial damage are found in sepsis-induced CRS.

Hemophagocytic lymphohistiocytosis and MAS share many clinical and laboratory features with CRS. Most patients with moderate-to-severe CRS have laboratory features that meet criteria for HLH/MAS as both CRS and HLH/MAS have activation of macrophages and the reticuloendothelial system that is initiated by T cell-mediated inflammation. Grading systems used to predict and assess the severity differ according to the cause of syndrome.

MANAGEMENT

The principle of management of CRS is as per severity grading (based on the cause).

Mild CRS is treated symptomatically with antipyretics, intravenous fluid with close monitoring of the symptoms and hemodynamics. The benefit–toxicity balance favors symptomatic treatment over immune modulation. In sever CRS, initial treatment with tocilizumab (IL-6 receptor blocker) plus corticosteroid achieves more rapid response to CRS control than either agent alone. The steroid (methylprednisolone up to 1 mg/kg/day or equivalents dexamethasone/hydrocortisone) should continue till improvement in CRS. Tocilizumab may be repeated after an interval of at least 8 hours in severe cases. Additionally, sever CRS requires intensive care unit management to receive aggressive management of hypotension, oxygenation (including mechanical ventilation), cardiac monitoring (especially arrhythmias), infections, and other anticipated clinical complication (especially heart failure/sepsis).

The clinical and laboratory status should be assessed regularly to determine the response to therapy. Resolution of fever and decrease/no need for oxygen supplementation and vasopressors indicate positive response to therapy. Steroid regimen should continue till no need for vasopressors and high flow oxygenation, thereafter steroids may be tapered off. A low threshold suspicion for coexisting infections and cardiac and thromboembolic complications should be kept especially in unresolving/partial response to therapy.

Those failing to improve, high-dose corticosteroid therapy has been used if there is no clinical improvement especially to oxygenation and hypotension within 24–72 hours, management for persistent or worsening CRS has been suggested. The possible treatments include alemtuzumab, ATG, cyclophosphamide, ruxolitinib, and ibrutinib have been tried for persistent and worsening CRS. There is a very limited response with other immune modulator agents such as monoclonal antibodies against IL-6 (siltuximab and clazakizumab), IL-1 blocker (anakinra), and TNF-α blocker (etanercept).

CONCLUSION

Though described earlier CRS has come out to be an important clinical entity in the modern medicine as it can be life-threatening. Mild secondary organ dysfunction during an inflammatory response is acceptable if it allows the host to overcome infection and survive. In short, CRS involves an immune response that causes collateral damage which may be greater than the immediate benefit of the immune response.

The strategy for CRS involves supportive care to maintain critical organ function, control of underlying disease with the targeted therapy, and elimination of triggers. Unfortunately, the outcomes of the disease in severe cases continue to be gruesome. Sufficient scientific progression is needed toward biomarker guided, individualized treatment of CRS. Further more reliable, quick, and accessible assays are needed to measure the soluble mediators of inflammation in plasma and tissues to determine the severity and/or progression of the disease. Nonetheless, given advances in multi-omic profiling and therapeutic modulation of the immune system as well as concerted efforts to work across the CRS umbrella, continued improvements in the outcomes can be expected.

RECOMMENDED READINGS

1. Fajgenbaum DC, June CH. Cytokine Storm. N Engl J Med. 2020;383(23):2255-73.
2. Lee DW, Santomasso BD, Locke FL, Ghobadi A, Turtle CJ, Brudno JN, et al. ASTCT consensus grading for cytokine release syndrome and neurologic toxicity associated with immune effector cells. Biol Blood Marrow Transplant. 2019;25:625-38.
3. Grupp SA, Kalos M, Barrett D, Aplenc R, Porter DL, Rheingold SR, et al. Chimeric antigen receptor-modified T cells for acute lymphoid leukemia. N Engl J Med. 2013;368:1509-18.
4. Lee DW, Gardner R, Porter DL, Louis CU, Ahmed N, Jensen M, et al. Current concepts in the diagnosis and management of cytokine release syndrome. Blood. 2014;124:188-95.

5. Diorio C, Shaw PA, Pequignot E, Orlenko A, Chen F, Aplenc R, et al. Diagnostic biomarkers to differentiate sepsis from cytokine release syndrome in critically ill children. Blood Adv. 2020;4:5174-83.
6. Hashimoto D, Chow A, Noizat C, Teo P, Beasley MB, Leboeuf M, et al. Tissue-resident macrophages self-maintain locally throughout adult life with minimal contribution from circulating monocytes. Immunity. 2013;38:792-804.
7. Zoller EE, Lykens JE, Terrell CE, Aliberti J, Filipovich AH, Henson PM, et al. Hemophagocytosis causes a consumptive anemia of inflammation. J Exp Med. 2011;208:1203-14.
8. Doherty GM, Lange JR, Langstein HN, Alexander HR, Buresh CM, Norton JA. Evidence for IFN-gamma as a mediator of the lethality of endotoxin and tumor necrosis factor-alpha. J Immunol. 1992;149:1666-70.
9. Cohen J. IL-12 deaths: explanation and a puzzle. Science. 1995;270:908.
10. Atkins MB. Interleukin-2: clinical applications. Semin Oncol. 2002;29:Suppl 7:12-7.
11. Kang S, Tanaka T, Narazaki M, Kishimoto T. Targeting interleukin-6 signaling in clinic. Immunity. 2019;50:1007-23.
12. Vercruysse F, Barnetche T, Lazaro E, Shipley E, Lifermann F, Balageas A, et al. Adult-onset Still's disease biological treatment strategy may depend on the phenotypic dichotomy. Arthritis Res Ther. 2019;21: 53.

CHAPTER

81

Envenomation: Snake and Scorpion

Dhruva Chaudhry, Diksha Tyagi

ABSTRACT

Snake and scorpion envenomation are the environmental and occupational hazards that commonly present as acute life-threatening emergency in the tropical and subtropical countries. Most of the bites are nonvenomous with patients presenting in fear and anxiety. Local symptoms are mild with no systemic involvement. Severe symptoms may develop because of the local and systemic absorption of toxins present in the venom. A snakebite patient may presents with any of the four clinical syndromes; i.e., progressive local symptoms, neurotoxic, vasculotoxic, and myotoxic envenomation or with overlapping features. Scorpion envenomation mainly present as autonomic hyperexcitation with cardiac complications. Early treatment with the antidotes namely anti-snake venom (ASV) in case of snake envenomation and prazosin (physiological antidote) with or without scorpion antivenom (SAV) in case of scorpion envenomation is the treatment of choice along the proper monitoring and intensive care.

"Understanding is the first step to acceptance, and only with acceptance can there be recovery"

—J K Rowling

SNAKE ENVENOMATION

INTRODUCTION

Snakes are one of the most venomous creatures known to humans. India is a country where snakes are worshipped and tamed since centuries. They share common habitat with humans in their houses and working areas leading to unintentional encounters. Hence, snakebite is a common medical emergency seen in the hospitals. The actual number of snakebites in India is not known because many patients still consults traditional healers (*Tantrik* and *Ojhas*) for the treatment. The estimated number of snakebites in India in 2015 was 1.11–1.77 million. Although the snake envenomation is a treatable condition, still 1.2 million snakebite deaths (average 58,000/year) has been reported from 2000–2019. About 25% of them are the children with age <15 years. The reason for this high fatality is due to the delay in diagnosis (in absence of history of snakebite), non-availability of ASV, delayed and inappropriate administration of ASV, lack of standard protocol for management, inexperienced doctors, and nonavailability of ventilators.

Till date, around 300 species of snakes are known in India. Out of these, only 52 species are venomous. The four species that are responsible for majority of the venomous bites are common cobra (*Naja naja*), Russell's viper (*Daboia russelii*), saw-scaled viper (*Echis carinatus*), and common krait (*Bungarus caeruleus*), collectively called as "Big four". Viper and cobra bites during the day or evening. On the other hand, kraits usually become active during night and bite a person while sleeping. An another species named hump-nosed pit viper (*Hypnale* species) has been recognized to cause severe systemic symptoms, mainly found in the Western Ghats of the South India. It has been found that neurotoxic envenomations are significantly higher in North India as compared to South India where vasculotoxic envenomations are prevalent. Data from our institute also showed that out of 185 cases of snakebite, 183 were Elapidae bites with neuroparalytic symptoms and two were viper bites with vasculotoxic manifestations.

SNAKE VENOM

Snake venom is a complex cocktail of different enzymes and nonenzymatic cytotoxins. Various enzymes are digestive hydrolase's, hyaluronidase, L-amino acid oxidase, 5'nucleotidase, DNAase, phospholipase A2, peptidase, nicotinamide adenine dinucleotide (NAD)-nucleosides and procoagulant enzymes. The venom of Indian cobra contains two neurotoxins (alpha-bungarotoxin and alpha-cobratoxin), cardiotoxin and phospholipase A2. The primary site of action of neurotoxins is neuromuscular junction. These toxins bind to acetylcholine receptors on postsynaptic membrane and prevent their interaction with acetylcholine. This, in turn prevent the opening of sodium channels and thus blocks the neuromuscular transmission. Cardiotoxin and phospholipase A2 has direct lytic action on cardiac, skeletal, and smooth muscles leading to severe inflammation and necrosis of local tissue. On the other hand, venom of Indian krait has both presynaptic (beta-bungarotoxin) and postsynaptic (alpha-bungarotoxin) neurotoxins. The predominant mechanism of action of neurotoxicity is the blockage of presynaptic receptors by beta-bungarotoxin preventing the release of acetylcholine in neuromuscular junction.

On the other hand, viper venom is hemotoxic in nature. It interferes in blood clotting by exhibiting both anticoagulant and procoagulant effects resulting in defibrillation syndrome or disseminated intravascular coagulopathy. Hemorrhagins-1,2 and metalloendopeptidase are responsible for acute bleeding in various organs of the body. Sea snake venom has myotoxins causing direct muscular damage.

CLINICAL MANIFESTATION

History of snakebite or visible fang marks are not always present. Therefore, a high degree of suspicion and experience is required in identifying a patient with clinical presentation similar to that of snake envenomation with no other obvious cause. A case of snake envenomation may presents with any of the four clinical syndromes; namely neuroparalytic, vasculotoxic (hemotoxic), myotoxic, and progressive local symptoms or with overlapping features. Any patient presenting with sudden onset of myasthenic symptoms in early morning or acute unexplained continuous bleeding should be suspected for snake envenomation. Always look for obvious evidence of a snakebite (fang puncture marks, bleeding, and swelling of the bitten part).

Most common symptoms are fear and anxiety with mild or no local symptoms. The severity of the symptoms depends upon the species of snake, amount of venom injected, season of the bite, whether snake is fed or unfed, site of bite, area covered or uncovered, dry or incomplete bite, multiple bites, venom injection in vessel, weight of the victim, and time elapsed between the bite and administration of ASV.

PROGRESSIVE LOCAL SYMPTOMS

Progression of local symptoms occurs most commonly in cobra bite followed by Russell's viper, saw-scaled viper, and hump-nosed pit viper bite. It occurs due to the direct action of venom on the tissues and vessels. Severe pain with sudden progression of swelling to involve the local area or limb along with erythema and blister formation are the typical features. Destruction of local blood vessels leads to ischemia and gangrene formation. Progressive increase in the pressure due to edema and necrosis may lead to compartment syndrome. The lymph nodes draining the affected area may become tender and enlarged.

SYSTEMIC ENVENOMATION

Systemic envenomation should be suspected in a patient of snakebite presenting with nausea, vomiting, pain abdomen, weakness, and drowsiness. Patients may present with any of the following syndrome.

Neuroparalytic envenomation: Neuroparalytic symptoms are characteristically seen in Elapidae bites (cobra and krait) due to the blockage of presynaptic and postsynaptic membrane of neuromuscular junction by neurotoxins (beta- and alpha-bungarotoxin). Symptoms typically appear within 30 minutes to 6 hours of cobra bite, but may be delayed in krait and hump-nosed pit viper bite for up to 12 hours. Neuronal involvement starts with blurring of vision due to paralysis of ciliary muscles of eyes and loss of accommodation followed by involvement of cranial nerves, bulbar palsy, and skeletal muscle paralysis. These are characterized by five D's, i.e., dyspnea, dysphonia, dysarthria, diplopia, and dysphagia and two P's, i.e., ptosis and paralysis (**Table 1**). The pattern of the neuromuscular weakness is descending in nature with involvement of facial muscles (mask like face), neck muscles (broken neck sign), and other skeletal muscles with loss of tendon reflexes.

TABLE 1 Signs and symptoms of neurotoxin envenomations: Five D's and two P's.

Five D's	Two P's
Dyspnea	**P**tosis
Dysphonia	**P**aralysis
Dysarthria	
Diplopia	
Dysphagia	

Subsequently, patient may lend into acute respiratory failure due to the involvement of respiratory muscles.

Locked-in syndrome is defined as a state of quadriplegia, complete ophthalmoplegia, and dilated pupils with retained consciousness. Patient may be misdiagnosed as brain dead or in the state of coma and hence leading to delay in treatment. This is a reversible condition that improves gradually with early initiation of mechanical ventilation and adequate treatment.

Vasculotoxic (hemotoxic) envenomation: Hemorrhagic manifestations are commonly seen in patients of viper bite (Russell's viper, saw-scaled viper, and hump-nosed pit viper). In addition to hemotoxicity, delayed appearance of neurotoxic symptoms is characteristic of Russell's viper bite. Bleeding usually starts within few hours of the envenomation due to the rapid consumption of coagulation factors leading to consumption coagulopathy. Spontaneous bleeding from various sites, i.e., gingival bleeding, epistaxis, ecchymotic patches, hematemesis, hemoptysis, bleeding per rectum, subconjunctival hemorrhages, continuous bleeding from the bite site, bleeding from pre-existing conditions, e.g., hemorrhoids, and bleeding from freshly healed wounds may occur. Patient may finally lend up in hypovolemic shock and acute kidney injury. Direct kidney injury may also occur due to the direct action of the venom on renal tubules resulting in acute tubular necrosis, interstitial nephritis, patchy cortical necrosis resulting in albuminuria, and presence of red cell casts in urine. Severe blood loss may also cause ischemic necrosis of pituitary gland resulting in amenorrhea and Sheehan's syndrome in females. Acute onset of shock in patients of viper bite may also occur due to the sudden release of bradykinin leading to anaphylactic reaction.

Capillary leak syndrome is a rare and serious complication seen in patients with Russell's viper bite. This is characterized by severe hypotension, hypoalbuminemia, and hemoconcentration without albuminuria due to the vascular endothelial damage resulting in leakage of plasma and proteins into the interstitial compartment.

Myotoxic envenomation: This type of envenomation is typically seen in sea snakebites. Patient presents with generalized muscle pain and tenderness with involuntary muscle contractions. Trismus may also be seen. Direct muscle injury due to the presence of myotoxins in the venom resulting in hyperkalemia and myoglobinuria with dark color urine and ultimately leading to acute kidney injury. Hyperkalemia may manifests as cardiac complications.

MANAGEMENT

FIRST AID TREATMENT—AT SITE

The treatment of snakebite begins at the site of the bite. This can be easily remembered by the mnemonic "CARRY NO RIGHT".

CARRY = Never allow the patient of a snakebite to walk, especially if the bite is on the lower limb. (To delay the systemic absorption of venom)

No—Tourniquets. It may lead to additional ischemic injury and gangrene of the limb.

No—Electrotherapy

No—Cutting/washing

No—Pressure immobilization

No—Venom sucking

R = Reassure the patient. Only 30% of the bites are from venomous species and out of the which, 50% are dry bites.

I = Immobilize in the same way as a fractured limb. Use bandages or cloth to hold the splints, not to block the blood supply or apply pressure.

GH = Get to Hospital immediately. Do not waste time in traditional remedies with no proven benefit. It will only delay the effective treatment.

T = Tell the doctor of any systemic symptoms that manifest on the way of hospital.

MANAGEMENT IN THE HOSPITAL

- Assess the circulation, airway, breathing, and consciousness level of the patient.
- Secure a large bore intravenous (IV) line.
- Look for the signs and symptoms of systemic envenomation. Patient may have tachypnea and tachycardia just because of anxiety and fear of death.
- Most of the times, the species of culprit snake is not known and could not be determined easily by the physical characteristic of the snake or fang marks. Therefore, it is always easier to look for the predominant type of envenomation by classifying the clinical features into four clinical syndromes (**Flowchart 1**).
- Immediate endotracheal intubation and mechanical ventilation will be needed in patients with respiratory failure due to neuromuscular paralysis (neurotoxicity).
- Resuscitate the patient in the presence of shock or cardiac arrest.
- In the absence of signs of envenomation, monitor the patient for at least 24 hours because appearance of symptoms may get delayed for some species.
- Tourniquets should be removed by slowly releasing the pressure with the help of blood pressure cuff. Always check the distal pulse before releasing the tourniquet. In the absence of pulse, treating physician should be ready to handle the complications due to sudden systemic release of venom leading to respiratory insufficiency and hypotension. In case of clinically confirmed venomous bite, tourniquet should be removed only after starting the loading dose of ASV.

INVESTIGATIONS

The 20-minute whole blood clotting test (20WBCT) is a most reliable test to assess the coagulability of the patient's blood and is recommended to be done in all patients of snakebite irrespective of the type of species. It is a simple test that can be easily performed at bedside by the physician on duty. 2–3 mL of fresh venous blood should be kept undisturbed in a fresh, clean, and dry glass test

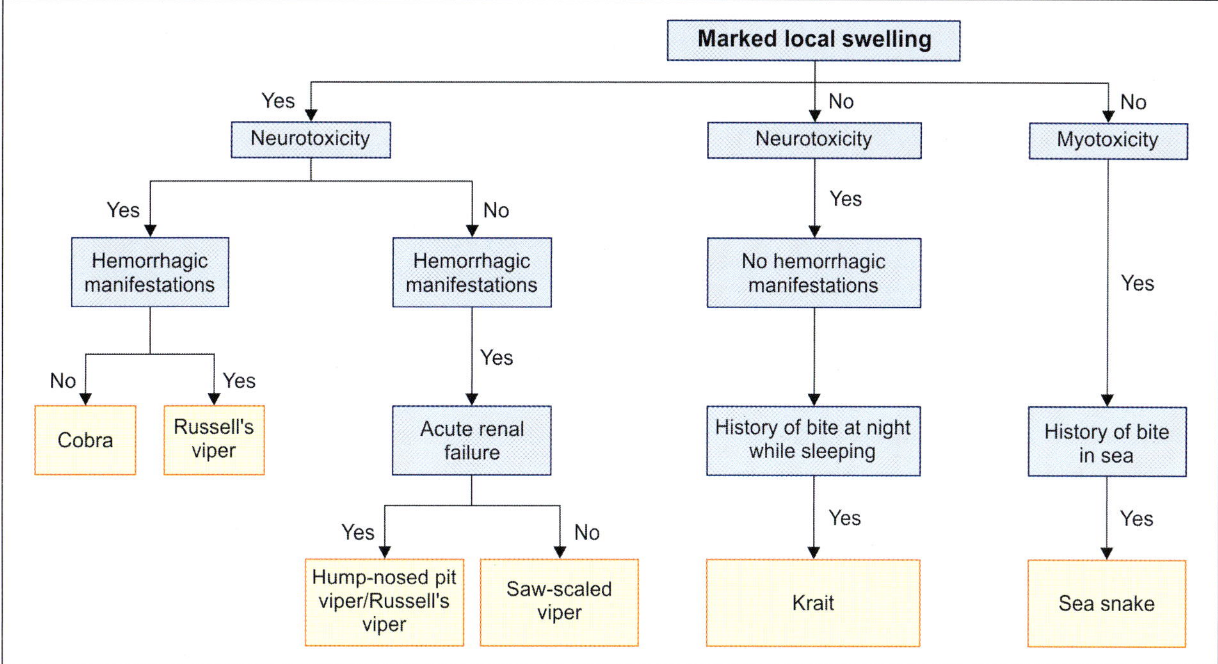

FLOWCHART 1: Identification of snake species on the basis of clinical syndrome.

tube for 20 minutes at the ambient temperature. Assess the coagulability of the blood by gently tilting the tube. If the blood is still liquid, that suggests the presence of consumption coagulopathy (test positive). The test should be repeated every hour for initial 3 hours and then 6 hourly for 24 hours until either the test result becomes positive or there is a clinical evidence of envenomation.

Supporting investigations:

- *Complete hemogram*: It may show transient elevation of hemoglobin due to the hemoconcentration (secondary to capillary leak) or anemia due to hemolysis along with neutrophilic leukocytosis. Thrombocytopenia may be seen in viper bites.
- *Coagulation profile*: Bleeding time, clotting time, and prothrombin time (PT)/activated partial thromboplastin time (aPTT)/fibrin degradation products (FDPs)/D-dimer.
- *Evidence of hemolysis*: Peripheral blood smear, urine for hemoglobinuria, hemosiderinuria, and elevated lactate dehydrogenase.
- *Liver function test and renal function test*: To look for the evidence of liver or kidney injury.
- *Urine complete examination*: Presence of albuminuria, hematuria, and red blood cell casts is suggestive of direct kidney injury due to venom.
- *Creatinine phosphokinase (CPK)*: Increased CPK along with myoglobinuria is suggestive of myotoxicity.
- *Arterial blood gas and electrolytes*: To assess the metabolic status.
- *Electrocardiogram (ECG) and echocardiogram*: To detect the presence of cardiac complications such as myocardial dysfunction (ischemia) and arrhythmias.
- *Chest radiograph*: To look for pulmonary complications such as acute pulmonary edema and secondary bronchopneumonia.

BOX 1 Important don'ts in the management of snakebite.

- Do not attempt to kill or catch the snake as this may be dangerous
- Do not allow the patient to walk
- Do not go for traditional remedies (*Ojhas* and *Tantrik*)
- Do not use any medical/herbal therapy
- Do not wash the wound
- Do not interfere with the bite wound (incisions, suction, rubbing, tattooing, vigorous cleaning, massage, application of herbs or chemicals, cryotherapy, and cautery)
- Do not tie tourniquets as it may cause gangrenous limbs
- Do not give ASV by intramuscular route or inject locally at the bite site

GENERAL TREATMENT

Important don'ts in management of snakebite (**Box 1**). Pain at the local site should be managed with paracetamol only. Use of nonsteroidal anti-inflammatory drugs (NSAIDs) is prohibited because of increased tendency to bleed. Snake contains aerobic and anaerobic bacteria in their mouth, therefore all the patients of snakebites should be administered a single dose of broad-spectrum antibiotic covering anaerobic bacteria and a booster dose of tetanus toxoid.

SPECIFIC TREATMENT

Anti-snake venom is the immunoglobulin against snake venom prepared by immunizing horses with the venom of poisonous snakes. Two types of ASV are available, i.e., monovalent (against a specific species) or polyvalent (against several species). The World Health Organization

(WHO) recommends the use of monovalent ASV as the treatment of choice, but is not usually administered because of the availability issues, high cost, and also, in most of the cases, the species of the snake is not known. It is available in two forms, namely liquid and lyophilized form. The latter is most commonly used in India as the liquid form requires a strict cold chain maintenance. The polyvalent ASV manufactured at Central Research Institute, Kasauli (Himachal Pradesh) is effective against all the four common venomous species found in India. However, the effectiveness of this ASV is questionable in other poisonous snakebites such as hump-nosed pit viper (*Hypnale hypnale*) and sea snakes.

Indications of anti-snake venom: Anti-snake venom therapy is not recommended in all the patients of snakebite. It should be administered in patients with symptoms and signs of systemic envenomation and severe local toxicity, i.e., rapid extension of swelling to involve more than half of the bitten limb and development of enlarged lymph node draining the bitten limb. It should be given as soon as possible, preferably within 4 hours but may be given up to 24 hours because it neutralizes only the unbound (free) toxin.

Dose of anti-snake venom: The dose of the ASV is determined by the amount of venom injected. One vial (10 mL) of polyvalent ASV neutralizes 6 mg of cobra, 6 mg of Russell's viper, 4.5 mg of krait, and 4.5 mg of *Echinus carinatus* venom. Therefore, based upon the amount of the venom injected in a fresh bite (about 63 ± 7 mg), it has been recommended to infuse 10 vials of ASV initially over 1 hour. In patients with neuromuscular paralysis, the second dose of 10 vials is to be infused after 1 hour if no clinical improvement is seen (**Flowchart 2**).

In cases of vasculotoxic envenomation, two regimens have been used, i.e., low-dose and high-dose regimen. Both of them have been found to be equally effective.

- *Low-dose infusion therapy*: Ten vials for Russell's viper or six vials for saw-scaled viper as infusion over

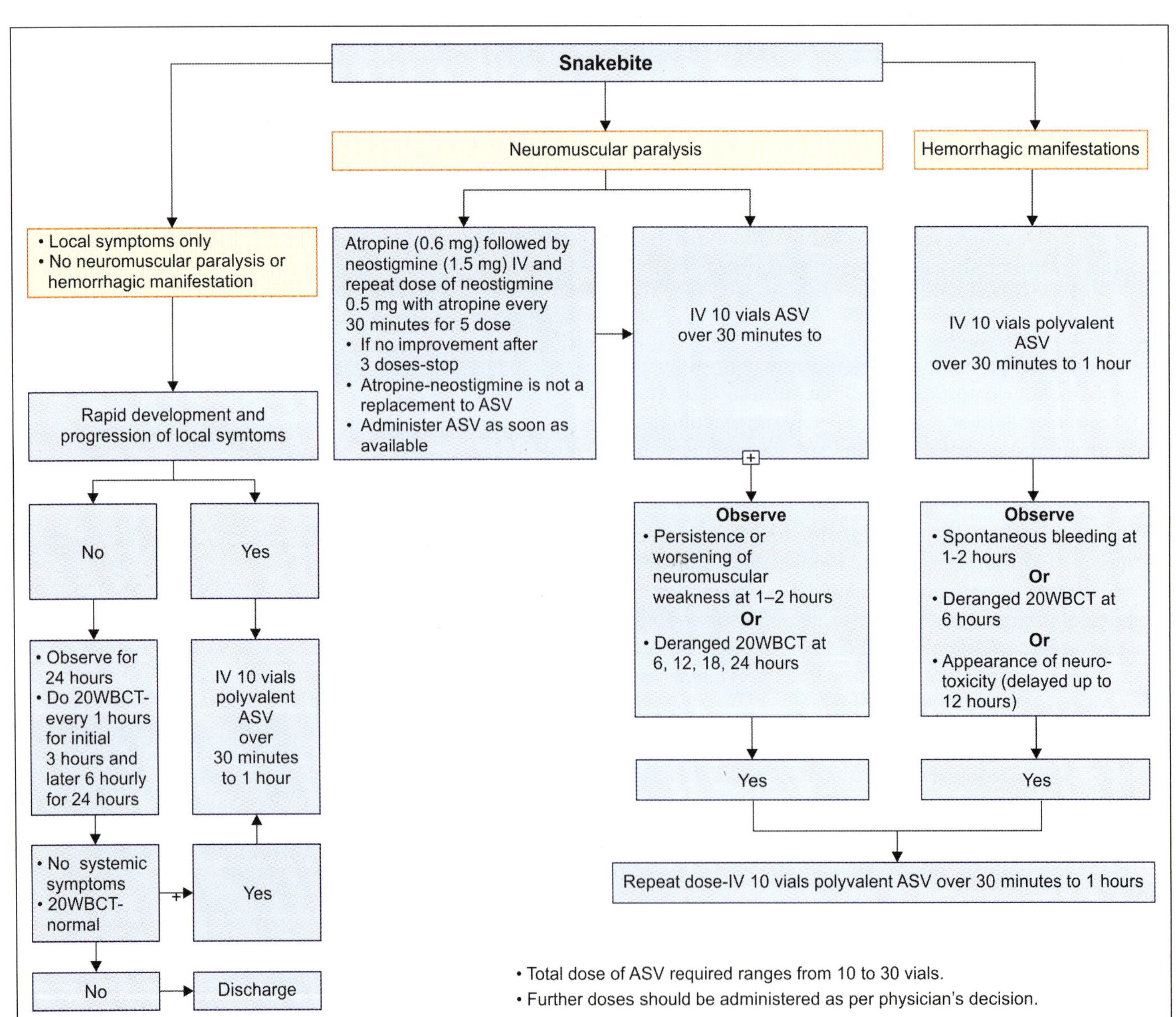

(ASV: anti-snake venom, IV: intravenous; 20WBCT: 20-minute whole blood clotting test)

FLOWCHART 2: ASV dose protocol in a patient of snake envenomation.

30 minutes followed by two vials every 6 hours as infusion in 100 mL of normal saline till clotting time normalizes or for 3 days whichever is earlier.

Or

- *High-dose intermittent bolus therapy*: Ten vials of polyvalent ASV over 30 minutes as infusion, followed by six vials 6 hourly as bolus therapy till clotting time normalizes and/or local swelling subsides.

The total required dose of ASV ranges between 10 and 30 vials but up to 50 vials has been used by physicians depending upon the clinical scenario. The experience at our institute also showed that the average dose required was 25.3 ± 0.93 vials. Local infiltration of ASV has not been found to be effective, on the contrary it is very painful and increase the chances of compartment syndrome in the limb.

Anti-snake venom dose in children and pregnant women: The dose of ASV in children and pregnant women is same as that of adult male as the amount of ASV required to neutralize the venom depends up on the amount of venom injected and not upon the age and sex of the patient.

Anti-snake venom reactions: Anti-snake venom is a foreign protein injected into the human body; therefore it carries a risk of hypersensitivity reactions. The spectrum of the reaction may range from mild to severe anaphylactic reactions.

- Pyrogenic reactions are caused by the pyrogens present in venom and are characterized by chills, rigors, and fever. They usually are reported after 1–2 hours of the infusion.
- Early anaphylactic reactions may present within 10 minutes to 2 hours of starting the infusion. The clinical features include itching, urticaria, dry cough, nausea and vomiting, abdominal colic, diarrhea, tachycardia, and fever. Life-threatening reactions such as hypotension, bronchospasm, and angioedema have also been reported.
- Late (serum sickness type) reactions are immune complex mediated (type III) hypersensitivity reactions that may develop between 24 hours and 7 days after the treatment. The patient may present with fever, nausea, vomiting, diarrhea, itching, recurrent urticaria, arthralgia, myalgia, lymphadenopathy, immune complex nephritis, and, rarely, encephalopathy.

Role of anti-snake venom sensitivity test: The ASV sensitivity testing is not recommended because it has been found that even a negative test does not exclude the occurrence of early or late reactions.

Prevention of anti-snake venom reaction—premedication:

- Use of prophylactic epinephrine in a dose of 0.25 mg of 0.1% solution by subcutaneous route (children 0.005 mg/kg body weight of 0.1% solution) is recommended just before the starting of ASV infusion for the prevention of the ASV reactions. The contraindications are the patients with cardiovascular disease and history of hypertension.
- No significant role of injectable hydrocortisone and H1 and H2 blockers has been found in preventing the ASV reaction.

Treatment of anti-snake venom reaction:

- *Early reactions*: Stop the infusion immediately at the very beginning of the reactions and administer epinephrine (1 in 1,000) 0.5 mg in adults and 0.01 mg/kg body weight in children intramuscularly. Repeat the dose every 5–10 minutes, if necessary. IV H1 antihistaminic (chlorpheniramine maleate 10 mg in adults and 0.2 mg/kg in children) and hydrocortisone (100 mg in adults and 2 mg/kg in children) should be given after subcutaneous epinephrine. In case of mild pyrogenic reactions, ASV may be restarted at slow infusion after the complete disappearance of symptoms (**Flowchart 3**).
- *Late (serum sickness-type) reactions*: Oral antihistamine (e.g., chlorpheniramine 2 mg 6 hourly in adults and 0.25 mg/kg/day in divided doses in children) for 5 days should be prescribed. In patients who do not respond, prednisolone (5 mg 6 hourly in adults and 0.7 mg/kg/day in divided doses in children) for 5 days is recommended.

SUPPORTIVE THERAPY

Neurotoxic envenomation: Patients suspected of neurotoxic envenomation should be closely monitored for progressive neuromuscular weakness. Protect the airway with early endotracheal intubation along with the initiation of invasive mechanical ventilation in patients with bulbar and respiratory muscle paralysis. Manual ventilation (self-ventilating anesthetic bag) will also save the patient's life in scarcity of ventilators. Mostly, the patients are weaned off within 24–48 hours, if the prompt infusion of ASV was done.

Neostigmine is an anticholinesterase that prevents the lysis and prolongs the action of acetylcholine on postsynaptic receptors at neuromuscular junction. Therefore, it causes the reversal of neurotoxic symptoms, especially in patients of cobra bites. A trial of anticholinesterase should be performed in every patient with neurotoxic envenomation. Atropine 0.6 mg followed by neostigmine (1.5 mg) to be given IV stat and repeat dose of neostigmine 0.5 mg with atropine every 30 minutes for five doses (in children, injection atropine 0.05 mg/kg followed by injection neostigmine 0.04 mg/kg IV and repeat dose 0.01 mg/kg every 30 minutes for five doses). A fixed dose combination of neostigmine and glycopyrrolate IV can also be used. 50% or more improvement in ptosis within 1 hour is considered as a positive response. Atropine and neostigmine should be stopped if any of the following has been seen:

- Complete recovery from neuromuscular paralysis.
- Side effects of atropine in form of fasciculations or bradycardia.
- No improvement after three doses (suspect krait bite).

Vasculotoxic envenomation: Prompt initiation of ASV reverses the coagulopathy in most of the cases, but in

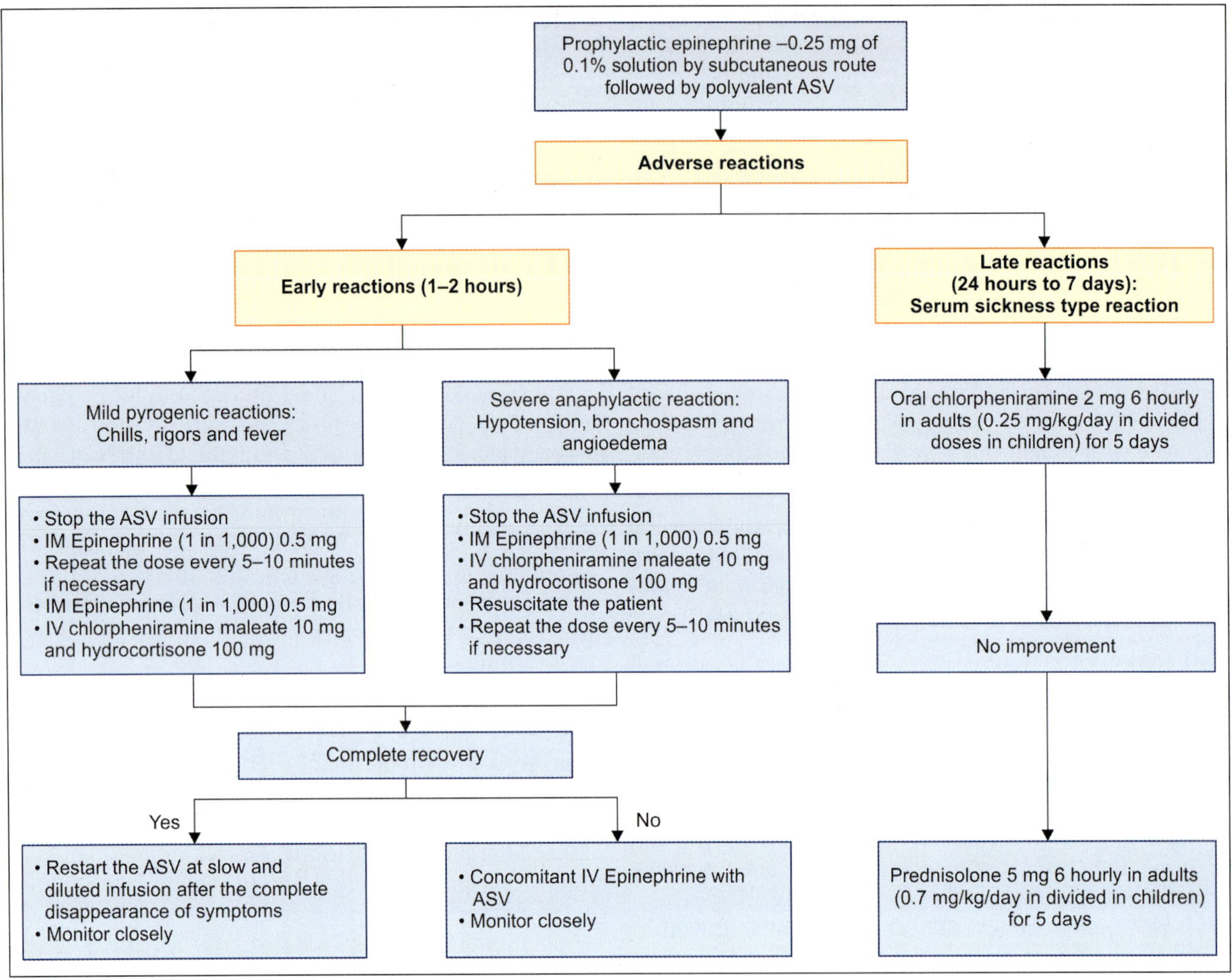

(ASV: anti-snake venom; IM: intramuscular; IV: intravenous)

FLOWCHART 3: Prevention and management of adverse reactions sue to ASV.

presence of severe hemorrhagic manifestations, fresh frozen plasma and cryoprecipitate are required to be transfused to stop the bleeding.

Hemodialysis may be required in patients with rhabdomyolysis and acute kidney injury caused due to hypotension, direct tubular, or glomerular injury.

Surgical intervention: Surgical debridement of the necrotic tissue and fasciotomy in case of compartment syndrome is required in patients of severe local envenomation to prevent limb ischemia and gangrene.

SCORPION ENVENOMATION

INTRODUCTION

Globally, around 1,500 species of scorpions has been reported. Out of which, > 100 species are known to exist in India and only 30 species are medically important. Annual incidence of scorpion bite is more than a million cases worldwide but in India, the data is lacking because of the underreporting of cases and ignorance among general population. Majority of scorpion bites are minor with no systemic manifestations. Severity of the symptoms depends upon the age of the patient (case fatality rate is 10 times more in children), size of scorpion, and the season of sting (hot and dry season). In India, the areas reporting the maximum number of cases are from Western Maharashtra, Karnataka, Andhra Pradesh, Saurashtra, and Tamil Nadu.

Scorpions belonging to Buthidae family are the most poisonous. In Indian subcontinent, *Hottentotta tamulus* (the Indian red scorpion) is the most notorious scorpion responsible for medical emergencies. The scorpion tail contains venom-secreting gland telson with sharp semi-curve stinger. Venom is injected deep under the subcutaneous tissue and it takes around 7–8 hours for complete absorption.

SCORPION VENOM

The venom is composed of numerous enzymes and toxins. Among these, the most important is alpha-toxin.

It is a neurotoxin that binds to the voltage gated Na+ channels present on cell membranes of neuronal tissue. This inhibits the inactivation of channel causing intense and prolonged depolarization and stimulation of postganglionic nerve endings of the sympathetic and parasympathetic nervous system resulting in massive release of acetylcholine, epinephrine, norepinephrine, and vasoactive peptide hormones such as neuropeptide-Y and endothelin-1. The other toxins that bind to potassium and calcium channels are of least importance in mammalian envenomation. The parasympathetic excitation usually occurs early and is less severe, followed by severe sympathetic activity with life-threatening complications such as myocardial injury, pulmonary edema, and cariogenic shock. The cardiac dysfunction may also occur due to direct myocardial toxicity of toxin in addition to catecholamine induced myocarditis (**Flowchart 4**).

Neuromuscular excitation may be seen due to the binding of toxin to neuronal sodium channels of somatic and cranial nervous system. On the other hand, involvement of central nervous system is rare because the toxins generally do not cross the blood brain barrier.

CLINICAL MANIFESTATION

Most of the scorpion bites are benign or dry with no systemic manifestations. Pain at the site of sting is the most common presentation. Severe excruciating pain radiating to respective dermatome with local edema, erythema, burning sensations, and fasciculations may be seen in 35% of cases. Sudden severe pain and withdrawal of the limb on tapping is diagnostic of scorpion bite and is called as TAP sign.

The systemic manifestations occur in less than one-third of cases and are characterized by neurotoxic excitation syndromes. The envenomation by the scorpions of *Centruroides* and *Parabuthus* family primarily manifests as neuromuscular toxicity. On the other hand, Buthidae scorpions envenomation presents with cardiovascular toxicity, which results from hyperstimulation of autonomic nervous system leading to the emergence of autonomic storm. There is an initial transitory release of acetylcholine manifested by increased salivation, sweating, vomiting, urinary incontinence, bronchial hypersecretion, diarrhea, abdominal distension, priapism, bradycardia, and hypotension. This is followed by prolonged hyperadrenergic

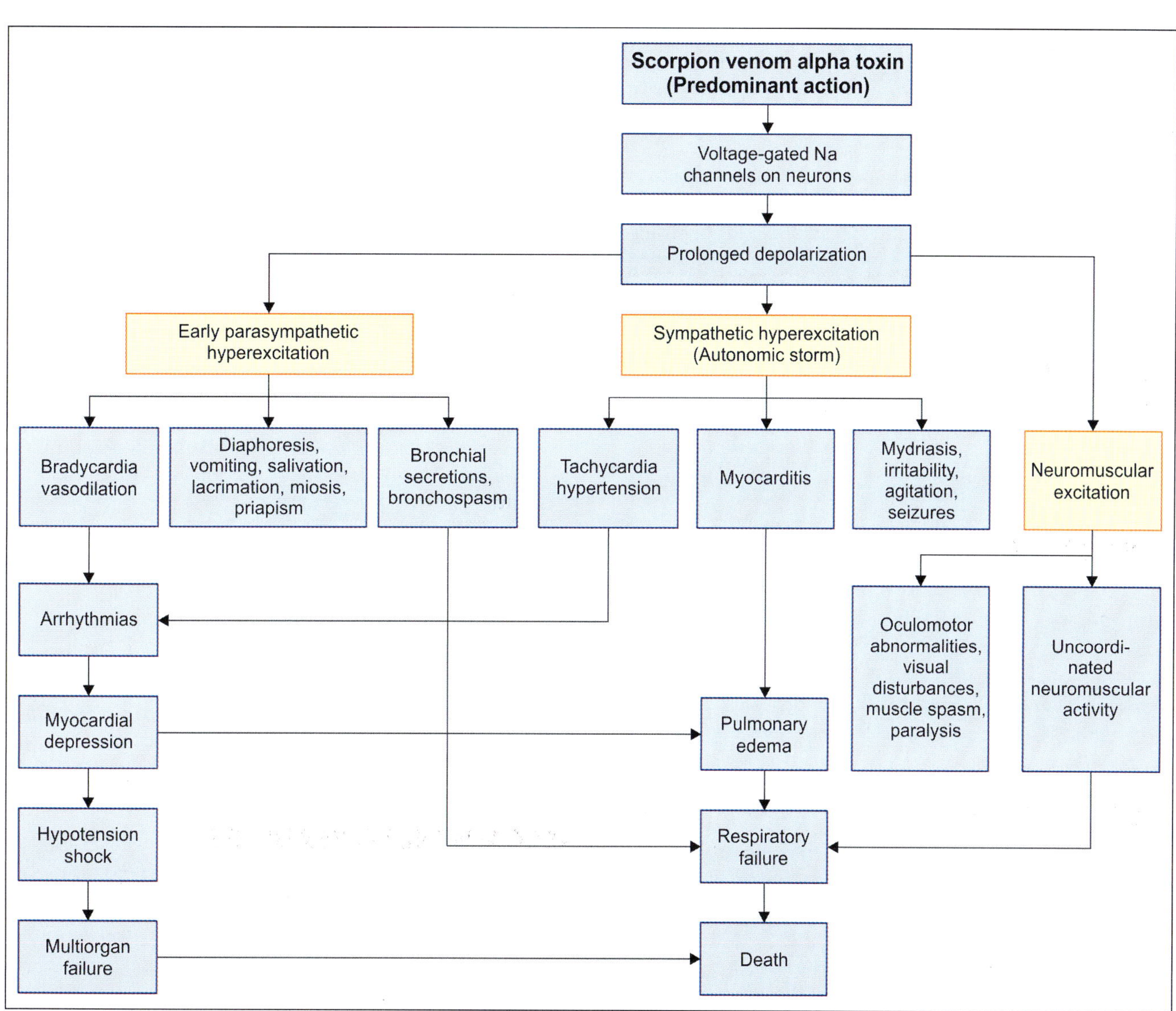

FLOWCHART 4: Pathophysiology of systemic scorpion envenomation.

state causing tachycardia, hypertension, mydriasis, hyperthermia, hyperglycemia, agitation, restlessness, and urogenital (bladder dilatation, urinary retention, priapism, and ejaculation in males). Increased autonomic stimulation leads to cardiac conduction abnormalities, i.e., atrial tachycardia, ventricular extrasystoles, T-wave inversion, ST-T wave changes, and, less frequently, bundle branch block. Hypertension is also present in most of the patients. Myocardial dysfunction, secondary to ischemia and toxic myocarditis, may complicates to cardiogenic shock and pulmonary edema.

Excitation of peripheral nervous system manifests as uncoordinated muscular activity leading to wild flailing, thrashing of the limbs, abnormal oculomotor movements (e.g., roving eyes), visual disturbances, muscle fasciculation, spasms of the face, tongue, and limbs, and ultimately involvement of respiratory muscles.

On basis of clinical manifestations, scorpion envenomation has been graded into four grades:

Grade 1: Local effects only

Grade 2: Autonomic excitation, agitation, and anxiety

Grade 3: Pulmonary edema, hypotension and cardiogenic shock, and severe neuromuscular excitation

Grade 4: Multiorgan failure including coma, seizures, and end-organ damage caused by hypotension

INVESTIGATIONS

No specific investigations are required for diagnosis of scorpion envenomation. They need to be done for the monitoring and detection of the associated complications. Leukocytosis is commonly seen. Hepatic and pancreatic involvement will lead to elevation in alanine transaminase, gamma-glutamyl transferase, alkaline phosphatase, lipases, and amylases. Serum creatinine levels should be measured to assess the presence of renal involvement. Increased creatine phosphokinase, troponin I, and aspartate transaminase are suggestive of myocardial ischemia. Electrocardiographic monitoring is required for early detection of arrhythmias.

TREATMENT

The treatment of scorpion envenomation requires symptomatic relief, specific therapy, and supportive management. Pain at the site of sting can be relieved by the use of ice packs and NSAIDs. Lignocaine ring block may also be used in cases of severe excruciating pain. In absence of systemic symptoms, patient should be monitored for at least 24 hours.

SPECIFIC THERAPY

Scorpion antivenom: Use of SAV has been a topic of discussion since decades. Initial studies showed no significant benefit, as quite a large number of patients included had no systemic features. Later studies revealed that in cases of systemic envenomation, SAV initiates binding to venom within 1 hour of IV therapy and showed marked improvement in neurotoxic symptoms within 4 hours. Therefore, SAV should be administered as soon as possible after the sting as it acts only on the unbound fraction of the toxin and can be used up to 6–8 hours after sting. The main hindrances in the use of SAV are the cost and poor availability.

Prazosin: Prazosin is known as poor man's SAV. It is a competitive inhibitor of postsynaptic alpha-1 adrenergic receptors with 1,000 times higher affinity to alpha receptors. Alpha receptors play an important role in the pathogenesis of myocardial dysfunction and acute pulmonary edema caused by scorpion envenomation. Alpha receptor antagonism reduces the preload and left ventricular impedance without causing tachycardia. It also inhibits phosphodiesterase enzyme and increases the levels of cyclic guanosine monophosphate (cGMP) which in turn enhances the nitric oxide synthesis. Venom induced inhibition of insulin secretion is also reversed and hence, prevent the development of hyperglycemia and hyperkalemia. Therefore, prazosin is a pharmacological and physiological antidote to the actions of scorpion venom and almost completely reverses the hemodynamic, hormonal, and metabolic effects of the venom. The recommended dose is 1 mg in adults (children 30 μg/kg) per orally or via nasogastric tube. Keep the patient in lying down position for at least 3 hours to avoid "first-dose hypotension". The dose may be repeated after 3 hours depending on the clinical response and later after every 6 hours to a maximum of five doses.

Prazosin and scorpion antivenom combination therapy: Two studies from India have compared the use of prazosin with combination of prazosin and SAV in the patients with severe envenomation. Out of which one was exclusively conducted in children. Both of the studies found that the patients who were treated with combination therapy showed a more rapid recovery and were less likely to undergo progression to severe envenomation syndrome. The dose of prazosin required was also less in the combination group.

SUPPORTIVE MANAGEMENT

Patients with severe envenomation should be managed in intensive care unit. Intubation and mechanical ventilation is required to be done in patients with respiratory depression. Patients developing pulmonary edema should be treated with propped up positioning, nasal oxygen, and IV loop diuretics. Other drugs that have been used to treat hypertension and pulmonary edema are nifedipine, nitroprusside, hydralazine, and dobutamine with variable results.

RECOMMENDED READINGS

1. Suraweera W, Warrell D, Whitaker R, Menon G, Rodrigues R, Fu SH, et al. Trends in snakebite deaths in India from 2000 to 2019 in a nationally representative mortality study. eLife. 2020;9:e54076.
2. Kumar V, Malik R, Chaudhary D, Garg M. Analytical study involving Neuroparalytic-snake Envenomation

cases reported to a North Indian tertiary care Hospital. J Indian Soc Toxicol. 2016;12(2):20-5.
3. NHSRC. (2017). Management of Snake bite. [online] Available from http://qi.nhsrcindia.org/sites/default/files/Management%20of%20Snake%20Bite.pdf.
4. Mohan G, Singh A, Singh T. Guidelines for the Management of Snakebites. Curr Trends Diagn Treat. 2018;2(2):102-8.
5. Bawaskar HS, Bawaskar PH. Management of Snake bite and Scorpion bite. Q Med Rev. 2009;60(4):4-47.
6. Isbister GK, Bawaskar HS. Scorpion Envenomation. N Engl J Med. 2014;371:457-63.
7. Cupo P. Clinical update on scorpion envenoming. Rev Soc Brad Med Trop. 2015;48(6):642-9.
8. Chippaux J-P. Emerging options for the management of scorpion stings. Drug Des Devel Ther. 2012;6: 165-73.

CHAPTER
82

Cardiopulmonary Resuscitation

Rakesh Kumar, Sunil Kumar

ABSTRACT

Over the years, the scope of cardiopulmonary resuscitation (CPR) has been expanded and the terms basic life support (BLS) and advanced life support (ALS) are used to accommodate this expanded vision. This expanded vision emphasizes on surveillance for identification of prearrest conditions and prevention of collapse on one hand and on the post-revival period in the form of postarrest care and recovery on the other hand. However, classically CPR implies the actions performed to revive a collapsed person. These actions include skills of both BLS and ALS, which this chapter covers. A systematic approach ensures a standardized way of dealing with the myriad situations that lead to collapse. The actions taken before the actual steps of CPR begin include scene safety, confirming collapse, and call for reinforcements. Thereafter, BLS assessment and management begins with basic skills and minimalistic equipment and continues as ALS (or advanced) assessment and management. A well-equipped trained team performs the advanced management by undertaking primary and secondary assessment and management, following the appropriate algorithm(s). The culmination of CPR depends on whether the resuscitative attempts have resulted in a positive or negative outcome.

"Confront chaos with discipline, treat tumult with calm. This is mastery of mind"

—Sun Tzu

INTRODUCTION

While the CPR guidelines have become quite broad over the years but CPR per se implies the sum total of the actions performed to revive a person after he has had a cardiorespiratory arrest. CPR is not a single skill but a series of assessments and interventions because cardiac arrest also is not a single problem and the steps of CPR may need to vary depending on the type or etiology of the cardiac arrest.

The usefulness of closed cardiac compression for CPR was confirmed by Kouwenhoven et al. in 1960 and almost simultaneously Redding and Pearson showed the role of epinephrine in CPR. The initial guidelines for CPR were published in 1966 by an ad hoc CPR Committee of the Division of Medical Sciences, National Academy of Sciences—National Research Council. Since then, the CPR guidelines have been reviewed and updated periodically by the International Liaison Committee on Resuscitation (ILCOR) and published by many associations around the world, including the American Heart Association (AHA). The present text is based mainly on the AHA guidelines, along with the enrichments from Our Team Life Support.

Over the past many decades, the CPR guidelines have expanded the thought process from only reviving the collapsed victim/patient to encompass *early recognition and prevention of collapse* and *postarrest care* and lately, *recovery* as well. To include this extended thought process, broader terms such as BLS and ALS or advanced cardiovascular life support (ACLS) have been used.

The present chapter will present the steps of BLS and ALS that constitute the actions recommended for managing a collapsed patient. The steps of CPR are somewhat simplified for lay rescuer, but this chapter will be devoted mainly to the outline of CPR for adult victims provided by healthcare providers (HCPs). The finer details of the involved skills can be accessed elsewhere.

SYSTEMATIC APPROACH

The *systematic approach* for CPR requires the HCP to first determine the level of consciousness of the patient after ensuring scene safety (**Flowchart 1**). Once it is ascertained that the patient is unresponsive, the HCP calls for emergency medical services (EMS) as he prepares for further management, which includes steps clubbed as *BLS assessment and management* and *ALS (primary and secondary) assessment and management* (**Flowchart 1**).

The term "basic" of BLS assessment and management denotes the actions that require either no or minimal and easy to use equipment and are summarized in **Flowcharts 2 A** and **B**. On the other hand, "advanced" of ALS assessment and management denotes the actions carried out by a well-trained team having advanced skills and equipment. The advanced CPR is continuation of high quality basic CPR with advanced (primary and secondary) assessment and management added to it, as shown in **Tables 1** and **2**.

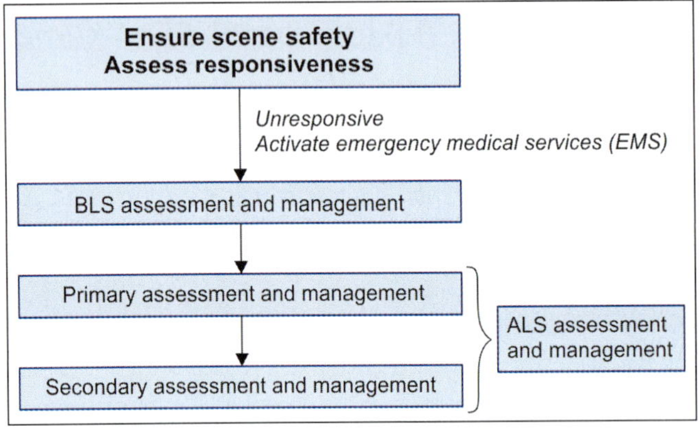

(ALS: advanced life support; BLS: basic life support)

FLOWCHART 1: Main steps of the systematic approach of cardiopulmonary resuscitation.

THE PROCESS

STEPS BEFORE BEGINNING

Prior to approaching any patient, *scene safety* must be ensured, both for the HCP and for the patient. For HCP, this means adhering to universal precautions that include safety measures taken to prevent transmission of diseases, based on the assumption that all body fluids of patient, which the HCP may come in contact with, might be infectious. The HCP should use some or all of the personal protective equipment (PPE) such as gloves, masks, gowns, specialized clothing, face shields, and protective eyewear, depending upon the need. Even in less than ideal situation and field situation, the HCP should do his best to prevent harm to himself so that he can be maximally useful as a rescuer. At the same time, the patient should also be protected from dangers lurking around him by keeping his immediate environment as safe as possible. After ensuring scene safety, the HCP *checks responsiveness* of the patient.

If the patient is unresponsive, the HCP immediately *activates EMS (or local emergency response system)*. In a hospital, this can be done by activating code blue at many centers and by calling a dedicated emergency phone number at others. In the field, EMS is called by asking a bystander to call a dedicated phone number (102 or 108 in India). Although, normally the code carts (emergency carts) and ambulances are supposed to carry automated external defibrillator (AED) or manual defibrillator, it is advisable that anyone activating the code blue/EMS also ensures that an AED or defibrillator is also brought along.

BASIC LIFE SUPPORT

After activating EMS, the HCP *assesses for pulse and breathing*. Carotid pulse and breathing are checked simultaneously for at least 5 seconds, but not > 10 seconds.

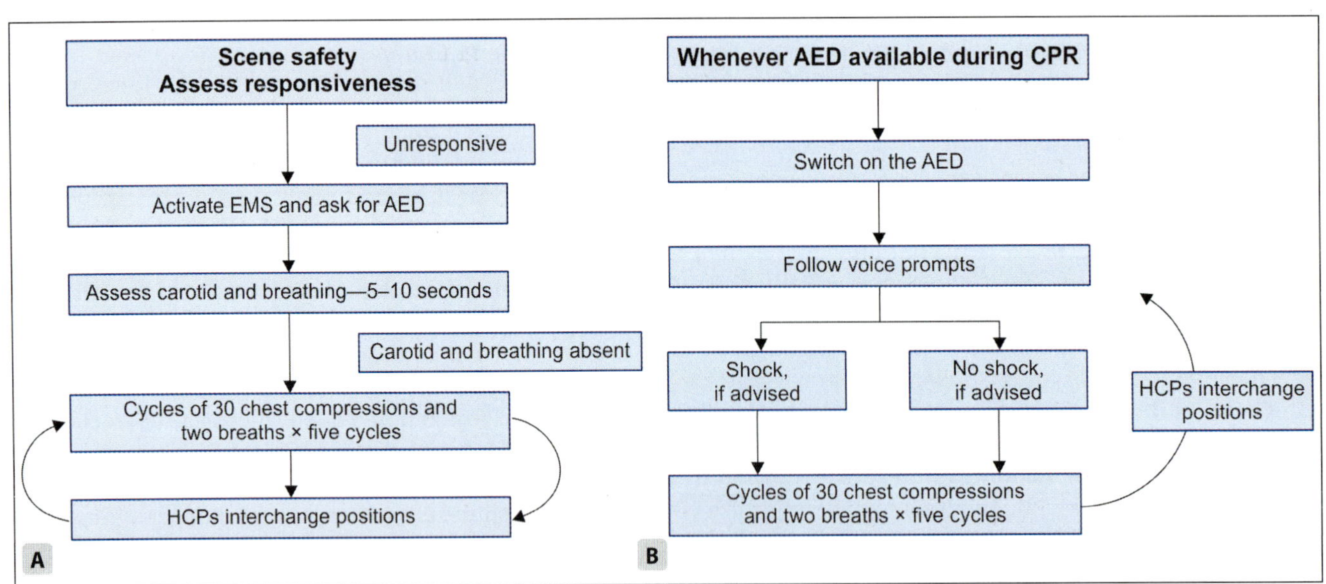

(EMS: emergency medical services; HCPs: healthcare providers)

FLOWCHARTS 2 A & B: Main steps of cardiopulmonary resuscitation (CPR) that are part of basic life support (BLS) without automated external defibrillator (AED) **(A)** and in the presence of AED **(B)**.

TABLE 1 The components of primary assessment and management aligned along ABCDE (Airway, Breathing, Circulation, Disability, and Exposure).

Component	Assessment of	Management
Airway	• Airway patency	• Open airway (manually or by suctioning) • If ineffective to ensure adequate mask ventilation, use supraglottic airway device (SAD), or endotracheal tube (ETT)
Breathing	• Efficacy of breaths being provided • Confirm position by $EtCO_2$ (after SAD or ETT placement)	• Provide ventilation with O_2 supplementation • Use bag mask or SAD or ETT (ETT only when expert is available). Secure SAD/ETT properly
Circulation	• Heart rate and rhythm • Quality of chest compression by $EtCO_2$ (if ETT or SAD placed)	• Maintain high-quality chest compression. Keep $EtCO_2$ >10 mm Hg, ideally >20 mm Hg • Follow the relevant cardiac arrest algorithm (**Box 1**) based on the arrest rhythm (**Fig. 1** and **Table 4**) • Infuse IV fluids and drugs as needed
Disability	Responsiveness	Monitor for any change from unresponsive status
Exposure	Medical alert bracelets; signs of any likely cause for patient's condition	Manage accordingly

($EtCO_2$: end-tidal carbon dioxide; IV: intravenous)

TABLE 2 The components of secondary assessment and management.

	Component	Management
SAMPLE history	***S***igns and ***S***ymptoms, ***A***llergies, ***M***edications, ***P***ast history, ***L***ast meal, and ***E***vents	Manage according to the most probable cause(s), especially the reversible cause(s)
H's and T's	***H***ypoxia, ***H***ypovolemia, ***H***ydrogen ions (acidosis), ***H***ypo/***H***yperkalemia, ***H***ypothermia ***T***ension pneumothorax, ***T***amponade (cardiac), ***T***hrombosis (cardiac), ***T***hrombosis (pulmonary), and ***T***oxins	

If definite carotid pulse and normal breathing are absent, *CPR* is started (**Flowchart 2**).

It is recommended that CPR should begin as soon as possible with emphasis on high-quality chest compression. To provide high-quality chest compression, place the patient face up on a firm, flat surface, and push hard (at least 2 inches or 5 cm in an adult, or at least one-third the anteroposterior diameter of the chest for all age groups) and fast [at the rate of 100–120 compressions per minute (30 compressions over 15–18 s)] over the lower half of sternum in the center of the chest (just below intermammary line) with both hands. Compressions become even more effective by allowing complete chest recoil (by taking the pressure off the chest at the end of each compression and avoiding leaning over the patient) and minimizing interruptions between two sets of 30 compressions to <10 seconds (to provide breaths).

After giving first set of 30 compressions, open patient's airway by head tilt-chin lift and give two breaths and then keep giving two breaths after each set of 30 compressions. Breathing is usually provided using bag-mask device or sometimes using pocket mask (in some field situations). Each breath (inspiration) should be of 1-second duration, with or without oxygen, and 1 second should be allowed for complete expiration. An effective breath causes a visible chest rise. Only two attempts are made to provide breath to an adult patient. Thereafter, the chest compressions are restarted, even if both the breaths have been ineffective.

If there is only one rescuer, he continues these cycles of 30 compressions and two breaths alone until another rescuer joins in. Once there is more than one rescuer available, the rescuers switch roles after every five cycles (nearly every 2 min) (**Flowchart 2 A**). This process continues until the patient shows signs of life or AED becomes available or advanced team takes over.

Once it has been ascertained that the patient is unresponsive, has no pulse and respiration, AED should be used as soon as it becomes available. AED is fully automated equipment and to use it, switch it on and then follow its voice-cum-visual prompts. The AED starts prompting as soon as it is switched on and then every 2 minutes to allow five compression-breathing cycles. Different models may have slight differences; however, most operate in basically the same way. AED prompts are different depending upon whether the AED detects shockable or nonshockable rhythm on rhythm analysis (**Flowchart 2 B**). Continue until advanced team arrives, or the patient vocalizes, or begins to breathe or move.

ADVANCED LIFE SUPPORT

Once the advanced team arrives with manual defibrillator-monitor and emergency cart (also called code cart) or the patient reaches an advanced facility, the *BLS assessment and management* and *advanced CPR* go on simultaneously. If six HCPs (ideal number) are available, then their recommended distribution is shown in **Table 3**.

Primary and secondary assessment and management: As mentioned before, the steps of CPR during ALS are clubbed

TABLE 3 Role allocation during advanced CPR.

HCP-1	Continues doing chest compression. *The HCP on compression must change every 2 min (or earlier if he is tired)*
HCP-2	Keeps managing the airway and breathing
HCP-3	Acts as the team coordinator and keeps the code running smoothly
HCP-4	Manages the defibrillator-monitor. Keeps an eye on the monitored parameters and checks rhythm every 2 min and gives shock, if there is shockable rhythm
HCP-5	Manages the IV line(s) and drug administration
HCP-6	He is the *record-keeper* who keeps the record of all the activities and updates the coordinator and the entire team every 2 min

- Once the roles are allocated and the advanced CPR is underway, *one of the HCPs interacts with the patient's attendants*, apprises them with the situation, elicits SAMPLE history (**Table 2**) and counsels them
- If there are five HCPs, then the team coordinator keeps a mental record of the advanced CPR. If there are 4 HCPs, then the coordinator manages the airway as well

(CPR: cardiopulmonary resuscitation; HCP: healthcare provider; IV: intravenous)

under primary and secondary assessment and management. Primary assessment and management consist of many advanced activities carried out by the advanced team. These activities are aligned along mnemonic ABCDE (Airway, Breathing, Circulation, Disability, and Exposure) (**Table 1**). Simultaneously, secondary assessment and management (**Table 2**) are conducted through SAMPLE history taking and analyzing the H's and T's to look for and treat any reversible cause(s) for the collapse.

Salient points of primary assessment and management: There are certain aspects of primary assessment and management mentioned in **Table 1** that need to be elaborated upon:

- Other than situations where early intubation is specifically indicated (e.g., anaphylaxis-induced cardiac arrest, inhalational burns, and pregnant victim), there is no hurry to introduce a definitive airway device such as supraglottic airway device (SAD) or endotracheal tube (ETT) if bag-mask ventilation (BMV) is adequate.
- Once a definitive airway device has been introduced, its position should be confirmed by five-point auscultation (over epigastrium, bilateral lower and upper axillae) and end-tidal carbon dioxide ($EtCO_2$), and the airway device should be secured properly.
- There is no need to alternate between 30 compressions and two breaths once a definitive airway device is in place. The compressions should now continue at the rate of 100–120 per minute and breaths should be provided at 10 per minute (one breath every 6 s).
- Circulation is maintained during ALS by continuing high-quality chest compression guided by monitoring and appropriate use of defibrillation, drugs, and fluids as described under algorithms later (**Table 4** and **Box 1**).

TABLE 4 Cardiac arrest rhythms or lethal rhythms.

Shockable	Nonshockable
• Ventricular fibrillation (VF) • Pulseless ventricular tachycardia (pVT)	• Asystole • Pulseless electrical activity (PEA)

Salient points of secondary assessment and management:

- Once the advanced CPR is underway, the team should be on the lookout for the likely differential diagnoses for the patient's condition. This is recommended to be done through two steps: (1) eliciting the history from patient's attendants in a structured manner, guided by the mnemonic "SAMPLE" (**Table 2**) and (2) an analysis of all the available information by the team to specifically look for the most common causes of collapse. These causes are tabulated as H's and T's (**Table 2**).
- It is also very important that the HCP who interacts with the patient's attendants apprises them of the patient's condition and counsels them.

Rhythms during cardiac arrest: Cardiac arrest rhythms are also called lethal rhythms (**Table 4**). Why is it "cardiac arrest" if there are rhythms during this period? Cardiac arrest is a condition where the heart is not able to generate any clinically relevant forward blood flow (detectable by a definitely palpable pulse in a large artery like the carotid or femoral). Thus, cardiac arrest does not necessarily mean that there is no electrical or physical activity in the heart. In fact, there is only one cardiac arrest situation in which there is no discernible electrical activity and that too in only some of the cases (asystole with a flat line). Similarly, there is a definite physical activity as well in two of the four cardiac arrest conditions. These two cardiac arrest conditions [ventricular fibrillation (VF) and pulseless ventricular tachycardia (pVT)] are shockable while the other two [asystole and pulseless electrical activity (PEA)] do not respond to defibrillation.

While VF and pVT are reasonably well understood by most HCPs, it may be worthwhile elaborating on PEA and asystole. PEA is a condition wherein there is an organized electrical activity of heart (ECG) at a rate of >6 beats per minute (bpm) *in the absence of carotid pulse*. On the other hand, a similar electrical activity of ≤6 bpm or an absence of any electrical activity (i.e., flat line on ECG) is labeled as asystole (**Fig. 1**).

Algorithms of cardiac arrest: The algorithms for the shockable and nonshockable cardiac arrest rhythms follow separate paths once rhythm check has confirmed the rhythm during advanced CPR (**Box 1**). While the algorithm for both the shockable rhythms is exactly the same, there is a subtle difference between the algorithms for the two nonshockable rhythms. Let us look at the salient features of these algorithms:

- High-quality chest compression (manual intervention) forms the core activity of these algorithms. To ensure this, the compressor should change every 2 minutes (or earlier, if tired).

BOX 1	Algorithms for management of cardiac arrest.

Algorithm 1: Algorithm for cardiac arrest with shockable rhythms (VF or pVT)

1. Continued high-quality CPR → 2. Advanced team arrives and starts advanced CPR

→ 3. [Rhythm Check—**Shockable**] → 4. Shock-1 delivered → 5. CPR × 2 minutes and IV/IO access

→ 6. [Rhythm Check—**Shockable**] → 7. Shock-2 delivered → 8. CPR × 2 minutes and epinephrine (then after every two cycles or after every 4 minutes)

→ 9. [Rhythm Check—**Shockable**] → 10. Shock-3 delivered → 11. CPR × 2 minutes and amiodarone or lidocaine

→ 12. [Rhythm Check—**Shockable**] → (BACK TO STEP 7).

If rhythm becomes nonshockable, go to Algorithm 2.

If there is return of spontaneous circulation (ROSC), postarrest management is initiated.

Algorithm 2: Algorithm for cardiac arrest with nonshockable rhythms (asystole or PEA)

1. Continued high-quality CPR → 2. Advanced team arrives and starts advanced CPR

→ 3. [Rhythm Check—**Nonshockable**] → 4. Look for a reversible cause → 5. CPR × 2 minutes and IV/IO access and epinephrine ASAP (then after every two cycles or after every 4 minutes)

→ 6. [Rhythm Check—**Nonshockable**] → 7. CPR × 2 minutes

→ 8. [Rhythm Check—**Nonshockable**] → 9. CPR × 2 minutes and epinephrine

→ 10. [Rhythm Check—**Nonshockable**] → (BACK TO STEP 7).

If rhythm becomes shockable, go to Algorithm 1.

If there is ROSC, postarrest management is initiated.

(ASAP: as soon as possible; CPR: cardiopulmonary resuscitation; IO: intraosseous; IV: intravenous; PEA: pulseless electrical activity; pVT: pulseless ventricular tachycardia; VF: ventricular fibrillation)

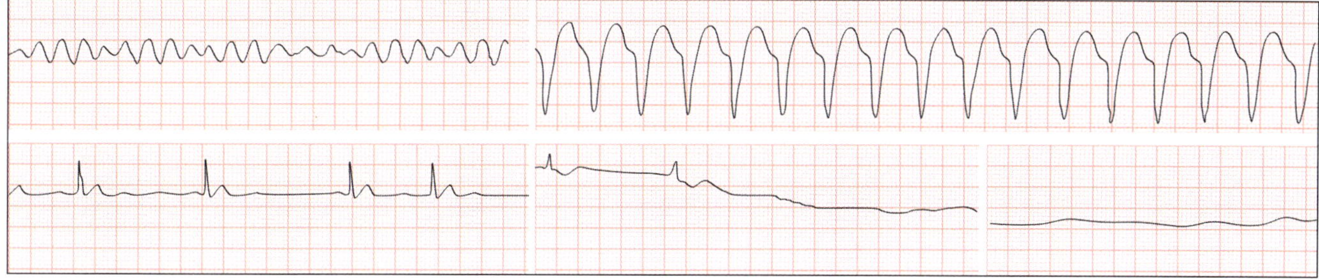

FIGURE 1: Cardiac arrest rhythms or lethal rhythms (carotid pulse absent). (Clockwise, from top left)—ventricular fibrillation, pulseless ventricular tachycardia, pulseless electrical activity, asystole with some electrical activity (≤6 bpm), and asystole with flat line.

- Although multiple markers [$EtCO_2$ of >10 mm Hg and ideally >20 mm Hg, diastolic invasive arterial pressure of >20 mm Hg, and central venous oxygen saturation ($ScvO_2$) > 30%] have been described to monitor the quality of compressions, only $EtCO_2$ in an intubated patient is universally accepted.
- In the algorithm for shockable rhythms (**Box 1, Algorithm 1**):
  - Defibrillation (electrical intervention) takes precedence over drugs (pharmacological intervention).
  - Epinephrine (1 mg in 1 mL diluted to 10 mL in saline) is injected intravenous (IV) [or intraosseous (IO)] after the second shock. Thereafter, it is repeated after every 4 minutes or two cycles.
  - For refractory VF/pVT, two bolus doses of amiodarone or lidocaine are recommended; amiodarone (300 mg) or lidocaine (1.5 mg/kg) after third shock and then repeated (in half the dose) after fifth shock.
- In the algorithm for nonshockable rhythms (**Box 1, Algorithm 2**):
  - Search and treat reversible cause(s) immediately because otherwise the outcome is very bleak.
  - Epinephrine (1 mg in 1 mL diluted to 10 mL in saline) should be given as soon as possible (so a quick IV/IO access is desirable). Thereafter, it is repeated after every 4 minutes or two cycles. The only other drugs that might be used in this algorithm are the antidotes for the causative factors.
  - If the rhythm is a flat line asystole, ensure that the flat line is not due to faulty electrode connection, mode selection, or very low gain (flat line protocol).
  - If the initial rhythm is PEA, then every rhythm check should be accompanied by a careful carotid pulse check because the rhythm in PEA can be deceptively organized right in the beginning and the only early clue of successful resuscitation [return of spontaneous circulation (ROSC)] may be a palpable pulse.

Use of extracorporeal CPR for advanced management of cardiac arrest: There is insufficient evidence to recommend the routine use of extracorporeal CPR (ECPR) for patients with cardiac arrest. ECPR may be considered for select cardiac arrest patients for whom the suspected cause of the cardiac arrest is potentially reversible during a limited period of mechanical cardiorespiratory support.

CULMINATION

If the CPR efforts are successful, there is ROSC. The patient is then considered for postarrest care and recovery depending upon is level of consciousness and cause of collapse. On the other hand, if the CPR attempts do not result in ROSC, then cessation of resuscitative effort is contemplated, based on multiple considerations such as the cause of arrest, presence of any reversible factor(s), delay in beginning of effective compressions and defibrillation, prearrest condition of the patient, availability of resuscitative aids and expertise, local protocols, and many more.

ACKNOWLEDGMENTS

We, the authors, thank all the members of Our Team Life Support for their inputs that we have put to use while preparing this manuscript.

RECOMMENDED READINGS

1. ECC Committee, Subcommittees and Task Forces of the American Heart Association. 2005 American Heart Association Guidelines for Cardiopulmonary Resuscitation and Emergency Cardiovascular Care. Circulation. 2005;112 (24 Suppl):IV1-203.
2. Kouwenhoven WB, Jude JR, Knickerbocker GG. Closed-chest cardiac massage. JAMA. 1960;173:1064-7.
3. Redding JS, Pearson JW. Resuscitation from Asphyxia. JAMA. 1962;182:283.
4. Pearson JW, Redding JS. The role of epinephrine in cardiac resuscitation. Anesth Analg. 1963;42:599-606.
5. National Academy of Sciences. Cardiopulmonary resuscitation. JAMA. 1966;198:372-9.
6. Kumar R, Sharma SD, Kumar S, Misra A, Gupta NR. Basic Life Support—An Atlas Based Approach, 2nd edition. Delhi: Arya Publication; 2017.
7. Kumar R, Sharma SD, Kumar S, Misra A, Gupta NR. "Basic Life Support—Kahani Jeevan Raksha Ki, 1st edition. Delhi: Arya Publication; 2020.
8. Field JM, Hazinski MF, Sayre MR, Chameides L, Schexnayder SM, Hemphill R, et al. Part 1: executive summary: 2010 American Heart Association Guidelines for Cardiopulmonary Resuscitation and Emergency Cardiovascular Care. Circulation. 2010;122(18 Suppl 3): S640-56.
9. Neumar RW, Shuster M, Callaway CW, Gent LM, Atkins DL, Bhanji F, et al. Part 1: Executive Summary: 2015 American Heart Association Guidelines for Cardiopulmonary Resuscitation and Emergency Cardiovascular Care. Circulation. 2015;132(18 Suppl 2):S315-67.
10. Merchant RM, Topjian AA, Panchal AR, Cheng A, Aziz K, Berg KM, et al. Part 1: Executive Summary: 2020 American Heart Association Guidelines for Cardiopulmonary Resuscitation and Emergency Cardiovascular Care. Circulation. 2020;142(16_Suppl_2):S337-57.
11. Hazinski MF, Travers HT, Eustice SK, Schoolfield B and the AHA BLS Project Team. Basic Life Support Provider Manual, ©2016 American Heart Association. Texas: Integracolor, Ltd.; 2016.
12. Donnino MW, Navarro K, Berg K, Brooks SC, Crider J, Hazinski MF, et al. Advanced Cardiovascular Life Support Provider Manual, ©2016 American Heart Association. Texas: Integracolor, Ltd.; 2016.

CHAPTER

83

Brain Death: Diagnosis and Management

Sunil Shroff, Mathew Joseph, Rahul Pandit

ABSTRACT

Organ transplantation is one of the greatest advances of modern science that has resulted in many patients getting a renewed lease of life. Transplantation would not be possible but for organ donation. Organs can be donated by a living person, after natural death, and after brain death. Brain death is a relatively new concept of death that was first recognized in Paris in 1959. The Government of India recognized brainstem death in the Transplantation of Human Organs (THO) Act that was legislated in 1994. This legislation was also enacted to streamline living donor transplants and made commercial dealings in organs illegal and a punishable offence. Since the THO Act came into being, it has been possible to undertake multiorgan transplant activity from brain-dead donors in India.

"The measure of life is not in its duration, but its donation"

—Peter Marshall

INTRODUCTION

The Transplantation of Human Organs Act was passed in 1994 in India to regulate organ donation and transplantation in the country and prevent commercial dealings in organs. It also defined "brainstem death" and permitted organ donation from brainstem-dead (brain-dead) donors and deceased donor organ transplantation. At any given time there are 8–10 brain-dead patients in different intensive care units (ICUs) in any major city of the country. India had 151,417 deaths from road traffic accidents in 2018 (Source: Ministry of Road Transport and Highways, Government of India). According to a study carried out in All India Institute of Medical Sciences (AIIMS), New Delhi, fatal traumatic brain injuries were seen in 68.73% of road traffic accident victims. In many instances, the traumatic brain injury leads to brain death. Therefore, there is a potentially large pool of brain-dead donors available in India. The critical care clinicians and nursing staff play an important role in facilitating deceased organ donation. The brain-dead patient is intrinsically a hemodynamically unstable patient. Therefore, once the family agrees to donate the organs, it is paramount to keep these patients stable and ensure that the organs are optimally functioning and are suitable for transplantation.

BRAINSTEM DEATH DIAGNOSIS AND CERTIFICATION

EVOLUTION OF THE CONCEPT OF BRAIN DEATH

History: Two French physicians in 1959 first recognized "Brain Death" on patients being ventilated in the ICUs and called it *"coma dépassé"* (a state beyond coma). In 1968, the Ad Hoc Committee of Harvard Medical School defined brain death as "irreversible coma with the patient being totally unreceptive and unresponsive with absence of all cranial reflexes and no spontaneous respiratory effort during a 3-minute period of disconnection from the ventilator." There are two differing concepts of what exactly constitutes brain death; whole brain death (predominantly in the US and Europe) and brainstem death (UK and India). This chapter will not attempt to explain the detailed difference between the two points of view, but it is important to know that the clinical testing in either system is identical, and that establishing whole brain death might require additional testing. Time is of the essence in organizing both procurement of organs and transplant of various organs and tissues to various patients as all organs have a critical time limit beyond which they cannot be stored.

Whole brain death project: In 2020, the Whole Brain Death Project (WBDP) developed consensus criteria on diagnosing Brain Death/Death by Neurological Criteria (BD/DNC) with the goal to harmonize practices across the world. The document recommends that BD/DNC be defined as "the complete and permanent loss of brain function as defined by an unresponsive coma with loss of capacity for consciousness, brainstem reflexes, and the ability to breathe independently." It should be primarily a clinical determination. It also recommends that BD/DNC determination be done by practitioners with training in this aspect and in counselling families at the end of life. Trainees in fields that manage patients with devastating brain injuries as well as students in all healthcare fields need to be educated about BD/DNC.

Legal framework in India for brainstem death: The THO Act, 1994 had the following aims:
- Regulation of removal, storage, and transplantation of human organs for therapeutic purposes
- Prevention of commercial dealings in human organs
- Legalized the concept of brainstem death; makes organ donation from brainstem dead donors possible

Some key definitions in the THO Act are:
- Brainstem death means the stage at which all functions of the brainstem have permanently and irreversibly ceased and is so certified.
- Deceased person means a person in whom permanent disappearance of all evidence of life occurs, by reason of brainstem death or in a cardiopulmonary sense at any time after live birth has taken place.
- Transplantation means the grafting of any human organs or tissue from any living person or deceased person to some other living person for therapeutic purposes.

The THO Act and the Rules, 1995 outlined the process for certification of brainstem death and consent from the family for organ donation from a brain-dead person. In 2011, the act was amended and was called THO (Amendment) Act 2011 and the accompanying Rules in 2014 brought the donation of tissues also under the ambit of this law and the rules are now called the Transplantation of Human Organs and Tissues Rules 2014 (THOTR).

Brainstem death certification is done by a panel of four doctors. Two clinicians who are experts in the field (like neurologists or neurosurgeons or intensivists) and are empanelled by the government are required for brainstem death certification. They are expected to do two sets of tests 6 hours apart to certify brainstem death. The legal time of death in these circumstances is taken as the end of the second set of brainstem death testing. The other two doctors required for the certification are the doctor looking after the patient and the head of the institute where the patient is being certified. The certification should be done as per the form laid out in the law (1995 THO regulations Form 8 and 2014 THOTR regulations Form 10). It is only after these formalities have been completed that organs can be retrieved or ventilatory support discontinued.

In a medicolegal case a forensic clearance is also required before proceeding. The certification should be done on laid out forms as per the act. The medical director or medical superintendent of the hospital should finally check the form before filing it in patient's notes (**Box 1**—Form 10. THOTR 2011).

BOX 1 Form 10 for Brain Death Certification [Transplantation of Human Organs and Tissues Rules (THOT) 2014].

Form 10 for Brain Death Certification (THOT rules 2014)
[See rule 4(3)(a) and (b)]

We, the following members of the Board of Medical Experts after careful personal examination hereby certify that Shri/Smt/Km .... aged about .... son of/wife of/daughter of .... resident of .... is dead on account of permanent and irreversible cessation of all functions of the brainstem. The tests carried out by us and the findings therein are recorded in the brainstem death certificate annexed hereto.

Date .... Signature ....

1. RMP-in-charge of the hospital in which brainstem death has occurred.
2. RMP nominated from the panel of names approved by the appropriate authority.
3. Neurologist/neurosurgeon nominated from the panel of names approved by the appropriate authority.
4. RMP treating the aforesaid deceased person

Brainstem Death Certificate

(A) Patient Details:

1. Name of the patient Mr/Ms ....
   S/O, D/O, W/O–Mr.......................... Sex ....Age..........................
2. Home address ....
3. Hospital number ....
4. Name and address of next of kin or ....
   person responsible for the patient (if ....
   none exists, this must be specified) ....
5. Has the patient or next of kin agreed to any transplant ....
6. In this a police case? Yes .... No ....

(B) Preconditions:

1. **Diagnosis:** Did the patient suffer from any illness or accident that led to irreversible brain damage?

Specify details ....

Date and time of accident/onset of illness ....

Date and onset of nonresponsive coma ....

2. Findings of Board of Medical Experts:

The following reversible causes of coma have been excluded:

Intoxication (alcohol)

Depressant drugs

Relaxants (neuromuscular blocking agents)

	First Medical Examination		Second Medical Examination	
	1st	2nd	1st	2nd
Primary hypothermia				
Hypovolemic shock				
Metabolic or endocrine disorders				
Tests for absence of brainstem functions				
Coma				
Cessation of spontaneous breathing				
Pupillary Size				
Pupillary light reflexes				
Doll's head eye movement				
Corneal reflexes (both sides)				

Continued...

Continued...

Motor response in any cranial nerve distribution, any responses to stimulation of face, limb, or trunk
Gag reflex
Cough (tracheal)
Eye movements on caloric testing bilaterally
Apnea tests as specified
Were any respiratory movements seen?
Date and time of first testing: ....
Date and time of second testing: ....
This to certify that the patient has been carefully examined twice after an interval of about 6 hours and on the basis of findings recorded above, Mr/Ms......................... is declared brainstem dead.
Signatures of:
1. Medical administrator-in-charge of the hospital .... 2. Authorized specialist ....
3. Neurologist/neurosurgeon........................ 4. Medical officer treating patient..............
Note:
I. The minimum time interval between the first testing and second testing will be 6 hours.
II. No. 2 and No. 3 will be co-opted by the administrator-in-charge of the hospital from the panel of experts approved by the appropriate authority.

DIAGNOSIS OF BRAINSTEM DEATH

PATHOPHYSIOLOGY

This situation of "physiological decapitation" that is implied by the declaration of brain death is usually caused by any pathology that increases the pressure within the confines of the cranium to a level that prevents adequate perfusion of the brain, and the resultant ischemia leads to irreversible dysfunction of the brainstem. In this situation the heart can continue to beat and keep the circulation of some of the other organs going, provided the patient is kept adequately ventilated and hemodynamic support is provided as required. However, this state can only be maintained temporarily and eventually cardiac asystole occurs in all the patients.

PREREQUISITES

The aim is to establish that the patient is:

- Unresponsive
- Absent brainstem reflexes, and is
- Apneic

There are certain preconditions that have to be fulfilled to make sure that the tests are performed on the right patient and at the right time. These are as follows: Cause of irreversible structural brain damage should be known.

- Functional reversible causes of a nonfunctioning brainstem should have been ruled out. These causes include.
  - Primary hypothermia
  - Alcohol intoxication
  - Neuromuscular blockade
  - Use of central nervous system depressant drugs like sedatives
  - Severe metabolic or endocrine disturbances
- Patient should have no circulating therapeutic levels of any drug/other compound that could cause coma.

CLINICAL TESTING AT THE BEDSIDE

Absence of brainstem function is essential for establishing the diagnosis of brain death (**Fig. 1**). In a brainstem dead patient cranial nerve reflexes (**Table 1**) are tested to observe their motor response to a sensory input. The absence of brainstem function is documented by conducting the following five tests:

1. Absence of pupillary reflex response to light
2. Absence of corneal reflexes
3. Absence of vestibulo-ocular reflex
4. Absence of cranial nerve response to pain
5. Absence of gag and cough reflexes

Unresponsive to pain: The patient should have no response to pain delivered by sternal pressure. Pain must also be delivered by supra-brow pressure to rule out the remote possibility that the unresponsiveness is due to a high cervical cord injury.

- Having established that the patient is unresponsive the following six tests of brainstem dysfunction are performed (they may be conveniently remembered as two eye, two ear, and two throat).

Pupillary light reflex: Shine a bright narrow beam of light should into each eye. No eye drops to dilate the pupils should have been used in the 4 hours previously. The pupils

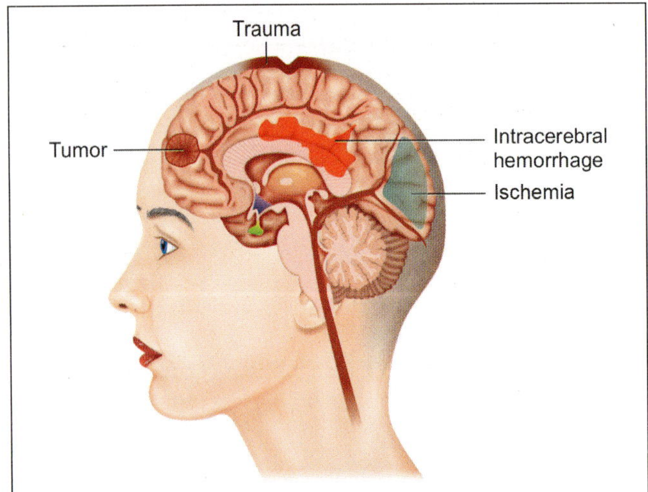

FIGURE 1: Common causes of brain death.

TABLE 1 Clinical testing for cranial nerves to diagnose absence of brainstem refexes.

Brainstem reflexes	Sensory cranial nerve	Motor cranial nerve
Absence of pupillary response to light	II	III (parasympathetic nerve fibers)
Absence of corneal reflexes	V	VII
Absence of cranial nerve response to pain	V	VII (and limb motor responses)
Absence of vestibulo-ocular reflexes	VIII	III and VI
Absence of gag and cough reflexes	X	IX

need *not* be dilated in the brainstem dead patients, but there should be no pupillary response to light.

Corneal reflex: A wisp of cotton should be teased off the tip of a moist cotton swab and should be used to lightly stroke the cornea without damaging it.

Vestibulo-ocular reflex: Also called the cold caloric test, this involves instilling a large volume of ice-cold water into the external auditory canal. This stimulates the lateral semicircular canal and causes tonic movement of the eyes to the same side (the fast component if nystagmus was present would have been to the opposite side). To maximize the stimulus flex the head to 30°—this will make the semicircular canal vertical. If there is no movement of the eyes (observe for at least 30 seconds after irrigation) the reflex is absent. Presence of ruptured eardrums prevents this test from being performed.

Oculocephalic reflex (doll's eye): Holding the eyes open, the patient's head is rapidly turned to one side. If the reflex is present the eyes will turn to the opposite side, giving the impression that the eyeballs have not moved. If the reflex is absent the eyes will move with the head. This movement (unlike the vestibulo-ocular reflex) is immediate and does not need sustained observation, and therefore may be repeated a few times in each direction. It is advisable to disconnect the ventilator before doing this as sudden movements of the head while connected to the ventilator might result in tube displacement.

Gag reflex: The same swab that was used for the corneal reflex can be used to firmly stimulate the posterior oropharynx on each side.

Cough reflex: This may be checked either by inserting a suction catheter through the endotracheal tube to stimulate the trachea, or may gently jerking the endotracheal tube itself to achieve the same stimulus.

Apnea test: The aim of the test is to establish death of the respiratory center in the medulla. This is the last test done as the rise in carbon dioxide could damage the brain of a patient who is not brain dead, and should therefore be done only after all other clinical tests for brain function are negative. The test itself involves disconnecting the ventilator for enough time for the partial pressure of oxygen (pCO_2) in arterial blood to rise to 60 mm Hg. The test has to be aborted if the patient develops hypoxia, hypotension, or cardiac arrhythmias. There are several preventable errors that are made during the performance of this test. Some hints for performing the test successfully are:

- Reduce the respiratory rate by about 30% and increase the fraction of inspired oxygen (FiO_2) to 100% when beginning to do the clinical testing. The pO_2 will be high and partial pressure of carbon dioxide (pCO_2) above 40 mm Hg at the beginning of the apnea test if this is done, minimizing the apnea time.
- To prevent hypoxia during the period of apnea, a catheter is inserted into the endotracheal tube to provide oxygen. The length of insertion should be measured so that the catheter just protrudes beyond the endotracheal tube—too short and the oxygen will flow back, too long and it will be delivered into a bronchus. A flow >8–10 L/min might produce an element of ventilation and slow the rise of carbon dioxide.
- The temperature should be as close to normal as possible (if not slightly above normal) and temperature of 36°C and above are very reasonable starting points. The general international consensus has been that adequate temperature is mandatory to test for brainstem function, but a temperature above the minimum required is preferred as the resultant higher metabolic rate generates carbon dioxide faster, shortening the apnea time.
- The patient's volume status must be good. Carbon dioxide is a powerful systemic vasodilator, and as the pCO_2 builds during the apnea test, the patient will develop hypotension if the patient is not adequately hydrated. In patients with chronic airway disease or severe chest trauma, the apnea test may be difficult to perform.

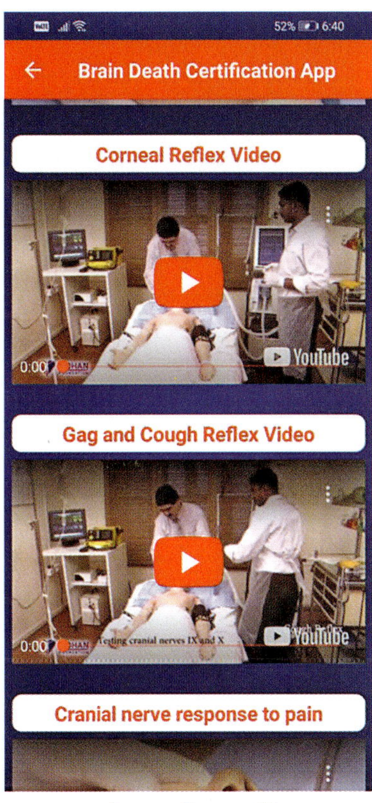

FIGURE 2: Brain Death Certification App.

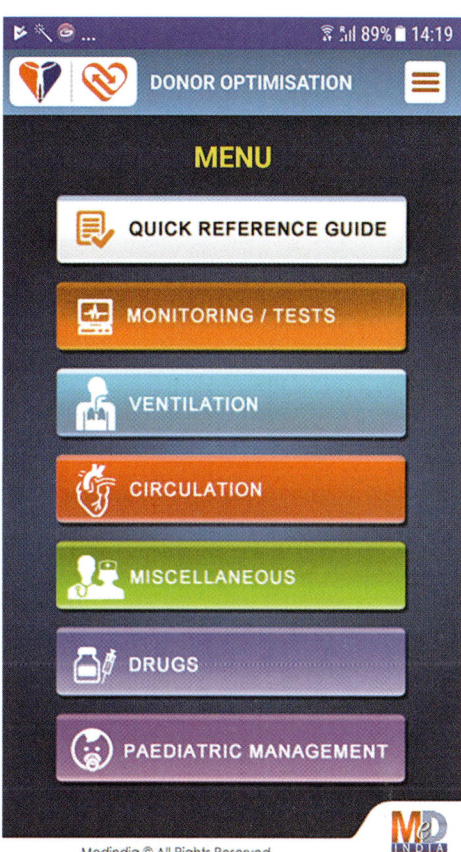

FIGURE 3: Donor Optimisation App.

The "Brain Death Certification" App developed by the MOHAN Foundation is a handy tool to understand the process (**Fig. 2**). It is extremely important for each institution to develop a written protocol; for the entire process. This makes sure the procedure goes smoothly, and also immunizes against change in personnel. An example of a protocol for the diagnosis of brain death is attached as **Annexure 1**.

POTENTIAL BRAIN-DEAD DONOR

Once there is confirmation of brainstem death the intensive care staff looking after the potential donor should switch their focus of the management from therapy for elevated intracranial pressure and brain protection, to preservation of organ function and optimization of tissue oxygen delivery. This will help to keep the organs in optimum condition for immediate functioning once they are transplanted. Supportive treatment should start as soon as brain death has been recognized irrespective of the consent process. The common problems encountered include hypotension, diabetes insipidus, hypoxia, pulmonary edema, arrhythmias, cardiac arrest, and renal hypoperfusion. The "Donor Optimisation" App developed by MOHAN Foundation and NHS Blood and Transplant, UK provides a handy, quick reference guide to handle these problems (**Fig. 3**). A sample summary of instructions for the medical management of a potential brain-dead organ donor is in **Annexure 2**.

REQUEST FOR ORGAN DONATION

The organ donation request is made either in the time interval between the first and second testing for brainstem death or after the second testing for brainstem death. If the relatives are agreeable the process of organ donation is undertaken and vital organs like heart, lungs, liver, pancreas, and kidneys are retrieved for transplantation.

The "Ramachandra Protocol"—to ask for organs: In the emotionally charged situation of a "brain-dead patient" the doctors or grief counsellors find it difficult to broach the subject of organ donation to the relatives. A protocol called the "Ramachandra Protocol" is now the accepted practice in many hospitals where eye donation is broached first with the relatives. Only if the relatives consent to eye donation is the request for solid organ donation made.

CONCLUSION

Early identification and certification of brain death and optimum management of the potential organ donor is necessary for a deceased organ donation program to be successful. The diagnosis of brain death as per the THO Act is based on simple clinical bedside tests. The passing of this Act in 1994 and its subsequent adoption by many Indian States has made the deceased organ donation and transplantation program possible in India.

ANNEXURE 1: Protocol used at the Christian Medical College, Vellore.

Protocol for Diagnosis of Brain Death for Organ Transplantation

Time from injury/ictus to first assessment:

A. Irreversible coma

Assessment	I	II
Date		
Time		
The answer to the following must be **YES**:		
Cause known (Accounts for the severity of the coma?)	Y/N	
Neuroimaging evidence of acute CNS catastrophe that is compatible with the clinical diagnosis of brain death	Y/N	
Toxic causes absent	Y/N	
Metabolic causes absent	Y/N	Y/N
Adequate core temperature (i.e., temperature > 35°C or 95°F)	Y/N	Y/N
The answer to the following must be **NO**:		
Alcohol consumed in last 6 hours	Y/N	
No history of recent treatment with sedatives, narcotics, or muscle relaxants. The following have/have not been given in the last 6 hours:		
• Muscle relaxants	Y/N	Y/N
• Sedatives	Y/N	Y/N
• Narcotics	Y/N	Y/N
• Phenobarbitone used as anticonvulsant	Y/N	Y/N
No response to pain delivered to body and face (suprabrow)	Y/N	Y/N

B. Absent brainstem reflexes

Pupils nonreactive	Y/N	Y/N
Absent **Doll's eye movement**	Y/N	Y/N
Cold caloric test:		
Tympanic membrane found intact	Y/N	
Ocular movement absent	Y/N	Y/N
Absent **corneal reflex** (use swab stick)	Y/N	Y/N
Absent **gag reflex**	Y/N	Y/N
Absent **cough reflex** (To suction catheter tip or ET tube movement)	Y/N	Y/N

C. Apnea test

Prerequisites at the time of testing:		
• Core temperature > 36°C or 97°F	Y/N	Y/N
• Systolic BP ≥ 90 mm Hg	Y/N	Y/N
• Positive fluid balance in the past 6 hours	Y/N	Y/N

Apnea test methodology: It is assumed that the patient is being ventilated at a pCO_2 between 30–35 mm Hg.

- Decrease respiratory rate to increase pCO_2 before disconnection, increase FiO_2 to 1.0
- Send ABG to confirm pCO_2 around 40–45 mm Hg (optional)
- Accurately measure length of oxygen catheter to reach 1 cm beyond the tip of the ET tube, insert up to the mark after disconnecting ventilator; set oxygen flow at 8 L/min
- Observe carefully for respiratory movements with hand on patient's chest
- Send ABG after at least 6 minutes (longer if patient stable) and reconnect to ventilator

Continued...

Abort the test if:

- Systolic BP drops below 90 mm Hg or
- SpO_2 drops below 91% or
- Significant cardiac arrhythmias develop

If the test has to be aborted repeat after 3–4 hours:

- The apnea test is **positive** if respiratory movements are absent, and arterial pCO_2 is ≥60 mm Hg.
  (A single incident of shrugging of shoulders or arching of back does not represent respiratory movements)
- The apnea test is **negative** if respiratory movements are present.
  (Watch for repetitive sustained movements)
- The apnea test is **indeterminate** if respiratory movements are absent, and arterial pCO_2 is <60 mm Hg.
- If indeterminate and there are strong clinical grounds to suspect apnea is present, correct parameters and repeat the test.

Apnea test I

pCO_2 after apnea: mm Hg

Result: Positive/Indeterminate/Negative

Apnea test II

pCO_2 after apnea: mm Hg

Result: Positive/Indeterminate/Negative

Diagnosis of brain death

Brain death is **present if yes** to all questions below on **both** assessments:

A.	All criteria for irreversible coma present	Yes/No
B.	All brainstem reflexes absent on neurological examination	Yes/No
C.	Apnea test is positive	Yes/No

Brain death is **absent** if the answer to any of these questions is **NO**.

Signature and designation of assessors:

Assessor A Assessor B

Steps to be followed when a diagnosis of brain death is being considered

1. Testing
   a. The **first series of tests** to be done at least 6 hours after stopping sedation.
   b. The second series to be done at least **6 hours** after the first in adults. In children the interval between tests must be at least **12 hours**.
2. Ensure that the following results are available (or at least have been sent) at the conclusion of the first series of tests:
   a. Blood for hepatitis B surface antigen
   b. Blood for HIV
   c. Blood for HCV
   d. Blood for blood group analysis
   e. Blood for liver function tests
   f. Blood for WBC, TC/DC
   g. Blood for PT, PTT, and platelets
3. Inform transplant coordinator about possible candidate after first positive test.
   (Note: The protocol is to be aborted if the transplant team examines the candidate, enquires about the candidate, or talks to the candidate's relatives before this)
4. The coordinator will:
   a. Interact with family and keep the ICU informed at all times
   b. Inform all other personnel of the transplant team (it is not the responsibility of the ICU to contact anyone other than the coordinator)
   c. Obtain all drugs and fluids necessary for the patient once the first test is positive
   d. Complete all legal formalities except for filling Form 8
5. If permission for harvesting organs is not granted, discontinue ventilation and certify death.
6. The time of death in all cases will be recorded as the time of the second positive test.

(ABG: arterial blood gas; BP: blood pressure; CNS: central nervous system; ET: endotracheal; HCV: hepatitis C virus; HIV: human immunodeficiency virus; ICU: intensive care unit; pCO_2: partial pressure of carbon dioxide; PT: prothrombin time; PTT: partial thromboplastin time; SpO_2: oxygen saturation; TC/DC: total count/differential count; WBC: white blood cell)

ANNEXURE 2: Medical management of the potential donor.

1. **Recognition of brain death:** The onset of any of the following should be an indication of possible brain death:
   - Diabetes insipidus (DI)
   - Hypotension requiring > 1 pressor/inotrope
   - Hypothermia
   - Patient not triggering the ventilator

   Pupils becoming nonreactive should not trigger the process.
2. **Stop drugs:** When the patient has not required muscle relaxants for at least 2 hours, check for a cough reflex. If absent, stop:
   - Sedation
   - Narcotics

   Restart at first sign that patient is not brain dead.
3. **Blood pressure:** Aggressive management—combination of volume, inotropes, pressors, and other drugs (as below) to maintain MAP between 70 and 80 mm Hg.
   - Begin support with noradrenaline then add adrenaline, if necessary. Other inotropes like dopamine and dobutamine may also be used.
   - The first choice of vasopressor is often vasopressin in a small dose of 0.02–0.03 units/kg/h which equates to 1–1.5 units/h. Keep pressor dose at a minimum. Early start of vasopressin helps use lower dose of other inotropes (CMC protocol does not follow this routinely).
   - Add levothyroxine bolus of 20 mcg followed by an infusion of 10 mcg/h, if it is readily available.
   - Start hydrocortisone at 50 mg q6h is optional—some units use it and others do not (CMC protocol does not follow this routinely).
   - Frequently before final brain death there is a surge in blood pressure; the MAP must be kept below 100 mm Hg at this time by:
     - Rapidly reducing dose of vasopressors
     - Metoprolol 5 mg IV boluses with 5 minutes intervals between doses or IV esmolol can be used as a single dose
4. **Fluid–electrolytes:** Recognize DI early—do not wait for fulfillment of output or serum sodium criteria as applicable for sellar-suprasellar lesions. Target sodium <150 mmol/L and potassium >3 mmol/L
   - A triple lumen line and a large bore peripheral line are mandatory.
   - Keep CVP over 10 cm.
   - If output very high, check and replace volume every 30 minutes.
   - Judge replacement fluid sodium concentration (normal saline, half normal saline, or plain dextrose) based on output and last serum sodium level.
   - High output states cause significant potassium depletion—remember to replace adequately.
   - Check electrolytes every 4 hours.
   - Once the patient develops DI begin a vasopressin infusion at 1–3 μg/h and titrate.
5. **Temperature:** If patient identified as potential donor keep covered with blanket at all times. If:
   - Patient develops hypothermia or
   - After first test completed

   Cover with warming blanket, cover scalp completely.

   If adequate measures are taken early there would be no requirement to use warm IV fluids to correct hypothermia.
6. **Ventilation:** Once the patient is suspected to be brain-dead and sedation has been stopped change ventilator settings to a tidal volume of 6 mL/kg predicted body weight.
7. **Family:** Once consent for donation is obtained, permit family to see patient in batches. This helps avoid congestion and obstruction on the way to the OR.
8. **Transfer to OR:** To be made only with the following criteria fulfilled.
   - Accompanied by consultant anesthetist who is aware of status of preparedness in the OR
   - Portable monitor and ventilator
   - Fully charged infusion pumps (stop thyroxine)
   - Fresh oxygen cylinder
9. Transfer patient onto trolley without disconnecting bedside monitor. Take as long as necessary to stabilize patient on the trolley before moving to the OR.
10. **Certification:** Cooperate with transplant coordinator to ensure that donor's family does not suffer any procedural delays in release of body.

(CVP: central venous pressure; MAP: mean arterial pressure; IV: intravenous; NG: nasogastric; OR: operating room)

RECOMMENDED READINGS

1. National Organ and Tissue Transplant Organization. Transplantation of Human Organs Act and Rules. [online] Available from www.notto.gov.in.
2. Greer DM, Shemie SD, Lewis A, Torrance S, Varelas P, Goldenberg FD, et al. Determination of Brain Death/ Death by Neurologic Criteria: The World Brain Death Project. JAMA. 2020;324(11):1078-97.
3. Wijdicks EF, Varelas PN, Gronseth GS, Greer DM; American Academy of Neurology. Evidence-based guideline update: determining brain death in adults: Report of the Quality Standards Subcommittee of the American Academy of Neurology. Neurology. 2010;74(23):1911-8.
4. A definition of irreversible coma. Report of the Ad Hoc Committee of the Harvard Medical School to Examine the Definition of Brain Death. JAMA 1968;205:337-40.
5. Mollaret P, Goulon M. [The depassed coma (preliminary memoir).] Rev Neurol (Paris). 1959;101:3-15.
6. Rosendale JD, Chabalewski FL, McBride MA, Garrity ER, Rosengard BR, Delmonico FL, et al. Increased transplanted organs from the use of a standardized donor management protocol. Am J Transplant 2002;2:761-8.
7. Shroff S, Navin S, Abraham G, Rajan PS, Suresh S, Rao S, et al. Cadaver Organ Donation and Transplantation—An Indian Perspective. Transplant Proc. 2003;35:15-7.
8. Kumar A, Lalwani S, Agrawal D, Rautji R, Dogra TD. Fatal road traffic accidents and their relationship with head injuries: An epidemiological survey of five years. Indian J Neurotrauma. 2008;5:63-7.
9. Vadi S, Shroff S. Redefining Death: Urgent Need to Evolve toward a Homogeneous Definition of Death in India. Indian J Crit Care Med. 2019;23(8):368-70.
10. Navin S, Suriyamoorthi S. Current state of acceptance of brain stem death and organ donation in India. Amrita J Med. 2020;16:87-94.

CHAPTER 84

End-of-life Care, Medico-legal Aspects, and Ethics in ICU

Raj Kumar Mani, Srinagesh Simha, Roop Gursahani

ABSTRACT

End-of-life care (EOLC) is one of the important quality measures of intensive care delivery. Toward the end of life, the focus of care must shift toward comfort and dignity in death. In the care of the dying, medical, ethical, sociocultural, and legal aspects intersect. This chapter begins with a description of a real-life scenario where an end-of-life decision was made. It briefly touches upon the ethical underpinnings of foregoing of life support. It provides definition of terms used around terminal care. It goes on to provide guidance on the clinical pathway to end-of-life decision-making that includes withdrawal (WD), withholding (WH) and do not attempt resuscitation (DNAR) orders. Legal developments in India are summarized and their practical application clarified.

"The end of life is to be like God, and the soul following God will be like Him"

—Socrates

CASE STUDY

Mrs JG was an 80-year-old mother of a well-loved and celebrated musician. She was admitted to the intensive care unit (ICU) with acute dyspnea and hypoxia that would need artificial ventilation. But her history pointed to futility of such support. She had metastatic pancreatic cancer for which she had no hesitation in declining treatment. She had said to her family that having had a full life she only wished for an end without struggle. The medical team also endorsed her wishes because it was clear that there would be more suffering from interventions with little prospects for cure. It was obvious that hooking her to a ventilator would only briefly postpone but not stop, her imminent death. We opened conversations around the goals of care with her daughters—it was plain to them she did not have long to live. The physician in-charge asked Mrs JG herself quietly whether it would be right if we used machines to support her life. She indicated to him and her daughters that she would not want that at all. The family and the intensive care team took a collective decision to withhold the ventilator and other interventions such as vasopressors and hemodialysis should the need arise. Her physician in-charge spent time with the family and by the bedside of Mrs JG. Respiratory distress was controlled with noninvasive support and opiates. Hypnotics were used judiciously for sleep. The team refrained from introducing a nasogastric tube for feeding. The family frequently looked for advice and support from physicians and nurses. They too, needed to be prepared emotionally to face the looming end. To ensure transparency and trust, the critical care team documented the gist of the conversations and the decisions taken with the family. In the ICU she was transferred to a single room to ensure privacy and quiet. The family was allowed to be with her all the time. They played music, talking to her about the life they had shared. The daughters, sons-in-law and grandchildren all would press her feet, share hugs, smiles and tears. All medicines other than analgesics and sedatives were stopped. Monitors were removed and frequent checking of vitals stopped. The team also stopped laboratory tests, bedside imaging and interventions, which had anyway lost any relevance. Nurses and doctors would enter the room only to check if she was in visible pain or distress, to ask if there was thirst and if motion was passed. The physician in-charge would stop by to offer a shoulder to the family who were often overcome with emotion. They asked for nothing but empathy and understanding. She passed away peacefully in a few days. The celebrity daughter we had admired always looked composed, even cheerful. A spiritual presence pervaded the scene. The family expressed gratitude for the support they had received from the team.

INTRODUCTION

The critical care unit, by virtue of its focus on critical illness is also an area of high mortality that ranges between 10 and 30%, depending on the case mix. Therefore, it has been viewed as an area for resuscitation, rescue, and salvage. The other side of the coin is early recognition of foreseeable death and the appropriate management of the dying process. This area that requires a paradigm shift in the clinical approach and bedside skills, has received much attention in the last two to three decades. There is increasing refinement of EOLC integrating ethical, medical, legal and sociocultural dimensions.

END-OF-LIFE CARE

End-of-life care aims to provide the patient and family care that focuses primarily on suffering—physical, emotional, psychosocial, and spiritual, around death and dying. Elisabeth Kübler-Ross, a Swiss-American psychiatrist first described the human response to the sense of loss in anticipated death. She described five stages of grief: (1) denial, (2) anger, (3) depression, (4) bargaining and finally, (5) acceptance. Time, skilled counseling, and empathetic support are needed to take the patient and the family through these stages. In the technology-driven ICU environment, there is another aspect of the burden of excessive, futile or nonbeneficial care that has, more often than not, come to precede death. In the impersonal environment of the ICU, where heroic medical measures have come to be the norm, the challenge is to facilitate a dignified death with as little of burdens as possible. Delivering a care that respects the patient's wishes and dignity brings up the questions of prognostic accuracy, ethics of foregoing life support (FLS), the legal requirements for such decisions, and the provision of adequate palliative care.

Recognition of terminal illness/situations unlikely to benefit from curative medical intervention is important.

There can be no absolute certainty in prognostication. However, reasonable predictions based on objective and subjective evaluations can be made. To minimize the chances of false positive conclusion of terminal illness some principles are to be followed:

- An iterative and deliberate method of evaluation
- Collective/collegiate assessment with a low threshold for second or multiple opinions
- Use of general and disease-specific scoring systems

With careful evaluation and open discussions over time, the risk of a "self-fulfilling prophesy" can be minimized.

ETHICS OF FOREGOING LIFE SUPPORT

The ethical foundations of FLS were enunciated by Beauchamp and Childress in the four well-known principles of autonomy, beneficence, nonmaleficence, and justice.

Autonomy: This principle is of respect for the patient as a person with values, wishes, and preferences. The patient must be empowered to exercise his/her free choice which must be respected by caregivers. Open, accurate, and understandable communication of the patient's condition and prognosis are imperatives to uphold this principle. Also, consistent with this principle, the patient has the unconditional right to consent or to refuse any medical intervention including life-sustaining treatment (LST).

Beneficence and nonmaleficence: These are the physician duties of care, to act for the benefit of the patient without subjecting him/her to unjustifiable or undue risks of harm. In case of tension between the two principles, i.e., substantial benefits without some harm appears difficult, potential benefits must always outweigh potential harm. The *principle of justice* indicates the duty to act fairly without discrimination on any basis.

With respect to FLS decisions, ethics require that these decisions are taken on the basis of the patient's informed refusal coupled with his/her best interests as judged by a team of physicians and caregivers. When a competent and informed patient refuses treatment over the physician's recommendation, it is an ethical and legal imperative that physicians act in accordance with the patient's choice. When autonomy cannot be exercised directly, it can be exercised through the agency of (1) Advance Medical Directives (AMD) with or without a legally appointed health care proxy; (2) Surrogates who may be family/next of kin/ significant other.

DEFINITIONS

Terminal illness: An irreversible or incurable disease condition from which death is expected in the foreseeable future (around 6 months or less).

End-of-life care: An approach to a terminally ill patient that shifts the focus of care to symptom control, comfort, dignity, quality of life, and quality of dying rather than treatments aimed at cure or prolongation of life.

Palliative care: Palliative care is a holistic approach to treatment that aims to improve the quality of life of patients and their families facing the problems associated with chronic or life-threatening illness through the prevention and relief of suffering, physical, psychological, emotional or spiritual.

Withholding of life sustaining treatment: A decision made not to initiate or escalate a LST in terminal illness in accordance with the expressed wishes of the patient or surrogate.

Withdrawal of life sustaining treatment: A decision made to cease or remove a life-sustaining intervention, without replacing it with an alternative intervention in terminal illness, in accordance with the expressed wishes of the patient or surrogate.

Euthanasia (or active euthanasia): Euthanasia is the intentional act of ending the life of a terminally ill patient on voluntary request, by the direct intervention of a physician for the purpose of the good of the patient (Active euthanasia is illegal in India.).

Medical assistance in dying (MAiD): An intentional act by the physician, on the voluntary request of a patient with terminal illness, providing the means or methods with which to help a person to end his/her life. (MAiD is illegal in India).

Double effect: A principle that distinguishes the adverse effects that are intended from those that are unintended though foreseeable.

Best interests: A concept that requires physicians to ensure potential benefits to outweigh harms before undertaking medical interventions.

Shared decision-making: A dynamic process with the responsibility for decisions on the medical care of a patient being shared between the health care team and the patient or surrogates.

Advance directives: A recorded statement made by a person with decision-making capacity stating his/her wishes regarding how to be treated or not treated at a stage when he/she loses such capacity.

Do not attempt resuscitation: A considered decision by the patient or by the medical team in her best interests, not to have cardiopulmonary resuscitation (CPR) performed in the event of an anticipated cardiorespiratory arrest.

MEDICAL PROCEDURE OF FOREGOING LIFE SUPPORT

Principles and procedures for FLS decisions have evolved over the last two to three decades. Several guidelines have been published by professional bodies at both national and international levels. Longitudinal surveys have estimated that in the United States (US) and Europe 70–90% of deaths in the ICUs are preceded by an FLS decision. There is a wide variability of the rates of FLS decisions preceding ICU deaths. The factors may be socioeconomic, cultural, religious or legal variations. It also depends on physician characteristics such as years of professional experience, training in ethics and EOLC, and personal beliefs.

BOX 1 Bedside checklist for initiating EOL discussions.

- Advanced age coupled with poor functional state due to one or more chronic debilitating organ dysfunction, e.g., end stage pulmonary, cardiac, renal or hepatic disease for which the patient has received/declined standard medical/surgical options
- Catastrophic illnesses with organ dysfunctions unresponsive to a reasonable period of aggressive treatment
- Coma (in the absence of brain death) due to acute catastrophic causes with nonreversible consequences such as traumatic brain injury, intracranial bleeding or extensive infarction
- Chronic severe neurological conditions with advanced cognitive and/or functional impairment with little or no prospects for improvement, e.g., advanced dementia, quadriplegia or chronic vegetative state
- Progressive metastatic cancer where treatment has failed or patient has refused treatment.
- Postcardio respiratory arrest poor neurological recovery after at least 3 days (7 days in case of therapeutic hypothermia)
- Comparable clinical situations coupled with a physician prediction of low probability of survival
- Patient/Family preference to limit life support or refusal to accept life support

Source: Mani RK, Amin P, Chawla R, Divatia JV, Kapadia F, Khilnani P, et al. Guidelines for end-of-life and palliative care in Indian ICUs: ISCCM consensus ethical position statement. Indian J Crit Care Med. 2012;16(3):166-81.

The guidelines by the Indian Society of Critical Care Medicine-Indian Association of Palliative Care (ISCCM-IAPC) joint statement comprise the following steps:

- Identifying terminal illness to consider transition from curative to palliative care. **Box 1** lists the contexts/triggers when the goals of care need to be reviewed.
- Consensus among the treating team. FLS decisions are to be initiated by a group of clinicians, rather than by an individual physician as per the current standards of end-of-life decision-making. When there is uncertainty in prognosis, curative treatments must continue.
- Opening up conversations with the patient/surrogates on prognosis and the unlikelihood of benefit from therapeutic interventions. In case of an incapacitated patient, the existence of an AMD should be asked for.

Early, open and complete disclosure of information is the key to fulfilling ethical principles. In the case of an incompetent patient in the absence of an AMD, conversations with surrogates are the means to identify patient's values and wishes. Quality communication requires time, skill, experience, and sensitivity. Structured training programs are found to be useful. A shared decision-making is the favored standard of care. This model combines and balances the principles of autonomy, beneficence and nonmaleficence. An FLS decision is made through the above steps (**Figs. 1** and **2**) and duly documented. Transparency is not only a legal requirement but also essential to keep public trust and to minimize the possibilities of misjudgment and misuse.

- Implementation of WD/WH/DNAR decisions. Shift from cure to care implies focus on the patient's comfort. Palliative care involves impeccable symptom assessment and control. It includes physical, emotional, and spiritual well-being of the patient. Palliative care is inclusive of support to the family in preparing them for the impending death of a loved one that extends to the bereavement period. Ensuring adequacy of symptom control may impose a foreseen but unintended effect of hastening the patient's death. However, this risk is widely regarded as ethically justifiable by the doctrine of "double effect". An unintended adverse effect during the course of treatment aimed at providing comfort, is not culpable, although largely foreseeable. In the US, under this concept, if due care is taken to identify terminal illness and palliation is applied according to standards of care, it is legally acceptable.
- Location of death and access to family. The option of dying at home should be discussed. Since in Indian culture as in others sanctity is attached to dying in one's home, such a request should be honored and enabled. If the location is the hospital, steps should be taken to ensure privacy and access to the family. Family presence around the dying hours should be facilitated. As far as possible requests for simple spiritual rites/rituals or the presence of priests should be allowed. A professional psychologist should be available if needed.
- *Family support*: The emotional stress of a loved one in the hospital, the uncertainties, stressful end-of-life decision-making and financial burdens all take their toll. Anxiety, depression and post-traumatic stress disorder (PTSD) are frequent among the family caregivers that can be mitigated by appropriate support. Support to the family should be provided in the immediate period after death and extended to bereavement, if required. Psychologist/psychiatric support may also be required.
- Oversight, assistance, dispute resolution, and quality control by a hospital EOLC committee.

LEGAL STATUS OF FOREGOING LIFE SUPPORT (WD, WH, AND DNAR) IN INDIA

Law by judicial precedence or common law has always existed even before the constitution of India came into force, for the right to protect bodily integrity and individual

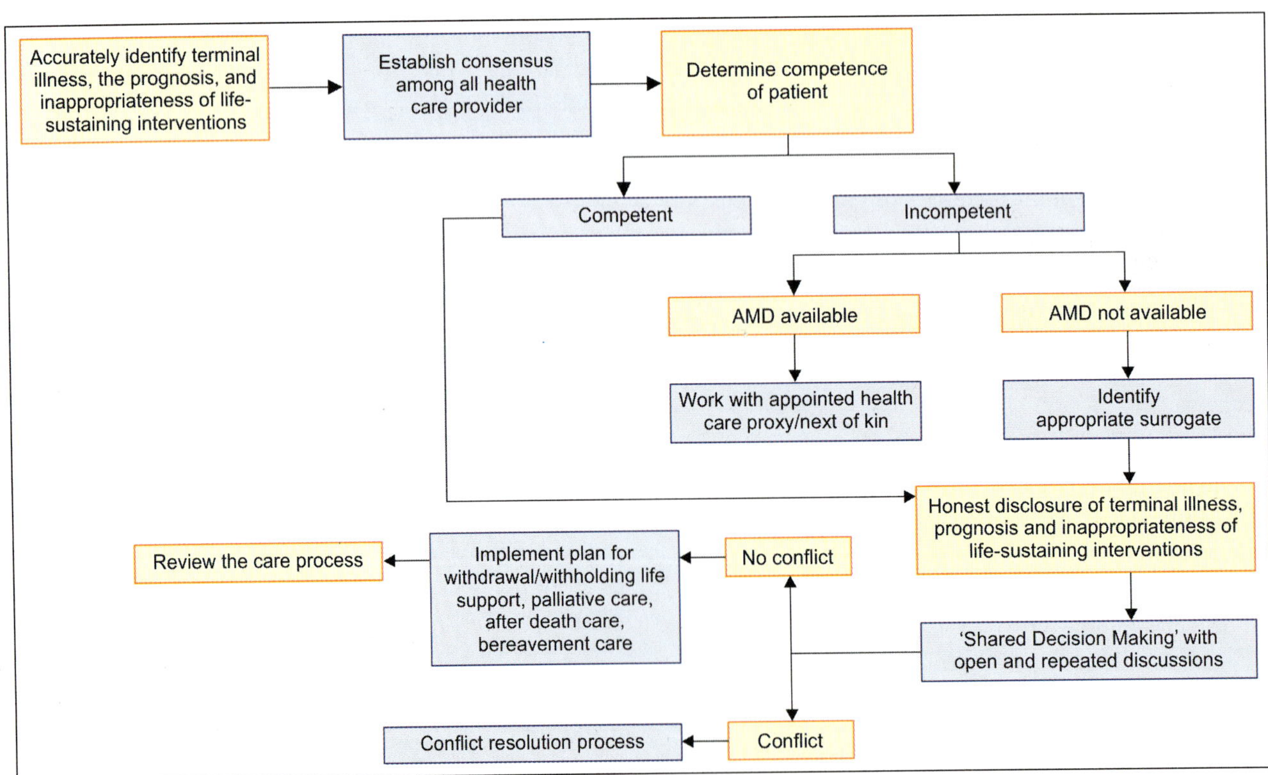

(AMD: Advance Medical Directives)

FIGURE 1: End-of-life care decision-making algorithm.

Source: Aggarwal KK. FICCI-ELICIT Guide to improving End of Life Care and Decision-making [online]. Available from http://kkaggarwal.com/Editorial/ficci-elicit-guide-to-improving-end-of-life-care-decision-making/[Last accessed April, 2021].

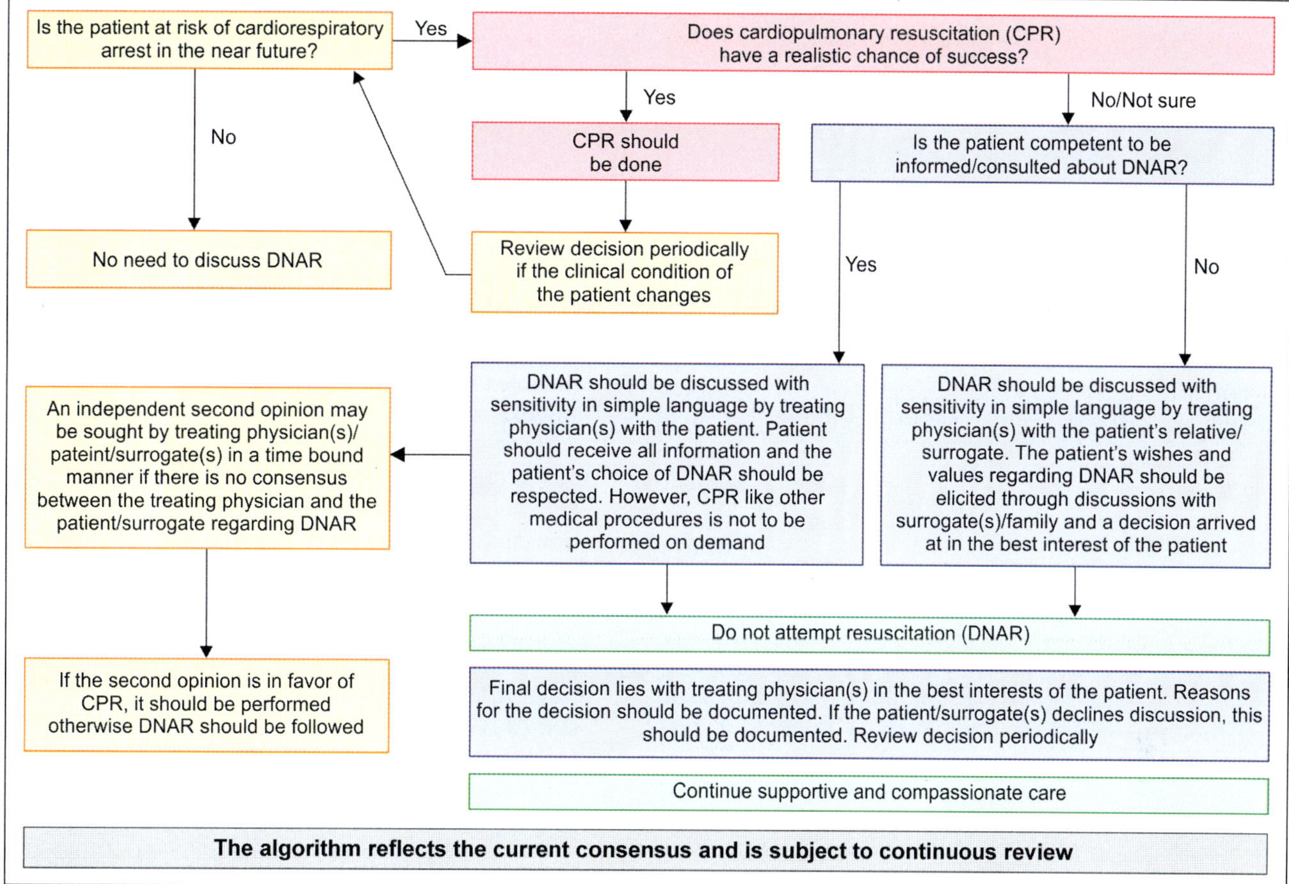

FIGURE 2: Do not attempt resuscitation decision pathway.

Source: Mathur R. ICMR Consensus Guidelines on 'Do Not Attempt Resuscitation'. Indian J Med Res. 2020;151(4):303-10.

autonomy. Implicit in it, there exists a common law right to refuse medical treatment, including the right to demand that a treatment ongoing be withdrawn. Not respecting refusal amounts to battery by the Indian penal code.

As per the constitution of India, the right to refuse treatment is further validated by three landmark judgments in the last decade. In the *Aruna Shanbaug versus The Union of India* (2012), WD of life support for an incompetent person was allowed under certain conditions that included a court procedure. The Amicus Curiae (a legal expert appointed by the court) had notably observed "several situations that are not subject to the restrictions of the law at all, because they are considered normal medical practice. These are: Stopping or not starting a medically useless (futile) treatment; stopping or not starting a treatment at the patient's request."

According to the judgment in *Justice (Retd). Puttaswamy versus Union of India (2017)* the right to privacy includes the right to refuse LST.

In the landmark judgment *Common Cause versus The Union of India, (2018)* AMD and WD/WH were clearly held to be legal. It unambiguously decriminalizes/allows all forms of FLS under certain conditions and safeguards. The prescribed procedure is as follows:

For AMD two attesting witnesses are required and countersigned by Jurisdictional Magistrate of the First Class (JMFC). Copies are to be sent to registry of the district judge, a competent officer of a local authority, and the family physician. The document will be valid only after the executor loses competency.

Implementation of FLS, with or without a valid AMD, involves a three-level system of oversight: An Internal Medical Board for a preliminary opinion, followed by a Board constituted by the District Collector, before final physical verification by the JMFC. The rules do not take into account the fact that most decisions in the ICU are required to be made under time pressure. More than half the FLS decisions are reported to be made within the first week of admission, as most situations are in the acute refractory or terminally acute stages of chronic incurable conditions. Recently, the ISCCM, along with the "Vidhi" center for legal policy has filed an application for clarification and modification of the procedure laid out in *common cause*.

TRANSLATION OF ESTABLISHED LEGAL PRINCIPLES IN EVERY DAY PRACTICE

- *Following the "spirit" of the law rather than the "letter"*: The Supreme Court (SC) judgment *common cause* establishes the fundamental right of autonomous choice to the patient. As an important safeguard against errors of judgment or misuse, the SC recommends a collegiate

BOX 2	Constituents of the hospital end-of-life care (EOLC) committee.
• The Director or his nominee of the ICU at a medical care facility who is not part of the team treating the patient	
• The Chief Administrator or his nominee of a medical care facility who is not part of the team treating the patient	
• An invited senior physician with relevant experience not on the staff or otherwise employed by the medical facility	
• A legal expert appointed by the medical facility	
• A lay person preferably involved in social service	

Source: VIDHI Centre for Legal Policy. (2019). End of Life Care in India Task Force, End of Life Care in India: A Model Legal Framework [online]. Available from https://vidhilegalpolicy.in/wp-content/uploads/2019/11/191031_-End-of-Life-Care-in-India-A-Model-Legal-Framework.pdf

as opposed to an individual physician decision-making. At least three physicians take part and sign off. As per the SC directives, all decisions should follow the principle of "shared decision" making with the patient, or with surrogates if the patient is incapacitated. Every hospital must have a standard EOLC policy with a standard operating procedure. A hospital EOLC committee should be set up and be available for review, consultation, verification of adherence to protocol and dispute resolution. Typical constituents of the committee are as per **Box 2**. Direct involvement of the committee is not required in most situations. This is because FLS decisions involve the building up of trust over time between treating teams and the family. Documentation and transparency should be reflected in the case records.

- *The refusal of consent for life sustaining treatment as basis for FLS decisions*: FLS decisions are viewed as exercising the right of informed refusal to continue an ongoing life support intervention once the treating team has conveyed its futility/nonbeneficial effects of medical interventions. By law no treatment can be initiated or continued when consent is refused.
- Precedence/practices around the world prescribe a process similar to that recommended by professional bodies/statutory organizations/institutions in India.
- The duty of care to respect autonomy and privacy includes dignity in death. Continuing with unwanted and unjustifiable burdens would violate these basic tenets of physician duties.

Documentation: Model forms for DNAR directives and for FLS are available by expert consensus. If forms are unavailable, the case records must document the disease diagnosis, prognosis in terms of life expectancy and quality of life, details of family meetings, individuals present in the meetings and the final consensus decision taken along with signatures.

CONCLUSION

End-of-life care is integral to intensive care delivery. For quality EOLC, the ethical, medical and legal aspects of patient care need to be addressed together. Formal training in ethics and EOLC for caregivers in intensive care is crucial. The last decade has seen significant legal reform relating to WD and WH of life support. It has also seen the emergence of advocacy groups for improving EOLC in India.

RECOMMENDED READINGS

1. Kübler-Ross E, Kessler D. On grief and grieving: finding the meaning of grief through the five stages of loss. New York: Scribner; 2014.
2. Downar J, Delaney JW, Hawryluck L, Kenny L. Guidelines for the withdrawal of life-sustaining measures. Intensive Care Med. 2016;42(6):1003-17.
3. Myburgh J, Abillama F, Chiumello D, Dobb G, Jacobe S, Kleinpell R, et al. End-of-life care in the intensive care unit: Report from the Task Force of World Federation of Societies of Intensive and Critical Care Medicine. J Crit Care. 2016;34:125-30.
4. Myatra SN, Salins N, Iyer S, Macaden SC, Divatia JV, Muckaden M, et al. End-of-life care policy: An integrated care plan for the dying: a joint position statement of the Indian Society of Critical Care Medicine (ISCCM) and the Indian Association of Palliative Care (IAPC). Indian J Crit Care Med. 2014;18(9):615-35.
5. Beauchamp TL, Childress JF (Eds). Principles of Biomedical Ethics, 7th edition. New York: Oxford University Press; 2013.
6. Jonsen AR, Siegler M, Winslade WJ. Clinical Ethics, 7th edition. A case-based approach to ethical decision-making. New York: McGraw-Hill; 2010.
7. Salins N, Gursahani R, Mathur R, Iyer S, Macaden S, Simha N, et al. Definition of Terms Used in Limitation of Treatment and Providing Palliative Care at the End of Life: the Indian Council of Medical Research Commission Report. Indian J Crit Care Med. 2018;22(4):249-62.
8. Mathur R. ICMR Consensus Guidelines on 'Do Not Attempt Resuscitation'. Indian J Med Res. 2020;151(4):303-10
9. Zulman DM, Haverfield MC, Shaw JG, Brown-Johnson CG, Schwartz R, Tierney AA, et al. Practices to foster physician presence and connection with patients in the clinical encounter. JAMA. 2020;323(1):70-81.
10. Curtis JR, Engelberg RA, Wenrich MD, Shannon SE, Treece PD, Rubenfeld GD. Missed opportunities during family conferences about end-of-life care in the intensive care unit. Am J Respir Crit Care Med. 2005;171(8):844-9.
11. Sprung CL, Ricou B, Hartog CS, Maia P, Mentzelopoulos SD, Weiss M, et al Changes in end-of-life practices in European intensive care units from 1999 to 2016. JAMA. 2019;322(17):1692-704.
12. Supreme Court of India. (2011). Aruna Shanbaug v Union of India [2011]2SCR869 [online] Available from https://indiankanoon.org/doc/235821/
13. Chandrachud DY. (2017). Reportable: In the Supreme Court of India Civil Original Jurisdiction. Writ Petition (Civil No. 494 of 2012. Justice KS Puttaswamy (Retd) versus Union of India, AIR 2017 SC 4161 [online]. Available from https://indiankanoon.org/doc/91938676/

14. (2018). Reportable In The Supreme Court of India Civil Original Jurisdiction. Common Cause versus The Union of India. Writ Petition (Civil) no. 215 of 2005 [online]. Available from https://indiankanoon.org/doc/184449972/
15. Aggarwal KK. FICCI-ELICIT Guide to improving End of Life Care and Decision-making [online]. Available from http://kkaggarwal.com/Editorial/ficci-elicit-guide-to-improving-end-of-life-care-decision-making/
16. VIDHI Centre for Legal Policy. (2019). End of Life Care in India Task Force, End of Life Care in India: A Model Legal Framework [online]. Available from https://vidhi-legalpolicy.in/wp-content/uploads/2019/11/191031_-End-of-Life-Care-in-India-A-Model-Legal-Framework.pdf

MULTIPLE CHOICE QUESTIONS

To access the multiple choice questions of this Section online, kindly scan the QR code.